CREATIVE ARTS AND PLAY THERAPY
FOR ATTACHMENT PROBLEMS

Creative Arts
and Play Therapy
for Attachment
Problems

Edited by

Cathy A. Malchiodi
David A. Crenshaw

THE GUILFORD PRESS
New York   London

© 2014 The Guilford Press
A Division of Guilford Publications, Inc.
72 Spring Street, New York, NY 10012
www.guilford.com

Chapter 11 © 2014 Richard L. Gaskill and Bruce D. Perry

Printed in the United States of America

This book is printed on acid-free paper.

Last digit is print number: 9   8   7   6   5   4   3   2   1

The authors have checked with sources believed to be reliable in their efforts to
provide information that is complete and generally in accord with the standards
of practice that are accepted at the time of publication. However, in view of the
possibility of human error or changes in behavioral, mental health, or medical
sciences, neither the authors, nor the editors and publisher, nor any other party
who has been involved in the preparation or publication of this work warrants
that the information contained herein is in every respect accurate or complete,
and they are not responsible for any errors or omissions or the results obtained
from the use of such information. Readers are encouraged to confirm the
information contained in this book with other sources.

Library of Congress Cataloging-in-Publication Data

Creative arts and play therapy for attachment problems / edited by
Cathy A. Malchiodi, David A. Crenshaw.
    pages cm. — (Creative arts and play therapy)
  Includes bibliographical references and index.
  ISBN 978-1-4625-1270-6 (hardback : acid-free paper)
  1. Attachment disorder in children.   2. Art therapy.   3. Play
therapy.   I. Malchiodi, Cathy A.   II. Crenshaw, David A.
  RJ507.A77C74 2014
  618.92'891653—dc23

                                                      2013031210

About the Editors

Cathy A. Malchiodi, PhD, ATR-BC, LPAT, LPCC, is an art therapist, creative arts therapist, and clinical mental health counselor, as well as a recognized authority on art therapy with children, adults, and families. She has given more than 350 presentations on art therapy and has published numerous articles, chapters, and books, including *Understanding Children's Drawings*; *Handbook of Art Therapy, Second Edition*; and *Creative Interventions with Traumatized Children*. Dr. Malchiodi is on the faculty of Lesley University and is a visiting professor at universities in the United States and internationally. She is also founder of the Trauma-Informed Practices and Expressive Arts Therapy Institute and has worked with a wide variety of community, national, and international agencies, particularly on the use of art therapy for trauma intervention, disaster relief, mental health, and wellness. The President of Art Therapy Without Borders, a nonprofit organization supporting international art therapy initiatives and service, Dr. Malchiodi is the first person to have received all three of the American Art Therapy Association's highest honors: Distinguished Service Award, Clinician Award, and Honorary Life Member Award. She has also received honors from the Kennedy Center and Very Special Arts in Washington, DC.

David A. Crenshaw, PhD, ABPP, RPT-S, is Clinical Director of the Children's Home of Poughkeepsie, New York, and Faculty Associate at Johns Hopkins University. He is a Fellow of the American Psychological Association and of its Division of Child and Adolescent Psychology. Dr. Crenshaw is Past President of the Hudson Valley Psychological Association, which honored him with its Lifetime Achievement Award, and of the New York Association for Play Therapy. He serves on the editorial board of the *International Journal of Play Therapy* and has published numerous journal articles, book chapters, and books on child therapy, child abuse and trauma, and resilience in children. Co-Chair of the board of directors of Astor Services for Children and Families and an advisory board member of the Courthouse Dogs Foundation in Seattle, Dr. Crenshaw has been a passionate advocate for legislative proposals to enhance children's rights. He is a frequent presenter at statewide and national conferences on play therapy.

Contributors

Jennifer N. Baggerly, PhD, Department of Counseling and Human Services, University of North Texas at Dallas, Dallas, Texas

Kira Boesch, BA, Doctoral Program in Clinical Psychology, City University of New York at City College, New York, New York

Phyllis B. Booth, MA, The Theraplay Institute, Evanston, Illinois

David A. Crenshaw, PhD, ABPP, RPT-S, Children's Home of Poughkeepsie, Poughkeepsie, New York

Christina Devereaux, PhD, Dance/Movement Therapy and Counseling Program, Department of Applied Psychology, Antioch University New England, Keene, New Hampshire

Teresa Dias, BA, Drama Therapy Master's Program, Division of Expressive Therapies, Lesley University, Cambridge, Massachusetts

Athena A. Drewes, PsyD, Astor Services for Children and Families, Rhinebeck, New York

Richard L. Gaskill, EdD, Department of Counseling, Educational Leadership, and Educational and School Psychology, Wichita State University, Wichita, Kansas

Eliana Gil, PhD, Gil Institute for Trauma Recovery and Education, Fairfax, Virginia

Jessica Gorkin, MEd, Doctoral Program in Clinical Psychology, City University of New York at City College, New York, New York

Eric J. Green, PhD, Department of Counseling and Human Services, University of North Texas at Dallas, Dallas, Texas

Henry Kronengold, PhD, Doctoral Program in Clinical Psychology, City University of New York at City College, New York, New York

Jennifer Lee, PhD, Columbia University College of Physicians and Surgeons, New York Presbyterian Hospital, New York, New York

Sandra Lindaman, MA, MSW, The Theraplay Institute, Evanston, Illinois

Cathy A. Malchiodi, PhD, ATR-BC, LPAT, LPCC, Division of Expressive Therapies, Lesley University, Cambridge, Massachusetts; Trauma-Informed Practices and Expressive Arts Therapy Institute, Louisville, Kentucky

Christen Pendleton, EdS, Department of Graduate Psychology, Combined–Integrated Program in Clinical and School Psychology, James Madison University, Harrisonburg, Virginia

Bruce D. Perry, MD, PhD, Child Trauma Academy, Houston, Texas; Department of Psychiatry and Behavioral Sciences, Feinberg School of Medicine, Northwestern University, Chicago, Illinois

Jacqueline Z. Robarts, MA, Nordoff Robbins Music Therapy Centre, London, United Kingdom

John W. Seymour, PhD, Department of Counseling and Student Personnel, Minnesota State University, Mankato, Mankato, Minnesota

Cynthia C. Sniscak, LPC, RPT-S, Beech Street Program, LLC, Carlisle, Pennsylvania

Anne Stewart, PhD, Department of Graduate Psychology, James Madison University, Harrisonburg, Virginia

Madeleine Terry, BA, Doctoral Program in Clinical Psychology, City University of New York at City College, New York, New York

Glade L. Topham, PhD, Department of Human Development and Family Science, Oklahoma State University, Tulsa, Oklahoma

Steven Tuber, PhD, Doctoral Program in Clinical Psychology, City University of New York at City College, New York, New York

Risë VanFleet, PhD, Family Enhancement and Play Therapy Center, Playful Pooch Program, Boiling Springs, Pennsylvania

William F. Whelan, PsyD, The Virginia Child and Family Attachment Center, University of Virginia, Charlottesville, Virginia

Marlo L.-R. Winstead, MSW, LSCSW, School of Social Welfare, University of Kansas, Lawrence, Kansas; Play Therapy Program, MidAmerica Nazarene University, Olathe, Kansas; The Theraplay Institute, Evanston, Illinois; Enriching Families, Tallahassee, Florida

Preface

The quality of parent–child interactions early in life has consistently been a focus in psychiatry, psychology, and the other mental health professions. More recently, leaders in the field of attachment theory have emphasized the crucial role of secure and positive early interpersonal relationships in human development. Much of our increased knowledge about attachment comes from greater understanding of neurodevelopment, the brain's responses to trauma, and how adverse events can result in disrupted, insecure, or disorganized attachment. As a result, there is now wide agreement that these findings support the idea that the quality of attachment during infancy and childhood significantly impacts emotional, cognitive, physical, and social development throughout the lifespan. We also know that nurturing, protective, and caring interactions between infants and primary caregivers not only are essential for attachment security, but also literally shape the structure and function of the child's developing brain. In particular, research and clinical findings pinpoint the central role of the right hemisphere of the brain in healthy attachment.

While there are many effective ways to treat attachment problems, we believe that there are specific, experientially based approaches that stimulate right brain activity and are important in reestablishing secure and positive attachment experiences. In particular, therapies that give young children ways to express their inner worlds through nonverbal communication are key. Additionally, the most effective approaches are those that are "user friendly" and come naturally to children.

We believe that the creative arts and play therapy have a natural affinity with attachment problems in children. Creative arts therapies (art, music, and dance/movement) and play therapy are approaches that capitalize on "right-brain-to-right-brain" connections between the child client and therapist. When early attachment experiences are disrupted by trauma, neglect, physical and sexual abuse, loss, separation from caregivers, or other factors, it becomes essential to use interventions that use forms of expression and processing to initiate and stimulate reparative processes in a brain-focused way. These experiential, sensory approaches are corrective experiences for the child even when the critical periods in early development are compromised. Through intensive, sequential, and repetitive play and creative arts therapy, child clients can successfully recapitulate and repair early sensorimotor, somatic, cognitive, and psychosocial experiences missed at earlier developmental junctures.

Creative Arts and Play Therapy for Attachment Problems is about that vital healing and reparative process, emphasizing a wide range of play therapy and creative arts therapy approaches. It is also the first volume in a new Guilford Press series, "Creative Arts and Play Therapy." As series editors, it is our privilege to bring theory, practice, and pragmatic applications of play therapy and creative arts therapies to a wide range of practitioners, including psychologists, social workers, mental health counselors, marriage and family therapists, play therapists, art therapists, music therapists, drama therapists, dance/movement therapists, psychiatric nurses, child life specialists, and health care professionals.

Finally, as mental health professionals who have worked with children with attachment problems, we are particularly excited and inspired by the work and depth of knowledge and expertise presented in this book. Each chapter in this volume provides clinical wisdom, specific interventions and approaches, and clinical applications that all practitioners who work with children can use in their work. We hope that these contributions not only form a foundation for greater understanding of play therapy and creative arts therapies with young clients, but also inspire readers to apply these methods in their own work with children.

CATHY A. MALCHIODI
DAVID A. CRENSHAW

Contents

8. Overcoming Complex Trauma with Filial Therapy   121

Glade L. Topham, Risë VanFleet, and Cynthia C. Sniscak

9. Theraplay in Reunification Following Relational Trauma   139

Phyllis B. Booth, Sandra Lindaman, and Marlo L.-R. Winstead

10. The Creative Use of Metaphor in Play and Art Therapy with Attachment Problems   159

Eliana Gil

11. The Neurobiological Power of Play: Using the Neurosequential Model of Therapeutics to Guide Play in the Healing Process   178

Richard L. Gaskill and Bruce D. Perry

III. Clinical Applications: Approaches to Working with At-Risk Populations

PART I

Introduction

CHAPTER 1

Creative Arts Therapy Approaches to Attachment Issues

Cathy A. Malchiodi

During the last several decades, attachment theory has significantly influenced the practice of psychotherapy; this has resulted in the acceptance of early bonding experiences as essential to well-being later in life. Attachment theory is not an approach in and of itself, but it has generated a whole range of therapeutic practices and models focused on increasing an insecurely attached or traumatized individual's ability to form secure relationships, regulate affect and behavior, and emotionally and physically attune to others. Attachment research emphasizes the psychobiological aspects of communication between caregiver and child, including interactive speech, vocalizations/sounds, body language/gestures, and eye contact. The overall goal of attachment work in therapy generally involves recreating experiences that recapture what the individual may have missed in early relationships.

The creative arts therapies include the purposeful application of visual arts, dance/movement, music, and dramatic enactment within a psychotherapeutic framework. Like play therapy, they are experiential, active approaches that capitalize on engaging individuals of all ages in multisensory experiences for self-exploration, personal communication, developmental objectives, socialization, and emotional reparation. This chapter defines and explains the basic foundations of the creative arts therapies, with an emphasis on the psychobiological and neurodevelopmental aspects of these sensory-based approaches to attachment work. It also explores how these therapies are used to treat disrupted or insecure attachment, and to enhance and support the development of secure attachment, particularly in children who have experienced multiple traumatic events or losses.

3

What Are the Creative Arts Therapies?

While many play therapists, counselors, and psychologists use one or more of the arts in their work with clients, the creative arts therapies emerged in the 20th century as distinct approaches with various theoretical and methodological frameworks. These approaches have been used to address a variety of emotional, behavioral, social, and physical disorders in individuals of all ages (Malchiodi, 2005; Warren, 2004) and are defined by psychology as "action therapies" (Weiner, 1999). Art and music making, dance and drama, creative writing, and play are experiential in nature. For example, art making, even in its simplest sense, can involve arranging, touching, gluing, constructing, painting, forming, and many other active experiences. All creative arts therapies encourage clients to become active participants in the therapeutic process, and can energize the clients, redirect their attention and focus, and influence emotions.

The creative arts therapies are most commonly defined as follows:

- *Art therapy* is the purposeful use of visual art materials and media in intervention, counseling, psychotherapy, and rehabilitation; it is used with individuals of all ages, families, and groups (Edwards, 2004; Malchiodi, 2012a).
- *Music therapy* uses music to effect positive changes in the psychological, physical, cognitive, or social functioning of individuals with health, behavioral, social, emotional, or educational challenges (American Music Therapy Association, 2013; Wheeler, Shultis, & Polen, 2005).
- *Drama therapy* is defined as an active, experiential approach to facilitating change through storytelling, projective play, purposeful improvisation, and performance (Johnson, 2009; National Drama Therapy Association, 2013).
- *Dance/movement therapy* is based on the assumption that body and mind are interrelated, and is defined as the psychotherapeutic use of movement as a process that furthers the emotional, cognitive, and physical integration of the individual and influences changes in feelings, cognition, physical functioning, and behavior (Goodill, 2005; National Dance Therapy Association, 2013; Payne, 2013).
- *Poetry therapy* and *bibliotherapy* are terms used synonymously to describe the intentional use of poetry and other forms of literature for healing and personal growth (Micozzi, 2011; National Association for Poetry Therapy, 2013).

The terms *expressive therapies* or *expressive arts therapies* are sometimes used interchangeably with the term *creative arts therapies*. However, the term *expressive therapies* is usually used in reference to a variety of creative methods and experiential approaches involving, but not limited to, all the arts therapies and various forms of play therapy (props, games, and sandplay). The *integrated arts approach* or *intermodal therapy* (also known as *multimodal therapy*) involves the use of two or more expressive therapies in an individual or group session. Intermodal therapy distinguishes itself from its closely allied disciplines of art therapy, music therapy, dance/movement therapy, and drama therapy by focusing on the interrelatedness of the arts. It is based on a variety of orientations, including arts as therapy, art psychotherapy, and the use of arts for traditional healing (Knill, Barba, & Fuchs, 2004).

In subsequent sections of this chapter, the relationship between attachment work and art, music, dance/movement, and drama therapies is explained within the context of attachment theory (Bowlby, 1988/2005; Schore, 2003), psychobiology and neurodevelopment (Perry, 2009; Siegel, 2012), and trauma-informed expressive arts therapies (Malchiodi, 2012a, 2012c). In order to explain how trauma-informed expressive arts therapy is used in the treatment of attachment, a brief case vignette is presented and used to illustrate key applications of creative arts therapies with attachment challenges. Specific applications of the creative arts therapies to support and enhance attachment are covered in more detail with case examples in other chapters of this book.

Creative Arts Therapies and the Brain

Just as attachment theory continues to be informed by the growing understanding of the brain, applications of the creative arts therapies are being clarified within the context of neuroscience and psychobiology. This section reviews five key areas in creative arts therapies and attachment work: (1) sensory-based interventions, (2) nonverbal communication, (3) right-hemisphere dominance, (4) affect regulation, and (5) relational interventions.

Sensory-Based Interventions

First and foremost, the creative arts therapies provide sensory experiences; that is, they are predominantly activities that are visual, kinesthetic, tactile, olfactory, and/or auditory in nature. In fact, each creative arts therapy is multisensorial; for example, music therapy not only involves sound, but also includes vibration, rhythm, and movement. Dramatic enactment may include vocalization, visual impact, and other sensory aspects. Dance/movement therapy encompasses a variety of body-oriented sensations, and art therapy is not limited to images because it also provides a variety of tactile and kinesthetic experiences.

Research on attachment disorders underscores the importance of sensory-based approaches in treatment that encourage active participation and include multisensory qualities. Perry (2008) presents a neurodevelopmental perspective: He describes the essential role of sensory-based experiences in early childhood, and discusses how they enhance secure attachment, affiliation with others, empathy, and self-regulation. He observes that our history as a human species has always included wellness practices such as holding each other; engaging in dance, song, image creation, and storytelling; and sharing celebrations and family rituals. These actions were used in early healing practices and, according to Perry, are now known to be effective in altering neural systems involved in stress responses and developing secure attachment. Similarly, the arts therapies are normalizing experiences for children and trauma-informed practices, in that they involve experiences that children in all cultures recognize (Malchiodi, 2008).

Siegel (2012) offers another perspective that clarifies the role of the creative arts therapies in treating attachment disorders from a sensory perspective. He cites the importance of "critical micromoments" of interaction with a client; these include the client's tone of voice, postures, facial expressions, eye contact, and motion, which Siegel believes provide clues to the individual's psychobiology. These sensory-based cues become particularly important in identifying and formulating strategies for addressing disrupted, insecure, or disorganized attachment. Siegel also proposes the use of experientially based methods such as drawing to help individuals become aware of sensations, emotions, images, and relationships.

Nonverbal Communication

Nonverbal communication is our most basic form of communication, and it is how caregiver and infant initially connect in the infant's first years of life (Schore, 2003). Although most creative arts therapies involve talk, they are also defined as nonverbal approaches because self-expression through an activity becomes a major source of communication. For children in particular, nonverbal means of communication are an important part of any therapy, because children do not always have the words to convey feelings and experiences accurately.

Because thoughts and feelings are not strictly verbal and are not limited to storage as verbal language in the brain, expressive modalities are particularly useful in helping individuals communicate aspects of memories and stories that may not be readily available through conversation. Memories in particular have been reported to emerge through touch, imagery, or carefully guided body movements (Rothschild, 2000). For some individuals, conveying a memory or story through one or more expressive modalities is more easily tolerated than verbalization. For example, children who have been severely traumatized may repeat experiences through play or art activity when the trauma memories are particularly complex or overwhelming (Gil, 2006; Malchiodi, 1997, 2008). In addition, nonverbal expression through a painting, play activity, imaginative role play, or movement may be a corrective experience in and of itself for some individuals.

Right-Hemisphere Dominance

In the field of attachment, it is widely accepted that what happens early in life in terms of relationships affects brain development and is essential to secure attachment (Perry, 2009). *Neuroplasticity* (also called *brain plasticity*) is the brain's ability to renew and, in some cases, even to rewire itself to compensate for deficits or injuries (Doidge, 2007). Brain plasticity is greater early in life—a fact underscoring the importance of appropriate intervention with young children in order not only to enhance attachment, but also to support the development of appropriate affect regulation, interpersonal skills, and cognition.

The right hemisphere of the brain is particularly active during early interactions between very young children and caregivers, and it stores the *internal working model* for attachment relationships and affect regulation (Klorer, 2008; Schore, 2003). Siegel (2012) and Schore (2003) note that interactions between baby and caregiver are right-brain-mediated, because during infancy the right cortex is developing more quickly than the left. Siegel (2012) also observes that just as the left hemisphere requires exposure to language to grow, the right hemisphere requires emotional stimulation to develop properly. He proposes that the output of the right brain is expressed in "non-word-based ways," such as drawing a picture or using a visual image to describe feelings or events.

Research on the impact of trauma proposes that highly charged emotional experiences are encoded by the limbic system and right brain as sensory memories (van der Kolk, 2006). Consequently, expression and processing of these memories on a sensory level are important parts of successful intervention (Rothschild, 2000; Steele & Malchiodi, 2012). Current thinking about trauma supports the effect of childhood trauma on integration of the hemispheres (Teicher, 2000), and it suggests that sensory-based interventions may be effective because they do not rely on the individual's use of left-brain language for processing (Klorer, 2008) and are predominantly right-brain-driven.

Affect Regulation

Hyperarousal is a common response in individuals whose attachment is insecure, disorganized, or disrupted; in particular, young clients who have experienced traumatic events have understandable difficulties with affect regulation. Children who have been victims of interpersonal violence are particularly at risk for problems with affect regulation, including hyperarousal and dissociation. On an implicit level, these children's worldviews include feelings of abandonment and lack of safety; in order to stay safe, they may often react with rage at anyone who is perceived as a threat, or may become disengaged from adults because they come to feel that caregivers abandon or hurt children.

The treatment of attachment difficulties begins with regulation of emotions, stress reduction, and restoration of feelings of safety. Fortunately, specific applications of the creative arts therapies can be used to activate the body's relaxation response. Depending on the individual, experiences with art making, music, and/or movement can have a comforting and calming affect that decreases anxiety or fear. For example, even simple activities such as drawing a picture of a pleasant time or hearing a soothing, familiar song, story, or rhyme are effective because of the imagination's capacity to recall sensory memories and details of positive moments (Malchiodi, 1997, 2008). Creative arts activities may stimulate the placebo effect through mimicking self-soothing experiences of childhood and inducing relaxation (Malchiodi, 2012a). A well-known example of affect regulation via mimicry is the child who strokes a blanket or toy in a way that mimics a caregiver's comfort. Creative arts therapies, especially with attachment disorders, seek to help individuals find activities that are effective in tapping positive sensory experiences, that can be practiced over time, and that eventually become resources for regulating overwhelming emotions. Repetition of pleasurable experiential activities can become a source of self-soothing, and as Gladding (2005) notes, the arts often allow people to experience themselves differently and in positive ways. Through carefully chosen opportunities for self-expression, individuals are able to exhibit and practice novel and adaptive behaviors, including the ability to induce calm feelings and self-soothe.

Relational Interventions

Interpersonal neurobiology (Badenoch, 2008; Siegel, 2012) refers to an overarching theory that weaves together many strands of knowledge, including attachment research, neurobiology, and developmental and social psychology. It is based on the idea that social relationships shape how our brains develop, how our minds perceive the world, and how we adapt to stress throughout the lifespan. In the field of counseling, the creative arts in counseling are defined as inherently "relational" approaches to treatment (Gladding, 2005). *Relational therapy* is historically defined as an approach that empowers individuals with the skills necessary to create productive and healthy relationships. In a broad sense, all psychotherapy and counseling are relational approaches, because the outcome of intervention is dependent on the core relationship between the therapist and client. Most therapy also addresses disruptions in relationships, such as acute or chronic trauma, loss, or attachment disruption.

Creative arts therapies are inherently relational therapies because they involve an active, sensory-based dynamic between practitioner and individual. All creative arts therapies are relational approaches to treatment that may involve mirroring, role play, enactment, sharing, showing, and witnessing (Malchiodi, 2005, 2012a). They may be helpful in repairing and reshaping attachment through experiential and sensory means, and may tap those early relational states that existed before words became dominant, allowing the brain to establish new, more productive patterns (Malchiodi, 2012b; Riley, 2002). In addition, being an attuned and focused witness to a child's efforts to complete a hands-on task, and assisting those efforts when appropriate, mimic the neurobiological relationship between a caring adult and a child. For some children, repetitive experiential and self-rewarding experiences that include a positive and attuned witness are central to repairing disrupted attachment and developing a sense of security and confidence (Perry, 2009). In brief, reparative enactments of secure attachment experiences, co-created by therapist and client, are fundamental to positive change.

Although all the creative arts therapies can be used with a goal of enhancing relationship, dance/movement therapy is most often used to address attachment issues, because it focuses on the body. For example, *mirroring* is commonly used to establish and enhance the relationship between the individual and the therapist. The goal of mirroring is not merely to have the client imitate movements, postures, facial expressions, and gestures, but to achieve a sense of connection and understanding between the client and practitioner. This is also a form of nonverbal, right-hemisphere communication that naturally occurs in secure attachment relationships through shared gestures, postures, and facial expressions between a caregiver and child. (For more information on dance/movement therapy, see Devereaux, Chapter 6, this volume).

Relational aspects are evident in art, music, and drama therapy also. In art therapy, a therapist is a provider of materials (nurturer), an assistant in the creative process, and an active participant in facilitating visual self-expression (see Malchiodi, Chapter 4, this volume). These are experiences that emphasize interaction through experiential, tactile, and visual exchanges, not just verbal communication, between the client and therapist. Music therapy (see Robarts, Chapter 5, this volume) provides similar experiences through interaction with music making; it also has the potential to tap social engagement and communication when collaboration or simultaneous playing of instruments is involved. Porges (2010) notes that vocalizations are particularly effective in stimulating a sense of affiliation and relationship, and that experiences involving specific music can inherently calm and self-regulate. Finally, drama therapy (see Gil & Dias, Chapter 7, this volume) offers multisensory ways to establish relationship through role play, mirroring, and enactment, and often includes other creative arts and play to support and enhance attachment.

Trauma-Informed Expressive Arts Therapy

Exposure to traumatic events is recognized as a significant factor in the development of attachment disorders (Oppenheim & Goldsmith, 2007). Freud (1920/1955) himself observed that traumatic experiences shatter the "protective shield" and threaten the core of the attachment relationship. Crises or loss disrupt parent–child dynamics and cause stress reactions in both the child and adult; these disruptions hinder the child's ability to find security from the caregiver, and may compromise the parent's ability to provide needed reassurance and comfort to the child. Insecure, disrupted, or disorganized attachment is often related to chronic traumatic experiences early in life. In general, these trauma experiences are encoded implicitly as sensory memories that are kinesthetic, auditory, olfactory, visual, and/or affective in nature. They influence relationships with caregivers and others, because individuals respond from lower-brain and limbic systems rather than from cortical areas (executive functions) of the brain.

Trauma-informed expressive arts therapy is one model for intervention that integrates neurodevelopmental knowledge and the sensory qualities of all the arts in trauma intervention, including attachment issues (Malchiodi, 2012a, 2012c). In brief, this approach takes into consideration how the mind and body respond to traumatic events; recognizes that symptoms are adaptive coping strategies rather than pathology; and helps individuals move from being "survivors" to becoming "thrivers" (Malchiodi, 2012c). Trauma-informed expressive arts therapy is based on the idea that the creative arts therapies are helpful in reconnecting implicit (sensory) and explicit (declarative) memories of trauma and in the treatment of post-traumatic stress disorder (PTSD) (Malchiodi, 2012a). In particular, it is an approach used to improve an individual's capacity to self-regulate affect and moderate the body's reactions to traumatic experiences to set the stage for eventual trauma integration and recovery.

Trauma-informed expressive arts therapy is also a means to address and enhance attachment, particularly in children who have experienced multiple traumas and losses. It includes a neurosequential approach that capitalizes on the expressive therapies continuum (Lusebrink, 2010) as a framework for applying appropriate creative arts therapies interventions (see Table 1.1). In attachment work, an emphasis is placed on arts-based experiences that reinforce a sense of safety through reconnection to positive attachment and self-soothing. The creative arts therapies are also used as ways to build strengths through experiences of mastery that normalize and enhance resilience. In brief, this means providing various opportunities for the individual to engage in creative experimentation that integrate experiences of unconditional appreciation, guidance, and support—experiences found in families with secure attachment relationships. In work with either a child or an adult, the goal is to help the individual recover the "creative

TABLE 1.1. Neurodevelopment and Arts Therapies

Area of brain	General functions	ETC level	Art therapy interventions
Brainstem	• Focus • Attunement to others • Attachment to others • Stress responses	Kinesthetic/sensory	• Sensory use of art materials • Texture and tactile elements • Self-soothing arts experiences (visual, music, movement) • Experiences of connection and approval • Rituals/structure in presentation
Midbrain diencephalon	• Motor skills • Coordination • Stress responses • Attunement to others • Attachment to others	Kinesthetic/sensory	• Physically oriented activities (cross the midline; engage body) • Learning skills via art and play • Self-soothing arts experiences (visual, music, movement) • Experiences of connection and approval • Rituals/structure in presentation
Limbic system	• Affect regulation • Pleasure • Relationships • Attunement • Attachment	Perceptual/affective	• Masks, puppets for projection and relational play • Arts and crafts for creative expression and skill enhancement • Group art therapy/family art therapy • Self-soothing arts experiences (visual, music, movement) • Rituals/structure in presentation
Cortex	• Cognition • Executive function • Self-image • Social competency • Communication	Cognitive/symbolic	• Cognitive-based methods possible, but sensory and affective methods may still be needed • Bibliotherapy with arts and play • Arts for skill enhancement and self-esteem • Teamwork in group art therapy • Problem-solving skills

Note. Based on the expressive therapies continuum (ETC) in Lusebrink (2010), Malchiodi (2012c), and Perry (2006). From Malchiodi (2012b). Copyright 2012 by The Guilford Press. Reprinted by permission.

life" (Cattanach, 2008), and to gain or regain a sense of well-being in oneself and in relationship to others.

In order to illustrate some of the key aspects of a trauma-informed expressive arts therapy approach with an attachment focus, the following brief case vignette is presented.

Case Vignette: Joanne, a Survivor of Multiple Traumas

Background and Early Sessions

Joanne, age 10, was referred to therapy after she witnessed her father beating her mother, Marie, on three occasions and was herself the victim of repeated physical abuse by her father. Marie did not report the incidents of child abuse or domestic violence until protective services removed Joanne and her younger brother Mark, age 5, from the home when their mother became unconscious due to a drug overdose. Joanne found her mother lying on the floor of their apartment and called the police, while Mark knelt screaming next to his mother's inert body. Although their mother recovered, social services felt it was in the children's best interests to stay at a residential treatment facility for the short term.

When I first visited Joanne at the facility, she was hypervigilant and unable to concentrate for very long. But she did like to draw and paint, and wanted to make a picture of her family because she missed her mother very much. When I asked Joanne to tell me more about the drawing, she said it was a picture of herself, Mark, and "my mommy." There were three human figures in the picture, each drawn appropriately for Joanne's age range (Figure 1.1). I asked, "Is there anyone else in the picture?" Joanne replied, "Well, I forget about my daddy a lot. He was mean to my mommy and hurt her all the time. He hit me and Mark, too."

Joanne's statement did not surprise me. Child abuse and domestic violence affect attachment relationships; children feel fearful that the violent parent or parental figure will cause injury or put them in danger. In order to resolve her difficult relationship with an abusive father, Joanne simply left him out of the picture. In subsequent art therapy sessions with Joanne, I also learned more about the complexities of her relationship with her mother: Joanne had increasingly become frightened and often angry at her mother, feeling abandoned during numerous incidents when Marie passed out from drug overdoses. In Joanne's case, attachment was also disrupted by Marie's neglect, indifference, or unresponsiveness; it shattered Joanne's trust that Marie would protect her from harm. Marie and Joanne both reported that Joanne was often anxious (hyperaroused) and also experienced sleep problems (nighttime anxiety and nightmares). In addition, Joanne's school counselor observed that she had difficulty with comprehension, focus, and attention, as well as with impulsively acting out (e.g., hitting other children or yelling at her classroom teacher).

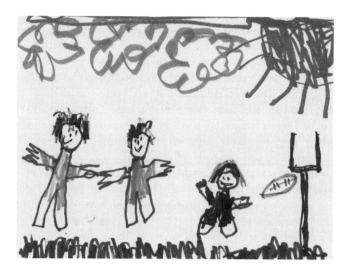

FIGURE 1.1. Joanne's drawing of her family, including her mother and younger brother but excluding her father.

Joanne's responses to me during our initial sessions mirrored her fear and anger about her primary caregivers. For example, she generally demanded my undivided attention when she was engaged in art making or play—particularly in the creative arts therapy group sessions, when she competed for attention with other child participants. On one occasion, she had a violent tantrum when I did not have enough clay on hand for her to complete a project; at another time, she scolded me for being a few minutes late for a session. It was easy to see that Joanne feared abandonment and had a difficult time self-regulating her emotions when confronted with situations she could not completely control or circumstances that felt unsafe.

In Joanne's case, the abuse by her father and a sense of abandonment by her mother both contributed to her attachment difficulties. Her attachment role also became disorganized because she had to assume the role of the caregiver when Marie's drug addiction prevented her from providing appropriate parenting to her children. In the art and play therapy room, Joanne often took on an adult persona, caring for other children and insisting on having a "helper" role during sessions.

A "Brain-Wise" Framework for Creative Intervention

In my work with Joanne, creative arts therapies interventions were guided by the five principles outlined in the earlier section on creative arts therapies and the brain, and by a trauma-informed expressive arts therapy framework. In brief, Joanne would benefit most from arts-based activities that addressed her emotional reactions and stress responses, create a sense of safety, and (to some extent) teach attunement to others and social awareness. She also would benefit from experiencing a positive relationship with me through sensory activities that recapitulated early attachment experiences via nonverbal and right-hemisphere interventions.

Initially, Joanne was able to show me easily through drawings that she felt detached from her abusive father by literally leaving him out of the picture. When working with children like Joanne, I generally start with arts experiences that are neurodevelopmentally related to lower parts of the brain (brainstem, midbrain, and limbic system) and designed to be self-soothing and self-regulating. Although Joanne was 10 years old, I introduced a few activities that I might use with much younger children, such as listening to various soothing rhythms, playing drums and percussion instruments together, and recalling favorite songs from preschool days. I introduced felt markers with different smells of familiar foods for drawing activities, as well as a variety of tactile materials for art making. In doing so, I took on the role of someone who provided materials for creative self-expression and accepted this self-expression with unconditional regard. At other times, I taught Joanne some child-friendly yoga poses, including ones that made us laugh because we enjoyed being "silly" together. We practiced deep breathing together, and I taught Joanne several child-appropriate mindfulness activities, such as balancing a long peacock feather on the tip of her finger and a colorful, self-created butterfly on the tip of her nose (Figure 1.2). All of these interventions were selected to support self-soothing experiences; in addition, I was making a "right-brain-to-right-brain" connection with Joanne by communicating with her through hands-on activities rather than words alone (the left hemisphere) and by using creative interventions to build a relationship.

Although it took many weeks before Joanne could engage in these initial sessions without angry or anxious feelings, she eventually began to feel safe in our relationship. She began to let me know what activities she enjoyed instead of communicating through tantrums, and even made suggestions indicating that she felt comfortable collaborating with me (e.g., asking if we could "make cookies together" or use materials "to build a house for a mother bird and her baby birds"). At this point in our relationship, I asked Joanne to share her feelings with me through art expression. She felt safe enough to respond with colors, lines, and shapes when I asked her "how your body feels when you worry" and "where in your body you feel worry, fear, and anger." I also introduced her to some simple musical instruments (drums, rattles, kazoo, and various percussion instruments) and encouraged her to make sounds to communicate feelings to me without words; Joanne began to use this activity as a way to convey to me how she was feeling at the beginning of each session. With my help, she was also able to begin to recognize situations when she felt these emotions and what types of situations caused her to become distressed.

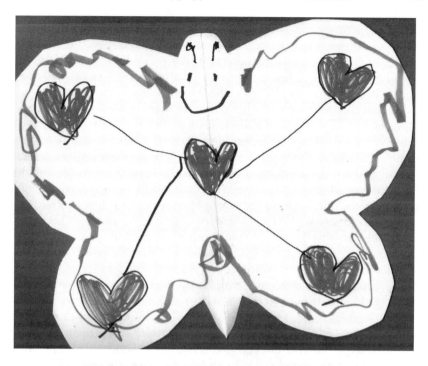

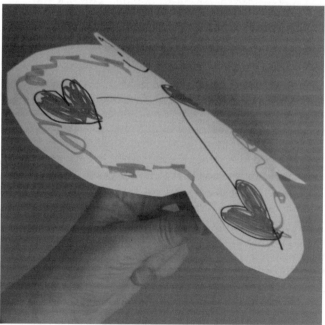

FIGURE 1.2 Two views of the butterfly Joanne created for use in a mindfulness activity.

My repetitive role as a provider of sensory means of self-expression, with unconditional positive regard for the outcome, became the bridge for Joanne to experience secure attachment with an adult. We made a good deal of progress in building a relationship before Joanne was moved to foster care in another town along with her brother, Mark. Her therapy continued for another year with another therapist after my work with her ended. However, before we terminated our sessions together, Marie was allowed to begin reestablishing her parenting role with Joanne and was asked to participate in several mother–child creative arts therapies sessions with us.

Because a trauma-informed expressive arts therapy approach applies to individuals of all ages, and particularly those who may be in need of trauma or attachment intervention, I repeated several of the activities I had used earlier with Joanne with Marie as a participant. For example, Marie herself was in need of self-regulation through other means than drugs; because she had been in a violent relationship with her husband for most of their married life, she understandably needed some self-soothing experiences as well. In particular, I focused on some simple self-soothing creative activities that Marie could initiate with Joanne at home, such as quiet times for drawing, scrapbooking pictures, and collage work. More importantly, I was able to introduce some experiences of collaborative, attachment-enhancing activities, such as building a dollhouse together from shoeboxes and making puppet families from socks. Although I do not know the ultimate outcome of our work together, I do know that Joanne, Mark, and Marie were eventually reunited, and that Marie, with the help of addictions counseling, has been able to maintain a drug-free existence.

Conclusion

With many child clients like Joanne and parents like Marie, we have a limited number of sessions to accomplish attachment goals that may or may not be retained over time. Despite the challenges of these types of situations, I believe that we do make an impact on the individuals we seek to help by using creative arts as part of therapy, for one key reason: The creative arts therapies are "brain-wise" interventions. When used in purposeful ways, these approaches are compatible with what we currently understand about the brain and attachment; they capitalize on nonverbal and right-hemisphere communication, active participation, and the self-soothing nature of creative expression through images, sound, movement, and enactment. Most importantly, the creative arts are a way to experience a secure relationship with a helping professional that resonates on a sensory level in both mind and body, and in a place within each of us where attachment is most authentically recognized, integrated, and appreciated.

REFERENCES

American Music Therapy Association. (2013). *About music therapy.* Retrieved February 25, 2013, from *www.musictherapy.org/about/musictherapy*

Badenoch, B. (2008). *Being a brain-wise therapist: A practical guide to interpersonal neurobiology.* New York: Norton.

Bowlby, J. (2005). *A secure base.* New York: Routledge. (Original work published 1988)

Cattanach, A. (2008). *Play therapy with abused children.* London: Kingsley.

Doidge, N. (2007). *The brain that changes itself.* New York: Penguin.

Edwards, D. (2004). *Art therapy.* Thousand Oaks, CA: Sage.

Freud, S. (1955). *Beyond the pleasure principle.* In J. Strachey (Ed. & Trans.), *The standard edition of the complete psychological works of Sigmund Freud* (Vol. 18, pp. 7–64). London: Hogarth Press. (Original work published 1920)

Gil, E. (2006). *Helping abused and traumatized children.* New York: Guilford Press.

Gladding, S. (2005). *Counseling as an art: Creative arts in counseling* (3rd ed.). Alexandria, VA: American Counseling Association.

Goodill, S. (2005). *Introduction to medical dance/movement therapy.* London: Kingsley.

Johnson, D. R. (2009). *Current approaches in drama therapy.* Springfield, IL: Thomas.

Klorer, P. G. (2008). Expressive therapy for severe maltreatment and attachment disorders: A neuroscience framework. In C. A. Malchiodi (Ed.), *Creative interventions with traumatized children* (pp. 43–61). New York: Guilford Press.

Knill, P., Barba, H. N., & Fuchs, M. (2004). *Minstrels of the soul: Intermodal expressive therapy.* Toronto: EGS Press.

Lusebrink, V. (2010). Assessment and therapeutic application of the expressive therapies continuum: Implications for brain structures and functions. *Art Therapy, 27*(4), 168–177.

Malchiodi, C. A. (1997). *Breaking the silence: Art therapy with children from violent homes* (2nd ed.). New York: Brunner-Routledge.

Malchiodi, C. A. (Ed.). (2005). *Expressive therapies.* New York: Guilford Press.

Malchiodi, C. A. (Ed.). (2008). *Creative interventions with traumatized children.* New York: Guilford Press.

Malchiodi, C. A. (2012a). Art therapy and the brain. In C. A. Malchiodi (Ed.), *Handbook of art therapy* (2nd ed., pp. 17–26). New York: Guilford Press.

Malchiodi, C. A. (2012b). Developmental art therapy. In C. A. Malchiodi (Ed.), *Handbook of art therapy* (2nd ed., pp. 114–129). New York: Guilford Press.

Malchiodi, C. A. (2012c). Trauma-informed art therapy with sexually abused children. In P. Goodyear-Brown (Ed.), *Handbook of child sexual abuse: Prevention, assessment, and treatment* (pp. 341–354). Hoboken, NJ: Wiley.

Micozzi, M. (Ed.). (2011). *Fundamentals of complementary and alternative medicine* (4th ed.). St. Louis, MO: Saunders/Elsevier.

National Association for Poetry Therapy. (2013). *National Association for Poetry Therapy.* Retrieved February 25, 2013, from *www.poetrytherapy.org/index.html*

National Dance Therapy Association. (2013). *About dance/movement therapy.* Retrieved February 25, 2013, from *www.adta.org/About_DMT*

National Drama Therapy Association. (2013). *What is drama therapy?* Retrieved February 20, 2013, from *www.nadt.org/what-is-drama-therapy.html*

Oppenheim, D., & Goldsmith, D. (Eds.). (2007). *Attachment theory in clinical work with children.* New York: Guilford Press.

Payne, H. (Ed.). (2013). *Dance movement therapy: Theory, research and practice.* New York: Routledge.

Perry, B. (2006). The neurosequential model of therapeutics: Applying principles of neuroscience to clinical work with traumatized and maltreated children. In N. B. Webb (Ed.), *Working with traumatized youth in child welfare* (pp. 27–52). New York: Guilford Press.

Perry, B. (2008). Foreword. In C. A. Malchiodi (Ed.), *Creative interventions with traumatized children* (pp. ix–xi). New York: Guilford Press.

Perry, B. (2009). Examining child maltreatment through a neurodevelopmental lens. *Journal of Trauma and Loss, 14,* 240–255.

Porges, S. W. (2010). Music therapy and trauma: Insights from the polyvagal theory. In K. Stewart (Ed.), *Symposium on music therapy and trauma: Bridging theory and clinical practice.* New York: Satchnote Press.

Riley, S. (2002). *Group process made visible.* New York: Taylor & Francis.

Rothschild, B. (2000). *The body remembers.* New York: Norton.

Schore, A. (2003). *Affect regulation and the repair of the self.* New York: Norton.

Siegel, D. (2012). *The developing mind* (2nd ed.). New York: Guilford Press.

Steele, W., & Malchiodi, C. A. (2012). *Trauma-informed practices with children and adolescents.* New York: Routledge.

Teicher, M. H. (2000). Wounds that won't heal: The neurobiology of child abuse. *Cerebrum, 2*(4), 50–62.

van der Kolk, B. (2006). Clinical applications of neuroscience research in PTSD. *Annals of the New York Academy of Sciences, 1071*(4), 277–293.

Warren, B. (2004). *Using the creative arts in therapy: A practical introduction* (2nd ed.). New York: Routledge.

Weiner, D. (1999). *Beyond talk therapy: Using movement and expressive techniques in clinical practice.* Washington, DC: American Psychological Association.

Wheeler, B. L., Shultis, C. L., & Polen, D. W. (2005). *Clinical training guide for the student music therapist.* Gilsum, NH: Barcelona.

CHAPTER 2

Play Therapy Approaches
to Attachment Issues

David A. Crenshaw

The need to explicate the role of play therapy and the creative arts therapies with attachment issues was vividly brought to my attention when
I searched the index of the often consulted and acclaimed second edition
of the *Handbook of Attachment* (Cassidy & Shaver, 2008). In this comprehensive volume of 1,020 pages, I found only four separate references to
page numbers in the index for play, and none for play therapy, art therapy,
creative arts therapy, or expressive arts therapy. I should note that the four
selections of page numbers in the index referring to play were important
ones, briefly detailing (1) the role of attachment security in social play rep-
ertoires; (2) the critical importance of attachment for the quality of play; (3)
the dependence of "play-mothering" and later caregiving capacity on the
experience of maternal care; and (4) the facts that exploratory behavior is
playful and that play only develops in a secure context. In spite of this lack
of attention until recently among attachment theorists and play therapy
researchers, there is a long history of play therapy approaches dedicated to
treating attachment problems.

Early Roots of the Focus on Attachment in Play Therapy

The crucial role of favorable early attachment was recognized and written
about extensively by the early psychoanalysts. A consensus in psychoanalytic writing from the earliest days was that human infants need unconditional love in order to develop in a healthy way what one analyst called

"non-obligating solicitude" (Bonime, 1989). The psychoanalyst Erich
Fromm (1947) expressed it eloquently:

> Motherly love does not depend on conditions which the child has to fulfill in
> order to be loved; it is unconditional, based only upon the child's request and
> the mother's response. No wonder that motherly love has been a symbol of the
> highest form of love in art and religion. (pp. 99–100)

Freud (1909/1959) also weighed in on the incomparable role of early attachment figures:

> For a small child his parents are the first and the only authority and the source
> of all belief. The child's most intense and most momentous wish during these
> early years is to be like his parents (that is, the parent of his own sex) and to
> be big like his father and mother. (p. 237)

Lili Peller (1946) understood that this love needs to come from those
with whom the infant is biologically bonded—a fact that has led to immeasurable heartbreak for children and parents in the foster care system. Peller
wrote:

> The child's greatest need is for love from the persons to whom he is attached,
> and not merely from persons who chance to be near him. 'Persons of his envi-
> ronment,' his teacher or nurse or a kind-hearted aunt, may offer this love
> amply to the child—yet he profits but little. We can assume that many foster-
> children have been offered love and affection to no avail. (p. 415)

The psychoanalyst Edward Edinger (1972) beautifully described the
gift enjoyed by recipients of unconditional love in infancy: "The sense of
innate worth prior to and irrespective of deeds and accomplishments is
the precious deposit that is left in the psyche by the experience of genuine
parental love" (p. 167).

Early roots of play therapy's focus on attachment and attachment
trauma can also be found in the writings of Donald Winnicott (1971), as
detailed by Tuber, Boesch, Gorkin, and Terry in Chapter 13 of this volume. Tuber (2008) has explained in an earlier publication that Winnicott
(1971) identified a tolerable window of infant distress when the mother
(primary caregiver) is absent; when this window is exceeded in duration, or
the infant undergoes emotional duress, the experience for the infant is one
of confusion and disorganization. Interestingly, nearly two decades later
the term *disorganized attachment* was introduced by Main and Solomon
(1990) to describe the effects of severe attachment trauma.

Winnicott became interested in attachment issues and the corollary
experiences of separation and loss during World War II. Winnicott, along
with John Bowlby, Anna Freud, and other prominent British and European
analysts, worked hard to resettle children in the countryside so that they

could escape the incessant bombings in London. In a letter written in 1939 to the *British Medical Journal* and titled "Evacuation of Small Children," Bowlby and Winnicott, along with the analyst Emanuel Miller, stated:

> It is quite possible for a child of any age to feel sad or upset at having to leave home, but . . . such an experience in the case of a little child can mean far more than the actual experience of sadness. It can in fact amount to an emotional "black-out" and can easily lead to a severe disturbance of the development of the personality which may persist throughout life. (Bowlby, Miller, & Winnicott, 1939, pp. 1202–1203)

Thus, in the midst of the horror of World War II, these early analysts described what we now consider *attachment trauma* and what is sometimes called in children *developmental trauma*.

What Is Attachment Trauma?

Attachment trauma is one of the terms intended to address the growing consensus that posttraumatic stress disorder (PTSD) does not adequately describe what happens to people when they suffer interpersonal trauma. This is especially true when the trauma ruptures relationships with primary attachment figures. PTSD—a diagnostic classification in the third, fourth, and now fifth editions of the American Psychiatric Association's (1980, 1994, 2013), *Diagnostic and Statistical Manual of Mental Disorders* (DSM-III, DSM-IV, and DSM-5 respectively)—describes a cluster of symptoms that tend to ameliorate in time (often in 3 months) and are responsive to evidence-based treatments, most notably cognitive-behavioral therapy. What the diagnosis of PTSD does not adequately detail is the often enduring relational impact when trauma intrudes into the interpersonal life of any person, but especially a child. If, for example, a child is abused by the very person(s) responsible for his or her well-being, safety, and nurture, the insidious effects on the capacity to trust, to risk closeness with another, and to envision a positive future are common enduring sequelae not addressed by the PTSD classification of symptoms; nor can they be addressed adequately in brief treatment models.

The inadequacy of the PTSD diagnostic criteria has long spurred a debate among some of the leading trauma researchers and clinicians. Judith Herman (1992) offered the term *complex trauma* to delineate trauma that involves repeated and chronic abuse, instead of a single traumatic event that can cause PTSD symptoms. Previously, Lenore Terr (1990) distinguished between *Type 1* and *Type 2* traumas. Type 1 represents single-event trauma, whereas Type 2 refers to repeated or chronic trauma and often multiple traumatic factors (such as growing up in poverty, exposure to abuse, and/or exposure to domestic or community violence). Herman also decried the use of what she considered demeaning diagnostic labels that are used to characterize the complexity of symptoms resulting from repeated exposure to trauma, such as borderline personality disorder. More recently, Bessel van der Kolk (2005) has offered the term *developmental trauma* to describe complex trauma in childhood, because of its potentially devastating impact on the course of the unfolding developmental process.

Allan Schore (2012) has written eloquently about *relational trauma*. Schore emphasizes the impact of unfavorable early attachments (during the first 18 months of life) on the development of the right hemisphere of the brain. Schore has demonstrated that ruptures and lack of repair of the attunement process between the infant and the primary caregiver result in impaired development of the right hemisphere. One of the major effects is the inability to regulate emotions adequately, and another is impaired relational capacity.

There was a time some 20 years ago when the work of attachment researchers and the work of clinicians in therapy rooms ran on separate tracks, with little collaboration between the two groups. All of that changed when the writings of two master integrators from the University of California at Los Angeles (UCLA), Daniel Siegel and Allan Schore, became widely read. Siegel's (1999, 2012) *The Developing Mind* opened the eyes of many to the possibilities of making use of attachment theory and research findings in therapeutic work. His development of the interpersonal neuro-biological approach not only combined attachment research with psycho-therapy theory and research, but added the contributions of neuroscience to our understanding of how attachment and psychotherapy change the structure of the brain. As noted above, Schore (1994, 2003a, 2003b, 2012) is the other UCLA researcher and clinician who has been able to synthe-size findings from psychoanalytic and attachment theory with neuroscience research to highlight the pivotal role of favorable early attachments in the proper development of the right hemisphere of the brain, which in turn critically influences the development of emotional regulation. Schore has also delineated the important implications of his work for psychotherapy, since emotional dysregulation is a key feature of most childhood and adult psychiatric disorders. This exciting work has not validated the concept of infantile determinism, because neuroscience research has demonstrated that new brain connections can be made throughout life, but it has affirmed the Freudian emphasis on early parent–child relationships and the critical periods for secure attachments coinciding with the incredible rate of brain development in the first 2 years of life.

Bruce Perry (Perry & Szalavitz, 2006), another key contributor to our understanding of the neurobiological underpinnings of emotional and rela-tional development, has explained that if critical periods in the early attach-ment process are missed, a child is not doomed; however, when repair is attempted later in development, it will take much longer and require much repetition of favorable experiences with attachment figures. The good news is that children possess impressive innate capacities for self-reparative and healing processes, combined with security in relationships with caregivers. The bad news is that if the healthy innate forces combined with favorable attachment experiences come later in the developmental sequence, it will take much more time to effect the positive changes.

Jon Allen (2013) is another seminal theorist and clinician; his work builds on the attachment research of British theorists, particularly Peter Fonagy (Fonagy & Target, 1997). Fonagy and his colleagues used the term *attachment trauma* to refer not only to trauma that takes place in the context of attachment relationships, but also to the damaging impact of such trauma on the capacity to develop secure attachment. Allen views *neglect* (defined as the lack of psychological attunement) as central to attachment trauma. Allen elaborates further that "trauma stems from being left *psychologically alone in unbearable emotional pain*" (p. xxii; emphasis in original).

In addition to the lack of consensus regarding the definition of attachment trauma and the controversies surrounding inclusion–exclusion of complex PTSD and developmental trauma disorder in DSM-5 (they were ultimately excluded), there is lack of agreement on variations of attachment disorders. Beginning with DSM-III, and followed by DSM-IV and DSM-IV-TR, reactive attachment disorder (RAD) was the only recognized attachment disorder included in this official diagnostic classification manual of the American Psychiatric Association. RAD is a rare form of attachment trauma suffered primarily by children who have been institutionalized in early life and/or severely abused. There were two recognized forms of this disorder: (1) the emotionally withdrawn/inhibited form, in which there is a failure to respond to comfort when offered and failure to seek comfort when distressed from a preferred attachment figure; and (2) the disinhibited/indiscriminately social type, in which the child is overly interested in interacting with and sometimes seeking affection from unfamiliar adults, without distinction. These more severe forms of attachment disorder are seen in some children in residential treatment centers, as well as in some (but certainly not all) cross-cultural adoptions of previously institutionalized children.

DSM-5 split the previously existing category of RAD into two separate diagnoses. Reactive attachment disorder is now defined as a lack of or incomplete formation of preferred attachments to familiar people, with a dampening of positive affect that resembles internalizing disorders (e.g., anxiety). Disinhibited social engagement disorder is the other diagnosis.

Play therapists may work with children with RAD in their private offices, clinics, or residential treatment center playrooms, but far more frequently play therapists see children with less severe problems of insecure attachment, and the goal is to increase attachment security. Even more advantageous are the prevention programs that can head off such relational problems by intervening early.

How Does Play Therapy Address Attachment Trauma?

Since the value of all psychotherapy rests on the foundation of the therapeutic relationship, play therapy, with its emphasis on the dyadic relationship, offers the possibility of greater attachment security for a child who has suffered interpersonal trauma. In addition, play therapy has a distinct advantage over other relationship therapies, in that one of the therapeutic powers of play is attachment formation (Schaefer, 1993; Schaefer & Drewes, 2014). Schaefer explains that secure attachment can be facilitated in children by replicating the positive parent–child relationship through sensory–motor play. Schaefer (1993) has observed, "Playful interactions involving touch and smiling are perhaps the most natural and enjoyable ways to form an attachment with a child in the playroom" (p. 11).

Theraplay

An early form of play therapy that preceded the seminal volumes on loss and attachment by Bowlby was a focused attachment process called Theraplay (Jernberg, 1979). In 1967, Ann Jernberg was appointed the director of the Head Start program in Chicago. She recruited Phyllis Booth as one of her assistants (see Booth, Lindaman, & Winstead, Chapter 9, this volume). Jernberg did not feel that referring the numerous children who needed intervention to existing crowded mental health clinics was an adequate solution; instead, she developed her own program. In order to meet the enormity of the need, she designed her program to make use of paraprofessionals working under the supervision of mental health professionals. Theraplay is a model of play therapy that is based on healthy parent–child interactions and draws partly on the work of Austin Des Lauriers (1962) and Viola Brody (1997). As a result of this pioneering work with Head Start, the Theraplay Institute was formed in 1971, and children from the community were referred for treatment. From this modest beginning in Chicago in the late 1960s, Theraplay is now practiced in over 36 countries around the world.

Filial Therapy

Filial Therapy (FT), developed by Bernard and Louise Guerney in the late 1950s, has considerable research support and has developed as a powerful family therapy and play therapy intervention (B. G. Guerney, 1964; L. F. Guerney, 2003; L. F. Guerney & Ryan, 2013; VanFleet, 2013). It has a specific focus on attachment and treating forms of insecure attachment, along with more severe cases of attachment trauma (see Topham, VanFleet, & Sniscak, Chapter 8, this volume). One of the compelling advantages of FT in the treatment of attachment trauma is the presence of the primary attachment figure(s) in the treatment. Attachment security is being built between the child and one or more primary caregivers even as the trauma is being addressed.

The Circle of Security

In addition to the attachment formation power of play, play enhances the relationship of the child not only with the play therapist but with others who may participate in the play therapy, such as the primary caregiver(s) in FT, in developmental play therapy (Brody, 1997), and in prevention programs like the Circle of Security (see Stewart, Whelan, & Pendleton, Chapter 3, this volume). The Circle of Security program specifically teaches parents to recognize when children need encouragement to explore and to move away from the parent, and to provide support and a secure base to return to when the child needs a safety net. The playful interactions combined with the sensitive attunement of the parent's empathic responding to the child's needs greatly enhances the attachment bonds. Schaefer (1993) has written: "The role of play in facilitating a positive relationship is related to the nature of playful interactions that are fun filled and concerned with enjoyment rather than achievement" (p. 12). The most effective way to build an attachment or enhance a relationship with a child is to create safe, trusting, and gratifying experiences with an adult, and play is an effective and natural medium to facilitate the process.

The Neurosequential Model of Therapeutics

As noted earlier, one of the pioneers in the neurobiology of attachment is Bruce Perry (Perry, 2009; Perry & Szalavitz, 2006), who has articulated the Neurosequential Model of Therapeutics. This model involves many play components, including sensory–motor play to help soothe the brainstem (see Gaskill & Perry, Chapter 11, this volume). The Neurosequential Model of Therapeutics has brought new understanding to the work of the play therapist in addressing disruptions of early attachments. Perry explains that what we do in therapy sometimes doesn't matter as much as when we do it. Timing and sequence are essential in addressing attachment trauma, and Gaskill and Perry offer a map to guide us.

Case Vignette: Play Therapy for Attachment Trauma

Individual Play Therapy Sessions

Jason, a 6-year-old boy constantly in trouble at school, entered the playroom and immediately headed for the plastic tubs of puppets. Puppets went flying in all directions until he found one that appealed to him. He finally settled on an alligator, with unusually sharp and long teeth; he then threw in the direction of the therapist a rather defenseless puppet, a beaver. Before the therapist was able to get his hand fully into the beaver puppet, Jason, with a startling roar, pounced on the beaver and locked him in a vise-like grip with amazing strength for such a young child. What were striking about the alligator's aggression were the intensity and the affect behind it. At one point, the therapist had to set a limit, because the viciousness of the attacks caused physical pain. To prevent injury to child and therapist, Jason was told, "It is OK for the alligator to be angry and attack the beaver, but it is not OK for either of us to get hurt, so you need to be not quite so rough." It was the only time that a limit was needed: Jason, while still expressing considerable rage in the alligator's attacks on the beaver in the remainder of that session and in subsequent sessions, always stopped short of inflicting pain on the therapist or causing injury to himself. The individual play sessions that followed were active, largely focused on the theme of aggression and revenge, but there was a gradual, nonlinear reduction in the intensity of the affect expressed as well as symbolized through the action of the play. Also, accurately depicting the pain of Jason's life situation, the alligator always acted alone. There were no companions or friends.

The rage expressed by this first-grade boy in the form of a vengeful, attacking alligator puppet accurately symbolized his internal inferno, stemming from multiple factors—most obviously the sudden death of his father, who had died of a heart attack while running a marathon 6 months earlier. Of the four children, Jason, the second-born, had experienced the most conflictual relationship with his father and carried the heaviest burden following his sudden death. Jason's attachment with his father had been insecure/ambivalent, and there was no longer an opportunity to make it more secure. Jason's father had been harder on him than on his two sisters and his younger brother. The paternal grandmother observed that Jason's father had had similar impulse and externalizing problems when he was Jason's age. Jason's mother had tried to protect Jason and thought her husband was truly too hard on him, but she surmised that her husband mostly had good intentions and didn't want Jason to have the same hard struggles that he had experienced as a child.

Although the father's intentions were probably good, the effect on Jason was to make him feel that he could never please his father, in spite of desperately wanting his approval. Jason experienced his father's concern more sharply as massive rejection. In addition, Jason struggled with neurodevelopmental challenges. His impulsivity was a component of his attention-deficit/hyperactivity disorder (ADHD), which made it hard for him to function without alienating his siblings or his peers at school and in sports. Whether with his siblings or his peers, he always was determined to be first and was quite willing to push others out of line if they were ahead of him. He was far more than a "rough-and-tumble boy" on the playground, sometimes hitting peers broadside at full speed, and occasionally causing injury (as well as alarm on the part of school officials and worried parents of other first graders). The play therapist attended frequent meetings with the mother and his teachers and school officials at his elementary school because of Jason's bullying, aggressive, and intimidating behavior. Behavioral plans were developed and implemented, with temporary improvements but no lasting change, because the underlying issues were complicated and would take time to work through adequately.

What Jason had experienced as a core part of his attachment trauma was a deep hurt shared by many children whose attachments are traumatically ruptured; it took the form of identification as a "child who does not fit." Jason "did not fit" in his family because of his dysregulated behavior associated with ADHD and his hostility stemming from his perception of rejection by his father. Jason "didn't fit" in school for the same reasons, plus his attempts to compensate for his lack of acceptance by becoming hypercompetitive. His extreme competitiveness further alienated his peers—not only in school, but when he played soccer or baseball. Jason always had to be captain, always win, and always be first, or else he would explode in anger. Any experience that symbolized "loss" in the slightest way triggered a huge emotional reaction, almost always taking the form of blind rage. James Garbarino (1999) has noted that the closest thing to a psychological malignancy is social rejection in childhood. When the rejection is perceived within a child's family as well as in his or her social world, the malignancy is particularly potent and often accompanied by the most profound forms of rage.

Jason shared another psychodynamic constellation with other children who suffer attachment trauma. Clinical experience indicates that anger/rage is experienced by children as an empowering emotion, whereas sorrow leaves them feeling vulnerable and exposed. Underneath Jason's burning rage was the far more delicate and vulnerable feeling of profound sorrow. The loss of his father was sudden and final, leaving him no opportunity to make amends or to resolve the struggle and conflict with his father. The wound was anything but clean, and healing would be complicated by the permanent absence of his father.

The individual play therapy sessions helped build trust in the therapist and enhanced the therapeutic relationship. Jason was able to displace safely, within the symbolism of the aggressive play (the alligator puppet's attacking the beaver and other defenseless animal puppets), the burning rage stemming from his unresolved loss and grief and from his social rejection. The play sessions allowed him to modulate his rage as he gave full expression to its intensity in a safe and controlled environment, and then, over a period of 10 subsequent sessions, exercised more conscious and safer control over different levels of intensity of affective expression. The individual play therapy, however, could not provide all of the ingredients needed for healing such a severe rupture in Jason's attachments. The play therapist needed to shift approaches to enlist the resources of the family system.

Focused Family Therapy Sessions

Although the play therapist would not have credibility in convincing Jason that there could be another meaning to his father's harshness, his mother, paternal grandmother, and aunts were in a more favorable position to do so. Basically, what Jason needed was a phase of cognitive work focused on modifying his belief that his father had never accepted him or loved him. The play therapist knew that it was going to take more than one person and more than one session to make a dent in his strongly held belief that his father "hated him," which he repeatedly stated. The play therapist decided to call on one family resource at a time. In the first session, his mother was invited to join with the therapist in talking with Jason about her belief that although Jason's father had been strict and tough on him, he did so because he loved him and he didn't want his son to get into trouble repeatedly, the way he had done himself. The play therapist primarily played the role of "silent witness" (Gil, 2010), but did amplify the alternative way of understanding the father's intention. When the mother stated her view of what the father was trying to do, the play therapist said, "Oh, that's a new way of looking at how your father felt about you. He was hard on you because he loved you, and he didn't want you to go through the hard times he went through." Jason was attentive but seemed skeptical.

Next the play therapist called on the paternal grandmother, who, in spite of her own considerable grief resulting from the death of her only son, did a remarkable job of sharing with conviction her belief that Jason's father had loved him and wanted to teach him lessons that he himself had had to learn the hard way. What seemed to intrigue Jason the most were the many examples his grandmother gave him of how his father had gotten into trouble when he was Jason's age. Some of them, like the time his father poured glue on his first-grade teacher's wooden chair, made him laugh. He seemed relieved that he was not the only "black sheep" in the family, and he also gained a sense of solidarity with his father. His mother's argument that his father had only been trying to straighten him out and keep him out of trouble seemed to gain more credibility with every story of misbehavior that the grandmother told.

Family Play Therapy

The final stage of Jason's therapy took the form of family play therapy (Gil, 1994), with the goal of restoring connections with his mother and siblings. In one quite poignant session with the mother and all four of her children, the children decided that the eagle puppet had a broken wing.

This was a powerful metaphor. Until the sudden, traumatic death of the father this had been an "all-American" type of family. The family members were all quite active, into sports and outdoors activities, but now they were grounded and having trouble getting airborne again. In the beginning, Jason refused to participate with his siblings. He sat next to his mother, but turned away from the other children. Jason was literally enacting in the session the destructive identity that he had embraced of "the child who did not fit—did not belong." His primary attachments had been disrupted not only by the unexpected death of his father, but by the alienation of his siblings and his peers. Jason enacted in the session the pattern that he doggedly enacted in his daily life, making sure that he was the "child who did not belong." His unspoken credo was "I will reject you before you will even get the opportunity to reject me." Yet beneath this maladaptive defensive pattern was the hunger that all humans share for acceptance and belonging.

The therapist recognized this as a critical moment in the family play therapy. Would everyone together—mother, siblings, and therapist—be able to convince Jason that he had an important place in the family, or would he choose to remain outside the circle of the family in his lonely, painful self-imposed exile? His mother expressed in a heartfelt way her wish for Jason to join the family and participate in the family play of the "eagle with a broken wing." Each of his siblings also tried their best to convince Jason to join them, but he still was holding out. The therapist then said to Jason, "We need you, Jason. We will not be able to heal the eagle's broken wing without you." The therapist then handed him the doctor's kit. Everyone in their room held their breath until Jason sprang to his feet and came over and began attending to the eagle, which was tenderly held by one of his sisters. This was a turning point. Jason finally was able to accept that he no longer had to be the "child who did not belong." His family had been convincing, and he was invested from that point on in the family play drama of healing the eagle's broken wing.

A particularly interesting feature of Jason's empathic attending to the eagle as a doctor with his various instruments of healing was singing to the eagle. Only a few weeks later, in a meeting with his mother, did I learn the significance of the singing. His mother told me that an important breakthrough had occurred at home in the week before the pivotal session. The loving and empathic mom had always gathered the children at bedtime and sung to them a song they all loved. After the death of the father, Jason in his anger would not tolerate his mother's singing. In the week prior to the "eagle's wing" session, Jason had come to his mom and asked her if he could sing the song that she had formerly sung before bedtime to the children. Jason did sing it and remembered all the words. This was part of the reparative movement toward reunion with his family, his acceptance of his father's death, and his willing to embrace the love of his family and perhaps for the first time enter into a heartfelt sense of belonging.

Conclusion

Play therapy has rich and enduring early roots in attachment theory, and some early work in attachment-focused play therapy even predates attachment theory. Not only did the early child psychoanalysts regard the parent–infant bond as a primary focus, but Theraplay—with its emphasis on enhancing attachment and bonding through playful interactions between primary caregivers and their babies—was launched in Chicago in the late 1960s, before the major writings of John Bowlby (who is most often identified as the pioneer of attachment theory) were published. Donald Winnicott, as an early analyst and pediatrician, used play therapy as a way of strengthening attachment, and collaborated later with Bowlby on projects during World War II to deal with the disrupted attachments of children evacuated from the bombings of London. More recently, the work of Allan Schore, Daniel Siegel, and Bruce Perry, grounded in the science of neurobiology, has greatly expanded our understanding of the neurobiology of early attachments; these researchers have shown how favorable consistent interactions are essential for infants to develop gradually the capacity for affect regulation, and how the timing of our interventions needs to be informed by new understandings of brain development. It is an exciting time to be a play therapist.

REFERENCES

Allen, J. G. (2013). *Restoring mentalizing in attachment relationships: Treating trauma with plain old therapy.* Arlington, VA: American Psychiatric Publishing.

American Psychiatric Association. (1980). *Diagnostic and statistical manual of mental disorders* (3rd ed.). Washington, DC: Author.

American Psychiatric Association. (1994). *Diagnostic and statistical manual of mental disorders* (4th ed.). Washington, DC: Author.

American Psychiatric Association. (2000). *Diagnostic and statistical manual of mental disorders* (4th ed., text rev.). Washington, DC: Author.

American Psychiatric Association. (2013). *Diagnostic and statistical manual of mental disorders* (5th ed.). Arlington, VA: Author.

Bonime, W. (1989). *Collaborative psychoanalysis: Anxiety, depression, dreams, and personality change.* Cranbury, NJ: Associated University Presses.

Bowlby, J., Miller, E., & Winnicott, D. W. (1939, December 16). Evacuation of small children [Letter]. *British Medical Journal, ii*(4119), 1202–1233.

Brody, V. (1997). *The dialogue of touch: Developmental play therapy.* Northvale, NJ: Aronson.

Cassidy, J., & Shaver, P. R. (Eds.). (2008). *Handbook of attachment* (2nd ed.). New York: Guilford Press.

Des Lauriers, A. (1962). *The experience of reality in childhood schizophrenia.* New York: International Universities Press.

Edinger, E. F. (1972). *Ego and archetype.* New York: Putnam.

Fonagy, P., & Target, M. (1997). Attachment and reflective function: Their role in self-organization. *Developmental Psychopathology, 9,* 679–700.

Freud, S. (1959). Family romances. In J. Strachey (Ed. & Tran.), *The standard edition of the complete psychological works of Sigmund Freud* (Vol. 9, pp. 235–242). London: Hogarth Press. (Original work published 1909)

Fromm, E. (1947). *Man for himself: An inquiry into the psychology of ethics.* New York: Rinehart.

Garbarino, J. (1999). *Lost boys: Why our sons turn violent and how we can save them.* New York: Anchor Books.

Gil, E. (1994). *Play in family therapy.* New York: Guilford Press.

Gil, E. (2010). Children's self-initiated gradual exposure: The wonders of post-traumatic play and behavioral reenactments. In E. Gil (Ed.), *Working with children to heal interpersonal trauma: The power of play* (pp. 44–63). New York: Guilford Press.

Guerney, B. G., Jr. (1964). Filial therapy: Description and rationale. *Journal of Consulting Psychology, 28,* 303–310.

Guerney, L. F. (2003). The history, principles, and empirical basis of Filial Therapy. In R. VanFleet & L. F. Guerney (Eds.), *Casebook of Filial Therapy* (pp. 1–19). Boiling Springs, PA: Play Therapy Press.

Guerney, L. F., & Ryan, V. M. (2013). *Group Filial Therapy: A complete guide to teaching parents to play therapeutically with their children.* Philadelphia, PA: Kingsley.

Herman, J. (1992). *Trauma and recovery: The aftermath of violence—from domestic abuse to political terror.* New York: Basic Books.

Jernberg, A. (1979). *Theraplay: A new treatment using structured play for problem children and their families.* San Francisco: Jossey-Bass.

Main, M., & Solomon, J. (1990). Procedures for identifying infants as disorganized/disoriented during the Ainsworth Strange Situation. In M. T. Greenberg, D. Cicchetti, & E. M. Cummings (Eds.), *Attachment in the preschool years: Theory, research, and intervention* (pp. 121–160). Chicago: University of Chicago Press.

Peller, L. E. (1946). Incentives to development and means of early education. *Psychoanalytic Study of the Child, 2,* 397–415.

Perry, B. D. (2009). Examining child maltreatment through a neurosequential lens: Clinical application of the Neurosequential Model of Therapeutics. *Journal of Loss and Trauma, 14,* 240–255.

Perry, B. D., & Szalavitz, M. (2006). *The boy who was raised as a dog: And other stories from a child psychiatrist's notebook.* New York: Basic Books.

Schaefer, C. E. (Ed.). (1993). *The therapeutic powers of play.* Northvale, NJ: Aronson.

Schaefer, C. E., & Drewes, A. A. (Eds.). (2014). *The therapeutic powers of play: 20 core agents of change* (2nd ed.). Hoboken, NJ: Wiley.

Schore, A. N. (1994). *Affect regulation and the origin of the self: The neurobiology of emotional development.* Hillsdale, NJ: Erlbaum.

Schore, A. N. (2003a). *Affect dysregulation and disorders of the self.* New York: Norton.

Schore, A. N. (2003b). *Affect regulation and the repair of the self.* New York: Norton.

Schore, A. N. (2012). *The science of the art of psychotherapy.* New York: Norton.

Siegel, D. J. (1999). *The developing mind: How relationships and the brain interact to shape who we are.* New York: Guilford Press.

Siegel, D. J. (2012). *The developing mind: How relationships and the brain interact to shape who we are* (2nd ed.). New York: Guilford Press.

Terr, L. (1990). *Too scared to cry: Psychic trauma in childhood.* New York: Harper & Row.

Tuber, S. (2008). *Attachment, play and authenticity: A Winnicott primer.* Lanham, MD: Aronson.

van der Kolk, B. A. (2005). Developmental trauma disorder. *Psychiatric Annals, 35,* 401–408.

VanFleet, R. (2013). *Filial Therapy: Strengthening parent–child relationships through play* (3rd ed.). Sarasota, FL: Professional Resource Press.

Winnicott, D. (1971). *Playing and reality.* London: Tavistock.

PART II

Clinical Applications: Approaches to Working with Attachment Issues

CHAPTER 3

Attachment Theory as a Road Map for Play Therapists

Anne Stewart
William F. Whelan
Christen Pendleton

> We are here concerned with nothing less than the nature
> of love and its origins in the attachment of a baby to his
> mother. . . . Attachment originates in a few specific patterns
> of behavior, some of which are manifest at birth and some of
> which develop shortly afterward. . . . Attachment is manifested
> through these patterns of behavior but the patterns do not
> themselves constitute the attachment. Attachment is internal.
> —AINSWORTH (1967, p. 429)

Attachment theory proposes that important behavior systems in all humans serve to maintain proximity between children and caregivers (Ainsworth, Blehar, Waters, & Wall, 1978; Bowlby, 1969, 1973, 1980). The Circle of Security (COS) is one of the most recent models expressing the therapeutic dimensions of attachment theory. The COS model helps illustrate the power of attachment theory to build secure relationships through sensitive everyday interactions. In this chapter, we describe the attachment-theory-based COS model; explain the major features of the COS; and provide a case vignette to illustrate the ways the COS may be used as a "roadmap" to guide play therapists' work. We first provide a brief introduction to the foundations of attachment theory and to major findings from field research. We then show the relationship between attachment theory and COS, and we share research supporting the importance of secure attachments in the lives of the children we serve as play therapists.

Overview of Attachment Theory and Findings from Field Research

According to the theory, children's *attachment behavior system* leads them to seek proximity to their caregivers in times of distress—whether the distress is mild or severe, momentary or long-standing. The caregivers, in turn, are prompted by their *caregiving behavior system* to serve as a safe haven of protection for their children, and as a secure base for children to use as they explore their world. The attachment and caregiving systems thus serve the biological functions in humans (as in other species), of ensuring protection in dangerous surroundings and promoting exploration and learning (Bowlby, 1969, 1982, 1988). Mary Ainsworth's innovative field and laboratory research, in the context of John Bowlby's theory, brought a scientific approach to the study of development (Ainsworth & Bowlby, 1991).

In 1954, Ainsworth set out for Kampala, Uganda, to begin her field studies in infant development, with special attention to the growth of attachment and the developmental pathway of bonding (see Ainsworth, 1967). What she found most often among the Ugandan babies and mothers, and later replicated in her famous Baltimore study (Ainsworth et al., 1978), was a predominant pattern of secure behavior. The pattern included the infant's increased differential responding toward the mother (as compared to other people) over time; exploration of the environment with the mother's support; contentment; returning to the mother for rest and refueling; and lower anxiety compared to other children.

Attachment Theory and the COS Model

Ainsworth (1967) summarized her findings by describing two distinct but related phenomena: the secure child's growing ability to use the caregiver effectively as (1) a secure base for exploration (of the social and physical environment) and (2) a haven of safety when tired or distressed. Over 30 years later, a graphic depiction of this summary was created, called the COS (Marvin, Cooper, Hoffman, & Powell, 2002)—and, along with it, an intervention for supporting the development of secure attachment–caregiving patterns (Marvin et al., 2002). This chapter extends these ideas and interventions to the child–therapist relationship in the context of play therapy. We illustrate how the use of the COS can enrich a play therapist's conceptualization of a child's needs, promote effective filial therapy and parent consultation, and enhance the healing benefits of the child's relationship experience with the play therapist. Let's consider the importance of a secure attachment for children's emotional well-being and learn how attachment relationships grow.

The Benefits of Secure Attachment

Why should we play therapists be concerned about the quality of a child's attachment? How can promoting more secure attachments benefit the children with whom we work? One compelling reason to use an attachment-based perspective like the COS is that when children come to us with behavioral and emotional problems, they are experiencing corresponding difficulties in their relationships with parents, teachers, or peers. In addition, many of the problems for which children are referred for treatment reflect basic difficulties in regulation of behavior, thoughts, and feelings. Disturbances in relationships and disruptions in regulation are central concerns addressed in the attachment-based COS approach and interventions.

Evidence Supporting the Importance of Secure Attachment for Child Outcomes

The secure pattern of relationship development is the attachment pattern most associated with resilience and positive outcomes in the childhood years and in adulthood (Grossmann, Grossmann, & Kindler, 2005; Sroufe, 2005). While secure attachment patterns do not ensure good outcomes across the lifespan, or protect individuals from all forms and levels of stress, children with secure attachments tend to have more effective and satisfying relationships with parents, friends, and teachers than children with nonsecure patterns do. They are better at social problem solving and the repair of relationship upsets, are more successful academically, have fewer behavior problems, are at lower risk for psychiatric problems and trouble with the law than their nonsecure peers, and are themselves more successful parents (e.g., Sroufe, 2005; Sroufe, Egeland, Carlson, & Collins, 2005).

Children with a secure pattern tend to send clear emotional cues to their parents (and play therapists) during times of mild to moderate arousal and stress, and their cuing tends to be robust. Their behavior usually fits the circumstances and clearly communicates their emotional needs, making it relatively easy for adults to perceive their cues correctly, make accurate inferences about their needs, and respond appropriately to those needs. During occasional moments of miscuing, when a child needs a parent but behaves as if there is no need or as if the parent is not important to him or her, parents of secure children are generally able to read through the miscue and address effectively the child's underlying need.

From a practical point of view, as well as an evolutionary one, the immediate outcome of this pattern is that the child's needs are usually correctly identified and met in the moment-to-moment emotional and behavioral episodes of the day. The longer-term outcome is that the child's brain builds an increasingly sophisticated structure of neural connections and subroutines—a structure that results in effective rhythms of soothing;

co-regulation of thoughts, emotions, and behavior; abilities for self-control; and behavioral and social competence (Schore, 2001, 2005).

Building Blocks of Secure Attachments

Our readers may have already deduced a remarkable discovery: Attachment patterns are built one interaction at a time, over time. This is good news for parents and play therapists. Indeed, it appears both from research (Dozier, 2005) and from our clinical practice that although caregivers with secure patterns cannot meet all their children's needs all of the time, they are able, through their own accurate perceptions and sensitivity to the children's emotional signals, to help the children form healthy attachment relationships through day-to-day interactions. This is a lovely and wonderful process to witness. Such caregivers, including birth parents, foster parents, teachers, and play therapists, provide an emotional environment that is sensitive, flexible, adaptive, and generally able to fine-tune itself to meet the needs of a particular child.

Children with histories of disturbed family relationships, interpersonal violence, and emotional and physical maltreatment tend to have nonsecure and usually high-risk (disorganized, disoriented, controlling, etc.) patterns of interaction. Compared to their secure peers, children with nonsecure patterns of attachment often exhibit underdeveloped abilities for co-regulation (i.e., little ability to make use of caregivers for regulation of emotion and behavior), for rhythms of soothing and self-control, or for effective partnership behavior. In this regard, and through no fault of their own, children with nonsecure attachment patterns provide fewer clear cues about their emotional and relationship needs in the moment. It is no wonder that caregivers often describe difficulty in developing relationships with these children, and often experience the children's behavior and emotions as enigmatic and unpredictable.

The COS Model

Attachment-based play therapy helps reorder and organize a child's emotional experiences through attuned and responsive interactions with a play therapist, so that the child's relationships and behaviors will become more satisfying, coherent, and rewarding. The COS helps the play therapist focus on meeting the child's basic relationship needs through play-based interactions (Stewart, Whelan, Gilbert, & Marvin, 2011).

Dimensions of the COS

In the COS model, the two basic dimensions are divided into top-of-the-Circle and bottom-of-the-Circle needs (see Figure 3.1). In the therapeutic

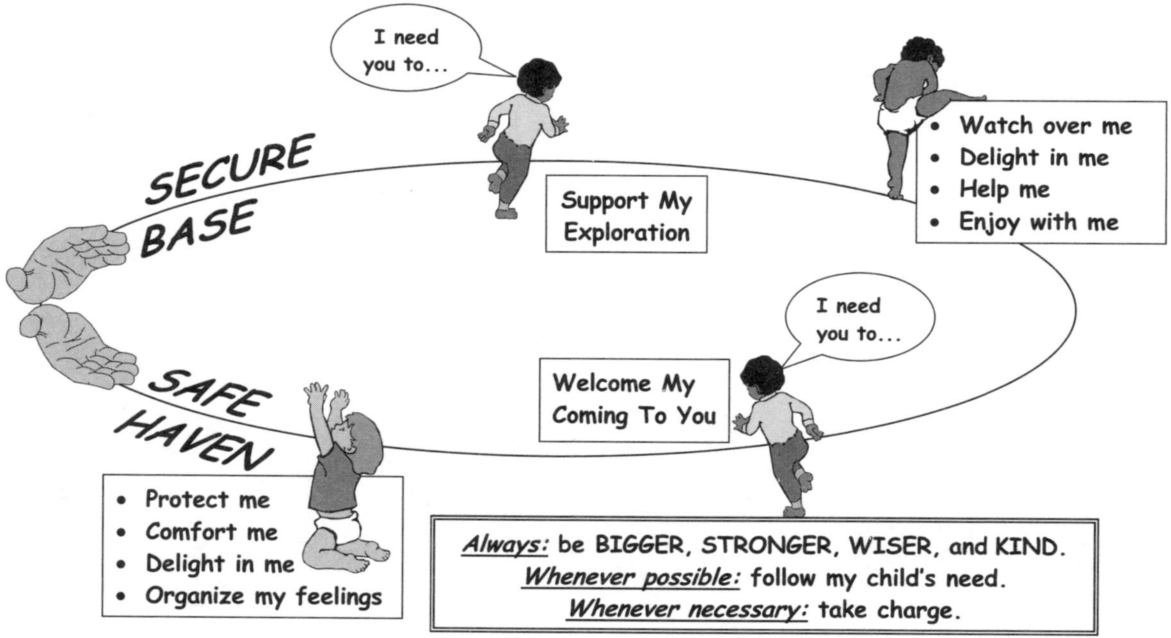

I need you to...
SECURE BASE
Support My Exploration
Watch over me
Delight in me
Help me
Enjoy with me
I need you to...
Welcome My Coming To You
SAFE HAVEN
Protect me
Comfort me
Delight in me
Organize my feelings
Always: be BIGGER, STRONGER, WISER, and KIND.
Whenever possible: follow my child's need.
Whenever necessary: take charge.

FIGURE 3.1. The Circle of Security: Caregiver attending to the child's needs. Copyright 1998 by G. Cooper, K. Hoffman, R. Marvin, and B. Powell. *circleofsecurity.org*. Reprinted by permission.

play relationship, *needs* are the child's needs from the therapist, in the moment, within the context of their growing relationship. Using this perspective, the therapist learns to ask the question "What does the child need from me?" rather than "Why is the child behaving this way?" The child's needs at the top of the Circle include *support my exploration, watch over me, help me, delight in me*, and *enjoy with me*. A child's needs at the bottom of the Circle include *welcome my coming to you, protect me, soothe me, organize me*, and *delight in me*.

The Importance of Observation

From a COS perspective, accurately observing interactions within an empirically supported theory is the foundation of understanding and helping. In this regard, identifying what the child's body is doing in interactions is initially more important for the therapeutic work than asking why it is happening. The therapist notices the child's body orientation, proximity, movement, physical contact, tone of voice, content of speech, body language, and feelings expressed. The therapist alters his or her behavior in the playroom from moment to moment according to the child's needs, and makes judgments about when to actively follow the child's needs versus when to take charge of the child's emotional experience and behavior in order to lead or protect the child. The result is that the therapist can use the COS to differentiate diagnosis and treatment of the child (Cooper, Hoffman, Powell, & Marvin, 2006). When the child's needs are met in a responsive, contingent manner, this helps to build neurological subroutines and abilities in the child and to generate patterns for soothing; co-regulation of emotion, thinking, and behavior; partnership behavior; and abilities for self-regulation and competence (Hoffman, Marvin, Cooper, & Powell, 2006; Whelan & Marvin, 2011).

As shown in Figure 3.1 and noted above, there are five primary needs at the top of the Circle:

1. *Support my exploration* refers to the child's need to experience support from the therapist to explore the playroom materials and activities— and, most importantly, to explore the relationship with the therapist. Encouragement for exploration is provided by the play therapist's affect, tone of voice, and body language, and is conveyed through attuned interactions and comments. Memories, worries, and fears, as well as past trauma, loss, and maltreatment, may be addressed in developmentally appropriate creative arts and expressive activities, in discussions, and of course in the context of imaginative play.

2. *Watch over me* reflects to the child's need for the therapist to make accurate observations of his or her behavior, so that accurate inferences and conclusions can be drawn about the child's needs. Given the charge to maintain the physical and psychological safety of the playroom, the

therapist must determine whether the child's actions reflect accurate emotional cuing or miscuing.

3. *Delight in me* concerns the positive emotional affect and acceptance the therapist communicates to the child. Delight can convey strength, safety, love, hope, and/or forgiveness—all in a well-timed reflection, gaze, or tone of voice. Delight is quickly lost in times of stress and is the only need to appear at both the top and the bottom of the Circle, due to its vital role in healing. Play therapists can promote healing through brief but genuine delight-filled interactions in the playroom, and in filial therapy through helping a caregiver experience delight in his or her child.

4. *Help me* refers to the play therapist's scaffolding the child's exploration of toys, play themes, emotions, and their relationship in the playroom.

5. *Enjoy with me* denotes the child's need for the therapist to convey how much the therapist simply enjoys the child's company and likes sharing activities with him or her. The child benefits by experiencing reciprocal and moment-to-moment partnership behavior, as well as the warmth and support inherent in relationships without conditions.

At the bottom of the Circle, there are also five primary needs:

1. *Welcome my coming to you* refers to accepting the child's uncertainty, distress, confusion, rudeness, rejection, sadness, aggression, misattributions, and poor judgments. Importantly, this does not mean approving of or reinforcing misbehavior, but rather welcoming whatever the child brings in order for the child to experience the therapist as being bigger, stronger, wise, and kind.

2. *Protect me* concerns the child's need for physical and emotional protection, including protection from events in the playroom, as well as from negative or overwhelming memories and emotions that become activated in the play therapy.

3. *Comfort me* includes the therapist's attempts to absorb and regulate the child's pattern of overarousal or inhibition and to soothe the child's anxiety and distress, without dismissing the child's upset.

4. *Delight in me* refers to sharing brief, playful moments of joy in the child, especially through interactions and activities that are fun and meaningful for both child and therapist. Expressing genuine pleasure at the presence of another person is one of the best ways to reassure children or adults that they are valued.

5. *Organize my feelings* refers to ways in which the therapist takes charge of the child's emotional experience, and sets the emotional tone to lead the child in a healthier interaction during times of upset. This is done via the therapist's presence and sensitivity, tone of voice and demeanor, body language, verbal expression, and physical movement. The therapist gives the child practice in the experience of having another person lead him or her through emotional arousal and distress, and helps the child

experience the safety and rest that comes in relying on the strength and security of one who is bigger, stronger, wiser, and kind.

Therapists who have the most success implementing the COS model have the ability to reflect on their own thoughts and feelings regarding a therapeutic relationship with the child, and to wonder how their thoughts, feelings, and behavior affect the child. They also exhibit the ability to see things kindly and empathically from the child's point of view and from a developmental standpoint, and to alter their own therapeutic caregiving behavior in the moment according to the child's changing needs. They are able to take charge and be bigger, stronger, wiser, and kind as needed. Importantly, this kind of therapeutic caregiving includes keen sensitivity not only to the child's cues, but also to the child's miscues (e.g., Marvin et al., 2002).

COS Cues and Miscues

In the COS model, *cuing* refers to behavioral and emotional signals from the child that, directly or indirectly, indicate the child's needs "around the Circle." *Miscuing* refers to behavioral and emotional signals from the child that point away from what the child actually needs at that time. Common examples of a child's miscues in relation to a therapist (or in relation to a parent or teacher) include anxious/avoidant behavior such as looking away, walking away, hiding his or her face, not responding to overtures, leaving the room, refusing to engage or collaborate, and rejecting the therapist's attempts at co-regulation. Miscues can also include behaviors such as rudeness, aggression, lying, stealing, or fire setting. For other children, common miscues include babyish behavior and exaggerated or overly bright affect; for still others, they include attempts to organize or take charge of interactions with the therapist or caregiver, attempts to take care of the adult, or punitive or bossy behaviors (i.e., role-reversed behaviors). Something all of these behaviors have in common is that they tend to push the therapist away or distract the therapist, at times when the child is otherwise clearly in need of adult help somewhere on the Circle. Such miscuing obscures the child's underlying relationship needs of the therapist around the Circle, and makes it more difficult for the therapist to identify them accurately. If these behaviors are not identified as miscues, then it is likely that the therapist will attempt to treat the miscues (or symptoms) and be led astray from the child's relationship needs in the therapy. From this point of view, a clue that important miscues may have been missed occurs when a target problem fails to improve with intervention, or when new problems continually pop up to replace the old ones. A way for a therapist to determine whether he or she has been chasing miscues, rather than meeting the child's needs (and thereby missing opportunities to shape the child's emotions and behaviors toward health), is that the emotional and behavioral problems do not improve or simply mutate over time rather than resolve. (Of course there are other reasons why things may not improve, including illness or the presence of stress or trauma in the child's life of which the therapist is not yet aware.) As one would expect, the therapist needs to reflect continually on the child's movement around the Circle, as well as on his or her own behavior and feelings, during interactions with the child.

Case Vignette: A COS-Informed Intervention

The COS as a Roadmap for Play Therapy

The COS helps play therapists conceptualize and meet a child's emotional needs by guiding how they intervene in the playroom. Here is an example of applying the COS model of observing the child's behavior, making inferences about where the child is on the Circle, inferring the child's needs, and responding in an individual play therapy format.

Malik was a 7-year-old child from a multistressed background. He was raised for the first 4 years of his life by his birth mother and father, who both struggled with substance abuse problems. Malik's childhood was marked by neglect, chaos, and domestic violence. Malik's parents frequently engaged in physical altercations in his presence, and although they tried to address his physical needs, they were often unavailable to provide for his emotional needs. At age 4, Malik was removed from his parents and was raised by relatives for the subsequent 3 years. Once he was removed from their care, Malik saw his parents only sporadically and was disappointed when they did not follow through with promises to attend family functions and holidays. The year Malik turned 7, his birth mother separated from his father, completed a drug rehabilitation program, and began working toward reunification with Malik. She started to engage in supervised visits with him and was completing court-ordered therapy as part of her reunification plan. Malik's relatives, who maintained physical custody of him, supported the reunification efforts and cooperated in assisting with supervised visitations. Therapy was arranged by child protective services for Malik, who exhibited unpredictable emotional reactions, such as aggression, defiance, difficulty separating, and clinginess with his mother. Malik's therapist, Laura, began by meeting individually with Malik for play therapy. As their work progressed, Laura engaged in filial therapy and consultation with Malik's biological mother and with the extended relatives who maintained physical custody. Laura used the COS as a roadmap to build her conceptualization of Malik's emotional needs, to guide her interactions with Malik in the playroom, and to guide her interactions and discussions with his caregivers.

During her initial sessions, Laura welcomed Malik by following his needs in the playroom, using the COS to guide her thinking about how to help him and make use of her to regulate his behavior. As Laura carefully observed Malik, she noticed that he engaged in more aggressive play with the dollhouse, banging the parent figures. When he was speaking for the figures, Malik's voice became louder and more pressured; his body tensed as he made the father and mother figures yell at one another and banged them together. Laura noticed that his language also became more violent than she had previously heard. Malik angled his body slightly away from Laura as he placed a young boy figure sitting in the corner of the dollhouse.

LAURA: I see that one is over there all alone. Maybe he is watching those two yelling.

MALIK: Yeah, they are always yelling and hitting. He doesn't wanna hear it.

LAURA: Ah, so he hears a lot of yelling and sees a lot of hitting. I wonder what he is thinking and feeling.

MALIK: Errrr-ow-ow-ow. (*Makes a low rumbling sound as his shoulders tense. He suddenly throws the dollhouse chair at the boy figure.*) He is bad, and that's why his mommy is leaving him there!

Although Laura was alarmed at the dramatic change in Malik's demeanor, she remained calm and close to him. She noticed that his breathing was shallow and rapid, and that tears sprang to his eyes as he toppled the rest of the furniture in the dollhouse. Using the COS, Laura understood how Malik's toppling of the furniture and threatening growl were miscues, fueled by his tendency to become dysregulated when enacting family scenes. Actually, his reaction made sense to her when she considered the chaotic and unpredictable nature of his first 4 years, coupled with the sense of abandonment he experienced at being removed from his parents' custody, shuffled among relatives, and repeatedly disappointed. Laura understood that Malik's sympathetic nervous system was activated and overburdened—something that had happened all too often as he witnessed verbal and physical aggression. From her observations, Laura knew that Malik was at the bottom of the Circle, and that his needs were for protection, comfort, and help with organizing his feelings.

Laura inferred that Malik was experiencing intense feelings that he could not make sense of by himself. Furthermore, she knew that this type of behavior often pushed away caregivers and peers, and elicited punitive or disciplinary responses from his parents and teachers. She could tell that Malik was feeling sad, vulnerable, scared, anxious, and angry, and his behavior conveyed to her, "I am overwhelmed and don't know what to do with the all the strong feelings that I am experiencing." Laura thus recognized Malik's need for welcoming and protection from his intense feelings, comfort to feel valued, and help in organizing his jumbled emotions. She also recognized that when he was this upset, assistance would be hard for Malik to accept. She understood that even though he needed her help, he was not used to getting help from adults, and that this would be a large part of their therapeutic work together. Laura offered her composed presence and a few calm but strongly stated (and nonjudgmental) comments, to let Malik know that his feelings would be accepted and that she would not be misled by miscues. She reflected, "It is so hard for him to know what to do! He feels so many big feelings all at the same time—the feelings all come out as throwing chairs and tables."

Since this was not the first time this kind of interaction had occurred, Laura's interaction demonstrated to Malik that she would consistently respond to his needs in a patterned way. Malik's shoulders eased slightly as he turned toward Laura. She leaned in toward Malik and inched a bit closer to him. Malik nodded slowly and relaxed slightly, looking up at Laura briefly as he began setting up the dollhouse furniture. Later in the session, Laura completed a drawing activity with Malik. On a gingerbread person outline,[1] Malik named four feelings the boy in the house might be feeling, matched colors with the feelings, and then drew where in his body he experienced those feelings. Laura and Malik talked about when Malik had feelings like the boy in the dollhouse, and what or who helped him feel better. After a few moments of talking, Malik began to crawl slowly around the playroom. He approached Laura, pretending to lick his hands.

MALIK: I'm a cat (*making purring sounds*).

LAURA: Oh, so you are a cat—a cat with a big motor for purring!

MALIK: You can pet my head if you want to. I am a friendly cat.

LAURA: You are a friendly cat, all comfy and safe, ready for some pats on your head (*patting Malik gently*).

MALIK: Yeah, and you can make me some milk, and then I'll take a nap here.

Laura observed that Malik's breathing had slowed, and that his face was relaxed as he crawled toward Laura and sat next to her legs. Laura recognized Malik's movement toward her and the content of his speech as cues that he needed her to welcome his coming and provide him caregiving within this play; she followed his needs and recognized that in doing so she was helping him at the bottom of the Circle. In this moment of interaction, his body had a chance to practice and experience what it felt like to bring some of his needs directly to her.

Malik lay down quietly at Laura's feet, which she recognized as a time of emotional refueling in the safe haven that she had provided him. After a few deep breaths, Malik opened his eyes, stretched his arms, and looked around at the toys across the room. Laura was able to see that her work in

---

[1]The gingerbread person drawing activity is based on an activity developed by Athena A. Drewes. (See Drewes, Chapter 12, this volume.)

attending to Malik's bottom-of-the-Circle needs had helped to co-regulate his emotions, and that he was feeling recharged and was moving toward the top of the Circle.

> LAURA: You are waking up from your nap and feeling better (*smiles*), and stretching your legs and paws and looking around at the toys. I'm so glad you took a nap here with me. Now there is so much to see in the playroom.

Malik eyed the trucks across the playroom and began to crawl toward them, but turned back to look at Laura midway, his eyes looking as if he wanted to make sure that she was still watching him. Laura recognized that Malik was now at the top of the Circle, as indicated by his calmer presence and his willingness to venture away from her. She understood his need for her to support his exploration.

> LAURA: I am still here, watching you. It looks like you have a plan as to what you might like to play with.
>
> MALIK: (*Smiles and crawls more rapidly this time to the trucks.*) I want to drive us! (*Faces Laura and moves toward her with the truck in his hand.*)

Laura smiled, delighting in Malik and moving in his direction to enjoy with him. Laura joined Malik on the carpet, sitting next to him and allowing him to direct their play as she remained attuned to his needs. She noticed that his relaxed body posture, his close proximity to her, his affect, and the content of his speech were all consistent and indicative of Malik's position on the top of the Circle. Laura sat next to Malik, pretended to buckle her seatbelt, and said, "You are going to take us for a ride. You know how to drive this truck!" She beamed back at Malik, reflecting his own look of delight. As Malik reached out and turned an imaginary steering wheel, Laura leaned slightly to the right, noting, "We are going around a curve." Malik giggled, leaning into Laura's shoulder in the same direction. They swayed in similar directions as he drove. Laura was able to meet Malik's top-of-the-Circle needs while co-regulating their body movements and emotions as Malik took them for a ride.

The COS as a Roadmap for Filial Work and Parent Consultation

The COS graphic (Figure 3.1) and approach can also guide filial work and parent consultation. Malik's case provides an illustration of how COS can be applied to these intervention formats.

As therapy progressed, Malik's mother and at times his extended relatives were invited to participate in therapy and receive consultation to learn about the COS dimensions and use the COS to think about Malik's needs. Using problem behaviors brought in by the caregivers, Laura helped them apply the COS to discover how Malik was communicating (and miscommunicating) his needs to them. Laura worked with Malik's mother and relatives to recognize, understand, and respond to his needs around the Circle with play-based interventions.

On the day that Malik's mother presented for their filial session, Laura invited her to the room, keeping in mind the ways in which the COS could also be used to welcome his mother and understand her needs in this new situation. As Malik and his mother entered the room, his mother hung back, looking nervous and unsure. Laura noticed the look of uncertainty on Malik's mother's face and determined that she was likely to be feeling out of place, vulnerable, and worried about what Laura would think of her.

LAURA: We are so happy to have you here today in the playroom. We've been talking about this special visit for a few weeks now. Malik and I talked about the different feelings that he might have today, and the way that people can feel nervous and excited all at once.

MALIK'S MOTHER: (*Smiles shyly and nods.*)

MALIK: Yeah, when I feel nervous in my tummy, like there are butterflies in there, I do balloon breathing to help calm down.

LAURA: Malik, you are remembering the balloon breathing that we learned in the playroom. (*To Malik's mother*) He is a real expert in using balloon breathing—taking deep breaths—to relax.

Malik beamed, looking at Laura and his mother. Laura modeled for his mother a response to his top-of-the-Circle needs, enjoying his skill and delighting in his demonstration of breathing skills. She noticed the way in which both Malik and his mother seemed to relax as they moved toward one another, sat down close together, and touched one another's stomachs as they engaged in the deep breathing technique. Laura also noticed the happiness on their faces as Malik taught his mother the technique, and the delight that his mother was able to convey as she and Malik breathed in tandem and laughed as they imagined balloons in their stomachs. As the demonstration ended, Laura noticed that both Malik and his mother looked to her with a "What's next?" expression. Laura took charge to lead the session by suggesting that they engage in a "reading and feelings identification" activity. She invited Malik's mother to read a story aloud, explaining that Laura and Malik would work to identify the feelings that the story characters were experiencing.

Laura pointed to the page that Malik's mother was reading, and wondered with Malik how the bear in the story was feeling and how they might be able to figure it out. She helped Malik notice what the bear was doing and saying.

MALIK: The bear is yelling 'cause he's mad (*in a tentative voice.*)

LAURA: Hmmm, it makes sense to you that when someone is yelling, they may be mad. That makes sense to me too. What about you, Mom?

MALIK'S MOTHER: Yes, and the story said that the bear's toys were taken away by the other animals, and I can imagine that that might make him feel mad.

LAURA: Well, Malik, it looks like you were right. You knew that this bear was feeling mad. I wonder how this bear's roar might sound when he is feeling so mad?

MALIK: I don't know. (*Giggles and looks up at his mother.*)

MALIK'S MOTHER: What do you think?

MALIK: Like this. Rooooaaarrr!

LAURA: Oh, wow! That was a big roar! (*Smiles at Malik and delights in his enthusiasm.*) I wonder if I can try one.

MALIK: Yeah, do it!

Malik giggled as Laura roared and then laughed with him. Laura was even more pleased when Malik's mother asked if she should try. The adults enjoyed the activity with Malik and delighted in him as he let out the final and loudest roar. Laughing, they agreed that they could continue with the story and could help each other to determine the bear's feelings. As they generated clues about the bear's feeling states, Malik inched closer to his mother and reached toward her to point to the book, letting his hand rest on her leg when it lowered. Laura recognized his need for his mother to enjoy the story with him and welcome his closeness, and she was pleased to see that his mother read his cues correctly and responded by placing her arm around him.

In a private meeting with his mother after the play session, Laura was able to point to this moment as a wonderful example of her reading his cues. She helped his mother notice the effect this had on Malik, how much he enjoyed it, and how this helped his exploration and experience of the story and his enjoyment with her. It also allowed Malik and his mother to continue to enjoy themselves together in the activity, delight in his ability to roar like a bear, and feel comfortable enough to engage in play by making animal noises together.

In a subsequent parent consultation session, Laura worked with Malik's mother on developing attunement and engaging with delight. Laura introduced and practiced an activity with Malik's mother in which she learned to face Malik directly, noticing and mirroring his facial expressions and body movements. She helped Malik's mother notice his facial expressions, body posture, movement, proximity, and tone of voice. Laura and Malik's mother practiced this activity several times before inviting Malik into the session to try it out. Malik's mother responded to his top-of-the-Circle need to be delighted in by asking him if he would like to play a game with her in which she would become his mirror. Malik giggled and said that he would. Laura explained that Malik's mother would stand opposite Malik and would mirror all of his expressions and movements for the next minute. As they engaged in the activity, Malik's mother remained affectively attuned with Malik. When the activity concluded, Malik's mother noted that she had enjoyed spending time playing with him and looked forward to playing again soon. Malik yelled, "Me too!" Laura again met privately after the session with Malik's mother to hear her experience of playing together and point out moments of co-regulation and attunement between her and her son. In this way, she helped his mother bask in the wonder of these small and powerful moments of connectedness and feel the reality of how important she was to her son.

The case of Malik and his mother is just one example of relationship healing in action—of the way little moments of intimacy can be guided to help a child and a parent experience (or awaken) the reality of their love and longing for each other. When this happens, the memory and experience will give the two a better chance of getting through difficult experiences ahead. The refueling, safety, and comfort they experience in small moments will protect them in times of trouble and make it more likely that they can stay with each other and practice rhythms of soothing, co-regulation, and forgiveness.

As the vignette illustrates, use of the COS in play therapy is not meant to be prescriptive, but rather employed as a relationship map to guide play therapists in recognizing and understanding children's needs. Play therapists are then in a better position to help shape a child's automatic patterns of thinking, feeling, and behaving toward security and resilience. Although security is characterized by resilience, buoyancy, emotional coherence, and competence, it is also robust, with a seemingly contrary (and wonderful) balance of dependence and independence. Isn't this what we wish for our children (and clients)? That is, we wish them to become strong and independent on the one hand, while also becoming connected in healthy and rejuvenating relationships on the other.

Conclusion

The COS graphic (Figure 3.1) portrays the way children move around the Circle with secure caregivers, smoothly venturing out from them to explore and returning to them for refueling and protection. Within a therapeutic relationship, the therapist attempts to be bigger, stronger, wiser, and kind, and seeks to follow the child's needs and take charge (to help, protect, and lead the child) as necessary. From an attachment perspective, the

COS can be used as a map to show how the power of attuned interactions comes through the therapist's ability to observe the child; arrive at developmentally sensitive inferences and conclusions about the child's needs; co-regulate the child's emotions, thinking, and behavior; and meet the child's needs within safe and sensitive relationship interactions. The healing power of this therapeutic relationship unfolds as the child experiences being safely held, organized, emotionally valued, and protected by the therapist at the bottom of the Circle, and effectively and delightfully supported in exploration at the top of the Circle.

We believe that the COS conceptual framework brings simplicity and direction to complex clinical situations. Therapists report feeling more confident, relaxed, and effective in their work when they employ the COS as a user-friendly map: They have many more experiences of feeling that they know what children need in various play therapy situations, and what to do to help them in the moment (i.e., in terms of welcoming the children's needs at the bottom of the Circle and supporting their exploration at the top). For these play therapists, the COS becomes an experiential, and eventually intuitive, template for developing the most secure and healing relationship possible with their child clients.

REFERENCES

Ainsworth, M. D. S. (1967). *Infancy in Uganda: Infant care and the growth of love.* Baltimore, MD: Johns Hopkins University Press.

Ainsworth, M. D. S., Blehar, M. C., Waters, E., & Wall, S. (1978). *Patterns of attachment: A psychological study of the Strange Situation.* Hillsdale, NJ: Erlbaum.

Ainsworth, M. D. S., & Bowlby, J. (1991). An ethological approach to personality development. *American Psychologist, 46,* 331–341.

Bowlby, J. (1969). *Attachment and loss: Vol. 1. Attachment.* New York: Basic Books.

Bowlby, J. (1973). *Attachment and loss: Vol. 2. Separation.* New York: Basic Books.

Bowlby, J. (1980). *Attachment and loss: Vol. 3. Loss: Sadness and depression.* New York: Basic Books.

Bowlby, J. (1982). Attachment and loss: Retrospect and prospect. *American Journal of Orthopsychiatry, 52*(4), 664–678.

Bowlby, J. (1988). *A secure base: Parent–child attachment and healthy human development.* New York: Basic Books.

Cooper, G., Hoffman, K., Powell, B., & Marvin, R. (2006). The Circle of Security intervention: Differential diagnosis and differential treatment. In L. J. Berlin, Y. Ziv, L. M. Amaya-Jackson, & M. T. Greenberg (Eds.), *Enhancing early attachments: Theory, research, intervention, and policy* (pp. 127–151). New York: Guilford Press.

Dozier, M. (2005). Challenges of foster care. *Attachment and Human Development, 7*(1), 27–30.

Grossmann, K., Grossmann, K. E., & Kindler, H. (2005). Early care and the roots of attachment and partnership representations. In K. E. Grossmann, K. Grossmann, & E. Waters (Eds.), *Attachment from infancy to adulthood: The major longitudinal studies* (pp. 98–136). New York: Guilford Press.

Hoffman, K. T., Marvin, R. S., Cooper, G., & Powell, B. (2006). Changing toddlers' and preschoolers' attachment classifications: The Circle of Security intervention. *Journal of Consulting and Clinical Psychology, 74*(6), 1017–1026.

Marvin, R., Cooper, G., Hoffman, K., & Powell, B. (2002). The Circle of Security project: Attachment based intervention with caregiver–pre-school child dyads. *Attachment and Human Development, 4*(1), 107–124.

Schore, A. N. (2001). Effects of a secure attachment relationship on right brain development, affect regulation, and infant mental health. *Infant Mental Health Journal, 22*(1–2), 7–66.

Schore, A. N. (2005). Attachment, affect regulation and the developing right brain: Linking developmental neuroscience to pediatrics. *Pediatrics in Review, 26*, 206–211.

Sroufe, L. A. (2005). Attachment and development: A prospective, longitudinal study from birth to adulthood. *Attachment and Human Development, 7*(4), 349–367.

Sroufe, L. A., Egeland, B., Carlson, E., & Collins, W. A. (2005). Placing early attachment experiences in developmental context. In K. E. Grossmann, K. Grossmann, & E. Waters (Eds.), *Attachment from infancy to adulthood: The major longitudinal studies* (pp. 48–70). New York: Guilford Press.

Stewart, A. L., Whelan, W. F., Gilbert, J., & Marvin, R. S. (2011, October). *Applying attachment theory and the Circle of Security model in play therapy.* Paper presented at the Association for Play Therapy International Conference, Sacramento, CA.

Whelan, W. F., & Marvin, R. S. (2011, April). *Caregiver patterns that moderate the effects of abuse and neglect.* Paper presenting results from the Virginia Foster Care study (NIH Award No. GC11456) at the biennial meeting of the Society for Research in Child Development, Montréal.

CHAPTER 4

Art Therapy, Attachment, and Parent–Child Dyads

Cathy A. Malchiodi

This chapter describes art-based approaches in work with parent–child dyads to build and enhance positive attachment. As defined in Chapter 1, *art therapy* is a creative approach that includes the purposeful use of art media (drawing, painting, and constructing) as an intervention for a variety of psychosocial, cognitive, and physical challenges in people of all ages (Malchiodi, 2005, 2012a). Art therapy is a somewhat different experience from play therapy, because the main goal is the creation of a tangible product to express perceptions, feelings, and imaginings.

The use of art therapy to address attachment issues is based both in concepts from object relations theory and in a contemporary understanding of neurodevelopment and neuroplasticity. These conceptual frameworks underscore that it is possible to revisit the window of opportunity for the development of secure attachment through sensory-based interventions and reinforcement of positive relationships. Art therapy is one way to engage the body and mind through experiential learning; when used as central to dyad work with parents and children, it provides opportunities for mutual *attunement*—a principle central to successful interpersonal relationship and attachment (Badenoch, 2008; Siegel, 2007). This chapter provides an overview of the importance of art therapy in attachment work with parent–child dyads, with an emphasis on why art therapy is an effective intervention and on recommended guidelines and approaches for its use to build secure attachment.

Art Therapy and Attachment

Historically, three main concepts are important in clinical applications of art therapy and attachment issues: (1) Donald Winnicott's *"good enough" parent*; (2) *transitional object* and *transitional space*; and (3) the art therapist's *third hand*. The first two concepts come from psychoanalytic and object relations theories; the third hand is an idea that originated from the field of art therapy (Henley, 1992; Kramer, 1993). In the 21st century, these concepts are being reframed through the growing understanding of the *developing mind* (Siegel, 2012) and *neurosequential development* (Perry, 2006; Perry & Szalavitz, 2006).

The "Good Enough" Parent

Winnicott (1965, 1971) was particularly interested in children's capability to be successfully with others as a prerequisite for being alone. He developed the concept of the *"good enough" mother* (referred to as the *"good enough" parent* in this chapter) who creates a relationship and environment that help the child internalize positive experiences, including secure attachment, without being overly protective. The "good enough" parent is also a way of explaining psychosocial aspects of any therapeutic relationship that model and reinforce experiences of basic comfort for an individual, with the purpose of reducing stress reactions and enhancing a sense of self-efficacy. Increased understanding of neurobiology now confirms that secure and positive relationships with adult figures are essential for children to thrive and flourish throughout life (Perry & Szalavitz, 2006; Steele & Malchiodi, 2012).

Art therapists who work with insecure or disrupted attachment in children often temporarily assume the role of "good enough" parent through their strategic use of art activities and their role as providers of creative materials (Malchiodi, 2012b). In brief, art therapists recapitulate positive relational aspects through purposeful creative experiences that offer sensory opportunities to reinforce secure attachment. In contrast to verbal counseling, art therapy engages not only the mind, but also the body in repetitive, rhythmic, tactile, auditory, olfactory, and other sensory aspects found in the early relationship between a child and parent.

Transitional Object and Transitional Space

Siegel (2012) discusses *evocative memory*, which children use to bring an image of attachment to mind. Winnicott (1953, 1971) is credited with the classic term *transitional object*, meaning an object (person, thing, or mental representation) or ritual that is used for self-soothing. In other words, a transitional object is something that helps children hold onto a representation of a parent or caregiver until they are able to do so on their own.

For example, when a parent and child take home artwork from a session, the artwork becomes the transitional object that contains the experience of their work together in art therapy. It also may be a representation of a specific experience shared in art therapy, such as a depiction of a family activity, a loss of a significant person, or some other event. Klorer (2008) notes that art expression itself functions as a transitional object, because it supports self-relationship, empowerment, and connection with the therapist and helps children to create a variety of metaphors through art that self-soothe and reduce internal conflict.

Transitional space is defined as an intermediate area of experience where there is no clear distinction between inner and outer reality (Winnicott, 1971). Art and play therapy use transitional spaces because they offer ways for individuals to bridge subjective and objective realities and to practice attachment and relationships. Transitional space is also a type of holding environment; in art therapy, the art therapist creates and facilitates a holding environment that includes a safe place where all creative expression is accepted, respected, and valued unconditionally.

The Third Hand

Art therapist Edith Kramer (1993) is credited with the concept of the *third hand* and its application to clinical work. In brief, the *third hand* refers to the art therapist's use of suggestion, metaphors, or other techniques to enhance the individual's progress in therapy. Kramer believes that an effective art therapist must have a command of the third hand to enhance a client's creativity without being intrusive, imposing the therapist's own style or artistic values, and/or misinterpreting meanings found in images. What Kramer calls the third hand in art therapy echoes what Siegel (2010) refers to as *mindsight*, a capacity for insight (knowing what one feels) and empathy (knowing what others feel). Thus third-hand interventions are provided nonintrusively (with insight and empathy), so that the therapist does not change the content of the client's art expression or inadvertently influence the individual. This stance also echoes the concept of the "good enough" parent, who supports the child's self-efficacy and sense of safety during exploration, experimentation, and learning.

There are many ways the third hand is used in art therapy to encourage attachment and demonstrate on a sensory level that the therapist is a "good enough" parent. For example, when working with a child client, I may begin a drawing for the child to complete as a way of establishing a relationship or communication. In another situation, I may prevent a child's clay figure from falling apart by showing the child how to reinforce the legs or armature. Sometimes an art therapist literally becomes the hands for an individual; for instance, a child with a debilitating medical illness may need me to help cut and arrange photos for a collage. At other times, I may make art during the session alongside a client if it is therapeutically helpful, or I may even communicate something nonverbally through an art expression rather than use words.

What Kramer defined as the third hand can also be defined as a form of attunement. *Attunement* is generally defined as a relational dynamic that helps to build a healthy sense of self in children and is a central feature of every caring relationship and secure attachment (Perry & Szalavitz, 2006; Siegel, 2012). It also refers to a parent's or caregiver's ability to respond with empathy to a child's emotions and moods. Well-attuned parents are able to detect what their children are feeling and to reflect those emotions back through sensory means, such as facial expressions, vocalizations, touch, and other behaviors; it helps children to recognize their own feelings and develop the ability to self-regulate. Perry implies that attunement is the capacity to be able to read the nonverbal communication and rhythms of others. In other words, it is not only perceiving what individuals say, but also attending to eye signals, facial gestures, tone of voice, and even breathing rate. In art therapy, it also means attending to the content of images and nonverbal cues, as reflected in how well the therapist uses the third hand in response to the client's creative process.

Dyad Art Therapy

Dyad art therapy refers to any application that includes two people (such as a parent and child or a couple) working on either individual artwork or co-created artwork during a session. The goal is to address various aspects of the dyad's relationship, including attachment issues, via creative expression and art-based directives. The concepts mentioned in the preceding section are central to applying art therapy in work with dyads, particularly parent–child dyads, to support healthy relationships and secure attachment. Dyad work also reflects the principles of interpersonal neurobiology (Badenoch, 2008; Siegel, 2007), which include empathy, attunement, and secure attachment.

Riley (2001) delineates how dyad art therapy helps to evaluate and reconstruct early attachment experiences, noting that "Learning about the interrelationship between neuronal growth and parent–child activities stimulated me to speculate if there were art therapy activities that could re-approach these bonding experiences in a manner that aroused interest between the parental/child dyad" (p. 35). Similarly, Klorer's (2008) work with children who have experienced chronic trauma and maltreatment and their parents also highlights the interconnection among neurodevelopment, art and play-based approaches, and attachment. She emphasizes that positive attachment as well as recovery from chronic trauma does not necessarily come about through a series of directives aimed at specific issues, but through the support and the creative environment provided by the art therapist.

Most of my clinical work with attachment is with parents and children who have experienced interpersonal violence, repeated traumas and losses, or lack of psychoeducation on parenting—all of which can disrupt bonding and successful parenting (Malchiodi, 1997, 2008, 2012c). In these cases, normal attachment is disrupted in many different ways, including developmental challenges, posttraumatic stress, dissociative reactions, and attention difficulties. For many, normal social and cognitive growth is halted because the parent–child focus is turned to personal safety and basic survival needs, especially in situations of interpersonal violence. The children may appear to have hyperactivity or an oppositional or conduct disorder, when in fact insecure or disrupted attachment may be the barrier to performance and affect regulation. In addition, some children adopt the role of parent within the family system—exchanging the normal role of child for one of caregiver, and thus missing experiences that contribute to appropriate attachment responses later in life.

When working with insecure, disrupted, or avoidant attachment, I see art therapy as an expressive approach to help children and parents revisit neurodevelopmental and psychosocial aspects of attachment to strengthen their relationship. It is also a way to capitalize on sensory learning to facilitate change. Engaging in art making together is not only a shared experience; it is an effective approach to learning, because creative expression is experienced on multiple sensory levels—visual, tactile, kinesthetic, olfactory, and auditory. Art therapy also sets up relational dynamics that are uniquely different from those in verbal psychotherapy and counseling. The relationship includes not only the parent–child dyad and the therapist; it also includes the art process itself and the art products created by the dyad. In work with a dyad, how a parent responds to a child's art expression and creative activity is an important part of the experience, in addition to the therapist's intervention. This provides the added opportunity for the art therapist to model and reflect being a "good enough" parent and appropriately using the third hand for the parent. Parents have the chance to learn important verbal and nonverbal responses to their children to strengthen communication, develop empathy, and build attachment (for more information on responding to art products and process, see below).

In the remainder of this chapter, I describe specific considerations and art-based approaches used in working with a parent–child dyad: 20-year-old Lisa and her 6-year-old son, John. Lisa became a single parent at the age of 14 and grew up in a home where she was physically and sexually abused by her father and brother. John's father was physically abusive to Lisa, and her pregnancy was difficult, resulting in a premature birth. Mother and child had a strained relationship from John's infancy through his preschool years, and her grandmother took over much of the caregiving. She and John were recommended for multiple sessions of individual and dyad art therapy to work on issues of attachment and chronic trauma.

Safety First

Without safety, there can be no attachment or relationship; it is also the first step toward setting the stage for successful art therapy. Therefore, initially anyone using art-based interventions must consider how to provide opportunities for creative expression in a consistent and predictable manner. This includes introducing parents and children to the art therapy room and its contents, which may include an array of materials for drawing, painting, and constructing, as well as props for creative play. In working with children and parents from violent homes and communities, I have also learned that establishing a well-organized space conducive to stress reduction and consistency is essential to successful intervention, including building attachment.

Safety also includes establishing rules for physical and emotional safety during art-making sessions, such as no verbal or physical violence in the therapy room or office, and no destroying of another individual's artwork. It also includes reinforcing the ideas that artistic talent is not necessary and that all efforts at creative expression are valued, important, and accepted. Communicating acceptance of all art expressions is particularly important, because it reflects a central principle in attachment: "I accept you for who you are, right now." This is a critical benchmark, because both a sense of trust and a sense of belonging are implicit within acceptance and invite positive attachment.

In the initial sessions of work with Lisa and John, I reinforced that unlike in an art class or classroom, it was not important for them to make "good art." I also emphasized that John in particular could benefit from hearing from Lisa that his creative work was unconditionally valued by her, without judgment or interpretation; I also knew that it would be important for me to be supportive of Lisa's participation in art therapy, because of her own insecurities and lack of an internal sense of safety. Because Lisa had not received the same unconditional regard and praise in her own childhood, I capitalized on strategic opportunities to model how to respond to John's efforts in art therapy, and to provide support for her own courage to participate in art activities.

Sensory Materials: Soothing Lower Parts of the Brain

Purposeful selection of art media that are multisensory, that are developmentally appropriate, and that stimulate creative expression in a variety of ways is essential to help recapitulate early experiences of exploration and mastery (Proulx, 2002). For dyad work with parents and children, it is important to have at least some drawing materials (crayons, felt markers, white paper, and colored paper), painting materials (finger paints, tempera paints, a variety of bristle and sponge brushes), collage materials (colored papers, fabrics, and yarn), and construction materials (Play-Doh, Model Magic clay, and spoons, forks, and other implements for making marks in clay). In particular, art activities that involve repetition and positive sensory sensations soothe the lower parts of the brain, reduce stress responses, enhance self-regulation, and slow down the sympathetic nervous system; they also nonverbally communicate that life is stable and consistent. (Therapists who are unfamiliar with the properties of art materials should consult Malchiodi, 2012a.) For example, pudding painting with one's fingers, blowing paint across a paper with straws, and modeling with soft clay often involve soothing repetition and engage the senses in pleasurable ways.

Therapists should identify what specific types of art-based experiences may be self-soothing and calming for both parents and children. In attachment-focused, trauma-informed work, asking participants about cultural preferences and any positive memories about creative activities can help guide choices of media and interventions (Malchiodi, 2012d). For example, when I asked Lisa about her previous experiences with art materials, she told me how she had always longed to have a brand-new box of crayons (the 64-color box in particular) and to have time to "just color" with her mother. This memory became a catalyst for planning a session when I presented both Lisa and John with new 64-color boxes of crayons. During the art therapy session, we spent time looking at the boxes, smelling the crayons, and practicing using them on different colored and textured papers. It was not only a time for Lisa and John to enjoy the same experience, but also a session when Lisa felt that she and John had a common bond with positive sensory memories that Lisa and her mother had never had the opportunity to enjoy. In brief, through this simple gesture I was able to help Lisa recapture and reframe a part of her life related to her own attachment issues.

Scribble Chase: Enhancing Reflective Convergence

Siegel (2007) emphasizes the importance of a parent's attunement to the internal world of a child or spouse. Attunement between parent and child or adult partners enhances feelings of happiness, mutual understanding, and trust. It is necessary for two people to "feel felt" by each other, and it literally reinforces the neural circuitry for attunement in the brain. According to Siegel, the mindful awareness of oneself and of another enhances the experience of *reflexive convergence* and promotes attunement, flexibility, and interpersonal attachment.

There are many ways to use art making as an approach to reinforce attunement. One of the first things I demonstrate to parent–child dyads when working with attachment issues is the so-called "scribble chase," or two-way scribble drawing. In brief, parent and child each choose a felt marker (markers that smell like a fruit or flower are a good choice) or crayon, and each has the opportunity to be the leader in a scribble drawing on a large piece of paper (Figure 4.1). For example, the child may be the leader of the first drawing, and while he or she scribbles with a pen on the paper, the parent follows the child's lines at the same time with his or her pen. Sometimes we reverse roles and the parent becomes the leader of the scribble, with the child following.

In many cases where insecure or avoidant attachment between parent and child exists, a parent may be unsuccessful in joining in the drawing; a child may scribble all over the parent's lines; or one or both may be unable or unwilling to make any marks at all. In coaching a parent to engage in this experience with a child, it is important to help the parent prepare the child with attachment difficulties for the activity. I often suggest to a mother, for example, that she make eye contact with her child and tell the child that they will be playing a game with crayons on paper. I also may suggest that she make some sort physical contact with her child, such as a light touch on an arm or the upper back, and to place their chairs as closely together as is comfortable for them at the table. In addition, I may model the activity with either the parent or child as co-scribbler, asking one of them to be the leader of the scribble drawing while I follow or vice versa. In essence, I am demonstrating ways to attune to another's behavior, particularly to sensory, nonverbal cues.

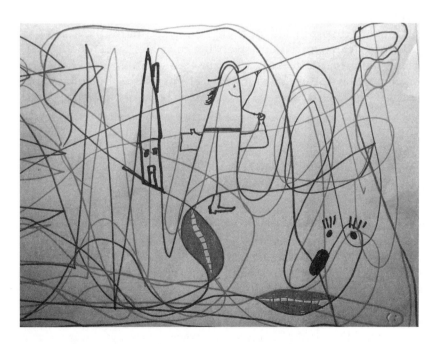

FIGURE 4.1. Example of the "scribble chase" activity.

This activity is sometimes called a "two-way conversation on paper," because many dynamics may emerge from this simple activity. For example, Lisa was eager to follow the lines scribbled by her 6-year-old son, John; however, she became immediately frustrated and angry when John was not able to follow her scribble and drew over her lines. She felt that John was doing this on purpose, and that he was being oppositional and defiant of what she thought were the rules of the scribble game. In this case, I helped Lisa understand that John's marks were not necessarily aggression toward her; they simply reflected the limited developmental motor skills of a young child who was challenged by trauma and loss. My third-hand intervention also involved ways to reframe the art experience, suggesting that perhaps John's marks were in part a positive action. I remarked that she could perhaps say to John, "I feel really happy when our lines touch. My lines are happy when your lines touched mine in the picture." My overall goal in this simple art activity is to create a sensory experience that reinforces positive relationship through tactile, visual, and physical contact and other aspects. In Lisa's case, I was able to help her start to attune to John and respond to his creative work in ways that she could carry over to other parts of the mother–child relationship to enhance positive bonding.

There is one other important aspect of a scribble chase that is also found in other art-based activities—*mirroring*. Art therapy is an approach that provides opportunities to witness another's creative expression; it also provides possibilities to introduce activities that can be imitated or learned through mirroring. As described by Gil and Dias in Chapter 7 on the integrative use of drama therapy within play therapy, mirroring is a key practice in building connection between the child and therapist; in dyad art therapy, children and parents learn through watching and interacting in similar ways. In all instances, aspects of interpersonal neurobiology are present in any shared sensory or expressive activities, including those in dyad art therapy.

The Bird's Nest Drawing and Three-Dimensional Construction

Working with a relevant metaphor through artistic expression is helpful in situations where there is insecure, disrupted, or avoidant attachment. One metaphor commonly used in art therapy is a "bird's nest." There is also an art-based assessment called the Bird's Nest Drawing (BND), which was developed to provide information about an individual's attachment security as depicted in a drawing of a bird's nest (Kaiser, 1996). The individual is asked, "Draw a picture with a bird's nest" (Figure 4.2). The BND is not a diagnostic tool per se, but a means to evoke representations of attachment, safety, and protection. Its originator, art therapist Donna Kaiser, hypothesized that the BND would encourage expression similar to that of family drawings, and that it would be less threatening to clients. Kaiser

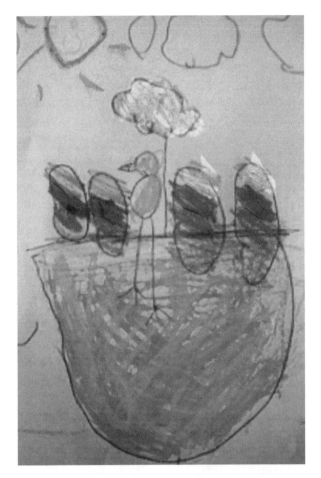

FIGURE 4.2. Drawing of a bird's nest by a child.

also developed a rating scale to measure specific graphic characteristics of secure and insecure attachment in BNDs (Francis, Kaiser, & Deaver, 2003; Kaiser & Deaver, 2009). Researchers have identified some consistent graphic elements and characteristics in these drawings that they believe are connected to attachment issues (Sheller, 2007).

Although a drawing of a bird's nest may be useful in evaluating attachment, children in particular respond positively to using a variety of art materials to create a bird's nest. In my experience, modeling clay, twigs, moss, leaves, tissue paper, and yarns have greater tactile and visual potential than drawing alone does, and they can engage children in more detailed representations. The sensory aspects of three-dimensional materials more closely approximate elements of a nest with eggs, parent birds, and baby birds, and dyads can use these more actively to express experiences of caregiving, security, and relationships through this metaphor. In dyad work, I may ask the parent and child to co-create a bird's nest together, using a variety of materials; I may also suggest that the parent allow the child to lead the way in designing the nest. I often arrange a separate session to coach the parent on ways to support the child's creative efforts for this activity, and also teach the parent about how to become a nonintrusive third hand in assisting. In addition, I use a variation of this activity that I call "creating a safe place for your duck," using a rubber duck toy that I provide as a prop.

In an individual session with Lisa, I explained to her that we would be working on a creative project on safety in an upcoming art therapy session with John, and that I would like her to try the project in advance so she could assist John. Lisa created her own "safe place" for a rubber duck on a paper plate, lining it with feathers and creating what she described as a "secure fort" for it (Figure 4.3). Without much prompting, she was quickly able to articulate her memories of fear and lack of a "safe place" as a child in a household where there was physical violence and sexual abuse. As she had observed in previous sessions, Lisa realized that these fear-based experiences compromised her own attachment to her mother, who she felt had not protected her from harm. Ultimately, Lisa's experience in creating a safe place for her duck taught her on a sensory level the importance of giving John a greater sense of safety through both actions and words. By their own mutual decision, they decided to co-create one safe place for two rubber ducks—a "Momma Duck" and a "Ducklet"—on a single paper plate (Figure 4.4).

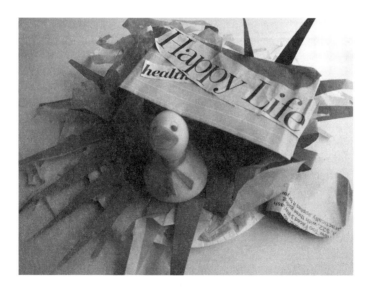

FIGURE 4.3. Lisa's construction of a safe place for a rubber duck.

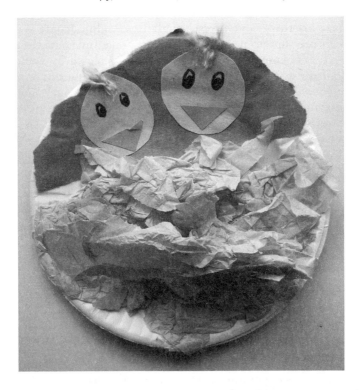

FIGURE 4.4. Lisa and John's co-created safe place for "Momma Duck" and "Ducklet."

Responding to Art Expressions

In my work with Lisa and John and with other parent–child dyads, I spend time coaching parents on what to say to their children about their art expressions rather than how to interpret their creative products. Therapists and counselors unfamiliar with art therapy often believe that it is important to be able to interpret the meaning of artwork. Although there may be visual metaphors in children's artwork that provide relevant information on trauma, loss, or other factors that may affect attachment, responding to the product and process through developmentally appropriate, "brain-wise" questions and supportive observations is much more important. Nonverbal responses are also important, including handling artwork with care and respect, and treating it with respect and value. Also, it is important to inform parents and children just how artwork will be stored between sessions if it is retained during an initial session; this can lead to a discussion of how the child's artwork that goes home should be treated or displayed. These actions reinforce a sense of safety, instill trust, and build the relationship among the therapist, parent, and child over time.

Because art therapy involves verbally responding to art expressions, practitioners can support positive attachment and attunement through their responses to art expressions, particularly those created by young clients. First and foremost, it is important not to place interpretations or judgments about the content or meaning of artwork; rather, it is much more helpful to demonstrate respect with both words and actions that art making is an important neurodevelopmental accomplishment for children. Here is a brief list of possible responses to children's creative work, which therapists can also teach parents to use when talking to their children about their art expressions:

> "I am really glad you can tell me about this and about how you feel through your drawings and artwork."
> "Your drawings and paintings helped me to understand how scary [sad, upset] you must have been. I get scared [sad, upset], too. It's OK to be scared [sad, upset]. I am glad that you can share these feelings through your artwork."
> "It doesn't matter what you draw [create]. I like watching you draw [create, play] and listening to your stories about your artwork."

In all cases, it is important to use nonverbal cues where possible and to attune these to the comfort level of clients, including eye contact, appropriate touch, and sincere gestures. Art therapy, like play therapy, provides a natural format for these attachment-building interactions, including active observation of expressive activities.

Conclusion

This brief chapter summarizes some key aspects of applying art therapy to attachment work with parent–child dyads. When art-based approaches are used to build or enhance attachment, sensory experiences that stimulate interaction and reinforce positive relationship between parent and child become the central strategies to initiate change. These sensory experiences also have the potential to recapture and restructure early experiences of bonding and attunement in both parent and child. Perry (2008) observes that "experience becomes biology" with reference to the impact of severe and recurrent trauma on attachment. Similarly, the experience of art therapy for those whose attachment has been compromised or disrupted may play a part in the recovery of what is most important to success throughout the lifespan—the experience of positive attachment and trust in secure relationships with others.

REFERENCES

Badenoch, B. (2008). *Becoming a brain-wise therapist: A practical guide to interpersonal neurobiology.* New York: Norton.

Francis, D., Kaiser, D., & Deaver, S. (2003). Representations of attachment security in the Bird's Nest Drawings of clients with substance abuse disorders. *Art Therapy: Journal of the American Art Therapy Association, 20*(3), 125–137.

Henley, D. (1992). *Exceptional children, exceptional art.* Worcester, MA: Davis.

Kaiser, D. (1996). Indications of attachment security in a drawing task. *The Arts in Psychotherapy, 23,* 333–340.

Kaiser, D., & Deaver, S. (2009). Assessing attachment with the Bird's Nest Drawing: A review of the research. *Art Therapy: Journal of the American Art Therapy Association, 26*(1), 26–33.

Klorer, P. G. (2008). Expressive therapy for severe maltreatment and attachment disorders: A neuroscience framework. In C. Malchiodi (Ed.), *Creative interventions and traumatized children* (pp. 43–61). New York: Guilford Press.

Kramer, E. (1993). *Art as therapy with children.* Chicago: Magnolia Street.

Malchiodi, C. A. (1997). *Breaking the silence: Art therapy with children from violent homes* (2nd ed.). New York: Brunner-Routledge.

Malchiodi, C. A. (Ed.). (2005). *Expressive therapies.* New York: Guilford Press.

Malchiodi, C. A. (2008). *Creative interventions with traumatized children.* New York: Guilford Press.

Malchiodi, C. A. (2012a). Art therapy materials, media, and methods. In C. A. Malchiodi (Ed.), *Handbook of art therapy* (2nd ed., pp. 27–40). New York: Guilford Press.

Malchiodi, C. A. (2012b). Psychoanalytic, analytic and object relations approaches. In C. A. Malchiodi (Ed.), *Handbook of art therapy* (2nd ed., pp. 57–74). New York: Guilford Press.

Malchiodi, C. A. (2012c). Art therapy and the brain. In C. A. Malchiodi (Ed.), *Handbook of art therapy* (2nd ed., pp. 17–26). New York: Guilford Press.

Malchiodi, C. A. (2012d). Trauma-informed art therapy and sexual abuse. In P. Goodyear-Brown (Ed.), *Handbook of child sexual abuse* (pp. 341–354). Hoboken, NJ: Wiley.

Perry, B. D. (2006). Applying principles of neurodevelopment to clinical work with maltreated and traumatized children: The neurosequential model of therapeutics. In N. B. Webb (Ed.), *Working with traumatized youth in child welfare* (pp. 27–52). New York: Guilford Press.

Perry, B. D. (2008). Foreword. In C. A. Malchiodi (Ed.), *Creative interventions and traumatized children* (pp. ix–xi). New York: Guilford Press.

Perry, B. D., & Szalavitz, M. (2006). *The boy who was raised as a dog.* New York: Basic Books.

Proulx, L. (2002). *Strengthening ties through parent–child dyad art therapy.* London: Kingsley.

Riley, S. (2001). *Group process made visible: Group art therapy.* New York: Brunner-Routledge.

Sheller, S. (2007). Understanding insecure attachment: A study using children's bird nest imagery. *Art Therapy: Journal of the American Art Therapy Association, 24*(3), 119–127.

Siegel, D. (2007). *The mindful brain.* New York: Norton.

Siegel, D. (2010). *Mindsight: The new science of personal transformation.* New York: Bantam.

Siegel, D. (2012). *The developing mind: How relationships and the brain interact to shape who we are* (2nd ed.). New York: Guilford Press.

Steele, W., & Malchiodi, C. A. (2012). *Trauma-informed practices with children and adolescents.* New York: Routledge.

Winnicott, D. W. (1953). Transitional objects and transitional phenomena. *International Journal of Psychiatry, 34,* 89–97.

Winnicott, D. W. (1965). *The maturation processes and the facilitating environment.* New York: International Universities Press.

Winnicott, D. W. (1971). *Therapeutic considerations in child psychiatry.* New York: Basic Books.

CHAPTER 5

Music Therapy with Children with Developmental Trauma Disorder

Jacqueline Z. Robarts

This chapter focuses on music therapy with children and adolescents living with unresolved attachment trauma, interpersonal violence, and/or neglect throughout early childhood, as well as high levels of stress in their homes. These children's physiological and emotional responses are affected at their core, inhibiting their psychological development and leading to *developmental trauma disorder*—an expansion of the posttraumatic stress disorder (PTSD) criteria for children with histories of complex trauma (van der Kolk, 2005). This chapter discusses music's power to affect intra- and interpersonal responses, and describes how music therapy can help children with early relational trauma. When applied with clinical perception and intent, musical improvisation and play within the therapeutic relationship can help regulate children's emotions and physiological responses, offer a wide range of sensory experiences, and encourage creative self-expression, thereby bringing about a more cohesive sense of self and continuity of being in the here-and-now.

This chapter also examines some aspects of music and *communicative musicality* (Malloch & Trevarthen, 2009; Trevarthen & Malloch, 2000), and their intrinsic *organizing* and *regulating* functions, as applied in music therapy (Robarts, 1998, 2009). From a synthesis of musical, developmental, and psychodynamic perspectives, the focus is on use of musical form as central to integrative processes of music therapy with young people whose foundations of self have been damaged by early relational trauma (Robarts, 2003, 2006, 2009).

Overview of Population

I have worked with children ages 3–18 years with attachment or early relational trauma—first during my early years as a music therapist in a music therapy department of a children's hospital with child and adolescent mental health and child development services; and later in a private music therapy center, where I specialize in this area of work with children and adults. Clinical supervision by child psychotherapists specializing in this field has supported and deepened my work, as have independent study and personal psychoanalysis.

The young people with whom I have worked in music therapy have been affected by a range of *traumatic* experiences: traumatic events preceding or surrounding a child's birth; repeated and prolonged separations in the first 3 years from a nonempathic mother; sexual abuse and neglect in early childhood; drug- and alcohol-abusing parents; witnessing violence between parents in the home; and/or successive and/or traumatic foster care and adoption processes. Persistent trauma in early childhood, where there have been overwhelming threats to basic safety and survival, may lead to developmental trauma disorder (van der Kolk, 2005). These children often present as pale and remote, yet hypervigilant; they are easily overaroused by ordinary movements, gestures, or sensory stimuli. The children may be so anxious that they will "shut down" their emotions or dissociate; become overly compliant; or become highly controlling and defensive, sometimes needing to withdraw physically from the situation (perhaps by hiding in a cupboard or a similar enclosed space). Their behavior and mood can change in a split second. In the occurrence of flashbacks of traumatic events, "the trauma is relived as isolated sensory, emotional and motoric imprints of the trauma, without a storyline" (van der Kolk, 2003, p. 183). Through its intrinsic sensory modalities and psychophysiological effects, music can be used in music therapy to help develop such children's continuity of self, capacity for sensory and symbolic play, and new narratives of being and being with others, untrammeled by trauma (Robarts, 2003, 2006, 2009).

Psychodynamic Music Therapy in the Field of Attachment Trauma

Psychodynamic music therapy has been well documented in collective and individually authored publications (Bruscia, 1998; Hadley, 2003; Wigram & De Backer, 1999). Music therapists specializing in trauma work are highly individual in their approaches or styles of working informed by a range of psychodynamic theories (Amir, 2004; Austin, 2008; Frank-Schwebel, 2002; Montello, 2003; Robarts, 2003, 2006, 2009; Scheiby, 2010; Schönfeld, 2003; Sutton, 2002). An essential aspect of all psychodynamically informed music therapy is receptivity to each client's internal world, particularly to musical and other aspects of transference and countertransference (nonverbal and verbal).

Musical and transference phenomena are complex visceral, emotional, and mental features of the therapeutic relationship. They are useful for understanding and working with a child's internal world and its constituent "object relations." They also present therapeutic challenges.

Holidays and any breaks in the children's therapy are prepared for, as is the ending of therapy. While children's confidentiality is strictly maintained except on a "need-to-know" basis, the music therapist works closely with parents and a multiagency team. This may include child protection, fostering, and adoption agencies.

In previous publications (Robarts, 2003, 2006, 2009), I have described some central aspects of music therapy that are particularly relevant to young people with unresolved early relational trauma and consequent developmental trauma disorder. In respect to attachment trauma, developmental psychology linked with affective neuroscience has emphasized the importance of the therapeutic attachment relationship in transforming interpersonal communicative relationships (Schore, 2001, 2003; Siegel, 2003; Stern, 2004; van der Kolk, 2003).

Issues and Challenges

Young people with unresolved attachment trauma present in music therapy with a wide range of issues that are challenging to both clients and therapists. This work requires heightened sensitivity; firm and highly adaptive therapeutic skills grounded in compassion; perceptive and creative use of mind and intuition; and a robust sense of reality. These young people present with the following, in various combinations: hypervigilance, hyperarousal, exaggerated startle response at the slightest trigger, disorganized or agitated behavior, withdrawal, a hardened or "hard-to-reach" demeanor, and emotional "tuning out." In such children, therapists are likely to meet a restricted range of feelings, impoverished capacity for play, and repetitive rituals in play (including self-harming or self-denigrating behavior or the reenactment of traumatic events). The more "acting-out" kind of behavior with poor capacity for play tends to be unsafe, because the children can easily become overexcited (and this may escalate into dangerous acts). It can be hard to maintain a vigilant stance while being open and receptive with such a child. To be firm yet relaxed requires a balance of skillful use of physical, verbal, musical, and spoken management in terms of boundaries to keep the child and the therapeutic relationship safe.

Added to these challenges is the scattered, fragmented, nonsequential nature of activity in the therapy room. Children may switch from screaming and kicking to remote, dissociative states. These switches are further complicated by the presentation of different stages of development in these children's behavior and their presymbolic and symbolic play. There is also the kind of "frozen" or "closed-down" child who presents with numbed responsiveness and a detached, avoidant style of relating and being. Often there is suicidal ideation or the exhibition of sexualized behavior in play. This may be accompanied by a controlling, intrusive style of relating, poor sense of physical interpersonal boundaries, physical and verbal abuse, and an unnaturally adult manner. In addition, there may be issues of shame and low self-esteem. Developmental delay and learning/attentional difficulties can all add to the attachment trauma and further affect the child's development.

All of these factors need careful understanding with regard to a child's feeling states and the symbolism in the child's play. The therapist needs to be able to understand where the child is developmentally at any given moment—and this may change from one moment to the next, with the child alternating between the coping strategies of a 6-year-old and those of the actual 14-year-old present in the room, all communicated either within the metaphors of symbolic play or more directly to the therapist. Features of the voice (such as volume and intonation), as well as the way in which the child is moving and generally behaving, inform the therapeutic process.

Avoiding Retraumatizing the Child

In working with children with PTSD and developmental trauma disorder in music therapy, the therapist needs to be aware of the impact that the sensory and interpersonal aspects of musical play and musical relationship may have, and the hyperarousal that even the slightest event may trigger. Frequently, the projections of an abused child's frightened and traumatized self make the therapist feel like one of the perpetrators of abuse. The therapist needs to develop a capacity to receive and then hold the intensity of transference feelings, along with any projections.

Mapping the Territory While Being Open to the New

Therapy processes are complex and multilayered, so that mapping the territory develops as part of one's craft (Robarts, 2000, 2003, 2009). Clinical experience is the most trustworthy route to theoretical understanding. My approach to music therapy sometimes embraces other art forms, such as drawing/painting, puppets, dance, and drama, in order to enrich the potential for children's symbolic play while affording a wide range of sensory experience. In my theory of symbolization, *poietic processes*, I elaborate the two-way channel between the preverbal and verbal self that allows integration to be nurtured in the therapy relationship (Robarts, 2003, 2009). The use of other expressive arts in music therapy sessions generally arises out of a child's spontaneous imaginative responses, and is developed within or alongside the music therapeutic process. Although I sometimes work solely in music (i.e., sound, instruments, voice), my clients constantly present all kinds of art forms, more accurately described by the Greek word for music, "mousike."

From a psychobiological perspective, the source of music and musicality has been described as "the intrinsic motive pulse" or "audible gesture" (Trevarthen, 1999, p. 175). "The essence of spontaneous musical expression is that it directly engages and activates the core of rhythmic and sympathetic impulses from which all human communication comes" (Robarts, 1998, p. 172). From the beginnings of life, music affects us. From 23 weeks of gestation, the fetus hears the intonation and timbre of its mother's voice, and recognizes this as its own mother's voice after birth (DeCasper & Carstens, 1981); this is the basis of prenatal attachment through sound. Parent–infant communication research shows our early intuitive emotional communication to be musical in all its dynamic forms—shaping and organizing the infant's developing brain, mind, and body through the parent's attuning to the infant in *protoconversational* forms, and thus building meaning and cultivating knowledge in relationships (Trevarthen, 1993). More recently, this process has been termed *communicative musicality*. It is a central, constructive feature of human relations and human development from the beginning of life and throughout the lifespan, and when it goes well, it lays the foundations of psychological health and well-being (Malloch & Trevarthen, 2009).

Conversely, if there are impairments or deficits in *intersubjectivity*, these will have a negative impact on the infant's core of rhythmic and sympathetic impulses, and thus on its developing brain connectivity and its self-regulatory and attachment capacities (Trevarthen, Aitken, Vandekerckhove, Delafield-Butt, & Nagy, 2006). In his descriptions of *affect attunement* in the infant–parent relationship, Stern (1985, 2004, 2010) has also described in musical terms the dynamic forms of vitality in early communication as a basis of attachment and emotional regulation in human psychosocial development. In music therapy, the regulating and shaping of musical–emotional communication are consistent with the constructs of communicative musicality and affect attunement.

Processes of Containment and Transformation in the Transference Relationship

I have found the psychoanalyst Wilfred Bion's concept of *containment* (Bion, 1962a, 1962b) very useful in music therapy. Bion developed this concept from Melanie Klein's original ideas of *transference* and the related intrapsychic processes of *projection, introjection,* and *projective and introjective identification.* To this, he added the idea of *transformation* to describe what happens when the mother/therapist receives the projections of infant/client, understands and thinks about them, and then gives them back in a useful form that can be felt with less anxiety and perhaps, at the right time, thought about—leading to his concept of the *container/ contained*. This has many parallels with the function of aesthetic form in the music therapy process described in this chapter. Bion emphasized not only the mother's receptivity to the infant's anxiety, but also her capacity to understand and give expression to the baby's unbearable feelings transforming them in ways that the baby can take in. If the baby's experiences are intolerable to its immature system, it then projects these feelings psychically into the mother, who then, identifying with the infant's emotional state and able to hold this state in her mind/feelings and understand it, gives the baby's feelings back transformed by her *understanding* response. In this way, Bion's explanation illuminates the processes of fragmentation and integration that take place in therapy as a client works toward creativity and well-being. This is helpful in considering the dynamic forms of the music therapy relationship.

Early object relations in terms of musical introjects and symbolization are also important (Robarts, 1994, p. 234). Regulatory processes in music involve the aesthetic creation of a space to think, and as such constitute a form of containment and transformation. Musical aspects of containment and transformation reside in the way the child is heard, listened to, and understood as much as being musically accompanied. This kind of "listening landscape" is the starting point and the point to which more active episodes in therapy return: The therapist remains open and receptive to what is arising in the moment, without expectation. Silence can enable a child to hear his or her own breathing, bringing the child a vital sense of being alive and present. A single tone, a sustained simple background of alternating harmonies (Austin, 2008), or a simple rhythm can be offered in a way that invites the child to respond if he or she wants to. Being with a traumatized child musically and affectively may center at first on letting the child explore the room and the instruments. It is important to let the child feel that he or she is in control and can check out everything, including the therapist!

While maintaining the boundaries of the therapeutic relationship, a therapist needs to respond sensitively and resourcefully to engage with a child's presenting developmental level(s). As explained earlier in this chapter, music is not necessarily the only form of engagement in music therapy; some children prefer to draw or play with toys, or roll on the mat. In music it is vital to create experiences of stability, often in the background of their other play preoccupations—such as a repeating melodic motive, an *ostinato* pattern, a shift in mood, a well-placed chord, a thickening or thinning of the harmonic texture, or a speeding or slowing of pace or tempo. All of these may offer some sense of connection, even without the child's response. Here the therapist's musical countertransference is akin to Bion's (1962a) maternal "reverie." Tuning into the *unsounded* music of the child's internal world is as important a process in music therapy as engaging in more overt modes of musical communication and play.

In a musical therapeutic relationship, children reveal their patterns of relating, motivations, and defenses, and often do so at varied developmental levels within a single therapy session. Augmenting positive and tolerable experiences of intersubjectivity through music is a primary concern, as is the assisting of emotional awakening and internalizing of experience when children's emotions are numbed or frozen. One only has to think of the physical pain of frozen limbs warming up to gain some appreciation of the pain of frozen emotions melting and beginning to flow. This is necessarily a slow and careful process. Music can engage children (and adults) at very early developmental levels when these are present in the therapy room. In adapting to the character and style that is likely to engage or respond to a particular client, simple musical form using musical techniques such as these can be used in infinitely flexible ways—from nursery songs to hip-hop, from blues to baroque.

In working with very disturbed children who have a fragile core sense of self, the therapist needs to be able to hold onto projected primitive anxieties for much longer than with clients whose ego function is stronger (Alvarez, 1992, 2010). Alvarez (1992) also describes the therapist's role in enlivening and engaging a child with significant developmental disorder and ego deficit. These facets of therapeutic work have importance in working with abused and traumatized children, whose self-protective defenses must be worked with sensitively by the therapist in order to build the children's capacity to trust, reflect on, and process experience. Working within the metaphors of children's songs, for instance, can enable maintaining much-needed defenses, while at the same time delicately bypassing these same defenses to address anxieties and nurture creative capacities.

Containing/Transforming Function of Improvised Songs: From Procedural Memory to Autobiographical Narrative

Song can bring forth emotions and images as autobiographical narratives from preverbal and visceral levels, from the procedural memory; this often integrates the dissociated, traumatized self-experiences in a freshly evolving here-and-now, supported by the music therapist. Developed in the early intimacy of infant–parent relating, the preverbal self is a social construction of implicit relational knowing (Siegel, 2012; Stern, 2004). When the preverbal self is traumatized in early development, the neural *template* of the intersubjective self is shattered, with lasting consequences. In music therapy, the underpinning of rhythm, pulse, or groove of the music increases the child's capacity for self-regulation, whereby a more secure and cohesive sense of self is experienced in musical coactivity. From this feeling of security and self-involvement, children with intelligence and language may begin singing their stories: autobiographical narratives or songs of self, often entirely in metaphor but clearly relating to themselves in a kind of borderland of half-conscious, half-unconscious.

One such child who improvised songs in music therapy was Lena (Robarts, 2003), whose case is described below. For the person who has suffered early trauma that has become embodied as part of the body–mind self, and is often beyond verbal recall, the power of music and singing can be a healing process (Austin, 2008). The preverbal, implicit, or procedural domain of the self is thought to function in quite a different way from the verbal self and declarative memory—the storehouse of our experiences that we can search and recollect consciously (Siegel, 2012). However, in my clinical experience, these two forms of memory or self-experiencing, implicit and explicit, can be bridged by art forms that *speak the language of the preverbal self*. In such cases, music can be used creatively not only in accessing the procedural domain of experience, but also in forging new relational experiences at that level, in musical interplay. These experiences are generally unplanned and arise spontaneously. The following case illustrations show how music therapy can bring new experiences of self into play, addressing unresolved trauma as well as developing normal healthy foundations of self.

Case Vignettes

The names of the children and the identifying features of their histories and therapy material have been changed to preserve confidentiality. For the same reason, songs and other material have been slightly altered, while retaining the salient therapeutic components.

Lena

Lena was an unwanted child who suffered severe neglect by her parents, and at the age of 2 years, during a traumatic separation from her mother, she was sexually abused by her grandfather. Throughout her early years, she was aggressive and provocative; as a result, she was excluded from nursery school. She then reported that she was being sexually abused by her brother and his friend. Lena felt she was "rubbish," a "throw-out," ugly, and unlovable. She was unable to learn effectively in school, and her bizarre behavior eventually raised sufficient concerns for her to be referred, at 9 years of age, to a child and adolescent mental health inpatient setting. There she stayed for 14 months. The unit staff was very conscious that she was being stigmatized by inpatient admission and made every effort to involve the whole family in regular therapy. Lena was also referred for music therapy once weekly (increasing to twice weekly after the first month), each session lasting 45 minutes.

Lena's music therapy fell roughly into three phases. The excerpts below (all described in the present tense, for greater immediacy) are drawn from Phase 1 and the very end of Phase 2. Phase 1 was characterized by listening; songs developing relationship and trust; idealization and self-protective defense; and symbolic use of musical instruments. In Phase 2, her defenses lowered: Her anxieties were expressed in song poems, later giving way to chaotic and eroticized play; flashbacks to early abuse; metaphors of the borderland between the unconscious and conscious in her improvised songs; and symbolic use of instruments. Phase 3 showed the beginnings of integration; expressions of sorrow at parting; and songs (again with power-ful metaphors arising from her unconscious) showing hope for the future in images of transformation.

Session 3 illustrates the use of nursery songs, as well as the defensive yet incipiently creative nature of her symbolic play and use of the instru-ments. Session 4 then shows my introduction of spontaneous, co-active song improvisation that helped reach beyond her "happy" mask to work with her defenses against sadness, and later her much more disturbed, chaotic feelings connected with early abuse. A much later session (Session 37) dem-onstrates her use of an improvised song to reach a new level of integration.

Session 3: Nursery Songs; the "Music House"; Symbolic Use of the Instruments as Containers

Today Lena arrives in what I now recognize to be her habitual superficially happy mood. After briefly playing the piano, Lena then chooses to surround herself with musical instruments, creating a "music house" on the far side of the room. This symbolic use of the instruments is extended in later ses-sions, but in this session, the instruments are arranged to form a physical barrier as much as a container. She demands that I listen attentively to her playing without joining in myself. From within her barricade, however, she now begins to permit some musical interaction through familiar nursery songs. She requests "Pop Goes the Weasel," "Hickory Dickory Dock," and "Ring a Ring of Roses." Lena jumps up and down like a 3-year-old as she plays inside her music house, especially enjoying the dramatic moments in each song.

I improvise music matching Lena's movements and vocalize in response to her squeals of excitement, which I am concerned may overwhelm her. However, her physical responses to the music show how efficiently the music is regulating her tendency toward overexcitement in shared play. By improvising clear phrase structures in music that matches her mood, I can not only meet but also *hold* and steady her feelings, musically trans-forming them into excitement and pleasure that she can tolerate without becoming avoidant or emotionally disturbed. The nursery songs offer her a certain predictability in which she can begin to trust our relationship. Nevertheless, her use of the songs is also quite defensive and controlling.

I introduce altered diatonic (nonconventional) harmonies in my accompaniment of the nursery songs, bringing different emotional qualities into the music to resonate with Lena's overt and underlying feelings, which I pick up in my countertransference and from her musical expression. I sing about her feeling safe inside her music house. I also introduce a *rondo* form (a musical form with the structure ABACAD, etc.) that uses her familiar tunes as a secure basis, from which she then engages in free vocalizing and improvisational–conversational exchanges. This style of refrain and episodic improvisational play develops in subsequent sessions, building new creative self-expression while also allowing Lena to work through her feelings and past experiences.

Session 4: A Happy–Sad Song That Brings Lena in Touch with Her Real Feelings and Builds a More Trusting Working Relationship

Lena wanders around the room rather distractedly. I play the "Child's Tune" motif (sol-mi-la-sol-mi) in unison, interspersed with close-textured diatonic harmonies. Lena repeats a question from Session 1: "What's music therapy for, anyway?" I answer her musings about music therapy by leading into a gentle I-Ib-IV-V accompaniment—a repeating sequence of a four-chord harmonic progression—banal in its predictability, wherein lies its therapeutic value in this instance. It becomes a refrain, to which we return when the musical development of emotional expression is more than Lena can bear:

> We can sing a happy song. Cheer us up, cheer us up;
> We can sing a happy song to cheer us up today.

Lena plays a countermelody on the metallophone, stopping intuitively at each cadence. I repeat the first phrase of the song. Lena joins in, singing and beating a conga drum and a cymbal so chaotically that her singing is almost inaudible. I then offer a contrasting idea (verbally and musically, shifting to a minor key, including dissonances and added 7ths, 9ths, and slightly slowing the tempo). I make these minimal changes to steady her beating and to begin to get in touch with her sadness. I sing, "We can sing if we're sad . . ." (ending on an open cadence in the hope that she will take over with the next line). I deliberately use "we" as a way of indicating that there is someone to share the "not happy" feelings and to avoid referring too directly to her (which might trigger her defense against sadness). The melody, previously characterized by ascending intervals, now is inverted as a descending phrase, in a minor key and in a slightly slower tempo. Lena does not respond, so I sing another phrase: "We . . . can . . . sing, if we're sa-a-ad. . . ." This time Lena echoes: "We . . . can . . . sing, if we're sa-a-ad. . . ."

Lena's singing now enters fully into the music's sadder mood, adding her own inflection of the melody. I continue singing and accompanying, to sustain this mood: "Sometimes we're sad. . . ." Lena interjects quickly: " . . . or happy . . . ," continuing: "Sometimes we're full of sorrow; sometimes we laugh with joy, full of joy. The sky's nice and bright; there's happiness in the air." My music reflects this idea with rippling impressionistic sequences in the upper registers of the piano. I hear a gentle sadness in my music (still in a minor key) with slightly increased harmonic tension and dissonance, thereby holding the two contrasting moods that Lena has expressed. The sadness is too much for her to bear getting in touch with. She sings rather wanly: "We can be so happy . . ." She then stops singing and chatters at such speed that I can barely grasp any of it, except to understand that she wishes to "get back to the bit about being happy."

Her verbal, cognitive defense against any feelings that might overwhelm her is evident; her desperation about being happy rather than sharing her real feelings is particularly poignant. I concur with a "happy" phrase, hoping to reengage Lena's singing and feelings rather than her verbal defenses against her emotions. I sing: "Happy, happy day," but in a minor key, continuing to the minor-key "bridge" section of the song. Here I reintroduce the mood and feeling states that Lena has seemed to deflect and split off (by way of dissociating), and which I am now feeling strongly in my countertransference, as I sing: "Sometimes . . . we feel sad. . . ." This time Lena takes over the song again, expressing her feelings more authentically, with the image of a lonely, upset child:

Sometimes we feel good;
Sometimes we feel like we're small and the world's against us;
Some days we feel joy, full of joy, and happiness in the air
And lovely smiley faces . . .
Children playing outside, happy and joy;
Someone sitting on their own, being upset . . .

Lena beats the cymbal and drum *sforzando*. She stops just as suddenly as she has begun and returns to her singing, reverting to the idea of happiness. She continues singing with a touching lyricism, while I accompany her, marking the pulse and harmonically coloring some of the emotive phrases:

Sometimes we're happy, sometimes we're sad,
Sometimes we're glad, sometimes we're ungra . . . a . . . a . . . ateful,
Sometimes we laugh, sometimes we sad
Sometimes we laugh, sometimes we . . . cough (*she coughs*),
Sometimes we laugh, sometimes we . . . grump,
Sometimes we sulk, sometimes we're sad, sometimes we're full of sorrow . . .
    again.

Holding on to the main issues of the narrative that pour from Lena in her songs and reflecting on them are central to this stage of therapy.

Session 37: A New Level of Integration

Lena's use of songs disappears almost entirely during a period when she presents highly disturbed behavior interspersed with dissociative states—remote, then chaotic and angry in turn. However, in Session 37 a new level of integration appears as she improvises a song about "The Haunted House." Many children imagine haunted houses, but this is a song poem that seems to be not just about any ghosts, but the ghosts in her life, in the home she grew up in. It contains powerful poetic images of resolution and integration, where good overcomes evil. All of this is communicated in metaphor, bringing experiences from the procedural realm to a half-consciousness—where I feel at this stage they should remain. Here is the hymn-like coda with its message of transformation in her song-poem, which Lena improvises while indicating to me (at the piano) what mood of accompaniment she wants, and encouraging me to repeat any motive or musical feature she finds *right* for her song as it evolves in the moment:

> As the world turns by, the house gets rottener and rottener;
> It gets uglier and creepier and ghostlier every day.
> And the people that spotted it have no desire
> And the people have noticed since it's been there.
> In a few years' time it's going to be knocked down
> Forever and ever and evermore.
> So one day a big bad windy storm—pshoo!—blows the house to bits . . .
> And the right notes (*Lena gestures to me to change the music*) make the next
>   day quiet . . .
> Nothing is left—just a chimney and half a door;
> The birds perch on what is left in there; the house is gone; no people in it.
> In a few years' time, the buildings there are shops and flats and houses,
> Forevermore . . . forevermore . . .

She then instructs me: "Ends! . . . End it!"

After a brief diversion, Lena continues singing, engaging easily with the new upbeat 5/4 meter or "groove" of my accompaniment:

> The house is forever gone; house is gone forevermore.
> Danger is nowhere in the world; bogey Martians have all gone.
> We have the joy of the sun; no badness on the earth.
> There is a goodbye today . . .
> There's a sun and come and wipe away evil.
> Evil has gone . . . when the house has been blown . . .
> The wind has gone . . .
> The evil has gone away from the derelict house. That's it, and it's gone.
> IT HAS GONE! (*Here Lena sings in an operatic style with great intensity.*)

Created in the moment with intensity of feeling coming from her soul, Lena's song-poems carried in metaphor aspects of autobiographical narrative, her past, the secrets in the family that haunted her and that were shaping her life. They represented the banishing of overwhelming evil, the transformation of shadowy ugliness with which she felt identified. Her music therapy drew to an end after 14 months when she moved to a residential school, before returning to live at home with family support from social services. Many years later I heard that she had married and had a child.

Laura

Laura presented as a pale, thin 7-year-old. Her clothes were old and dirty and hung on her bony body like rags. Intelligent but emotionally withdrawn, she presented as a "closed-down" and "frozen" child, with numbed feelings—unable to talk, much less smile. Laura seemed unreachable, just standing limply, then compliantly engaging in what she thought I expected of her. From babyhood and through the first 5 years of her life, Laura was repeatedly placed in foster care. During periods when her parents were living together (there were frequent separations), they were frequently unconscious from drug abuse; when conscious, they were arguing and attacking each other. By the time Laura was 6, she was used to looking after her parents and trying to survive in a highly stressful, unsafe home. She found safety in a cupboard beneath the stairs, or in her bedroom where she developed obsessive organizing and tidying types of play. At 7 years of age, she was taken permanently into foster care. Her new school then referred her to music therapy. For several years, I saw her twice weekly during school term time. The music therapy room was a space that Laura solemnly arranged to her liking. I noticed that she did not chatter to herself while she played; she was completely silent.

Initially, Laura engaged in some familiar, clearly patterned, improvised black-note piano duets. She seemed to be developing a sense of safety and trust in the clear phrasing and patterns of the music, and in the ways in which I accompanied her melodies. I noticed her body sometimes moving to the pulse of the music, enjoying its predictability and equally the very slight variations of the melodic and rhythmic patterns as she began to respond spontaneously. At the time I remembered Frances Tustin's account of "the rhythm of safety" in the infant–mother relationship as well as the therapeutic relationship, where new rhythmic experiences of self and other are created through the adapting of one to another in a shared, reciprocal experience (Tustin, 1986, pp. 268–275). However, I soon found that the piano duets became increasingly perfunctory, and that music making itself was being used by Laura as a defense against feeling—a means of blocking out unbearable feelings. I soon learned that it was her habit to switch off her spontaneous feelings to their safely numb state whenever they arose as she became engaged in her play.

In later sessions, it was encouraging to see this entrenched state shifting. Laura's play became fragmentary and disorganized, but more authentic; in many ways, it represented the patterns of her early experiences of frequent abandonment and uprooting from one foster home to another. I felt it was important to wait, attend, listen, and accept however she wished to use her sessions. Equally, it felt important to enliven and *lift* the mood of the sessions in some way by injecting some energy into the room. I am reminded of Alvarez's (1992) thoughts on the therapist's sometimes needing to alert and enliven the child. My offering her a sudden idea (with an intake of breath, raised eyebrows, and a sense of excitement) engaged her briefly, but was then rejected.

Rejecting me and music and controlling her world were central themes in Laura's therapy—just as, undoubtedly, she had been rejected and neglected as a child. Yet Laura came every week and, later, twice weekly. Laura found ever-inventive ways of disappearing and hiding during the sessions, much as she had evaded the violence between her parents. It also showed me how she erected barriers to provide physical safety. Inside her room at home, she had rearranged its contents almost daily, creating her own world over which she had control. She began to treat the therapy room in much the same way, except that she now used a large instrument cupboard in which to create her own private space, where she busily drew and labeled everything. (I had to preserve these labels from week to week—and in doing this I felt I was helping with the continuity of her play, which she had previously seemed incapable of maintaining.)

One day, from inside the cupboard, Laura began to tap. From the other side, I tapped back. An exchange of rhythmic patterns developed. This recurred in the following sessions; at last, there was some continuity of play that felt meaningful and spontaneous, coming from her own motivations. I wondered if my whistling instead of tapping in response might lead to Laura to use her voice expressively (she spoke barely audibly in the sessions). To my surprise, an exchange of whistled phrases ensued with dramatic melodic swoops up and down, in patterns and varying phrase lengths, questioning and answering each other. In her whistling, there were the first signs of spontaneous play and emotional expression, which were never heard in her speaking voice or instrumental play.

In this way, I encountered for the first time her sense of humor and playfulness. However, these musical exchanges lasted only briefly, returning to quiet tapping games and a guessing game she invented: I had to guess where her hand was on the other side of the wooden cupboard door. This felt like a very controlled game of hide-and-seek, where she definitely had the advantage. But it was also a game in which the purpose or goal was for me to *find/locate* the very spot where her hand was on the other side of the door. It grew to be a reciprocal game in which some real communication took place. Toward the end of one session, I heard her quietly singing a song to her parents: "I miss you, I'm sorry." From these tentative, simple musical exchanges, our therapeutic relationship grew in a more real way—working through the many painful experiences that had numbed her feelings, and bringing new experiences that opened the door to new possibilities in her life. This was a five-year-long therapeutic process.

Conclusion

This chapter presents an overview of music therapy with children with unresolved attachment trauma or developmental trauma disorder. I have described the nature of music and communicative musicality, and have linked these to early relational phenomena from developmental psychology and psychotherapy. Music therapy can provide a "listening landscape," as well as a "sounding of the self." Being musically and clinically resourceful, receptive, and open to the new, and serving as an actively responsive participant, are vital qualities in the music therapist. Working with children, especially those with developmental trauma disorder, I have learned much about the essence of what it is to be human, to be heard, to sound, to find one's voice, and to forge new experiences of self and well-being within and beyond the musical-therapeutic relationship.

ACKNOWLEDGMENTS

I would like to thank Dr. Barbara Wheeler for her helpful advice on this chapter. I would also like to thank Barcelona Publishers for their kind permission to include here in a revised form some excerpts from my chapter in *Psychodynamic Music Therapy: Case Studies* (Robarts, 2003).

REFERENCES

Alvarez, A. (1992). *Live company: Psychoanalytic psychotherapy with autistic, borderline, deprived and abused children.* New York: Routledge.

Alvarez, A. (2010). *The thinking heart: Three levels of psychoanalytic therapy with disturbed children.* New York: Routledge.

Amir, D. (2004). Giving trauma a voice: The role of improvisational music therapy in exposing, dealing with and healing a traumatic experience of sexual abuse. *Music Therapy Perspectives, 22*(2), 96–103.

Austin, D. (2008). *The theory and practice of vocal psychotherapy: Songs of the self.* London: Kingsley.

Bion, W. R. (1962a). A theory of thinking. *International Journal of Psycho-Analysis, 43,* 306–310.

Bion, W. R. (1962b). *Learning from experience.* London: Heinemann.

Bruscia, K. E. (1998). *The dynamics of music psychotherapy.* Gilsum, NH: Barcelona.

DeCasper, A. J., & Carstens, A. A. (1981). Contingencies of stimulation: Effects on learning and emotion in neonates. *Infant Behavior and Development, 4,* 19–35.

Frank-Schwebel, A. (2002). Developmental trauma and its relation to sound and music. In J. P. Sutton (Ed.), *Music, music therapy and trauma: International perspectives* (pp. 193–207). London: Kingsley.

Hadley, S. (Ed.). (2003). *Psychodynamic music therapy: Case studies.* Gilsum, NH: Barcelona.

Malloch, S. N., & Trevarthen, C. (Eds.). (2009). *Communicative musicality: Exploring the basis of human companionship.* Oxford: Oxford University Press.

Montello, L. (2003). Protect this child: Psychodynamic music therapy with a gifted musician. In S. Hadley (Ed.), *Psychodynamic music therapy: Case studies* (pp. 299–318). Gilsum, NH: Barcelona.

Robarts, J. Z. (1994). Towards autonomy and a sound sense of self. In D. Dokter (Ed.), *Arts therapies and clients with eating disorders* (pp. 229–246). London: Kingsley.

Robarts, J. Z. (1998). Music therapy and children with autism. In C. Trevarthen, K. Aitken, D. Papoudi, & J. Z. Robarts (Eds.), *Children with autism: Diagnoses and interventions to meet their needs* (pp. 172–202). London: Kingsley.

Robarts, J. Z. (2000). Music therapy and adolescents with anorexia nervosa. *Nordic Journal of Music Therapy, 9*(1), 3–12.

Robarts, J. Z. (2003). The healing function of improvised songs in music therapy with a child survivor of early trauma and sexual abuse. In S. Hadley (Ed.), *Psychodynamic music therapy: Case studies* (pp. 141–182). Gilsum, NH: Barcelona.

Robarts, J. Z. (2006). Music therapy with sexually abused children. *Clinical Child Psychology and Psychiatry, 11*(2), 249–269.

Robarts, J. Z. (2009). Supporting the development of mindfulness and meaning: Clinical pathways in music therapy with a sexually abused child. In S. N. Malloch & C. Trevarthen (Eds.), *Communicative musicality: Exploring the basis of human companionship* (pp. 377–400). Oxford: Oxford University Press.

Scheiby, B. B. (2010). Analytical music therapy and integrative medicine: The impact of medical trauma on the psyche. In K. Stewart (Ed.), *Music therapy and trauma: Bridging theory and clinical practice* (pp. 74–87). New York: Satchnote.

Schönfeld, V. (2003). "Promise to take good care of it!": Therapy with Ira. In S. Hadley (Ed.), *Psychodynamic music therapy: Case studies* (pp. 207–224). Gilsum, NH: Barcelona.

Schore, A. N. (2001). The effects of early relational trauma on right brain development, affect regulation, and infant mental health. *Infant Mental Health Journal, 22,* 201–269.

Schore, A. N. (2003). Early relational trauma, disorganized attachment, and the development of a predisposition to violence. In M. F. Solomon & D. J. Siegel (Eds.), *Healing trauma: Attachment, mind, body, and brain* (pp. 107–167). New York: Norton.

Siegel, D. J. (2003). An interpersonal neurobiology of psychotherapy: The development mind and the resolution of trauma. In M. F. Solomon & D. J. Siegel (Eds.), *Healing trauma: Attachment, mind, body, and brain* (pp. 1–56). New York: Norton.

Siegel, D. J. (2012). *The developing mind: How relationships and the brain interact to shape who we are* (2nd ed.). New York: Guilford Press.

Stern, D. N. (1985). *The interpersonal world of the infant: A view from psychoanalysis and developmental psychology.* New York: Basic Books.

Stern, D. N. (2004). *The present moment in psychotherapy and everyday life.* New York: Norton.

Stern, D. N. (2010). *Forms of vitality: Exploring dynamic experience in psychology, the arts, psychotherapy, and development.* Oxford: Oxford University Press.

Sutton, J. P. (Ed.). (2002). *Music, music therapy and trauma: International perspectives.* London: Kingsley.

Trevarthen, C. (1993). The self born in intersubjectivity: The psychology of an infant communicating. In U. Neisser (Ed.), *The perceived self: Ecological and interpersonal sources of self-knowledge* (pp. 121–173). New York: Cambridge University Press.

Trevarthen, C. (1999). Musicality and the intrinsic motive pulse: Evidence from human psychobiology and infant communication. *Musicae Scientiae* (Special Issue 1999–2000), 155–215.

Trevarthen, C., Aitken, K. A., Vandekerckhove, M., Delafield-Butt, J., & Nagy, E. (2006). Collaborative regulations of vitality in early childhood: Stress in intimate relationship and postnatal psychopathology. In D. Cicchetti & D. J. Cohen (Eds.), *Developmental psychopathology: Vol. 2. Developmental neuroscience* (2nd ed., pp. 65–127). Hoboken, NJ: Wiley.

Trevarthen, C., & Malloch, S. N. (2000). The dance of wellbeing: Defining the musical therapeutic effect. *Nordic Journal of Music Therapy, 9*(2), 3–17.

Tustin, F. (1986). *Autistic barriers in neurotic patients.* London: Karnac.

van der Kolk, B. A. (2003). Posttraumatic stress disorder and the nature of trauma. In M. F. Solomon & D. J. Siegel (Eds.), *Healing trauma: Attachment, mind, body, and brain* (pp. 168–196). New York: Norton.

van der Kolk, B. A. (2005). Developmental trauma disorder: Towards a rational diagnosis for children with complex trauma histories. *Psychiatric Annals, 35*(5), 401–408.

Wigram, T., & De Backer, J. (Eds.). (1999). *Clinical applications of music therapy in psychiatry.* London: Kingsley.

CHAPTER 6

Moving with the Space between Us
The Dance of Attachment Security

Christina Devereaux

Significant research findings have underscored nonverbal parent–child interaction as an important collaborative exchange that supports healthy development and enhances positive social relationships (Ainsworth & Bell, 1970; Beebe & Lachmann, 1998; Bowlby, 1969, 1988; Schore, 2001; Siegel, 2012; Tronick, 2003, 2007; Tronick & Beeghly, 2011). *Attuned* interactions between parent and child are nonverbal communications that assist individuals in building empathy/understanding and developing healthy attachment relationships. This attunement involves all of the physical senses and also depends on the awareness of sound, tone of voice, and nonverbal rhythms of communication. However, when there is consistent disengagement or disruption in this dance of interaction, both parent and child can be affected, influencing the security of the attachment relationship.

Attachment theory, an approach emphasizing parent–child interaction (Ainsworth, Blehar, Waters, & Wall, 1978; Bowlby, 1969, 1988), has been incorporated into a variety of theories providing many implications for clinical application and developmental research. Its core construct is a biologically based predisposition for physical proximity and connection between mother (or other primary caregiver) and child (Bowlby, 1988); the security of this attachment predicts later functioning. These theoretical constructs are widely applicable in assessment and intervention for individuals, groups, and families, especially within nonverbal psychotherapeutic disciplines such as dance/movement therapy (DMT).

This chapter first discusses how attachment, viewed as a metaphorical dance, can be enhanced through nonverbal attunement and body-based intervention. A more in-depth look into the discipline of DMT through the theoretical lens of attachment theory follows. Examples from DMT interventions with individuals with attachment needs support this discussion.

Theoretical Foundations: Attachment Theory and the Body

Bowlby (1969) emphasized the importance of a behavioral system that equips a child with body-based signal behaviors (i.e., smiling, crying) designed to keep the primary caregiver in reach. These signal behaviors are complemented by an exploratory system that allows the child to crawl away from the primary caregiver and explore the world, once a "secure base" (Bowlby, 1988) is established. In times of distress (e.g., separation from the primary caregiver or other stress), a child tries to resort to comfort by moving into closer proximity to the caregiver, resulting in the deactivation of the exploratory behavior. This emphasis on both the biological drive for proximity seeking when distressed, and the drive to explore out into the world when internalized security is established, highlights the importance of attending to nonverbal, body-based, interactive cues when one is examining attachment relationships.

Attachment research has proposed that a primary caregiver and infant have a goal to achieve a state of reciprocity, consisting of connectedness, intimacy, oneness, synchrony, and mutual delight, and that "to attain it they jointly regulate the interaction with interactive behaviors" (Tronick, 2007, p. 178). This is demonstrated in research (Brazelton, 1982; Tronick, 1980, 2007; Tronick & Beeghly, 2011) highlighting how infants, when faced with interactive ruptures, activate a number of predictable strategies designed to repair the mismatch or to cope with the failure via self-soothing or withdrawal. For example, Tronick's "still-face" research and subsequent studies (Tronick, 1980, 2003, 2007) obtained significant findings suggesting that when a caregiver disengages from the interactive cycle with an infant, the infant responds by attempting to reengage the connection through various strategies. Tronick and Beeghly (2011) discuss how an infant's capacity to make meaning out of the interaction with a primary caregiver occurs primarily through nonverbal cues, such as affect and movements. This strongly indicates that attachment security develops as a result of body-based nonverbal communication. They also suggest that the dyadic attachment relationship is a mutually regulating system of communication.

Tronick's research is highly significant to DMT, as it stresses the value and importance of the infant–caregiver relationship for the infant's socio-emotional behavior, and shows how disruptions in the interactive exchange activate the attachment behavioral system. Schore and Schore (2008) have discussed how these attachment relationships are formed through nonverbal, body-based attunement (i.e., eye gaze, vocal tone, and facial expressions). Therefore, therapists can rely on nonverbal communication to form attachment relationships within the therapeutic alliance, since such communication acts as a mechanism to support interactive regulation with clients. These constructs are some of the core principles of the discipline of DMT.

Assumptions and Principles of DMT

Dance/movement therapists view movement of the body as both expressive and communicative, and utilize it both as a method of assessing individuals and as the mode for clinical intervention. DMT is based upon the belief that there is a fundamental interconnection between the mind and body; it is assumed that whatever is having an impact on the body will have a reciprocal impact on the mind. Therefore, a core principle of DMT is that healthy overall functioning relies upon the integration of mind and body (Levy, 2005). When there is a lack of mind–body integration, individuals may suffer from a variety of psychological disorders. Similarly, there is a foundational belief that examining one's movement vocabulary or range "opens a door to the study of patterns of early development, coping strategies, and personality configurations" (Kestenberg Amighi, Loman, Lewis, & Sossin, 1999, p. 2). An increased integration of a person's body parts and awareness of others expands the individual's movement vocabulary, thus increasing his or her ability to communicate needs and desires.

DMT focuses directly on movement behavior as it emerges out of the developed therapeutic relationship. A DMT pioneer, Marian Chace, emphasized that "the therapeutic relationship is core to the meaning of movement structures that evolve between the dance therapist and those with whom he/she works and it is the interactive process that enables change" (Fischer & Chaiklin, 1993, p. 138). Furthermore, because "movement is a universal means of communication" (Erfer, 1995, p. 196), it is an especially useful therapeutic approach that can both provide a direct link to feelings and build a connection or relationship with others. Finally, because people's early attachment influences affect their later development of healthy relationships (Ginot, 2012; Schore, 2003; Schore & Schore, 2008; Siegel, 2012; Stern, 1985; van der Kolk, 2006), movement can serve as the common language for building communication and establishing secure attachment relationships.

DMT and Attachment Theory

Behrends, Müller, and Dziobek (2012) have discussed the evolving connections between different disciplines such as neuroscience and DMT. They suggest that it is "cructial to integrate the bodily dimension of perceptive and expressive processes as part of social interactions in diagnostic procedures and treatment plans for patients with problems with . . . social relationships" (p. 114), such as those with attachment difficulties. van der Kolk (2006) also emphasizes that effective treatment of developmental trauma must involve the traumatized individual's "learning to tolerate feelings and sensations . . . [and] learning to modulate arousal" (p. 277). Subramaniam's (2010) qualitative study examined how attachment theory and work within the attachment and relational framework informs the work of dance/movement therapists. The results of her interviews with attachment-oriented dance/movement therapists "demonstrated linking what the field of attachment-oriented psychotherapy has been calling for—an integration of more body-based and nonverbal interventions" (p. ii). Her results also suggested that approaches in DMT can "provide significant benefit for clients with disrupted attachment experiences . . . [by] working with the preverbal experiences of the self, which are in turn influenced by our early attachment relationships" (p. ii).

Other literature has highlighted the use of DMT to support, develop, enhance, or "rechoreograph" areas important to attachment relationships, such as emotional regulation (Betty, 2013; Hervey & Kornblum, 2006; Kornblum, 2002, 2008; Koshland & Wittaker, 2004), socioemotional development (Thom, 2010), body awareness (Moore, 2006), the bonding between infants and caregivers (Loman, 1998; Tortora, 2006), and attachment relationships within the family structure (Devereaux, 2008). However, a firmer scientific foundation and further research are needed to support and strengthen this evidence-base.

DMT does have a unique set of processes for promoting the emergence of bodily experience within the therapeutic movement relationship. The development of kinesthetically attuned interactions will support a client in establishing emotional regulation and a healthy attachment relationship. It is particularly important that clinical interventions include a "rechoreography" of new embodied patterns, so that "repair work" of insecure attachment relationships can occur through the body and become integrated on a bodily level.

The following sections address some concepts used in clinical intervention to support this focus, such as mirroring, attunement, mutual regulation, spatial exploration, and the use of connective tools. A case vignette follows this discussion.

Mirroring, Attunement, and Empathy

The DMT relationship begins with the process of *attunement* or "matching" (Tortora, 2006, p. 259), in which the dance/movement therapist experiences the qualitative aspects of a client's movement through reflecting back and conveying understanding of the client's communicative gestures.

In DMT, this is accomplished through relational dances and movement interactions such as trying on various body shapes, exaggerating or exploring various movement dynamics, and engaging in heightened moments of rhythmic synchrony. Indeed, the interactive movement relationship is essential in the dance/movement therapy treatment process (Berrol, 2006).

Through the use of the traditional DMT technique called *mirroring* or *empathic reflection* (Chaiklin & Schmais, 1993), the therapist reflects an individual's body rhythms, movement patterns, and/or vocalizations to begin the process of relationship formation. The goal is to attune to the client where he or she is, both physically and emotionally, and to establish a trusting therapeutic movement relationship that builds an awareness of the self and other. Because most of these attuned interactions occur on a nonverbal level, DMT can be an ideal treatment intervention in supporting the development of a safe therapeutic relationship emphasizing consistency, trust, and empathy—an experience that clients who exhibit severe attachment needs may not have had (Bowlby, 1988, Devereaux, 2008; Schore, 2003; Siegel, 2012). Because of these clients' challenges, establishing a therapeutic relationship can be extremely difficult. According to Chaiklin and Schmais (1993),

> There is a fine line between empathy on a movement level and mimicry. Mimicry involves duplicating the external shape of the movement without the emotional content that exists in the dynamics and in the subtle organization of the movement. . . . Empathy meant sharing the essence of all nonverbal expression resulting in . . . direct communication. (p. 86)

Therapeutic interactions that include imitation or reflection of a client's movements or actions and attunement to the individual's emotional state send the nonverbal message "I hear you, I understand you, and it's OK." Trust is established through nonverbal recognition and response to the client. Therefore, DMT can support healthier attachment relationships through the therapist's and client's participating in shared movement experiences and engaging in shared focus. These joint experiences can assist a client in feeling seen and joined with, and in reexperiencing attuned nonverbal interactions—all of which are imperative to establish a secure attachment.

The process of moving with someone through the art of dance empathically connects the therapist with the attachment-disordered individual, so that the experience of attunement can begin (Berrol, 2006; Fischman, 2009; Devereaux, 2012). "Knowing [the child's] rhythm, affect, and experience by metaphorically being in its skin . . . goes beyond empathy to create a two-person experience of connectedness by providing a reciprocal affect and/or resonating response" (Erskine, 1998, p. 236). In DMT, attunement is communicated not just by what is said, but also by facial or body movements; these signal to the child that his or her affect and needs are perceived, are significant, and make an impact on another (Devereaux, 2008, 2012). Schore (2003) asserts that to enter into this communication, one must be psychobiologically attuned not so much to the child's overt behavior as to the reflections of the rhythms of the child's internal state. These affective attunements, which are both spontaneous and nonverbal, are "the moment-to-moment expressions of [one's] regulatory functions occur[ing] at levels beneath awareness" (Schore, 2001, p. 14).

In DMT, once an initial attuned relationship is established, the therapist then serves as "a catalyst, gradually assisting in the expansion and elaboration of the patient's movements until they reach full expressivity— yet always watching the patient's emotional and kinesthetic reactions to this change and adjusting their empathic movements accordingly" (Merna, 2010, p. 111).

Mutual Influences in the Attachment Relationship

Another purpose of attachment lies in the experience of psychological containment of difficult and threatening affective states. Such containment is required for the development of a coherent self (Siegel, 2012). Fuertes, Lopes-dos-Santos, Beeghly, and Tronick (2009) emphasize that coping with strong affect (affect regulation) and caregiver behavior both seem to influence the formation of the attachment relationship, suggesting that attachment interactions have the capacity to be mutually regulating. These mutual influences, called *interactive/mutual regulation*, occur during times of shared affective moments where caregiver and child can become attuned in a synchronistic nonverbal exchange (Stern, 1985). According to Beebe and Lachmann (1998), during these shared experiences "contingencies flow in both directions between partners. That is, the behavior of each partner is contingent upon (influenced by) that of the other" (p. 485). Studies in infant mental health clarify the importance of mutuality and interactive movement relationship between the dance/movement therapist and the individual with an attachment disorder. Fischer and Chaiklin (1993) state:

> The dance therapist in the role of participant observer must have a clear realization and responsibility for his or her own dance in relation to the other individual. Just as the tension of any existing anxiety present in the mother induces anxiety within the infant, such tension in the therapist will affect the interaction. The meeting in movement of the therapist and the client assumes that both are part of the dialogue, even though one is identified as helper and the other as needing help. (p. 139)

As previously discussed, attunement and mirroring are of prime importance in order to establish a safe therapeutic relationship for clients in DMT, especially for clients who exhibit severe attachment needs and have not had feelings of security in past relationships (Baudino, 2010; Betty,

2013; Devereaux, 2008; Tortora, 2006). The therapist must also attend to his or her own embodied responses (i.e. countertransference) to serve as guideposts in the development of empathy (Subramaniam, 2010).

Spatial Exploration as Metaphor

Kossak (2009) has emphasized that attunement is a dynamic relationship where "the [client] begins to learn about relational space and safety" (p. 14). Spatial exploration as a metaphor for this safety of the relational space is an essential tool for therapists to utilize in DMT interventions. Dance/movement therapists give important attention to the full range of spatial exploration—such as moving on different levels (moving from the floor to standing) and maintaining physical distance between self and other—that occurs when they are moving with clients. This active exploration of the physical holding environment also allows a client to physically experience moving out and away into the movement space (widening the distance between therapist and client) or moving toward another (narrowing the distance between therapist and client). Interventions that emphasize the actual physical distance between self and other parallel the healthy development of the exploratory system (Bowlby, 1988). Other body-level interventions also provide opportunities for a client to reexperience a healthy sequence of movement development (Kestenberg Amighi, Loman, Lewis, & Sossin, 1999). For example, moving in the *horizontal* plane surrounding one's body involves spreading to open and reveal the body and reach to the furthest rim of ones's *kinesphere*, or personal space. This way of moving can be an expansive opening movement, while the opposite way of moving in the horizontal plane is generally enclosing or gathering oneself together, as if closing oneself off from the outside world. Ascending to the upright stance of the *vertical* plane provides a client with possibilities of rising and falling. Movement along this vertical plane is one of display: "Here I am!" Movements that explore advancing forward or moving backward through space, on what is referred to as the *sagittal* plane, directly highlight the exploratory system that Bowlby (1988) discusses. Therefore, when the therapist assists the client in using explorations that support the physical awareness of the kinesphere, or the awareness and expansion of multidimensional uses of the client's own body space, this can "facilitate the formation of complex relationships" (Kestenberg Amighi et al., 1999, p. 175).

When a client begins to internalize a secure base within the therapeutic alliance, the client has a safe opportunity to reexperience moving away out into space in the sagittal plane from the attachment figure, and then coming back in closer proximity in a new spatial configuration. The therapist can continue to attune to these relational dynamics by narrating the movement patterns as they are literally occurring. For example, "I noticed that when I came closer, you moved your body away. I wonder, how far do I need to go for you to feel comfortable? I am all the way in the corner, and

I'm still too close." Or, conversely, "You seem to be almost on top of me, and it's still not feeling close enough for you." When the therapist reflects back to the client the active, in-the-present-moment processes occurring within the attachment relationship, together the client and the therapist (through the movement metaphor) can make sense of and rechoreograph the attachment dynamics.

Bridging the Space with Connection Tools

Dance/movement therapists also emphasize the exploration of the physical space via the use of props (e.g., stretch fabrics, scarves, balls, and music) during sessions. These props serve as connective and communicative tools. They can provide a less threatening way to make various connections: from a client to others in a group, from one client to another, from therapist to client, from client to therapist, or from client to imagination and exploration. In particular, these connection tools can assist in providing a bridge of contact between therapist and client, and can also serve as a means "to express feelings and thoughts, which [create] an outlet for imagination and exploration" (Baudino, 2010, p. 126). For example, if the therapist initiates connection and joining to a client through the use of a scarf or a flexible piece of stretch fabric, the prop can create connection and provide a visual representation for the attachment relationship. The client can experience pulling against the therapist, joining in a less threatening way, or feeling the self as separate by carving out his or her own kinesphere or personal space bubble. The use of connective tools provides opportunities to play with the flexibility of distance, to experience resistance to or desire for closeness, and to dance and move the attachment relationship through an active and metaphorical process (Devereaux, 2012).

The use of music as an auditory external holding environment can support the sense of connection through rhythm to support and attune the individual to the energetic tone of the session. As therapist and client dance together to same rhythm with music, there is an embodied sense of connection. In addition, Erfer (1995) notes that "rhythm is a meaningful organizer of impulses" (p. 201).

In summary, a client who has experienced insecurity in the space around him or her may benefit through actual movement explorations that involve establishing a physical therapeutic container, defining a personal kinesphere, and bridging the relational or intermediate area of space between client and therapist. Such interventions can support the establishment of a relationship in a less intimate way than the use of touch, direct movement matching, or even verbalization can do.

In the following section, I describe a case in which the concepts described above are integrated with a clinical example. Specifically, I discuss how the DMT process came to assist an individual child client with rechoreographing his attachment insecurity and internalizing the capacity to regulate strong affect, healthy coping strategies, and experience an attuned secure base via the therapeutic alliance.

Case Vignette: Joey

Joey, an 8-year-old child, worked with me in once-a-week 50-minute DMT sessions in an outpatient clinic. His mother referred Joey to treatment after becoming severely concerned about his acting-out behavior at school (refusing to complete homework, angry outbursts, aggression with other peers, increasing fear of trying new things, and disrupting class) and his escalating behavior at home (verbal and physical aggression toward his older sibling and his mother).

Joey witnessed consistent verbal and physical abuse from his father toward his mother. His father was now inconsistently present in his life, and was involved in a new relationship where there was a baby on the way. Joey would come to DMT sessions and both verbally and nonverbally express his own underlying feelings of low self-worth. He appeared to be ambivalent about his relationship with his father, and this ambivalence seemed to be carried over into his patterns of interactions with his mother, sibling, and peers. His mother reported that at times, he would become clingy, sleep with her in her bed, and refuse to leave the house. At other times, when he would get angry, it appeared as if nothing could soothe him. He also began to be less comfortable with taking risks and exploring new things at school. His exploratory system was often deactivated, as he was often under stress, and his capacity for self-regulation was limited. My approach with him in DMT sessions was first to establish a trusting therapeutic alliance through attuned reflective relational experiences, where his nervous system could become regulated and he could internalize healthier coping strategies for expressing his underlying feelings, especially during times of heightened affect. Through this approach, Joey could begin to rechoreograph his coping strategies when under stress by internalizing a sense of embodied security.

In the beginning of our work together, Joey would often project his own insecurities onto me, both verbally (e.g., "You never do anything right") and nonverbally (e.g., when I would attempt to mirror his movements, he would reject these connections by moving away or placing an object between us to create more spatial distance). At the same time, he appeared to crave connection with me as his therapist. His mother reported that he would become anxious if they might be late to a session, and would request phone sessions if his mother could not bring him to therapy. Through the use of a connection tool, he began to use his sessions to explore his ambivalent feelings more deeply. The active and metaphorical processes of DMT allowed a secure attachment relationship to form, develop, and serve as a reparative experience.

Fairly early in the treatment process, Joey became invested in engaging me in a ritual game through the use of a soft foam ball. Rather than using the ball to connect directly with me, he would actively throw the ball against the wall and explore various ways to make it difficult for me to catch it. This initial stage of relating allowed me to see metaphorically how strong his defenses were in direct attuned-movement relationships. Instead of trying to change this spatial position of relating, I joined with him, moving in parallel, and narrated out loud verbally the challenges that he set forth for me. I attuned to his movement dynamics by matching his intensity with sound. He would not tolerate any direct movement mirroring or matching, but he did allow me to reflect his movements through the tone of my voice. Slowly, he also began to experiment with moving at varied intensity levels, and would attend carefully to how I would adjust my sound so that he could match and attune to the change in intensity. If I didn't "do it right," he would tell me. He was clearly telling me through his movement presentations that he wanted a relationship with me, but that it needed to developed at his own pace and in his own way. Furthermore, it was important that I tell him both verbally and nonverbally, through my own interactions, that I could accept all intensities of him, regardless of his ambivalence. This was the start of our relational dance.

As our sessions continued, I assisted Joey in movement involving different spatial relationships with me (i.e., beside each other, back to back, and eventually facing each other directly). We also engaged in dance explorations through imagery, where we would move at varied intensity levels and work on the acceleration and deceleration of these intensities (i.e., moving in "slow motion"; having an "instant replay" and starting again; speeding up to "hyper speed"; and finding a "relaxed place, like being on a desert island and just chilling"). At times, Joey would take charge of the speed and intensity at which we would move, but slowly he allowed me to have some ideas, and invited cues to help his body adjust to a different intensity. At other times, we engaged in a sort of "freeze dance," where we took turns being in charge of creating the music to make one person move and the other person freeze into a creative shape. Joey took joy in experimenting with different ways to keep his body in control even in a still position. His increasing capacity to share the leadership with me indicated increasing trust that I would follow his pace, and that I could be with him in all his affective states. In addition, his movements, regardless of their intensity, were accepted and attuned to. He began to take more and more risks with his body, while taking pride that he could stay in control when required to on a given cue. He was beginning to feel less ambivalent in the therapeutic relationship.

On one particular day, during the middle phase of treatment, Joey came into session very angry, but was not verbalizing any feelings. His body appeared tense, and his posture was enclosed. He was emotionally shut down and unresponsive to my attempts to engage him in verbal dialogue, yet I had a strong sense that he was craving some connection with me. It was clear that he needed to discharge and release his feelings; therefore, I engaged him solely through the body. I invited him to be the leader in a dance and to move his body as it needed to move. My intention was to observe closely to see whether he wanted me either to move with him or to watch him. To my surprise, he quickly started his dance. His movements were strong and direct, with high intensity. His body was showing his emotional state, but his rejections of my joining with him were heightened. I attempted several ways to find a way in to attune to him (verbally, nonverbally, and through sound), but most of these attempts were rejected. He continued to intensify his dance, but became emotionally dysregulated and began to become physically destructive in the therapy room (throwing objects, tearing things from the walls). It appeared as if what he needed to do at that moment in our attachment relationship was to actively test the boundaries of our secure relationship. I reflected back to him the safety guidelines of the therapy room, but also that I could see that he was "needing to make a mess." He watched me intensely as this occurred as if to see whether I could accept and contain the strong affective experience that he was holding. In this moment, I felt that he needed me to see physically how "messy" he felt inside. As I inquired about this physical representation of his emotional feeling, I watched his body relax, as if he felt me understanding him in a new way. He was able to leave the "mess" in the therapy room for me to "hold." In the following weeks, this was somewhat of a ritual ending for each session where he would decide how to "leave a mess," but slowly we began to collaborate during the closure. He would watch me assist him in cleaning up parts of the "mess," and he would care for other parts. Week after week, he left the therapy room in less of a "mess." It appeared as if he started to internalize that all intensities of his feelings (all of his "messiness") could be accepted, and that there was a container to express it. Most importantly, the rechoreography of his patterns of expression (aggression and outbursts) was starting to become embodied, and he was starting to develop emotional regulation.

After several more months, Joey was able to put feeling words to his emotion dances and make some insightful connections about his family situation and his underlying feelings. He appeared to have internalized the therapeutic alliance as a secure relationship that could hold all parts of him.

During our final session, Joey was drawn to a small, smooth, grayish stone that was in a bowl in the dance/movement therapy room. He picked up the stone and began to tap it on a table, in a clear rhythm. In order to attune to him, I picked up another stone and joined with his rhythm, engaging with him in a little "stone dance." At one point during this synchronistic nonverbal exchange, Joey's stone broke open, revealing the stone's "insides." Ironically, the inside of this stone was crystal-like. In awe and amazement, Joey examined the insides with intrigue. It was a perfect symbolic reflection of his own therapeutic process that I chose to reflect directly to him, "Isn't it amazing that on the outside it appeared so gray, dull, and ugly, but now that we can see the inside it has revealed all of its beauty?"

Discussion

Over the course of therapy, as I used Joey's movements to attune with his body state, a co-created, improvised dance of relationship emerged through the nonverbal exchanges in the movement process. This dance assisted Joey in modulating his own impulses and empowered him to activate his own regulatory capacities. As I engaged Joey in an attuned-movement communicative dialogue, our formerly insecure relationship developed into a dance of listening and reflecting back, allowing Joey to take full mastery over his own movement impulses. I would constantly look at my own countertransference, and would attune to him and to myself simultaneously. I focused on being mindful of Joey's pace and readiness to make connections between his movement presentations that were occurring through our relationship and his own underlying struggles. I could not say, "You're so angry because your father is inconsistently in your life, and hence you are creating messes." He was not ready—he did not have the internal working models, so to speak—to be able to internalize this. Over time, however, through the consistency, trust, and nonverbal attunement we developed, he was able to take in more and more and allow an attachment relationship to feel nourishing. The expansion of his movement vocabulary through his experiments with movement modulation assisted him in being able to translate this into affect regulation. His outbursts decreased. He was able to be more verbal about his feeling states, rather than holding them in until he exploded. He used healthier outlets to channel his underlying feelings and used his body as a resource to discharge and release tension.

The quality of the therapeutic relationship with Joey focused first on the need for me as the therapist to provide a consistent and uninterrupted psychological containment for the affective experiences that he could not verbally express. After this secure base was established and internalized, it allowed Joey to express the intensity of the affective experiences that he was holding inside. These were reflected in his movement presentations. His readiness to allow for regulation and connection with me as a secure base became evident when he began to explore a different spatial relationship with me: He was now moving with, facing, and in collaboration with me. This also informed me that he was tolerating the stronger affect that was being stimulated by his family situation, and that he felt he had an adequate emotional container to discharge and process these feelings.

Conclusion

As discussed in this chapter, the embodied experiences of individuals are essential to examining attachment behavior. Specifically, because movement is communication, it can provide information about a client's emotional state. In the context of the DMT relationship between client and therapist, intervention takes place in a relational and moving context that opens opportunities for attunement and reparative attachment relationships to happen.

The therapeutic process requires careful pacing, adequate holding, and accurate mirrored reflection within a trusting therapeutic relationship in order to allow for repair of ruptured attachment relationships. Once consistent and secure attachment is reexperienced within the therapeutic alliance and internalized, it can become a blueprint for new behaviors. Therefore, the new internalized relational dance can serve as a rechoreography of past attachment relationships, and the client can be influenced by the newly developing relationship with the therapist.

Repeated experiences of attuned and empathically reflected movement through the therapeutic movement relationship during the DMT sessions can provide a reparative secure base to assist clients in developing healthier attachment relationships with others. According to Siegel (2012),

> When attuned communication is disrupted, as it inevitably is, repair of the rupture can be an important part of reestablishing the connection. Repair is healing as well as important in helping to teach the child that life is filled with inevitable moments of misunderstandings and missed connections that can be identified and connection created again. (p. 51)

Therapeutic approaches such as DMT that work directly with the body provide new avenues for assisting clients with attachment needs through simultaneous physical and metaphorical processes. Dance/movement therapists have a unique capacity to approach and rechoreograph these clients' interactive struggles into healthier attachment relationships.

REFERENCES

Ainsworth, M. D. S., & Bell, S. M. (1970). Attachment, exploration, and separation: Individual differences in strange-situation behavior of one-year-olds. *Child Development, 41,* 49–67.

Ainsworth, M. D. S., Blehar, M. C., Waters, E., & Wall, S. (1978). *Patterns of attachment.* Hillsdale, NJ: Erlbaum.

Baudino, L. (2010). Autism spectrum disorder: A case of misdiagnosis. *American Journal of Dance Therapy, 32,* 113–129.

Beebe, B., & Lachmann, F. M. (1998). Co-constructing inner and relational processes. Self and mutual regulation in infant research and adult treatment. *Psychoanalytic Psychology, 15*(4), 480–516.

Behrends, A., Müller, S., & Dziobek, I. (2012). Moving in and out of synchrony: A concept for a new intervention fostering empathy through interactional movement and dance. *The Arts in Psychotherapy, 39*(2), 107–116.

Berrol, C. F. (2006). Neuroscience meets dance/movement therapy: Mirror neurons, the therapeutic process and empathy. *The Arts in Psychotherapy, 33*(4), 302–315.

Betty, A. (2013). Taming tidal waves: A dance/movement therapy approach to supporting emotion regulation in maltreated children. *American Journal of Dance Therapy, 35*(1), 39–59.

Bowlby, J. (1969). *Attachment and loss: Vol. 1. Attachment.* New York: Basic Books.

Bowlby, J. (1988). *A secure base: Parent–child attachment and healthy human development.* New York: Basic Books.

Brazelton, T. B. (1982). Joint regulation of neonate–parent behavior. In E. Tronick (Ed.), *Social interchanges in infancy: Effect, cognition, and communication* (pp. 7–22). Baltimore, MD: University Park Press.

Chaiklin, S., & Schmais, C. (1993). The Chace approach to dance therapy. In S. Sandel, S. Chaiklin, & A. Lohn (Eds.), *Foundations of dance/movement therapy: The life and work of Marian Chace* (pp. 75–97). Columbia, MD: Marian Chace Memorial Fund of the American Dance Therapy Association.

Devereaux, C. (2008). Untying the knots: Dance/movement therapy with a family exposed to domestic violence. *American Journal of Dance Therapy, 30*(2), 58–70.

Devereaux, C. (2012). Moving into relationship: Dance/movement therapy with children with autism. In L. Gallo-Lopez & L. Rubin (Eds.), *Play-based interventions for children and adolescents with autism spectrum disorders* (pp. 333–351). New York: Routledge.

Erfer, T. (1995). Treating children with autism in a public school system. In F. Levy (Ed.), *Dance and other expressive arts therapies* (pp. 191–211). New York: Routledge.

Erskine, R. (1998). Attunement and involvement: Therapeutic responses to relational needs. *International Journal of Psychotherapy, 3*(3), 235–244.

Fischer, J., & Chaiklin, S. (1993). Meeting in movement: The work of therapist and client. In S. Sandel, S. Chaiklin, & A. Lohn (Eds.), *Foundations of dance/movement therapy: The life and work of Marian Chace* (pp. 136–153). Columbia, MD: Marian Chace Memorial Fund of the American Dance Therapy Association.

Fischman, D. (2009). Therapeutic relationships and kinesthetic empathy. In S. Chaiklin & H. Wengrower (Eds.), *The art and science of dance/movement therapy* (pp. 33–53). New York: Routledge.

Fuertes, M., Lopes-dos-Santos, P., Beeghly, M., & Tronick, E. (2009). Infant coping and maternal interactive behavior predict attachment in a Portuguese sample of healthy preterm infants. *European Psychologist, 14*(4), 320–331.

Ginot, E. (2012). Self-narratives and dysregulated affective states: The neuropsychological links between self-narratives, attachment, affect, and cognition. *Psychoanalytic Psychology, 29*(1), 59–80.

Hervey, L., & Kornblum, R. (2006). An evaluation of Kornblum's body-based violence prevention curriculum for children. *The Arts in Psychotherapy, 33,* 113–129.

Kestenberg Amighi, J., Loman, S., Lewis, P., & Sossin, K. (1999). *The meaning of movement.* New York: Brunner-Routledge.

Kornblum, R. (2002). *Disarming the playground: Violence prevention through movement and pro-social skills training manual and activity book.* Oklahoma City, OK: Wood'N'Barnes.

Kornblum, R. (2008). Dance/movement therapy with children. In D. McCarthy (Ed.), *Speaking about the unspeakable: Non-verbal methods and experiences in therapy with children* (pp. 100–114). Philadelphia: Kingsley.

Koshland, L., & Wittaker, J. W. B. (2004). PEACE through dance/movement: Evaluating a violence prevention program. *American Journal of Dance Therapy, 26*(2), 69–90.

Kossak, M. S. (2009). Therapeutic attunement: A transpersonal view of expressive arts therapy. *The Arts in Psychotherapy, 36,* 13–18.

Levy, F. (2005). *Dance movement therapy: A healing art.* Reston, VA: American Alliance for Health, Physical Education, Recreation, and Dance.

Loman, S. (1998). Employing a developmental model of movement patterns in dance/movement therapy with young children and their families. *American Journal of Dance Therapy, 20*(2), 101–115.

Merna, M. (2010). *Compiling the evidence for dance/movement therapy with children with autism spectrum disorders: A systematic literature review.* Unpublished master's thesis, Drexel University.

Moore, C. (2006). Dance/movement therapy in the light of trauma: Research findings of a multidisciplinary project. In S. C. Koch & I. Bräuninger (Eds.), *Advances in dance/movement therapy: Theoretical perspectives and empirical findings* (pp. 104–115). Berlin: Logos Verlag.

Schore, A. N. (2001). Effects of a secure attachment relationship on right brain development, affect regulation, and infant mental health. *Infant Mental Health Journal, 22,* 7–66.

Schore, A. N. (2003). *Affect regulation and the repair of the self.* New York: Norton.

Schore, J. R., & Schore, A. N. (2008). Modern attachment theory: The central role of affect regulation in development and treatment. *Clinical Social Work Journal, 36,* 9–20.

Siegel, D. (2012). *The developing mind: How relationships and the brain interact to shape who we are* (2nd ed.). New York: Guilford Press.

Stern, D. (1985). *The interpersonal world of the infant.* New York: Basic Books.

Subramaniam, A. (2010). *Moving towards a secure base: The role of attachment theory in clinical dance movement therapy.* Unpublished master's thesis, Lesley University.

Thom, L. (2010). From a simple line to expressive movement: The use of creative movement to enhance social emotional development in preschool curriculum. *American Journal of Dance Therapy, 32*(2), 100–112.

Tortora, S. (2006). *The dancing dialogue.* Baltimore, MD: Brookes.

Tronick, E. (1980). On the primacy of social skills. In D. B. Sawin, L. O. Walker, & J. H. Penticuff (Eds.), *The exceptional infant: Psychosocial risks in infant environmental transactions* (pp. 144–158). New York: Brunner/Mazel.

Tronick, E. (2003). Things still to be done on the still-face effect. *Infancy, 4*(4), 475–482.

Tronick, E. (2007). *The neurobehavioral and social-emotional development of infants and children.* New York: Norton.

Tronick, E., & Beeghly, M. (2011). Infants' meaning-making and the development of mental health problems. *American Psychologist, 66*(2), 107–119.

van der Kolk, B. (2006). Clinical implications of neuroscience and PTSD. *Annals of the New York Academy of Sciences, 1071*(1), 277–293.

CHAPTER 7

The Integration of Drama Therapy and Play Therapy in Attachment Work with Traumatized Children

Eliana Gil
Teresa Dias

This chapter focuses on the application of drama and play therapies to advance therapeutic goals involving attachment issues in traumatized children. In particular, this chapter addresses work with children who have suffered complex interpersonal trauma during early development, and whose social, physical, emotional, and psychological functioning may have become disturbed or compromised. Contemporary wisdom about the treatment of childhood trauma is ample (D'Andrea, Ford, Stolbach, Spinazzola, & van der Kolk, 2012; Osofsky, 2011; Shaw, 2010) and provides a blueprint for clinical interventions for attachment issues associated with such trauma. Specifically, we (1) present a brief overview of the interface between drama and play therapies; (2) discuss the relevance of doing attachment work with traumatized children; and (3) describe drama and play therapy approaches that indirectly or directly address attachment issues with such children.

Drama Therapy and Play Therapy

Play therapy theories, techniques, and approaches are varied and unique (O'Connor & Braverman, 1997, 2009) and have shown to be effective in helping resolve a variety of psychosocial difficulties (Bratton, Ray, & Rhyne, 2005). Drama therapy likewise has diverse methodology, particularly in its clinical applications and clinical impact (Jones, 2010; Weber

& Haen, 2005). Drama therapy utilizes various aspects of dramatic performance and physical movements in order to encourage affective expression and its therapeutic benefits. Drama therapy and its companion discipline, psychodrama, emphasize spontaneity, creative expression, and affect enhancement. In general, drama therapists may begin as "theater people" with theatrical training and then receive specialized drama therapy and psychotherapy training. Psychodramatists tend to be psychotherapists first, who then train intensely in J. L. Moreno's psychodramatic method. Moreno (1934) defined *psychodrama* as "the science which explores the 'truth' by dramatic methods. It deals with interpersonal relations and private worlds" (p. 13).

Jones (1996) describes core processes of drama therapy similar to Schaefer's (1993, 1994) curative factors. These include dramatic projection; drama therapeutic empathy and distancing; role playing and personification; interactive audience and witnessing; embodiment (dramatizing the body); playing; life–drama connection; and transformation. Drama therapy has the potential to access constricted energy and cause release, to oxygenate the body, and to allow for self-initiated personal momentum to lead the way into discovery of internal concerns. As Jones (1996) states, "play enables the client in drama therapy to create within the session a playful relationship with reality" (p. 93). As suggested by Irwin (1983), there are developmental levels of play. Similarly, Jones (1996) conceptualizes a continuum, which includes the following key aspects: "sensory motor play, imitative play, pretend play, dramatic play, and drama" (p. 177).

It is difficult to take the play out of drama therapy or the dramatic component out of play therapy. Thus the merging of play and drama therapies is a natural and easy partnership, one that equips practitioners with a much richer repertoire for work with attachment and trauma. Drama and play therapies have several factors in common—specifically, playing, dramatic projection and distancing, and empathy building. In addition, many children naturally use embodiment as they "try on" and "act out" characters as they role-play and pretend, using their creative imaginations. Both play and drama therapies encourage expression through varied holistic activities that elicit physical, emotional, sensory, spiritual, and cognitive engagement, thereby evoking introspection, reflection, and change. In brief, play and drama therapy are *whole-brain activities*, which, according to Siegel and Bryson (2011),

> help our children become better integrated so they can use their whole brain in a coordinated way. For example, we want them to be horizontally integrated, so that their left-brain logic can work well with their right-brain emotion. We also want them to be vertically integrated, so that the physically higher parts of their brain, which let them thoughtfully consider their actions, work well with the lower parts, which are more concerned with instinct, gut reactions, and survival. (p. 7)

When utilizing therapeutic play in an environment of specially selected therapeutic toys, children make internal associations, project thoughts and perceptions, and attribute and delegate affective specificity to their toys and their stories. These projected externalizations, embedded with personal meaning, are kept at a safe enough distance for children to view them from afar, in order to permit gradual approaches to feared thoughts or emotions. In cognitive-behavioral terminology, children organically use their own projections to achieve *gradual exposure*—a way to desensitize themselves to or inoculate themselves against specific, intolerable sensations, cognitions, or feelings (Cohen, Mannarino, & Deblinger, 2006).

Children, Complex Trauma, and Attachment

The term *complex trauma* suggests a layering of difficulty that can have a major impact on general functioning, especially with more vulnerable populations such as children. Complex psychological trauma is defined by Courtois and Ford (2009) as "including traumatic stressors that (1) are repetitive or prolonged; (2) involve direct harm and/or neglect and abandonment by caregivers or ostensibly responsible adults; (3) occur at developmentally vulnerable times in the victim's life, such as early childhood; and (4) have great potential to compromise severely a child's development" (p. 1). The most significant aspect of complex trauma is that it is often caused by those who are most important in children's lives and who are supposed to meet their early needs for nurturing and survival. Probably the most insidious lesson of abuse is that "people who love you hurt you," and this early association can have a negative impact on a child's view of the world from that point forward. As Herman (2009) notes, the trauma is occurring within a *relational matrix* in which "the strong do as they please, the weak submit, caretakers seem willfully blind, and there is no one to turn to for protection" (p. xiv). She goes on to state that children may then develop self-loathing, as well as pervasive distrust of the abusive caregivers and others. In fact, abused children have myriad responses, including fierce loyalty to their abusive caregivers, anxious or insecure attachments to them, or fear or avoidance of them. But most importantly, since their primary caregiving relationships serve as their templates for future relationships and expectations (internal working models), complex trauma has huge implications for children's relational experiences with others. In addition, when abuse continues uninterrupted, children will develop more refined coping mechanisms and defenses that can keep them emotionally shut down, disconnected from others, and unable to negotiate their important needs.

Cook et al. (2005) describe six core components of treatment for complex trauma: safety, self-regulation, self-reflective information processing, integration of traumatic experiences, relational engagement, and enhancement of positive affect. Although these consensus-based areas provide a uniform direction to help children (and their families) recover from early trauma, clinical approaches by definition must remain relationally based, developmentally sensitive, evocative, trauma-informed, "brain-based," and engaging.

There has been consistent advocacy in the last decade for incorporating evidence-based practices into all clinical settings; this trend challenges clinicians to remain attentive to research studies that provide effective treatment outcomes. In the forefront of evidence-based treatment models for working with traumatized children is trauma-focused cognitive-behavioral therapy (TF-CBT). TF-CBT provides a structured and well-articulated model that emphasizes critical areas of care and provides guidance about the treatment trajectory with abused children and their families. Recently, TF-CBT's developers have emphasized the potential use of play activities to advance trauma-focused goals in ways that might engage younger children and their families in fuller participation (Cohen, Mannarino, & Deblinger, 2012). There are several other evidence-based models for working with childhood trauma (domestic violence, physical abuse) that include play-based interventions based on psychoanalytic principles of play therapy (see, e.g., van Horn & Lieberman, 2009, and Eyberg, 1988). Other evidence-based practices in working with children and families are emerging (Ford & Cloitre, 2009).

This past decade has also been one of innovation, technological advances, and great excitement as the field of neuroscience has gained great relevance in clinical work. Several threads of valuable and critical neuroscientific data now provide support for the theoretical foundation that has been laid since the 1970s. Leaders in the field of neuroscience have repeatedly noted the impact of trauma on the development of children's brains, pointed to the plasticity of the brain, and emphasized the fact that the brain repairs itself best in the context of relational health (Ludy-Dobson & Perry, 2010; Siegel, 2012).

Treatment of Complex Trauma in Children

When children enter treatment as a result of complex trauma, several key issues need immediate attention, particularly the pivotal concern of establishing safety and trust. Because children have by definition been hurt in the context of trusted relationships, their attachments to primary caregivers have been severely compromised, disrupted, or damaged. This happens when the predictable, repetitive patterns of caregiving and responding to children's basic needs are not consistently provided. Such children are never fully soothed, may associate caregiving with disappointment or anxiety, and have difficulty in developing self-regulation. When children cannot trust that their needs will be met, they develop anxiety and mistrust, and attempt to adjust their needs in a variety of ways. Children may learn to avoid eye contact; they may even learn to cry weakly or stay quiet; or they may exhibit a range of symptoms associated with stress, such as an acute or delayed startle response. Given an impaired caregiver–child attachment system, a child remains vulnerable and may develop anxious, avoidant, or disorganized interactions with caregivers.

In a therapy context, when therapists make themselves available for personal interactions, the therapist–child relationship can provoke anxiety; children may manifest that anxiety by exhibiting either overly compliant (fear-based) behaviors, or emotional or behavioral dysregulation (nervousness and hyperactivity). Moreover, children may become anxious when asked to "talk" to therapists about traumatic events. Decreasing and managing young clients' anxiety, and establishing a safe therapeutic environment, are therefore critical to meaningful progress.

A beginning therapeutic goal is to attend to child clients in a conscientious and reflective way, which will give these children the experience of collaborative communication. Alert observation can be learned and practiced in individual or group therapy settings through various drama and play therapy activities.

A Selection of Integrative Drama and Play Therapy Exercises

As noted earlier, the integration of drama and play therapy is one of the most natural, refreshing, and logical mergers that can occur. Play therapy already includes an appreciation for children's natural physicality; their mimicking through pretend play; their exaggerated emotional expression at times; and their availability for and engagement with fantasy, creative imagination, and enactments through story and play. Applying principles of drama therapy is good common sense and is inherently a good fit: Pretend play often spontaneously occurs within drama therapy. The following sections illustrate how specific treatment goals in work with traumatized children can capitalize on the blending of play and drama interventions. These individual and group exercises have two central therapeutic elements: focused attention and mirroring, which are the primary ways children learn and explore their worlds in the early years.

Individual Exercises

Synchronized Water Breaths

Synchronized water breaths are slow full-body breaths done side by side or face to face; the therapist can move from a side-to-side position to a face-to-face position over several sessions as the client's comfort grows. On the in-breath, arms go out to sides and then scoop down to ground (as if scooping water) and lifting over the head. During the out-breath, the overhead hands flow back down to the body and cross in front. Together, the therapist and child bring a subsequent breath in and bring arms out to sides again (the synchronization is more important than the choreography of arms).

This activity provides a co-regulating metaphor in which a therapist and a child client work in tandem, while at the same time the child is encouraged to oxygenate the body, is helped to decrease his or her anxiety, and is taught the breathing skills so necessary to self-regulation. This exercise can be even more engaging when child and therapist choose animal masks to wear; the mask provides the child with a buffer against feeling too exposed. Also, the movement itself suggests picking up water and gently allowing it to spill and wash over the body. The therapist can use a variation on the idea of "picking up water" and collaborate with the client at the beginning or end of a session to intentionally "pick up" a feeling, color, or attribute, and allow this to wash over the pair. For example, anxious children may benefit from scooping and pouring a feeling of "calm" over themselves, or the "love" of a favorite person. This exercise can become an opening or ending ritual that establishes predictability and delineates boundaries in the session.

Mirroring

As an exercise, mirroring has its roots in theater and is used in training actors to hone observation skills and character development (Boal, 1992; Spolin, 1986). It must be kept in mind that clients can experience face-to-face activities as intimate and intense, so in order to respect initial boundaries, clinicians are encouraged to use peripheral mirroring to establish therapeutic trust gradually. Recent research in neurobiology (e.g., Iacoboni, 2008) shows that mirror neurons may be critical neural elements in the evolution of language.

The classic, face-to-face mirroring exercise (Boal, 1992; Spolin, 1986) has value for building attunement, trust, and shared leadership. Therapists who are face to face with child clients without touching them can begin to move their bodies slowly, making faces and moving their arms while maintaining loose eye contact. Therapists encourage clients to follow their movements exactly, and then give the children the opportunity to lead while the therapists copy the clients' movements. As children engage in this exercise, they learn to regulate their physical and emotional states, and they have the opportunity to develop attunement by sharing resonating neurons in which physical states are mirrored and emotional states are conveyed.

"Healer" or "Wise Person"

Another drama therapy exercise can follow mirroring and is particularly useful in introspection and exploring inner strengths and self-empathy. In this exercise, the therapist facilitates the creation of a real or imagined character by asking the client to think of a "healer," or a "wise person," or "a person who knows a lot," or "a person who knows a lot about helping others." The child imagines a person with full detail, standing in front of the child or sitting in an empty chair. The child is encouraged to look over the imagined character from head to toe, noticing everything about how he or she looks, smells, and seems. Once the image is clear, the client can sit in the chair or stand in the place of the wise person (the moment of changing places or sitting in the empty chair is an important point, because the client literally and figuratively steps into the role of the other). The therapist suggests that the client take a minute to become the character, asking questions like "How does the wise person stand?" Once it is clear that the client is ready, the therapist interviews the "wise one." The following vignette illustrates the use of this exercise.

Case Vignette: Carla

Carla was 16 years old and had disclosed her brother's sexual abuse of her when she was 10 or so. For whatever reasons, this disclosure was met with minimization by her parents, and even a school guidance counselor had questioned whether she had imagined the abuse. Her mother's response, in particular, had made her skeptical about therapy in general and whether anyone would really believe her or be capable of helping her. The abuse had apparently continued for a while, until she was able to ask for and get a lock on her bedroom door; her brother also became more socially active and started spending much of his time away from home. Carla felt lonely in her home and spent most of her time in her room. She became depressed in her junior year of high school; she had been unable to make close friends, stating that she felt different from others her age. In the last few months prior to the referral, Carla's grades had also begun to plummet, partly due to her lack of motivation and disinterest in her current classes, teachers, and homework. Her parents opted to bring her to therapy at the point when her grades became a problem to them, and Carla was somewhat reluctant to invest much of herself in therapy.

Carla and I (Eliana Gil) had just moved into the end of the initial phase of treatment, and therapeutic trust had been established. Carla was now feeling happy to come see me and prioritized her appointment time, often insisting that her parents bring her even when their schedule was problematic. We had developed a fairly good therapy relationship, and I had worked hard to be viewed as trustworthy. I had told her that if I had seen her when she was 10, the whole family would have been asked to come to therapy, and everyone would have had to acknowledge how painful and confusing her brother's alleged abuse had been to her. She smiled when I told her that he would have been court-ordered into therapy right away, because what he was doing was not "normal"; in fact, it was abusive. (I had stated precisely the same to the parents when they came in to see me.)

Carla was hesitant to talk about the abuse or her brother, although she was agreeable to doing some focused work on what had happened, since it often "haunted her" and "came into her mind." I had assessed that she was having intrusive flashbacks, which are not unusual for individuals with unresolved complex trauma. I opted to use the "wise person" technique to begin to connect Carla with the part of herself that had been wise enough to report what she knew to be wrong, and wise enough to know that her parents had not done all they could to help her at that time. In addition, I thought it important to strengthen her coping strategies and inner resources prior to doing more specific trauma work. Without assigning blame, we proceeded with the "wise person" interview. Carla had established her receptivity to symbol work, metaphorical language, guided imagery, and role playing by using miniatures in our early sessions, so she easily went into the role of "wise person."

THERAPIST: What is your name?

CARLA: (*as the wise person*) Clementine.

THERAPIST: How do you feel about your name, Clementine?

CARLA: (*as Clementine*) It suits me perfectly.

THERAPIST: How so?

CARLA: (*continuing as Clementine*) I am small, I am sweet, and people are surprised at what a good fruit I am, even when they are looking for an orange and picked me by mistake.

THERAPIST: How old are you?

CARLA: I am without an age. I can look different ways, but where I live, there are no young or old—only beings who float in time.

THERAPIST: What are you wearing?

CARLA: Just robes, lavender robes, that don't pull or push anywhere. They just float with me as I go.

THERAPIST: How do you know Carla?

CARLA: Oh, I've been knowing her since she was about 5 years old.

THERAPIST: Five years old! You've known her 11 years. That's a long time!

CARLA: Yes, indeed, she and I are old friends—old souls, I mean, connected and bonded and very close.

THERAPIST: What can you tell me about your friend as a little girl?

CARLA: She was wise beyond her years, quiet, spent a lot of time in her room. She is very kind, kind-hearted, and spirited, like a wild horse galloping through a leafy forest.

THERAPIST: Kind and spirited. I see. How else would you describe her as a little girl?

CARLA: Loving, very loving—looking to be loved, really. She was always wanting hugs and kisses, but her parents were always busy, and her dad traveled a lot.

THERAPIST: So she wanted hugs and kisses, like most little girls do, but her parents seemed busy a lot of the time. So what did she do?

CARLA: Well, that's when she first started talking to me. She loved her brother a lot and he was only a few years older, and they spent a lot of time alone together. But he started hugging her too tight, and she didn't like it and told him so. But he just kept pushing and started doing other stuff she didn't like.

THERAPIST: So she turned to you for advice with this problem? What a smart girl to turn to you for help!

CARLA: Yes, she could see that this was not OK, that her brother seemed mean and angry some of the time, and that he wasn't being nice to her. So I asked her to tell her mother what was going on.

THERAPIST: Oh, so you were wise enough to give this important advice?

CARLA: Yes, and she listened right away, and tried two or three times to tell her mother.

THERAPIST: This is a very hard thing to do, to keep trying when her mother was not able to hear.

CARLA: Yes, but she managed it because she has a lot of "stick-to-it-veness"!

THERAPIST: And it sounds like she got support from you the whole way, even when her mother and father thought she was making a mountain out of a molehill.

CARLA: She knew she was right. She was there. She could see that something was wrong with her brother, especially when he kept trying to do more and more bad things to her.

THERAPIST: She was lucky to have you when it sounds like she was feeling very alone.

CARLA: Oh, yes, she was very alone, and that's when she started feeling that no one understood her—except for myself, of course. We had many, many long conversations, and she understood that parents sometimes do the best they can with difficult situations. She even thought, when she got a little older, that her parents were worried about him and wanted to hope and pray that she was exaggerating so that they wouldn't need to worry so much.

THERAPIST: Wow, she really is very kind . . . she tried hard to understand why her parents would want to think of this as normal. She surely was kind to them, but I wonder, wise one, how you felt about her being so lonely and not having anyone in her family believe her.

CARLA: She is truly amazing. She found a way to keep herself safe, and she kept telling other people outside the home, which I also thought was the right thing to do.

THERAPIST: How do you think she got through all this on her own and with your help?

CARLA: She is a very special, kind, and strong girl. She has lost her way a little now, but she knows deep down that what doesn't kill you makes you stronger.

THERAPIST: So she has gotten "strong at the broken places?"

CARLA: Yeah, that's right. She's tougher than she looks, and as I said, she's forgotten a little about all she went through to come out on the other side, but I think she'll remember a little. I know that I do.

THERAPIST: So what would you most like her to know from you today?

CARLA: I'd tell her, "Carla, you've been through rough times. You've had good times too. You need to find your compass again, like I've seen you put in the sandtray pictures over and over. You can do it. There are lots of important paths for you in the future."

THERAPIST: What's the one thing you think would help her the most right now?

CARLA: To know that her mother still loves her and doesn't blame her for what happened.

THERAPIST: That sounds like an important thing for her to know. All kids like to know that their parents love them and don't blame them. And, by the way, what is it that she thinks she's blamed for?

CARLA: She thinks they blame her for her brother's drinking problem and his getting into trouble after she told.

THERAPIST: Oh, I think it might be important to check that out with her parents and find out what they think instead of guessing.

CARLA: (*as Clementine*) That might be good. (*as herself*) I think I want to stop now.

THERAPIST: OK, wise one, just one last question: What surprises or delights you most about Carla?

CARLA: (*as Clementine again*) That she remains kind and expects the best from others.

THERAPIST: That sounds great. How did you get to be so wise?

> CARLA: I talk to a lot of kids who need my help. I listen to them and learn from them too.
>
> THERAPIST: Sounds great. OK, I'd like for you to begin to imagine your friend Carla and begin to step back into her shoes, so that Carla can come back into the room.

When Carla was reoriented to time and place, we debriefed a little by talking about the experience of her wise person and what she had learned from her today. She told me that she had not "seen her" in a long time and had forgotten how calm she felt when she talked with her. I told Carla that I was impressed by how much the two of them had in common. "I know," she said quietly. Subsequent sessions were guided by some of what had been disclosed in this conversation and included family therapy sessions.

This dramatic role play was quite revealing, showing when Carla's attachment disruption began. It was clear that at the age of 5, she had turned to her mother and father, who were unable or unwilling to hear her disclosure. In an effort to protect themselves from the truth, they minimized what Carla said, and turned away from her obvious need to be heard and believed. They did not do this maliciously; they were simply unequipped to know how to be of help to their daughter. But in turning away from Carla's disclosure and spoken need for protection, the mother in particular had also turned away from her emotional connection to her daughter, and from that point on functioned to avoid what was before her. Carla became a reminder of what the mother considered her failure, and this perception led to years of loneliness for them both. Now, 11 years later, it was not only relevant but crucial to bring them together to attempt an attachment reparation, a foundation that was necessary if more growth was possible for them in the future.

So I gingerly approached Carla about having joint family sessions with her parents, in an attempt to have them respond more appropriately to her initial disclosure. Although Carla thought it was too late (and not necessary) to have these sessions, we consulted with the wise one, Clementine, who agreed it was worth making the effort. We talked to Clementine often, and in so doing allowed Carla to tap into her own impressive internal resources and access the wisdom or advice she already possessed. Wisdom and knowing are elusive for many young clients. Many have suffered physical or emotional blows, and their positive identity formation has been compromised. This exercise can be changed to create someone who is a fan, cheerleader, or champion of a child and thinks positively of him or her. It may be the family dog, a teacher, or a favorite aunt. In using role reversal with these characters, children are able to see themselves more positively through the eyes of a trusted other. They are able to stand within the love that is available to them, and perhaps feel it more fully—embodied self-love is very powerful.

Group Exercises

Stop–Walk–Run

Groups can work toward group awareness and cohesion through Stop–Walk–Run (Zapora, 1995), which allows children to be anonymous leaders from within a group. While the group is instructed to mill around (to walk in a designated space, zigzagging in an unpredictable pattern, without touching), someone can initiate a "freeze" by simply stopping. The other children must follow the lead of any child who freezes first and must freeze until the whole group has stopped. Next, a new member initiates movement, which cues the group to resume. Without planning, the group members are invited to take the leadership role and are challenged to respond to the group as a whole. As the group has opportunities to practice moving together, members develop their ability to use peripheral vision while strengthening their sense of cohesion. Through this activity, children learn to be attuned and sensitive to each other and to behave in respectful ways. They also learn to be both leaders and followers, and can experiment with being in and out of control without fear. This exercise also builds group cohesion, because it allows children to feel a part of something larger than themselves, and is safe and mutually created.

Mirroring within a Group

Mirroring can also encourage acceptance in a group, in that it gives children the sense of being seen and accepted by others. Mirroring exercises may be expanded as groups become more cohesive. For example, as a circle group game, an embodied check-in can be mirrored back. Older kids can be given a prompt such as "How are you feeling about being in group?" or "How was your day before group?" In a circle, children take turns choosing a sound and movement to reflect their check-in—for example, a frustrated body shake accompanied by a growl if they are feeling annoyed or irritated. Then the whole group is encouraged to mirror back the check-in as a validating experience. The person who has demonstrated an embodied feeling is usually pleased to have been heard, and the group has made way for each member to be the focus of brief attention.

Emotional Statues

In a group setting, children are asked to mill around, and the therapist calls out the name of an emotion such as "Sadness." The children are asked to walk while embodying that emotion (embedding the emotion physically), and the therapist then notices and highlights the physical attributes in the children. For example, the therapist can say, "I see many heads are hung down, and shoulders are slumped," or "People are walking slowly and sighing a lot." Then on the count of 3, the therapist calls a "freeze," and children are asked to create a statue of the emotion. For some children, holding still is already addressing their issues of impulse control. Once children have created their affective statues, the therapist introduces the idea of "turning up the volume" as on a radio. With each clap, children are encouraged to exaggerate the sadness (or other emotion) into a new sculpture.

Therapists determine how much to turn the intensity up or down, depending on children's reactions to the exercise and their ability to stay in control and involved with the exercise. On a scale of 1–10, the emotional intensity can be escalated from a 3 to a 5, back down again, then up to 10, then back down to 3. As closure for this activity, children are asked to mill around again and shake off their feelings, restoring their bodies to a normal walk. The therapist can bring attention to common physical signs of emotions, such as fist clenching or holding breaths, so that children learn to associate their somatic experience and their affective states. One of the interesting outcomes to this exercise is that children begin to develop an understanding of affective scaling (i.e., the concept that their feelings can be smaller or larger) and that they have some degree of control over increasing or decreasing their emotions. (The clinical use of affective scaling has become quite popular—e.g., the Subjective Units of Distress Scale.)

Another variation of this exercise is family sculpting, popularized by Papp, Silverstein, and Carter (1973) and originated by Virginia Satir. One family member is asked to "sculpt" family members to represent his or her perceptions of family relationships—how close or distant they feel, or how they view others on an emotional level. For example, family members can be shaped into positions that manifest affect, such as crossed arms and pursed lips for anger, or open arms and smiles for welcoming. Clearly, this exercise can quickly identify attachment concerns and give family members a chance to identify them in a graphic and physical way—not only as they currently exist, but as they might be imagined or desired. Drama therapists consider sculpting a pivotal way for clients to activate their bodies and physically *try on* the positive attributes that they seek.

Big–Bigger–Biggest

Big–Bigger–Biggest is adapted from a Playback Theater exercise by Salas (1993). The therapist selects three group members to be the "actors" on stage. The other group members become audience members, and the roles are rotated throughout the group therapy session. The three actors stand side by side. A group member calls out an emotion, and each actor steps forward to show the emotion in a sculpture, with increasing intensity. After the third actor has finished, the audience claps for all three of them enthusiastically. Each actor has had a chance to express embodied emotion in a unique way; to amplify the intensity of each emotion; to watch two other group members do their renditions; to be visible to the audience; and to be acceptable to and accepted by the audience.

In drama therapy, the goal is to expand every client's repertoire of affect identification, modulation, and expression. Therefore, children participating in this exercise are challenged to try on a muted or more expressive affect in order to expand their own emotional repertoire. A "de-role" (which can be as simple as a physical brush-off) can be built into this and other more emotionally intense exercises, to allow the children to disengage from acting out troubling emotions and to attain regulatory closure. The creation of the "stage" can be as simple as asking the audience to sit in one area as the actors come onstage in another area; using this language sets the tone without fuss.

Specific Activities for Addressing Attachment Issues in Complex Trauma

There is a general consensus that childhood trauma is best addressed directly, in order to give clients the opportunity to integrate the experience in a healthy way; however, *processing* is a term that means different things to different people. As mentioned previously, Cook et al. (2005) provide guidance about specific aspects of processing trauma, including self-reflective information processing and the integration of traumatic experiences. What becomes clear is that the intended goals include some type of self-reflection, opportunities to correct cognitive distortions, affective release, and eventual restoration of personal power through controlled recall. All of these will eventually allow the person to integrate the experience as one of many—one that does not hold undue power and influence over future choices and options. Central to future choices and options are the selection and management of interpersonal relationships, which can be compromised by a lack of trust and by negative expectations of relationships as harmful rather than potentially rewarding.

It is also considered crucial to help clients create accurate trauma narratives. Memories of the trauma become less intensely felt as clients have repetitive exposure to and reevaluation of such narratives. One of the questions in work with young children is whether their narratives have to rise to the experience of full consciousness, or whether their narratives can be conducted through play, art, or other means of self-expression (Gil, 2010). This debate is likely to continue.

Drama and play therapies provide many mechanisms for reflection that can help with the goals of trauma processing (which we suggest will include reflection, improved management, and transformation of some type, as well as the capacity to regard past events with decreasing emotional intensity). Below, we describe some activities that have the potential to help accomplish goals associated with trauma processing within an increasingly trusted therapeutic relationship.

Integrating the Social Atom and the Play Genogram

J. L. Moreno, the founding father of psychodrama, originated the activity known as the *social atom* in the 1930s (Moreno, 1934). The social atom is similar to a *genogram* (McGoldrick & Gershon, 1986), in that it serves as a graphic representation of a relational map that can be drawn on paper. The major difference between a genogram and a social atom is the emphasis on the subjective world of the client. With a social atom, the client maps out connections to those people or institutions that have an impact on his or her life at the present time. Moreover, proximity and distance are used to indicate the sense of closeness or distance in each relationship. Because this activity focuses primarily on a client's subjective perceptions of important relationships, and particularly on whether these relationships are viewed as sources of emotional nurturance and support, it is relevant to the work of resolving traumas occurring in an interpersonal context.

Gil (2003) has developed a *play genogram* that uses miniatures to enliven the paper-and-pencil genogram (McGoldrick, Gerson, & Petry, 2008). We suggest these adaptations: (1) a paper-and-pencil social atom, animated with miniatures; and (2) a social atom with brightly colored circles and squares of different sizes. Both of these approaches help elicit children's fuller participation in these therapeutic strategies, and decrease their resistance to following a path of self-contemplation. Children, in particular, may find it less threatening to miniaturize or play out their concerns or problems than to discuss them verbally. These processes can eventually lead to verbal conversations that might not have been available in other ways. In addition, the act of *choosing* miniatures is a projective technique that communicates rich metaphoric information to the therapist without words. Drama therapy adaptations may include an "interview" of the characters on the social atom, conducted in the same way that the director would interview the auxiliary characters in an enacted psychodrama (Dayton, 2005).

Social Atom with Miniatures

The therapist first provides the child with a large sheet of paper with several concentric circles drawn on it, and invites the client to draw him- or herself in the center, using a circle if the client is female or a square if the client is male. Next, the client adds images (shapes or colors) of the people, institutions, and pets that are important to him or her. The child is instructed to put the people and places that play a big role in his or her life closer to the symbol in the center representing the child. The purpose is to create a relational map from the client's point of view. Once the client seems to have added the significant people and institutions, he or she can then pick a miniature to represent each shape in the social atom, placing them directly on the page at proximities representing their actual closeness or distance to the child. (See Figure 7.1 for two different examples.)

Once the miniatures are selected and placed, and depending on the child's age and propensity for verbal communication, the therapist can initiate an exploratory dialogue by signaling the child to "say as much or as little about the things you have chosen and their closeness to your circle." These conversations should be explorative, and should stay within metaphorical language unless the child shifts to first person. For example, it may be better to ask, "The owl seems to be facing in this direction. What does it see?" than "I see the object you've chosen for your mother is looking away from you." The first question is explorative, and the second is interpretive; the latter can have the effect of causing the child to feel self-conscious or self-protective. Processing any metaphorical work must be carefully approached, in order to maximize the child's engagement rather than inadvertently cause defensive responses (Gil, 2010). The social atom map can be photographed and discussed at later times; or the child can be asked to embody one of the chosen miniatures to bring it more to life; or the child can be asked to take one miniature and give it a voice (dialogues between two or more miniatures can even be elicited).

As mentioned above, a drama therapy adaptation of this activity can include an interview with some of the characters chosen. For example, the therapist can ask specific miniatures an array of questions, such as these:

"Who are you?"
"How long have you known [the client]?"
"How did you first meet [the client]?"
"What did you first notice about [the client]?"
"What one thing have you learned about [the client] that you didn't know at first?"
"What kinds of things do you and [the client] like to do together?"
"What kind of things do you say to [the client]?"
"What's the best advice you have ever given [the client]?"

The questions can be designed to gain information, but can also serve as a warm-up for dramatic play. An important element to remember is always to guide the child to end the explorations in the role of him- or herself. Even when other characters are animated, the exercise needs to be finished with the client as him- or herself.

If a child spontaneously includes, or is asked for therapeutic purposes to include, the abuser in the atom, it is not advisable to have the child role-play that particular role. In the case of a known abuser, a conversation could occur about him or her from others' point of view. This is a subtle and important difference that the therapist controls for obvious reasons.

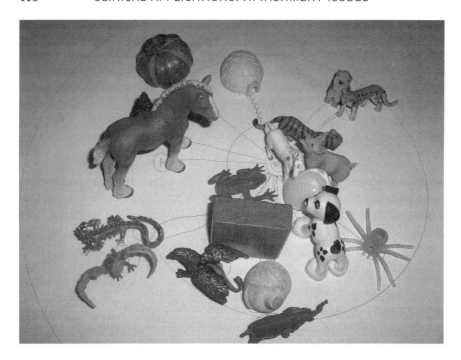

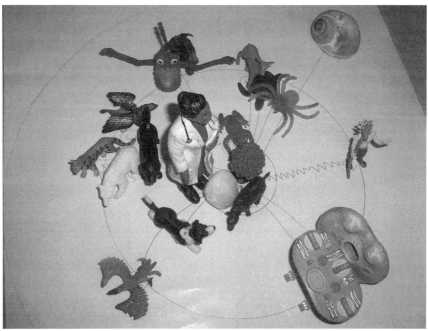

FIGURE 7.1. Two examples of a social atom with miniatures.

The social atom can also be enhanced and explored by using art materials or miniatures to represent the *types* of relationships that are drawn on the paper. For example, a child may choose to represent a rocky relationship between two characters in an atom by drawing a zigzagged line. The line may be blocked or broken in some relationships that have been discontinued. Once the line representing the connection is added, the line itself can be animated with art materials. Miniatures may provide additional information and metaphors to the relational line, such as a rock that blocks a connection or a snake that threatens a path.

Social Atom with Circles and Squares

Another adaptation of the social atom is to have a child draw a large circle on a large sheet of paper and place the sheet on the floor in an ample area. Then the child picks a circle or square to represent the self (as in the previous exercise, a circle if the child is female and a square if the child is male). The child next picks other sizes and colors of circles and squares for people in his or her life, and places them close to the central circle/square or far away (see Figure 7.2). Once this graphic social atom is created, the

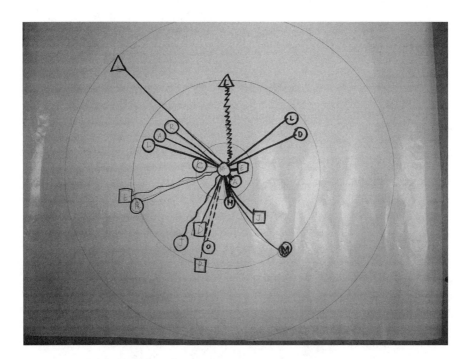

FIGURE 7.2. A re-created example of a social atom placed on concentric circles. The circle and square symbols represent females and males, while the triangles represent significant institutions.

child can step into the circles/squares of others, in order to be interviewed by the therapist. Each circle or square in and of itself carries important information—for example, how "big" or "small" this person is to the child, and in terms of color, how intense, muted, bright, and so on the energy that the child sees in this person is. A drama therapist is obviously interested in the actual embodying of the person that the child can portray as he or she takes the role of each person, while an art or play therapist may be more interested in the spaces between the circles/squares and how to interact playfully with those spaces, or how the colors convey their own meaning about the child's experience of each person.

Conclusion

Play and drama therapists have much in common: Both play and drama are free and natural phenomena that emerge spontaneously in childhood, and yet therapists who make use of both have struggled to establish their disciplines as credible mental health practices with legitimate potential to advance therapeutic goals. Both play and drama therapists believe that emotions can become unavailable for expression for a variety of reasons, and both provide ample opportunities for release that are not restricted to verbal communication. Much more holistic by definition, play and drama engage the mind and body in attempts to cause internal movement and transformative experience through reflection and expression.

Childhood trauma has traditionally been described as overwhelming a person's perceived capacity to cope with external stressors, and its treatment is generally thought to include expression of affect, cognitive and perceptual shifts, assimilation of fragmented memories, and sensory and physical release. Traumatized children can feel isolated, stigmatized, and compromised in their ability to establish or maintain important relationships. In addition, their attachment to others can feel frightening and necessary at the same time, causing them to feel dysregulated in the presence of caregivers. Trauma must be addressed directly or indirectly in order for these children to move forward and create new and more positive future options for themselves. Drama and play therapists are in a unique position to advance the goals of trauma resolution by providing clients with tools that give them the necessary combination of resources and safety to reflect, give voice, express affect, make shifts in perception and thinking, and eventually feel a greater sense of mastery and control.

REFERENCES

Boal, A. (1992). *Games for actors and non-actors*. New York: Routledge.
Bratton, S. C., Ray, D., & Rhine, T. (2005). The efficacy of play therapy with

children: A meta-analytic review of treatment outcomes. *Professional Psychology: Research and Practice, 36*(4), 376–390.

Cohen, J. A., Mannarino, A. P., & Deblinger, E. (2006). *Treating trauma and traumatic grief in children and adolescents.* New York: Guilford Press.

Cohen, J. A., Mannarino, A. P., & Deblinger, E. (Eds.). (2012). *Trauma-focused CBT for children and adolescents: Treatment applications.* New York: Guilford Press.

Cook, A., Spinazzola, J., Ford, J. D., Lanktree, C., Blaustein, M., Cloitre, M., . . . van der Kolk, B. (2005). Complex trauma in children and adolescents. *Psychiatric Annals, 35,* 390–398.

Courtois, C. A., & Ford, J. D. (2009). Defining and understanding complex trauma and complex traumatic stress disorders. In C. A. Courtois & J. D. Ford (Eds.), *Treating complex traumatic stress disorders: An evidence-based guide* (pp. 13–30). New York: Guilford Press.

D'Andrea, W., Ford, J., Stolbach, B., Spinazzola, J., & van der Kolk, B. (2012). Understanding interpersonal trauma in children: Why we need a developmentally appropriate trauma diagnosis. *American Journal of Orthopsychiatry, 82*(2), 187–200.

Dayton, T. (2005). *The living stage: A step-by-step guide to psychodrama, sociometry and experiential group therapy.* Deerfield Beach, FL: Health Communications.

Eyberg, S. (1988). PCIT: Integration of traditional and behavioral concerns. *Child and Family Behavior Therapy, 10,* 33–46.

Ford, J. D., & Cloitre, M. (2009). Best practices in psychotherapy for children and adolescents. In C. A. Courtois & J. D. Ford (Eds.), *Treating complex traumatic stress disorders: An evidence-based guide* (pp. 59–81). New York: Guilford Press.

Gil, E. (2003). Family play therapy: "The bear with short nails." In C. E. Schaefer (Ed.), *Foundations of play therapy* (pp. 192–218). New York: Wiley.

Gil, E. (2010). Children's self-initiated gradual exposure: The wonders of posttraumatic play and behavioral reenactments. In E. Gil (Ed.), *Working with children to heal interpersonal trauma: The power of play* (pp. 44–66). New York: Guilford Press.

Herman, J. (2009). Foreword. In C. A. Courtois & J. D. Ford (Eds.), *Treating complex traumatic stress disorders: An evidence-based guide* (pp. xiii–xvii). New York: Guilford Press.

Iacoboni, M. (2008). *Mirroring people: The new science of how we connect with others.* New York: Farrar, Straus & Giroux.

Irwin, E. C. (1983). The diagnostic and therapeutic use of pretend play. In C. E. Schaefer & K. J. O'Connor (Eds.), *The handbook of play therapy* (pp. 148–173). New York: Wiley.

Jones, P. (1996). *Drama as therapy: Vol. 1, Theory, practice and research.* New York: Routledge.

Ludy-Dobson, C. R., & Perry, B. (2010). The role of healthy relational interactions in buffering the impact of childhood trauma. In E. Gil (Ed.), *Working with children to heal interpersonal trauma: The power of play* (pp. 26–43). New York: Guilford Press.

McGoldrick, M., & Gerson, R. (1986). *Genograms in family assessment.* New York: Norton.

McGoldrick, M., Gerson, R., & Petry, S. (2008). *Genograms: Assessment and intervention* (3rd ed.). New York: Norton.

Moreno, J. L. (1934). *Who shall survive?: A new approach to the problem of human interrelations.* Washington, DC: Nervous and Mental Disease Publishing.

O'Connor, K. J., & Braverman, L. M. (1997). *Play therapy theory and practice: A comparative presentation.* New York: Wiley.

O'Connor, K. J., & Braverman, L. M. (2009). *Play therapy theory and practice: Comparing theories and techniques* (2nd ed.). Hoboken, NJ: Wiley.

Osofsky, J. D. (2011). *Clinical work with traumatized young children.* New York: Guilford Press.

Papp, P., Silverstein, O., & Carter, E. (1973). Family sculpting in preventive work with "well families." *Family Process, 12*(2), 197–212.

Salas, J. (1993). *Improvising real life: Personal story in Playback Theater.* Dubuque, IA: Kendall/Hunt.

Schaefer, C. E. (Ed.). (1993). *The therapeutic powers of play.* Northvale, NJ: Aronson.

Schaefer, C. E. (1994). Play therapy for psychic trauma in children. In K. J. O'Connor & C. E. Schaefer (Eds.), *Handbook of play therapy: Vol. 2. Advances and innovations* (pp. 297–318). New York: Wiley.

Shaw, J. A. (2010). A review of current research on the incidence and prevalence of interpersonal childhood trauma. In E. Gil (Ed.), *Working with children to heal interpersonal trauma: The power of play* (pp. 12–25). New York: Guilford Press.

Siegel, D. (2012). *The developing mind: How relationships and the brain interact to shape who we are* (2nd ed.). New York: Guilford Press.

Siegel, D., & Bryson, T. P. (2011). *The whole-brain child: Revolutionary strategies to nurture your child's developing mind.* New York: Delacorte Press.

Spolin, V. (1986). *Theater games for the classroom: A teacher's handbook.* Evanston, IL: Northwestern University Press.

van Horn, P., & Lieberman, A. F. (2009). Using dyadic therapies to treat traumatized young children. In D. Brom, R. Pat-Horenczyk, & J. Ford (Eds.), *Treating traumatized children: Risk, resilience, and recovery* (pp. 210–224). New York: Routledge.

Weber, A. M., & Haen, C. (Eds.). (2005). *Clinical applications of drama therapy in child and adolescent treatment.* New York: Brunner-Routledge.

Zapora, R. (1995). *Action theater: The improvisation of presence.* Berkeley, CA: North Atlantic Books.

CHAPTER 8

Overcoming Complex Trauma with Filial Therapy

Glade L. Topham
Risë VanFleet
Cynthia C. Sniscak

Children experiencing complex trauma offer significant challenges to their parents or other caregivers, as well as to the therapeutic process. Their histories are interwoven with maltreatment and attachment disruptions, leaving these children with serious emotional, behavioral, and social difficulties, further complicated by a decreased ability to trust the adults in their lives. Because their behaviors can be extreme and sometimes destructive, children with complex trauma can become a source of significant frustration to those who care for them. A negative interaction pattern can exacerbate the problems, yielding even greater stress and exasperation for all involved.

Filial Therapy (FT) has been used successfully with many children with attachment trauma—within the care system (foster care, kinship care), with adoptive families, and during the reunification process with their own biological parents (VanFleet, 2006b; VanFleet & Sniscak, 2003; VanFleet & Topham, 2011). There are a number of reasons why FT is an extremely valuable treatment for these children, and these are discussed in this chapter, along with case illustrations of how the FT process works to resolve emotional, behavioral, and relational problems while resolving the trauma and attachment issues that fuel children's maladaptive behaviors.

This chapter begins with a description of FT and some of its variations, followed by a discussion of the relevance of FT in meeting the needs of these children and the families that care for them. A section that highlights the research evidence for the efficacy of FT is followed by case vignettes illustrating its use with child victims of interpersonal trauma and attachment disruption.

Filial Therapy

FT was the brainchild of Drs. Bernard and Louise Guerney in the late 1950s, and they have guided its research and development as a powerful family therapy intervention from the beginning, nearly 50 years ago (B. G. Guerney, 1964; L. F. Guerney, 2003; L. F. Guerney & Ryan, 2013; VanFleet, 2013). It is a deceptively simple approach that fully integrates play therapy and family therapy, with a foundation and methods that draw from all the major schools of psychological thought (Ginsberg, 2003; L. F. Guerney & Ryan, 2013; VanFleet, 2011a, 2011b, 2011c, 2013). FT engages parents or caregivers as the primary change agents for their children; this was a novel idea when FT was created, and it remains so today. Therapists who are fully trained in FT's psychoeducational framework teach parents to conduct special 30-minute nondirective play therapy sessions with their own children. The therapists directly supervise the early parent/caregiver–child play sessions until the parents master the necessary skills, after which the therapists provide continuing support as the family members hold the play sessions at home unsupervised (or are supervised indirectly by video).

Overview

To avoid cumbersome language, the term *caregivers* is used from here on to refer to whichever parents, grandparents, kinship caregivers, foster parents, or adoptive parents are involved with a child during the FT process.

FT was developed for children ages 2½ to 12—the ages at which children use imaginary play the most to express their feelings, wishes, and dilemmas—but we have extended its use to children with complex trauma as old as 16. Because of their developmental disruptions, children who have experienced trauma and attachment disruptions often function socially and emotionally as if they were younger, thereby making it possible to apply FT with some adolescents with little variation.

In FT, a therapist teaches caregivers four basic skills for use within the caregiver–child play sessions. These play sessions are nondirective in nature, following the principles and practices of child-centered play therapy (CCPT) (Axline, 1969; Cochran, Nordling, & Cochran, 2010; Landreth, 2012; VanFleet, Sywulak, & Sniscak, 2010; Wilson & Ryan, 2005). The caregivers conduct a 30-minute play session with the child each week, and in cases where there are other children in the family, it is desirable that they each have a 30-minute play session with the caregivers as well. This prevents a singling-out effect on the target child, while facilitating the development of healthy attachment relationships within all of the dyads in the family (VanFleet, 2013). Furthermore, all adult caregivers in the household are strongly encouraged to participate.

In FT, the therapist first demonstrates one or more CCPT sessions for the caregivers (usually one with each child in the family), and discusses each session thoroughly with the caregivers. The therapist then takes approximately three 1-hour sessions to train the caregivers to conduct the play sessions. This is done using an empathic, positive, and playful approach, culminating in mock play sessions in which the therapist role-plays a child while a caregiver practices all of the skills. The therapist gives encouraging feedback to caregivers as they do this. After this, each caregiver conducts approximately four to six play sessions with the child that are directly supervised by the therapist. Each of these sessions includes a feedback segment, in which the therapist provides skill feedback and discusses play themes and daily concerns with the caregivers. Only after caregivers have mastered the skills of the play sessions and understand how to identify and understand play themes do they begin unsupervised play sessions at home. They continue to meet with the therapist to discuss the home play sessions and to begin generalizing the skills they've learned to daily life. When conducted with individual families, FT typically takes between 15 and 20 hourly sessions, although the number of sessions can easily be extended as needed for families dealing with serious trauma and attachment issues.

The Skills Taught to Caregivers

Therapists teach four basic play session skills to the caregivers: *structuring, empathic listening, child-centered imaginary play*, and *limit setting* (see VanFleet, 2006a, 2012, and 2013, for details). *Structuring* includes the messages given to a child to establish the relatively permissive climate of the playroom upon entry, as well as 5-minute and 1-minute warnings that the play session is ending. *Empathic listening* refers to brief descriptions of what the child is doing (tracking) and reflections of the child's feelings, as expressed either directly by the child or indirectly through the imaginary characters in the child's play. *Child-centered imaginary play* requires the caregiver to play out roles that are assigned by the child, and to play them in a manner that follows the child's lead. The child is viewed as both the director and an actor in the play, and the caregiver is an actor under the child's direction. *Limit setting* is used to establish safety and boundaries in the play; in FT, caregivers learn to state a limit, to give a warning, and to carry out the consequence if the child disregards the limit. In all cases, if a child breaks the same limit three times during a session, the session ends. This quickly reestablishes caregiver authority, since most children enjoy the play sessions and do not wish them to end. The skills of empathic listening and imaginary play foster a permissive environment in which the child can explore, express, and enjoy. This permissiveness is balanced by the skills of structuring and limit setting to ensure safety and establish ultimate caregiver authority.

Training Adjustments for Children with Complex Trauma

In work with children with complex trauma, adjustments are sometimes made to the usual FT process (VanFleet, 2006b; VanFleet & Sniscak, 2003). Caregivers need more information about trauma, attachment processes, and the relationships of these to child behaviors and well-being. For example, they need to understand how past trauma and attachment disruptions can result in extreme behaviors and emotional reactions over which children seem to have little control. A better understanding of the importance of secure attachment and how it is fostered provides a framework for the FT that the therapist is recommending. Furthermore, these children are more likely to play in aggressive or sexualized ways because of their histories, so it is sometimes advisable to add an extra mock play session to show the caregivers how to respond to emotionally difficult material during the play sessions.

Didactic and Dynamic Elements of FT

FT consists of a blend of didactic and dynamic elements that unite to create positive change for both children and caregivers. The didactic element involves the training process to prepare caregivers to conduct the play sessions and master the CCPT play session skills. The dynamic element includes the discussions that therapists hold with caregivers to help them recognize and understand children's play themes, as well as empathic explorations of the caregivers' own feelings and reactions to the play and the process. Play sessions frequently trigger caregiver reactions that can prevent the caregivers from being responsive to the child. The skilled FT practitioner processes these reactions in a manner that helps caregivers develop understanding and make their own changes as needed.

Formats and Variations

FT was initially developed as a family group intervention, which is an efficient and cost-effective format for FT. This approach is detailed in L. F. Guerney and Ryan (2013); the 20-week group model described there can be shortened or lengthened as needed. VanFleet (2006a, 2013) has described the use of FT with individual families in detail, as well as a number of other group formats and resources. VanFleet, Sniscak, and Faa-Thompson (in press) describe a 14- to 18-week group FT format for use specifically with foster parents and adoptive parents. When therapists are properly trained and adhere to the values, principles, and process of FT, the method has great flexibility for effectively meeting the complex needs of families of children with serious trauma and attachment problems. The section that follows discusses an integrated model for treating attachment trauma, and provides the rationale for using FT with these children and their caregivers.

Targets of Treatment for Attachment Trauma

Attachment and trauma are intertwined for children. When children experience trauma, it threatens the attachment relationship, as well as children's trust that they are safe and that attachment figures will protect them. Furthermore, children with insecure attachments may have more trouble recovering from the effects of trauma and may also be more vulnerable to the effects of future trauma, because they may lack both the internal and external resources and supports to deal with overwhelming experiences. Therefore, the treatment of child trauma and of attachment disruption needs to be informed by both attachment and trauma theories (Busch & Lieberman, 2007).

A useful framework for guiding treatment of chronic interpersonal trauma or complex trauma in children that integrates attachment and trauma theories is the *attachment, self-regulation, and competency* (ARC) treatment framework (Blaustein & Kinniburgh, 2010; Kinniburgh, Blaustein, Spinazzola, & van der Kolk, 2005). The ARC model is not a treatment protocol, but rather a framework that highlights key areas and targets of treatment for child complex trauma, based on the existing body of research on the effects of child trauma. Below we list the three areas and 10 components or targets of the ARC model, as well as the associated challenges commonly seen in children who have experienced complex trauma. Then we use the ARC framework to describe how FT addresses the key caregiver and child targets of effective treatment for complex trauma.

Attachment

The four target areas of *attachment* in the ARC framework are *caregiver management of affect*; *attunement*; *consistency of response*; and *routines and rituals*. In the case of complex trauma, caregivers, who in the past have failed to provide proper protection and care for their child, frequently have poor emotional awareness and poor emotion regulation skills; these deficits significantly impairing their ability to be responsive and available to their child. Furthermore, even in cases where there is no history of maltreatment or neglect with current caregivers, it is frequently difficult for caregivers to manage their emotional experiences in response to the sometimes volatile behavior and emotions of a child who has experienced complex trauma. Furthermore, children who have experienced complex trauma are frequently accustomed to chaos in their family systems, leaving little sense for consistency, predictability, and safety (Arvidson et al., 2011).

Self-Regulation

The three target areas of child *self-regulation* in the ARC framework are *affect identification, affect modulation*, and *affect expression*. Children who have experienced trauma often experience overwhelming negative emotions, with limited awareness of these emotions or their origins; have few strategies for modulating their inner experience; and are frequently unable to communicate effectively with others about their inner experience (Kinniburgh et al., 2005).

Competency

The two target areas of developmental *competency* in the ARC framework are *executive functions*, and *self-development and identity*. Children who have experienced trauma often feel little sense of influence over their environments and have difficulty with problem solving and persevering with challenging tasks. They also commonly experience an internalized negative self-concept as a result of traumatic experiences and inconsistent care from attachment figures. Furthermore, trauma commonly interferes with children's development and may result in a delay in developmental competencies. The final building block of the ARC model is *trauma experience integration*. Children who have experienced trauma frequently have a fragmented internal experience that is overwhelming, leaving the children with little ability to make sense out of the internal experience and the associated events (Arvidson et al., 2011).

FT and Treatment of Complex Trauma

FT is well suited for the treatment of complex trauma in children because a child is treated within the context of the caregiver–child relationship; treatment focuses simultaneously on improvement in the child, the caregiver, and the caregiver–child relationship; treatment attends to all of the key targets of treatment as specified in the ARC model; treatment can be flexibly applied with biological, foster, or adoptive parents; treatment is structured and time-limited; the nondirective nature of the caregiver–child sessions allows FT to be utilized to treat a wide range of child symptoms and caregiver–child relationship problems; and treatment is positive and strength-based. Below we describe how FT addresses the targets of the ARC model in the areas of attachment, self-regulation, and competency.

Attachment

Caregiver Management of Affect

While developing and refining the four FT skills, caregivers learn to manage their own internal experiences in interaction with their child. The empathic listening and child-centered imaginary play skills challenge caregivers to set aside (i.e., regulate) their own personal needs, fears, and reactions in order to be fully present for their child. In setting limits, caregivers learn to manage their reactions in order to stay emotionally present and avoid shaming or rejecting their child. An important component of the work in helping caregivers improve self-regulation happens in the feedback sessions that follow play sessions. There the therapist helps caregivers identify points of emotional reactivity during the play session, helps caregivers identify and talk through possible reasons for their reaction from their own backgrounds, and helps caregivers understand the child's behaviors from trauma and attachment perspectives. Through these discussions, caregivers become more self-aware and more intentional about self-regulation.

Attunement

At the core of the empathic listening and child-centered imaginary play skills is caregiver attunement. A focus on these skills pushes caregivers to attune to and reflect the child's inner experience, including feelings, desires, and intentions. Child-centered imaginary play causes caregivers to flex their attunement "muscles" as they strive to play in the ways they sense the child wants or needs them to play. During the postplay feedback sessions, the therapist fosters caregiver attunement by engaging caregivers in reflective discussions regarding the meaning of the child's play and what might be going on for the child (as viewed through developmental and trauma lenses). Furthermore, the therapist models attunement in interaction with caregivers by attending to the caregivers' internal experience.

Consistency of Response, and Routines and Rituals

Utilizing the structuring skill, caregivers learn to create consistency and predictability during play sessions by providing the same introduction and concluding statement to play sessions and by providing a 5-minute and a 1-minute warning before concluding the session. Furthermore, the playroom is set up in the same way with the same toys for each play session. Caregivers are taught to generalize the structuring skills outside of play sessions by creating consistency and predictability in the child's schedule and environment, and to be particularly attentive to trauma triggers for the child when doing so. For example, children who have experienced complex trauma frequently become anxious and fearful at bedtime. In addition to common bedtime rituals, caregivers might do a bedroom check with a child to be sure the room is "safe," turn on extra night lights, leave the door open a crack, and give the child a stuffed animal to watch over him or her (Arvidson et al., 2011).

Self-Regulation

Affect Identification

Using the empathic listening skill, caregivers verbally reflect a child's feelings, intentions, and desires throughout play sessions, helping the child become attuned to and accepting of his or her own internal experience.

Affect Modulation

In play sessions, children are provided with various toys that tend to lead to up-regulation of arousal (e.g., bop bags, swords, aggressive animals) and various toys that tend to lead to down-regulation of arousal (e.g., a sandtray, baby dolls, bottles). In the safety of the play session, children who may initially be fearful of particular states of arousal are able to experiment gradually with different arousal states, and to experience an increasing sense of mastery over those states. Caregiver-imposed limits provide children with opportunities to regulate behavior and emotion; caregiver reflections reinforce the children's emerging regulation abilities (e.g., "You are really mad that you can't color on the wall, but you figured out something that you could color on").

Affect Expression

As children become increasingly aware of and accepting of their emotional experience as a result of caregiver reflections, it becomes easier for children to express their feelings. In many cases, as children become accustomed to caregiver reflections, they begin to provide their own narrations of thoughts and feelings in later stages of FT. In generalizing the empathic listening skill, caregivers are taught how to continue to assist their children in understanding, modulating, and expressing emotions in conjunction with everyday experience.

Competency

Executive Functions

The nondirective play sessions in FT provide a fertile context for children to develop problem-solving skills. In this context, children experience control over their environment and can take on simple problems at first (e.g., building a basic tower), then increasingly difficult problems (e.g., putting a dart correctly in a dart gun) as they gain confidence. Large barriers to problem solving for children who have experienced trauma are poor frustration tolerance and a limited ability to persist in the face of challenge. In FT, caregivers' reflections help scaffold children's problem solving, helping the children regulate frustration and sustain focus and effort. Furthermore, esteem-building reflections by caregivers (e.g., "It was so hard to figure out how to get the dart to go into the gun, but you turned it until you figured it out, and now you got it to work!") help children consolidate their emerging skills and develop confidence.

Self-Development and Identity

Caregivers' reflections about children's internal experience help children develop a sense of being unique, as well as an internal acceptance of their uniqueness. A positive sense of self is also fostered as children gain mastery over their environment, reinforced by caregiver reflections of their positive feelings (e.g., "You are really proud you were able to make that tower so high").

Trauma Experience Integration

A central objective of FT is to create a context in which children can "play through" past traumatic and distressing experiences. Within the context of the caregiver–child play sessions, a child is able to play through and gain mastery over previously overwhelming memories, experiences, and emotions, and by so doing to integrate fragmented internal experience.

Supportive Research

A number of positive child outcomes have been demonstrated in FT treatment programs, including increased emotional expression, decreased depression and anxiety, increased self-confidence, and decreased behavioral problems. Additional positive outcomes include increased caregiver sensitivity, empathy, and acceptance; decreased caregiver stress; and improved caregiver–child relationships (see VanFleet, Ryan, & Smith, 2005, for a review). A recent study (Topham, Wampler, Titus, & Rolling, 2010) examining the predictors of treatment success in FT found that higher levels of caregiver distress and poorer child emotion regulation at pretest were predictive of significant reductions in child behavior problems across treatment. Similarly, poor caregiver emotion regulation at pretest was predictive of significant increases in caregiver acceptance across treatment. Although research has not yet examined whether FT leads to improvement in caregiver and child emotion regulation, this study indicates that caregivers and children with poorer emotion regulation (as is commonly the case with children who have experienced complex trauma) are likely to experience positive gains in FT, leading to speculation that the positive changes are a function of improving emotion regulation.

Case Vignettes

The identifying information in the case illustrations that follow has been changed, and the illustrations may represent composites of several families. All of them represent realistic depictions of the FT process at work, however.

Tory

Tory was 3 years old when she was removed from the care of her biological mother. She had been burned on the bottom half of her body by a hot bath, and had been in a major medical facility for many months healing from the effects of this abusive experience. Tory was referred for play therapy due to the trauma of sustaining her injuries, the numerous painful medical procedures related to those injuries, her lengthy hospital stays, and the loss of her primary caregiver. More surgeries were expected in her future. In addition to the abuse, Tory's primary caregiver, who had cared for her since she was an infant, died of a heart attack when Tory was alone with her. Furthermore, her dependency placement took her away from her two siblings.

Tory met her new foster family when she was still in the hospital. When she presented for treatment, she was a shy, introverted, and withdrawn child who had considerable developmental delays in most areas of functioning. She had significant communication problems and was very difficult to understand when she attempted to speak. The treatment plan focused on three goals: (1) assisting the family with developing a secure attachment, (2) helping Tory to heal from the past trauma, and (3) helping her with her developmental issues. At the time the family presented for outpatient psychotherapy, Tory was fitting into the foster family quite well. There were no significant behavioral problems, except that she seemed to have nightmares related to her prior trauma, and she often cried with frustration if she could not master things. Tory was described by her foster mother as lovable, persistent, resilient, and independent. It was mutually decided that FT would be the primary intervention to promote a healthy relationship and attachment, while working on developmental and trauma issues. After the FT process was well established, a number of additional directive play therapy interventions were woven into the treatment to work on some of her more specific issues.

Tory's play was delayed for her age, most likely as a result of her history. She moved from toy to toy without any consistent themes or sequence. She did not engage her foster mother or father during play sessions with them, but kept her back to them. The therapist encouraged the foster parents, during their respective play sessions with her, to move to a position at her side where they were better able to see her play and make eye contact with Tory as they empathically listened.

Trauma themes emerged early in the parent–child play sessions. Without talking, Tory played very roughly with the baby dolls. She shook the babies repeatedly and hit them. She held them down and pressed on them. She threw them across the room and piled them on top of each other. She then hit the bop bag and aggressively pushed everything away from her. Themes seemed to be related to power, control, aggression, and prior trauma.

As FT play sessions with her foster parents continued, Tory's play became less chaotic and more focused on developmental and trauma mastery and on relationship building. As the play expanded, Tory showed patterns and themes related to exploration, trust building, mastery, problem solving, developmental play, relationship, nurturance, and self-identity. She became interested in making sure the doll babies always had enough food and were well cared for. She then moved to water play, pouring water into different containers and spilling it. Although this play often represents developmental mastery, it was especially significant for Tory, because she had initially been afraid of the sounds of water being poured. This fear may have been related to her traumatic experience.

As Tory expanded her interest in the toys in the playroom, she put on many masks, trying to trick her foster parents. She then removed them to show her parents that it was really her underneath, saying, "It's *me*!" Hiding behind and trying on different identities constitute a common theme among children who are working on developing a secure attachment. At first, Tory had been afraid of all the masks in the playroom, but her tolerance of them and other "scary" toys grew as her anxiety decreased within the relationships with her foster mom and dad.

Tory eventually found the emergency vehicles and the hospital set. She began putting figures inside the ambulances. After the play sessions switched to the home setting, she began playing with the medical kit. At first she played with these items by herself, giving herself shots. After a couple of sessions like this, she hesitantly began treating her foster mom.

As the play sessions continued and Tory worked through her traumatic experiences, the attachment with her foster parents grew, and Tory's play resembled what one would expect of a child at her developmental level. She was then able to attend preschool, and was adopted by her foster parents. Later, the family also adopted her two siblings, and the parents held regular one-to-one filial play sessions with all three children. The mother called 9 months after discharge to report that everyone in the family looked forward to their continuing weekly play sessions. The play sessions, coupled with the parents' use of their now-generalized skills in daily life, were still yielding excellent results.

Lilly

Lilly was removed from her young mother's care for neglect and was placed in the foster care system. This first placement was found to be abusive, and the child was removed and then placed in kinship care with her grandmother. Most unfortunately, for a second time, Lilly had been placed in an abusive home; this time, she received such severe injuries that she had to be hospitalized for several months. Lilly suffered brain injury so severe that part of her brain had to be removed to allow for swelling. When she was well enough to be released, she was unable to walk and had lost the use of one of her arms and a hand. The grandmother who had perpetrated the abuse was found guilty and sentenced to many years in prison.

Given Lilly's history of attachment disruption, severe abuse, inconsistent care, and medical trauma, it was not surprising that she had become a child with challenging behaviors. She was introduced to her new foster mothers while still in the hospital. One of her new parents had to be out of town for the first several months of her placement, further interfering with the development of a secure attachment. Moreover, Lilly's medical treatment continued, with numerous additional hospital stays and difficult treatments.

When Lilly presented for therapy, she had already been adopted by the foster mothers, who reported concerns relating to anxiety, temper tantrums, fearfulness, oppositional behaviors, and defiance. Lilly constantly tested limits and tried to triangulate her parents. Her well-intentioned adoptive parents invited her birth mother, her other grandmother (not the perpetrator of the abuse), and her half-brother to share vacations with them once a year. After these visits, Lilly became especially dysregulated and difficult to manage. The adoptive family asked for help to assist Lilly in resolving her trauma-related issues, regulating her emotional reactions, and controlling her maladaptive behaviors. They also requested assistance with attachment issues. FT was the primary intervention used with this family, although other play interventions were used as well to facilitate progress.

Both parents attended every training and therapy session. It took Lilly several weeks of parent–child play before she trusted that she could actually do "almost anything you want." Her early play involved frequent checking to make sure the parent playing with her was happy with what she was doing—a common theme in children who have anxious attachments. Soon Lilly started to take risks related to aggressive play, such as shooting guns and trying some disrespectful words.

Once Lilly began to trust that her mothers meant what they said and were accepting of her play, she expanded her play themes. She began to play aggressively with the bop bag, beating it and then pretending to shoot one or the other of her moms repeatedly, telling her she was a bad person. Within just a couple of play sessions, she began asking her moms to join her in fighting the "bad people" together. There was soon evidence of behavioral improvement, and the parents developed confidence in generalizing some of the play session skills to daily life.

Just as the significant improvements seemed to be consolidating, Lilly had to attend a rehabilitation program that seemed to trigger her sensory memory of her traumatic experiences, resulting in a huge escalation of her problematic behaviors. The therapist helped the parents, who were confused by the escalation, understand Lilly's extreme reactions and behavioral regression in the context of her trauma. Together, they developed strategies for showing understanding of Lilly's triggered emotions while managing her behaviors.

During this period, Lilly had a particularly difficult week. She had numerous outbursts and tantrums, was oppositional much of the time, and showed great fear at bedtime. The parents, with the clear understanding of trauma gained from FT, discovered that the time of year coincided with Lilly's initial traumatic hospitalization and her entry into her new family. They suspected that another powerful sensory memory had been awakened.

The therapist suggested a more directive play therapy activity to assist Lilly with discharging some of the distress she felt about her frequently mentioned abusive grandmother. In this family play intervention, Lilly drew a large picture of the perpetrator. Lilly, her mothers, and the therapist threw wet wads of toilet paper at the perpetrator, simultaneously shouting at the symbolic perpetrator that she could no longer hurt children and that she would be in jail for a long time. Lilly's parents also let Lilly know that they would never let the perpetrator near her again. Lilly started yelling at the symbolic perpetrator she had drawn, telling the paper representation of her grandmother what she would no longer tolerate from her, and at the same time talking about what her grandmother had done to her. Lilly exclaimed loudly, "She almost killed me!" As her moms joined in, she got bolder and more intense, using three complete rolls of toilet paper.

After this 20-minute activity, Lilly had an FT session with one of her mothers. Interesting themes after the directive play emerged. She asked this mom to help her build a double-thick wall of large cardboard blocks, indicating that they would be safe in there. She said that there was only one way in and one way out. Lilly proclaimed that she was the boss of that place and no one was welcome except her two moms. Her mother accurately reflected that it was a safe place; they were all together; and nothing bad could happen to them within those double walls. When Lilly left the playroom, after giving her mom a hug, she seemed relaxed and calm. The parents reported seeing a huge improvement in her affect and behavior after this session. Lilly's play became less intense, and she focused on mastery, problem solving, and her relationship with her mothers. She seemed happy, laughing frequently both during her play sessions and in daily life. The gains were maintained for the duration of her therapy and thereafter.

Joshua

At age 4, Joshua was removed from his mother's home for neglect and placed in the custody of child protective services. When he was referred to therapy 6 months later, Joshua had been removed from several foster homes due to behavioral problems. There was a possibility that he had been exposed to drug and alcohol abuse by adults in the mother's home. It was definitely known that Joshua had been exposed to pornographic material and had witnessed parental sexual activity, including incest: He told the therapist that he had tried to stop his grandfather from having sex with his mother, but he had been unable to stop it. He also described being sexually abused by two men who frequently visited his home. Joshua told his therapist that he "was kicked out of school for being 'bad.' "

Joshua had been diagnosed with attention-deficit/hyperactivity disorder, oppositional defiant disorder, and reactive attachment disorder; his diagnosis also included a notation for "neglect of child." His first foster mother had identified issues related to impulsivity, aggressiveness, oppositional behavior, and destructive behaviors. She reported that Joshua seemed to exhibit a lack of conscience and cause-and-effect thinking, and that he had been cruel to animals in their home.

The school had reported that Joshua was urinating on things and exhibiting inappropriate sexualized behaviors. At home, he played with dolls and stuffed animals in a sexualized way, and his caseworker reported that he inappropriately touched other children. He wet his pants and masturbated frequently.

Initially, the therapist attempted to involve Joshua's foster parents in FT, but his placements were too unstable; his behavior was so dysregulated that the first few foster families would not keep him in their homes. The therapist used individual CCPT until there was more stability in his placements and relationships. From the start, Joshua's play was extremely trauma-based, including lots of aggression and sexualized play, especially after visits with his biological mother and grandfather. His play was chaotic and intense. He was often very agitated as he played. Joshua's play themes related to sex, protection, danger, anxiety, safety, rescue, power, control, aggression, good versus evil, limit testing, exploration, relationship, and loss. Limit setting was frequently needed during the play sessions to keep Joshua safe and regulated.

After 6 months of weekly CCPT sessions and disrupted placements, Joshua was placed in an appropriate foster home. His newest foster mother was eager to learn and conduct FT play sessions with him. During the training phase, the therapist added an additional mock training session to assist her with the expectation and management of traumatic play. Two FT play sessions were conducted on a weekly basis—one at home and the other in the playroom under the therapist's supervision, because Joshua's play was very trauma-based, intense, and disturbing to the mom. She needed the therapist's support and feedback to help her understand the play themes and their relationship to his traumatic experience and behavioral issues.

Joshua's play sessions often focused on a bad or dangerous situation, like a robbery or catastrophe of giant proportions. Often his foster mother was the victim in the imaginary play. He played the role of the strong and powerful "good guy" who dispatched the villain or put him in jail. For several sessions at the beginning of the parent–child play sessions, Joshua shifted between the roles of victim and victimizer. This is a frequent theme for children who have been traumatized, as they try to work out and make sense of their experience. For several sessions, Joshua tied up the "bad guy" (bop bag) with a rope and pretended to cut off his private parts, asking him, "Now how do you like that?" He then covered the bop bag's wounds with many Band-Aids. After this he put the bad person in "jail" and asked his foster mother to help him get "bad people." Together they made sure the world was a safe place.

FT was very beneficial for this child. There were positive changes in behavioral self-regulation, attention, focus, peer relationships, and general well-being. Joshua became closer and more trusting as his attachment with his foster mother grew.

Joshua's play themes greatly expanded as his trust grew. At the beginning of his therapeutic work, his play was chaotic, disorganized, and non-sequential. Sexual themes were a frequent focus in his behaviors and his play. Almost immediately after beginning FT, there was a reduction in sexual acting out and sexual play themes, as well as a reduction in sexually inappropriate language both in and out of the playroom.

As Joshua's play in the playroom became less hyperactive, impulsive, and chaotic, and more organized, so did his general functioning, with a few exceptions. He was now capable of playing out themes that were intentional and focused. His play themes became more sequential and healthier.

As FT sessions continued, Joshua's play themes focused on relationship, attachment, mastery, and self-esteem. Some play themes that are common to children with histories of trauma and attachment disruption were still evident; however, they were now accompanied by positive themes, including nurturance, healing, family and problem solving. For example, Joshua often asked his mother to become the mother of the doll babies, and together they cared for them—giving them bottles and food, and making sure they were tucked in for naptime. He also prepared food for his mom, asking her what she would like and making sure that she had everything that she needed.

As FT play sessions continued at home, more directive play therapy sessions were conducted in the office. These focused on safe and appropriate touch; understanding what to do when touch is not safe; peer relationship issues; impulse control and self-regulation; attention and focus; understanding foster placement and the loss of his mother and extended family; feelings identification; and sharing feelings appropriately. There was also work on stress management, relaxation techniques, and relationship and attachment issues. Several sessions of canine-assisted play therapy focused on creating relationships and treating animals kindly. In one of their last office sessions, Joshua and his foster mom painted each other's faces with face paint, looking into each other's eyes, smiling, laughing, and asking the therapist to take a picture. Shortly afterward, Joshua's foster mom became Joshua's adoptive mom. FT sessions continued at home, with ongoing benefits for the mom, the child, and the relationship.

Conclusion

Children whose lives have been marred by maltreatment and attachment disruptions struggle with a variety of maladaptive emotional reactions, behaviors, and relationship patterns. Their caregivers face significant challenges as they try to create a safe environment in which to overcome trauma and build secure attachments. FT offers an ideal intervention to address the complex needs of both children and their caregivers. Under the supervision of an appropriately trained FT practitioner, caregivers learn to conduct special nondirective play sessions with children, creating the safety and understanding needed for children to process and overcome prior trauma and gradually develop healthy attachments with caregiving adults.

In this chapter, we have provided a brief description of FT, which integrates family therapy with play therapy. We have shown how FT fits within the ARC treatment framework for complex trauma by addressing caregiver management of affect, attunement, consistency of response, and routines and rituals. After an overview of the relevant research, we have concluded with case vignettes of FT in action. Because FT addresses both child and family needs so thoroughly and effectively, it should be considered a leading therapeutic modality for children with complex trauma and their caregivers.

REFERENCES

Arvidson, J., Kinniburgh, K., Howard, K., Spinazzola, J., Strothers, H., Evans, M., . . . Blaustein, M. (2011). Treatment of complex trauma in young children: Developmental and cultural considerations in application of the ARC intervention model. *Journal of Child and Adolescent Trauma, 4,* 34–51.

Axline, V. M. (1969). *Play therapy* (rev. ed.). New York: Ballantine Books.

Blaustein, M. E., & Kinniburgh, K. M. (2010). *Treating traumatic stress in children and adolescents: How to foster resilience through attachment, self-regulation, and competency.* New York: Guilford Press.

Busch, A. L., & Lieberman, A. F. (2007). Attachment and trauma: An integrated approach to treating young children exposed to family violence. In D. Oppenheim & D. F. Goldsmith (Eds.), *Attachment theory in clinical work with children: Bridging the gap between research and practice* (pp. 139–171). New York: Guilford Press.

Cochran, N. H., Nordling, W. J., & Cochran, J. L. (2010). *Child-centered play therapy: A practical guide to developing therapeutic relationships with children.* Hoboken, NJ: Wiley.

Ginsberg, B. G. (2003). An integrated holistic model of child-centered family therapy. In R. VanFleet & L. F. Guerney (Eds.), *Casebook of Filial Therapy* (pp. 21–47). Boiling Springs, PA: Play Therapy Press.

Guerney, B. G., Jr. (1964). Filial Therapy: Description and rationale. *Journal of Consulting Psychology, 28*, 303–310.

Guerney, L. F. (2003). The history, principles, and empirical basis of Filial Therapy. In R. VanFleet & L. F. Guerney (Eds.), *Casebook of Filial Therapy* (pp. 1–19). Boiling Springs, PA: Play Therapy Press.

Guerney, L. F., & Ryan, V. M. (2013). *Group Filial Therapy: A complete guide to teaching parents to play therapeutically with their children.* Philadelphia: Kingsley.

Kinniburgh, K., Blaustein, M., Spinazzola, J., & van der Kolk, B. A. (2005). Attachment, self-regulation, and competency. *Psychiatric Annals, 35*(5), 424–430.

Landreth, G. L. (2012). *Play therapy: The art of the relationship* (3rd ed.). New York: Routledge.

Topham, G. L., Wampler, K. S., Titus, G., & Rolling, E. (2011). Predicting parent and child outcomes of a Filial Therapy program. *International Journal of Play Therapy, 20*, 79–93.

VanFleet, R. (2006a). *Introduction to Filial Therapy* [DVD]. Boiling Springs, PA: Play Therapy Press.

VanFleet, R. (2006b). Short-term play therapy for adoptive families: Facilitating adjustment and attachment with Filial Therapy. In H. G. Kaduson & C. E. Schaefer (Eds.), *Short-term play therapy interventions for children* (2nd ed., pp. 145–168). New York: Guilford Press.

VanFleet, R. (2011a). Filial Therapy: What every play therapist should know. Part One of a series. *Play Therapy: Magazine of the British Association of Play Therapists, 65*, 16–19.

VanFleet, R. (2011b). Filial Therapy: What every play therapist should know. Part Two of a series. *Play Therapy: Magazine of the British Association of Play Therapists, 66*, 7–10.

VanFleet, R. (2011c). Filial Therapy: What every play therapist should know. Part Three of a series. *Play Therapy: Magazine of the British Association of Play Therapists, 67*, 18–21.

VanFleet, R. (2012). *A parent's handbook of Filial Therapy: Building strong families with play* (2nd ed.). Boiling Springs, PA: Play Therapy Press.

VanFleet, R. (2013). *Filial Therapy: Strengthening parent–child relationships through play* (3rd ed.). Sarasota, FL: Professional Resource Press.

VanFleet, R., Ryan, S. D., & Smith, S. K. (2005). Filial Therapy: A critical review. In L. A. Reddy, T. M. Files-Hall, & C. E. Schaefer (Eds.), *Empirically based play interventions for children* (pp. 241–264). Washington, DC: American Psychological Association.

VanFleet, R., & Sniscak, C. C. (2003). Filial therapy for attachment-disrupted and disordered children. In R. VanFleet & L. F. Guerney (Eds.), *Casebook of Filial Therapy* (pp. 279–308). Boiling Springs, PA: Play Therapy Press.

VanFleet, R., Sniscak, C., & Faa-Thompson, T. (in press). *Filial Therapy group program for foster and adoptive families: A practitioner's manual* [working title]. Boiling Springs, PA: Play Therapy Press.

VanFleet, R., Sywulak, A. E., & Sniscak, C. C. (2010). *Child-centered play therapy*. New York: Guilford Press.

VanFleet, R., & Topham, G. (2011). Filial Therapy for maltreated and neglected children: Integration of family therapy and play therapy. In A. Drewes, S. C. Bratton, & C. E. Schaefer (Eds.), *Integrative play therapy* (pp. 153–175). Hoboken, NJ: Wiley.

Wilson, K., & Ryan, V. (2005). *Play therapy: A non-directive approach for children and adolescents* (2nd ed.). London: Elsevier.

CHAPTER 9

Theraplay in Reunification Following Relational Trauma

Phyllis B. Booth
Sandra Lindaman
Marlo L.-R. Winstead

Isaiah, a 6-year-old boy living in a low-income, chronically violent neighborhood, was found looking for food in the garbage. When the police took him home, they found his mother incoherent and high on crack. The child was immediately placed in foster care and had no contact with his mother. One month later, the foster mother contacted a therapist; she was concerned about Isaiah's aggression, defiance, unresponsiveness to affection, and extremely controlling behavior at home and school. Theraplay with Isaiah then began. Over the course of the next 6 months, the biological mother abstained from drugs, and her life became more stable. The court allowed supervised visits with the goal of reunification. Although Isaiah was calmer in his foster home, he fell back into patterns of aggression, defiance, opposition, and intense mood swings during visits with his mother. His mother was attempting to regain custody and to use the new strategies she was learning in parenting class, but could not seem to get control of the situation. The therapist started to include the biological mother in therapy, and discovered that she had been in foster care herself. In both her biological and her foster families, she had experienced attachment disruptions and severe abuse.

As therapists planning treatment for the relational trauma sustained by Isaiah's family, we asked ourselves:

- What impact had the lack of safety and responsive caregiving had in the lives of Isaiah and his mother?
- What would help this foster mother meet Isaiah's needs during placement?
- Would it be possible to support Isaiah's biological mother enough to make reunification feasible?
- What kinds of treatment would facilitate socioemotional health and healing for this mother and her son?

The Theraplay®[1] model would answer these questions in this way: Because the mother had not received responsive caregiving or felt safe as a child, she was unable to play her part in the healthy interaction that would have led to a secure attachment and long-term mental health for her son. Both she and Isaiah needed to share new experiences that would change their views and expectations, and to create relationships that would meet their needs for safety, intersubjectivity, regulation, mutual enjoyment, and ongoing healthy development. The first step would be to provide these experiences for Isaiah and his foster mother. The question of whether Isaiah's mother could achieve the stability and mental health needed to make reunification possible would depend on the quality of support she receives and on her own inner strength.

In this chapter, we describe the Theraplay approach to working with children and parents who have suffered relational trauma. We start by discussing the nature, impact, and treatment of relational trauma; we then present the Theraplay model, its history, its theoretical basis, and a typical treatment plan. An account of the Theraplay treatment with Isaiah, his foster mother, and his biological mother concludes the chapter. Theraplay was supplemented at crucial points by other modalities, but contributed in large part to the success of the family's treatment.

The Impact and Treatment of Relational Trauma

The mental health field has begun to look at the significant effect of trauma on the relationships and ongoing neuroaffective development of young children. Terms commonly used to describe this new view of trauma are: *developmental trauma*, referring to the interpersonal and developmentally adverse nature of child trauma (van der Kolk, 2005); *complex trauma*, describing seven domains of impairment of critical developmental experiences (Cook, Blaustein, Spinazzola, & van der Kolk, 2003); and *relational trauma*, acknowledging that the source of neglect or abuse is often the primary caregiver (Schore, 2001). In this chapter, we use *relational trauma* to

---

[1]Theraplay is a registered service mark of The Theraplay Institute, Evanston, Illinois.

describe the experience of Isaiah and his biological mother. In their child-hoods, each of them was faced with the paralyzing dilemma that the very caregivers who should have been the source of comfort and protection were instead the source of neglect and pain.

Allan Schore (2003) describes how the preverbal emotional communi-cation between parent (or other primary caregiver) and infant in a healthy attachment relationship shapes the maturation of the infant's right brain. The parent attends closely to the child and follows the minute facial, vocal, and gestural cues of the infant. As the parent attunes to the ups and downs of the infant's bodily arousal, the two gradually learn each other's rhythms and together create a new, specific shared rhythm. Through this moment-to-moment dance of attunement, they come to understand each other. Any misstep in this process creates a moment of stress, which the sensitive par-ent repairs with a return to synchrony. Through this process, the child becomes capable of regulating positive and negative emotions as he or she grows.

The emotional communication of the abusive and/or neglectful par-ent is less synchronized and less playful. Reactions to the infant's stressful emotions are minimal, unpredictable, inappropriate, or rejecting. Schore (2003) notes,

> Instead of modulating, she induces extreme levels of stimulation and arousal, and because she provides no interactive repair the infant's intense negative states last for long periods of time. Prolonged negative states are toxic for infants and although they possess some capacity to modulate low-intensity negative affect states, these states continue to escalate in intensity, frequency and duration. (p. 124)

When a caregiver does not connect with a child's active bid for attunement, the child experiences shame. When that shameful reaction is paired with a caregiver's sustained anger or lack of repair, the child experiences a humili-ation that is damaging to the developing brain and to the regulation of emotion. This child enters a hyper- or hypoaroused physical and emotional state outside the autonomic nervous system's window of tolerance, result-ing in reduced ability to function adaptively and flexibly (Siegel, 2012). In summary, when early trauma alters the development of the right brain the child's ability to process socioemotional information, regulate body states, and cope with emotional stress is impaired, leading to serious consequences for the development of the bodily and emotional self (Schore, 2003).

How should we treat such relational trauma? Schore and Schore (2008) advise that therapists must understand the importance of early dyadic regulation, right-hemisphere development, and the formation of implicit procedural memory. Effective intervention should focus on the preverbal, facial, vocal, and gestural communications that occur within the healthy attachment relationship. This focus will lead to optimal development of the limbic system and right-brain functions, and ultimately of the child's affect regulation (Schore, 2003).

Theraplay treatment, as described in this chapter, is a re-creation of the positive emotional communication of the securely attached parent and child through its emphasis on attuned, synchronous, and reciprocal right-brain-based interaction, appropriate up- and down-regulating to widen the window of tolerance, attention to bids for attunement, opportunities for repair in the here-and-now, and reflection with and guidance of the parent to move into a healthier relationship with the child. Appropriate modifications of Theraplay for trauma have been expanded in the third edition of the Theraplay text (Rubin, Lender, & Miller, 2010).

The Theraplay Model

Theraplay takes as its model the sensitive, responsive, playful give-and-take that occurs naturally between parents and their healthy young children— the kind of interaction that creates secure attachment, supports healthy brain development, and leads to long-term mental health. The goal is to develop regulation, social skills, positive internal working models for parents and child, and secure attachment through the emotional communication of reciprocal right-brain interaction.

History of Theraplay

Theraplay, developed in the early 1970s as a mental health treatment for preschoolers, has a history of meeting attachment needs before the term *attachment* was widely used and understood. In 1969, Ann Jernberg, a clinical psychologist, was awarded the contract to provide psychological services to the Head Start program in Chicago. In that first summer, our team identified a large number of children who needed help; we also found that there was little chance of meeting their needs within existing treatment centers. Jernberg came up with a simple solution for this problem: We would train lively young people to engage in one-on-one play with each troubled child. We had no toys, no games, and no play therapy tools. In each case, there was just an unhappy child and a lively adult who was prepared to pay full attention to the child and to entice him or her into interactive play.

We found that this kind of play worked magic. Soon, unhappy, withdrawn children become livelier, more outgoing, and more responsive; angry, aggressive, acting-out children settled down and began to interact appropriately with others. It was obvious that these children felt much better about themselves and were ready to engage with others in friendly interaction. They became lively, alert youngsters who did well in school (Jernberg, 1979; Jernberg & Booth, 1999).

John Bowlby's just-published theory of attachment (Bowlby, 1969/1982) offered us a partial explanation for our success: In his terms, we had changed the children's *internal working models*. Children learn about themselves and what they can expect from others in the repeated face-to-face experience of interaction with important adults in their world. The unhappy children we were working with came to us with negative views of themselves and fears that they couldn't count on a caring response from adults. By presenting such a child with a new experience of feeling safe and being responded to, admired, and enjoyed, a caring adult had created a new and more hopeful internal working model for that child.

Presently, mental health and education professionals in the United States and 37 other countries in a variety of settings practice Theraplay with children ranging in age from infancy to adolescence. Current best practice is described in the third edition of the Theraplay text (Booth & Jernberg, 2010). The Group Theraplay model was developed (Rubin & Tregay, 1989) and expanded and described in further publications (Munns, 2000, 2009). Sunshine Circles (Schieffer, 2012) is a classroom application for conveying the Theraplay principles of connection, cooperation, and socioemotional growth. Theraplay training and certification programs are administered by The Theraplay Institute (*www.theraplay.org*). In 2009, Theraplay was rated as demonstrating "promising research evidence" by the California Evidence-Based Clearinghouse for Child Welfare (2012). Its rating of 3 on a 5-point scale indicates that Theraplay meets the following standards: No empirical or theoretical evidence exists that Theraplay has a substantial risk of harming clients, as compared to its possible benefits; a manual is available; two peer-reviewed studies utilizing some form of control have been published (Siu, 2009; Wettig, Coleman, & Geider, 2011); and the outcome data support the benefits of Theraplay.

In addition, applications published since 2000 include Theraplay in residential care for youth with severe behavior problems (Robison, Lindaman, Clemmons, Doyle-Buckwalter, & Ryan, 2009), in a domestic violence shelter (Bennett, Shiner, & Ryan, 2006), in the Finnish SOS Village long-term fostering project (Mäkelä & Vierikko, 2004), with substance-abusing mothers (Salo, Lampi, & Lindaman, 2010), in adoption (Booth, 2000), and with children on the autism spectrum (Bundy-Myrow, 2012). The Theraplay model has been compared favorably to other parent–child interaction methods (Mäkelä & Salo, 2011). Combinations of Theraplay and other treatment modalities include Theraplay and dyadic developmental psychotherapy (DDP; Becker-Weidman & Schell, 2005), Theraplay and eye movement desensitization and reprocessing (EMDR; Gomez & Jernberg, 2013), and Theraplay and play therapy trauma treatment (Booth & Gil, 2011).

Dimensions of Theraplay

We turn now to describe the basic concepts of Theraplay and the research and theory that explain its effectiveness. We distinguish four basic dimensions of healthy parenting that we use to assess and to plan treatment, based on the specific needs of the parents and child: *structure, engagement, nurture,* and *challenge.*

Structure

Guidance and structure provide a sense of safety, organization, and regulation for both the child and the parents. We respond to the child's need for dyadic regulation of his or her experience, and for having an adult who can be counted on first to keep the child safe and later to set limits and provide a model for appropriate behavior. We structure simple, playful activities—such as blowing cotton balls back and forth, popping bubbles, and making a stack of hands together—using signals for when to start and variations in pacing and predictability to meet the child's need for regulation. We help parents (who may themselves be dysregulated) to experience the comfort of being guided in their interactions with their child, and in turn to learn to take the lead. In the case of neglect/trauma, establishing safety is particularly important. Many traumatized children exhibit controlling behavior, which comes from a need to be safe rather than from a need to be oppositional. We consider a young child's efforts to be prematurely autonomous and in charge of interactions to be a burden that the guided interaction of Theraplay can relieve.

SUPPORTING RESEARCH AND THEORY

The development of a healthy relationship requires the presence of a caring adult who can make the baby feel that this adult can provide safety, support, and guidance (Bowlby, 1988). Innate capacities exist in both parent and child to keep them close in order to be safe. If it were not so, babies could never survive (Bowlby, 1969/1982). During the first 2 years of life, repeated patterns of interaction create neural circuits and their corresponding internal working models of attachment relationships. As the child enters the second year of life, adult guidance and clear rules provide the foundation for self-regulation, resilience, and self-confidence (Baumrind, 1991; Grotberg, 1997). Rather than creating dependency, adult guidance and secure relationships are the foundation of self-reliance; "autonomy grows out of attachment" (Shahmoon-Shanok, 1997, p. 38).

In order to change the negative patterns of a child who has experienced relational trauma and to create mature neural circuits, it is necessary to provide a similarly direct, interactive, and sensitive emotional experience that challenges the old patterns and expectations (Hart, 2008; Schore, 2003).

New understanding of experience-dependent brain development and of the effects of neglect and trauma on the developing brain supports our focus on meeting the child's younger emotional needs, on finding ways to calm the dysregulated child, and on creating feelings of safety for the traumatized child (Perry, 2006; van der Kolk, 2005). Brain research places affect regulation at the center of healthy development (Schore, 1994).

Engagement

Engaging activities—such as peek-a-boo, clapping games, decorating each other with feathers, or "flying" the child on the adult's knees—create connection, optimal arousal, and shared joy. This playful, responsive interaction gives the child a new experience of his or her body and how to interact with others in a lively, coordinated manner. Theraplay treatment is geared to the child's current state of arousal and makes use of the nonverbal language of the right brain—facial expression, eye contact, movement, rhythm, and touch—to create the deep levels of neural integration that must be developed before it is possible to communicate on the mentalizing and narrative levels later on. We create "now moments" of intense connection and shared meaning, which lead to a major shift in internal organization and sense of self (Mäkelä, 2003; Tronick et al., 1998). We respond in an attuned and reflective manner to both the parent and child; in turn, we help the parent respond with synchrony and affective resonance to the child's readiness for interaction. If there has been relational trauma, the parent and child may never have experienced this joyful companionship. It is therefore particularly important that the therapist guide the parent in creating such experiences. In order to respond sensitively, parents must be able to reflect on their own and their children's internal states, and to understand the link between the children's behaviors and underlying mental states; parents who have little positive experience with emotional communication and connection in their own lives find this difficult to do (Fonagy, Gergely, Jurist, & Target, 2002; Slade, 2002).

SUPPORTING RESEARCH AND THEORY

When babies seek interaction and parents delight in the smiles and laughter they share with their children, a second innate capacity is demonstrated: the drive to share meaning and the joy of companionship. The process of *intersubjectivity* occurs in face-to-face human interaction resulting in a shared state of feelings and actions, making it possible for two people to synchronize their movements and to resonate with one another's feelings (Trevarthen & Aitken, 2001). In responding to a child, a sensitive parent attunes to the level and tone of the child's emotion, or "vitality affect" (Stern, 1985). An infant learns about his or her own feelings by seeing them mirrored in a parent's face (Winnicott, 1971). This sharing of emotional experience leads to empathy and a sense of connection (Stern, 1995). Mirror neurons also contribute to our understanding of the intentions of others (Iacoboni, 2008).

Stephen Porges's (2011) *polyvagal theory* provides insights into the way the human autonomic nervous system unconsciously mediates social engagement, trust, and intimacy. Well-defined neural circuits—particularly the vagal system, connecting facial, throat, heart, and stomach muscles involved in communication and emotional processing—support shared social engagement behaviors and the defensive strategies of fight, flight, or freeze. All of these capacities make it possible for babies and their responsive parents to establish an intimate, intersubjective experience in which they are present to each other and share meaning and companionship (Hughes, 2007; Siegel, 2006; Trevarthen & Aitken, 2001). Feeling safe, as discussed above in regard to the structure dimension, is essential to the activation of the social engagement system. Children who feel anxious and fearful do not readily enter into rhythm, resonance, and synchrony, and therefore find it difficult to understand the intentions of others and join in the interactive dance (Hart, 2008). Members of families who are not securely attached become hesitant to engage in intersubjective experience with one another because it does not feel safe or rewarding (Hughes, 2007).

Nurture

Nurturing experiences—such as caring for hurts, feeding, singing a lullaby, or making powder handprints—help calm and regulate the child and create feelings of self-worth. When adults respond empathically to a child's need for comfort and reassurance, they create a safe haven that is vital to the child's sense of being valued and protected. Touch is an essential ingredient in most nurturing experiences. We provide many opportunities for safe and appropriate therapist–child and parent–child physical contact and stimulation of all the senses. If a parent has difficulty touching a child gently, the therapist first demonstrates such touch with the child; next he or she practices with the parent; and finally the therapist guides the parent with the child. If a child or parent has experienced neglect or abuse, as Isaiah and his mother had, we introduce safe touch gradually and are very sensitive to both the parent's and the child's responses. Our goal is that they will be able to experience the benefits of healthy touch throughout their lives together.

SUPPORTING RESEARCH AND THEORY

Attachment research (Ainsworth, Blehar, Waters, & Wall, 1978) indicates that the sensitive, contingent responses of a caring parent are an important factor in the development of secure attachment. "Nurturing interactions form the basis of secure relationships" (Goldsmith, 2007, p. 211). Tender, comforting responses create an atmosphere of acceptance that helps the child feel that he or she has a safe haven to return to in times of stress. Touch is fundamental to human experience, first for survival and then for meaning (Brazelton, 1990). An infant requires the warmth of body contact to support the immature regulatory system. Touch and warmth raise the levels of the hormone oxytocin, which is calming to adult and child alike (Mäkelä, 2005). Human infants who are not touched and handled sufficiently at an early age may develop a distorted body image (Weiss, 1990). A large body of animal and human research supports the value of touch in stimulating development of premature infants (Field, 1995), creating the capacity to relate to others (Harlow, 1958), and reducing stress (Tronick, Ricks, & Cohn, 1982).

Challenge

Challenging activities—such as balancing on a stack of pillows, punching a newspaper, or keeping a balloon in the air—help a child experience feelings of competence, mastery, and playfulness. We choose the activities carefully so that the child can experience success. We also pay attention to the child's level of arousal, providing interludes of calm that regulate the experience. The child learns not only to expand his or her horizons, but to count on adults to be there when needed. Challenge activities are also used to respond to a child's resistance with acceptance and interest in the child's abilities. Attending to the appropriate level of challenge can help a parent who expects too much or too little from a child, or who finds it hard to focus on positive accomplishments. In working with a child who has experienced neglect or trauma, gentle, well-chosen challenge activities can help the child feel strong and free to act.

SUPPORTING RESEARCH AND THEORY

The lively, playful interaction between parents and their young children provides stimuli to all the senses. Tactile, vestibular, and proprioceptive systems are involved in the sense of self and the ability to interact in healthy ways with others (Williamson & Anzalone, 1997). The shared joy of interactive play creates a strong emotional bond and programs the brain to be fully social. Play episodes provide opportunities for affective synchrony and for co-regulation, which enhance the development of brain synapses (Hart, 2008). When the excitement of physically active play is co-regulated by an attuned caregiver, the child develops the capacity to regulate high states of arousal (Stern, 1974). As noted neuroscientist Jaak Panksepp (2009) suggests, "Any therapist who can capture the therapeutic moment in mutually shared play episodes will have brought the client to the gateway of happy living" (p. 17).

The Theraplay Treatment Process

The complexity of the family's needs in the case of Isaiah made the treatment process longer and involved more treatment segments than the typical Theraplay sequence. Over the course of treatment with this family, parts of the program described below were repeated with the different caregivers; other treatment modalities were added as needed. Theraplay treatment for children or parents with developmental problems may also be longer and involve other modalities.

Families experiencing mild to moderate difficulties in relationship and behavior typically participate in a series of 18–26 weekly sessions, with 2–4 follow-up sessions at quarterly intervals over the next year. The first session is an information-gathering interview with the parents. The second and third appointments are observation sessions using the Marschak Interaction Method (MIM; Theraplay Institute, 2011), in which the child and one parent perform a series of tasks together. The interactions are video-recorded and later analyzed by the therapist in preparation for a fourth session with the parents. In that session, the therapist and parents discuss their observations of the interaction and agree on a plan for treatment. In the fifth session, the therapist demonstrates Theraplay activities with the parent, and they discuss the purpose of the activities, the child's potential reactions, and the parent's reflections on the experience.

Sessions 6–25 involve direct Theraplay with the family, adapting to the child's developmental needs the kind of playful interactions that parents and young children naturally engage in together. The interaction includes structuring, engaging, nurturing, and challenging activities in combinations geared to the specific needs and problems of the individual child and family. The therapist and the parents meet after every third session without the child, to discuss progress and goals.

Parents observe all Theraplay sessions, and when they are ready, join in the activities with the therapist and child. The Theraplay model ideally involves two therapists—one who interacts with the child, and one who works with the parents. When two therapists are present, the parents' therapist observes with the parents and discusses the rationale for the activities (e.g., encouraging the development of trust and self-esteem, building a sense of self as lovable, developing confidence, permitting pleasurable experiences, encouraging intimacy, developing a positive body image, strengthening perceptual–motor coordination). This discussion includes ways in which the parents can implement these ideas at home. If only one therapist is involved, these discussions take place with the parents at the end of each session, by phone, or at a separately scheduled time.

The final treatment session ends with a goodbye party. The parent–child interaction assessment and any standardized tests are readministered and discussed with the parents to reflect on progress and make recommendations. Two to four follow-up sessions are scheduled with parents and child over the next 12 months.

Case Vignette: Theraplay in Isaiah's Journey Home

Additional Background

Child welfare first became involved with this family when Isaiah was 2 years old. The day care staff reported that they witnessed the mother repeatedly spanking Isaiah very hard on the bottom and aggressively flicking his mouth. The report was confirmed, and family preservation services were provided. For the next 4 years, the child welfare system received a number of reports related to the mother's behavior, but Isaiah stayed in the home until he was found looking for food in the garbage. At this point, the caseworker supported termination of parental rights and wrote that Isaiah had "no attachment" with his mother, Tonya. The case reports did not contain any reference to the biological mother's history in foster care as a victim of abuse and trauma.

Treatment with the Foster Family

The first step in Isaiah's journey was the Theraplay work with him and his foster parents.

Referral

The desperation in the voice of the foster mother, Cynthia, was clear as she described her struggles with Isaiah:

> "I have no idea what to do. I try to talk to him, and he covers his ears; I try to hug him, and he punches me; I give him gifts, and he breaks them on purpose; I ask him to be patient, and he pees all over my bed. He cries for his mama, so I let him call his mama; then he throws the phone on the floor and cusses at her, me, my husband, and anyone else around. I thought I could do this, but I'm not so sure. He acts the same way at school, and he has no friends. His teacher doesn't even like him. The caseworker says that this is normal, and it will stop, but I think Isaiah is in real trouble and I don't know how to help him. I don't know everything he's been through, but something has made him the way he is. Can you please, please, please help us?"

Assessment

I (Marlo Winstead) met with the foster parents, Cynthia and Kirk, for an intake interview. They were committed to doing their very best with Isaiah, but they felt completely unsupported by the child welfare system and very inadequate as caregivers. I administered a variety of child behavior scales and projective measures to learn about Isaiah. I also administered the MIM to learn more about Isaiah's healthy and unhealthy relational strategies.

He was easy to engage and enjoyed being playful. He exhibited anger and aggression during challenge and structure tasks, however, and he tried very hard both overtly and subtly to gain control of the tasks. During nurture tasks, he was ambivalent and fearful of receiving nurture, but wanted to care for his foster parents.

Theraplay with the Foster Mother and Child

Because the foster mother was the primary caregiver and the foster father was less available, I began Theraplay sessions with Isaiah and Cynthia in the foster home. The goals were to foster positive, relational, and experiential interactions that would result in shared joy and healing, while simultaneously targeting Isaiah's difficulty with adult direction (structure), his initial response of defeat when presented with a new activity (challenge), and his aversion to being cared for (nurture). I planned on incorporating Tonya, the biological mother, into treatment when she gained her visitation privileges.

As we see with many traumatized children, Isaiah was suspicious, easily dysregulated when touched, and hypervigilant. Similar to his presentation in the MIM, he was the most uncomfortable during tasks that focused on the dimensions of structure and nurture. Out of respect for his trauma history, I slowed down and made attunement my primary goal, reminding myself that I was seeking affective resonance, synchrony, and cooperation. I spoke in a clear, confident, and calm way and asked permission to make physical contact during our sessions. Cynthia was present during our first two sessions, observing and taking note of the successful and less successful techniques.

During Session 3, Cynthia watched as Isaiah bopped a balloon back and forth with me—first with his hands, and then, as I gradually increased the challenge, with his knees, feet, elbows, and head. Isaiah was initially reluctant, but my praise and encouragement helped him feel supported and confident in his ability to be the "best balloon bopper" ever. The success he experienced helped him to accept structure when Cynthia joined the session and decided which body part we would use to hit the balloon, and when the activity would start. Accepting Cynthia's direction and guidance during enjoyable activities increased the likelihood that Isaiah would accept her direction not only in sessions, but outside of sessions when they were not engaged in fun activities.

Little by little, Isaiah became more comfortable; he was less inhibited, he smiled a bit more, and he began to engage in playful ways. In Session 6, we had a "moment of meeting." Isaiah was feeling very confident after punching through three sheets of newspaper I was holding. Together we wadded the paper tightly into little balls to throw into the hoop I then made with my arms. I said, "When I say, 'Ready, set, go,' I want you to throw the ball into my arms. Ready . . . set . . . ," but before I said "go" he released the ball. In an accepting manner, I picked up the ball and said, "Wow, you have a great shot on 'set,' so let's see you throw the ball on 'set' this time.

Ready . . ." He threw the ball as hard as he could at my face, with a seeming intent for harm. I calmly picked up the ball, gently held his hand, and said, "We don't have any hurts when we're playing. I'm not for hurting, *and* I am not going to hurt you." Isaiah looked up and locked eyes with me. After intently scrutinizing me in a very no-nonsense, "I'm looking deep into your soul" kind of way, he said, "OK, then." It was as if we made a pact not to hurt one another. He seemed to absorb the fact that I was there to help him.

In Sessions 4–10, Cynthia started to participate actively in the Theraplay activities under my guidance and direction. She gradually moved from co-leading to leading activities like "blow me over, pull me up," copying each other's movements, and tracing shapes on Isaiah's back. My role became that of coach, teacher, and supporter, in order to focus the work on the relationship between Isaiah and Cynthia instead of me. Cautiously, Isaiah allowed himself to be vulnerable and accept Cynthia's structure and nurture. His maladaptive behaviors at home and school decreased, and positive behaviors (i.e., sharing and helping) took their place. Isaiah settled into the rituals of Theraplay, and looked forward to the sessions as well as to the Theraplay "homework" that Cynthia was doing with him between our sessions.

Sessions 10–14 proved to be difficult for Isaiah because of out-of-session changes in his life. Since his biological mother, Tonya, was getting stronger, completing her service plan, and maintaining sobriety, Isaiah began weekly 2-hour supervised visits with her. It seemed that Isaiah's tumultuous and traumatic early years with her made it difficult for him to believe that she was actually "better." Isaiah wanted to see his mother but was defiant, oppositional, and aggressive during the visits; she was very hurt and discouraged. In the sessions with the foster mother, I added DDP (Hughes, 2007) techniques into our Theraplay sessions, to provide a safe space to process the mixed emotions Isaiah was feeling toward his mother; he wanted to be with her and hoped for her to love him, but he was also distrustful, hurt, and angry because of her actions in the past. The foster mother continued to provide comfort and care in the difficult moments both in therapy and outside of sessions. With the biological mother's visitation granted, and the continued goal of reunification, it was time to transfer the work of strengthening relationships and increasing capacity for attachment to Tonya and Isaiah.

Theraplay with Both the Foster and Biological Mothers and the Child

An MIM between Isaiah and Tonya revealed Tonya's desire to be in relationship with Isaiah, and her commitment to using the new parenting skills she was learning. Isaiah engaged with Tonya for fleeting moments throughout the assessment, but he was very controlling and did not respond to her attempts to structure or nurture him. During the MIM feedback session with Tonya, she shared her own history of relational trauma, which included physical and sexual abuse, foster care, and numerous romantic relationships in which she was the victim of domestic violence. Before including Tonya in Theraplay sessions, I spent time connecting with her through providing education and support in regard to her history and how it was informing her parenting.

Sessions 15–18 included both Tonya and Cynthia, in order to help everyone make the transition and to generalize the growth, development, and acquisition of skills to Isaiah's "new" relationship with Tonya. Isaiah initially regressed to mild resistance, dysregulation, and hypersensitivity to touch. I attuned closely to his verbal and especially to his nonverbal signals, and worked hard to support everyone. It was both confusing and helpful for Isaiah to see his mother and foster mother endorse each other and work together. Over time, the content of the sessions implicitly gave him permission to love and care about both of them without feeling that he was betraying one or the other. The continued integration of DDP techniques gave Isaiah explicit permission to care about and to be cared for by both women.

The primary goal was attunement and affective resonance among all members of the session. At one point, Cynthia hid a dot of powder on Isaiah's elbow, and Tonya found and rubbed it in. This simple activity led to natural giggles and shared smiles that demonstrated cooperation among the three, trust as Isaiah's muscles relaxed when his eyes were closed, and progress with Isaiah's capacity for accepting nurture and Cynthia's provision of nurture in a healthy and safe way. It was a bittersweet session when Cynthia finally made the transition out of the therapeutic work. Isaiah and Tonya both missed Cynthia's presence, but after this, Tonya seemed to come out of her shell and was more confident in her participation.

Theraplay and Other Treatment with the Biological Mother and the Child

Over the next 8 months, treatment included Theraplay sessions as well as DDP (Hughes, 2007) techniques as described above, EMDR (Lovett, 2007), sandtray therapy (Homeyer & Sweeney, 2010), and projection through narrative work with puppets (Johnson & Clark, 2001). Outside of sessions, Tonya vacillated between her old methods of interaction (i.e., shouting, spanking, harsh discipline, unrealistic expectations, and rejecting behavior) and the new skills and strategies she was learning. She sometimes reported feeling hopeless because her "case" lingered on in the child welfare system, but she gradually became more powerful and competent to raise her child with new ideas and a fresh outlook.

Theraplay Session: Saying Goodbye to the Foster Parents

Seventeen months after placement and more than 65 therapy sessions later, Isaiah was going home, but not before experiencing a very healthy goodbye with his foster parents. Opportunities to honor the time spent with Cynthia and Kirk were maximized throughout the session. After measuring Isaiah's growth since coming into foster care by measuring his hands and feet with crepe paper strips, we made a "circle of love" out of a long strip of paper to provide a visual image of the relationship shared with his foster parents. I used a teddy bear as my foster son, "Ralph," who visited and shared his story (Johnson & Clark, 2001). This technique resonated on a very deep level, but also created sufficient psychological distance and safety for Isaiah. Questions such as "If you love me, why am I moving?", "Did I do something bad, and is that why I am moving?", and "Will you still love me?" were answered. At the close of a difficult session, Isaiah received lots of nurture, a shared snack, a story (*I Love You Through and Through*; Rossetti-Shustak, 2005), and a special song ("Twinkle Twinkle Little Star, what a special boy you are . . ."; Booth & Jernberg, 2010, p. 538). The message of a deep, warm, genuine, and sincere desire for relationship was conveyed through laughter, shared joy, acceptance, attuned and positive interactions—and tears. The foster parents allowed themselves to be vulnerable, which was not surprising, but Isaiah mirrored that vulnerability and did not use his unhealthy adaptive strategies to avoid or dismiss his feelings.

Outcome

Tonya was able to overcome innumerable hurdles from her past and her present in order to bring her child home; it took almost 2 years of hard work, which included a total of approximately 100 therapy sessions. There are still areas of growth for Tonya, but she has captured the essence of Theraplay within her parenting. She truly "sees" Isaiah for who he is, and her level of acceptance has significantly increased. Tonya no longer employs physical punishment; her capacity for providing nurture has improved; and as a result, she has more success in helping her son regulate his affective, emotional, and physical states. Isaiah's aggressive outbursts decreased significantly while his verbalization of feelings increased. He accepted structure and nurturing from his mother similar to other children his age, and he started taking risks, like trying out for a basketball team. For Isaiah, Theraplay provided an opportunity to experience the depth of love that his mother felt for him and to start to heal the deep wounds of neglect and abuse.

Conclusion

In this chapter, we have presented a vignette illustrating the use of Theraplay as a major part of the treatment for a young boy and his mother, both of whom had suffered relational trauma. The attachment-based approach provided a forum for relational repair and healing, as well as the necessary guidance and support to enter into the hard work of mending wounds and rebuilding trust.

The therapeutic journey with this family included the following steps:

- Helping the child form a safe connection with his foster parents, in order to reduce his violent behavior and prepare him to be open to a healing experience with his biological mother.
- Creating a safe and supportive experience for the biological mother, in which she could begin to reflect on her own feelings and those of her son.
- Giving the biological mother an opportunity to work together with the foster mother, so that she could benefit from her experience, use her support to understand her child's needs, and gain confidence in her own ability to respond appropriately.
- Collaboratively creating a well-planned transition for this child from the foster home back to living with his mother.

AUTHORS' NOTE

We dedicate this chapter to the case vignette families (foster and biological), all families in the child welfare system, all foster parents, and especially to our colleague Mary Pat Clemmons, LCSW, who died in 2012 while writing her doctoral dissertation about Theraplay and reunification. Her passion for her clients and for life continues to inspire us.

REFERENCES

Ainsworth, M. D. S., Blehar, M. C., Waters, E., & Wall, S. (1978). *Patterns of attachment: A psychological study of the Strange Situation.* Hillsdale, NJ: Erlbaum.

Baumrind, D. (1991). The influence of parenting style on adolescent competence and substance use. *Journal of Early Adolescence, 11*(1), 56–95.

Becker-Weidman, A., & Schell, D. (2005). *Creating capacity for attachment: Dyadic developmental psychotherapy in the treatment of trauma–attachment disorders.* Oklahoma City, OK: Wood'N'Barnes.

Bennett, L. R., Shiner, S. K., & Ryan, S. (2006). Using Theraplay in shelter settings with mothers and children who have experienced violence in the home. *Journal of Psychosocial Nursing and Mental Health Service, 44*(10), 38–47.

Booth, P. (2000). Forming an attachment with an adopted toddler using the Theraplay approach. *The Signal: Newsletter of the World Association for Infant Mental Health, 8*(3), 1–9.

Booth, P., & Gil, E. (2011). *Integrating Theraplay techniques into trauma treatment.* Paper presented at the 28th Annual International Play Therapy Conference, Sacramento, CA.

Booth, P., & Jernberg, A. (2010). *Theraplay: Helping parents and children build better relationships through attachment-based play* (3rd ed.). San Francisco: Jossey-Bass.

Bowlby, J. (1982). *Attachment and loss: Vol. 1. Attachment.* New York: Basic Books. (Original work published 1969)

Bowlby, J. (1988). *A secure base: Parent–child attachment and healthy human development.* New York: Basic Books.

Brazelton, T. B. (1990). Touch as a touchstone: Summary of the round table. In K. E. Barnard & T. B. Brazelton (Eds.), *Touch: The foundation of experience* (pp. 561–566). Madison, CT: International Universities Press.

Bundy-Myrow, S. (2012). Family Theraplay: Connecting with children on the autism spectrum. In L. Gallo-Lopez & L. C. Rubin (Eds.), *Play-based interventions for children and adolescents with autism spectrum disorders* (pp. 73–96). New York: Routledge.

California Evidence-Based Clearinghouse for Child Welfare. (2012). *Theraplay.* Retrieved from *www.cebc4cw.org/program/-2*

Cook, A., Blaustein, M., Spinazzola, J., & van der Kolk, B. (Eds.). (2003). *Complex trauma in children and adolescents: White paper from the National Child Traumatic Stress Network.* Retrieved from *www.nctsnet.org/nctsn_assets/pdfs/edu_materials/ComplexTrauma_All.pdf*

Field, T. (1995). *Touch in early development.* Mahwah, NJ: Erlbaum.

Fonagy, P., Gergely, G., Jurist, E. L., & Target, M. (2002). *Affect regulation, mentalization, and the development of the self.* New York: Other Press.

Goldsmith, D. F. (2007). Challenging children's negative internal working models: Utilizing attachment-based treatment strategies in a therapeutic preschool. In D. Oppenheim & D. F. Goldsmith (Eds.), *Attachment theory in clinical work with children* (pp. 203–225). New York: Guilford Press.

Gomez, A. M., & Jernberg, E. (2013). Using EMDR therapy and Theraplay. In A. M. Gomez, *EMDR therapy and adjunct approaches with children* (pp. 273–297). New York: Springer.

Grotberg, E. H. (1997). The International Resilience Project: Findings from the research and the effectiveness of interventions. In B. Bain (Ed.), *Psychology and education in the 21st century: Proceedings of the 54th Annual Convention of the International Council of Psychologists* (pp. 118–128). Edmonton, Alberta, Canada: IC Press.

Harlow, H. F. (1958). The nature of love. *American Psychologist, 13,* 673–685.

Hart, S. (2008). *Brain, attachment, personality: An introduction to neuroaffective development.* London: Karnac Books.

Homeyer, L. E., & Sweeney, D. S. (2010). *Sandtray: A practical manual* (2nd ed.). New York: Routledge.

Hughes, D. A. (2007). *Attachment-focused family therapy.* New York: Norton.

Iacoboni, M. (2008). *Mirroring people: The science of empathy and how we connect with others.* New York: Farrar, Straus & Giroux.

Jernberg, A. (1979). *Theraplay: A new treatment using structured play for problem children and their families.* San Francisco: Jossey-Bass.

Jernberg, A., & Booth, P. (1999). *Theraplay: Helping parents and children build better relationships through attachment-based play* (2nd ed.). San Francisco: Jossey-Bass.

Johnson, S. P., & Clark, P. (2001). Play therapy with aggressive acting-out children.

In G. Landreth (Ed.), *Innovations in play therapy: Issues, process, and special populations* (pp. 239–256). Philadelphia: Brunner-Routledge.

Lovett, J. (2007). *Small wonders: Healing childhood trauma with EMDR*. New York: Free Press.

Mäkelä, J. (2003, Fall–Winter). What makes Theraplay effective: Insights from developmental sciences. *Theraplay Institute Newsletter*, pp. 9–11.

Mäkelä, J. (2005). Kosketuksen merkitys lapsen kehityksessä [The importance of touch in the development of children]. *Finnish Medical Journal, 60*, 1543–1549.

Mäkelä, J., & Salo, S. (2011). Theraplay—vanhemman ja lapsen välinen vuorovaikutushoito lasten mielenterveysongelmissa [Theraplay—Parent–child interaction treatment for children with mental health problems]. *Duodecim, 127*, 29–39.

Mäkelä, J., & Vierikko, I. (2004). *From heart to heart: Interactive therapy for children in care. Report on the Theraplay Project in SOS Children's Villages in Finland 2001–2004*. Espoo, Finland: SOS Villages Finland Association.

Munns, E. (Ed.). (2000). *Theraplay: Innovations in attachment-enhancing play therapy*. Northvale, NJ: Aronson.

Munns, E. (Ed.). (2009). *Applications of family and group Theraplay*. Lanham, MD: Aronson.

Panksepp, J. (2009). Brain emotional systems and qualities of mental life: From animal models of affect to implications for psychotherapeutics. In D. Fosha, D. J. Siegel, & M. F. Solomon (Eds.), *The healing power of emotion: Affective neuroscience, development & clinical practice* (pp. 1–26). New York: Norton.

Perry, B. D. (2006). Applying principles of neurodevelopment to clinical work with maltreated and traumatized children: The neurosequential model of therapeutics. In N. B. Webb (Ed.), *Working with traumatized youth in child welfare* (pp. 27–52). New York: Guilford Press.

Porges, S. W. (2011). *The polyvagal theory: Neuropsycholgical foundations of emotions, attachment, communication and self-regulation*. New York: Norton.

Robison, M., Lindaman, S., Clemmons, M. P., Doyle-Buckwalter, K., & Ryan, M. (2009). "I deserve a family": The evolution of an adolescent's behavior and beliefs about himself and others when treated with Theraplay in residential care. *Child and Adolescent Social Work Journal, 26*(4), 291–306.

Rossetti-Shustak, B. (2005). *I love you through and through*. New York: Cartwheel.

Rubin, P., Lender, D., & Miller, J. (2010). Theraplay for children with histories of complex trauma. In P. Booth & A. Jernberg, *Theraplay: Helping parents and children build better relationships through attachment-based play* (3rd ed., pp. 359–403). San Francisco: Jossey-Bass.

Rubin, P., & Tregay, J. (1989). *Play with them—Theraplay groups in the classroom: A technique for professionals who work with children*. Springfield, IL: Thomas.

Salo, S., Lampi, H., & Lindaman, S. (2010). Use of the Emotional Availability Scales to evaluate an attachment-based intervention—Theraplay—in substance abusing mother–infant dyads in Finland. *Infant Mental Health Journal (Supplement), 32*, 77.

Schieffer, K. (2012). *Sunshine Circles(r): Interactive playgroups for social skills development and classroom management.* Evanston, IL: Theraplay Institute.

Schore, A. N. (1994). *Affect regulation and the origin of the self: The neurobiology of emotional development.* Hillside, NJ: Erlbaum.

Schore, A. N. (2001). The effects of early relational trauma on right brain development, affect regulation, and infant mental health. *Infant Mental Health Journal, 22*(1–2), 201–269.

Schore, A. N. (2003). Early relational trauma, disorganized attachment, and the development of a predisposition to violence. In M. F. Solomon & D. J. Siegel (Eds.), *Healing trauma* (pp. 107–167). New York: Norton.

Schore, J. R., & Schore, A. N. (2008). Modern attachment theory: The central role of affect regulation in development and treatment. *Clinical Social Work Journal, 36,* 9–20.

Shahmoon-Shanok, R. (1997). Giving back future's promise: Working resourcefully with parents of children who have severe disorders of relating and communicating. *Zero to Three, 17*(5), 37–48.

Siegel, D. J. (2006). An interpersonal neurobiology approach to psychotherapy. *Psychiatric Annals, 36*(4), 248–256.

Siegel, D. J. (2012). *The developing mind: How relationships and the brain interact to shape who we are* (2nd ed.). New York: Guilford Press.

Siu, A. F. Y. (2009). Theraplay in the Chinese world: An intervention program for Hong Kong children with internalizing problems. *International Journal of Play Therapy, 18*(1), 1–12.

Slade, A. (2002). Keeping the baby in mind: A critical factor in perinatal mental health. *Zero to Three, 22*(6), 10–16.

Stern, D. N. (1974). The goal and structure of mother–infant play. *Journal of the American Academy of Child Psychiatry, 13*(3), 402–421.

Stern, D. N. (1985). *The interpersonal world of the infant: A view from psychoanalysis and developmental psychology.* New York: Basic Books.

Stern, D. N. (1995). *The motherhood constellation: A unified view of parent–infant psychotherapy.* New York: Basic Books.

Theraplay Institute. (2003). *Marschak Interaction Method (MIM): Manual and cards* (3rd ed.). Chicago: Author.

Trevarthen, C., & Aitken, K. J. (2001). Infant intersubjectivity: Research, theory, and clinical applications. *Journal of Child Psychology and Psychiatry, 42*(1), 3–48.

Tronick, E. Z., Bruschweiler-Stern, N., Harrison, A. M., Lyons-Ruth, K., Morgan, A. C., Nahum, J. P., . . . Stern, D. N. (1998). Dyadically expanded states of consciousness and the process of therapeutic change. *Infant Mental Health Journal, 19*(3), 290–299.

Tronick, E. Z., Ricks, M., & Cohn, J. F. (1982). Maternal and infant affective exchange: Patterns of adaptation. In T. Field & A. Fogel (Eds.), *Emotion and early interaction* (pp. 83–100). Hillside, NJ: Erlbaum.

van der Kolk, B. (2005). Developmental trauma disorder: Towards a rational diagnosis for children with complex trauma histories. *Psychiatric Annals, 35,* 401–408.

Weiss, S. J. (1990). Parental touching correlates of a child's body concept and body sentiment. In K. E. Barnard & T. B. Brazelton (Eds.), *Touch: The foundation of experience* (pp. 425–432). Madison, CT: International Universities Press.

Wettig, H. G., Coleman, A. R., & Geider, F. J. (2011). Evaluating the effectiveness of Theraplay in treating shy, socially withdrawn children. *International Journal of Play Therapy, 20*(1), 26–37.

Williamson, G. G., & Anzalone, M. (1997). Sensory integration: A key component of the evaluation and treatment of young children with severe difficulties in relating and communicating. *Zero to Three, 17*(5), 29–36.

Winnicott, D. W. (1971). *Playing and reality.* London: Tavistock.

CHAPTER 10

The Creative Use of Metaphor in Play and Art Therapy with Attachment Problems

Eliana Gil

Many practitioners have long regarded metaphor as a pivotal and central focal point in therapy. Specifically, clinical interest persists in the manner in which clinical metaphor takes center stage, and therapists listen for, invite, or explore metaphor in order to assist clients toward positive therapeutic gains. Play and art therapists consider metaphor work a natural part of their field of study. These expressive therapists have a profound recognition of the importance of clients' having the emotional distance and the inherent safety that they can enjoy as a result of having something stand in the place of something else. In addition, play and art therapists are taught to "stay with" the metaphors created, rather than making jarring verbal interpretations of similarities between the metaphors and real life.

This chapter discusses and presents various ways of working with metaphors—both inviting and responding to clinical material highlighted in metaphorical language or images. Metaphor work is likely to be helpful with any client, but I focus on the use of metaphor to enhance parent–child attachment in dyads where such attachment is confused, hurtful, or ambivalent. These situations can occur because of parental inability or unwillingness to provide consistent and empathic care or children's compromised receptivity.

Defining *Metaphor*

Metaphor is defined in different ways, but common ground exists among these definitions. It is usually considered something that is used to represent something else, a symbol. The word comes from the Greek word *metapherein*, which means "to carry over" or "to transfer." A symbol can be broadly understood as a representation, a mark, a pictogram, or a sign. Symbols can be toys, images in art, or physical signs such as a peace sign, but they can also be conveyed through language, and this happens often. Consider how often we hear terms such as "I'm running on half-empty," or "My cup runneth over," or "His boat hasn't docked yet." Our language is rich with metaphors that are used as shorthand for other, more complex concepts.

My adult client Doug started talking to me about what was going on in his life, and as he did so his affect became flat and his words sing-song and monotonous, to say nothing of vague. I felt disconnected from him, as if he were trying to "keep a lid" on what was really bothering him. At one point, he said, "The clearest way I can describe it is that I feel like I'm sinking in quicksand." Now I felt immediately connected, because his metaphor captured his sense of desolation, despair, and urgency completely. Metaphors often present the listener with a mental picture of something conceptual that resonates on a deeper level.

The clinical use of metaphor has been widely discussed. It probably gained its greatest visibility with the brilliant work of Milton Erickson (Erickson & Rossi, 1979), who is credited with inspiring hundreds of clinicians to place their trust in the innate value of metaphors, created by clients and clinicians alike. Erickson earned great reverence through his brilliant use of metaphors with clients, who, he felt, could create their own meaning. He felt that in this way, clients would learn lessons that might otherwise be too painful for their conscious minds to tolerate; he believed that the stories could get in "sideways," while more direct interventions might be denied entry. Erickson was truly a master at creating provocative, insightful, and powerful metaphors that his clients listened for intently and that are still remembered in the clinical community (Lankton, 2004). In the play therapy field, these traditions have been well continued by Joyce Mills (*www.drjoycemills.com*) and Nancy Davis (1990).

Esparza (2012) describes therapeutic metaphors as among the most elegant tools for assisting people in the process of personal transformation and growth. He further describes them as communicating from and with the subconscious mind, bypassing the critical faculties of the conscious mind. In therapy, a metaphor can represent a client's problem and often provides up a solution to the problem in an indirect way. My client Doug, for example, in presenting the "sinking in quicksand" metaphor, had to address whether to allow himself to "sink" or whether to gather resources for the fight to get out. Ricoeur (1967) states that metaphors work as an intermediary element between the languages of logic and of emotion, imagination, and affection.

Onnis et al. (2007) state that "The metaphor, because of its 'evocative' and not explicative power has the advantage [of] allud[ing] to the preverbal and unconscious level, without pretending to make it explicit; in this way on the one side it can elude some defensive mechanism, [and] on the other side it opens spaces for a more free and 'creative' translation by [whoever] receives it" (p. 2). Guiffrida, Jordan, Saiz, and Barnes (2007) encourage clinical use of metaphors because they can promote several therapeutic functions, including relationship building with clients, accessing and symbolizing emotions, uncovering and challenging clients' tacit assumptions, and introducing new frames of reference. Surely these functions greatly increase clients' receptivity to clinical interventions. Esparza (2012) finds therapeutic stories useful in that they can stimulate creativity (energy); they can illustrate points; they can open up possibilities; they can introduce doubt in the mind of a client who sees a position in only one way; and they can suggest options and possibilities.

Child Maltreatment and Attachment

The topics of child maltreatment and its effects on attachment are addressed throughout this book. For purposes of this chapter, it is important to emphasize that early disruptive, violent, or neglectful parental interactions will create internal working models that have far-reaching implications for young children. Specifically, children seem to learn the lesson that "people who love you will hurt you, reject you, or want sexual contact with you," and thus their efforts to get their needs met for affection, attention, protection, or nurturance are confused and compromised. These issues are exhibited whenever children interact with others—and given the intimate nature of the therapist–child relationship, they seem to be activated particularly strongly in the therapy process.

Case Vignette: Christine and Sarah

The case of Christine and her mother, Sarah, illustrates clinical work with metaphors.

Background

Christine was referred for treatment after having been placed in foster care a year earlier, at the age of 4. When she was removed from her mother, Sarah, 24, she had many signs of physical abuse at the hands of her aggressive father, Mike.

Christine was interviewed by a child protective services worker in tandem with a juvenile police officer, and she refused to respond to any questions. The officers had more luck with her mother, who, upon hearing the extent of Christine's injuries, told them about Mike's alcohol/drug abuse and what sounded like a classic history of domestic violence, including both physical and emotional abuse of Sarah and Christine. Sarah insisted that she had gone to great lengths to protect her daughter—locking her in the closet when Mike was drinking or using drugs, and telling her to run next door when Mike was beyond her control. She also talked about long hours of huddling together in the closet, waiting out Mike's explosive tirades. Sarah was under the impression that if Christine did not *see* her mother being beaten, she would be spared any emotional distress. Little did Sarah know that young children are seriously affected by a climate of fear and anxiety, by listening to their parents being beaten, and most definitely by being hidden or shoved out the door by their parents. In addition, Sarah was surprised to learn that children experience a unique type of distress at seeing their parents unable to protect themselves, and guilt at their own inability to help them.

When Christine was taken into the county's custody and was placed in foster care, Sarah fell into a deep depression and became homeless; without her daughter, she temporarily lost her will to live. But Sarah was a true survivor. In her shelter for the homeless, she was receptive to kind guidance from a social worker, and slowly but surely she revealed a predictable history of her own witnessing of violence and chaos when she was a child. She had run away from home after being sexually abused by one of her mother's boyfriends, and had never looked back.

Sarah met Mike at a dance club when she was 17, and she became pregnant almost immediately. She hinted that their first sexual encounter was not consensual and that he moved in immediately after meeting her. She noted that he acquired large quantities of money sporadically, and Sarah soon discovered that he sold drugs. Mike moved Sarah's roommate out quickly and was emotionally abusive from the start, but Sarah's first beating occurred when the baby was about 3 weeks old and she could not quiet her. Mike was intolerant of the child's screaming from the beginning, and he would take his anger out on Sarah. Sarah described her relationship to Mike as "weird," adding, "I don't think we ever liked each other."

After the unpredictable and violent environment with Mike, the shelter provided Sarah with a deep sense of relief. She would later tell me, "I woke up in the morning and knew it would be a good day. I would work hard to get back my daughter, and now I believed that it was possible for me to work for things I wanted. I felt like a fog was lifted and I could make decisions for myself." Her life had taken a wrong turn when she was young and vulnerable. Mike was 18 years older than she was, and he was obviously very self-involved, impulsive, and dangerous. He had held her captive for years, and once Sarah was born, she too was exposed to a chaotic and unsafe existence. Sarah consistently stated that she loved Christine and would do whatever it took to get her back. She had a lot of obstacles to overcome in order to achieve this goal: She had to get a job, find a place to live, and show some kind of stability in her life. Her motivation was palpable, however, and it was as if she was positioned to make a significant growth spurt in her emotional maturity. My job was to help Sarah and Christine establish a warm and safe attachment with each other, since their attachment had been so deeply disrupted from the outset.

Just as Sarah was thriving in a safe environment, Christine had made a positive attachment to her new foster parents, Dan and Gerttie. Although I was grateful that Christine was feeling secure, I recognized the challenges of divided loyalties for her, so I quickly asked Gerttie to encourage Christine to call her "Gerttie" rather than "Mom," and to remind Christine about her mom, Sarah, whenever she could. Gerttie had already tried to correct her foster child when Christine called her "Mom," and Christine's compromise was to call her "Grandma Gerttie," which several of Gerttie's grandchildren called her as well.

Dan and Gerttie were in their 50s; they were grandparents to a number of young children and excellent caregivers. They had been married during their first year in college. They were quiet and warm individuals, and they chose to be foster parents to give back some of their good fortune. Their children were either in college or married, and they had decided together that they could offer a good temporary home to a child in need. Christine was the third foster child they had taken into their home.

They described a frightened, shy, anxious child when Christine first arrived at their home. She still had some physical injuries that needed tending and rest. Gerttie settled Christine into her oldest daughter's room, which had a canopy bed, a small vanity table, pictures of puppies and kittens, and a beautiful night light that made stars on the ceiling and had soft music playing. Gerttie stayed with Christine all night the first few nights so that the child could rest. Christine kept asking for her mother and wondered whether Sarah had died. Gerttie reassured her and tried to make her comfortable. Once in the first week when Gerttie came to see her in the morning, Christine was under the bed and appeared cold and shaking. Her eyes were open, and she was sucking her fingers. Gerttie was concerned about Christine and made an investment of time and attention to ensure her adjustment to her new home. Gerttie didn't know that Christine had often slept in a closet, that she had never had a room of her own, and that her sleep was often interrupted by violent outbursts from Mike or Mike's friends. Sarah also volunteered that her own fears and worries caused her to be "nervous and worried" all the time, and thus she did not eat or sleep well herself.

It took Gerttie a full 2 months to get Christine settled into her new environment. After that, Christine followed her around the house, wanted to hold her hand, and called her "Mommy" despite Gerttie's encouragement to do otherwise. She still asked after her own mother, continually asking whether Sarah was dead. She was allowed to see her mother after 3 months, once Sarah was back on her feet emotionally. Sarah was anxious to see her daughter and was surprised to see Christine shy away from her and cling to Gerttie when she first saw her. This caused Sarah to cry and be sad, at which point Christine would no longer look at her. The social worker had tried to prepare Sarah for a wide array of possible responses in Christine, and although she had heard that sometimes children take a while to warm up, she was also shocked and disheartened by Christine's clinginess to her foster mother.

Christine Comes to Therapy

The presenting concerns of the social worker were Christine's anxiety, clinginess, and ambivalence toward her mother. In addition, Gerttie wanted guidance about how to prepare Christine for supervised visits, and how to help Christine when she became dysregulated after visiting with her mother. These visits had just begun, but they seemed to destabilize Christine.

When she arrived for her first therapy session, Christine sat in Gerttie's lap and looked away when I said hello. She seemed acutely anxious, but she appeared to relax a little when I told her that she and Gerttie could both come into my play therapy office. I told her there might be some things in my room that she would like. I showed Gerttie and Christine around, saying that I wasn't sure what she would like to play with, but she could look around and decide what to do. For the first four meetings, Christine stayed in Gerttie's lap while Gerttie and I sat together and played with different toys, hoping to interest Christine, who seemed a comfortable fixture in this warm foster parent's lap. I noticed a glimmer of interest in Christine as Gerttie and I played with a baby girl doll, fed her a baby bottle, and changed her diapers. At the end of this session, I decided to put the doll, diapers, and baby bottle in a bag; I told Christine that I wanted her to take the doll home this week, play with her, take good care of her, and bring her back the following session. Slowly but surely, this technique began to yield results as Christine became more and more comfortable in the play therapy office and with me. I asked Gerttie to begin to give Christine opportunities to tolerate more and more time without her, so Gerttie would take longer and longer bathroom breaks during the sessions. When she returned to the office, she would sit on a couch and be present while Christine and I played together. Eventually Christine began to enter the play therapy office easily by herself, although she would sometimes go to the door, open it, and make sure that Gerttie was still waiting for her in the waiting room.

Sandtray Scenario: **Up a Tree without a Ladder**

Christine had liked the feel of the sand in the sandtray from about the 10th session forward. She put her little fingers in the sand with great hesitation at first, but when Gerttie covered her own hand and asked Christine to find it, Christine finally smiled a little as she uncovered Gerttie's hand. This session (about 3 months into therapy) was the first time Christine put miniature objects in the tray. The metaphor she created became pivotal to our understanding of her perceptions of her life, and it also provided us with a way of helping her with her current ambivalence about her mother.

As shown in Figure 10.1, Christine placed a large, sturdy tree in the center of the tray. This tree had a cavity on the bottom, and she filled that cavity with a porcupine. She then placed a mother and a baby deer in the branches, high inside the tree. Behind the tree, she placed a very large and sturdy house on the right side. On the left side of the tray, she placed a structure that appeared to be a rock formation (the sort of thing that usually goes inside fish tanks) and had openings in several places. There was a dolphin in the corner. She also placed another tree in the front, on the left side. Finally, she placed a small cat in front of the sturdy house, and the cat was turning its head and looking forward. She then spent time making little uplifts in the sand with her small hands—sometimes patting the sand

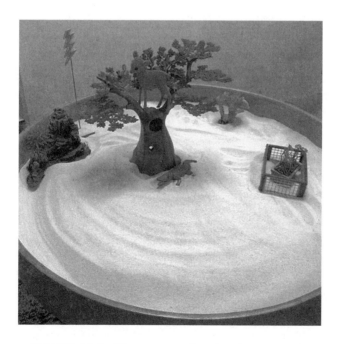

FIGURE 10.1. The quiet mother deer keeps guard.

down, at other times lifting it ever so slightly. She seemed very engaged in the process of creating the sandtray scenario, and she did not speak throughout. I sat facing her, but far enough away that I was not intruding. She looked up frequently to see what I was doing, and she saw me looking patiently at her tray.

Christine did not speak throughout this process, but we had long since broken silence in general and become comfortable with each other. Up to this point, though, Christine had not volunteered very much information except about her present-day activities: where she had gone on the weekend, how her cat was purring and hissing at her foster home, how she and her next-door neighbor were learning to ride bikes, and so forth. Sometimes I would ask whether she'd seen her mom, Sarah, and she would nod her head but offer nothing more. In the second session, we had started doing some work on affect identification, and she was able to point to feelings she had at different times (we used a poster with faces showing different emotions). Gerttie had led the way, pointing to how she was feeling at the moment or how she had felt at different situations. We first engaged Christine in show-ing us how she thought the baby doll was feeling, and later how she herself was feeling about different things. Eventually Christine was able to correct Gerttie and specify how she was feeling; later on, she could also say what size each feeling was, using a worksheet that shows feelings in smaller or bigger circles (Gil, 2013).

After Christine finished her sandtray, she stood up, and so did I. I walked around the sandtray, encouraging her to see it from different angles, and she followed me around the tray. I said, "The sandtray looks different from different sides." She stood at each of the four sides of the wooden box and stared at what she had made. I waited for spontaneous communica-tion, but none happened. I asked her whether I could take a picture, and she agreed; she also wanted me to take a picture of her "holding it," with her arms thrown around the box. I took both pictures and gave her copies at our next meeting (these days, I send the .jpg files via email when kids ask for copies).

Given this child's usual withdrawal, and her anxiety and ambivalence, I decided to keep the sandtray intact and rolled it into another room. I had another sandtray in the room that other children could use during the week. By the time Christine returned for her next session, I would have processed the metaphor and prepared myself to invite her to "work the metaphor" with me—but I knew much would depend on how Christine reacted when she came into the office and found that her sandtray was intact and waiting for her.

My basic approach to "working the metaphor" is to consider it an externalization of very important and relevant material that cannot yet be addressed directly. In other words, I consider that if a client could tell me his or her problem explicitly, the client would do so. The metaphor is a way to tell without talking, and it is equally important that the client is telling him- or herself in tandem with telling someone who serves as an unconditional witness. Thus my exploration of the client's metaphor is done gingerly, in complete recognition of the trust that has been placed in me.

In order to prepare for engaging children in metaphor work, I first allow myself to spend time with the work that has been produced in therapy. When the work is a sandtray scenario, this means spending time taking in "the life of the tray"—looking at a photo, transcribing dialogues, whatever it takes to properly chronicle the therapy work of the client. In this particular situation, I sat in front of the tray after Christine had left (luckily, my next appointment was canceled, so I had ample time for reflection). I allowed myself to make free associations as I looked at the objects in the tray; I identified *points of entry* (target spots that aroused my curiosity); and I wrote down about six to eight pithy questions for three entry points. I also wrote comments and observations about the child's process in making the tray, as well as the content presented, and I crafted my language carefully to avoid eliciting defensive or distracting responses. My primary goal was to encourage Christine to reflect on what she had created, and to help her explore and amplify her own metaphor, which so clearly centered on attachment between the mother and baby deer (i.e., her mother and herself).

Amplifying the Metaphor

When metaphors appear in stories, art images, verbal language, or movements, some may be obvious, visible, and distinctive; others may be vague and convey a hint of something else. When we give children an opportunity to create sandtrays, we give them a chance to create metaphors by using miniatures to create tangible stories. These scenarios include important information about children's internal worlds.

I have stated elsewhere (Gil, 2011) that something important seems to happen when children externalize internal images, pictures, feeling states, and perceptions into a container (in this case, the sandtray). Children can be reassured by having the experience of placing miniatures in a contained space with firm boundaries (such as those provided in traditional wooden sandtrays). In addition, this externalization creates the "safe enough distance" that play therapists value immensely. In other words, children find a way to talk about themselves without taking risks that they may not yet perceive as possible (although this perception may not be a conscious, cognitive process, but a sensory and affective one in which they hesitate or feel uncomfortable). They begin to look at what is going on in their worlds in a way that allows them to maintain safety while approaching what they fear. In this fashion, children often use play to initiate gradual exposure—a way to expose themselves to feared or complex material in such a way that affect can be gradually tolerated and results in the feared material's losing its power.

It is of great importance to treat an externalized metaphor as just that—something that is standing for something else. As I have stated previously, if children felt comfortable discussing difficult experiences spontaneously, they would do so. I have had experiences in which children seem to be anxious to communicate verbally about what their parents did to them, or state openly how they feel, or make it clear that they want to go home. But when children seem reluctant or unable to commit to verbal language, an externalized metaphor provides them with an alternative method of approaching their traumatic experiences in a way that makes sense to them, and as such it often carries greater possibilities for integration of something that has changed.

Our first steps in this process are to encourage children's curiosity about what they have created, to redirect their attention back to what they've made, and to stimulate some introspection. We model therapeutic curiosity, and by doing so, we engage them in amplifying the metaphor in order to expand their awareness of their creation. The trick is to avoid interpretations and suggestions of things that our child clients have not already named or told us. As therapists, we may feel tempted to solve problems that appear in metaphors, to provide a reassuring ending, or to bring in a resource prematurely. Amplifying metaphors does not mean moving or manipulating them in any way. It means accepting what has come forward and simply attending to what is present, not necessarily to what it means narrowly or to what it could become. It means focusing on problems or worries or concepts that are presented, not those that we surmise or interpret as something else. When a child is describing a vulnerable deer, for example, it is less useful to wonder about who might be feeling vulnerable or afraid, and more useful to understand the deer's experience of vulnerability or safety (or whatever) as it is created by the child.

Identifying Points of Entry

Points of entry are areas of a story, sandtray, artwork, or the like with one or more identifiable objects that can serve as ways of entering the metaphor. For example, in Christine's sandtray, the house on the right, the tree in the front, and the cat looking forward were all entry points, as were the other animal objects. Clinicians can decide which entry point to work with in different ways:

1. They can consider the sequence in which the tray was made. Christine placed the large tree in the center of the tray first, so some clinicians might choose that; others might choose the last object placed to explore.
2. Clinicians may try to identify what are the most and least threatening aspects of the tray, and to start with the point of least resistance.

3. Clinicians can select a point of entry based on emergent issues, phase of treatment, or relationship to the client—in other words, intangible variables unique to each therapy case.

However the point of entry is selected, clinicians then develop some questions, comments, and observations in order to refocus the child's attention on a specific aspect of the tray (like using a wide lens on a camera and then focusing on the forefront or background). In spite of the fact that talking will occur and the left hemisphere of the brain is now activated, it is important to note that staying within the metaphor itself actually pulls for a *whole-brain* response, in which the left and right hemispheres are equally engaged and active (Siegel, Payne, & Bryson, 2012). If the child was being asked to answer questions related to real life, or to indicate how the metaphor stands for something other than what we see, the child might have to revert to left-hemisphere activity that could cause defensive mechanisms to come into play. The goal here is to have the child remain open and receptive, rather than need to use defenses because the material is crossing the "safe enough" threshold and begins to feel threatening.

Pithy Questions to Amplify Metaphors

In my clinical experience, careful and purposeful therapeutic language is the most challenging part of amplifying metaphors. Although there are only a few rules that guide this process of asking or commenting, clinicians are encouraged to "practice, practice, practice" creating these questions, because they do not come easily.

The rules are as follows:

1. Do not ask questions that require a "yes–no" answer (e.g., "Do you want to tell me about this?").
2. Do not ask "why" questions (e.g., "Why did you pick this particular miniature?").
3. Do not make interpretive comments (e.g., "So it seems that you might be feeling scared of your mom").
4. Do not rush ahead or go beyond what is presented to you by the child (e.g., "So how will this bear decide what to do next?").

Some ideas that may be helpful in creating amplifying questions are as follows:

1. Express your therapeutic curiosity about the object/metaphor.
2. Be patient and spend some time with the identified point of entry.
3. Questions are fine, but once you can see that the child is not responsive, try making comments or observing things instead, and take the emphasis off expecting the child to respond verbally.

When Christine returned to the next session after making her tray, she let out a huge sigh and covered her mouth with her hands as she walked over to the sandtray. "It's still here," she said with apparent excitement and pleasure. "I knew it would be here!" I responded by saying, "I thought we might take a longer look at it together." She seemed completely receptive as she started dusting sand off the house, making more fingerprints in the sand, and slightly rearranging how things were in the sandtray. Her first movement was to anchor the tree deeper in the sand and move more sand to surround its roots.

Here are the questions I prepared prior to this session for Christine's sandtray, after spending some time allowing myself to explore the tray. I identified three possible entry points and then created questions designed to amplify the metaphors in the tray:

Entry Point 1: The Cat in Front of the House

"I notice there is a cat in front of the house. What is the cat doing?"
"I wonder if the cat has been in the front of this house before?"
"If the cat were to turn his head the other way, what would he see?"
"What's the cat's favorite part of this house?"
"If the cat could use words, what would he say to the house?"
"When the cat is not in front of the house, where is the cat?"
"What does the cat see as he looks out?"

Entry Point 2: The Tree in the Center of the Tray

"What kind of a tree is this?"
"How long has the tree been in this place?"
"What's it like for the tree to be exactly in the place it is?"
"I notice this tree has a little open space. How does the tree like having that space there?"
"It seems there is something inside the tree. I wonder what that is?"
"If the tree could speak to that creature, what would it say to it?"
"I wonder how long that creature has been in that space?"

Entry Point 3: The Mother Deer

(Christine had placed two deer, a mother and a baby, in the branches of the tree. She had also placed another creature inside the tree, a porcupine "with needles.")
"What is the mother doing on the branch of the tree?"
"I notice there is a baby next to the mother deer. What's it like for the mother to be near the baby?"
"What's it like for the baby to be atop the tree?"
"What is the mother/baby thinking?"
"What is the mother/baby doing?"

"I wonder if they could speak to each other, what they would say?"

"I wonder if they know there is a porcupine nearby?"

"What do they think about the porcupine being nearby?"

"How do the branches feel about having company up high?"

"If the mother could be heard by the cat, what would she want the cat to know?"

Here is the dialogue that I had with Christine, based on some of the questions that I had prepared.

THERAPIST: What is the mother doing on the branch of the tree?

CHRISTINE: She's trying to be very quiet.

THERAPIST: So she's trying to be very quiet.

CHRISTINE: Yeah, she doesn't want to make too much noise.

THERAPIST: What will happen if she makes too much noise?

CHRISTINE: She'll get caught hiding, and then she'll be in trouble.

THERAPIST: So the mother deer is hiding right now.

CHRISTINE: Yep, right in the branches . . . but she's also watching, you know, keeping guard.

THERAPIST: Oh, so Mom is keeping guard.

CHRISTINE: Yeah, she's a good guard, too!

THERAPIST: It's great when moms can be good guards, and sometimes they hide so they don't get in trouble.

CHRISTINE: Yeah, you have to be really quiet.

THERAPIST: How does the baby feel when the mom is guarding and hiding?

CHRISTINE: She holds her breath. She is really quiet. She doesn't say anything and keeps real still.

THERAPIST: Oh, so the baby knows what to do. She's real quiet, holds her breath, keeps still.

CHRISTINE: Yep, she doesn't want to get caught because bad trouble comes . . .

THERAPIST: What kind of trouble comes?

CHRISTINE: You know, the porcupine. He has very sharp needles, and he shoots them out and hurts the mommy deer.

THERAPIST: Oh, so the porcupine has sharp needles and hurts Mom.

CHRISTINE: Yeah, we don't like him. He's mean all the time.

THERAPIST: What does the porcupine do when he's not being mean and shooting needles?

CHRISTINE: I don't know.

THERAPIST: How is the porcupine mean to the baby deer?

CHRISTINE: He hurts her mommy and screams at her too.

THERAPIST: I'm so sorry to hear that. I'm so sorry that the porcupine hurts and scares the mommy and baby. . . . What's it like for the baby to be atop the tree?

CHRISTINE: She likes it there. Her mommy likes it there too, because she's tricking the porcupine.

THERAPIST: So being away from the porcupine feels safe to the baby and mommy?

CHRISTINE: Yeah.

THERAPIST: I wonder if the baby and mommy deer can feel safe anywhere else?

CHRISTINE: Only if the porcupine isn't there. Sometimes the police take him far away, but he always comes back and finds them.

THERAPIST: Sounds like he's a very persistent porcupine. . . . I wonder if the mommy and baby could speak to each other, what they would say?

CHRISTINE: Just "I love you."

THERAPIST: The mommy and baby love each other.

CHRISTINE: Yep.

THERAPIST: How do the branches feel about having company up high?

CHRISTINE: They like the deer being there. That's funny . . . deers don't climb trees, but sometimes they do. And squirrels do, and caterpillars do.

THERAPIST: If the mother could be heard by the cat, what would she want the cat to know?

CHRISTINE: The mommy would thank the cat for being a good pet and tell her that we'll be back home soon, as soon as we can find a new place to live. Mommy says we're going to have a new home with a cat.

THERAPIST: I see you and your mom are going to live together in a new home with a cat.

I had chosen and prepared my questions in order from least to most difficult (at least, I surmised that it might be most difficult for Christine to talk about the experiences with domestic violence that I believed were being represented in the center of the tray). We spent about four sessions exploring her metaphor, and she developed more and more comfort as we spoke.

By the time we got to the third question, Christine was willing, even eager, to stay with the metaphor and answer questions or comments from that vantage point; however, she was almost always reluctant to say anything about her father and his violent behavior. It was almost as if she thought talking about it would be discovered by him and put her in danger. Christine's subsequent trays were typically developmentally appropriate, with princesses and fairylands. Apparently, the tray that first slipped out (the mother and baby deer up a tree) was closer to reality than she could tolerate for very long.

Dyadic Work with Sarah and Christine

One of the central aspects of our work was attachment-based. It was clear that the violence in the home had caused profound disruptions in the parent–child relationship. Specifically, Christine had experienced an environment of tension and violence, which increased her stress level and affected her ability to soothe or self-regulate. Her mother's attention was constantly diverted, and although Sarah was making her best efforts to protect Christine from harm, Christine was often neglected, pushed away, or simply left alone to fend for herself. Even when Sarah held or fed Christine, she did so in an anxious, frightened state that was visible in her eyes, her facial tension, her skirted glances, and the constricted muscles in her arms. In addition, Christine had learned that her mother was unable to protect herself from harm, and by extension, unable to protect her. The child's basic safety and security had been severely compromised, and this damage needed to be addressed in therapy.

This work had two stages: having mother and child share and reflect on the story that Christine had told in the sand, and having them use Christine's metaphor to rework the issue of safety.

When I first told Christine that I'd like her mother to see the sandtray she had made about the mother and baby deer and the porcupine, she looked a little uncertain. She wondered whether her mother might get mad at her for telling me the story. I told Christine that her mother and I had talked about the sandtray story, that her mother was looking forward to hearing about it from Christine, and that Sarah might even want to add to the story and might have some ideas about it. Christine was hesitant to show the tray to her mother, but quickly became excited about telling her the story that she had told me, adding some of the things she had discovered when she and I had talked together. Here is a paraphrase of what Christine told her mother and how Sarah responded to her child:

CHRISTINE: (*pointing to the recreated scenario in the sand tray*)
Mommy, look, the mommy deer and the baby are high, high on the tree. And the porcupine is there, but he can't climb up the tree; he can't come scare them. Mommy, look, the baby and mommy

love each other, and they live together in a tall tree where the porcupine can't get them!

SARAH: (*asking Christine to sit on her lap and holding her*) I see the
mommy and the baby, and I am so sorry that they feel afraid of
the porcupine.

CHRISTINE: (*stepping off and facing mother*) But he can't climb up the
tree, Mommy, so the mommy and baby are safe now.

SARAH: (*putting her back on her lap and hugging her*) The mommy
went up the tree because it was the only thing she could think to
do, because she was afraid of the porcupine. But now the mommy
deer has learned a lot—a lot about taking care of herself and getting away from the porcupine. I think this mommy and baby deer
deserve to live on the ground, where they can find food for themselves, and they can build a house with a roof, so they don't get
wet when it rains. And you know what else? The mommy deer has
to stretch her legs and stand up straight, and help her little deer
learn how to stretch too! What I'd like to do now, sweetie, is put
that porcupine somewhere else, so that the mommy and baby deer
can come down and see how much fun it is to be on the ground!

And with that, Sarah set the context for more attachment work as she
began to present herself as capable (no longer a victim) to her child. She
took the porcupine, held it in her hands, and in a firm voice stated, "I'm
not afraid of you any more, and you are never allowed to come around us
again!" She placed it in a box in the office and said, "You are out of our
lives forever. I have a little deer who has a lot of safe living to do, and she
and I are going to explore our nice forest together!" Christine looked at
her mother with big eyes, and kissed her on the cheek. "Come on, Mom,"
she said, "come over and let's make a new world for them." They played
together and moved things around, and the mother and baby deer made
tracks in the sand as Sarah said, "They're on firm ground now. They are
flexing their muscles now, kind of like you and me. I'm getting a place
ready for us that will be safe and cozy. You'll see."

Reintroducing the Metaphor

Another option for amplifying the metaphor is to reintroduce it to the child
in some other medium or in some other way. In this particular case, after
the wonderful work Sarah and Christine did in the sandtray, I reintroduced
the story of the mother and baby deer hiding from the porcupine by doing
an art therapy project called the Safe Environment Project (Sobol & Schneider, 1998). Sarah and Christine did this work together, and I provided a
paper plate, some paints and markers, and the mother and baby deer miniatures. I then asked them to create a safe environment for the two deer.

Mother and daughter produced an environment with foliage, color, a protective fence, a small covered area, food, water, and a friend for the deer.

This reintroduction of the mother and baby deer, in a completely different activity, allowed Christine to interact once again with the metaphor she had created earlier and to find ways to engage with the metaphor further on another level of resource building, now introduced by the clinician (myself), at this advanced phase of therapy. My integrated approach is documented elsewhere (Gil, 2006), but suffice it to say that therapy can include the purposeful integration of directive and nondirective strategies. In addition, consensus exists on the importance of integrating dyadic work with young children and their parents into play therapy with the children, and "attachment therapies" have been developed and well articulated in the last decade (Berlin, Ziv, Amaya-Jackson, & Greenberg, 2005; Booth & Jernberg, 2010; Greenspan & Lieberman, 1988; Hughes, 2000, 2007; Schore, 1994).

Conclusion

The use of clinical metaphor has been encouraged throughout the clinical literature on hypnotherapy as well as family therapy. Expressive therapists have long considered metaphor work pivotal to what they do; they recognize that children in particular find play and art natural ways of communicating and expressing themselves.

Art and play therapists understand the myriad benefits of valuing children's metaphors, and often engage children by creating clinical metaphors and introducing these into their own work with the children. Whether the metaphors are initiated by clients or their clinicians, they serve as projections or representations of something that cannot always be acknowledged or verbalized. Thus it behooves clinicians to learn to decipher the camouflaged communications imbedded in metaphors, and to help clients reflect, explore, and amplify these in order to become more interested in and curious about their creations and themselves.

Metaphors are, by definition, opportunities for transition, and clinicians using metaphor work believe in the potential of processed or managed metaphors to be reintegrated on a deeper level—taken back in, as it were, with new acquired meaning. Metaphors also offer opportunities for healing through processing of difficult experiences.

This chapter summarizes the importance of giving children (and their parents) the opportunity to do metaphor work, and it gives suggestions for amplifying metaphors in ways that facilitate self-reflection and exploration. An integrative approach allows for processing the metaphors both symbolically and verbally; therapists help children to externalize their thoughts and feelings by staying within their metaphors, rather than drawing too-quick correlations between the metaphors and real life. In fact, if children were feeling able or willing to speak about their distress, they would do so. Instead, they seem to find it much easier to "speak" through metaphor and amplification of their work. In the case described in this chapter, attachment-based work was central to improved health in the mother–child relationship, and both Christine and Sarah were able to stay with Christine's metaphors and receptive to guidance about deepening their understanding of their symbolic communication. In addition, it is important to note that no attachment work is complete without direct interventions with the parent–child dyad, and these can be delivered in a playful, energetic, and creative manner within an integrated (directive and nondirective) model. This case example illustrates a fluid methodology of individual and conjoint work, as well as a natural continuum from nondirective to directive work.

REFERENCES

Berlin, L. J., Ziv, Y., Amaya-Jackson, L., & Greenberg, M. T. (2005). *Enhancing early attachments: Theory, research, intervention, and policy.* New York: Guilford Press.

Booth, P. B., & Jernberg, A. M. (2010). *Theraplay: Helping parents and children build better relationships through attachment-based play* (3rd ed.). San Francisco: Jossey-Bass.

Davis, N. (1990). *Therapeutic stories that teach and heal.* Burke, VA: Author.

Erickson, M. H., & Rossi, E. L. (1979). *Hypnotherapy: An exploratory casebook.* New York: Irvington.

Esparza, D. P. (2012). Therapeutic metaphors and clinical hypnosis. *Purpose-driven hypnotherapy: A method for positive change.* Retrieved from *www.pdhypnosis.com/index.php/weblog/articles/181*

Gil, E. (2006). *Helping abused and traumatized children: Integrating directive and nondirective approaches.* New York: Guilford Press.

Gil, E. (2011). *Working with children to heal interpersonal trauma: The power of play.* New York: Guilford Press.

Gil, E., & Shaw, J. (2013). *Working with children with sexual behavior problems.* New York: Guilford Press.

Greenspan, S. I., & Lieberman, A. F. (1988). A clinical approach to attachment. In E. J. Blesky & T. Nezworski (Eds.), *Clinical implications of attachment* (pp. 387–424). Hillsdale, NJ: Erlbaum.

Guiffrida, D. A., Jordan, R., Saiz, S., & Barnes, K. L. (2007). The use of metaphor in clinical supervision. *Journal of Counseling and Development, 85,* 393–400.

Hughes, D. A. (2000). *Facilitating developmental attachment: The road to emotional recovery and behavioral change in foster and adopted children.* Northvale, NJ: Aronson.

Hughes, D. A. (2007). *Attachment-focused family therapy.* New York: Norton.

Lankton, S. (2004). *Assembling Ericksonian therapy: The collected papers of Stephen Lankton.* Phoenix, AZ: Zeig, Tucker, & Theisen.

Onnis, L., Bernardini, M., Giambartolomei, A., Leonelli, A., Menenti, B., & Vietri, A. (2007). *The use of metaphors in systemic therapy: A bridge between mind and body languages.* Paper presented at the Congress of the European Family Therapy Association, Glasgow, Scotland. Retrieved from *www.eftacim.org/doc_pdf/metaphors.pdf*

Ricoeur, P. (1967). *The symbolism of evil.* New York: Beacon Press.

Schore, A. N. (1994). *Affect regulation and the origin of the self.* Hillsdale, NJ: Erlbaum.

Siegel, D. A., & Payne Bryson, T. (2012). *The whole-brain child: 12 revolutionary strategies to nurture your child's developing mind.* New York: Bantam Books.

Sobol, B., & Schneider, K. (1998). Art as an adjunctive therapy in the treatment of children who dissociate. In J. L. Silberg (Ed.), *The dissociative child: Diagnosis, treatment, and management* (2nd ed., pp. 191–218). Lutherville, MD: Sidran Press.

CHAPTER 11

The Neurobiological Power of Play

Using the Neurosequential Model of Therapeutics to Guide Play in the Healing Process

Richard L. Gaskill
Bruce D. Perry

Children, like all human beings, are best understood in a social context. We humans are healthiest and most productive when we are born, grow, live, work, and raise our families in social groups (Ludy-Dobson & Perry, 2010). We have existed and thrived for thousands of years because of our neurobiological drive to form safe, nurturing, mutually rewarding, and lasting attachments (Szalavitz & Perry, 2010). In normative attachment relationships, children can safely explore new experiences and master developmental competencies, including the ability to regulate themselves cognitively, affectively, behaviorally, physiologically, and relationally (Blaustein & Kinniburgh, 2005). Secure attachments ultimately become the basis of resiliency in children exposed to distressing experiences (Shapiro & Levendosky, 1999). When these important attachment systems are compromised through multiple and chronic lapses within caregiving systems, crucial neural systems can be altered. This alteration negatively affects key competencies, such as the ability to regulate emotions and experiences. These effects in turn can contribute to neuropsychiatric problems and result in enduring social and emotional difficulties across the lifespan (Blaustein & Kinniburgh, 2005). Zeanah et al. (2004) have reported the prevalence of attachment-disordered children to be as high as 35% of children entering foster care, and as high as 38–40% of high-risk infant and toddler populations. Such demographics suggest the need for play therapy intervention techniques that can appropriately target the neural networks involved in self-regulation and relational functioning.

Any discussion of the role of play in neurodevelopment must first address one core question: What is *play*? What are the key elements that distinguish play from other activities? For the purposes of this chapter, we use the three elements used by Burghardt (2005) to define play in animals. First, play mimics or approximates a common or important purposeful behavior; second, play is voluntary, is pleasurable, and has no immediate survival role or obvious "purpose"; and, finally, play takes place in a non-threatening, low-duress context. These key elements are often at odds with many well-intended (and typically ineffective) therapeutic experiences. It is no surprise that the core elements of play echo some of the essential ingredients of successful therapeutic interactions with maltreated and traumatized children—perceived control, reward, and manageable stress (see Perry & Szalavitz, 2006). Bringing play into therapeutic work, therefore, not only makes sense; it is often an essential element for therapeutic progress. Yet it is important to appreciate that "play" for the toddler looks different from "play" for the adolescent. Play is an effective therapeutic agent when it provides a developmentally appropriate means to regulate, communicate, practice, and master. As with other therapeutic approaches, however, we often select the manner of "play" that we bring into therapy according to a child's chronological age and to our specific training as therapists; there are thus times when the expectations we bring into the therapeutic relationship are unrealistic. The resulting mismatch between a therapist's expectation and a child's capability undermines the potential for true play (i.e., the interaction is not spontaneous or pleasurable for the child), and thereby therapeutic progress. When the therapist (or parent, caregiver, or teacher) understands the real developmental capabilities of the child and the child's current state (e.g., calm, alert, fearful), realistic expectations and developmentally appropriate activities (including the manner of play) can be used to help the child heal. This crucial awareness of the "stage" and the current "state" is informed by an understanding of neurobiology. This chapter provides an introduction to some neurodevelopmental principles that inform play therapy practice.

Play Therapy: Overview, Context, and Efficacy

Historical Overview and Scope of Play Therapy

The developmental importance of children's play has been recognized for hundreds if not thousands of years, beginning with the thoughts of Plato (427 B.C.–347 B.C.) and continuing later with Rousseau's (1762/1930) notions. In the 20th century, Freud (1924), Gesell and Ilg (1947), Erikson (1964), Piaget (1962), Kohlberg (1963), Vygotsky (1967), and other developmental theorists defined, articulated, and advocated for the role of play during childhood. Developmental theorists generally have viewed play as an essential experiential element of social, emotional, physical, intellectual, and psychological development. The somatosensory experiences in some play activities have been viewed as the neurological foundations for later advanced mental skills, such as creativity, abstract thought, prosocial behavior, and expressive language. Furthermore, Zigler, Singer, and Bishop-Josef (2004) have cited a growing body of research finding that "Vygotskian-type" play promotes development of self-regulation, a cornerstone of early childhood development across all domains of behavior (social, emotional, cognitive, and physical). Play has been considered so critical to healthy development that the United Nations recognizes it as a specific right for all children (Office of the United Nations High Commissioner for Human Rights, 1989). Since the period from birth to age 6 establishes the foundation for learning, behavior, and health throughout the lifespan, the United Nations has accorded play equal importance with nutrition, housing, health care, and education.

Landreth (2002) has suggested that talk and cognitively oriented therapies are inappropriate for children through much of their development, due to the relative underdevelopment of complex cognitive capacities in childhood. The powerful role of play in children's growth, and the slow attainment of adult mental and verbal abilities, both suggest play as a developmentally appropriate strategy for treating children's emotional and behavioral difficulties. Accordingly, play has been incorporated into therapies with children for years. Freud's treatment of "Little Hans" incorporated play into therapy at the turn of the last century (Bratton & Ray, 2000; Bratton, Ray, Rhine, & Jones, 2005; Landreth, 2002). From this time on, there has been significant growth of play therapy theory and practice—from psychoanalytic play therapy in the 1920s, to release play therapy in the 1930s, to relationship play therapy also in the 1930s, and finally to nondirective play therapy beginning in the 1940s and 1950s (Landreth, 2002). Play therapy variations continued to expand through the end of the 20th century with the development of Adlerian play therapy (Kottman, 1995), Jungian play therapy (Allen, 1988), gestalt play therapy (Oaklander, 1994), ecosystem play therapy (O'Connor, 2000), object relations play therapy (Benedict, 2006), experiential play therapy (Norton & Norton, 1997), cognitive-behavioral play therapy (Knell, 1995), developmental play therapy (Brody, 1997), Filial Therapy (Guerney, 1964), and others.

Studies have described play therapy strategies for social maladjustment, maladaptive school behavior, self-concept, anxiety, conduct disorder, aggression, oppositional behavior, emotional maladjustment, fear, developmental disabilities, physical and learning disabilities, autism, schizophrenia, psychoticism, posttraumatic stress disorder, sexual abuse, domestic violence, depression, withdrawal, alcohol and drug abuse, divorce, reading disorders, speech and language problems, and multicultural issues

(Bratton & Ray, 2000; Bratton et al., 2005; LeBlanc & Ritchie, 2001). Recent research has begun to address the efficacy of play therapy versus other treatments, using randomized controlled studies with large sample sizes (Bratton & Ray, 2000; Bratton et al., 2005; Pearl et al., 2012; Tsai & Ray, 2011).

Efficacy of Play Therapy

Over the past 30 years, a number of meta-analytic studies examining multiple play therapy studies have found play therapy to be effective with a wide variety of problematic issues. These studies demonstrated that children had improved prosocial behavior and decreased symptomatic behavior (Bratton et al., 2005; Casey & Berman 1985; LeBlanc & Ritchie, 1999, 2001; Ray, Bratton, Rhine, & Jones, 2001; Weisz, Weiss, Alicke, & Klotz, 1987). The treatment effect sizes ranged from a high of 0.80 (Bratton et al., 2005) to a low of 0.66 (LeBlanc & Ritchie, 2001), with most falling between 0.71 and 0.79. These results indicate that children receiving play therapy interventions performed much better than children who did not receive play therapy, and that play therapy demonstrated a large effect on children's behavior, social adjustment, and personality (Bratton et al., 2005; Ray et al., 2001).

Play therapy interventions appear to be equally effective, regardless of the presenting problem. Play therapy is effective across modalities, ages, genders, and theoretical schools of thought (Bratton et al., 2005; LeBlanc & Ritchie, 1999; Ray et al., 2001). Several studies suggest that the maximum effect size is achieved after 30–40 sessions, whereas shorter or longer treatment durations are less effective (Bratton et al., 2005; LeBlanc & Ritchie, 1999, 2001). LeBlanc and Ritchie (1999, 2001) suggest that short-term play therapy treatment models may obtain negative outcomes because children are acting out previously unexpressed feelings in the early stages of such treatment and have insufficient time to resolve these issues. These authors have observed that children participating in play therapy appear to take considerably more time to process information and make effective changes in thinking or behaving, compared to adults in conventional therapies.

Multiple studies (Bratton et al., 2005; LeBlanc & Ritchie, 1999, 2001; Ray et al., 2001) point to the importance of parental involvement as an essential predictor of positive outcome. When parents received structured play therapy supervision or guided interactions between themselves and their children, effectiveness rose dramatically. Bratton and colleagues noted that the Filial Therapy model (Guerney, 1964) and the child–parent relationship theory model (Landreth, 2002) yielded larger effect sizes than other studies. This is not surprising, given that play therapy with humanistic interventions produced a larger effect size than nonhumanistic treatments. Children learn through play, and this often requires a patient, supportive, and caring adult to scaffold that process (Vygotsky, 1967).

The Developing Brain and the Vulnerability of Childhood

The human brain is organized in a hierarchical manner. The higher regions in the brain mediate the more complex and executive functions, while the lower areas mediate the simpler, more regulatory functions. There are four developmentally distinct regions (brainstem, diencephalon, limbic, and cortical) that are woven together by multiple neural networks, some of the most important being the well-studied monoamine (i.e., norepinephrine and dopamine) and other related (e.g., serotonin, acetylcholine) systems. These networks originate in lower areas of the brain; have widespread distribution (collectively to all brain areas and the body); and have a direct impact on all motor, social, emotional, and cognitive functioning, as well as the stress response. When these networks develop normally, there is smooth functional integration. When these networks are impacted by intrauterine insults (e.g., prenatal alcohol or drug exposure), early life attachment disruptions, or traumatic stress, these networks will be dysregulated, resulting in compromise in all in the functions impacted by their wide distribution. These crucial networks play a role in integrating, processing, and acting on incoming patterns of information from the primary sensory networks (such as touch, vision, and sound), which monitor the external environment; somatic networks (such as motor–vestibular, cardiovascular, and respiratory), which monitor the internal environment; and cerebral networks (such as cortical modulating networks), which monitor the brain's internal environment.

The continuous input from the brain, body, and world, coupled with their widespread distribution, provides these networks with a unique role in the stress response—and in stress- or trauma-related dysfunction. Furthermore, as neurodevelopment progresses from lower (i.e., brainstem and diencephalon) to higher (i.e., limbic and cortical) areas, these regulatory neural networks play a key role in the development of the brain from the intrauterine period through adolescence. The timing and pattern of activation of these regulatory neural networks play a crucial role in shaping the functional capacity of all brain and body areas (see Perry, 2001).

Neurons and neural networks change in response to activity. In the case of the stress response networks, predictable, moderate activity leads to flexible and capable stress response capacity (with a potential for demonstrating resilience), whereas extreme, unpredictable, or uncontrollable activation leads to a sensitized, overly reactive set of stress response networks (see Perry, 2008, 2009; Ungar & Perry, 2012). Any developmental insult—such as prenatal alcohol or drug exposure, or extreme, prolonged activation of the stress response (such as that seen in maltreatment or other traumatic experience)—will alter the development of these crucial neural networks, and thereby disrupt functioning in all of the areas these regulatory networks innervate.

The resulting alterations in the regulation and functioning of both central and peripheral autonomic neural networks (as well as the neuroendocrine and the neuroimmune systems) will result in increased risk of significant and lasting emotional, behavioral, social, cognitive, sensory–motor, and physical health problems (Anda et al., 2006; Felitti et al., 1998; Perry, 2006, 2008, 2009; Perry & Dobson, 2013; Perry & Pollard, 1998; Perry, Pollard, Blakley, Baker, & Vigilante, 1995). Manifestations of the resulting sensitized stress response systems have been well documented. They include intrusive recollections; persistent avoidance of associated stimuli or numbing of general responsiveness; and arousal symptoms of hyperarousal, hypervigilance, increased startle response, sleep difficulties, irritability, anxiety, and physiological hyperactivity. Maltreated and traumatized children may exhibit behavioral impulsivity, increased muscle tone, anxiety, a fixation on threat-related cues, affect regulation, language disorders, fine and gross motor delays, disorganized attachment, dysphoria, attention difficulties, memory problems, and hyperactivity (Perry et al., 1995). Furthermore, these physical, emotional, psychological, and intellectual effects may persist across the lifespan (Anda et al., 2006; Spinazzola, Blaustein, & van der Kolk, 2005). Nearly two-thirds of traumatized children exhibit physical signs and symptoms indicating dysregulation in brainstem or diencephalic functions, such as inhibition of gastrointestinal processes, cardiac activity, blood pressure, respiration, anxiety, and hypervigilance (Hopper, Spinazzola, Simpson, & van der Kolk, 2006; Perry, 2001, 2008). The specific physical signs and symptoms will depend upon a multitude of contributing factors, including genetics, epigenetics, intrauterine environment, early bonding experiences, history of developmental adversity, and attenuating relational buffers (see Ungar & Perry, 2012). This creates a confusing clinical picture that does not fit neatly into our current inadequate model of categorization. The comorbidity of neuropsychiatric diagnoses associated with childhood maltreatment is so pervasive that it encompasses nearly all diagnoses in the new fifth edition of the *Diagnostic and Statistical Manual of Mental Disorders* (DSM-5; American Psychiatric Association, 2013), resulting in the inability of current diagnostic labels to capture the complex heterogeneous dysfunction adequately (Perry, 2008; Perry & Dobson, 2013).

Although traumatic experiences may have a negative impact on adult functioning, the same adverse experiences have a much more deleterious impact on children because of the pervasive impact on development. Traumatic stress in adulthood affects a developed and functioning brain; trauma in childhood affects the organization and functioning of the developing brain. Adults suffering a traumatic event have been found to attain asymptomatic posttreatment status 75% of the time, but children suffering a traumatic event have been found to achieve asymptomatic status only 33% of the time (van der Kolk et al., 2007).

The Stress Response and State-Dependent Functioning

The crucial regulatory neural networks involved in the stress response (and multiple other functions) are themselves modulated through patterned, repetitive, and rhythmic input from both bottom-up (i.e., somatosensory) and top-down (i.e., cerebromodulatory) systems. The brain processes (and acts) on incoming input at multiple levels; although the brain is essentially an open and interactive system, this multilevel process of sensing, processing, and acting on the environment basically begins at the site of initial input of sensory, somatic, or cerebral input to the lower areas of the brain. The primary regulatory systems that originate in the lower areas of the brain begin to sort, integrate, interpret, store, and respond to incoming stimuli long before conscious portions of the brain receive the information, if they receive it at all (Marteau, Hollands, & Fletcher, 2012; Perry, 2006). Primary somatosensory processing takes place below the level of consciousness, and only novel, significant, or potentially threatening stimuli are passed on to higher cortical centers for further processing (Perry, 2008; Sara & Bouret, 2012). When the input to these regulatory networks is unfamiliar (novel), disorganized (chaotic), or associated with potential threat (i.e., reexposure to a cue from a previous traumatic experience), there will be alterations in the activity of these systems. In the crucial norepinephrine-containing networks originating in the locus coeruleus, for example, a complex and graded response that is proportional (in typically functioning individuals) to the level of threat (Sara & Bouret, 2012) will begin. A key part of that response is a shift of "control" from higher, cortical systems to limbic, then diencephalic systems. Neuroimaging during highly emotional states demonstrates increased activation of subcortical regions and significant reduction of blood flow to the frontal lobe during intense arousal (van der Kolk, 2006). This shift in activation alters cognitive, social, emotional, and motor functioning. In other words, novelty, chaos and threat change the "state" of the individual. This shift in state involves shutting down the cortical modulatory networks that could typically be recruited and involved in conscious, intentional modulation of the feelings of anxiety, hunger, thirst, anger, and other "primitive" feelings and perceptions. The result is that less mature, more poorly regulated, more impulsive behaviors will result under perceived threat. And if child's developmental experiences have been such that they have fewer cortical-network-building experiences (e.g., neglect- or chaos-related poverty of touch, words, relationships), their cortical modulation networks will be relatively underdeveloped as well. The combination of a sensitized set of regulatory neural networks (i.e., the stress response systems are "locked into" a persisting state of fear) with a "shut-down" and underdeveloped cortex will result in a very impulsive, globally dysregulated child. This is worth remembering when one is interpreting trauma-related and attachment-related behavioral problems with maltreated children; exhausted and frustrated caregivers, teachers, and therapists are quick to personalize and infer deliberate intention to automatic, elicited behaviors. The capacity for self-reflection, planning, and intentional behavior requires a relatively organized, regulated, and accessible cortex.

Another crucial aspect of this shift is its impact on the capacity to feel pleasure. Release of dopamine in the two regions of the brain—the nucleus accumbens and the ventral tegmental area—can provide a sensation of pleasure. These "reward" areas can be stimulated in many ways, ranging from cortically mediated, intentional behaviors that are consistent with an individual's beliefs or values (e.g., sharing candy with someone) to primarily limbic mediated relational interactions (e.g., a laugh with a friend) to diencephalon-mediated appetitive experiences (e.g., eating sweet, salty, or fatty foods) to brainstem-mediated regulatory behaviors that decrease physiological distress (e.g., drinking cold water when dehydrated). As the individual moves down the arousal continuum, the reward "options" shrink. In a state of high arousal or fear, delayed gratification is impossible. Future consequences or rewards of behavior become almost inconceivable to the threatened child. Reflection on behavior is impossible for the child in an alarm state, and cognitive strategies to modify behavior (even if previously internalized and mastered) cannot be recruited in an efficient way because the cortex is relatively inaccessible under threat. Cut adrift from the internal regulating capabilities of the cortex, the individual acts impulsively to any perceived threat. The key to helping the child begin to move back to a more regulated state, making the child feel safe and thereby more available for cognitive engagement and therapeutic change, is to utilize the direct somatosensory routes and provide patterned, repetitive, rhythmic input. Therapeutic change starts from a sense of safety; in turn, the sense of safety emerges from these regulating somatosensory activities.

Finally, these complex children will be very resistant to traditional therapeutic (i.e., primarily cognitive-behavioral or cognitive-relational) interventions (see the case vignette below). Traditional psychodynamic or cognitive-behavioral play therapies that support the development of cognitive regulatory control are likely to fail when the lower brain networks are disorganized, underdeveloped, or impaired. A neurodevelopmentally informed assessment process and therapeutic strategy can help the clinical team better understand such a child's developmental stages and state reactivity; to be effective, the clinician must *know the stage and watch the state.*

Implications for Play Therapy

We (Gaskill & Perry, 2012) have previously outlined the primary challenges of integrating a neurodevelopmental perspective with traditional play therapies. Child mental health treatment models, including play therapy, evolved out of adult psychodynamic and cognitive-behavioral therapies that use primarily cognitive and verbally mediated (i.e., top-down) inter-actions focusing on executive processing, insight, understanding, plan-ning, and decision making. Ultimately, maltreated children will need to address cognitive issues such as guilt, shame, self-esteem, grief, and loss, and to gain understanding of, acceptance of, and a new perspective on their experiences—but these cortically mediated issues must be addressed in a developmentally sensitive sequence, and only after some modulation of the primary regulatory networks has been established (Perry, 2001, 2006, 2008, 2009; Cook et al., 2005).

Accordingly, the play therapists will often need to use bottom-up modu-latory networks (somatosensory) to establish some moderate self-regulation prior to the implementation of insightful reflection, trauma experience inte-gration, narrative development, social development, or affect enhancement. Doing so will require therapeutic methods to access and provide reorganiz-ing input to the regulatory networks of the lower brain areas (Kleim & Jones, 2008; Perry, 2008, 2009). The key to treatment is to be sure that the child is regulated and that relational and cognitive expectations are appropriate for the child's developmental age. Furthermore, this requires rethinking traditional "dosing" and context of therapy.

Complex, deeply troubled children need more than the traditional once-a-week play therapy model. They will require therapeutic environ-ments that immerse them in positive, repetitive rehearsals of healthy inter-actions and activities. These interactions and activities often need to be regressive in nature, requiring low adult-to-child ratios (often 1:1) and activities frequently associated with much younger children, as many foun-dational experiences (neural networks) have been missed or are incomplete (Perry, 2006, 2009, in press; Perry & Dobson, 2013). The numbers of inter-actions required to change ingrained low-brain patterns call for extensive commitment from parents, teachers, therapists, and extended family, as the time required exceeds the capabilities of a single individual (Perry, 2009).

Fortunately, many playful activities that provide the activation nec-essary to modulate and reorganize these regulatory neural networks can be integrated into play therapies and playful therapeutic experiences (most therapeutic change happens outside of therapy). Play therapists should never forget that if something is not fun, it is not play, and that it is impossible for a child to have pleasure in a relational interaction if the child's brain is in an alarm state. The key, therefore, to being true to the "play" in play therapy is helping the child become regulated and thereby safe. Once basic state regulation has been established, more traditional play therapies will be effective. Bottom-up interventions for children with state-regulatory dif-ficulties will consist of some variety of somatosensory activity (e.g., music, dance, walking, drawing). Although language will undoubtedly be neces-sary in the process of working with these children, play therapists must realize that in dysregulated children it will not be likely that words, rea-soning, or ideas will change the primary regulatory networks in the lower areas of the brain. Rather, regulatory organization and creation of normal homeostatic states depend more on the "primal language" of gentle tones of voice; comforting, repetitive sensory experience; and soothing repetitive and patterned movements by patient, safe adults. Providing this "primal language" may take the form of child-directed free play; repetitive, patterned sensory integration activities carried out at home, school, and clinic; or fine and large motor activities. All such activities will require an atmosphere of enjoyment, safety, and attunement between adults and children. As noted above, this work must often be done in very low adult-to-child ratios that match a child's functional age, often 1:1 (see Gaskill & Perry, 2012). For a child with severe dysregulation, the play therapist may need to restrict the environment as well, to control environmental stimuli to match the child's developmental age; otherwise, overstimulation of the child is likely to produce frustration, irritability, tantrums, aggression, and withdrawal (including dissociation).

Finally, the unique aspects of each child's history, genetic endowment, and epigenetic influences preclude a "one-size-fits-all" treatment model (Ungar & Perry, 2012). Such multifaceted symptomatology requires play therapists to incorporate neurobiological principles, comparing play therapy techniques, delivery methods, treatment frequencies, optimal numbers of treatment sessions, and outcome measures (Bratton et al., 2005; Perry & Dobson, 2013; Ray et al., 2001). A crucial element in any therapeutic approach with these children is patience. Neural plasticity is a primary neurophysiological process underlying therapeutic change; expressed plasticity (i.e., changing a neural network) requires adequate (sometimes thousands of) repetitions (Kleim & Jones, 2008). Play therapists, family members, teachers, and other caregivers who are not aware of this can often become frustrated/confused and give up (Perry, 2009).

The Neurosequential Model of Therapeutics

The Neurosequential Model of Therapeutics™ (NMT) is a developmentally sensitive, neurobiology-informed approach to clinical problem solving. NMT is not a specific therapeutic technique or intervention. As described by Brandt, Diel, Feder, and Lillas (2012),

> The Neurosequential Model of Therapeutics™ (NMT) (Perry, 2006) provides an integrated understanding of the sequencing of neurodevelopment embedded in the experiences of the child, and supports biologically informed practices, programs, and policies. As a global evidence-based practice (EBP) and coupled with the NMT's brain mapping matrix, the model supports providers in identifying specific areas for therapeutic work and in selecting appropriate therapies, including evidence-based therapies (EBTs), within a comprehensive therapeutic plan. Organized NMT-based intervention models, such as NMT therapeutic child care, can be EBTs. (p. 43)

A key component of the NMT is an assessment process that informs a clinician about a child's broad set of brain-mediated strengths and vulnerabilities. From this assessment process, the general direction for therapeutic, educational, and enrichment expectations and opportunities can be determined. In the case of play therapy, simply stated, the NMT can help the therapist appropriately design the most developmentally appropriate forms of play to bring into the therapy. The following case vignette illustrates the power of play in the therapeutic process. It also illustrates the specific value of selecting developmentally appropriate forms of play in a relationally safe context, and of using adequate "dosing" in a patterned, repetitive, rhythmic, and rewarding manner.

Case Vignette: Tom

History

Tom is a 7-year-old boy who has been living with a foster family for the last 13 months. He was the only biological child born to an 18-year-old mother who actively used multiple drugs (marijuana, nicotine, alcohol, and cocaine) during her pregnancy. He was born addicted to cocaine and spent 2 weeks in a pediatric intensive care unit following his birth at 36 weeks' gestation. Both of his biological parents had extensive family histories of mental health problems, substance abuse, and criminal behavior. The parents split up when Tom was 2 months old, due to domestic violence; he lived with his mother, who was described as "disengaged, withdrawn, and flat." Multiple reports of abandonment and neglect were made, and at 14 months child protective services placed Tom with his biological father. The father lived in a violent, drug-filled, chaotic world, with no stable housing. Visitations (both formal and informal) with the mother continued during this time. The father tended to drop Tom off when he was involved in a criminal activity or drug binge. During visits, Tom witnessed his mother having sex and being beaten up by various men; Tom was also physically (and possibly sexually) abused by several of these men. His mother locked him in a bedroom, only episodically feeding him and rarely interacting with him. At age 5, Tom was removed and placed in foster care after his father was arrested for armed robbery of a convenience store; the father had walked into the store with Tom and used him as a decoy during the robbery.

Original Presentation

At the time of removal, Tom demonstrated abnormalities in functions mediated by all areas of the brain, from brainstem to cortex. He had excessive salivation and blinking. He was extremely fearful, anxious, and hypervigilant; he had an increased startle response, as well as sleep difficulties and frequent nightmares. He was also aggressive and threatening: He lashed out at other children in placement and was cruel to the pets; he "plotted to trap and kill" the carers. Tom was violent to peers, strangers, and especially all of his foster parents (hitting, kicking). He demonstrated a wide range of primitive and unsocialized behaviors, including growling and snarling; smearing feces; urinating while standing and having meals; gorging food; and consuming soap, shampoo, and dishwater. He had extreme tantrums that could last for 3 hours. He picked skin to the point of bleeding when upset. Tom misread signals; he found smiles threatening. He tried to control others, would lie to do so, and would blow up when he did not get what he wanted. He had articulation problems, pressured speech, and echolalia. Finally, his cognition was very primitive: He could not demonstrate either literacy or numeracy (i.e., he could not recognize letters or numbers).

Clinical Course

Tom's difficult behaviors resulted in five disrupted placements over 14 months; all of the carers felt he was too dangerous (at age 6) to keep in their homes. During this time, he was in weekly therapy at a local mental health authority and had two therapists over this period. The notes indicated that "evidence-based" trauma-focused cognitive-behavioral therapy was used by one therapist (with no apparent improvement), and that play therapy was used by the second therapist. The play therapy was conducted in the office of this therapist, who primarily attempted to use sandtray work as part of the process. The therapist expressed frustration at Tom's limited "capacity for insight" and his "unwillingness" to share his fears or concerns. She documented that in the majority of the sessions he refused to sit and "do therapy," but insisted on standing, walking around, jumping, and making many attempts to leave the office. Tom did not seem to be having a lot of fun in the form of "play" that this therapist wanted to integrate into therapy.

NMT Assessment and Recommendations

Tom was ultimately placed with foster parents who were familiar with the NMT. Clinicians certified in the NMT consulted with the play therapist working with Tom. An NMT assessment was conducted (see Perry & Dobson, 2013 for more details). As part of the NMT assessment process, a brain map was constructed indicating functional status (fully developed and typically functioning relative to a mature adult brain, emerging or precursor capability or mild to moderate compromise, undeveloped or severely dysfunctional). Brain functions are localized to the brain region mediating the specific function (e.g., cardiovascular regulation is a brainstem function; sleep is a diencephalon function; attachment is a limbic function; and abstract cognition is a cortex function). This oversimplification attempts to localize function to the brain region that is the final common mediator of the function, with the knowledge that all brain functions are the product of complex, transregional neural networks. This approximation, however, allows a useful estimate of the developmental/functional status of the child's key functions, establishes the child's "strengths and vulnerabilities," and determines the starting point and nature of enrichment or therapeutic activities most likely to meet the child's specific needs. The map becomes a comparison with a typical, same-age child. The graphic representations allow a clinician, teacher, or parent to quickly visualize important aspects of a child's history and current status. The information is key in designing developmentally appropriate educational enrichment and therapeutic experiences to help the child. Not surprisingly, this assessment demonstrated that while Tom was chronologically 6 years of age, he was developmentally functioning below the level of a toddler in some domains, and in others at or below the level of an 18 month old. He was extremely dysregulated, and it was estimated that his baseline level of arousal was high alarm. This meant that he would have minimal access to any cortically mediated functions and would have minimal cerebromodulatory capability. In short, words were not going to change Tom's behavior. A shift in therapeutic strategy was recommended. The foster parents, Tom's teachers and the play therapist were willing to shift their expectations and interactions with Tom away from cognitive-predominant to an enriched somatosensory schedule. Therapy took place while Tom and his therapist walked, in parallel, in a park. The school allowed Tom to avoid small-group activities (for which he was not yet developmentally ready), and to pursue a schedule of primarily somatosensory activity with a 1:1 aide (walking, playing with clay, finger painting, rocking in a chair, swinging, kicking a soccer ball, etc.). In the home, time with caregivers was spent walking, running, helping groom the pets, giving and receiving hand massages, and sitting side by side in a rocking bench (while his foster mother read to another of the children). The number of "intentional" (i.e., scheduled) somatosensory regulatory and therapeutic hours in the week was increased from 3 (which had been somewhat random) to 18 in the first 3 months of placement, and then to 30 (set up in a more scheduled, predictable pattern).

This regulating set of activities had the effect of minimizing Tom's dysregulated, impulsive, and aggressive behaviors. The positive impact on his state resulted in improved relational functioning, with a corresponding decrease in the anxiety that the teachers and carers felt when Tom was around. The confidence and positive affect of the adults contributed to additional regulation and reward. The positive feedback cycle led to a remarkable cascade of improved functioning that reflected a shift in his baseline state (from high arousal at baseline to low arousal/high alert). This shift in state "unmasked" some previously unexpressed functional capability; moreover, there was improved internalization of new cognitive and relational experiences, which contributed to the building of new functional capabilities. Most remarkable was that Tom passively learned to read (and now loves to read) by sitting next to his foster mother as she read to another child. Certainly Tom has far to go. But prior to the 8 months (at this writing) of the developmentally targeted regulatory interventions, he had 14 months of traditional therapeutic work with minimal impact. Of primary interest to a play therapist is the joy Tom now feels while he is succeeding; play therapy is most effective when it can capture the core elements of true play. The neurobiological power of play can only be fully expressed, however, when the types of adult-imposed play activities match the developmental needs and strengths of the regulated child.

Conclusion

Children who have experienced trauma, chaos, and neglect exhibit complex functional compromise in multiple domains, including physiological, motor, emotional, social, and cognitive. The specific nature and presentation of this multidomain functional compromise will vary, depending upon such factors as genetics and epigenetics, as well as the timing, nature, and pattern of both stressors and relational "buffers" in a child's life. A central finding in these children is a sensitized set of regulatory neural networks that originate in lower areas of the brain and have a wide distribution in the brain and body. By integrating a neurobiology-informed clinical approach, play therapists can select and sequence developmentally appropriate play activities that will help regulate these children and facilitate therapeutic efforts to enhance their relational and cognitive capabilities. The NMT is an evidence-based practice that can provide a practical and useful clinical framework to help play therapists identify the strengths and vulnerabilities of maltreated children, and implement developmentally appropriate therapeutic, educational, and enrichment services.

REFERENCES

Allen, J. (1988). *Inscapes of the child's world: Jungian counseling in schools and clinics.* Dallas, TX: Spring.

American Psychiatric Association. (2013). *Diagnostic and statistical manual of mental disorders* (5th ed.). Arlington, VA: Author.

Anda, R. F., Felitti, V. J., Bremner, D. J., Walker, J., Whitfield, C., Perry, B. D., . . . Giles, W. G. (2006). The enduring effects of abuse and related adverse experiences in childhood. *European Archives of Psychiatric and Clinical Neuroscience, 256*(3), 174–186.

Benedict, H. E. (2006). Object relations play therapy: Applications to attachment problems and relational trauma. In C. E. Schaefer & H. G. Kaduson (Eds.), *Contemporary play therapy: Theory, research, and practice* (pp. 3–27). New York: Guilford Press.

Blaustein, M. E., & Kinniburgh, K. M. (2005). Providing the family as a secure base for therapy with children and adolescents. In K. Blaustein, M. Spinazzola, & B. van der Kolk (Eds.), *Attachment theory into practice* (pp. 48–53). Brookline, MA: Justice Resource Institute.

Brandt, K., Diel, J., Feder, J., & Lillas, C. (2012). A problem in our field. *Journal of Zero to Three, 32*(4), 42–45.

Bratton, S., & Ray, D. (2000). What the research shows about play therapy. *International Journal of Play Therapy, 9*(1), 47–48.

Bratton, S., Ray, D., Rhine, T., & Jones, L. (2005). The efficacy of play therapy with children: A meta-analytic review of treatment outcomes. *Professional Psychology: Research and Practice, 36*(4), 376–390.

Brody, V. (1997). *The dialogue of touch: Developmental play therapy.* Northvale, NJ: Aronson.

Burghardt, G. M. (2005). *The genesis of animal play: Testing the limits.* Cambridge, MA: MIT Press.

Casey, R., & Berman, J. (1985). The outcome of psychotherapy with children. *Psychological Bulletin, 98*(2), 388–400.

Cook, A., Spinazzola, J., Ford, J., Lanktree, C., Blaustein, M. B., Cloitre, M., . . . van der Kolk, B. (2005). Complex trauma in children and adolescents. *Psychiatric Annals, 35*(5), 390–398.

Erikson, E. (1964). *Childhood and society* (2nd ed.). New York: Norton.

Felitti, V. J., Anda, R. F., Nordenberg, D., Williamson, D. F., Spitz, A. M., & Edwards, V. (1998). Relationship of childhood abuse and household dysfunction to many of the leading causes of death in adults: Adverse Childhood Event Study. *American Journal of Preventive Medicine, 14*, 245–258.

Freud, S. (1924). *A general introduction to psycho-analysis.* London: Boni & Liveright.

Gaskill, R. L., & Perry, B. D. (2012). Child sexual abuse, traumatic experiences, and their impact on the developing brain. In P. Goodyear-Brown (Ed.), *Handbook of child sexual abuse: Identification, assessment, and treatment* (pp. 30–47). Hoboken, NJ: Wiley.

Gesell, A., & Ilg, F. (1947). *Infant and child in the culture of today.* New York: Harper.

Guerney, B. (1964). Filial Therapy: Description and rationale. *Journal of Consulting Psychology, 28*, 304–310.

Hopper, J. W., Spinazzola, J., Simpson, W. B., & van der Kolk, B. A. (2006). Preliminary evidence of parasympathetic influence on basal heart rate in posttraumatic stress disorder. *Journal of Psychosomatic Research, 60*, 83–90.

Kleim, J. A., & Jones, T. A. (2008). Principles of experience-dependent neural plasticity: Implications for rehabilitation after brain damage. *Journal of Speech, Language, and Hearing Research, 51*, S225–S239.

Knell, S. M. (1995). *Cognitive behavioral play therapy.* Northvale, NJ: Aronson.

Kohlberg, L. (1963). Moral development and identification. In H. W. Stevenson (Ed.), *Child psychology* (pp. 277–332). Chicago: University of Chicago Press.

Kottman, T. (1995). *Partners in play: An Adlerian approach to play therapy.* Alexandria, VA: American Counseling Association.

Landreth, G. (2002). *Play therapy: Art of the relationship* (2nd ed.). Muncie, IN: Accelerated Development.

LeBlanc, M., & Ritchie, M. (1999). Predictors of play therapy outcomes. *International Journal of Play Therapy, 8*(2), 19–34.

LeBlanc, M., & Ritchie, M. (2001). A meta-analysis of play therapy outcomes. *Counseling Psychology Quarterly, 14*(2), 149–163.

Ludy-Dobson, C. R., & Perry, B. D. (2010). The role of healthy interaction in buffering the impact of childhood trauma. In E. Gil (Ed.), *Working with children to heal interpersonal trauma: The power of play* (pp. 26–43). New York: Guilford Press.

Marteau, T. M., Hollands, G. J., & Fletcher, P. C. (2012). Changing human behavior to prevent disease: The importance of targeting automatic processes. *Science, 337*(6101), 1492–1495.

Norton, C. C., & Norton, B. E. (2002). *Reaching children through play therapy: An experiential approach.* Denver, CO: White Apple Press.

Oaklander, V. (1994). Gestalt play therapy. In K. O'Connor & C. E. Schaefer (Eds.), *Handbook of play therapy* (Vol. 2, pp. 144–146). New York: Wiley.

O'Connor, K. (2000). *The play therapy primer* (2nd ed.). New York: Wiley.

Office of the United Nations High Commissioner for Human Rights. (1989, November 20). *Convention on the rights of the child* (General Assembly Resolution No. 44/25). Retrieved from *www2.ohchr.org*

Pearl, E., Thieken, L., Olafson, E., Boat, B., Connelly, L., Barnes, J., et al. (2012). Effectiveness of community dissemination of parent–child interaction therapy. *Psychological Trauma: Theory, Research, Practice, and Policy, 4*(2), 204–213.

Perry, B. D. (2001). The neuroarcheology of childhood treatment: The neurodevelopmental costs of adverse childhood events. In K. Franey, R. Geffner, & R. Falconer (Eds.), *The cost of maltreatment: Who pays? We all do* (pp. 15–37). San Diego, CA: Family Violence and Sexual Assault Institute.

Perry, B. D. (2006). Applying principles of neurodevelopment to clinical work with maltreated and traumatized children. In N. B. Webb (Ed.), *Working with traumatized youth in child welfare* (pp. 27–52). New York: Guilford Press.

Perry, B. D. (2008). Child maltreatment: The role of abuse and neglect in developmental psychopathology. In T. P. Beauchaine & S. P. Henshaw (Eds.), *Textbook of child and adolescent psychopathology* (pp. 93–128). New York: Wiley.

Perry, B. D. (2009). Examining child maltreatment through a neurodevelopmental lens: Clinical application of the Neurosequential Model of Therapeutics. *Journal of Loss and Trauma, 14,* 240–255.

Perry, B. D. (in press). Applications of a developmentally sensitive and neurobiologically-informed approach to clinical problem solving: The Neurosequential Model of Therapeutics (NMT) in young maltreated children. In K. Brandt, B. D. Perry, S. Seligman, & E. Tronick (Eds.), *Infant and early childhood mental health.* Arlington, VA: American Psychiatric Publishing.

Perry, B. D., & Dobson, C. L. (2013). Application of the Neurosequential Model of Therapeutics (NMT) in maltreated children. In J. D. Ford & C. A. Courtois (Eds.), *Treating complex traumatic stress disorders in children and adolescents* (pp. 249–260). New York: Guilford Press.

Perry, B. D., & Pollard, R. (1998). Homeostasis, stress, trauma, and adaptation: A neurodevelopmental view of childhood trauma. *Child and Adolescent Psychiatric Clinics of North America, 7*(1), 33–51.

Perry, B. D., Pollard, R., Blakley, T., Baker, W., & Vigilante, D. (1995). Childhood trauma, the neurobiology of adaptation, and "use-dependent" development of the brain: How "states" become "traits." *Infant Mental Health Journal, 16*(4), 271–291.

Perry, B. D., & Szalavitz, M. (2006). *The boy who was raised as a dog: And other stories from a child psychiatrist's notebook.* New York: Basic Books.

Piaget, J. (1962). *Play, dreams, and imitation in childhood.* New York: McGraw-Hill.

Ray, D., Bratton, S., Rhine, T., & Jones, L. (2001). The effectiveness of play therapy: Responding to the critics. *International Journal of Play Therapy, 10*(1), 85–108.

Rousseau, J. (1930). *Emile.* New York: Dent. (Original work published 1762)

Sara, S. J., & Bouret, S. (2012). Orienting and reorienting: The locus coeruleus mediates cognition through arousal. *Neuron, 76,* 130–141.

Shapiro, D., & Levendosky, A. (1999). Adolescent survivors of childhood sexual abuse: The mediating role of attachment and coping in psychological and interpersonal functioning. *Child Abuse and Neglect, 11,* 1175–1191.

Spinazzola, J., Blaustein, M., & van der Kolk, B. A. (2005). Post-traumatic stress disorder treatment outcome research: The study of unrepresentative sample. *Journal of Traumatic Stress, 18*(5), 425–436.

Szalavitz, M., & Perry, B. D. (2010). *Born for love.* New York: HarperCollins.

Tsai, M., & Ray, D. C. (2011). Play therapy outcome prediction: An exploratory study at a university-based clinic. *International Journal of Play Therapy, 20*(2), 94–108.

Ungar, M., & Perry, B. D. (2012). Violence, trauma and resilience. In R. Alaggia & C. Vine (Eds.), *Cruel but not unusual: Violence in Canadian families* (2nd ed.). Waterloo, Ontario, Canada: Wilfrid Laurier University Press.

van der Kolk, B. A. (2006). Clinical implications of neuroscience research in PTSD. *Annals of the New York Academy of Science, 107*(IV), 277–293.

van der Kolk, B. A., Spinazzola, J., Blaustein, M. E., Hopper, J. W., Hopper, E. K., Korn, D. L., et al. (2007). A randomized clinical trial of eye movement desensitization and reprocessing (EMDR), fluoxetine, and pill placebo in the treatment of posttraumatic stress disorder: Treatment effects and long-term maintenance. *Journal of Clinical Psychiatry, 68*(1), 37–46.

Vygotsky, L. S. (1967). Play and its role in the mental development of the child. *Soviet Psychology, 5*(3), 6–18.

Weisz, J., Weiss, B., Alicke, M., & Klotz, M. (1987). Effectiveness of psychotherapy with children and adolescence: A meta-analysis for clinicians. *Journal of Consulting and Clinical Psychology, 55*(4), 542–549.

Zeanah, C. H., Scheeringa, N. W., Boris, N. W., Heller, S. S., Smyke, A. T., & Trapani, J. (2004). Reactive attachment disorder in maltreated toddlers. *Child Abuse and Neglect, 28*(8), 877–888.

Zigler, E. F., Singer, D. G., & Bishop-Josef, S. J. (2004). *Children's play: The roots of reading.* Washington, DC: Zero to Three Press.

PART III

Clinical Applications: Approaches to Working with At-Risk Populations

CHAPTER 12

Helping Foster Care Children Heal from Broken Attachments

Athena A. Drewes

This chapter addresses the impact of attachment difficulties that children and teens in the foster care system experience with their caregivers, and describes how therapists can utilize a prescriptive/integrative approach to treat them. Play therapists and other child therapists will be helped to understand the unique challenges these children/teens and their foster caregivers confront in forming attachments; ways to utilize play-based techniques that will directly address complex trauma suffered through loss of the biological parents, broken attachments, and other subsequent abuses; and ways to work with a caregiver and family in understanding a foster child's special emotional needs. I describe the need for both directive and nondirective treatment approaches in working with foster care children, as well as how and what expressive arts techniques can be successfully utilized to help heal the emotional hole in the heart of such a child.

Challenges to Attachment Formation in Foster Care

Children in foster care often have histories of complex trauma (primarily attachment-based trauma), which results in increased externalizing and internalizing problems. Those foster care children with externalizing behaviors are at particular risk for placement disruptions, resulting in multiple placements over time and creating a vicious cycle of breaks in attachment. Consequently, they are not likely to trust authority figures and other adults around them, and are guarded and disengaged (Earl, 2009). Engaging such children in treatment involves confronting a series of challenges.

Emotional walls are put up as inner fortifications, and these defenses make it extremely difficult to gain access to these angry young persons in therapy. However, we as play and child therapists play an important role as attachment figures and can be agents of change in reaching troubled attachment-disordered foster children and teens.

After an initial "honeymoon" period in treatment (and in the foster home), a foster child with a history of disrupted attachment generally begins testing limits, looking for vulnerabilities and weak spots within the foster parents to see how long they will tolerate the child's behaviors before sending him or her away again, as all the other foster parents have done. Difficulties with affect regulation; problems with feelings identification, expression, and integration; limited coping strategies; hoarding of food; poor hygiene; destruction of property; low self-esteem; and hypercontrol soon begin to manifest themselves. These behaviors in the foster home cause the foster parents, and even the therapist, to feel helpless, demoralized, emotionally exhausted, angry, frustrated, and hostile. In turn, these feelings lead to deeper feelings of inadequacy and guilt.

Moreover, treatment may need to involve not only the foster child and foster parents, but also the child's siblings, both biological and foster. These siblings can feel terrorized in their own home both physically and through verbal assaults by the foster child, along with feeling resentful that the foster child is getting more attention through negative behaviors than they do. Even family pets are not immune from negative actions by the foster child. Pets can be poked, kicked, teased, dropped, fed too much or too little, or even killed by a foster child.

Many foster parents have the mistaken view that "love will conquer all." Although in part this is true, since a caregiver's unconditional love is of course essential, other factors are needed as well: stability and security of the home, clear expectations, and concise directions, along with nurturance and encouragement of the caregiver by the therapist to remain in control. However, these factors do not create the most comfortable environment for the foster child, who will resist and engage in control battles that will spill into the therapy sessions. It is important for the therapist to work individually not only with the foster child on attachment issues, but with the foster caregiver, who may in time become the adoptive parent.

Treatment Approaches

Within the safety of the therapy room, much as in the safety of the new foster home, the foster child can feel secure enough to explore, identify, and make sense of thoughts, feelings, wishes, and intentions, along with discovering strengths and seeing him- or herself from a new perspective (Hughes, 2009). It is therefore critical for the therapist to sincerely accept and respect the inherent worth and dignity of the foster child, while offering a safe and genuinely supportive environment. This will be especially important when the foster child begins testing the therapist and the limits of therapy, and resists getting emotionally attached during treatment. We therapists need to give foster children control over their physical environment—allowing them to determine how close to or distant from us they want to be, whether they need a physical barrier (e.g., a hoodie pulled over the head, a pillow or stuffed animal to hug), and at what pace they wish to engage with us or try to navigate the intensity of the one-to-one relationship (Earl, 2009). Indeed, the child-centered play therapy philosophy of following a child's/teen's lead and pace allows the young client to feel that personal boundaries and protective defenses are being respected.

Offering invitational expressive arts and directive play-based activities within the sessions not only will allow the child or teen to experience fun, but will give him or her a sought-after sense of control. The use of expressive arts materials allows the therapy to move at the level of the foster child's emotional rather than chronological age. It also allows the therapist time to get to understand and respect the vulnerable foster child's avoidant, withdrawn, or aggressive defensive behaviors, which were created to protect the child from perceptions of an unsafe and betraying world (Earl, 2009). In addition, the play therapist offers through the shared activities an emotional nurturance, or what Miller (2005) terms "nourishing communication." Through the therapist's playfulness, acceptance, curiosity, and empathy, the foster client begins to experience *intersubjectivity*, feeling nourished and enhanced by another person—experience lacking while the client was an infant. Child-centered, play-based therapy sessions can offer the child/teen the necessary time, space, and choice to begin exploring the treatment relationship along with his or her personal issues, in an atmosphere of unconditional acceptance. Such therapy sessions with an attachment-disordered foster child can also reduce verbal demands on the child through the use of expressive arts materials (e.g., sandtray work, drawing, collage making, clay work, painting, music, movement, drama, mask making, etc.). Working with expressive arts allows for communication to stay within a metaphor while the child or teen explores intimate and often painful material nonverbally. The creation can contain what has been experienced without causing the young client to feel exposed.

It is particularly critical for us as therapists to convey to foster children that we are equally interested in all aspects of their lives, not just the problems. We are not merely interested in "fixing" them, but are genuinely interested in their interests, worries, strengths, challenges, and successes, as well as the past and future, with all on an equal level. Through attunement to and matching of a foster child's or teen's affective state, along with a shared focus of attention, a relationship and a dialogue can begin to develop.

Treatment Issues

Issues that surface in working with foster care clients include grief and bereavement over the loss of their biological parents (at birth or later in their lives), difficulties with affect regulation (particularly anger), and difficulties with forming and keeping relationships and friendships. Consequently, the treatment of choice can be dyadic therapy with the foster parent/caregiver (if possible) or family therapy, but often it is individual therapy with collateral contact with this caregiver. For younger foster care children (especially those under the age of 10 for whom therapists are trying to build a relationship with their foster caregivers), the use of developmental play, Theraplay, parent–child interaction therapy, the Circle of Security, dyadic developmental psychotherapy, child–parent relationship therapy, or Filial Therapy can be most helpful, along with individual therapy as needed.

Once a safe environment is established in therapy, and trust begins to develop between a foster care client and a therapist, use of a prescriptive/integrative approach should be considered for individual therapy. In such an approach, the therapist takes responsibility for guiding the therapy process and for challenging the foster care client to address specific concerns. An integrative approach uses both directive and nondirective approaches—respecting the traumatized foster child's competing drives for mastery and control, while they may at the same time want to suppress and avoid painful and conflicted material that needs to be dealt with. The therapist assesses prescriptively what treatment approach and techniques should be utilized, based on the client's symptoms and current concerns. As treatment progresses, the therapist may change treatment modalities (e.g., may bring in dyadic work more or may move more into individual work) as indicated by the needs of the client. Therefore, treatment is custom-made for each client and evolves over time.

The use of play-based techniques and expressive arts interventions is often the most successful method of engaging a foster care client and working through many issues. The way I handle an integrative session is to use the first 5 minutes as a "check-in" on issues or homework from the last session, reports from the school or foster parent, unfinished issues from the last session, and so on. Then we spend the next 15–20 minutes on directive expressive arts and play-based techniques that address various issues facing the foster child. The remaining time is left for nondirective play, in which the child can choose an activity or use the playroom in any way he or she would like (as long as safety and other basic requirements are respected). The foster parent can be brought in during any of these time slots to join in the activities, or alternate sessions may include dyadic work with the foster parent, or a once-monthly session can be held alone with the foster parent to work on parenting skills, as needed.

Addressing Allegiance Issues

Allegiance is a big topic that often arises with regard to foster children or teens and their current caregivers versus their biological parents. Often a foster child has ambivalence about connecting with or loving another "mother," which results in difficulty bonding with the current caregiver or future adoptive parent. Loyalty to the biological mother remains, regardless of how much or little a foster child or teen knows about the birth parent or of the treatment the child received from that parent. Some foster clients may not want to be adopted because of their strong feelings of allegiance to their birth parents. Therefore, it is always critical that the foster caregivers not force the teen or child into calling them "Mom" and "Dad" upon entering their home. It is also crucial that the foster caregivers not speak poorly of either birth parent, as the foster client has 50% of each birth parent within him or her! Any negative comments that are made about the birth parent(s) are interpreted as though they are made about the client and become integrated into the child's sense of self, further decreasing his or her already low self-esteem.

Expressive Arts and Play-Based Techniques

Letters to Birth Parents

In addressing foster children's loss of and grief for their birth parents, I explore with them whether they ever wonder about their birth parents. Do they ever wonder if they look like them? On their birthdays, do they wonder if their birth parents are thinking about them? Foster caregivers are encouraged to ask these questions too, and to make statements such as "Your birth parents would be proud of you, just as we are," or "I wonder if your birth mom has curly hair like you," or "I'm so glad they gave you to us!" (Eldridge, 1999).

I also wonder (and encourage foster parents to wonder) to the foster clients about the various confusions that could arise from having two sets of parents, the biological and the foster parents; or about their mixed-up feelings on birthdays when they remember their birth parents; or what questions they might have about why their birth mothers placed them for foster care or adoption. It is important to normalize the common feeling among foster children that they should not love another mom. Many children and teens feel anger at their birth mothers and want to punish them for abandonment, while at the same time they are crying from the depths of their broken hearts for a reunion. But I assure my foster clients that their hearts are big enough for two moms.

I often work with a foster client on writing a letter to a birth parent (whether or not the child knows anything about this parent) that the client can then keep. The letter can be short or can elaborate on such issues as these:

> "Why didn't you keep me? Is it because you didn't like me? What is your name, and what do you look like? I feel really mad because I didn't get to know you. Is there something wrong with you? Is that the reason I can't see you? Is there something wrong with me?"

Case Vignette: Candace's Letter to the Court and Grief Box

Sometimes children do not want to be adopted and want to stay in foster care. Advocating for their right to decide is an important job of the therapist. Here is an example of one foster teen's feelings about allegiance issues. Candace was 12 years old, and recounted that she had been in seven foster homes and two group homes prior to coming to our program to be in a therapeutic foster home. She had initially been placed in regular foster care at around 4 years of age; she numbered only three of her homes as favorites. Her birth mother was involved in drugs, and her parental rights were terminated. Candace was removed from her last foster home (with her sister) because she kept running away, mainly to be able to have contact with her mother. In therapy, she wrote the following for the judge:

> "I have been living with [the foster family] about one year and a couple of months. Many of my foster parents are the type of parents that I wouldn't mind being adopted by them. The only problem is that I only have one mother, and I don't want anyone else to be my real mother. She is my birth mother. Many people also tell me that just because you get adopted doesn't mean you can't go looking for your birth mother. But the way I feel is that you could only have one real mother. And only one. But that is my very own opinion. I don't mind living with a foster parent for a couple of years or so, but for me, I don't want to be adopted by anyone. I have a mother. But I am thankful for those who think of me as their child. And I think of them as my parents, but not my real parents."

Being able to tell the judge her feelings helped Candace to feel empowered.

Our sessions were spent on Candace's grief for and loss of her biological mom. Candace made up collages of things she remembered about her biological mother, as well as things she could enjoy about her foster mother. We also created a "grief box" (Eldridge, 1999). This is a box that can be decorated on the outside. We made a list of the various losses she had in her life: the loss of her birth parents, her personal medical history, her birth family's history, a sense of belonging, and a sense of having a continuous life narrative. Candace was encouraged to select from magazines pictures of a mother and child and of a father and child to represent the loss of her birth parents; to use a Band-Aid for loss of her full medical history (she often could not answer questions the doctor would ask about allergies and medical history of her family); to draw a picture of a tree or to find a blank family tree chart for the loss of her birth family's history; to use a drawing or magazine photo of someone who looked sad for her loss of belonging; and to use a broken cord or string for the loss of a continuous life story. Throughout treatment, we referred back to the grief box and the various objects, decorating it, and we sometimes added other things to it. This box became the storage place for all the emptiness Candace felt and the hole in her heart that was created by the loss of all these things.

I became the caretaker of these heavy burdens and losses, and we kept exploring them gently and slowly throughout treatment. Throughout our work together, through expressive art and play-based techniques, we explored ways to fill the hole in Candace's heart. At various points in treatment, I would repeatedly stress how her parents had done the best they could with the abilities they had at the time they were living together. Her birth mom's own problems got in the way of being the parent Candace wanted her to be, so she just could not be the parent she needed her to be. I stressed to Candace that she was lovable and was born lovable. Unfortunately, however, there was no magic to be able to make her parents into the people she needed them to be and wanted desperately for them to be.

Wall around the Heart

Daniel Hughes (1997) writes of a technique that Foster Cline (1991) has developed for therapy with foster children. Cline draws sequential pictures of babies from birth, at the age of their broken attachment and their placement in foster care, and then at their current age, to help emphasize how they create a "wall around the heart." I have adapted this technique and prefer to use drawings of hearts, but I use the same time sequence. In the first picture, I have the foster client draw a small heart and write under it his or her name, with "One day old" next to it. I ask the child, "Do you know what the heart is for?" Most kids say that it is necessary to keep them alive. I agree that it helps the blood to keep moving, but that it also is for loving and feeling love, an emotional heart. I suggest that when a child was born, his or her heart worked quite well, and the child was probably pretty good at being able to give and receive love. Then the next picture drawn is a somewhat larger heart, again with the child's name, and then with the child's age at about the time the child was neglected or the parent(s) abandoned him or her. I speak briefly about the pain of being treated that way and indicate that such pain hurts the heart. We then draw cracks on the heart. Drawing a third heart, larger still, I talk about how the pain in the heart is so great that the child has worked out a very smart way of saving the heart from any further pain. We then draw a wall around the heart. We create arrows of pain by crumpling up paper and then throwing it at the heart, but it all bounces off the wall and cannot cause any more cracks. I praise the child for saving his or her heart from breaking further by creating that strong wall. Then the child is asked to draw a fourth heart and date it at a time since he or she has been living in the current foster home. I ask the child to draw the cracks again, but to make many of them smaller; we also put Band-Aids over several of the bigger cracks (see Figure 12.1), representing how the cracks are healing or have healed. I then have the child draw the wall around the heart again in pencil. I tell him or her,

> "You no longer need the wall. And in fact, the wall stops love from reaching your heart. You may not be sure that your foster parents really do love you, but there is no way to experience the love, because the wall is there. The best solution is for us to find a way to take down the wall. Instead of the wall being a fort that helped to keep pain out, it has now changed into a prison wall. Now it keeps you from getting the love that you want."

I tell the child that the foster parents and I are willing to help him or her learn how to take down the wall. I ask for suggestions on how we can do this, and we then can start to erase the wall a little at a time.

Letter from the Biological Mother

As noted earlier, many foster children feel that they cannot love two mothers. In such cases, I reflect that their birth mothers would want them to

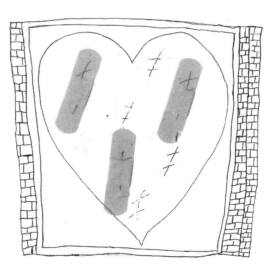

FIGURE 12.1. A re-created example of the fourth heart in the Wall around the Heart exercise, showing the partial healing of earlier cracks/wounds.

have mothers who loved them, since they could not raise them, and that the children's hearts are big enough to love two mothers. I ask them, "What would you imagine your birth mother saying to you, if she found out when you were 18 years old that you had continued to fight your foster or adoptive parents and refused to be close to anyone during your entire childhood?"

Then I make up a letter:

"[Child's name], I am so sad that you were unhappy and angry during your whole childhood. I know that I was not able to provide you with a good childhood. I could not be the parent you needed me to be. But I also wished that you had let yourself get close to another mom who could have loved you, laughed with you, taught you and kept you safe. I know that [the foster mother's name] could have been that mom. I'm sad that you did not let yourself get close to her. You could have loved her and me too your whole life."

The child can then write his or her own letter from the birth mother, or even a letter back to the birth mother. It is important to help the child get in touch with the grief for and loss of the hoped-for parent—the idealized parent.

Techniques for Affect Identification and Regulation

Allan Schore (2003a, 2003b) writes that the most far-reaching effect of relational trauma is the loss of the ability to regulate the intensity of affect. Therefore, I usually work with foster children on building up a feelings vocabulary, being able to physically identify where they have their feelings, and learning how to integrate their feelings with better choices for problem-solving and coping skills when they are angry and upset. The Gingerbread Person Feelings Map (Drewes, 2001) is a variation of the Color Your Life technique (O'Connor, 1983), but uses drawing of a gingerbread person with arms outstretched, and with eyes, nose, and smile. It can be used with teens, as well as younger children, and in caregiver/parent–client dyads. The technique is used in order to assess (1) the overall range of feelings the client has and can verbally identify; (2) how aware the client is of where he or she physiologically feels these emotions; and (3) how well integrated the client's emotions are. The Gingerbread Person Feelings Map allows this information to be gathered in a nonthreatening and play-based way; it only takes a few minutes and can be used as an icebreaker in a first session, or at any time during treatment when appropriate.

Next to the shape of a gingerbread person, I add the words, *happy, sad, angry, worried, afraid*, and *love*, one under the other (see Figure 12.2). I then ask the foster child or teen to choose a few other feeling words to add. (I am often surprised at what children include, such as *petrified, stupid,*

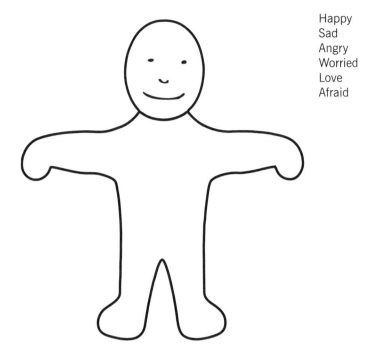

Happy
Sad
Angry
Worried
Love
Afraid

FIGURE 12.2. Gingerbread Person Feelings Map.

anxious, wishing I was somebody else, etc.) I write these words underneath the standard emotion words. This helps the child to expand his or her "emotional vocabulary." It also helps to give the child some control over the task and a feeling of being an active participant in the process. Next, I have the child choose a color for each feeling. It does not matter what colors are chosen (sometimes I get black for happy!). I also have the child or teen put a little line using the color chosen next to each of the feeling words, like creating a legend for a map.

Then I ask the client to use each color to indicate where inside the gingerbread person he or she may physically experience each feeling listed. The client can shade the colors in, scribble, draw hearts, or the like. Next, I go through each feeling and have the client imagine where he or she feels each one (so that none are left out). Once this task is completed (usually after less than 5 minutes), we process the drawing together. I pay particular attention to where in the body anger is expressed and how this might play out in the foster child's or teen's world in responding to situations, and I point this out to the client. I also look for how many feelings are integrated, and for how much color is used and where. In addition, I look for discrepancies: for instance, the child may have colored in happy feelings on the face, but anger in the hands, feet, or body; or may have placed a spot of color

representing anger outside of the figure (possibly signifying difficulty tolerating that emotion). In such a case, I process how the client may present to
others as calm, but inwardly he or she is seething, or perhaps is manifesting
anger through hitting others or restlessness in the legs. Also, where does the
child or teen put love (often drawn as a heart), and is it "walled off" by layers of scared, hurt, or angry feelings? If so, I explain how we each can have
more than one feeling at a time within us; sometimes we feel ambivalent
(e.g., angry and loving) at the same time toward someone. And sometimes
one feeling is so strong that it can hide other feelings that we are feeling too,
making us feel confused and unsure of what we are feeling.

This technique can be used with a foster parent and the teen/child
together, with each working independently of the other. At the end, the parent and child/teen can share their finished products and compare similarities and differences in the ways anger and other emotions are felt. Another
adaptation of this technique involves using two gingerbread figures (Gil,
2006). The child or teen colors in each figure according to the various feelings experienced when with each parent, either foster parent or biological
parent.

Young clients who may be uncomfortable thinking about their bodies and using a person-like shape (especially if they were sexually abused)
may prefer using a heart shape. Heartfelt Feelings Coloring Card Strategies (Crenshaw, 2008) are preprinted cards, each with a drawn heart and
feelings words to add colors to, in order to help children identify, label,
and express their feelings about "heartfelt" issues and relationships with
the important people in their lives. As with the Gingerbread Person Feelings Map or Color Your Life, a teen or child picks colors to match various
feelings listed and fills in the amount of each feeling he or she has, thereby
quantifying how he or she is feeling at the moment or at some other point
in time. The client can also write on the card a response to a time when
he or she had this feeling. Color Your Heart (Goodyear-Brown, 2010) is
another variation utilizing a heart shape, which is colored in proportion to
the amounts of feelings in the child's heart.

Use of Clay as a Metaphor for Clients' Lives

I ask foster clients to take a small piece of Play-Doh or oogly clay (*www.
theooglykit.com*), which is easily malleable and softens up quickly; to close
their eyes (or, if they do not feel safe enough to do that, to stare off at
something across the room); and, without looking or speaking, to create
something within a 2-minute time period. Once the time is up, I have them
look at what they created. Is it as they had imagined it would be? Did it turn
out the way they expected?

I then process with the clients how their clay creations are much like
their lives. Things happen in their lives, many of which are beyond control
(being put into foster care, having parents who were unable to care for

them, being unable to magically change their lives, having other abuses happen to them, etc.). But just as they are now able to change their creations, improve on them, make them more like how they want them to look, or start all over, so too they can do that with their lives. Some things may take until they are 18 years old or older, such as living on their own or looking for their biological parents. But they can make changes in other things now, such as how they react when they are angry, how they cope, whether they want to let others into their hearts and trust them, or whether they can keep from being sent away to another home. And just like their creations at this moment, they too can decide whether they want to continue with what has turned out or be an active force in making a difference in their lives and in the lives of those with whom they come in contact.

Magical Smiles

I teach my foster clients that they have magic within themselves. This is something that no one can take from them, that is within them and with them all the time, and that is so magical it can make others do things. Intrigued, the foster clients inevitably become interested. I tell them, "It is your smile. You have the most beautiful smile." (And, truly, I have not met anyone who does not have a beautiful smile that makes me respond in turn with a smile!) Of course, once I say this, a bright smile forms on every client's face! I then challenge the clients with homework of going out in the next week and smiling at three people that they choose (and we talk about people they know that they might try this with). The catch is that the clients need to look each person in the eye, so the other person knows they are looking at him or her. Then, when eye contact is made, they smile and see what happens. I always start the next session by checking on this homework and seeing the results of their smiles. Inevitably, even if they only tried it once, magic occurred in making another person smile back!

Case Vignette: Kayla's Jenga Session

Jenga is a game that taps physical and mental skills and can be played by children ages 5 and up, as well as by teens and adults. It is played with 54 small wooden blocks stacked in groups of three, which are criss-crossed to create 18 levels. Moving in Jenga consists of taking one and only one block from any level (except the one below the incomplete top level) of the tower, and placing it on the topmost level in order to complete it (see Figure 12.3). The game ends when the tower falls. The child/teen can go first, but it does not matter if the foster parent or therapist goes first, at the child/teen's request. Usually the client wants to go first, but if the client is unsure of the game and how to play it, it is sometimes helpful for the therapist to go first to model how it is played.

Kayla, age 9, was placed in foster care at age 5. Kayla's biological mother had a history of psychiatric problems, along with alcoholism, and

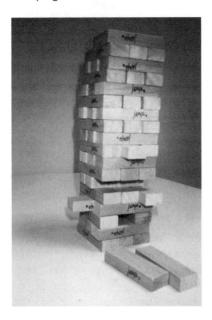

FIGURE 12.3. A Jenga session in progress.

there was no known history on the biological father. Kayla entered therapy because of attachment and bereavement issues related to the loss of significant people in her life, as well as systemic family issues in her foster home that were affecting her emotional and behavioral functioning.

After several sessions, Kayla spontaneously decided to use the Jenga game and wanted to go first after setting up the tower. Kayla carefully removed each of her blocks, putting them on the top and building the tower up. She was proud of her ability to build up the tower without making it fall. When it finally did fall, after many layers, it was due to my removal of a block. Kayla was delighted, clapping and laughing with glee when this happened. She quickly built up the tower to play another game. At this point, I decided to use Jenga metaphorically to help represent Kayla's losses and begin to address her attachment and loss issues. After about five or six blocks had been removed, leaving holes in the tower, and being placed on top with the tower higher, I began a discussion:

THERAPIST: You know, Kayla, when each block gets taken out, there is a hole that remains behind that makes the tower not very solid and strong. It reminds me of losses children experience and how it feels like there are emotional holes in their heart, which make their reactions to people and situations off balance. It makes me think of the experiences that you have had in your life.

KAYLA: Yeah?

THERAPIST: Yep. You have had many losses in your life. Let's see, each hole could represent your bio-mom, your bio-dad, and your foster dad, along with Tim, Fred, and now John.

KAYLA: My foster mom has a lot of boyfriends.

THERAPIST: And each time you make a friendship, then they leave. It must be hard to trust and try to get close to people, like the next boyfriend.

KAYLA: Yeah. Mom wants me to call them Dad, but I don't like that. And sometimes they act like they are the boss of me.

THERAPIST: So sometimes it makes you angry and maybe even confused. And then when they leave, sometimes you are left with a feeling hole in your heart, missing the people you cared for. And then there are some important people that you didn't even get to know well, like your bio-mom and bio-dad, who put you into foster care. (*Kayla appears interested and is actively watching and listening.*) So when you take out the block from Jenga and it makes a hole, it results in an unstable foundation. And the tower can fall down. Just like when people leave your life, they make a feeling hole in your heart, which results in not trusting others and acting out your feelings.

KAYLA: Yeah!

THERAPIST: But then you can rebuild the Jenga tower again the way you want it to be. You can take blocks from the top to make a secure base. Just like in therapy, we can help to start to fill in the holes in your heart by talking about all your feelings and missing your bio-parents and your foster dad. And we can find out who in your life could help give you what you need when you are feeling upset. So for this first block, if we were to put it back in to make the tower stronger, who would it represent? Who in your life now could be there for you and help you feel better when you are upset?

KAYLA: My foster mom. Even though she makes me angry sometimes, I can talk to her, and she gives lots of hugs.

THERAPIST: Great. Let's think of another person.

KAYLA: This one can be Miss Higgins, my teacher. She always knows the right thing to say when I am feeling sad. And this other one is for you, because you are a good listener and care about how I feel. And this last one is for my best friend, Maria. I can share my worries with her, and she shares hers.

THERAPIST: Great. Let's now take some of the blocks out and write different feelings on them. I'll write *angry* on this one. What feeling do you want to put on this one?

KAYLA: *Happy.*

THERAPIST: I'll put down *sad.*

KAYLA: *Frustrated. (This process continues until about 15 of the blocks have been given different feeling words, sometimes with help from the feelings poster on the wall.)*

THERAPIST: Now let's play Jenga again, but this time let's mix up the blocks with these feeling words on them with those that don't have anything written. Each time we pull out a block, we can talk about a time we had the feeling, and what we did to feel better or show our feeling.

Kayla and I continued to play Jenga, talking about the various people who had left an emotional hole and ways that it could be filled. We then went on to discuss feelings that came up in particular situations, along with ways the feelings were handled successfully or not so successfully. Toward the end of the session, I took a few of the fallen tower blocks and showed Kayla how thoughts, feelings, and behaviors are connected, and how one action can lead to another and perhaps to a not-so-beneficial outcome.

I selected seven blocks and placed them in a row near each other, standing up. Using a recent example of something that happened in school that got Kayla in trouble, I identified each block as representing each step of the situation.

THERAPIST: So first the girl bumps into you while you are near your desk, which is this first block. Then the second block represents you feeling angry and yelling back at her. The third block is when you push the girl back. The fourth block is when the teacher comes over. The fifth block is when you get upset at the teacher and yell at her for telling you to quiet down. The sixth block is when you kick over your chair. And the last block is when your teacher tells you to go down to the principal's office. So if we push over this first block *(the therapist does this)*, see how it quickly knocks down each of the other blocks to the end.

But now we can set them up a bit differently. *(The therapist stands two blocks close together, and the remaining five blocks much further apart from each other, so they will not knock each other down if they fall.)* This first block is where the girl knocks into you and you feel angry. The second block is where you feel angry but decide instead to do something else, like take a deep breath and say, "Hey, don't push me," instead of pushing her back. If we knock over the first block, it hits the second block, but all the rest of the blocks still remain standing, and you don't get sent to the principal's office.

Our work together in therapy is going to help you in identifying your feelings and figuring out other ways to react early on, so that you don't get yourself in trouble. How does that sound to you?

KAYLA: Great. Thanks! I don't like getting in trouble in school. This is fun. See you next week!

By using the Jenga game in these ways, a therapist can help explain attachment deficits and their impact on a client's emotional life, explore the resources available to the client, and increase the client's feelings vocabulary. The therapist can also expand the game to include coping strategies that could go with angry and sad feelings, and the blocks can be used to match up feelings with strategies. Also, the therapist can write sentence stems on pieces of paper (these stems may reflect misperceptions about being in foster care, questions about why the birth parents gave the client up, self-esteem statements, etc.). Some examples of sentence stems are "Only bad children get adopted," "I am lovable," "Parents always love their children," "The color of my hair is ugly," and "I am beautiful and smart." Each time a block is taken out (leaving a hole behind), the child/teen or therapist chooses one of the slips of paper and reads it. The therapist can then explore which thoughts are helpful and accurate and which are unhelpful and inaccurate by asking, "How does that sentence make you feel?" or "What if your best friend said that? What would you say back?" The child is then encouraged to come up with alternative statements that are more helpful or accurate: "What could you say that would help to make you feel better?"

In Kayla's particular case, Jenga was used to help understand the child's view of being in foster care; to access her deep feelings of loss, bereavement, and broken attachment; and to assess resources in her life, along with the depth of Kayla's feelings and her ability to make use of feelings vocabulary. However, Jenga can also be used for assessing and developing fine motor skills, increasing impulse control and task-oriented behavior, building self-esteem and competence, encouraging acceptance of rules, and modeling losing as well as winning. My hope in this session and subsequent ones was that Kayla would be able to better understand and visually grasp the concept of having "emotional holes in her heart" with regard to her losses and multiple placements, and the related feelings associated with the experiences. The foster parent could also be invited in to play the game and also help fill in the missing information to make the tower stronger.

Guided Relaxation

To aid children with deep breathing/relaxation and to help them avoid acting out when angry, the guided relaxation exercise known as Safe Place

(Drewes, 2011a, 2011b; James, 1989) is an effective tool they can use at any time. As clients sit with eyes closed, they imagine being a movie director. They are directed to breathe slowly in and out and to think of a time and place when they felt safe. It could be lying in the sun at the beach, hiding under their covers, snuggling with a favorite pet, or the like. They are told to zoom in their camera and film the location, taking in all that there is. Then they freeze the camera shot. As they continue to breathe slowly in and out, they look around and notice what they see, smell, hear, and feel, and whether or not there are any people or animals there. As they continue to breathe slowly in and out, they are instructed to feel how safe they are and how relaxed they feel in their bodies while in their safe space. Next they give their special safe place a name, preferably one word. It is the key that will get them back to their safe place any time they wish to go. All they have to do is remember the name. The clients continue to breathe in and out slowly, focusing on how relaxed and safe they feel. Then after a few minutes, they are directed to move the camera slowly back, and in another minute they will be back in the room with the therapist with their eyes open. The goal is to use operant conditioning to link the deep breathing with the experience of feeling safe and with the word chosen. Then, when the clients are upset or anxious, they can remember the word and their bodies will automatically begin to relax.

Conclusion

In general, the important key to entering the world of an attachment-disordered foster child or teen is integrative use of directive and nondirective expressive arts and play-based techniques that are both enjoyable and engaging, and that prescriptively meet the needs arising from the child/teen's symptoms and issues at the moment. It is also important to work on the issues of loss/bereavement resulting from separation from the biological parents, along with affect regulation and expression to help in dealing with underlying attachment and allegiance issues. Inclusion of the foster parent(s) is also critical in reinforcing gains and helping to generalize learned techniques for coping, as well as in building the bond of a new attachment.

REFERENCES

Cline, F. W. (1991). *Hope for high risk and rage filled children*. Evergreen, CO: Evergreen Consultants in Human Behavior.

Crenshaw, D. A. (2008). Heartfelt Feelings Coloring Cards Strategies. In L. Lowenstein (Ed.), *Assessment and treatment activities for children, adolescents, and families* (pp. 80–81). Toronto: Champion Press.

Drewes, A. A. (2001). Gingerbread Person Feelings Map. In H. G. Kaduson & C. E. Schaefer (Eds.), *101 more favorite play therapy techniques* (pp. 92–97). Northvale, NJ: Aronson.

Drewes, A. A. (2011a, April 29). *A skill-building workshop: Effectively blending play-based techniques with cognitive behavioral therapy for affect regulation in sexually abused and traumatized children.* Workshop presented at the Annual Conference of the Canadian Association for Child and Play Therapy, Guelph, Ontario, Canada.

Drewes, A. A. (2011b). Working with attachment disordered teens in foster care. *Play Therapy: Magazine of the British Association for Play Therapy*, No. 68, pp. 6–9.

Earl, B. (2009). Exterior fortresses and interior fortification. In A. Perry (Ed.), *Teenagers and attachment: Helping adolescents engage with life and learning* (pp. 97–121). Richmond, UK: Worth.

Eldridge, S. (1999). *Twenty things adopted kids wish their adoptive parents knew.* New York: Dell.

Gil, E. (2006). *Helping abused and traumatized children: Integrating directive and nondirective approaches.* New York: Guilford Press.

Goodyear-Brown, P. (2010). *Play therapy with traumatized children: A prescriptive approach.* Hoboken, NJ: Wiley.

Hughes, D. (1997). *Facilitating developmental attachment: The road to emotional recovery and behavioral change in foster and adopted children.* Northvale, NJ: Aronson.

Hughes, D. (2009). Principles of attachment and intersubjectivity. In A. Perry (Ed.), *Teenagers and attachment: Helping adolescents engage with life and learning* (pp. 123–140). Richmond, UK: Worth.

James, B. (1989). *Treating traumatized children.* Lexington, MA: Lexington Books.

Miller, P. W. (2005). *Body language: An illustrated introduction for teachers.* Munster, IN: Patrick W. Miller and Associates.

O'Connor, K. J. (1983). Color-Your-Life technique. In C. E. Schaefer & K. J. O'Connor (Eds.), *Handbook of play therapy* (pp. 251–258). New York: Wiley.

Schore, A. (2003a). *Affect regulation and the repair of the self.* New York: Norton.

Schore, A. (2003b). *Affect dysregulation and disorders of the self.* New York: Norton.

CHAPTER 13

Chronic Early Trauma as a Childhood Syndrome and Its Relationship to Play

Steven Tuber
Kira Boesch
Jessica Gorkin
Madeleine Terry

As Donald Winnicott described so beautifully (Winnicott, 1971; see also Tuber, 2008, 2012), the capacity for play is both an exalted hallmark of human development and yet something that is not an automatic out-growth of the developmental process. A "good enough" degree of reliable, predictable, nontoxic caregiving must occur for an infant to develop the "luxury" of being able to take the caregiver for granted while beginning to show curiosity and playfulness in the world around him. When children experience chronic neglect or abuse, the effects are often devastating and far-reaching in restricting or even preventing this capacity for play. van der Kolk et al. (2009) propose the term *developmental trauma disorder* (DTD) to capture the comprehensive clinical picture of these children. DTD is an overarching concept intended to subsume the numerous consequences for a child who has suffered chronic deprivation, neglect, and/or abuse in the context of inadequate caregiving. In this chapter, we place DTD within a specific context: describing how these afflicted children's patterns of affect and defense, neurological functioning, and burgeoning self-concept are all drastically disrupted, and in turn disrupt the children's capacity to play.

Affect and Defense in DTD

The experience of trauma, by definition, implies intolerable distress and a resulting affective overload that can easily become overwhelming. In the case of children who endure chronic traumatic stress, the development of tools necessary for the seamless regulation of emotion is especially affected. When caregivers are absent or are unable to tolerate distress themselves, children are not helped to attend to their internal states and therefore do not learn to differentiate among them or label them. Research has shown that abused and neglected children evidence deficits in their ability to detect and accurately label emotional states in experimental vignettes (Pollack, Cicchetti, Hornung, & Reed, 2000). The children's inability to understand emotion in these external situations also reflects their difficulty in comprehending their own internal emotional landscape. When children do not learn to differentiate among internal states, they do not learn to associate their bodily sensations with affect and cognition (van der Kolk, 2005). As such, van der Kolk et al. (2009) propose that DTD is, at its core, a disorder of affective dysregulation. Traumatic stress overwhelms maltreated children's ability to regulate, effectively preventing the retrieval of relevant sensations, affects, and cognitions, and thereby prohibiting the children from understanding or acting upon what is happening to them (van der Kolk, 2005).

Pearlman (1997) describes feelings as "the underpinnings of needs" (p. 22). Without adequate affect regulation, children with DTD are likely to have difficulty identifying and accepting their needs. At the same time, children who cannot verbalize and make sense of their own emotional responses cannot rely on affect states to serve as accurate signals (Krystal, 1978). The result is that many children with DTD may suffer from an inability to distinguish threatening from nonthreatening situations, and may consequently present with emotional lability caused by an extreme, excessive response to minor stressors (Cook et al., 2005). Indeed, children exposed to violence have been shown to exhibit higher levels of mood and behavioral problems than children in control groups (Liberman & Knorr, 2007). However, as van der Kolk (2005) points out, many of the behavioral manifestations associated with DTD can be understood as efforts to minimize objective threat and to regulate emotional distress.

Defenses are cognitive strategies that alter veridical perception to protect an individual from overwhelming affect (Cramer, 2006). Given their difficulty in labeling affect and their tendency to overreact to even trivial stimuli, it follows that children with DTD mobilize defense configurations that are also impaired and subject to distortion and disruption. Like other cognitive abilities that emerge early in life, defenses develop from more primitive to more nuanced over the course of development (Tuber, 2012). Most children are able to use increasingly advanced defenses characterized by flexibility and discreteness of focus as they move toward adulthood.

However, the experience of chronic interpersonal trauma inherent to DTD disrupts the development of defenses, so these children may not learn to utilize more sophisticated and advanced defenses flexibly. Instead, during the first years of life (when boundaries between self and other are not yet fully differentiated), children may come to overrely on so-called "primitive" defenses, which appear anew at times when overwhelming experiences must be completely evaded (Tuber, 2012).

Although evasive defenses serve to protect children with DTD from overwhelming negative affect, the overuse of such defenses can result in affective numbing. Furthermore, primitive defenses are rarely able to protect the children completely from negative emotions. Rather, blocked affects such as terror, betrayal, and pain are likely to return in uncontrolled bursts or reenactments, which further contribute to the chronically traumatized children's affect regulation difficulties (Hegeman & Wohl, 2000). When children are not able to learn to use more sophisticated defenses to regulate affects, it is not uncommon for affects to be discharged through action such as aggression (Pearlman, 1997).

Children with DTD may learn to employ higher-level, more advanced defenses, but often in maladaptive ways. For example, identification is considered to be a higher-level defense and a developmental achievement. In their use of this defense, children with DTD may identify with their aggressors. Identification with the aggressors involves role reversal in fantasy, which may then be enacted in behavior, allowing the children (victims) to gain mastery by transforming themselves into the persons who create the threat. Thus even high-level defenses such as identification may come to be used in ways that are ultimately counterproductive for children with DTD.

DTD is also characterized by the use of dissociative defenses. Unlike denial or identification, dissociation is not considered part of a normal developmental process; it serves to automatize behavior, compartmentalize negative affects, and allow the individual to detach from awareness (Blum, 1987). Dissociation involves alterations in the capacity to integrate identity, memory, consciousness, and perceptions of the environment (Waller, Putnam, & Carlson, 1996). As we discuss further in the section on the development of selfhood, dissociative defenses are often essential in an environment of chronic trauma in order to protect the self from overwhelming and damaging affects. However, use of dissociation also robs children of an adaptive strategy with which to contain strong feelings. In such a situation, children tend to alternate between blocking affects entirely and becoming flooded by painful feelings (Hegeman & Wohl, 2000).

It is important to remember that defenses, which operate as protective mechanisms, may interfere with the development of emotional closeness, attachment, imagination, and readiness to learn (Lieberman & Knorr, 2007). This is of crucial importance in its impact on the capacity to play, stunting its arrival and linking it to fears of becoming overwhelmed if imaginary musings should become all too real.

Neuropsychological Implications of DTD

Particular adjustments at the neuropsychological level constitute a foundation for the aforementioned difficulties with disrupted affect regulation and maladaptive patterns of defense seen in children with DTD. These changes structurally diminish the capacity for play. Structural changes in the brain allow a growing child to interpret new sensory input, and to perceive, process, and integrate new experiences (van der Kolk, 2003). When complex developmental trauma invades and disrupts the maturational process, brain function is drastically affected (D'Andrea, Ford, Stolbach, Spinazzola, & van der Kolk, 2012).

The changes to the course of neurodevelopment that occur in complex developmental trauma are part of the immature brain's adaptation to a malevolent or neglectful environment, and constitute an alternative pathway that prioritizes survival behavior (Ford, 2005; Teicher et al., 2003). Experiencing chronic maltreatment or inevitable repeated traumatizations during sensitive stages leads to particular stress-induced changes in the mind and brain that render children vulnerable to reexperiencing early maltreatment in several ways (van der Kolk, 2005). A tendency toward dysregulation predominates. An examination of current neurobiological and neuropsychological research situates developmentally traumatized children within a context of struggle and disorientation. Difficulty with integrating sensory, emotional, and cognitive information can be traced to particular neurological structures and pathways that fail to facilitate the construction of meaning and grounding of experience so desperately needed by these children (van der Kolk, 2003, 2005).

Chronic trauma causes a breakdown in communication between the brain's two hemispheres. It is thought that this ongoing exchange of information can be disrupted by early trauma (Teicher et al., 2003). Teicher and colleagues assert that early exposure to high levels of stress hormones eventually results in deformities in the bundle of neural fibers called the corpus callosum, which connects the two hemispheres to facilitate their communication.

Children who have suffered abuse and neglect show impaired cognitive functioning by late infancy when compared with children who have not been maltreated, and the sensory and emotional deprivation associated with neglect seems to be particularly detrimental to cognitive development. Traumatized children are bombarded by excessive subcortical activation. This hyperactivity is compounded by decreased cortical inhibition, which leads them to disregard incoming information. High levels of the neurotransmitter norepinephrine, a catecholamine that acts as a stress hormone and neurotransmitter, add to the difficulties these children have in exerting executive control. Their perception of incoming information is distorted by deficient capacities to modulate and achieve the calm that is necessary to formulate a response (van der Kolk, 2003). As such, neglected infants and toddlers show delays in expressive and receptive language development, as well as deficits in overall IQ (Cook et al., 2005). According to O'Neill, Guenette, and Kitchenham (2010), children who have experienced chronic abuse and neglect in early childhood will struggle to learn across the lifespan, due in large part to the environment in which they were raised.

The noradrenergic alarm system is activated when children feel threatened. This is the system that organizes the release of norepinephrine; it has been associated with arousal and impaired prefrontal cortex activity. Activation of this system engages the "fast tracks" of the limbic system, which fire before the gradually responding prefrontal cortex has time to evaluate the stimulus and engage in planning action (van der Kolk, 2003). When a developmentally traumatized child becomes hyperaroused, activation of the orbitofrontal cortex (another structure of the limbic system that is necessary for discriminating stimuli) is disrupted, so that the child not only struggles to learn and assess, but also may lose control over behavior (van der Kolk, 2003). Chronic abuse and neglect may also be detrimental to the electrophysiology and development of the limbic system by leading children to experience excessive neural activation when faced with minor stimuli. This produces the extreme, emergency response patterns in reaction to minor stressors that we have discussed in the section on affect regulation (van der Kolk, 2003).

Different rates of maturation in the amygdala, hippocampus, and prefrontal regions also affect posttraumatic reactions in the developing child. The amygdala starts to function just after birth, so that infants rapidly become able to experience fear and assess danger. The hippocampus, which puts danger in a spatial context in a child's mind, matures comparatively slowly over the first 5 years of life (van der Kolk, 2003). As a result, children under normal conditions gradually acquire the capacity to identify and organize the nature of a threat, whereas victims of early abuse lack these cognitive skills at the time of severe trauma (van der Kolk, 2003).

As previously described, chronically traumatized children are also prone to dissociation and alterations in consciousness. Dissociative states are likely to arise from imbalances in cerebrospinal fluid levels of neurotransmitters and their metabolites; over time, chronic trauma exposure perpetuates neurochemical imbalances and may lead to a dependence on dissociation as a way to cope with emotional arousal.

When a chronically traumatized child experiences unrelenting threat, whether actual or perceived, physiological changes unfold to affect the body and brain, slowing brain growth and suppressing the immune system (Cook et al., 2005). Children with DTD are affected at multiple levels, but perhaps most strikingly in terms of their physical, somatic experience. Given that successful development can be thought of as the "transformation of external into internal regulation" (Schore, 2003, p. 180), these children must ultimately learn to notice and reflect on their bodies as a means of access to their internal selves. It is here that the impact on the capacity to play is most dramatically engendered. Play is perhaps children's greatest tool for learning to understand their bodies and themselves. Helping these children to identify, understand, and trust the connections among bodily sensations, inner feelings, and thoughts constitutes the foundation from which they can make sense of and master their own unique, human experience. Furthermore, their bodies act as containers of experience. Despite the terrifying and chaotic nature of their surroundings, these children may be helped to gain a sense of the divide between the body and the outside world, fostering a newfound capacity to differentiate within the play setting. It is this body–self unity that forms a critical foundation for ego integration. When a child presents with a deficient or nonexistent capacity for play, a premium is placed on the part of the play or art therapist to act as a catalyst in the reparation of the child's impaired ability to link mind, body, affect, and behavior. Through play and imagination, the therapist can foster the child's sense of and trust in the integrity of the self within the matrix of internal and external worlds.

The Development of a Self in DTD

As mentioned above, children with DTD lack a sense of coherence among their bodily perceptions, feelings, and thoughts. Another way of conceptualizing this is to consider the impairments in DTD at the level of the development of a viable sense of self. A coherent and consistent sense of self is a developmental achievement that depends upon early relationships with specific characteristics (Williams, 2004). The first of these characteristics is the caregiver's contingent response to an infant's expression of need (Fonagy, Gergely, Jurist, & Target, 2002). A second crucial aspect of caregiver behavior is consistency. A caregiver's consistent response patterns help the infant to experience the caregiver as an organized and cohesive other who is separate from him- or herself, even as the caregiver plays a major role in the infant's self-regulation. Finally, in infancy and beyond, development of the self is facilitated by caregivers who mirror and reflect children's inner states and behaviors, thus reinforcing the children's emerging self-states (Pearlman & Courtois, 2005).

Children who have suffered early relational trauma are deprived of many of the optimal circumstances for selfhood development described here. Caregivers who are themselves traumatized or experiencing extremely adverse life circumstances may not be able to reflect their children's emerging self-states back to them accurately and reliably. In the subsequent absence of having their bodily sensations acknowledged, symbolized through language, and regulated by their caregivers, the children miss opportunities for becoming aware of their agency and having their experience of themselves symbolized and represented to them by a close other.

In some situations of relational trauma, children are in the position of becoming attached to adults whom they perceive to be dangerous or negligent. It is a ubiquitous part of development that representations of the other are internalized before the self fully forms, laying the groundwork for identification. These alien parts within the self-structure are universal precisely because no caregiver is perfectly sensitive to a child's mind (Fonagy & Target, 2006). However, especially in response to caregivers who project their own unsymbolized feelings and thoughts onto their infants, traumatized children may more insidiously incorporate the invasive objects' characteristics, including malignant aspects, as part of their own selves and identities (Williams, 2004).

As a result, traumatized children can lose awareness of the boundary between internal and external reality, slipping into what is called *psychic equivalence mode*—the belief that their own thoughts are no different from external reality. In this state of mind, these children can easily come to feel that their memories of trauma are real, and come to fear their own minds. It is easy to imagine the consequences of such a state on the capacity for play. If one's mind is above all else to be feared, than how can one afford to let it "wander" playfully? Indeed, the avoidance of imagination becomes paramount in such a scenario, creating a vicious cycle of concrete thinking in the face of concrete, all-too-real adversity. This vulnerability often results in dissociation and shame, which in turn pose further threat to a cohesive sense of self and to adaptive relationships with others.

As we have discussed in both prior sections, the prevalence of dissociation in DTD is rampant. Here we highlight its impact on the growth of a sense of self. Dissociation is seen as the opposite of an integrated self and has been described as a void of subjectivity (Schore, 2002), such that in moments of dissociation both self and other cease to exist. This is exemplified by case studies of complex trauma survivors, in which patients are frequently represented as needing and wanting regulation from the outside (West, 2011) and seeking external references as a source of self-organization (Pinheiro & Viana, 2011).

Victims of relational trauma frequently cannot fully avoid a sense of responsibility for what has been inflicted upon them. Self-blame can even be a coping mechanism that allows these children to preserve a more positive image of their parents and preserve their attachments to them. However, the shame that results from this approach can become part of a growing child's very personality structure and sense of self (Herman, 1992).

The profound shame resulting from early traumatic experience not only becomes part of the self-structure, but also exerts a profound effect on relationships with others. This is because shame implies an imagined judgment of the self on the part of the other. The ubiquity of shame as a major threat to the self is striking in case studies focusing on adults with a history of relational trauma (Grossmark, 2009; Pinheiro & Viana, 2011). Pinheiro and Viana (2011) suggest that traumatized individuals may in fact organize their subjective experience around shame.

In sum, the formation of a secure sense of self is hindered in the phenomenon of developmental trauma, both because of deprived early relational experiences and because of challenges to the nascent sense of self that are above and beyond the trials of normative experience. In developmental trauma, an infant is faced with a sensory and emotional overload that cannot be processed within the caregiver–infant dyad. As a result, emotions cannot be symbolized, and behaviors, feelings, sensations, and cognitions are dissociated from one another, so that a unified personality cannot be fully formed. As we have discussed, children with DTD may lack the capacity to play for several reasons. Playing increases children's sense of agency in the world and helps them master how their own feelings and thoughts affect their external world. Children with DTD who have already been deprived of opportunities for self–other differentiation and agency thus continue to be deprived through their inability to engage in play. However, through play therapy, they can learn to differentiate self from other and experience validation of their feelings and nonverbal traumatic experiences (Young, 2008).

Case Vignette: Chang

Perhaps a clinical vignette from the treatment of a child whose history featured many components of DTD would be relevant to our discussion. I (Steven Tuber) met the patient (whom I will call Chang) very early in my training at an adolescent residential treatment center. Chang was 15 years old at the time, and as a consequence of his parents' substance dependence difficulties, he had spent the bulk of his early years in and out of multiple foster homes. Random separations from parental figures, and episodic, unpredictable violence both witnessed and felt by this child, were also marked features of his early life. I met him the day before treatment would formally begin, shook his hand as I introduced myself, and told him we would meet the next day. Chang had sufficient privileges on his unit to walk to treatment on his own the following day, and he came to my opened door with an excited, hopeful look on his face and a card in his hand. It was an 8½- by 11-inch piece of colored paper, folded in half, to which he had painstakingly glued scallops of aluminum foil around the edges. In elaborate italics was written *"To Steve"* on its cover, and when opened, in equally detailed italics was written: *"Would you be my friend?"* I was completely blindsided by this elaborate gesture of "love," and my bewildered, indeed frightened facial expression must have made this all too apparent to Chang. When I looked up and began to stammer some faint disclaimer, his face turned floridly enraged and he leapt at my throat, knocking me over and landing on top of me, forcing his hands around my neck in an effort to choke me. I reacted with panic, threw him off me, pinned his arms and legs with mine, and screamed at him, "Back off!" After a few tense moments, he calmed down, I calmed down (somewhat!), and I could let go of him. He quickly returned to his unit.

What had happened in that exchange? To use some of the prior wording of this chapter, Chang had taken my warm greeting of the previous day and turned it into an "all-or-none" expectation of deeply longed-for symbiosis, hoping for some way in which our possible "friendship" could replace his history of neglect, chaos, and abuse. He had apparently worked for hours on the unit making this card and telling his peers and counselors that "someone" was going to "really help" him this time. The precariousness of this longing, precisely because it had never been reliably fulfilled in any sustaining way, could not withstand even the slightest of disappointments. When he saw my frightened, overwhelmed reaction to the presentation of his "gift," his capacity to modulate or defend against his rage surrounding abandonment could not be accessed. Within a true "psychic equivalent" mode, I became the embodiment of all who had ever attacked and rejected him, leaving him with no alternative, in his mind, but to kill before being killed. As described above, Chang's thinking became concrete; his shameful rage became omnipresent; his limbic system became overwrought; his defenses became nearly nonexistent; his need to act rather than think or feel became mandatory; and the cycle of attack and counterattack became manifest within our first moments together.

It is crucial to emphasize, both for Chang and for other patients suffering from DTD, the intertwining nature of DTD's impact on affect–defense configurations, infant and child neurophysiology, and the development of the sense of self and other. Self–other experience occurs within a "bath" of affect; affects in turn inevitably evoke defenses to modulate them; all of these manifestations cause and are reciprocally caused by shifts in brain chemistry and physiology. For children with DTD, the resulting combination of difficulties stifles the use of imagination and play—usually the two great allies of children who are wrestling with psychological conflicts. The now feared capacity for play is atrophied in such children, furthering a cycle of maladaptation. This creates a toxic concoction that wreaks havoc on the child, the family, and society at large. For Chang, the result was a sudden, violent enactment of his need to destroy before being destroyed.

A Brief Nod to History

This chapter has sought to reorganize a great deal of research and theory on the impact of chronic early abuse and neglect into the burgeoning literature on DTD as a new, overarching syndrome in child psychopathology. As with all "new" diagnostic concepts, however, it is crucial to note its historical antecedents, since indeed there is nothing new under the sun. In the case of DTD, its roots lie squarely in the theoretical writings of Win-nicott (1971; see also Tuber, 2008). In his seminal paper "On the Location of Cultural Experience," Winnicott wrote of the baby's experience:

> The feeling of the mother's existence lasts x minutes. If the mother is away more than x minutes, then the imago fades, and along with this, the baby's capacity to use the symbol of the union ceases. The baby is distressed, but this distress is soon *mended* because the mother returns in $x + y$ minutes. In $x + y$ minutes the baby has not become altered. But in $x + y + z$ minutes the baby has become *traumatized*. In $x + y + z$ minutes the mother's return does not mend the baby's altered state. Trauma implies that the baby has expe-rienced a break in life's continuity, so that primitive defenses now become organized to defend against a repetition of 'unthinkable anxiety' or a return of the acute confusional state that belongs to disintegration of nascent ego structure. (1971, p. 97)

What we (and others) are calling DTD as a syndrome is thus a recon-ceptualization of Winnicott's depiction of $x + y + z$ time. Note how he dis-cusses the impact in terms of self, other, affect, and defenses, which we mir-ror in the discussion above. Crucially, Winnicott also provides DTD with a temporal, phenomenological dimension. If the child's attempts at affect regulation (defenses) do not permit sufficient self-soothing while waiting for the caregiver's arrival in $x + y$ time; if brain chemistry and physiol-ogy "conspire" to reduce the child's capacity for cognitive and emotional flexibility during this time frame; if the child's experience of self has been linked to hopelessness regarding the reemergence of "good enough" care-giving by an attuned "other"; and if the "other" cannot be attuned enough to return to the child's needs within these all-too-real time constraints, then the child will indeed experience $x + y + z$ time—a time of trauma. In Win-nicott's words, confusion and disintegration become the child's primary experience. In our present attempt to make sense of the child's experience, we are calling the manifestations of this $x + y + z$ state DTD. In Chang's experience, we can see how it played out all too violently and chaotically. We believe that this notion of DTD does diagnostic justice both to the remarkable distress of such a child's early experience and to the often life-long adverse sequelae of this experience. We thus are in favor of using DTD as an appropriate term to describe children who have experienced chronic early trauma, but we encourage practitioners to link this "new" syndrome to its earlier theoretical antecedents for the best understanding of its etiol-ogy and prognosis.

It should also be noted how adversely DTD can affect the capacity to use play therapy. If the very capacity for playfulness has been made toxic by the aftermath of DTD, then the experience of being encouraged to "play out" one's feelings can create a milieu of dread and panic instead of a forum for repair and replenishment. Chang's first session can be seen as a dramatic example of the consequences that occur when a child has no access to play and thus experiences dread with no buffer or respite. In the terminology used in this chapter, such a forum can overpower affect regulation, engender the rigid use of primitive defenses of avoidance and expulsion, and wreak havoc with the fragments of selfhood that may exist. For such children, the play therapy experience must be presented with great caution, often with a specific structure, and always with a strong sense by the therapist of how terrifying being alone with one's feelings may be for these children, across the domains of intrapsychic, neurophysiological, and interpersonal experience.

REFERENCES

Blum, H. P. (1987). The role of identification in the resolution of trauma: The Anna Freud Memorial Lecture. *Psychoanalytic Quarterly, 56*, 609–627.

Cook, A., Spinazzola, J., Ford, J., Lanktree, C., Blaustein, M., Cloitre, M., . . . van der Kolk, B. (2005). Complex trauma in children and adolescents. *Psychiatric Annals, 35*(5), 390–398.

Cramer, P. (2006). Coping and defense mechanisms: What's the difference? *Journal of Personality, 66*(6), 919–946.

D'Andrea, W., Ford, J., Stolbach, B., Spinazzola, J., & van der Kolk, B. A. (2012). Understanding interpersonal trauma in children: Why we need a developmentally appropriate trauma diagnosis. *American Journal of Orthopsychiatry, 82*(2), 187–200.

Fonagy, P., Gergely, G., Jurist, E. L., & Target, M. (2002). *Affect regulation, mentalization, and the development of the self.* New York: Other Press.

Fonagy, P., & Target, M. (2006). The mentalization-focused approach to self pathology. *Journal of Personality Disorders, 20*(6), 544–576.

Ford, J. D. (2005). Treatment implications of altered affect regulation and information processing following child maltreatment. *Psychiatric Annals, 35*(5), 410–419.

Grossmark, R. (2009). The case of Pamela. *Psychoanalytic Dialogues, 19*(1), 22–30.

Hegeman, E., & Wohl, A. (2000). Management of trauma-related affect, defenses, and dissociative states. In R. H. Klein & V. L. Schermer (Eds.), *Group psychotherapy for psychological trauma* (pp. 64–88). New York: Guilford Press.

Herman, J. (1992). *Trauma and recovery.* New York: Basic Books.

Krystal, H. (1978). Trauma and affects. *Psychoanalytic Study of the Child, 33*, 81–116.

Lieberman, A., & Knorr, K. (2007). The impact of trauma: A developmental framework for infancy and early childhood. *Psychiatric Annals, 37*(6), 416–422.

O'Neill, L., Guenette, F., & Kitchenham, A. (2010). 'Am I safe here and do you like me?': Understanding complex trauma and attachment disruption in the classroom. *British Journal of Special Education, 37*(4), 190–197.

Pearlman, L. (1997). Trauma and the self. *Journal of Emotional Abuse, 1*(1), 7–25.

Pearlman, L., & Courtois, C. A. (2005). Clinical applications of the attachment framework: Relational treatment of complex trauma. *Journal of Traumatic Stress, 18*(5), 449–459.

Pinheiro, T., & Viana, D. (2011). Losing the certainty of self. *American Journal of Psychoanalysis, 71*(4), 352–360.

Pollack, S., Cicchetti, D., Hornung, K., & Reed, A. (2000). Recognizing emotion in faces: Developmental effects of child abuse and neglect. *Developmental Psychology, 36*(5), 679–688.

Schore, A. N. (2002). Advances in neuropsychoanalysis, attachment theory, and trauma research: Implications for self psychology. *Psychoanalytic Inquiry, 22*(3), 433–484.

Schore, A. N. (2003). *Affect dysregulation and disorders of the self.* New York: Norton.

Teicher, M. H., Andersen, S. L., Polcari, A., Anderson, C. M., Navalta, C. P., & Kim, D. M. (2003). The neurobiological consequences of early stress and childhood maltreatment. *Neuroscience and Biobehavioral Reviews, 27,* 33–44.

Tuber, S. (2008) *Attachment, play and authenticity: A Winnicott primer.* Lanham, MD: Aronson.

Tuber, S. (2012). *Understanding personality through projective testing.* Lanham, MD: Aronson.

van der Kolk, B. (2003). The neurobiology of childhood trauma and abuse. *Child and Adolescent Psychiatric Clinics of North America, 12,* 293–317.

van der Kolk, B. A. (2005). Developmental trauma disorder: Towards a rational diagnosis for children with complex trauma histories. *Psychiatric Annals, 35*(5), 401–408.

van der Kolk, B., Pynoos, R., Cicchetti, D., Cloitre, M., D'Andrea, W., Ford, J. D., . . . Teicher, M. (2009). *Proposal to include a developmental trauma disorder diagnosis for children and adolescents in DSM-V.* Unpublished manuscript.

Waller, N., Putnam, F., & Carlson, E. (1996). Types of dissociation and dissociative types: A taxometric analysis of dissociative experiences. *Psychological Methods, 1*(3), 300–321.

West, M. (2011). Attachment, sensitivity and agency: The alchemy of analytic work. *Journal of Analytical Psychology, 56*(3), 354–361.

Williams, P. (2004). Symbols and self preservation in severe disturbance. *Journal of Analytical Psychology, 49*(1), 21–31.

Winnicott, D. (1971). *Playing and reality.* London: Tavistock.

Young, M. E. (2008). Play therapy and the traumatized self. *Psychology and Education: An Interdisciplinary Journal, 45*(1), 19–23.

CHAPTER 14

The Princess and *Dal Bhat Tarkari*

Play Therapy with Children of Cross-Cultural Adoption

Henry Kronengold

ABBY: OK, here's what we're doing. You're trying to find the princess. She was taken captive by the witch, who locked her in the castle. The witch is hiding her there. You try to save her. But be careful, the witch has guards all around.

ME: OK. Here I go. (*I adopt a brave posture and head toward the castle.*) I'm coming to save the princess, I'm coming to save the princess. (*Abby looks at me and puts her finger to her mouth, gesturing that I should be quieter. My voice lowers to a whisper.*) Right. Now to find the entrance. Ah-ha, I think it's over here. (*I point to a small room inside my toy castle, and I pretend to burst in.*) Princess, are you here? I've come to save you!

ABBY: Thank heavens you made it. Now let's get out of here quick. We have to get past the witch's guards. Come on! This way!

ME: OK, let's go. (*We run out of the castle, heading toward freedom. We keep running, pursued by guards and a very angry dragon. At last, we make it out of the castle, where I pause to catch my breath and plan our next move.*) Princess, we're out of there, but we need to find a safe place to rest before we continue the journey back home. (*I pause for a second, but there's no response.*) Princess, did you hear me? (*Still no response. Concerned, I start to look around.*) Princess, Princess, where are you? Did you go for

227

a walk somewhere? Princess? (*I start to look around some more, but I don't know where she is. My face takes on a look of worry; my voice is now rising and more pressured.*) Princess? Princess?

ABBY: She's gone, you know. She's disappeared.

ME: What? What do you mean? How? She was just here!

ABBY: Not any more. She's disappeared, and you need to find her again. Did you hear that sound? The laughing?

ME: Yes. It's . . . (*My voice slows now.*) It's. The. Witch.

ABBY: (*Looks at me with a knowing glance.*) It wasn't going to be that easy you know.

As Abby would remind me repeatedly in our sessions, trying to find her and her constantly shifting identities in our sessions was definitely not going to be easy. In the dialogue above (and in many others), a princess was captured by a witch, whose motives were never clear. Despite repeated attempts to rescue the princess, she would mysteriously disappear, leaving the heroic prince both hapless and helpless in his efforts to rescue her. Play with Abby was rich, stimulating, and often confusing as she kept developing stories with missing and disappearing characters who would often transform themselves within a single scene (see Kronengold, 2010, for a detailed description of Abby's case). Interestingly, she wasn't the only child who presented with this sort of play. In a strikingly similar scene, Alma created and directed me in her own story involving a prince and a princess.

ME: Princess, Princess, I'm here to rescue you! (*I pretend to barge into the castle dungeon.*)

ALMA: Hi, Prince. Quick, we have to get out of here. The witch is nearby, and her guards are everywhere. I know a good spot we can hide. C'mon, let's go (*as she points toward the side of the castle*).

ME: OK, are you all right? I missed you.

ALMA: Yeah, I'm fine. But hurry, we've got to get away from here.

ME: Right, let's go. Umm, where are we going?

ALMA: To the inn. It's in the middle of the forest. We can hide there for the night and then head back home tomorrow.

ME: (*I pause to consider the idea. I also have a feeling that I know where this is heading as I nod my assent to Alma's plan.*). To the inn! Let's go. (*We hurry to the inn, have a seat, and make plans to get some food.*) I'll go to the innkeeper and bring back some food for us to eat. What would you like?

ALMA: Anything. I'm starving.

ME: OK, I'll be back in a minute. (*I walk over to talk to the pretend innkeepers; get some pretend bread, chicken, and water; and head back to the princess.*)

ALMA: (*Gestures to me to come over to the side of the room, as she wants to tell me something. She leans toward me and speaks in a whisper.*) Henry, you come back, but the princess is gone.

ME: (*whispering*) Gone? Where did she go?

ALMA: She's gone. Just gone. You have to figure that out. She disappears. The witch's guards must have found her, or the witch cast a spell and brought her back to the castle.

ME: Seriously?

ALMA: Seriously. She's gone again.

Although Alma's storyline was similar to Abby's, Alma's princess was more assertive, and her role in the play differed from Abby's. Whereas Abby took great pleasure in my confusion, Alma broke character to tell me about the scene, almost joining me in wondering what might have just happened. As I thought of this scene alongside the one from Abby, my mind wandered to yet another scene played out with Sarah, a child I had seen some years earlier.

SARAH: Henry, you're the brother. Now look, you see this house over here. There are five different rooms. Each one is used for something special in the house. The sister's bedroom is here, and you go looking around for her, but she's not there. You have to try to find her, but she's not around. OK?

ME: OK. What do I do once I can't find her?

SARAH: You get very worried and start calling the police.

ME: Do they find her?

SARAH: No. And anyway, you have to play the game. OK, now let's start. You start looking for me.

ME: OK, I'm looking. (*I look searching around the room.*) Hmm, I wonder where she could be? Hello! Where are you? Are you in the house? (*I search the area.*) She's not there. Where could she be? Where has she gone? I hope she's OK.

SARAH: Now you call the police.

ME: (*I pick up an imaginary telephone.*) Hello, police? I need some help. I can't find my sister. I've looked everywhere.

SARAH: (*Takes on the deep voice of an imagined police officer on the other end of the line.*) Hello. This is the police.

ME: Hi, can you help me? I can't find my sister. She's supposed to be home, but she's gone, and I can't find her. (*My voice becomes more plaintive*.) I've looked everywhere.

SARAH: You have to keep looking for her.

ME: (*surprised*) Yes, but I'm calling for help. I need some help finding my sister. You see, she's disappeared.

SARAH: I can't really help. Sorry. You need to find her. But don't worry. You will.

ME: I'm glad you think so. I just don't know where she is. Well, OK, then. I'll keep looking. (*I hang up the phone and resume searching. As I look, Sarah motions for me to look near the closet area of the office, next to a large brown desk chair where she's hiding*.) Hmm. I think I saw something moving over there. Maybe it's her? Sister, Sister, is that you? It's me.

SARAH: Yeah, hi. I was wondering when you were going to find me.

ME: Well, I didn't know where to look. What were you doing here, anyway?

SARAH: I had to get away. I'll explain it all later, but for now, let's just get back home.

ME: OK, let's head back. I can't wait to hear the whole story. (*As we walk back, Sarah whispers to me*.)

SARAH: She disappears again.

ME: Again? But she was just with me. How did she disappear?

SARAH: She just does. Then you have to go find her again.

ME: That's a lot of searching.

SARAH: Yeah, I know. You'll find her again.

The three dialogues above are rich and evocative, each reflecting a child's journey as she tries to make sense of where she comes from, where she is going, and how she got there. What is also remarkable about these dialogues is that, on appearance, they could have involved the same child. Instead, the stories and themes were voiced by three different children, whom I worked with at different times over a period of 13 years. The similarity of the children's play speaks volumes about common themes among children, as well as the role of play in helping children better understand and explore questions and feelings about their past.

My discussion about the three children in this chapter is not meant to be exhaustive regarding therapy with children who have been adopted across cultures, or the attachment difficulties that pose a challenge to their families and therapists alike. Rather, it is meant to consider an element of working with children that frequently arises within play. In this case, I discuss excerpts from my work with Sarah, Abby, and Alma, with an eye toward how play (along with other expressive media) can serve as a powerful vehicle to foster a child's development and healthy transition to his or her adopted family.

When Sarah first began treatment, she was nearly 4 years old; she was living with her adopted parents as well as another child her parents had adopted, a brother. Her brother, 9 years old, struggled with explosive behavior. Sarah was an unusually verbal child who regularly spoke to her mother about her brother's challenges and used to watch him like a hawk, lest he lose control without anyone noticing. Sarah's precociousness had served her well in life, and she was often praised for her maturity and intelligence. Of course, there was another side to staying so vigilant: Sarah was highly controlled, rarely expressed her feelings to other people, and (as can be seen in the dialogue above) was most comfortable directing others.

Alma walked into my office as an extremely poised, verbal, and precocious 4-year-old. She played, chatted, painted, danced, and smiled. In short, she did everything one could imagine to be a good play partner. She was incredibly charming, funny, and creative. At the end of our first meeting, I thought how much I enjoyed our session and how much fun it was to spend time with Alma. As I explored my own reaction, I recalled other children who had made such an impact in our first meeting. Prominent among this group were, of course, Sarah and Abby. Abby had made herself at home almost as soon as she walked into my office, immediately announcing her playful presence as we began our work together. How unusual it was for these children to occupy this particular place in therapy and in my own mind. Working with each of them was great fun; their sessions were both creative and rich. At the same time, I wondered: Was the very reason they were coming to see me connected to their ability to connect so easily in their initial sessions? Other children would begin sessions warily, careful not to stray too far from their parents. But Alma, Sarah, and Abby were so different.

The answer seemed connected to their attachment histories and to the changes in each child's early experience. In a healthy situation, children born to biological parents typically become attached to those parents, depending on them for nurturance and support, while enjoying their time with each parent in a way that is both loving and reciprocal. There are of course lapses in a child's attachment to his or her parents—but in a typically developing and healthy child, there is what we refer to as a *secure* attachment (Ainsworth, Blehar, Waters, & Wall, 1978; Bowlby, 1969/1982, 1973), where the child feels safe in the presence of the parents and gradually internalizes that feeling of safety to explore the world. In a child's younger years, he or she is most comfortable with caregivers and is careful when meeting new people. In Alma's case, however, she hadn't developed this sort of connection at a younger age. She had been raised first in an orphanage and then by a loving foster family in the Himalayan Mountains. Alma's unusual ability to solicit attention, to lodge herself into another person's world, and to make that person want to get to know her had probably contributed to her winding up with a new loving mother in New York City. Her ability to engage others with such impressive skill and fearlessness stood out, just as it did for Abby and for Sarah. Each of them had come from a different part of the world, and each had developed a capacity to stand out from other children. These skills proved most useful on first impression, making initial sessions and meetings memorable. Based on my own experience in my initial session with Alma, I can only imagine how her adopted mother felt during and after their first meeting. Alma's adaptive abilities were extraordinary. But at what cost? What happened after the shine of the first meeting wore off? This little girl worked so hard to impress and engage others, presenting more as a young adult than a small child. What happened when she needed to be a child again? Could she? Perhaps there was a reason why Alma also couldn't sleep at night, calling as a younger child might for her mother's comfort. Perhaps there was a reason why when Alma became upset and her mother didn't respond with perfect empathy, Alma would say that she shouldn't have been adopted and didn't deserve to have a mommy. Whereas some of Alma's statements may have had a manipulative element, others suggested her lingering insecurity, manifested by the inconsolable flow of tears at those difficult moments.

Then there was Abby, playful and fun but struggling with her behavior. Abby acted out at home and at school, with frequent tantrums and difficulty following classroom routines. In our early sessions, she wished to control my every move, from how I played to where I stood in my office. The ever-vigilant, mature, and articulate Sarah was less overtly controlling, but she kept watch over everyone and everything in her home. At school Sarah adopted the role of a teacher's assistant, with a particular eye on helping struggling classmates. Once she personally referred a preschool classmate of hers who was struggling with tantrums. At the same time, Sarah also complained of headaches, stomach pain, and various other bodily ailments. For a highly verbal child, she was very uncomfortable expressing her feelings; when upset, she would become overwhelmed and shut down. In one memorable episode, Sarah became upset at school and fell to the floor, seemingly unconscious. Her teachers, worried that Sarah had had a concussion or possible seizure, immediately sought medical attention as attendants tried to figure out what happened and why Sarah was unresponsive. It was only an hour later, when her mother came to the doctor's office and spoke to her daughter, that Sarah opened her eyes, picked up her head, grabbed her backpack, and calmly walked out the door to head home. She had been awake the entire time.

In the cases of these three girls, their play offered details as to what they were struggling with, in terms of both their attachment and their confusion over their early experiences. Alma's play began quickly, as did Sarah's and Abby's. In our early sessions, Alma directed a version of her story about a princess who had been captured by an evil witch, was saved by the prince, was recaptured by the witch, was saved again by the prince, and so on and on. Alma played this game repetitively at home, although she maintained her enthusiasm no matter how many times she played out the drama.

ALMA: I'll be the princess and you'll be the prince. Oh, and I'll be the witch also, and you can play some of the guards, OK?

ME: OK.

ALMA: (*In a most industrious mode, she sets up the castle and characters in exact positions.*) OK, I'm the princess now, and you're the prince, and we're about to get married. Ready, OK?

ME: OK. What I am supposed to do?

ALMA: (*in a friendly but assertive voice*) You're supposed to ask the princess to marry her, and then you'll walk back to all the people to tell them you're getting married, and they'll start to get everything ready for the big wedding, but before they have the wedding, the witch, she's going to set up a trap for them, and she'll capture the princess, and she'll bring the princess back to her house and keep her there. OK?

ME: Yup, I think I have that. (*I'm impressed but also surprised by Alma's strength and efficiency.*)

ALMA: Good, let's go. OK, c'mon.

ME: Right, oh, yes. Hello, Princess, it is so wonderful to see you today. My princess, my princess, would you like to marry me?

ALMA: (*Maintains her friendly voice.*) No, no, you're supposed to do that in this part of the castle, and you don't say, "Would you like to marry me?" You say, "Come, Princess, let's get married."

ME: OK. Come, Princess, let's get married.

ALMA: Right, but you do that when we start the play, not yet.

ME: I was just practicing.

ALMA: OK, let's start.

ME: Oh, hello, Princess. (*I look back at Alma to make sure I'm getting this right.*) Princess?

ALMA: Yes (*expectantly, waving with her hand to cue me.*)

ME: Come, let's get married.

ALMA: OK. (*She now gives me directions about where we're supposed to go to prepare for the wedding.*) Now we move over to this part of the castle, but the witch is going to be waiting for us.

ME: OK, let's walk over there to get married, my princess.

ALMA: (*Continues directing.*) We walk over here (*she points to the back of the castle*), and then the witch pops out and gets the princess.

ME: Got it.

ALMA: OK, now we're walking.

ME: Yes, we're walking. Soon, Princess, we shall be married.

ALMA: (*She now takes on the scary voice of the witch, who has appeared near the castle walls.*) Not so fast. Ha, ha! Away, Prince, the princess is mine! (*She goes back to her regular voice as Alma.*) The witch takes the princess away and disappears. Now you're supposed to go look for her. Everyone is looking for her. But they can't find her.

ME: Where has the princess gone? This is the work of that evil witch! Ah, I must find her. I must find my princess. I shall look over there, in the mountains (*as I point to the sofa in my office*).

Alma's play was notable for its theme of a missing princess, a witch who wanted the princess for herself, and a beloved prince who was looking to rescue her. Her play was also notable for its great detail and for precise stage and dialogue directions. At the same time that Alma gave me instructions as to what I was supposed to say, there hadn't been too much actual dialogue in our scenes. In the process, Alma hadn't given much of a clue as to the emotions behind our scenes and characters. Perhaps Alma was trying very hard to control these emotions, reflecting various degrees of loss and longing, or maybe she wasn't yet aware of them. In any event, the lack of emotional content may have been why Alma kept repeating this story in our early sessions and in her play at home with her mother. Maybe she was trying to locate the feelings that were likely to be resonating in her own experience, but so far she wasn't able to. Instead, she had latched onto this familiar fairy tale as a sort of proxy for her own experiences. I saw our play as an opportunity for Alma to begin either to better understand her emotional world or allow it to register. Now that I was the prince doing the searching, I had a bit more space to operate in our session. I expected that while Alma would offer direction, I could begin to narrate my own experience of looking for the princess, and in the process start to introduce more emotional themes into our play.

ME: Princess, Princess! Oh, Princess! My beloved princess, where are you? Where could you be? Where did that wretched witch take you? What has she done? (*I search around unsuccessfully.*) Ahh! (*I let out a sound that tries to capture both sadness and anger.*) Princess? (*I look around the sofa/mountain area longer.*) She's not here. This used to be the witches' lair. She must have moved and is holding my princess somewhere else. I will check back near the castle. Maybe there is some sort of magic area she has come up with. Those witches. Terrible creatures!

ALMA: He's going to look for her over there. But she's not there either. But then he goes to the forest and he hears a sound, and he realizes the princess is close by, so he looks over here (*she points near a playhouse in my office*), and then he sees the witch's house and he rescues the princess. But then they run away, and they stop at a place where they get something to eat and drink, and the witch's guards are there looking for them, and the guards recognize the prince and the princess and they have to run, and some people at the place try to help the prince and princess, but other people try to stop them.

ME: Got it.

ALMA: OK. Csshh! (*She makes a noise to show me the princess is nearby.*)

ME: Wait a second. I'm still over here near the castle. I haven't even walked over to the forest yet. (*I do this as I'm trying to slow this scene down—to allow it to simmer and resonate, rather than just playing out the details so quickly.*)

ALMA: OK. Well, go over there, then.

ME: I'm going to head over to the forest. Maybe I can find the princess over there. Oh, Princess! Princess! Where are you?

ALMA: (*Looks at me.*) OK, now I'm going to make the sound, and you'll go and realize it's the princess.

ME: (*I nod my head.*) Yes, I remember. I've got it. Go ahead, do the "Csshh" sound thing.

ALMA: (*Smiles.*) Csshh! Csshh!

ME: Two sounds!

ALMA: Just go ahead.

ME: What was that? A squirrel? A rabbit? An owl flying in the forest? Or, maybe it was a sign, a message! Perhaps the princess is nearby. I'm looking for her. (*My voice starts to slow down and lowers to a whisper.*) Maybe I'll hear another clue.

ALMA: (*in a faint, tiny voice*) Help! Help!

ME: I hear her. She's out there. Shh. I'll walk quietly and listen. (*I put my hand to my ear and walk carefully through the office.*)

ALMA: In here. Over here. It's me. She stuck me in the dungeon.

ME: Here I come. (*I arrive at the dungeon.*) Princess, it's me! I'm here to rescue you!

ALMA: (*Starts directing me.*) Now they escape and run back to the castle.

ME: (*Here I decide to nudge Alma to stay in our play—to stay with the emotion of the story rather than its direction.*) Wait a minute. I was in character.

ALMA: They escape.

ME: Yeah, but I was ready to act the whole thing out.

ALMA: So they try to get married again.

ME: But the escape?

ALMA: (*Looks at me sympathetically.*) OK. Let's go ahead.

ME: (*in a pleased voice*) Great. OK, um, where were we?

ALMA: You were rescuing the princess.

ME: Right, OK, back to our places. I'm . . .

ALMA: You're outside the dungeon, and I'm in the dungeon, and you rescue me, and then we run away, but the witch chases after us with her guards. We get to this inn where there's a place to eat and drink and stay there, but the guards find us and then . . .

ME: (*I playfully put my hands up, urging Alma to slow down a bit.*) I was kind of "in the rescue moment," you know. Like, this whole thing is a little way ahead here. Can I just, well—I mean no disrespecting the story, which of course is quite fascinating—but can we get back to the rescue? I feel like I'm kind of focused on that part right now, and then we can get to the rest of the story.

ALMA: Well, OK. Go ahead. Just remember where they go next.

ME: Totally. I got it. Clear on this. After the rescue, they go to the inn, get chased, the whole thing.

ALMA: Good. OK, go ahead.

ME: OK. (*I pause for a minute, as I'm feeling we went a little far afield. I also want to make sure I haven't lost Alma in my wish to keep the keep the scene going.*)

ALMA: Well?

ME: Sorry, just taking a second to get back into the scene. I was looking for you. I just found you in the dungeon after you called out, and now I'm trying to rescue you. Just getting back into the feeling.

ALMA: Can we just go ahead?

ME: Yes, yes. Just a second more. I'm the prince, and I just found you. Kind of a mix of excitement and, and . . .

ALMA: You're happy to find me, but you were also scared.

ME: (*My eyes open wider.*) That's good. That works.

ALMA: (*Sighs.*) Let's go.

ME: Ready. (*My voice rises.*) Princess, I'm here, I'm here to rescue you.

Oh, I thought I'd never find you again. (*I look around.*) We need to figure out a way out of here.

ALMA: The lock on the door is on the side. Open the lock, and I can get free. But beware of the witch.

ME: (*I fumble with the lock, making a few sounds of annoyance as I work at it.*) Almost got it, Princess. Almost. Getting there.

ALMA: Try turning it (*she motions with her hand*) that way.

ME: Got it. C'mon, Princess, let's get out of this place before the witch finds out and tries to catch us.

ALMA: OK, so now they run to the inn and . . .

ME: (*I sigh.*) We're in character, here you know.

ALMA: Oh, all right. All right.

ME: Let's go, Princess, through the forest. There's an inn at the edge of the forest. We can stop there to rest and eat something before we return to the castle. Princess, I can't believe I found you. I was worried the witch had made you vanish or put some sort of spell on you.

ALMA: She tried to. (*Now Alma is using her hands to gesture as she talks.*) She tried to put this spell on me to make me fall asleep forever, but I wouldn't let her, because I had learned magic to keep her from being able to put me under a spell.

ME: Magic? Hmm, what form of powerful magic is this that you learned, Princess?

ALMA: Just magic. I learned it from the fairies in the forest when I was younger.

ME: Remarkable. Very powerful, this magic is. Fairies, huh?

ALMA: (*Points to one of the chairs in the office.*) There's the inn.

ME: Yes, there it is. It will be good to get a chance to rest. All this running around has left me tired.

ALMA: I know, me too. And I'm more tired and hungry, because I was stuck in the dungeon all that time, you know. Let's go inside. (*She gives me some more information as to our setting.*) OK, so there are a lot of people inside and it's noisy, and we sit down to have something to eat and drink, but then the witch's guards come in, and they're looking for us.

ME: OK. (*I go back into character. I take a bit of pretend food and a drink from a pretend glass.*) Oh, it's good to eat something. I'm sorry, Princess, you must be really hungry and tired. Are you OK?

ALMA: Yes, I'm OK now. (*Starts to look worried.*) But look over there, I know those two guys. They work for the witch! We've got to get out of here!

ME: Uh-oh! C'mon, let's go out this way. (*We run to the side of the castle, trying to elude our pursuers.*)

ALMA: They're getting closer. I can hear them.

ME: I know, me too. Let's hide in those trees. (*We run over to the floor lamp in my office. Alma looks up at me, and I put my finger to my mouth.*) Sshh. (*I whisper, as Alma nods and we stand perfectly still for a minute. Alma makes an exaggerated gesture to show that she's not moving at all as she stands silently, almost holding her breath. Then I wave with my hand for her to peek out of the trees with me.*) I think they missed us.

ALMA: They could be back or close by.

ME: True. Let's head this way, but stay close to the trees in case we need to hide again. And let's be very, very quiet.

ALMA: OK. Let's go. This way. I'll lead. (*Alma starts to walk as I follow. We continue silently until she suddenly stops.*) I heard something!

For Alma, play was an opportunity to grapple with her prior attachment history and her fears. Her controlling, grown-up behavior belied her reality as a young and vulnerable child who had already experienced the helplessness that comes from confronting loss and confusion. Born in a small village, raised first in an orphanage and then in a foster home, Alma ultimately met a woman who would adopt her and become her mom. Dazzling on first impression, Alma grew bossier and moodier as she got to know people. As her play illustrates, she was also in a regular state of anxiety about how secure she could feel in her new home. I found that as Alma became able to use the play not just to make up stories, but to embody characters representing a range of feelings (such as anxiety, sadness, loss, and longing), she became calmer both in our sessions and at home. This was also the case with Sarah and Abby, who also created stories with trapped or missing characters who would pop in and out of the stories and transform themselves at any moment. All three children had been stuck in a loop of repeating the same story in their play. In Alma's case, she reenacted the same scenes when playing with her mother at home. Not surprisingly, her mom tired of this play and perhaps experienced some discomfort with Alma's focus on being kidnapped and taken by an evil witch. Alma's mother was certainly not such a person and was trying to create a loving and stimulating life for Alma in New York. But for Alma, there was still the fear that perhaps something could happen and she could be cast aside once more. When Alma first played out her stories with me, she was relatively removed from her play: She was happy to tell me about what was going to happen in the princess story, and was even happier to direct me. But I wanted Alma to become an actor in the story. I wanted her to be able to embody the emotions that had come with her experiences. I wanted Alma to have the opportunity to tell her story, and the fears it embodied, in a safe place with a degree of emotional investment that would allow her to begin to move forward and develop her attachments and relationships.

As play with Alma continued, she began to branch out with her themes. The prince and princess gave way to other stories, characters, and expressive media, as Alma enjoyed my castle, action figures, paints and markers, and particularly my fake food and kitchen utensils.

Food has played a role in understanding attachment since Harlow's (1958) early attachment research with rhesus monkeys. Influenced by Bowlby's (1951/1977) early theories of attachment emphasizing nurturance over biological sustenance as the most important factor in the relationship between a child and his or her primary caregiver, Harlow decided to test some of these theories in research with primates. He set up two groups of baby rhesus monkeys and put them in two separate cages. In one cage was a "mommy monkey" that was made of wire, but that had a feeding tube connected to it to provide milk. In the other cage was a "mommy monkey" also made of wire, but covered with a soft cloth material suited for cuddling. Harlow was interested in testing out how the baby monkeys developed and how they related to their respective "mommies." He found that the baby monkeys in the cage with the cloth monkey became attached to the "mommy monkey," and demonstrated improved health effects (e.g., they were better able to digest the milk dispensed to them). So began much of modern attachment research, as developmentalists started to focus on the nature of the relationship between mother and child and how that relationship was based on emotional attachment and psychological attunement rather than on a purely biologically based need for sustenance, as had previously been believed (Bowlby, 1969/1982). Since then, countless studies have been devoted to exploring the relationship between children and parents, with an eye on the importance of secure attachment in a child's healthy development.

But, as anyone who has ever felt comforted with a warm bowl of soup or a refreshing bowl of ice cream can attest, food still holds a certain sway in the world of psychological meaning. It certainly did for Alma, who had quickly developed a sophisticated palate, along with a near-compulsive need to finish her food and try out the dishes of her fellow diners. Alma was always hungry. I wondered what this hunger was about, as Alma ate as if she was worried that each meal might be her last for some time. Certainly this was an understandable stance for a child who had been through so many twists and turns in life. Not surprisingly, food started to make an appearance in our play as well, as Alma and I began to work on pretend recipes and kitchen organization.

ALMA: Let's take out the food. Do you have any kitchen things?

ME: Some. Take a look in that bin. (*I point to a blue bin in my toy closet.*)

ALMA: Hmm. (*She rummages through the bin, finding some small plates, utensils, cups, a tea kettle, and an egg beater.*) Do you have any big plates? Any more pots? There isn't that much here.

ME: Well, look, here's a pot, some plates, forks, and stuff. (*I pick up another utensil.*) And a teapot.

ALMA: (*Sighs.*) We'll use that stuff. You should really get a kitchen. (*She looks around the room, her eyes settling on a space near my bookcase.*) You could put it right over there. Then we could play with it.

ME: It's an idea. What kind of kitchen?

ALMA: You know, a kitchen.

ME: Yes, yes, but what should I have? I'm detecting a feeling that I may not have quite what I need here in the kitchen department, so I'm just looking for some input here.

ALMA: You'd have more pots and pans, and an oven, and an area for cutting stuff. Also a sink. You could have lots of pretend food. Even more than you have.

ME: Sounds impressive.

ALMA: Oh, and it should be pink.

ME: Pink.

ALMA: Yeah, that would look really pretty. C'mon, let's play.

ME: You want me to put a pink kitchen right over there, next to the nice rug.

ALMA: Uh-huh. We have to make the food now. C'mon.

ME: What are we making?

ALMA: Lunch.

ME: What's for lunch?

ALMA: We're making it. (*She starts to set up the tops of the bins as if they're trays, and with my help starts to use a couple of empty bins as an oven and a sink. I help her put things in place, noting her creativity and resourcefulness in using these everyday items to arrange nearly the same kitchen she has just recommended.*) I'm going to start cooking things. Let's see, let's make some pasta, some chicken, some vegetables. Oh, there's some steak. (*Alma notes the items as she begins to proceed through each and every food item in the bin. There are about 25 items in total, and Alma goes through each one, occasionally pausing to express her satisfaction with a smile and lingering gaze when she gets to a favorite item, such as ice cream or a piece of pretend pink frosted chocolate cake. Finally, every piece of food is sitting somewhat precariously, yet neatly, atop a flat blue plastic tray.)*

ME: Wow, that's a lot of food.

ALMA: *(with a satisfied look on her face)* Everything is there!

I looked at the platter, and I suddenly remembered similar play with Sarah over 13 years ago. I was in a different office with different toys. I also had pretend food, which Sarah would arrange carefully, and a large number of pretend animals, which she used to spend time arranging so that each animal was set up properly near its neighbor and no animals were ever left behind. Sarah had been particularly careful to make sure that all the baby animals were placed right atop one of their parents; this kept the babies safe and prevented the babies and the parents from getting separated. Sarah had accounted for every animal and every food item, perhaps to avoid leaving anything behind. Once everyone was lined up properly, the animals could partake of the food or go on adventures, but always together. Over time, Sarah had allowed the animals to separate from one another for periods of time. As the animals grew more adventurous, Sarah's anxiety and hypervigilance had cooled as well. Interestingly, as she became less anxious, she was better able to rely on her parents to take care of any issues at home with her brother or at school, while Sarah allowed herself to act more like a child. As I remembered the array of the animals and the food, another voice was calling out to me.

ALMA: Hello, are you listening?

ME: Yes. Sorry. My mind wandered for a second there.

ALMA: That was funny. I daydream sometimes, too. OK, let's make some food. Let's see, for breakfast we can eat . . . *(Alma looks over the food and starts picking items. As she does this, I start to associate to what she may have been eating back in her birth country before the adoption. I wonder about this association—is it my own projection, or is it connected to our play?)* We'll have some eggs, and some peaches . . . *(Alma is listing food again. As she does so, I'm still wondering about this girl who has only been in New York City for about a year and who's completely focused on arranging a meal that looks like the breakfast buffet at the Courtyard Marriott.)*

ME: What did you used to eat in India?

The question of when to stay in and when to step out of play is one of the most perplexing ones for any therapist. Staying in play allows the richness and fullness of a metaphor to take hold, uninterrupted by a therapist's need to make the metaphor linear. Linearity is comforting for adults and can make a therapist feel that he or she is being "therapeutic," but such linearity may not honor how a child comes to understand or manage his or her world (Engel, 2005; Kronengold, 2010). On the other hand, there are times when stepping out of a metaphor can deepen a child's capacity to reflect on experience and can allow the metaphor to take on a fuller shape (Carnochan, 2010). It would be wonderful to have a clear decision-making tree for when to wonder about a child's metaphor and when to follow it. But such decisions generally fall into the province of clinical judgment, which may vary considerably for any given child.

Abby had used all sorts of metaphors, as we played prince and princess, teddy bears, or brother and sister, and went on journeys and adventures. In her case, I trusted staying in the metaphor—what some may refer to as "trusting the process"—rather than stepping out and connecting her play to her life in any explicit way. But with Alma, I felt I was dealing with a different child. Abby was always younger in her style, always playful, rambunctiously so. Stepping out of her play felt inauthentic to how she approached the world. Alma, on the other hand, was another story. She was tremendously verbal and very comfortable expressing herself; she just didn't use words to express her feelings. With Alma, I wanted to help her reconnect to a developmentally appropriate place by using her capacity for fantasy and play—but I also realized that staying completely in play could in fact negate an important part of Alma. So I decided to ask my question and with it, perhaps open another world for us to explore: "What did you used to eat in India?"

ALMA: What do you mean?

ME: Well, what did you used to eat? Back in India, it must have been different from this food.

ALMA: Oh, yeah. We didn't have all this. No hamburgers or hot dogs like in here. It's different there.

ME: I can imagine. (*As we talk, we keep working on our pretend meal—arranging some food, putting dishes in our imaginary oven, and setting the table.*)

ALMA: We ate *dal bhat tarkari.* (*She says this very fast, as if swallowing the name of the dish in one gulp.*)

ME: What is it?

ALMA: *Dal bhat tarkari.* (*She repeats herself very fast, at least to my untrained ears.*)

ME: Huh?

ALMA: (*slightly annoyed*) *Dal bhat tarkari.*

ME: (*I still haven't actually heard what Alma was saying very well. I give it my best, knowing that I'm about to fail.*) *Dabat taka. Taka, taka?*

ALMA: (*laughing*) No, no. *Dal bhat tarkari.*

ME: (*I still don't know what she's saying, so I protest good-naturedly.*) Could you slow this down a little? I'm having a hard time here. (*As we slow down our pronunciation, I notice that our work in the pretend kitchen is moving more slowly as well, and Alma seems to be working on a dish unlike the ones I've seen her arrange before. She has a pretend fish in a bowl and only a couple of other ingredients near it.*)

ALMA: OK.

ME: Let's go piece by piece. What's the first part?

ALMA: *Dal.*

ME: *Dal.*

ALMA: *Bhat.*

ME: *Bhat.*

ALMA: *Tarkari.* (*She says this so it sounds more like "tree."*)

ME: What? (*I scrunch my face and look at her hopefully.*)

ALMA: *Tar-ka-ri.*

ME: Ah! *Tar-ka-ri.* I've got it. *Da,* umm, wait. (*I'm trying to remember the first parts of the name now, but I'm having a hard time.*) I can do this. Um, *da, ba, tarkari?*

ALMA: (*Rolls her eyes and laughs again.*) No, silly. *Dal bhat tarkari.*

ME: You do realize I really can't keep up when you say that. *Dhal, tak, tak, tak,* umm, I don't know.

ALMA: I'm working on dinner now.

ME: Yeah, I'll help.

Alma and I kept on preparing dinner. I made some vegetables, and it became clear to me that Alma was working on a particular dish rather than just using every ingredient in the office. As we talked about her home country and the food she used to eat, her relationship to the pretend food shifted. Alma was now comfortably moving back and forth between play and talking—or, better yet, imagination and reality. In fact, she appeared to be integrating the two. Our conversation shifted what Alma was making, and as she prepared the salmon, a dish with an added emotional resonance, our conversation shifted in turn. The humor between us allowed a playful quality to our back-and-forth, and the added connection between Alma and me allowed us to talk about a snippet of her life in India.

ME: Do you ever miss the food from your old home?

ALMA: Not really. I think about it sometimes. We have a lot of food here.

ME: Oh, OK. I was just wondering. You know like that dish, the . . . (*I'm still having trouble with the pronunciation. I feel at first a bit silly, but then I realize that there's an opportunity here, as my difficulty means that Alma gets to be my guide to entering this part of her world.*) . . . *bhak* something or other.

ALMA: (*Laughs.*) *Dal bhat tarkari.* We thought of making it. But then we didn't. One day we will. OK, this dinner is almost ready, I'm making salmon in a pot. There's salmon, and I cook it in soy sauce.

ME: (*I'm intrigued by how different this dish is from other pretend food creations.*) Salmon and soy sauce.

ALMA: Yeah, we're making a salmon bowl. We need to make the soy sauce, and we need some rice. Hmm. Do you have any soy sauce?

ME: No, but we can make some of our own.

ALMA: How?

ME: We can draw it.

ALMA: Good idea. (*She and I turn our attention to a drawing pad and art supplies. I start sketching little grains of rice, while Alma draws the soy sauce. We spend a few minutes checking our designs and cutting out the pieces that we'll use for our dish.*) Can you make some more of those? We need a lot of rice. Just drop them in the pot; it's already cooking. (*Alma surveys the salmon pot.*)

ME: Sure. I'll make some more. (*I take a whiff.*) Smells good.

ALMA: Yup, it's going to be very delicious.

ME: I never made this sort of dish before.

ALMA: Really? Oh, I make it all the time. You should try it; it's really good.

ME: I'm sure.

We worked on our salmon dish, at an almost meditative pace. Our play was quieter. We talked with each other, but our exchanges, both verbally and nonverbally, were not as busy. There was a calm to Alma's play, as for the first time it felt as if she had plenty of time and didn't need to rush as much information and content as possible into a session. It was hard to miss the connection between Alma's talking about her life back in India, the shift in how her food play moved from arranging items to creating something of her own, and her increasing calm in the session.

For Alma, and for Sarah and Abby as well, our work was about finding a voice within the support of a therapeutic relationship. Alma could certainly hold her own, and was one of the most formidable 4-year-olds I've ever met. But some of what seemed like a strong voice to others could be a smoke screen; her regular chatter and poise served to obstruct a view of a child who had been through so many transitions and so much uncertainty. Alma needed to play out the dramas of the disappearing princess to connect with her earlier experiences. She needed to play out the making of the food, to reclaim a part of herself that would allow her to make a full transition to her new life in New York City with her adopted mother. In the same way, Abby needed to lead me on adventures to faraway places with characters who began to emerge from the shadows, and Sarah needed to bring me into her own family dramas and her desire to be found and never again lost.

Each of these children used play, in the context of a therapeutic relationship, to explore and understand elements of her past. All three of them created vignettes that were strikingly similar in their depiction of missing princesses, forlorn princes and mothers, and ambiguously evil witches. Each child was unusually controlling in her play, working very hard to maintain direction over scenes that in an earlier time, had been far out of their control. Of course there were clear differences among Abby, Sarah, and Alma in the content of their play, their relationships to me, and their own personalities. But their shared presentations and predilections spoke loudly of their shared experiences and attachment histories. And their play revealed a shared longing to understand, to connect, and to give voice to what had happened to them. It is precisely this longing that can be addressed and honored in giving such children an opportunity to engage and in treatment find their voices.

REFERENCES

Ainsworth, M., Blehar, M., Waters, E., & Wall, S. (1978). *Patterns of attachment: A psychological study of the Strange Situation*. Hillsdale, NJ: Erlbaum.

Bowlby, J. (1973). *Attachment and loss: Vol. 2. Separation: Anxiety and anger*. New York: Basic Books.

Bowlby, J. (1977). *Maternal care and maternal health*. New York: Aronson. (Original work published 1951)

Bowlby, J. (1982). *Attachment and loss: Vol. 1. Attachment*. New York: Basic Books. (Original work published 1969)

Carnochan, P. (2010). Earning reality. *Journal of Infant, Child, and Adolescent Psychotherapy, 9*, 26–33.

Engel, S. (2005). *Real kids: Creating meaning in everyday life*. Cambridge, MA: Harvard University Press.

Harlow, H. (1958). The nature of love. *American Psychologist, 13*, 573–685.

Kronengold, H. (2010). Hey Toy Man. *Journal of Infant, Child, and Adolescent Psychotherapy, 9*, 3–17.

CHAPTER 15

Turning Back the Clock

Life before Attachment Trauma

David A. Crenshaw
Jennifer Lee

Googling the phrase *turning back the clock* yielded some surprises to me (David A. Crenshaw), and I spent several hours perusing the search results. One surprise was the overwhelming number of results related to sports. Particular games were referenced where the outcome would have been totally different if someone had not fumbled a ball or not struck out, or had scored a goal or a basket. There were, of course, a number of references to *turning back the clock* at the times during the year when daylight savings time in the United States begins and ends. Another large number of results were related to loss of health, particularly in life-changing spinal cord injuries or accidents causing brain injury. There were also a number relating to regrets, sadness about the natural aging process, and loss of physical vitality. However, I was surprised that there were relatively few results related to posttraumatic stress disorder (PTSD) and traumatic events, which are the focus of this chapter. The few references to PTSD in the Google search hits were primarily related to combat injuries and the psychological fallout from such devastating experiences as loss of limbs or memory due to brain trauma. *Turning back the clock* in this chapter refers to the powerful wish of a child or family members to reclaim the life they once lived before a traumatic event occurred (or, in the case of attachment trauma, more often a series of traumatic events).

Usually the image of play therapy consists of a young child engaged with a therapist in imaginative play where the child's life dramas and sometimes traumas are played out in symbolized form that allows safe distance from the actual events. Over time, the child gains mastery over these experiences and becomes able to continue onward with his or her developmental path. Older school-age children and adolescents who find it hard to talk with a therapist may sometimes engage in various expressive arts therapies, such as artwork, sandtray work, storytelling, poetry writing, or work with symbols, but they don't typically engage in fantasy play. There are exceptions, however, when older children (even adolescents) get down on the floor, play in the family dollhouse, and enact events that need to be processed at the same cognitive and emotional levels that pertained at the time of attachment trauma. One such severely traumatized teen was 14 when he got down on the floor, began playing with the family dollhouse, and enacted scenes of traumatic events that took place when he was only 4 (Crenshaw & Hardy, 2007). The extremely limited cognitive and emotional processing that he was capable of at age 4 required him to revisit these events therapeutically via symbolic play—the natural language of the preschool child. This case is discussed in more detail in the next section.

Longing for the Pretrauma State

Play therapists and family therapists are familiar with a child or family enacting patterns of behavior and interaction more appropriate to an earlier developmental stage in the life of the child or family (Crenshaw & Hardy, 2007; Fussner & Crenshaw, 2008). Interpersonal trauma can result in developmental arrest for a child (Billings, Hauser, & Allen, 2008; Hennighausen, Hauser, Billings, Schultz, & Allen, 2004), as evidenced by stunted ego development. A review of the research literature revealed that terms like *developmental arrest* were far more prevalent in the literature of the 1970s and 1980s, but have rarely been discussed in more recent literature except by the above-cited researchers. The paucity of literature on ego or developmental arrest may coincide with the declining popularity of psychodynamic approaches in recent decades. This is surprising in light of Shedler's (2010) meta-analytic review of the research indicating not only that psychodynamic therapy compared favorably with other evidence-based treatments, but, importantly, that its benefits lasted longer. Shedler explained the greater duration of benefits as probably due to increased insight, which resulted in improved adjustment after therapy ended.

An alternative or additional explanation for the striking enactments of behavior reflective of earlier developmental norms is the compelling longing in a child or even in a whole family to turn back the clock to the time before the trauma occurred. Consider this example: Janice (fictitious names are used throughout the chapter), age 14, in a session with the Reese family, was acting more in keeping with the developmental norms of a 10-year-old child. The therapist noticed that the other family members were also treating her as if she were 10. What was happening in this family? The therapist was curious about the developmental history of the family. In this instance, Janice was 10 when her mother went into a substance abuse rehabilitation program. Since then, there had been frequent crises and relapses requiring further inpatient treatment for the mother, and the family had been struggling to regain a stable footing for the past 4 painful years. The adolescent girl and her entire family burned with desire to turn back the clock to before the family trauma occurred. In time, they were able to express this longing in words and grieve together for the loss of the earlier happy times as a family.

In the case of severe attachment trauma previously described (Crenshaw & Hardy, 2007) and referred to above, a 14-year-old boy, Roberto, left his chair, sat down on the floor, and pulled the toy family house off the shelf. For close to a year, neither Roberto nor the therapist returned to their chairs in the office they had occupied during the first 6 months of the therapy. Roberto enacted the horrific violent scenes that he and his family had experienced at the hands of his alcoholic father, who had since been imprisoned for killing Roberto's mother. It is highly unusual that Roberto at age 14 would spontaneously take to the floor and play out his earlier experiences, but Roberto had been "incubated in terror" (Perry, 1997). Roberto processed the traumatic events in the experiential mode characteristic of children age 6 and under, which coincided with the time in his life when these horrifying events occurred. At age 6, finding words to tell any painful story would have been difficult; it was particularly so when the events were so terrifying in nature. The therapist served as a respectful and mostly "silent witness" (Gil, 2010) during the enactment of trauma scenes, except when Roberto became stuck in *revivification* rather than progressive mastery of the trauma events (Gil, 2006). It is essential for the therapist to intervene in the case of revivification, where the anxiety is increased rather than reduced by the enactments of the traumatic play. Gil (2010) has distinguished between *dynamic* and *toxic* posttraumatic play. Dynamic posttraumatic play displays movement, even if gradual, toward a sense of mastery. Toxic posttraumatic play indicates a stalemate: The child is stuck in repetitious play that does not relieve anxiety. When the child is stuck in posttraumatic play (Terr, 1990), intervening actively in a manner outlined by Gil (2006) is recommended. In the case of repetitively violent scenes, for example, when the character that Roberto was most closely identified with was immobilized by terror, the therapist would take command and call in the police and rescue vehicles to halt the violence and attend to the injured.

Creating the Trauma Narrative through Play

Roberto used the language of play that was available to him at the developmental age of 6 to create his trauma narrative, which allowed him to move forward with his development and become more invested in age-appropriate adolescent interests and concerns. After he achieved a sense of mastery through the play enactments, Roberto and the therapist returned to their chairs, and he focused largely on appropriate concerns for a 14-year-old (such as worries about girls liking him, body image, and academic pressures). Among the most striking features of symbolic therapeutic play are its compelling value when a child's issues remain to be resolved, and the complete loss of interest once the child can move on to other concerns.

In recent decades, the value of a narrative approach has been embraced in much of psychotherapy, including family therapy. Attachment research has revealed that narrative coherence is an important index of resolution of previous trauma and loss and leads to increased attachment security (van IJzendoorn, 1995). In the Reese family described above, multiple steps were required for the family to move forward. The mother's stopping her drinking was a crucial one, but also essential was the creation of a coherent family narrative that would allow them to grieve together for the loss of the pretrauma family life that they all in their own ways wanted to reclaim.

Work with trauma narratives in adult psychotherapy has received considerable attention in recent years (Schore, 2012; Siegel, 2012). Creation of trauma narratives in play therapy through developmentally appropriate language (the right-hemisphere language of play, symbol, and metaphor) has received less attention. It is helpful in the service of generalization for children to be able to verbalize their trauma narratives eventually, and play therapists can facilitate verbalization as they narrate and reflect on the children's play and its possible meaning. Although verbalization will be the ultimate goal many younger children—and older children who have suffered severe attachment trauma—will need to rely initially on creating meaning, perspective, and coherence of the narrative through the safe haven provided by the symbolism in play.

Developmental Kaleidoscopes

A serious drawback to the concept of developmental arrest (which has largely gone out of favor, as noted earlier) is that rarely is development blocked across the board at the point of the onset of attachment trauma. Typically children will present with a wide variety of developmental configurations, which are more reminiscent of a kaleidoscope than the linear developmental progression we expect to see. An adolescent boy may be an accomplished athlete and an adequate student academically, but when it comes to emotional regulation, he may be so variable in his control that his explosive behavior reminds his teachers of a preschool child. An adolescent girl may be abusing alcohol/drugs and may be sexually promiscuous, but she may only be able to sleep with a night light and a host of stuffed animals arranged in a specific order, which would be more common for a 3- or 4-year-old girl. In both cases, the symptomatic behavior results from poor emotional regulation that may stem from attachment trauma, but passes more easily for adolescent rebellious behavior than the more dependent longings expressed by the teenagers' actions. The actions point to the approximate age of the developmental trauma.

In the case of the 14-year-old girl, Jaime, her father left the family when she was 5 and gradually disappeared from her life. Her mother had a series of relationships with alcoholic and abusive men, which led to the mother's psychiatric hospitalization when Jaime was 13; this pushed Jaime into a kind of exaggerated pseudoindependence, because she no longer felt she could depend on anyone.

Jaime was immediately drawn to the family playhouse in the therapist's office with no detectable self-consciousness. The therapist, aware of the presenting problems, was initially taken aback that this would happen in the first session. Jaime engaged in ordering and organizing play in the first session, setting up the house, the furnishings, and the people in just the way she wanted them. She was quite decisive and didn't deliberate or agonize over her placements of people or furniture. The therapist asked whether he could join her on the floor, and she nodded approvingly. He sat at a distance that seemed comfortable and not intrusive to Jaime. He simply joined her as a silent, interested witness in the emotional space she inhabited upon entering the therapeutic context.

Over time, Jaime enacted numerous scenes that reflected the harrowing losses she had experienced when the parents separated and divorced, followed by the chaos stemming from her mother's choice of abusive partners, and finally her mother's depressive collapse and subsequent psychiatric hospitalization. She played out early memories of family picnics and vacations when she was quite, young before the divorce. Some of these scenes were actual memories; others may have been longings for and idealized images of the family she had hoped for but never really experienced. Unresolved grief and anger accompanied these unmet longings, along with the wish to turn back the clock to before things started to unravel in the family.

Necessary Grieving

Since the clock can't be turned back except in fantasy, in order for developmental progress to resume in the emotional life of a traumatized child, the long-avoided but necessary grieving needs to be undertaken. Since the pain of recognizing that one will never have what one longs for is so intense, it is no wonder that children and adults alike avoid the necessary grieving for as long as possible. The difference is that adults usually have more cognitive and psychological resources available to them for undertaking grief work. In order for the grief process to be fully therapeutic, it needs to be holistic. All child therapists encounter children who are able to talk about the sudden death of a sibling in a detached, nonemotional way. In these instances, there is cognitive awareness of the death, and the children are able to talk about the death in an intellectual way, but the affect is detached. The opposite can also occur: A child may experience waves of intense sadness, without a clue as to what the sadness is about. This is an example of internal emotional attunement without the cognitive awareness. If either the cognitive or emotional awareness is detached, the therapeutic benefit of talking about the grief will be limited.

The death of a parent for a young child can result in attachment trauma, but the rejection, neglect, abuse, or abandonment of a child by a parent can also constitute attachment trauma and in some ways may be more challenging to resolve. Although the death of a parent is exceedingly painful, it is also final and clear. In the case of rejection, neglect, abuse, or abandonment, the loss is sometimes ambiguous. Parents may come in and out of the lives of their children, for example, in cases of substance addiction. An abusive parent may at times be engaged with a child in positive ways. Perhaps the hardest to grieve for is a parent who rejects or neglects a child. As long as the parent is still alive, the child may hold out hope that the parent will someday be the parent the child needs. Disconnection can be harder to grieve for than death; it is a more confusing loss.

Children in the foster care system are particularly likely to experience disenfranchised grief (Crenshaw, 2002; Doka, 2002). Foster children carry within them a huge burden of unattended grief. The trail of disrupted attachments and broken-off relationships may be so long that no one loss can be adequately addressed in terms of its meaning and impact on a child. Unattended, often never grieved-for losses can be the emotional underpinnings of rage externalized, and profound sorrow internalized. A typical case history of children suffering from severe attachment trauma is replete with loss and repeated interpersonal injuries (often rejections, neglect, and abandonment).

In some instances, the effort to turn back the clock is driven by self-reparative attempts to recapture needed stimulation of the brain during an earlier critical period. A poignant example of such a child has been provided by Bruce Perry (Perry & Szalavitz, 2006) in his description of Connor, a 14-year-old boy who rocked and hummed to himself; was socially isolated, lonely, and depressed; failed to make eye contact; and had violent temper tantrums typical of a 3- or 4-year-old boy. Perry discovered that this child had suffered a history of early neglect by a caregiver hired by the family, who left him alone in the dark repeatedly for hours each work day. Perry saw the rocking, humming, and tantrums as desperate attempts by Connor to seek the stimulation that his brain had needed during the early months of life. As in many other cases of children who seek to turn back the clock because of neurobiological reparative needs, it was not one event that caused the damage but a cumulative deprivation suffered over time.

Case Vignette: Kai

When Kai, a 15-year-old girl, came to the office for her initial therapy sessions, she was immediately drawn to fantasy play activities expected of a much younger child. She eagerly played with dolls, created jungle scenes with plastic animal figurines, and held tea parties with her loyal cadre of teddy bears. She excitedly arrived to subsequent sessions bringing pictures of animals, many of which adorned her bedroom walls, or stuffed animals from her personal collection to incorporate into her play.

Kai and I (Jennifer Lee) consciously chose a pseudonym for her that reflected her background and history. The name Kai is somewhat ambiguous to reflect her cultural and mixed racial identity. It is symbolic of her complex history and those layers of identity and personal experiences that are not immediately apparent to others. Upon first appearance, Kai's heritage is not immediately apparent until one inquires about the meaning and significance of her name. This was symbolic of the deeper levels of Kai's personal history and the underlying vulnerability beneath her behavioral difficulties. Among these layers were the immeasurable losses and traumas she suffered, which led to her placement in residential care. Yet even after I worked with Kai for close to a year, there were many unknown layers, leaving an incomplete narrative that brought up more questions than answers.

Kai's early childhood was significant for multiple losses and disrupted attachments. When Kai was 4, her mother left the family (for reasons unknown) and had limited, sporadic contact with her children thereafter. Several years later, at the age of 8, Kai was orphaned when she lost both parents in the same year: Her father drowned in a boating accident, and her mother died of chronic illnesses. The death of her mother followed the death of her father by 3 months. Throughout her early childhood, moreover, Kai had had periodic psychiatric hospitalizations because of her dangerous behaviors in the home—specifically, temper tantrums, acts of self-harm, and extreme mood lability. It appears that Kai demonstrated an early vulnerability toward emotional instability, which was further compounded by the mother's abandonment, the death of both parents, and subsequent placements in foster care. Her foster placements were numerous and short-lived prior to her referral to residential care.

Kai rarely spoke about her parents and tended to avoid any discussions about her family. It was a rare clinical moment when she shared a lucid childhood memory; these moments, cobbled together, provided a hazy portrait of her early family life. Kai recalled endearing times at home with her mother, who was a weaver and made beautiful rugs and shawls. She also fondly recollected times listening to her father as he played a piano. Perhaps as a way to honor her father's memory and preserve an elusive yet heartfelt connection, Kai studied the piano as a teenager, taking lessons and practicing with patience and determination.

Necessary Grieving

Kai's clinical team was aware of upcoming dates that held personal significance, such as her parents' birthdays and the anniversaries of their deaths. Kai was able to articulate that these were important dates, but she could rarely find the words to express the depths of her sadness and longing. As we have discussed earlier, necessary grieving is critical for developmental progression in the emotional life of a child. Kai, however, had understandably limited cognitive, emotional, and psychological resources to process the multitude of her complex losses. As a child in foster care with severe attachment trauma, she was particularly vulnerable to disenfranchised grief (Crenshaw, 2002; Doka, 2002). With this seemingly endless list of disrupted attachments and splintered relationships, the meaning and impact of each of these losses were impossible to address. Working through unresolved grief in one relationship was likely to trigger a traumatic grief reaction from another disrupted relationship. The cascading effect of grief upon more grief felt insurmountable. Yet the impact of the avoidance of necessary grieving was manifested in Kai's repeated hurt and rejection in interpersonal relationships. She desperately wanted to have friends, but found that her desire for connection with same-age peers was not often reciprocated. While she struggled to fit in with other teenagers, she found camaraderie with younger children whose play interests were more compatible with hers. The absence of necessary grieving was further evident in the ambivalent way Kai related to adult figures in her life. Kai typically grew attached to staff members, sometimes requesting extra time for sessions and seeking as much contact as she could get. At other times, she would be inconsolable and unreachable, yelling at staffers to go away and insisting that she be left alone.

Developmental Kaleidoscope

With her intense interest in fantasy play with dolls and stuffed animals, Kai might be mistaken for a child of latency age or younger. At other moments, however, she was eager to talk about the fashion trends, her new hairstyle, and the boys at school like a typical teenager. Although it might appear as if Kai was stuck in the vacillation between her developmental and chronological ages, we are reminded that development for children like Kai does not necessarily progress in a linear fashion. As discussed earlier, their developmental configurations are more dynamic and complex, like the view through a kaleidoscope. There were strong variations in Kai's capacity for emotional self-regulation and interpersonal relatedness. She sometimes demonstrated adequate ego strengths when handling conflict and stressful interactions with her peers, yet she could immediately unravel into tantrum-like behavior at the slightest stressor without warning. At times, she would not know how to reciprocate in social interactions, being consumed by her own needs at the expense of ignoring important social cues. At other times, she would show genuine concern for the well-being of others and do whatever she could (e.g., bring food or offer personalized artwork) to ease their apparent suffering. Her ongoing tension between independence and dependence could readily be contextualized as typical adolescent behavior. Yet through the developmental kaleidoscope, we need to recognize the underlying longings for protection and security that were most likely unavailable when Kai was a young child. Similarly, her tension between fulfilling self-needs and the needs of others probably reflected a deeper desire for nurturance stemming from emotional deprivation from early caregivers. Although it would be convenient to embrace a global view of arrested ego development, a kaleidoscopic perspective allows for a deeper and expanded understanding of adolescent development for traumatized youth.

Creating the Trauma Narrative

The dollhouse was a central apparatus in Kai's play therapy sessions. She constructed a household of an extended family consisting of a single mother, her three young children, and elderly grandparents. Kai typically took on the role of the youngest boy, whom she named "Ted." In fact, Kai was so identified with Ted that she became visibly upset when she wasn't able to find the boy figurine at the beginning of one session. Once she located the figurine, she expressed great relief and was able to move forward in her play. Kai sometimes referred to this character as Teddy, a 5-year-old boy, Ted, a 15-year-old teenager; once she described him as "a 5-year-old boy who thinks that he is 15." This age confusion aptly reflected Kai's developmental arrest, perhaps indicating actual or recollected trauma occurring at or about the age of 5.

Whether Kai was Teddy or Ted, there was consistency in her character's behavioral issues. In one of her early sessions, Ted was charged with assaulting his grandmother and was sent to a group home because his behaviors were "too difficult" for the family to manage. In the course of Kai's play, Ted was often described as being aggressive with his siblings, running away from home, being sent to the psychiatric emergency room, or being removed from the home to live with another family. In the beginning, when her therapist alluded to exploration of the character's feelings, Kai's play became increasingly aggressive. It became clear that she did not possess the language or the verbal capacity to express her emotions safely. Her therapist adapted to the situation and learned to communicate with Kai through symbolic play and representation—the intuitive language of a much younger child.

Although Kai played out repetitive themes of removal, there was often a resolution through reunification with the family. This engagement in dynamic posttraumatic play compared to toxic posttraumatic play (Gil, 2010) suggested a gradual movement toward mastery of past trauma. These positive outcomes of being reunited with family members appeared to represent Kai's wish and longing to be with those she had loved and lost. Furthermore, it was a hopeful sign that Ted could always be contained by either caring grandparents or compassionate mental health professionals, who were often played by the therapist. Perhaps this was Kai's intuition that no matter how frequently she tested the limits and acted aggressively, her primary caregivers in her residential placement were not going to abandon her.

Kai generally demonstrated an ambivalent relationship with caregivers and authority figures through her play. She characterized "Cary," the mother, as a neglectful and incompetent parent with virtually no authority over her own children. Cary would often leave the house unannounced to spend time with her boyfriend, leaving the elderly grandparents to care for her young children. This enactment probably represented Kai's actual mother's physical and emotional abandonment of the family when Kai was 4 years old. Kai also personified ancillary authority figures as distrustful, dishonorable characters with ulterior motives. For example, a burglar masqueraded as a uniformed police officer in order to gain access into the family's home. A lawyer presiding over Ted's trial was later found to have an extensive criminal history. A worker from the ASPCA was an imposter who kidnapped and abused animals for his own amusement. However, her therapist, playing the role of the benevolent, empathic grandparents, was able to soothe Ted during an emotional crisis; the grandparents were strong and resourceful enough to contain the family unit and protect the children from outside threats and dangers.

A central theme in therapy was Kai's search for a safe place. In one dramatic scene, wild animals surrounded the house, leaving the family trapped inside and unable to escape. Impingements on the family's security were often dramatized with aggressive, violent overtones. The resolution of these scenes usually involved rescue to a secure location with outward expressions of love, gratitude, and belonging among family members. Again, Kai's engagement in dynamic posttraumatic play not only helped relieve tension and decrease anxiety, but was a hopeful indicator of her continued movement toward mastery of her past trauma.

About 6 months into treatment, there was a notable shift in Kai's play. She requested that she and her therapist switch characters and stances from the ones they normally played. When Kai took on the role of the mother, she embodied a different posture as a caregiver who loved and nurtured her children. This was in contrast to Cary's typically hostile, angry demeanor and her frequent abandonment of her young children. With greater frequency, Kai created family-oriented scenes (e.g., the adults baked holiday cookies and the children helped decorate the Christmas tree). Rather than the usual scenes of being chased by wild animals or running away from home, Kai became interested and invested in cultivating domestic scenes where the family was participating in everyday activities such as playing games and going out for ice cream. These scenes, either real or idealized perceptions of family life, reflected a deeper longing for quiet moments of connection and belonging.

Kai engaged in less posttraumatic play for several sessions, but this shift was temporary. At this time, Kai began to experience greater difficulties in school and in her residential placement. The next few months were marked by periodic hospitalizations and school suspensions, which also disrupted her course in therapeutic treatment. The causes or precipitants of this shift were unclear. Kai vehemently expressed her desire to leave her residential placement and merely explained that she did "not want to be here." Although Kai's request to be transferred to another facility was granted, there were lingering concerns about her eventual disappointment when faced with similar circumstances. When the therapist tried to process this transition with Kai, there was no sense of attachment or grief over the attachments already made. It was as if Kai was sealing herself off from any more loss, because loss in itself, as familiar as it was, felt unbearable. In the days before her discharge, Kai could be heard intermittently screaming and running away from staff members. It was as if she were trying to run away from her own shadow. If she ran fast enough, her shadow would go away. If she screamed loud enough, her shadow would leave her alone. She often reported not feeling safe, and yet it appeared little to do with her external environment. Her experiences and perceptions seemed to reflect an internalized fear and profound lack of safety she felt deeply within herself.

During her final session, Kai created a scene where the children were involved in a car accident and kidnapped by an unsavory character and his accomplices. The perpetrator, initially thought to be the mother's boyfriend, turned out to be the boyfriend's "evil twin brother." The real boyfriend was a kind and loving man who wanted nothing more than to care for the family. The split between "good" and "evil" appeared to reflect Kai's internalized dilemma between needing closeness and distance—wanting to stay in care and wanting to leave, and her desire to be compliant but having no real choice but to act out in defiance. Her characterization of the "good, real" brother might represent her desire to repair and salvage personal relationships, yet in the end, she left abruptly without saying goodbye.

During Kai's course in treatment, she was able to utilize the language of play to construct the beginnings of a trauma narrative. It appeared to be a safe avenue for her exploration to delve into the symbolism of play, where she could direct the actions of her characters and work toward some resolution of prior losses. Although it was an incomplete narrative, her treatment team can only hope that it was an initial step in the important process of her healing and recovery.

Conclusion

In our work with children who suffer from severe attachment trauma, we may also long to turn back the clock and help them reclaim their lives before the series of traumatic events began. As therapists, we may feel overwhelmed by the magnitude of the losses that our clients have suffered; these losses often seem like a seemingly impossible mountain to traverse before any real therapeutic outcome can be achieved. We may feel as helpless as the children we treat, and may fear that no amount of therapeutic work can resolve the tremendous, inconsolable grief they experience deep within themselves. And yet we can never magically turn back the clock, reverse the sequence of traumatic life events, or have the power to change any preexisting vulnerabilities. Nevertheless, we may be able to help our clients access a safe, symbolic language through play to help reach the inner recesses of their emotional life.

The developmental kaleidoscope is a dynamic, multifaceted process. As mentioned earlier, one configuration may show us a competitive athlete. Another configuration may reveal a dedicated student who takes pride in academic achievements. Yet another formation may unveil a gifted artist, musician, or writer. With each turn of the kaleidoscope, another image appears, and another perspective is realized. We may recognize developmental arrest in areas of emotional regulation, the capacity to tolerate distress, and interpersonal relatedness; yet these delays are part of a broader landscape. In the words of Robert Brooks (1993), we can faithfully search for "islands of competence" in the children we serve. As clinicians, we can adopt a strengths-based approach and honor the resilience our clients have demonstrated to make it through to this moment in time. We certainly don't have the power to turn back the clock, but we can remain sure-footed in our efforts to work through complicated grief and trauma by building on our clients' strengths and holding onto hope for their necessary healing and growth.

REFERENCES

Billings, R. L., Hauser, S. T., & Allen, J. P. (2008). Continuity and change from adolescence to emerging adulthood: Adolescence-limited vs. life-course-persistent profound ego development arrests. *Journal of Youth and Adolescence, 37,* 1178–1192.

Brooks, R. (1993). *The search for islands of competence.* Paper presented at the Fifth Annual Conference of CHADD, San Diego, CA.

Crenshaw, D. A. (2002). The disenfranchised grief of children. In K. J. Doka (Ed.), *Disenfranchised grief: New directions, challenges, and strategies for practice* (pp. 293–306). Champaign, IL: Research Press.

Crenshaw, D. A., & Hardy, K. V. (2007). The crucial role of empathy in breaking the silence of traumatized children in play therapy. *International Journal of Play Therapy, 16*, 160–175.

Doka, K. J. (Ed.). (2002). *Disenfranchised grief: New directions, challenges, and strategies for practice*. Champaign, IL: Research Press.

Fussner, A., & Crenshaw, D. A. (2008). Healing the wounds in a family context. In D. A. Crenshaw (Ed.), *Child and adolescent psychotherapy: Wounded spirits and healing paths* (pp. 31–48). Lanham, MD: Aronson.

Gil, E. (2006). *Helping abused and traumatized children: Integrating directive and nondirective approaches*. New York: Guilford Press.

Gil, E. (2010). Children's self-initiated gradual exposure: The wonders of post-traumatic play and behavioral reenactments. In E. Gil (Ed.), *Working with children to heal interpersonal trauma: The power of play* (pp. 44–63). New York: Guilford Press.

Hennighausen, K. H., Hauser, S. T., Billings, R. L., Schultz, L. H., & Allen, J. P. (2004). Adolescent ego-development trajectories and young adult relationship outcomes. *Journal of Early Adolescence, 24*, 29–44.

Perry, B. D. (1997). Incubated in terror: Neurodevelopmental factors in the "cycle of violence." In J. D. Osofsky (Ed.), *Children in a violent society* (pp. 124–149). New York: Guilford Press.

Perry, B. D., & Szalavitz, M. (2006). *The boy who was raised as a dog: And other stories from a child psychiatrist's notebook*. New York: Basic Books.

Schore, A. (2012). *The science of the art of psychotherapy*. New York: Norton.

Shedler, J. K. (2010). The efficacy of psychodynamic psychotherapy. *American Psychologist, 65*, 98–109.

Siegel, D. J. (2012). *The developing mind: How relationships and the brain interact to shape who we are* (2nd ed.). New York: Guilford Press.

Terr, L. (1990). *Too scared to cry: Psychic trauma in childhood*. New York: Harper & Row.

van IJzendoorn, M. H. (1995). Adult attachment representations, parental responsiveness, and infant attachment: A meta-analysis on the predictive validity of the Adult Attachment Interview. *Psychological Bulletin, 117*, 387–403.

CHAPTER 16

Integrated Play Therapy with Childhood Traumatic Grief

John W. Seymour

Many children at some point in their lives will experience some sort of potentially traumatic event (Copeland, Keeler, Angold, & Costello, 2007). Much less commonly, one of those traumatic events involves a child's loss of a loved one, increasing the child's risk of complicated bereavement and persistent trauma symptoms. Cohen and Mannarino (2010; Mannarino & Cohen, 2011), have summarized the recent history of efforts by researchers and clinicians to define this combined experience, and have suggested the term *childhood traumatic grief* (CTG), defined as "a condition in which children whose loved ones die under traumatic circumstances develop trauma symptoms that impinge on the children's ability to progress through typical grief processes" (Mannarino & Cohen, 2011, p. 24). The combined experience of grief and trauma can become very challenging for children, families, support systems, and child mental health professionals.

With CTG, as a traumatized child moves through the grief process, thoughts and feelings of the loved one trigger trauma memories and symptoms, making it difficult for the child to sustain the experience of grieving sufficiently to achieve resolution. The grieving child becomes stuck in grief, blocked by what can become an increasing list of trauma symptoms, such as hypersensitivity, avoidance of trauma and grief cues, and withdrawal from supportive relationships. Trauma symptoms disrupt the grieving process, leading to further distress for the child, family, and support system, and hampering their ability to address either the trauma or the grief (Gil, 2006, 2010; Mannarino & Cohen, 2011).

There are strong interactions between a child's attachment pattern and the experiencing of CTG, as both the child and probably the parent(s) and/or other close caregivers will also be experiencing the trauma and loss (Blaustein & Kinniburgh, 2010; Crenshaw, 2007; Dozier, Bick, & Bernard, 2011; Mannarino & Cohen, 2011). Children and families with histories of loss, grief, or attachment injury will be particularly vulnerable to the effects of CTG. When the lost loved one is a parent or caregiver, the child has lost a proven resource for coping from the past as well as for the future. The surviving parent(s) or other key caregiving adults face the challenge of managing their own responses to trauma and loss, as well as trying to respond to the child's needs (Crenshaw, 2007). Typically, the younger the child, the more the child will be affected by the well-being of these grieving adults. Assessment and treatment approaches for CTG will need to include a thorough understanding of the attachment histories of the child, parent(s), and close caregivers, which will be a part of the recovery period (Crenshaw, 2007; Dozier et al., 2011).

Child therapists working with these families can find it very difficult to make basic and ongoing decisions within the assessment and therapeutic process: what exactly is happening (trauma, grief, or both); who is being most affected (child, parent, other caregiver); and how to make wise choices among therapeutic relational responses and techniques (trauma-based, grief-based, directive, nondirective, child-focused, parent-focused, child- and parent-focused, etc.). Cohen, Mannarino, and Deblinger (2006) suggest a layered approach to the therapy process—one that alternates between grief and trauma work. Gil (2006, 2010) has pointed out that this layered approach will require a child therapist at any given moment to be both highly attuned to the child's needs and flexible in responding to those changing needs.

The child therapist will need to have a working knowledge of the current literature on childhood grief and trauma, and of the assessment and treatment methods most effective for the combination of both (Gil, 2006, 2010; Mannarino & Cohen, 2011; Webb, 2010). In this chapter, current research on child development and on best child therapy practices in grief work, trauma recovery, and attachment repair are first reviewed for applicability to CTG. To illustrate the challenges and opportunities in providing child mental health services to this special population, the reader is then introduced to Gail and her family, who experienced the traumatic loss of a family member. Gail's story is a distillation of therapeutic work with several children and their families who had similar experiences of grief combined with trauma. Her story will not be every child's story, so the reader is referred to more detailed resources for a broader understanding of the range of how children experience grief, trauma, and recovery, with examples from Gail's treatment narrative of specific therapeutic assessment points and therapeutic techniques. Finally, suggestions regarding further professional study and professional self-care are included, to support the child therapist in maintaining continued effectiveness in this type of therapeutic work.

Trends in Child Research Influencing the Treatment of CTG

In the past 20 years, there has been a surge of research and clinical interest in childhood bereavement, trauma, development, and psychotherapy. These recent findings have some common themes particularly applicable to the assessment and treatment of traumatic grief. The complexity of CTG suggests that child therapists will need a range of approaches adaptable to the changing features of the recovery process. Kazdin (2009) has pointed out that while there is a wealth of research literature on child psychotherapies, our empirical understanding of their processes and outcomes is still limited. There continue to be debates regarding the best methods of research and practice to support convincing research, but efforts have intensified to determine precisely which therapeutic processes are the most effective for particular problems of childhood (Reddy, Files-Hall, & Schaefer, 2005; Steele, Elkin, & Roberts, 2008). Until there is more clarity in the outcome research, child therapists looking for guidance on the best practices for addressing CTG can be informed by these recent trends in clinical research.

Childhood Bereavement

In *Helping Bereaved Children: A Handbook for Practitioners*, Webb (2010) has reviewed the historic and current trends in childhood grief research, which can serve as an excellent resource to a child mental health professional wanting to update skills in assessment, treatment, and serving special populations of grieving children. Contemporary models of childhood grief and recovery have moved beyond earlier understandings of childhood grief, which were frequently couched in the modernist assumptions of psychoanalysis and other early theories of psychotherapy. These models understood grief work as a fairly linear process of stages, with the assumptions that children lack some capacity for grief work, and that the goal of grief work should be autonomy of the bereaved from the loved one lost.

More recent studies, such as the ones summarized by Klass, Silverman, and Nickman (1996), have built on qualitative research in childhood grief and development. In these studies, grief work is understood as being a more circular process, with the goal of being more interdependent with memories of the deceased as well as the living support system. In this model, "maintaining an inner representation of the deceased is normal rather than abnormal" (p. 349). Therapeutic interventions focus on facilitating ways that children can maintain bonds with their living community while creating bonds with the deceased. These connections "are not based on physical proximity but with memories, dreams, internal conversations, and cherished objects" (p. 350). This approach assumes that children do have the capacity for grief work, encourages a more open and inquiring approach toward grieving children, and values each child's perspective and coping style. It also promotes a strengths-based approach that builds on the capacities of the child, family, and support system.

Webb (2010) has adapted several crisis assessment protocols for children into a tripartite assessment for a bereaved child, focusing on three areas (individual factors, factors related to the death, and family/social/religious/cultural factors), with particular attention to details that will best inform clinical work with the child. Suggestions are made for specific assessment tools, and sample interview questionnaires are provided. Individual factors include age-related factors; past coping and adjustment; medical history; and prior experience with death and/or loss. Death-related factors include the type of death; details of the child's prior contacts with the deceased and the time of death; prior relationship to the deceased; and grief reactions experienced. Family/social/religious/cultural factors include the grief responses of the immediate and extended family; school and peer responses; religious affiliation, traditions of grieving in the family, faith, or culture; sociocultural meanings of the loss; and cultural expectations for children's involvement in the grieving process.

Whereas earlier studies of grief identified a more linear stage model for the grief process (Webb, 2010), current research emphasizes tasks that will be completed in more of an ebb-and-flow model, particularly for children. Although there will be a great deal of variation from child to child, a general understanding of the grief process can help normalize the experience for the child and family members. Worden's (1996) four common tasks of the grief process—(1) accepting the reality of the loss; (2) working through the pain of grief; (3) adjusting to life without the loved one; and (4) finding a way to hold on to memories of the loved one while moving ahead with life—have been frequently used to help give people a better understanding of what they are experiencing. Wolfelt (1996), describing a process of reconciling the loss, has identified these tasks: acknowledging the reality of the death; embracing the pain of loss; remembering the person who died; developing a new self-identity; searching for meaning; and reaching out to receive support from others.

A thorough assessment not only will prepare the child mental health professional to deal with the expected grief process resulting from the loss of a loved one, but will provide an important baseline of information for understanding a child's trauma responses when the grieving process becomes disrupted. The assessment phase is also a time of establishing the therapeutic relationship, and creating a safe and trusting environment for the challenging work that will be ahead.

Childhood Trauma

The trauma-focused cognitive-behavioral therapy (TF-CBT) model has been widely used and studied in the treatment of child abuse and trauma (Cohen & Mannarino, 2010; Mannarino & Cohen, 2011). TF-CBT is a manualized treatment that uses trauma-sensitive cognitive-behavioral interventions to assist children, parents, and families. Building on TF-CBT, Mannarino and Cohen (2011) have proposed and begun researching a traumatic grief cognitive-behavioral therapy (TG-CBT) model, created by adding a specific grief recovery component for the treatment of CTG to the earlier model. Initial trials of TG-CBT have shown the integrated grief and trauma model to be effective in reducing the symptoms of children and adolescents with CTG.

Cognitive-behavioral approaches incorporated into play therapy can be used to structure more specific alternatives for emotional expression, changes in perspective, or the rehearsal of new risk-limiting skills (Drewes, 2009; Knell, 2011). Despite the demonstrated success of cognitive-behavioral models for trauma treatment, however, a growing body of trauma literature is now suggesting that the affective, sensory, and relational dimensions need to be included along with the cognitive dimension in understanding the dynamics of trauma and the methods of treatment (Gil, 2006, 2010; Malchiodi, 2008; Shelby, 2010; Shelby, Avina, & Warnick, 2010; Shelby & Felix, 2005; Steele & Malchiodi, 2012; Stien & Kendall, 2004). Steele and Malchiodi (2012) have summarized this concern in their recent book, *Trauma-Informed Practices with Children and Adolescents*; they explain that "trauma is a predominately sensory process for many children and adolescents that cannot be altered by cognitive interventions alone" (p. xix), and they argue for a more balanced approach to trauma treatment. Along with comprehensive assessment, they identify the importance of developing self-regulation, providing trauma integration, and building child resiliency as other important aspects of trauma treatment. Sutton-Smith (2008) describes the origins of natural play as the child's first efforts to regulate personal responses to real conflicts, and notes that play continues to be the major means of handling conflict throughout childhood. Gil (2006), noting that sensory experiences of trauma are processed primarily through the right hemisphere of the brain, has suggested that more emphasis be placed on treatment strategies with sensory and experiential components.

Child Development

Recent research in child development has focused on the growing understanding and appreciation of neurodevelopment and neurobiology. Schore (2012) and Siegel (2012) have chronicled this surge of research, which has been made possible in part by advances in biotechnology and imaging technologies that have provided new tools for understanding the interactions of brain and body as humans interact in and with their environments. These findings have deepened our understanding of the attachment process in the developing child, providing us with new insights on how trauma and loss disrupt normal development and how strong attachment relationships moderate the effects of trauma. Some of these findings have particular applicability to child therapy. Perry and colleagues (Barfield, Dobson, Gaskill, & Perry, 2012; Perry, 2006; Perry & Hanbrick, 2008) have developed the Neurosequential Model of Therapeutics, which describes a progressive process of providing therapeutic interventions in the order of brain development, moving from the brainstem to the frontal cortex. Initial therapeutic interventions, then, should be based more on sensory integration and self-regulation, and these interventions should lead into higher-order affective, cognitive, and relational work. When grief work is complicated by trauma symptoms related to the loss of a child's loved one, the child therapist will need to be prepared to address the more sensory-based trauma symptoms with interventions designed to help with calming and self-regulation.

The human brain has come to be understood as dependent on social experience for development (Perry, Pollard, Blakley, Baker, & Vigilante, 1995). Accordingly, greater emphasis is now being placed on emotional and relational aspects of development—a shift from a more strictly cognitive-behavioral approach. Siegel (2012) suggests that therapeutic models should be experientially and relationally based, aimed toward promoting integration of body and brain through relationships. Since this integration first begins as children form attachments with caregivers, Schore (2012) suggests that the work of psychotherapy "is not defined by what the therapist does for the patient, or says to the patient (left brain focus). Rather, the key mechanism is how to be with the patient, especially during affectively stressful moments (right brain focus)" (p. 44). The combination of attachment threat with the death of a loved one and the sense of danger from the trauma surrounding the loss can create a great deal of disruption in the brain, as it tries to make sense of the overwhelming fight–flight–freeze response of CTG. In Siegel's (2012) model of interpersonal neurobiology (IPNB), the child therapist "seeks to create an understanding of the interconnections among the brain, the mind, and our interpersonal relationships" (p. 3). These findings in IPNB add detail to our understanding of the effects of the therapeutic relationship in reducing trauma symptoms, as well as the therapeutic effects of relational-based psychotherapies that enhance the child's relationships with parent(s) and other close caregiving adults. Internal human development is mirrored in the interactions of children through their experiences and relationships, which are commonly mediated through natural play.

Child Psychotherapy

Recent developments in child psychotherapy have closely paralleled developments in the broader field of psychotherapy, which has been gradually shifting away from model-specific treatments to more integrated and prescriptive models (Drewes, 2011a, 2011b; Osofsky, 2004, 2011). These models focus more on the qualities that establish and maintain the therapeutic relationship; on multimodal methods of assessing children's needs; and on matching these needs with interventions based on an understanding of the therapeutic mechanisms common in most models of child therapy. These integrative approaches are well matched for addressing the complexities of CTG.

Crenshaw (2007) has reviewed the recent research in neurobiology and child therapy and has proposed a seven-stage IPNB-informed treatment model for CTG. This model moves from an initial stage of establishing safety, through steps of grieving, to finding meaning and a coherent narrative to understand the traumatic loss. Dozier et al. (2011) have developed and pilot-tested an attachment and biobehavioral catch-up (ABC) model for teaching parents of a young child how to (1) recognize the child's problematic coping strategies; (2) encourage the child to practice better coping strategies; (3) overcome any attachment and trauma issues of their own that may get in the way of their current relationship with their child; and (4) help promote the best setting for their child to achieve better self-regulation.

Stien and Kendall (2004) have proposed an integrative three-stage model for addressing childhood trauma, building on Herman's (1997) trauma model for adults, and incorporating recent research in neurodevelopment. In Stage One, safety and stabilization, the therapist works to create a safe and predictable environment for the therapy, and to address issues of safety and predictability beyond the therapy room. The children and parents are provided with basic psychoeducation on the effects of trauma and steps toward recovery. In Stage Two, the therapist focuses on the symptom list with interventions to reduce arousal, transform the affective state of the child and family members, reduce avoidance behaviors, and improve current functioning. In addition, memory work is done to help the child and family members reinterpret the experience of trauma in such a way as to build self-efficacy. Cognitive techniques may be used, along with teaching healing imagery. In Stage Three, the therapist addresses developmental skills of appropriate connectedness and relatedness with family and support system members, helping to develop better problem-solving skills, to develop or reestablish social skills, and to highlight common values. Therapeutic work in this model includes experiential and expressive therapies to help with self-awareness and self-regulation.

Applying the Research to a Child Experiencing CTG

Complexities of CTG and the Benefits of Play

A common thread through the recent research has been the role of play-based techniques in addressing the complex components of CTG. Play-based techniques constitute a key element in TG-CBT (Cohen & Mannarino, 2010; Mannarino & Cohen, 2011) for children experiencing CTG. Play is a crucial part in the natural development of a child's abilities to relate to others and respond to challenges in life; it promotes self-regulation and self-mastery in the face of these challenges (Brown, 2009; Sutton-Smith, 2008). Play includes a certain randomness and uncertainty, and when it is used in child therapy, it provides opportunities to reinforce successful ways of relating and problem solving, as well as opportunities to expand a child's personal repertoire of coping skills. Play therapy, along with other experiential and expressive child therapies, can provide an approach that incorporates cognitive, affective, and relational components for trauma recovery (Steele & Malchiodi, 2012). In play therapy, the play becomes transformative in providing a new perspective on self and environment. Physical activity, personal expression, interpersonal relating, and meaning making with symbols and metaphors in play can all be utilized in the therapeutic setting for dealing with CTG.

The integrative play therapy (IPT) model (Drewes, 2011a, 2011b) is a strengths-based model, focusing on qualities inherent in play that can enhance the therapeutic relationship, match therapeutic interventions to clients served, and be informed by research on the therapeutic mechanisms shared by various play therapy models. Schaefer (1993) originally identified 14 change mechanisms common in all play therapy models, and recently expanded the listing to 20 in a coedited book, *The Therapeutic Powers of Play: 20 Core Agents of Change* (Schaefer & Drewes, 2014). IPT allows the child therapist to be nimble in responding to the changing directions in psychotherapy when grief and trauma are co-occurring (Gil, 2010), since interventions are chosen according to a child's immediate needs, rather than the outline of a particular theory's model. It allows the therapist to choose between more and less directed approaches, to better match the ebb and flow of the child's ability to sustain the intense feelings needed to address CTG (Gil, 2006, 2010; Shelby, 2010; Shelby & Felix, 2005; Webb, 2007, 2010). In IPT, the child therapist can implement therapeutic interventions that fulfill all four of the broad functions of natural play identified by Russ (2004): providing a means of expression for the child; enhancing communication and relationship building; facilitating insight and working through; and allowing the child to practice new forms of expression, relating, and problem solving.

Gail's Journey through CTG Begins

One summer afternoon, Gail (age 11) and her brother Matt (age 6) were swimming and playing in the family's backyard pool, a favorite gathering place for family and friends. Mom watched from a nearby pool chair, chatting on the phone with Dad, who soon would be home from soccer practice with brother Sam and Sam's best friend, Russell (both age 9). Mom suddenly noticed that the pool had gotten very quiet. To her right, she saw Gail in the center of the pool, swimming a slow backstroke, enjoying the cool water on a hot afternoon. To her left, she spotted Matt, motionless, near the bottom of the deep end. She dove in, pulled Matt out of the pool, and began efforts to revive him. Gail grabbed Mom's cell phone and made a 911 call for help, next called Dad, and then went to help Mom with Matt.

The family home was in a rural area, some distance from the main road. As Gail and Mom attended to Matt, they heard a siren in the distance, seeming to come closer and then go farther away. Minutes passed, and they continued to hear the siren moving back and forth through the countryside as the driver desperately searched the back roads for the right address. Finally, they saw the ambulance coming down their dirt road, with a cloud of dust billowing behind. The emergency personnel went right to work attending to Matt, loaded him in the ambulance, and sped off to the hospital, just as Dad arrived home with Sam and Russell.

Gail and Mom jumped into the car with them and headed for the hospital. When they rushed into the emergency room, hospital staffers brought them to the family consultation room. Russell's parents joined them at the hospital to wait for news. Soon a somber-faced physician and nurse came to the consultation room to give them the news that they had done everything they could do to help Matt, but even their best efforts had not been able to revive him. Matt had died. Russell's parents took him home, and Gail and Sam remained with their parents at the hospital to view Matt's body and begin the paperwork and phone calls related to funeral preparation.

Each of these persons shared this moment of loss together, yet they came to this moment with very different life histories and their own unique experiences of the events surrounding Matt's death. Although they would continue to have much in common in their grief, their individual grief experiences would vary widely as time went on. Each would have experiences that significantly affected their future well-being, and the ups and downs of their grief experiences would significantly affect each of them. This part of the chapter primarily describes the experience of Gail, Matt's 11-year-old sister, who over the coming weeks began demonstrating several signs of distress as a result of Matt's death.

At home, Gail's sleep was disrupted with nightmares that often related to the drowning. She avoided being outside near the pool, and developed a routine in the house that would keep her from being anywhere that she might see the pool. She avoided Matt's room and was bothered by the many reminders of his life that were around the house. Always a good student, she was now struggling in school. Teachers reported that she did not have her usual enthusiasm for learning and being with friends. She often seemed distracted from class interactions, and began making occasional trips to the school nurse for stomachaches and headaches. Her energy level was low and her appetite poor. Now and then, she would have brief outbursts of tears or temper, and on several occasions she made tearful statements that she felt responsible for not watching out for Matt in the pool that day.

Gail was fortunate to have an existing caring support system of family, friends, and school personnel, as well as other helpful adults in her life, such as her pastor and Scout leader. Even with everyone's best efforts, however, Gail's distress worsened, and her parents made an appointment with a child mental health professional to seek further help.

IPT with Gail

The IPT sessions with Gail were held in a therapy room designed for family therapy and play therapy, consistent with the primary training of the child therapist providing the care. One corner of the room anchored a small sitting area arranged in a living room style; the opposite corner of the room anchored a play therapy area with a small set of chairs and table, and rows of shelves with a variety of play materials. Additional sensory-based and developmentally based play materials, along with a portable sandtray table with figures, were stored close by for use when needed. The play materials available reflected Webb's (2007) listing of materials for grief work, including art techniques, doll play, puppet play, storytelling, sandtray play, and board games.

Gail's mom had already begun seeing a psychotherapist a few weeks after Matt's death, concerned that she would not be able to care properly for her other two children while experiencing this terrible loss. Gail's mom had confided to her therapist that she was concerned with Gail's behaviors at home and school, and even though Sam seemed to be doing fairly well, she did not feel confident about knowing that for sure. The therapist encouraged Gail's mom to make an appointment for Gail to be seen. Gail's mom scheduled a first visit so that both parents could meet with the child therapist and give an overview of their concerns.

Gail's mom and dad had met with their pastor several times since Matt's death, so it was not a new experience for them to be together discussing that terrible day. However, it was a first visit with a new professional, and initially the conversation was fairly matter-of-fact—relating the basic story of Matt's death, providing details of the family's and children's histories, and explaining their observations and concerns (primarily about Gail, but secondarily about Sam). They saw themselves as still reeling from the experience, and experiencing some significant highs and lows, though they had both been able to return fairly quickly to their jobs and daily routines (not that anything seemed routine at that point). Later in the interview, the therapist provided some basic pointers on childhood grief, trauma, and the recovery process, to normalize the experiences they were having and to give them some predictability concerning what to expect next from both the grief/trauma and the therapeutic approaches to working with children to address these concerns. As Gail's parents turned their attention to the play area of the room and a sampling of some of the play materials, they grew quiet and tearful. The quietness of the play area and the array of unused toys reminded them of Matt's now very quiet bedroom at home. Some time was taken to allow them to grieve and reflect before completing the session. The agreed-upon plan was to begin work with Gail, accompanied by one of her parents, and later to consider including Sam if it was decided that this would be helpful for Gail or him.

Gail arrived for her first session with her mom, and for the next several sessions alternated between coming with her mom and her dad. She seemed reassured that her parents had already met me, and had a little curiosity about the play materials. She was not eager to talk directly about Matt's death, but she was able to acknowledge that she knew that was why her parents wanted her to come, so the therapist focused on getting to know about her interests, abilities, friends, and activities. Spotting a Connect Four game, she asked to play. Soon after play began, she reported that she was worried because "since Matt [no verb]," she had been feeling "hyper" and "creeped out." She also gave details of what were intrusive memories of the day Matt died. The therapist and Gail talked about what she called the "pictures in my mind," her observations of when they had been worse or better, and anything she had found that would make them stop and leave her feeling better. She had used some simple techniques of distraction, such as reading and watching TV; to build on those successes, a number of simple techniques were demonstrated for Gail and her mother to try and then implement at home. Near the end of the first visit, Gail spotted a large bin of Legos in the play area. She said that Legos were Matt's favorite toy, and that she knew what she would play with next time.

During the next several visits, each time Gail came in the room, she would scan the room for any new play materials. At a few points, the therapist provided some additional psychoeducation on the grief process and trauma recovery, and reviewed and expanded on the anxiety reduction skills that Gail was using (sometimes on her own, and sometimes when prompted by her mom or dad). She enjoyed starting sessions with a brief game, but then her attention would turn to the Legos and she would begin to build. For three sessions during her play, she carefully and thoughtfully built a deep, four-sided structure of Legos, never saying a word. The third time she built it, she made a slow, barely audible "woo" sound that went up and down in pitch. The therapist and her dad thought that this was a siren sound, but neither interrupted her play to ask, and she seemed not to notice that she was even making the sound. At the end, she asked the therapist to keep the Legos object until her next visit, and it was stored safely away.

She returned the next week and immediately asked for the four-sided Legos object. She took it over to the play area, and after pulling out and arranging the dollhouse, she placed the box in the back yard of the doll-house. After choosing a number of small doll figures and vehicles, she solemnly said, "I'm going to show you what happened," and went through the entire sequence of events of Matt's death. As suggested by Gil (2010), she had in her own way used the play materials to expose herself gradually to her traumatic experience, in such a way that she was able to manage her traumatic symptoms. Over the course of her sessions, she would periodically pair more challenging play enactments (repeating parts of the story of Matt's death and events surrounding the funeral) with self-nurturing and calming elements (e.g., playing quiet games, caring for a baby doll, or gathering up the stuffed animals to be cared for at her farm) or more energized play (e.g., rhythm games, ball toss games) that would release some tension through active play. At other times, the therapist, discerning her need, might suggest one or the other of these activities for her to try, or engage Gail and her parents in a conversation of choices on how she could achieve better self-regulation through her choice of play at home.

Gail had predictable ups and downs in her progress. As could be predicted, family events would sometimes trigger both grief and trauma responses. Holidays were particularly challenging, and the therapist worked with Gail and her parents to develop special play remembrances (usually referred to as *rituals* when used with adults and families) that gave them the opportunity to acknowledge both Matt's loss and his continuing presence with them. The arrival of winter, and the placement of the winter pool cover, seemed to help Gail feel that this part of their home had fewer unpleasant reminders of Matt's death. By the spring, Gail's parents had incorporated enough information about grief and trauma that they initiated a conversation prior to removing the pool cover for the season, to brainstorm ways that they might prepare themselves and the children for a new season of swimming. Their preparations made the day less stressful than expected, and gradually, they returned to their warm-weather routines around the pool. By then Gail was coming only for occasional check-in visits, and then she and her parents ended play therapy, with the option to reconnect if there were concern in the future.

Over the course of play therapy with Gail and her family, all the elements of the IPT model of directive and nondirective play therapy (Shelby & Felix, 2005) were implemented. This approach included the parents' involvement in both parent education and Gail's play therapy sessions. It was developmentally informed, matching Gail's age and abilities. Thorough evaluation of Gail and her family setting guided the work throughout. The therapist had specific training in play and family therapy, as well as in applications to grief and trauma. Finally, the course of treatment, while well defined by shared goals and by Gail's progress, was matched to her timetable of managing her recovery rather than arbitrarily defined by a therapeutic protocol.

Many other techniques were used over the course of Gail's care, with every effort made to match her interests and the timing of her recovery process. Play therapists seeking additional resources for techniques for the grief process are referred to books by Fiorini and Mullen (2006) and Webb (2010). For techniques for the trauma recovery process, play therapists are referred to books by Stien and Kendall (2004) and Steele and Malchiodi (2012). For incorporating the therapeutic powers of play into therapeutic work for CTG, see Schaefer and Drewes (2014) as well as Seymour (2009, 2014).

Self-Care of the Child Therapist and CTG

Whatever the therapeutic model used with children experiencing CTG, child therapists wanting to remain effective with this population will need to continue professional development to stay abreast of new trends in treatment approaches. Child therapists trained in one particular approach, such as play therapy or art therapy, will benefit from learning other expressive and experiential approaches, to provide themselves with the widest repertoire of therapeutic options. There are also many personal challenges for child therapists who do ongoing work with CTG, and so these therapists need to maintain good personal and professional care to reduce the likelihood of vicarious traumatization (Gil, 2010). Ryan and Cunningham (2007) have described 10 strategies that enable child therapists to help themselves. These include continued professional training; supervision and professional peer support; balancing the types of clients seen; using team treatment models; and practicing good self-care of physical, emotional, and relational needs.

Child therapists will find working with clients experiencing CTG both challenging and rewarding. The complexity of the symptoms, the wide range of feelings, and the sense of unpredictability will affect both children and therapists. Child therapists who are able to maintain personal and professional care will have for their use with clients like Gail a number of beneficial approaches to CTG, supported by a growing body of research efforts in child development and psychotherapy.

REFERENCES

Barfield, S., Dobson, C., Gaskill, R., & Perry, B. D. (2012). Neurosequential Model of Therapeutics in a therapeutic preschool: Implications for work with children with complex neuropsychiatric problems. *International Journal of Play Therapy, 21,* 30–44.

Blaustein, M., & Kinniburgh, K. (2010). *Treating traumatic stress in children and adolescents: How to foster resilience through attachment, self-regulation, and competency.* New York: Guilford Press.

Brown, S. (2009). *Play: How it shapes the brain, opens the imagination, and invigorates the soul.* New York: Avery.

Cohen, J. A., & Mannarino, A. P. (2010). Bereavement and traumatic grief. In M.

K. Dulcan (Ed.), *Textbook of child and adolescent psychiatry* (pp. 509–516). Washington, DC: American Psychiatric Association.

Cohen, J. A., Mannarino, A. P., & Deblinger, E. (2006). *Treating trauma and traumatic grief in children and adolescents.* New York: Guilford Press.

Copeland, W. E., Keeler, G., Angold, A., & Costello, E. J. (2007). Traumatic events and posttraumatic stress disorder in childhood. *Archives of General Psychiatry, 64,* 577–584.

Crenshaw, D. A. (2007). An interpersonal neurobiological-informed treatment model for childhood traumatic grief. *Omega, 54,* 319–335.

Dozier, M., Bick, J., & Bernard, K. (2011). Attachment-based treatment for young vulnerable children. In J. D. Osofsky (Ed.), *Clinical work with traumatized young children* (pp. 75–95). New York: Guilford Press.

Drewes, A. A. (Ed.). (2009). *Blending play therapy with cognitive behavioral therapy: Evidence-based and other effective treatments and techniques.* Hoboken, NJ: Wiley.

Drewes, A. A. (2011a). Integrative play therapy. In C. E. Schaefer (Ed.), *Foundations of play therapy* (2nd ed., pp. 349–364). Hoboken, NJ: Wiley.

Drewes, A. A. (2011b). Integrating play therapy theories into practice. In A. A. Drewes, S. C. Bratton, & C. E. Schaefer (Eds.), *Integrative play therapy* (pp. 21–35). Hoboken, NJ: Wiley.

Fiorini, J. J., & Mullen, J. A. (2006). *Counseling children and adolescents through grief and loss.* Champaign, IL: Research Press.

Gil, E. (2006). *Helping abused and traumatized children: Integrating directive and nondirective approaches.* New York: Guilford Press.

Gil, E. (Ed.). (2010). *Working with children to heal interpersonal trauma: The power of play.* New York: Guilford Press.

Herman, J. L. (1997). *Trauma and recovery: The aftermath of violence—from domestic abuse to political terror* (2nd ed.). New York: Basic Books.

Kazdin, A. E. (2009). Understanding how and why psychotherapy leads to change. *Psychotherapy Research, 19,* 418–428.

Klass, D., Silverman, P. R., & Nickman, S. L. (1996). *Continuing bonds: New understandings of grief.* Washington, DC: Taylor & Francis.

Knell, S. M. (2011). Cognitive-behavioral play therapy. In C. E. Schaefer (Ed.), *Foundations of play therapy* (2nd ed., pp. 313–328). Hoboken, NJ: Wiley.

Malchiodi, C. A. (Ed.). (2008). *Creative interventions with traumatized children.* New York: Guilford Press.

Mannarino, A. P., & Cohen, J. A. (2011). Traumatic loss in children and adolescents. *Journal of Child and Adolescent Trauma, 4,* 22–33.

Osofsky, J. D. (Ed.). (2004). *Young children and trauma: Intervention and treatment.* New York: Guilford Press.

Osofsky, J. D. (Ed.). (2011). *Clinical work with traumatized children.* New York: Guilford Press.

Perry, B. D. (2006). The Neurosequential Model of Therapeutics: Applying principles of neuroscience to clinical work with traumatized and maltreated children. In N. B. Webb (Ed.), *Working with traumatized youth in child welfare* (pp. 27–52). New York: Guilford Press.

Perry, B. D., & Hanbrick, E. P. (2008). The Neurosequential Model of Therapeutics. *Reclaiming Children and Youth, 17,* 38–43.

Perry, B. D., Pollard, R. A., Blakley, T L., Baker, W. L., & Vigilante, D. (1995).

Childhood trauma, the neurobiology of adaptation, and "use-dependent" development of the brain: How "states" become "traits." *Infant Mental Health Journal, 16,* 271–291.

Reddy, L. A., Files-Hall, T. M., & Schaefer, C. E. (Eds.). (2005). *Empirically based play interventions for children.* Washington, DC: American Psychological Association.

Russ, S. W. (2004). *Play in child development and psychotherapy: Toward empirically supported practice.* Mahwah, NJ: Erlbaum.

Ryan, K., & Cunningham, M. (2007). Helping the helpers: Guidelines to prevent vicarious traumatization of play therapists working with traumatized children. In N. B. Webb (Ed.), *Play therapy with children in crisis: A casebook for practitioners* (3rd ed., pp. 443–460). New York: Guilford Press.

Schaefer, C. E. (Ed.). (1993). *The therapeutic powers of play.* Northvale, NJ: Aronson.

Schaefer, C. E., & Drewes (Eds.). (2014). *The therapeutic powers of play: 20 core agents of change* (2nd ed.). Hoboken, NJ: Wiley.

Schore, A. N. (2012). *The science of the art of psychotherapy.* New York: Norton.

Seymour, J. W. (2009). Resiliency-based approaches and the healing process in play therapy. In D. A. Crenshaw (Ed.), *Reverence in the healing process: Honoring strengths without trivializing suffering* (pp. 71–84). Lanham, MD: Aronson.

Seymour, J. W. (2014). Resiliency as a therapeutic power of play. In C. E. Schaefer & A. A. Drewes (Eds.), *The therapeutic powers of play: 20 core agents of change* (2nd ed., pp. 241–263). Hoboken, NJ: Wiley.

Shelby, J. S. (2010). Cognitive-behavioral therapy and play therapy for childhood trauma and loss. In N. B. Webb (Ed.), *Helping bereaved children: A handbook for practitioners* (3rd ed., pp. 263–277). New York: Guilford Press.

Shelby, J. S., Avina, C., & Warnick, H. (2010). Posttraumatic parenting: A parent–child dyadic treatment for young children's posttraumatic adjustment. In C. E. Schaefer (Ed.), *Play therapy for preschool children* (pp. 39–87). Washington, DC: American Psychological Association.

Shelby, J. S., & Felix, E. D. (2005). Posttraumatic play therapy: The need for an integrated model of directive and nondirective approaches. In L. A. Reddy, T. M. Files-Hall, & C. E. Schaefer (Eds.), *Empirically based play interventions for children* (pp. 79–103). Washington, DC: American Psychological Association.

Siegel, D. J. (2012). *The developing mind: How relationships and the brain interact to shape who we are* (2nd ed.). New York: Guilford Press.

Steele, R. G., Elkin, T. D., & Roberts, M. C. (Eds.). (2008). *Handbook of evidence-based therapies for children and adolescents: Bridging science and practice.* New York: Springer.

Steele, W., & Malchiodi, C. A. (Eds.). (2012). *Trauma-informed practices with children and adolescents.* New York: Routledge.

Stien, P. T., & Kendall, J. (2004). *Psychological trauma and the developing brain: Neurologically based interventions for troubled children.* New York: Haworth Press.

Sutton-Smith, B. (2008). Play theory: A personal journey and new thoughts. *American Journal of Play, 1,* 82–125.

Webb, N. B. (Ed.). (2007). *Play therapy with children in crisis: A casebook for practitioners* (3rd ed.). New York: Guilford Press.

Webb, N. B. (Ed.). (2010). *Helping bereaved children: A handbook for practitioners* (3rd ed.). New York: Guilford Press.

Wolfelt, A. D. (1996). *Healing the bereaved child: Grief gardening, growth through grief, and other touchstones for caregivers.* Fort Collins, CO: Companion Press.

Worden, J. W. (1996). *Children and grief: When a parent dies.* New York: Guilford Press.

CHAPTER 17

Mending Broken Attachment in Displaced Children

Finding "Home" through Play Therapy

Jennifer N. Baggerly
Eric J. Green

> But to penetrate the darkness we must summon all the
> powers of enlightenment that consciousness can offer.
> —JUNG (1931/1969, p. 389)

"All my toys are in the garbage where we used to live." "I don't have any friends in this new place." "My dad had to go to another city to find work." These are common expressions of loss and grief for children who have experienced homelessness or displacement due to natural or human-made disasters. These responses could be temporary or could become complicated grief, contributing to attachment difficulties. What determines the outcome? In some cases, it may be a skilled and empathetic child therapist.

In this chapter, we show how mental health professionals using art therapy and play therapy can contribute to healing for children suffering from these types of displacement. First, we create a context by describing characteristics and challenges of children displaced by homelessness or by natural or man-made disasters. Second, we discuss how to use play therapy to help children who are homeless. Finally, we discuss how to use Jungian art therapy to help children who are displaced by disasters. Play and art therapy can help children create a new sense of "home" within their own hearts that will strengthen current and future attachments.

275

Characteristics and Challenges

Homelessness

Children who are *homeless* lack a fixed, regular, and adequate nighttime residence intended for ongoing shelter (National Coalition for the Homeless [NCH], 2009a). It is important to understand that homelessness is not due to moral inadequacy of a parent. Reasons why a family may be homeless are complex; they may include poverty, lack of affordable housing, low wages, cutoff of public assistance, lack of affordable health care, domestic violence, mental illness, or addictions. Overall, "homelessness results from a complex set of circumstances which require people to choose between food, shelter, and other basic needs" (NCH, 2009b, p. 7). Understanding these causes of homelessness will increase play therapists' empathy for families who are homeless and will help the therapists recognize children's play reenactment of events leading to homelessness.

In the United States, young children in families are the fastest growing segment of the homeless population (NCH, 2009a). As of 2007, children made up 39% of the homeless population. There are 1.35 million children who are homeless each year in the United States, which is approximately 1% of the general population (NCH, 2009a). The average age of a homeless child is 6 years old (Institute for Children and Poverty [ICP], 2007).

Disasters

Children who are displaced by a natural or man-made disaster have experienced an event that met the following criteria: It (1) caused destruction of property, injury, or loss of life; (2) had an identifiable beginning and end; (3) was sudden and time-limited; (4) adversely affected a large group of people; (5) was a public event that affected more than one family; (6) was beyond the realm of ordinary experience; and (7) was psychologically traumatic enough to induce stress in almost anyone (Rosenfeld, Caye, Ayalon, & Lahad, 2005). According to the World Health Organization Centre's for Research on the Epidemiology of Disasters, in 2010 "a total of 385 natural disasters killed more than 297,000 people worldwide, affected over 217 million others and caused \$123.9 billion of economic damages" (Guha-Sapir, Vos, Below, & Ponserre, 2010, p. 1). In a representative sample survey of 2,030 U.S. children ages 2–17, Becker-Blease, Turner, and Finkelhor (2010) found that approximately 14% reported a lifetime exposure to a disaster, and 4.1% to a disaster in the past year.

Impact of Homelessness and Disasters on Children

Both children who are homeless and children who have been displaced by a natural or man-made disaster have experienced loss of physical and emotional safety, which can affect them in numerous ways. Neurodevelopment in children who are homeless can be hindered because of multiple losses and trauma (Kagan, 2004; Perry, 2001). Homelessness results in attachment disruption to children's important relationships, such as those with grandparents, teachers, and friends (NCH, 2009b). Attachment disruption may also occur between a child and a parent who is no longer emotionally or physically available because of stress from poverty, mental illness, drug addiction, or incarceration (NCH, 2009b).

Trauma, such as physical or sexual abuse, neglect, and domestic violence, is also common among children who are homeless (NCH, 2009b). In fact, Buckner, Bassuk, Weinreb, and Brooks (1999) found that homeless children are three times more likely than poor but housed children to have witnessed violence in their neighborhoods or schools, to have mothers with alcohol or drug problems, or to have mothers who have been arrested. Homeless children compared with poor but housed children are also twice as likely to have been in foster care. Of 777 homeless parents surveyed, 22% said that domestic violence was the primary reason for being homeless (NCH, 2009b).

It comes as no surprise, then, that emotional and psychological development in children who are homeless can be negatively affected. Children who are homeless tend to experience more depression and anxiety than children who are housed (Buckner et al., 1999). Approximately 47% of children who are homeless have been found to have clinically significant internalizing problems, such as depression and anxiety, compared with only 21% of children who are poor but housed (Buckner et al., 1999). Socially, children who are homeless have been found to have less social support and fewer coping behaviors than children who have never been homeless or were previously homeless (Menke, 2000).

Behaviorally, homeless children also tend to exhibit more externalizing problems, such as delinquent and aggressive behavior, than normative samples (Buckner et al., 1999). As early as preschool, children who are homeless have been found to have more behavior problems than children who are not homeless (Koblinsky, Gordon, & Anderson, 2000). Youngblade and Mulvihill (1998) found that the longer preschool children stayed at a homelessness shelter, the more negative their social behavior became. Many of these behavioral problems stem from losses and trauma experienced as a result of homelessness. "The fearful child cannot concentrate in school; will misinterpret comments; and will sometimes regress to immature behavior (a young child may start to bed-wet) or self-destructive coping behavior" (Perry, 2001, p. 36).

Cognitive development in children who are homeless can be affected as well. Flores (2007) found that children who were homeless and attended Head Start programs possessed less conventional knowledge about time than their peers who attended university day care centers. Academic achievement problems have been reported for children who are homeless (Masten et al., 1997; Ziesemer, Marcoux, & Marwell, 1994). Rubin et al. (1996) found that elementary school children who were homeless performed significantly more poorly on academic tests than children who were not homeless. According to the ICP (2007), 75% of homeless children perform below grade level in reading.

These neurological, social, emotional, psychological, behavioral, and cognitive impacts on children who are homeless hinder their developmental growth and place them at risk for ongoing mental health problems. Children who are homeless need mental health interventions to facilitate their developmental growth and resolve mental health problems.

Play Therapy with Children Who Are Homeless

Definitions

Child-centered play therapy (CCPT) is one mental health intervention that has provided positive results for elementary school children who are homeless (Baggerly, 2003, 2004; Baggerly & Borkowski, 2004). CCPT is defined by Landreth (2012) as

> a dynamic interpersonal relationship between a child and a therapist trained in play therapy procedures who provides selected play materials and facilitates the development of a safe relationship for the child to fully express and explore self (feelings, thoughts, experiences, and behaviors) through play, the child's natural medium of communication, for optimal growth and development. (p. 16)

Rationale

The evidence base for the effectiveness of CCPT has been well established by Baggerly, Ray, and Bratton's (2010) description of 12 quantitative treatment control group studies. In addition, a meta-analysis of 93 play therapy and filial therapy studies (Bratton, Ray, Rhine, & Jones, 2005) showed that humanistic, nondirective play therapy had a large treatment effect ($d = 0.92$). In research specific to displaced populations, CCPT has been shown to be effective in reducing symptoms in children who were homeless (Baggerly, 2004; Baggerly & Jenkins, 2009), children exposed to domestic violence (Tyndall-Lind, Landreth, & Giordano, 2001), children who were refugees (Schottelkorb, Doumas, & Garcia, 2012), and children exposed to natural disasters (Shen, 2002).

Self-Reflection

CCPT with a child who is homeless begins with building a safe therapeutic relationship based on the core conditions of unconditional positive regard, empathy, and genuineness (Landreth, 2012; Rogers, 1951). To convey these core conditions effectively to children who are homeless, play therapists must engage in ongoing self-reflection. Concerning unconditional positive regard, the following questions can be illuminating: "Do I deeply believe that every person is worthy of respect, regardless of economic status—even if it is a parent who was evicted in part because of drug abuse? Do I feel guilty over my own economic security when I know that my child client will go hungry tonight in a cold setting?" This type of self-reflection can help therapists determine whether they harbor any disdain or guilt, and can thereby help them avoid a "blame the victim" attitude that diminishes warmth and acceptance of children.

Genuineness, or openness to feelings and attitudes, is enhanced when therapists "listen to self and accept without fear their own complexity of feelings and experiences" (Rogers, 1951, p. 53). When working with children who are homeless, therapists need to monitor their own feelings and experiences related to their racial, cultural, and socioeconomic identity developmental level (Sue & Sue, 2013). Since most play therapists are white and middle-class (Ryan, 2002), it is imperative for such therapists to progress through the white racial identity development stages of resistance, introspection, and integrative awareness (Sue & Sue, 2013). This progression can be accomplished by implementing strategies such as self-exploration, development of friendships with diverse people, and commitment to community change (Sue & Sue, 2013). Genuineness is also strengthened when play therapists reevaluate their foundation for hope: Is it based on financial gain, or on faith and healthy relationships? A therapist whose sense of hope is based on money will inadvertently communicate hopelessness to children who are poor and homeless. Conversely, a therapist whose sense of hope is based on faith and healthy relationships will communicate hopefulness whenever faith and healthy relationships are available, regardless of financial status.

Empathy is conveyed when therapists "sense the feelings and personal meanings which clients experience in each moment and communicate that understanding to clients" (Rogers & Stevens, 1967, p. 54). To develop empathy for children who are homeless, it can be helpful to ponder two questions: "What does it mean to be middle-class?" and "What is it like to live in poverty?" The differences between being middle-class and living in poverty include (1) an intense daily struggle for survival, such as choosing between medicine for a sick family member and a meal for the other family members (NCH, 2009b); and (2) a mistrust of helping professionals who appear judgmental and condescending (Sue & Sue, 2013). Therapists who face the harsh reality of poverty and who accept social responsibility for mitigating its effects on children will begin to understand the struggle of homelessness and empathize with children who are homeless.

Procedures

After a critical self-reflection, we recommend implementing the standard CCPT procedures of (1) allowing the child to lead the play session;

(2) tracking play behavior; (3) reflecting content and feelings; (4) returning responsibility; (5) providing encouragement and building self-esteem; (6) facilitating understanding; and (7) setting therapeutic limits (Landreth, 2012). In work with homeless and displaced children, these procedures are best described in the framework of Maslow's hierarchy of needs: physiological survival; safety; love and belonging; self-esteem; and self-actualization (Daniels, 1992; Maslow, 1968).

The physiological survival need of children who are homeless is met by providing snacks, such as fruit, crackers, and juice, as well as a comfortable place to rest. Such children will arrive at the playroom hungry and physically exhausted, and will not be able to engage in meaningful play until these needs are met. The safety need of children who are homeless is met by creating a safe, private therapeutic setting within the playroom—perhaps the ideal home they are missing (Walsh & Buckley, 1994). Providing play therapy in a quiet setting at the homeless shelter or school adds to children's sense of safety and alleviates transportation concerns. Confidentiality should be explained to children in a concrete manner, such as the following: "This is a confidential or private time for you. If you want to tell others what you did or said, you can, but I will not tell unless you or someone else is being hurt a lot." Personal space and privacy can be emphasized by posting a privacy sign on the door.

A safe therapeutic environment is also created by providing children with carefully selected toys in the following categories: (1) real-life items such as a bendable doll family, a cardboard box top with rooms indicated by strips of tape, a nursing bottle, plastic dishes, a small car, a small plane, and a telephone; (2) aggressive release items, such as handcuffs, a dart gun, a rubber knife, toy soldiers, and an inflatable plastic punching toy; and (3) creative expressive items, such as Play-Doh, a small plain mask, papers, crayons, and blunt scissors (Landreth, 2012). Given the limited budgets of homeless shelters and schools, the least expensive ways to obtain these toys are through garage sales, thrift stores, or dollar stores, or in a play therapy tote bag (available through play therapy toy vendors). However, if funding is available, Landreth's (2012) more extensive list of therapeutic toys is preferable.

Since over 60% of homeless children are African American or Hispanic (NCH, 2009b), ethnically appropriate dolls, artwork, and play food items should be added to the playroom (Glover, 2001). In addition, play therapists are advised to seek understanding of children's cultural backgrounds, beliefs, and values through discussions with parents, reading ethnic literature, and attending ethnic community events. However, play therapists should respect the uniqueness of each child by avoiding stereotypes and overculturalization (i.e., attributing characteristics to ethnicity rather than poverty) (Glover, 2001; Sue & Sue, 2013).

Safety within play sessions is also established when play therapists appropriately and consistently set therapeutic limits to protect people and toys (Landreth, 2012). Therapeutic limit setting through a three-step "A-C-T" process of acknowledging children's feelings or intentions, communicating the limit, and targeting an alternative provides a caring and consistent structure for children to self-regulate their behavior. For example:

> RICHEY: Give me that money. I need it. (*Grabs money from Andy and runs to the other side of the room.*)
>
> ANDY: I'll get you. (*Loads dart gun and aims it at Richey.*)
>
> PLAY THERAPIST: Andy, I know you are mad at Richey for taking your money, but people are not for shooting. You can choose to pretend the Bobo is him and shoot Bobo or tell him you're mad.

The need for love and belonging in children who are homeless is met by consistently implementing Axline's (1969) eight basic principles:

> 1) developing a warm, friendly relationship, 2) accepting children exactly as they are, 3) establishing a feeling of permissiveness, 4) reflecting children's feelings, 5) maintaining a deep respect for children's problem solving ability, 6) allowing the child to lead the session, 7) being patient with the process, and 8) only setting limits as needed. (pp. 73, 74)

Through these principles, play therapists communicate an attitude of love and create an atmosphere of belonging that reaffirm children's inherent value as important persons in society. If children are selected for group play therapy (Sweeney & Homeyer, 1999), they experience a sense of belonging with other children who are homeless, and gain the added therapeutic benefit of universality. These benefits are observed in the following dialogue between 6-year-old Mark and 6-year-old Darron, who both resided at a homeless shelter:

> MARK: I'm going to work so I can have money to pay the rent.
>
> DARRON: Yeah, me too. I don't want to get kicked out of my house.
>
> MARK: I'm going to be a banker to make lots of money for my family.
>
> DARRON: I'm going to be a doctor.
>
> PLAY THERAPIST: You're both excited to make money and keep your family safe.

In this group interaction, the boys validated each other's fear of losing their homes and encouraged each other in finding solutions. The need for self-esteem in children who are homeless is met as play therapists return responsibility to children, encourage them through a difficult process, and give them credit for succeeding on their own (Landreth, 2012). For example, consider the following dialogue between Mark and his play therapist:

MARK: I can't get these [bowling pins] to stand up. (*Grimaces.*)

PLAY THERAPIST: You're frustrated, but you're still trying. [Reflects feeling; encourages.]

MARK: You do it.

PLAY THERAPIST: Mark, I know you're frustrated, but that's something you can keep on trying.

MARK: Well, I got this row up. (*Continues working.*) I got them all up. (*Smiles.*)

PLAY THERAPIST: You're proud you did it on your own!

Through such interactions, children who are homeless learn mastery of situations that seem hopeless and develop the self-esteem they need to overcome future challenges.

Children's highest need, as identified by Maslow, is "a basic human drive toward growth, completeness, and fulfillment" (Corsini & Wedding, 2000, p. 469). The self-actualization of children who are homeless is facilitated through consistent implementation of play therapy procedures such as following children's lead, avoiding judgmental statements, reflecting feelings and content, facilitating decision making, enhancing self-esteem, setting therapeutic limits, and enlarging the meaning of children's play to increase insight (Landreth, 2012). Glimpses of an 8-year-old boy's self-actualization process are seen in the following transcript:

ANDY: I have handcuffs, a cop's badge, a cop's license, and a cop's ID. I have everything I need to be a cop.

PLAY THERAPIST: You have everything you need to be an important person.

ANDY: Now you can't arrest me.

PLAY THERAPIST: You're safe.

ANDY: I'm going to put on my battery charger. Going turbo. Zoom. (*Twirls around and then stands with hands on his hips.*)

PLAY THERAPIST: Now you're powerful!

ANDY: Now that I'm turbo, I may look the same, same clothes, but I'm different. I'm super strong. You can't mess with me. Pow! (*Punches down Bobo doll.*)

PLAY THERAPIST: You're different now. You feel strong and protected.

Through his play, Andy was in the process of changing his self-concept from feeling unimportant and powerless—a common feeling among homeless children—to becoming important and powerful. In the safe, supportive, permissive, and therapeutic environment of play therapy, Andy empowered himself rather than relying on someone else. Ideally, as he incorporated these positive experiences into his self-concept, he would see himself as possessing positive power and a bright future, which would lead him toward self-actualization.

Play Themes and Facilitative Responses

The growth and development of children who are homeless is greatly enhanced as play therapists implement the procedure of enlarging the meaning of children's play. Using toys for their words and play as their language (Landreth, 2012), children symbolically reenact common experiences to resolve conflicts and compensate for unsatisfied needs (Piaget, 1962). To expedite this process, play therapists should enlarge the meaning of children's play by identifying common play themes; linking these themes to children's experiences; and verbally reflecting this understanding of feelings, beliefs, and desires to children. Doing all of this will increase children's awareness and insight. Two unique play themes of children who are homeless appear to be eviction and "I'm rich." However, children who are homeless also display common play themes, such as power and control; aggression; and nurturing (Benedict et al., 1995; Holmberg, Benedict, & Hynan, 1998).

Eviction

Homeless children frequently reenact the experience of being evicted from their homes during their play. Feelings of helplessness, anger, confusion, and loss become evident as children use the toys to relive their eviction. This theme is illustrated in the play of 7-year-old Tyronne, who resided in a homeless shelter and was referred for play therapy by his mother because of his frequent anger outbursts and low self-esteem. During Tyronne's first several sessions, he created disorganized and chaotic battles between toy soldiers and animal families, frequently throwing all the toys together. Therapeutic responses of reflecting his feelings and play content included "The soldiers and animals are so angry that they are fighting," and "They are confused about what to do."

During the 10th session, Tyronne's story became more organized, with the following distinct scene. He carefully set up the furniture and a family of people in the playhouse. He pretended the people were going about the daily routine of cooking, eating, and sleeping, when suddenly the soldiers entered the house, knocked over furniture, and threw the people out of the house. The animals helped the people by checking to see if they were safe and bringing the family back together. Then the animals tried to fight the soldiers to regain the house, but the soldiers prevailed. The play therapist enlarged the meaning of Tyronne's play by recognizing the play theme of eviction, linking it to his experience, and verbalizing reflections such as "The family is scared that the soldiers are kicking them out of the house.

You know what that's like," and "The animals are helping the people, just like you are helped here."

The progression of Tyronne's play themes from disorganized aggression to specific reenactment of eviction reflected identifiable stages of therapeutic progress from general hostility to specific symbolization (Hendricks, 1971; Moustakas, 1955). In his play, Tyronne appeared to be reliving the fear and frustration of his family's eviction, the perceived hostility of the landlord's (soldiers') actions, the nurturance he received from the homeless shelter staff (animals), and the reality of not being able to return home. Providing therapeutic responses along with core conditions helped Tyronne (1) become aware of repressed emotions and beliefs that were clamoring for his attention; (2) reprocess intrusive memories of the traumatic event; (3) gain a sense of mastery and control over his overwhelming experiences; (4) integrate these experiences into his self-structure; and (5) become a more organized whole, thereby moving from maladjusted incongruence to adjusted congruence (Landreth & Sweeney, 1997; Rogers, 1951).

"I'm Rich"

Another common play theme of children who are homeless is called "I'm rich," because children count play money or toss it up in the air and exclaim, "I'm rich!" Children who are homeless appear to be intensely aware of their family's lack of money. For example, one 10-year-old girl stated, "I didn't get to have a birthday party and I only got one present, because we didn't have a house or money." Children who are homeless introject into their self-structure their parents' statements about money, such as "If we just had enough money for rent, we'd be OK,"or "If only we won the Lotto, we wouldn't have to worry." In an attempt to gain in fantasy what they do not have in reality, children use the play money to pretend they are rich. Therapeutic responses of enlarging the meaning for the "I'm rich" theme include "You feel happy and powerful with all that money!" and "You really wish you had lots of money so you could have your own home."

Children who are homeless often reveal inaccurate perceptions about money, however. Some children believe that money can only be obtained in unconventional manners. For example, some children toss money up in the air as if it magically falls from the sky, rather than pretending to obtain it through working. Other children pretend to sell drugs to get money so that they can buy sodas and fast food. In addition, some children who are homeless seem to believe that money is more reliable and valuable than relationships. For example, during play, some children may pretend to trick or "kill" a friend to steal the friend's money. Their value of money over relationships may reflect their experience of unreliable parents or other relatives who have left them without basic necessities, and their consequent desperation for survival. Play therapists should communicate this understanding through empathic, nonjudgmental therapeutic responses such as

"You were so hungry you decided to steal the money," or "You know one way to get money fast. Perhaps you've seen that before." Play therapists can also address this complex issue by consulting with parents, teachers, and community leaders about family dynamics, money management, career planning, and social justice.

Power and Control

Children who are homeless have even less power and control over themselves and their circumstances than children who have homes. When children live at homeless shelters, they have little control over when, what, and where they will eat, when they will go to bed, and where they can play. Since a child at a shelter usually resides in one dormitory-type room with the parent(s) and siblings, privacy and space is limited. In addition, prior to becoming homeless, many children have experienced a lack of power and control within communities where drugs, prostitution, and crime are rampant. Consequently, a play theme of power and control is common among children who are homeless. Therapeutic responses of enlarging the meaning help children gain a sense of power and control, as illustrated in the following scenario:

> TRAY: I'm a secret agent for the president.
>
> DAVID: I'm a bodyguard for the princess.
>
> PLAY THERAPIST: You're both someone real important!
>
> TRAY: I'll shoot the bad guys! They can't get me!
>
> DAVID: Me, too. I'll get them first!
>
> PLAY THERAPIST: You're both powerful and in control now!
>
> TRAY: Yeah, we're in charge!

Through such play, children who are homeless assert their sense of innate power and develop their identity as powerful people. Thus, even when their current experience at the shelter limits their power, children will find hope for the future in their strengthened sense of self. Children's empowerment can be facilitated further by encouraging parents and teachers to offer their children as many choices as possible, such as "Do you want to go outside before or after doing your homework?"

Aggression: Abuser/Victim/Protector Roles

Since many children who are homeless have witnessed domestic and community violence (NCH, 2009b), aggression is a common play theme. Children frequently reenact violent scenes by playing the role of the abuser, victim, and/or protector. During this type of play, it is crucial that play therapists maintain a nonanxious presence so as to create a sense of safety for children, as such play can be emotionally overwhelming. As play therapists reflect children's feelings, motives, and physiological responses, such as rapid heart rate and clenched muscles, children begin to associate physiological responses with feelings and to learn to self-regulate. Consider the following scenario:

> MARTY: Don't be messin' with my wife. (*Punches and jumps on top of bop bag.*)
>
> PLAY THERAPIST: You're protecting your wife! You're angry. Your muscles are tight.
>
> MARTY: (*Punches bop bag for several minutes.*) I'm letting you have money to buy a house. But when I see you, you owe me. (*Stands over bop bag and jumps on it.*)
>
> PLAY THERAPIST: You're helping him out, but you're tough and in control.
>
> MARTY: (*Picks up money.*) This money is for my family. You think I'm going to get kicked out of my house? No way! (*Kicks and punches bop bag.*)
>
> PLAY THERAPIST: You're mad! You don't wanna get kicked out of your house. You wanna provide for your family.

Through such therapeutic responses, children will learn to differentiate the feelings of aggression (e.g., anger and rage) from the motives of aggression (e.g., protection and safety). As children become aware of their motives, they can begin to explore alternative, nonviolent strategies for being safe and protected.

Nurturing

Nurturing is another common play theme for children who are homeless. Since basic needs of food and a safe, comfortable bed have not been consistently met for such children, they often symbolically meet this need through play activities such as feeding baby dolls, cooking meals, making beds, and doctoring each other. Consider the following scenario:

> MARY: I'm giving the baby her oatmeal.
>
> PLAY THERAPIST: You're making sure she has enough to eat.
>
> MARY: Here's a blanket, so she won't get cold while she sleeps.
>
> PLAY THERAPIST: You know it's important to keep her warm.
>
> MARY: Time for her checkup from the doctor.
>
> PLAY THERAPIST: You're making sure she's well. You like taking care of the baby.

Through such play, children who are homeless satisfy their own desire for such care; experience the power and pleasure of positive caregiving; and affirm themselves as nurturing persons, thereby integrating nurturing values into their self-structure. Occasionally, however, children will reenact failed nurturance by activities such as pretending to spank a crying baby rather than comforting the baby. When they project feelings of distress and helplessness through this play, therapeutic responses such as "The baby is scared and sad when she doesn't get what she needs" will increase children's awareness of their feelings and affirm that their needs are legitimate. Thus, rather than introjecting the experience of failed nurturance as indication of their lack of worth, they will begin to accept their need for nurturing as an indication of their worth.

Serial Drawings with Children after a Natural Disaster

Serial drawing is a therapeutic approach based on Jungian concepts. It involves having a child produce artwork over time, thereby providing a view of the child's inner world to the therapist (Green, 2007). After a therapeutic relationship and trust are formed between the therapist and child, problems are expressed symbolically in the artwork and healing, and resolution of inner conflicts occurs (Allan, 2004; Green, 2007). The serial drawing technique involves a therapist meeting with a child regularly and asking the child to "draw a picture while we talk." Jung (1931/1969) believed that in times of significant crisis, children can turn inward toward the unconscious for dreams and images that carry within them the potential for healing—otherwise known as the *self-healing archetype*. From Green's (2007) perspective, the play therapist does not analyze the child's images, but rather (1) encourages the child to make the images freely, with little to no direction from the therapist; (2) allows the child to absorb the images fully, so that the images can lead the child wherever he or she may need to go (toward self-healing); and (3) links the meaning of the symbols with the child's outer world at the point the child's ego can accept, and helps the child to build a bridge between "transitional spaces." To reiterate, the serial drawing alone does not heal broken attachment. Rather, the self-healing archetype in children is activated by a curative alliance with a nonjudgmental therapist (Green, 2007). The serial drawing provides for safe expression and exploration of feelings associated with the children's traumatic experiences and dissipated sense of secure attachment.

According to Walsh and Allan (1994), a therapist may employ three different therapeutic styles when utilizing the serial drawing technique with a child: (1) directive (the therapist gives the child specific images to draw related to the trauma); (2) nondirective (the therapist simply says, "Draw whatever you'd like"); and (3) semidirective (the therapist intermittently requests the child to redraw a specific symbol already produced to further explore its inherently healing capacities). In addition to a tolerance for ambiguity, therapists should provide an atmosphere that contains unconditional positive regard, trust, genuineness, warmth, and empathy, all of which may assist children to draw freely in a protected space. To process the serial drawing and amplify its symbols, Allan (2004) suggests that the therapist ask the child one or more of the following questions:

> "Does this picture tell a story?"
> "I'm wondering if you can tell me what is happening in this scene?"
> "If you could give this picture a title, what would it be?"
> "If you were inside this picture, what would it feel like?"
> "What went on in the story before this scene occurred? What happens next?"
> "Could you tell me what you were thinking or feeling as you drew this?"
> "What does this [identify a certain object or symbol in the picture] mean to you?"

During the processing (or resolving) of drawings, it is important for a therapist to remember that all verbal and nonverbal communications to the child should reflect support, so the child will come to realize that both good and horrible feelings are acceptable to convey in the therapeutic relationship. Through this acceptance and mutual understanding, feelings of secure attachment slowly begin to emerge as children's feelings, however horrendous, are seen as acceptable; thereby they feel accepted not as *damaged*, but as *whole* psychological individuals.

Case Vignette: Keisha's Serial Drawing

Keisha, a 7-year-old African American female, and her impoverished single mother lived in a dilapidated Section 8 housing unit in a low-lying part of the deep South. As a major hurricane came closer to shore, rising floodwaters seeped into their living room through the home's front door. Riding out the storm overnight, they believed the worst was behind them. Yet the rain and wind continued to pummel the city into the next day. The levees were breached as floodwaters rose to the floor of the attic, completely inundating their house with water and debris. Keisha was to be indefinitely homeless following this massive destruction.

In the days following the storm's passing, Keisha exhibited uncontrollable fits of crying and panic. At night, her mother indicated she would wake up screaming periodically, waking others up at the temporary shelter they were placed in. Keisha was eventually referred to a play therapist for counseling, as she was not coping well with being permanently displaced by the storm. Keisha enjoyed drawing and painting; therefore, the therapist's aim was to sit quietly and allow her to create whatever she wanted.

Keisha moved directly toward the art supplies, which consisted of plain white paper and sharpened colored pencils. These and other art materials, such as paper, glue, and paints, allow children to create free images of what is going on in their lives and express themselves comfortably within the therapeutic dyad. As Keisha drew, the play therapist remained relatively quiet, not wanting to take the focus away from her artistic creation. During play therapy sessions, while a child is drawing, a play therapist does not initiate conversation or take any notes. Instead, the therapist observes the child; the way the child approaches the drawing; the placement of figures; and the types of images, symbols, and themes that emerge in the child's pictures.

In each of the first two sessions, Keisha spent approximately 15–25 minutes drawing a scene. The two scenes looked very similar to each other: The paper was largely covered by dark water, and within the water was a broken vessel with dead fish strewn about. The therapist asked her whether she could describe what it would be like if she was on the boat in the scene. She said, "It would be scary, 'cause it's sunk and everyone's dead." In the third session where the serial drawing technique was utilized, the play therapist asked Keisha whether there was any way the people in the boat could find a life raft or save themselves, and she responded, "Yes, maybe if the sun comes up and saves them." With all of this macabre imagery, the play therapist noticed a bright, shining sun at the top of the scene. Keisha commented how the sun might be a source of healing, and how she missed playing in her backyard in the sunshine with her soccer ball.

After the fifth and sixth play therapy sessions with serial drawing, Keisha began to draw a less macabre scene. She drew and commented that the boat was almost at land, where it would be safe. In children's drawings, the sun can represent a healer, a restorer, or a provider of warmth and understanding for development (Allan, 2004). The ocean or water typifies primordial water, which is the one of the four elements responsible for sustaining life. In a child's drawings, water can represent life and death, or can illustrate the vast, formless unconscious of the child's nascent ego attempting to regenerate.

In one of the last sessions where Keisha used the serial drawing technique, she drew a boat located at the shoreline. Also, people appeared in this scene, all of whom were positioned in the sand with smiley faces. This drawing seemed to reflect Keisha's ongoing sense of coping with her displacement. Her final serial drawing was a bright yellow-and-orange mandala (Figure 17.1). She commented that the sun was happy in this drawing and that she felt happy too. When asked whether she would be OK living in a new home because her old one was no longer there, she responded, "Yes, I'll be OK. We'll find a new home, and it will be OK." Toward the end of the treatment, her affect dysregulation had completely dissipated. She was engaging in regular play with her peers, and the nightmares had stopped.

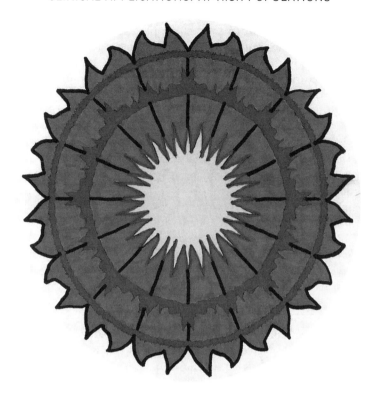

FIGURE 17.1. Sun (a re-creation of Keisha's final drawing).

Conclusion

Play therapy can help children create "home" within their own hearts, thereby giving them the courage to invite others in. Through sensitive and carefully timed interventions within the central arc of a stable, secure relationship with a trained adult, traumatized children begin to abreact the feelings of abandonment and loss that have resulted from homelessness or displacement by a disaster. Through the safe space afforded by a play therapist, many children begin to rediscover a sense of hope and wonder about their world, and begin to develop (or redevelop) healthy, secure attachments with their immediate caregivers and other caring adults surrounding them.

REFERENCES

Allan, J. (2004). *Inscapes of the child's world: Jungian counseling in schools and clinics.* Dallas, TX: Spring.
Axline, V. M. (1969). *Play therapy.* New York: Ballantine Books.

Baggerly, J. N. (2003). Play therapy with homeless children: Perspectives and procedures. *International Journal of Play Therapy, 12*(2), 87–106.

Baggerly, J. N. (2004). The effects of child-centered group play therapy on self-concept, depression, and anxiety of children who are homeless. *International Journal of Play Therapy, 13*(2), 31–51.

Baggerly, J. N., & Borkowski, T. (2004). Applying the ASCA national model to elementary school students who are homeless: A case study. *Professional School Counselor, 8*(2), 116–123.

Baggerly, J. N., & Jenkins, W. (2009). The effectiveness of child-centered play therapy on developmental and diagnostic factors of children who are homeless. *International Journal of Play Therapy, 18*, 45–55.

Baggerly, J. N., Ray, D. C., & Bratton, S. C. (Eds.). (2010). *Child-centered play therapy research: The evidence base for effective practice.* Hoboken, NJ: Wiley.

Becker-Blease, K. A., Turner, H. A., & Finkelhor, D. (2010). Disasters, victimization, and children's mental health. *Child Development, 81*, 1040–1052.

Benedict, H. E., Chavez, D., Holmberg, J., McClain, J., McGee, W., Narcavage, C., . . . Wooley, L. (1995). *Benedict play therapy theme codes.* Unpublished manuscript, Baylor University.

Bratton, S., Ray, D., Rhine, T., & Jones, L. (2005). The efficacy of play therapy with children: A meta-analytic review of the outcome research. *Professional Psychology: Research and Practice, 36*, 376–390.

Buckner, J. C., Bassuk, E. L., Weinreb, L. F., & Brooks, M. G. (1999). Homelessness and its relation to the mental health and behavior of low income school-age children. *Developmental Psychology, 35*, 246–257.

Corsini, R. J., & Wedding, D. (2000). *Current psychotherapies* (6th ed.). Itasca, IL: Peacock.

Daniels, J. (1992). Empowering homeless children through school counseling. *Elementary School Guidance and Counseling, 27*, 104–112.

Flores, R. L. (2007). Effect of poverty on urban preschool children's understanding of conventional time concepts. *Early Child Development and Care, 177*, 121–132.

Glover, G. J. (2001). Cultural considerations in play therapy. In G. L. Landreth (Ed.), *Innovations in play therapy: Issues, process, and special populations* (pp. 31–41). New York: Brunner-Routledge.

Green, E. (2007). The crisis of family separation following traumatic mass destruction: Jungian analytical play therapy in the aftermath of Hurricane Katrina. In N. B. Webb (Ed.), *Play therapy with children in crisis: Individual, group, and family treatment* (3rd ed., pp. 368–388). New York: Guilford Press.

Guha-Sapir, D., Vos, F., Below, R., & Ponserre, S. (2010). *Annual disaster statistical review 2010: The numbers and trends.* Brussels: Centre for Research on the Epidemiology of Disasters. Retrieved from *http://cred.be/sites/default/files/ADSR_2010.pdf*

Hendricks, S. (1971). A descriptive analysis of the process of client-centered play therapy (Doctoral dissertation, North Texas State University, 1971). *Dissertation Abstracts International, 32*, 3689A.

Holmberg, J. R., Benedict, H. E., & Hynan, L. S. (1998). Gender differences in children's play therapy themes: Comparisons of children with a history of attachment disturbance or exposure to violence. *International Journal of Play Therapy, 7*(2), 67–92.

Institute for Children and Poverty (ICP). (2007). *Quickfacts.* Retrieved August 22, 2007, from *www.icpny.org/index.asp?CID_7*

Jung, C. (1969). The stages of life. In H. Read (Ed.) & R. F. C. Hull (Trans.), *The collected work of C. G. Jung, Vol. 8. The structure and dynamics of the psyche* (2nd ed., pp. 387–403). Princeton, NJ: Princeton University Press. (Original work published 1931)

Kagan, R. (2004). *Rebuilding attachments with traumatized children: Healing from losses, violence, abuse, and neglect.* New York: Haworth Press.

Koblinsky, S. A., Gordon, A. L., & Anderson, E. A. (2000). Changes in the social skills and behavior problems of homeless and housed children during the preschool year. *Early Education and Development, 11,* 321–338.

Landreth, G. L. (2012). *Play therapy: The art of the relationship* (3rd ed.). New York: Routledge.

Landreth, G. L., & Sweeney, D. S. (1997). Child-centered play therapy. In K. J. O'Connor & L. M. Braverman (Eds.), *Play therapy: Theory and practice* (pp. 17–45). New York: Wiley.

Maslow, A. H. (1968). *Toward a psychology of being* (2nd ed.). Princeton, NJ: Van Nostrand.

Masten, A. S., Sesma, A., Si-Asar, R., Lawrence, C., Miliotis, D., & Dionne, J. A. (1997). Educational risks for children experiencing homelessness. *Journal of School Psychology, 35,* 27–46.

Menke, E. M. (2000). Comparison of the stressors and coping behaviors of homeless, previously homeless, and never homeless poor children. *Issues in Mental Health Nursing, 21,* 691–710.

Moustakas, C. (1955). Emotional adjustment and the play therapy process. *Journal of Genetic Psychology, 86,* 79–99.

National Coalition for the Homeless (NCH). (2009a). *How many people experience homelessness?* (NCH Fact Sheet No. 2). Retrieved from *www.nationalhomeless.org/publications/facts/How_Many.pdf*

National Coalition for the Homeless (NCH). (2009b). *Why are people homeless?* (NCH Fact Sheet No. 1). Retrieved from *www.nationalhomeless.org/publications/facts/Why.pdf*

Perry, B. (2001). Children and loss. *Academic Search Premier, 110,* 36.

Piaget, J. (1962). *Play, dreams, and imitation in childhood.* New York: Norton.

Rogers, C. (1951). *Client-centered therapy, its current practice, implications, and theory.* Boston: Houghton Mifflin.

Rogers, C., & Stevens, B. (1967). *Person to person: The problem of being human.* Lafayette, CA: Real People Press.

Rosenfeld, L. B., Caye, J. S., Ayalon, O., & Lahad, M. (2005). *When their world falls apart: Helping families and children manage the effects of disasters.* Washington, DC: NASW Press.

Rubin, D. H., Erickson, C. J., Agustin, M. S., Cleary, S. D., Allen, J. K., & Cohen, P. (1996). Cognitive and academic functioning of homeless children compared with housed children. *Pediatrics, 97,* 289–294.

Ryan, S. (2002). *Who are we?: Findings from the Association for Play Therapy membership survey.* Paper presented at the 19th Annual Association for Play Therapy International Conference, St. Louis, MO.

Schottelkorb, A. A., Doumas, D. M., & Garcia, R. (2012). Treatment for childhood refugee trauma: A randomized, controlled trial. *International Journal of Play Therapy, 21*(2), 57–73.

Shen, Y. J. (2002). Short-term group play therapy with Chinese earthquake victims: Effects on anxiety, depression and adjustment. *International Journal of Play Therapy, 11*, 43–64.

Sue, D., & Sue, D. (2013). *Counseling the culturally different. Theory and practice* (6th ed.). New York: Wiley.

Sweeney, D. S., & Homeyer, L. E. (1999). *The handbook of group play therapy: How to do it, how it works, whom it's best for.* San Francisco, CA: Jossey-Bass.

Tyndall-Lind, A., Landreth, G. L., & Giordano, M. A. (2001). Intensive group play therapy with child witnesses of domestic violence. *International Journal of Play Therapy, 10*(1), 53–83.

Walsh, D., & Allan, J. (1994). Jungian art counseling with the suicidal child. *Guidance and Counseling, 10*(1), 3–10.

Walsh, M. E., & Buckley, M. A. (1994). Children's experiences of homelessness: Implications for school counselors. *Elementary School Guidance and Counseling, 29*(1), 4–15.

Youngblade, L. M., & Mulvihill, B. A. (1998). Individual differences in homeless preschoolers' social behavior. *Journal of Applied Developmental Psychology, 19*, 593–614.

Ziesemer, C., Marcoux, L., & Marwell, B. (1994). Homeless children: Are they different from other low-income children? *Social Work, 39*, 658–668.

Index

True False 16. Alternative treatments such as acupuncture and meditation can be effective treatments for chronic pain.

True False 17. Alcohol is an important contributor to both intentional and unintentional injuries.

True False 18. "No pain, no gain" is true for receiving health benefits from exercise.

True False 19. The lower a person's cholesterol, the lower his or her risk of dying.

True False 20. Eating a high-protein diet is a healthy choice.

True False 21. Totally eliminating alcohol from one's life is a healthy choice.

True False 22. People who experience chronic pain have underlying psychological disorders that are the real basis of their pain problem.

True False 23. Only viruses and germs trigger activation of the immune system.

True False 24. African Americans are more likely than European Americans to develop and to die of heart disease.

True False 25. Both positive and negative events may produce stress.

True False 26. Psychologists have found that lack of willpower is the primary reason why smokers cannot quit.

True False 27. Sugar pills (placebos) can boost the effectiveness of both psychological and medical treatments.

True False 28. People with a minor illness are about as likely as people with a serious illness to seek medical treatment.

True False 29. People who live with a smoker have about the same risk for cancer and heart disease as do cigarette smokers.

True False 30. Sick people who have a lot of friends usually live longer than sick people who have no close friends.

The answers to these questions appear on the back endpapers. You can also find an answer key on the website for this book: www.cengagebrain.com.

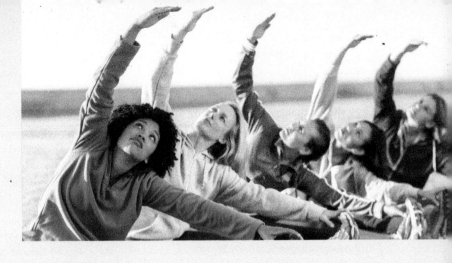

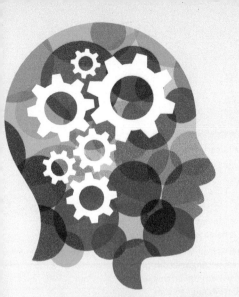

HEALTH
Psychology

An Introduction to Behavior and Health

NINTH EDITION

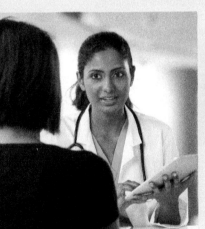

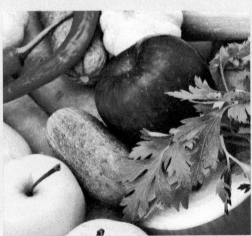

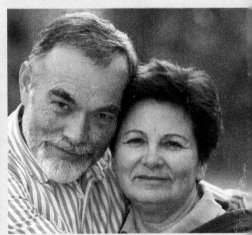

Linda Brannon
McNeese State University

John A. Updegraff
Kent State University

Jess Feist

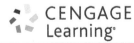

CENGAGE
Learning®

Australia • Brazil • Mexico • Singapore • United Kingdom • United States

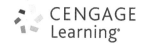

Health Psychology: An Introduction to Behavior and Health, Ninth Edition
Linda Brannon, John A. Updegraff, and Jess Feist

Vice President, General Manager: Social Science & Qualitative Business: Erin Joyner

Product Director: Marta Lee-Perriard

Product Manager: Star Burruto

Production Manager: Brenda Ginty

Content Developer: Linda Man

Product Assistant: Katie Chen

Manufacturing Planner: Karen Hunt

Art and Cover Direction, Production Management, and Composition: Lumina Datamatics, Inc.

Cover Images: Serg64/Shutterstock, Alexander Raths/Shutterstock, Stuart Jenner/Shutterstock, wavebreakmedia/Shutterstock, Iterum/Shutterstock

Interior images: Titima Ongkantong/Shutterstock, Felicity.S/Shutterstock.com

Intellectual Property
Analyst: Deanna Ettinger

Project Manager: Reba Frederics

For product information and technology assistance, contact us at
Cengage Learning Customer & Sales Support, 1-800-354-9706

For permission to use material from this text or product, submit all requests online at **www.cengage.com/permissions**
Further permissions questions can be emailed to
permissionrequest@cengage.com

Library of Congress Control Number: 2016957429

Student Edition:
ISBN: 978-1-337-09464-1

Loose-leaf Edition:
ISBN: 978-1-337-09468-9

Cengage Learning
20 Channel Center Street
Boston, MA 02210
USA

Cengage Learning is a leading provider of customized learning solutions with employees residing in nearly 40 different countries and sales in more than 125 countries around the world. Find your local representative at **www.cengage.com**.

Cengage Learning products are represented in Canada by Nelson Education, Ltd.

To learn more about Cengage Learning Solutions, visit **www.cengage.com**.

Purchase any of our products at your local college store or at our preferred online store **www.cengagebrain.com**

Printed in the United States of America
Print Number: 02   Print Year: 2017

BRIEF CONTENTS

CONTENTS

CHAPTER

PREFACE

ealth is a far different phenomenon today than it was just a century ago. Most serious diseases and disorders now result from people's behavior. People smoke, eat unhealthily, do not exercise, or cope ineffectively with the stresses of modern life. As you will learn in this book, psychology—the science of behavior—is increasingly relevant to understanding physical health. *Health psychology* is the scientific study of behaviors that relate to health enhancement, disease prevention, safety, and rehabilitation.

The first edition of this book, published in the 1980s, was one of the first undergraduate texts to cover the then-emerging field of health psychology. Now in this ninth edition, *Health Psychology: An Introduction to Behavior and Health* remains a preeminent undergraduate textbook in health psychology.

The Ninth Edition

This ninth edition retains the core aspects that have kept this book a leader throughout the decades: (1) a balance between the science and applications of the field of health psychology and (2) a clear and engaging review of classic and cutting-edge research on behavior and health.

The ninth edition of *Health Psychology: An Introduction to Behavior and Health* has five parts. Part 1, which includes the first four chapters, lays a solid foundation in research and theory for understanding subsequent chapters and approaches the field by considering the overarching issues involved in seeking medical care and adhering to health care regimens. Part 2 deals with stress, pain, and the management of these conditions through conventional and alternative medicine. Part 3 discusses heart disease, cancer, and other chronic diseases. Part 4 includes chapters on tobacco use, drinking alcohol, eating and weight, and physical activity. Part 5 looks toward future challenges in health psychology and addresses how to apply health knowledge to one's life to become healthier.

What's New?

The ninth edition reorganizes several chapters to better emphasize the theoretical underpinnings of health behavior. For example, Chapter 4 focuses on adherence to healthy behavior and presents both classic and contemporary theories of health behavior, including recent research on the "intention–behavior gap." Readers of the ninth edition will benefit from the most up-to-date review of health behavior theories—and their applications—on the market.

The ninth edition also features new boxes on important and timely topics such as

- Why is there a controversy about childhood vaccinations?
- Do online social networks influence your health?
- Could acupuncture benefit animals as well as humans?
- How much of your risk for stroke is due to behavior? (Answer: nearly *all*)
- Does drug use cause brain damage?
- Can sleep deprivation lead to obesity?
- Can exercise help you learn?

Other new or reorganized topics within the chapters include:

- Several new Real-World Profiles, including Hope Solo, Ricky Gervais, Danny Cahill, Rajiv Kumar, and big city taxi drivers.
- Illustration of the evolving nature of health research in Chapter 2, through examples of studies on the link between diet and colon cancer.
- New research on the role of **stigma** in influencing people's decision to seek medical care, in Chapter 3.
- The role of **optimism** and **positive mood** in coping with stress, in Chapter 5.
- **Mindfulness** as a useful technique for managing stress (Chapter 5), managing pain (Chapter 7), and as a promising therapy for binge eating disorder (Chapter 14).

- Stress and its influence on the length of **telomeres**, in Chapter 6.
- **Marriage** as a key factor in predicting survival following cancer diagnosis, in Chapter 10.
- The use of **dignity therapy** as a means to address psychosocial issues faced by terminal patients, in Chapter 11.
- The use of **smartphone "apps" and fitness trackers** in promoting physical activity, in Chapter 15.

What Has Been Retained?

In this revision, we retained the most popular features that made this text a leader over the past two decades. These features include (1) "Real-World Profiles" for each chapter, (2) chapter-opening questions, (3) a "Check Your Health Risks" box in most chapters, (4) one or more "Would You Believe …?" boxes in each chapter, and (5) a "Becoming Healthier" feature in many chapters. These features stimulate critical thinking, engage readers in the topic, and provide valuable tips to enhance personal well-being.

Real-World Profiles   Millions of people—including celebrities—deal with the issues we describe in this book. To highlight the human side of health psychology, we open each chapter with a profile of a person in the real world. Many of these profiles are of famous people, whose health issues may not always be well-known. Their cases provide intriguing examples, such as Barack Obama's attempt to quit smoking, Lance Armstrong's delays in seeking treatment for cancer, Steve Jobs' fight with cancer, Halle Berry's diabetes, Charlie Sheen's substance abuse, and Ricky Gervais' efforts to increase physical activity. We also include a profile of "celebrities" in the world of health psychology, including Dr. Angela Bryan, Dr. Norman Cousins, and Dr. Rajiv Kumar, to give readers a better sense of the personal motivation and activities of those in the health psychology and medical fields.

Questions and Answers   In this text, we adopt a *preview, read, and review* method to facilitate student's learning and recall. Each chapter begins with a series of *Questions* that organize the chapter, preview the material, and enhance active learning. As each chapter unfolds, we reveal the answers through a discussion of relevant research findings. At the end of each major topic, an *In Summary* statement recaps the topic. Then, at the end of the chapter, *Answers* to the chapter-opening questions appear. In this manner, students benefit from many opportunities to engage with the material throughout each chapter.

Check Your Health Risks   At the beginning of most chapters, a "Check Your Health Risks" box personalizes material in that chapter. Each box consists of several health-related behaviors or attitudes that readers should check before looking at the rest of the chapter. After checking the items that apply to them and then becoming familiar with the chapter's material, readers will develop a more research-based understanding of their health risks. A special "Check Your Health Risks" appears inside the front cover of the book. Students should complete this exercise before they read the book and look for answers as they proceed through the chapters (or check the website for the answers).

Would You Believe …? Boxes   We keep the popular "Would You Believe …?" boxes, adding many new ones and updating those we retained. Each box highlights a particularly intriguing finding in health research. These boxes explode preconceived notions, present unusual findings, and challenge students to take an objective look at issues that they may have not have evaluated carefully.

Becoming Healthier   Embedded in most chapters is a "Becoming Healthier" box with advice on how to use the information in the chapter to enact a healthier lifestyle. Although some people may not agree with all of these recommendations, each is based on the most current research findings. We believe that if you follow these guidelines, you will increase your chances of a long and healthy life.

Other Changes and Additions

We have made a number of subtle changes in this edition that we believe make it an even stronger book than its predecessors. More specifically, we

- Replaced old references with more recent ones
- Reorganized many sections of chapters to improve the flow of information
- Added several new tables and figures to aid students' understanding of difficult concepts
- Highlighted the biopsychosocial approach to health psychology, examining issues and data from a biological, psychological, and social viewpoint
- Drew from the growing body of research from around the world on health to give the book a more international perspective

- Recognized and emphasized gender issues whenever appropriate
- Retained our emphasis on theories and models that strive to explain and predict health-related behaviors

Writing Style

With each edition, we work to improve our connection with readers. Although this book explores complex issues and difficult topics, we use clear, concise, and comprehensible language and an informal, lively writing style. We write this book for an upper-division undergraduate audience, and it should be easily understood by students with a minimal background in psychology and biology. Health psychology courses typically draw students from a variety of college majors, so some elementary material in our book may be repetitive for some students. For other students, this material will fill in the background they need to comprehend the information within the field of health psychology.

Technical terms appear in **boldface type,** and a definition usually appears at that point in the text. These terms also appear in an end-of-book glossary.

Instructional Aids

Besides the glossary at the end of the book, we supply several other features to help both students and instructors. These include stories of people whose behavior typifies the topic, frequent summaries within each chapter, and annotated suggested readings.

Within-Chapter Summaries

Rather than wait until the end of each chapter to present a lengthy chapter summary, we place shorter summaries at key points within each chapter. In general, these summaries correspond to each major topic in a chapter. We believe these shorter, frequent summaries keep readers on track and promote a better understanding of the chapter's content.

Annotated Suggested Readings

At the end of each chapter are three or four annotated suggested readings that students may wish to examine. We chose these readings for their capacity to shed additional light on major topics in a chapter. Most of these suggested readings are quite recent, but we also selected several that have lasting interest. We include only readings that are intelligible to the average college student and that are accessible in most college and university libraries.

MindTap® Psychology: We now provide *MindTap®* in the 9th edition. *MindTap for Health Psychology 9th Edition* is the digital learning solution that helps instructors engage and transform today's students into critical thinkers. Through paths of dynamic assignments and applications that you can personalize, real-time course analytics, and an accessible reader, MindTap helps you turn cookie cutter into cutting edge, apathy into engagement, and memorizers into higher-level thinkers. As an instructor using MindTap you have at your fingertips the right content and unique set of tools curated specifically for your course all in an interface designed to improve workflow and save time when planning lessons and course structure. The control to build and personalize your course is all yours, focusing on the most relevant material while also lowering costs for your students. Stay connected and informed in your course through real-time student tracking that provides the opportunity to adjust the course as needed based on analytics of interactivity in the course.

Online Instructor's Manual: We provide an online instructor's manual, complete with lecture outlines, discussion topics, suggested activities, media tools, and video recommendations.

Online PowerPoints: Microsoft PowerPoint® slides are provided to help you make your lectures more engaging while effectively reaching your visually oriented students. The PowerPoint® slides are updated to reflect the content and organization of the new edition of the text.

Cengage Learning Testing, powered by Cognero®: Cengage Learning Testing, Powered by Cognero®, is a flexible online system that allows you to author, edit, and manage test bank content. You can create multiple test versions in an instant and deliver tests from your LMS in your classroom.

Acknowledgments

We would like to thank the people at Cengage Learning for their assistance: Marta-Lee Perriard, Product Director, Star Burruto, Product Team Manager, Katie Chen, Product Assistant, and Reba Frederics, Intellectual Property Manager. Special thanks go to Linda Man, our

Content Developer and to Joseph Malcolm who led us through the production at Lumina.

We are also indebted to a number of reviewers who read all or parts of the manuscript for this and earlier editions. We are grateful for the valuable comments of the following reviewers:

Sangeeta Singg, Angelo State University

Edward Fernandes, Barton College

Ryan May, Marietta College

Erin Wood, Catawba College

Linda notes that authors typically thank their spouses for being understanding, supportive, and sacrificing, and her spouse, Barry Humphus, is no exception. He made contributions that helped to shape the book and provided generous, patient, live-in, expert computer consultation and tech support that proved essential in the preparation of the manuscript.

Linda also acknowledges the huge debt to Jess Feist and his contributions to this book. Jess was last able to work on the sixth edition, and he died in February, 2015. His work and words remain as a guide and inspiration for her and for John; this book would not have existed without him.

John also thanks his wife, Alanna, for her support throughout the process and his two children for always asking about the book, even though they rarely comprehended what he told them about it. John thanks all of his past undergraduate students for making health psychology such a thrill to teach. This book is dedicated to them and to the future generation of health psychology students.

Linda Brannon is a professor in the Department of Psychology at McNeese State University in Lake Charles, Louisiana. Linda joined the faculty at McNeese after receiving her doctorate in human experimental psychology from the University of Texas at Austin.

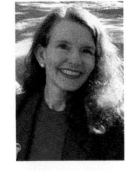

Jess Feist was Professor Emeritus at McNeese State University. He joined the faculty after receiving his doctorate in counseling from the University of Kansas and stayed at McNeese until he retired in 2005. He died in 2015.

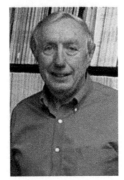

In the early 1980s, Linda and Jess became interested in the developing field of health psychology, which led to their coauthoring the first edition of this book. They watched the field of health psychology emerge and grow, and the subsequent editions of the book reflect that growth and development.

Their interests converge in the area of health psychology but diverge in other areas of psychology.

Jess carried his interest in personality theory to his authorship of *Theories of Personality,* coauthored with his son Greg Feist. Linda's interest in gender and gender issues led her to publish *Gender: Psychological Perspectives,* which is in its seventh edition.

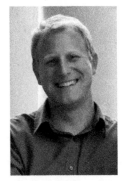

John A. Updegraff is a professor of social and health psychology in the Department of Psychological Sciences at Kent State University in Kent, Ohio. John received his PhD in social psychology at University of California, Los Angeles, under the mentorship of pioneering health psychologist Shelley Taylor. John then completed a postdoctoral fellowship at University of California, Irvine, prior to joining the faculty at Kent State.

John is an expert in the areas of health behavior, health communication, stress, and coping, and is the recipient of multiple research grants from the National Institutes of Health. His research appears in the field's top journals.

John stays healthy by running the roads and trails near his home. John is also known for subjecting students and colleagues to his singing and guitar playing (go ahead, look him up on YouTube).

CHAPTER 1

Introducing Health Psychology

CHAPTER OUTLINE

- Real-World Profile of Angela Bryan
- *The Changing Field of Health*
- *Psychology's Relevance for Health*
- *The Profession of Health Psychology*

QUESTIONS

This chapter focuses on three basic questions:

1. How have views of health changed?

2. How did psychology become involved in health care?

3. What type of training do health psychologists receive, and what kinds of work do they do?

Real-World Profile of **ANGELA BRYAN**

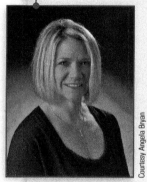

Courtesy Angela Bryan

Health psychology is a relatively new and fascinating field of psychology. Health psychologists examine how people's lifestyles influence their physical health. In this book, you will learn about the diverse topics, findings, and people who make up this field.

First, let's introduce you to Angela Bryan, a health psychologist from the University of Colorado Boulder. Angela develops interventions that promote healthy behavior such as safe sex and physical activity. Angela has won several awards for her work, including recognition that one of her interventions is among the few that work in reducing risky sexual behavior among adolescents ("Safe on the Outs"; Centers for Disease Control and Prevention [CDC], 2011b).

As an adolescent, Angela thought of herself as a "rebel" (Aiken, 2006), perhaps an unlikely start for someone who now develops ways to help people to maintain a healthy lifestyle. It was not until college that Angela discovered her passion for health psychology. She took a course in social psychology, which explored how people make judgments about others. Angela quickly saw the relevance for understanding safe sex behavior. At this time, the HIV/AIDS epidemic was peaking in the United States, and condom use was one action people could take to prevent the spread of HIV. Yet, people often resisted proposing condoms to a partner, due to concerns such as "What will a partner think of me if I say that a condom is needed?" Angela sought out a professor to supervise a research project on perceptions of condom use in an initial sexual encounter.

Angela continued this work as a PhD student and developed a program to promote condom use among college women. In this program, Angela taught women skills for proposing and using condoms. This work was not always easy. She recalls, "I would walk through the residence halls on my way to deliver my intervention, with a basket of condoms in one arm and a basket of zucchinis in the other. I can't imagine what others thought I was doing!"

Later, she expanded her work to populations at greater risk for HIV, including incarcerated adolescents, intravenous drug users, HIV+ individuals, and truck drivers in India. She also developed an interest in promoting physical activity.

In all her work, Angela uses the biopsychosocial model, which you will learn about in this chapter. Specifically, she identifies the biological, psychological, and social factors that influence health behaviors such as condom use. Angela's interventions address each of these factors.

Angela's work is both challenging and rewarding. She works on a daily basis with community agencies, clinical psychologists, neuroscientists, and exercise physiologists. She uses solid research methods to evaluate the success of her interventions. More recently, she has started to examine the genetic factors that determine whether a person will respond to a physical activity intervention.

Although she views many aspects of her work as rewarding, one aspect is especially worthwhile: "When the interventions work!" she says. "If we can get one kid to use a condom or one person with a chronic illness to exercise, that is meaningful."

In this book, you will learn about the theories, methods, and discoveries of health psychologists such as Angela Bryan. As you read, keep in mind this piece of advice from Angela: "Think broadly and optimistically about health. A health psychologist's work is difficult, but it can make a difference."

The Changing Field of Health

"We are now living well enough and long enough to slowly fall apart" (Sapolsky, 1998, p. 2).

The field of health psychology developed relatively recently—the 1970s, to be exact—to address the challenges presented by the changing field of health and health care. A century ago, the average life expectancy in the United States was approximately 50 years of age, far shorter than it is now. When people in the United States died, they died largely from infectious diseases such as pneumonia, tuberculosis, diarrhea, and enteritis (see Figure 1.1). These conditions resulted from contact with impure drinking water, contaminated foods, or sick people. People might seek medical care only after they became ill, but medicine had few cures to offer. The duration of most diseases—such as typhoid fever, pneumonia, and diphtheria—was short; a person either died or got well in a matter of weeks. People felt very limited responsibility for contracting a contagious disease because such disease was not controllable.

Life—and death—are now dramatically different than they were a century ago. Life expectancy in the United States is nearly 80 years of age, with more Americans now than ever living past their 100th birthday. Over 30 countries boast even longer life expectancy than the United States, with Japan boasting the longest life expectancy at 84 years of age. Public sanitation for most citizens of industrialized nations is vastly better than it was a century ago. Vaccines and treatments exist for many infectious diseases. However, improvements in the prevention and treatment of infectious diseases allowed for a different class of disease to emerge as today's killers: chronic diseases. Heart disease, cancer, and stroke—all chronic diseases—are now the leading causes of mortality in the United States and account for a greater proportion of deaths than infectious diseases ever did. Chronic diseases develop and then persist or recur, affecting people over long periods of time. Every year, over 2 million people in the United States die from chronic diseases, but over 130 million people—almost one out of every two adults—live with at least one chronic disease.

Furthermore, most deaths today are attributable to diseases associated with lifestyle and behavior. Heart disease, cancer, stroke, chronic lower respiratory diseases (including emphysema and chronic bronchitis), unintentional injuries, and diabetes are all due in part to cigarette smoking, alcohol abuse, unhealthy eating, stress, and a sedentary lifestyle. Because the major killers today arise in part due to lifestyle and behavior, people have a great deal more control over their health than they did in the past. However, many people do not exercise this control, so unhealthy behavior is an important public health problem. Indeed, unhealthy behavior contributes to the escalating costs of health care.

In this chapter, we describe the changing patterns of disease and disability and the increasing costs of health care. We also discuss how these trends change the very definition of what health is and require a broader view of health than in the past. This broad view of health is the biopsychosocial model, a view adopted by health psychologists such as Angela Bryan.

Patterns of Disease and Death

The 20th century brought about major changes in the patterns of disease and death in the United States, including a shift in the leading causes of death. Infectious diseases were leading causes of death in 1900, but over the next several decades, chronic diseases such as heart disease, cancer, and stroke became the leading killers.

During the first few years of the 21st century, deaths from some chronic diseases—those related to unhealthy lifestyles and behaviors—began to *decrease*. These diseases include heart disease, cancer, and stroke, which all were responsible for a smaller proportion of deaths in 2010 than in 1990. Why have deaths from these diseases decreased in the last few decades? We will discuss this in greater detail in Chapter 9, but one major reason is that fewer people in the United States now smoke cigarettes than in the past. This change in behavior contributed to some of the decline in deaths due to heart disease; improvements in health care also contributed to this decline.

Death rates due to unintentional injuries, suicide, and homicide have increased in recent years (Kung, Hoyert, Xu, & Murphy, 2008). Significant increases also occurred in Alzheimer's disease, kidney disease, septicemia (blood infection), liver disease, hypertension, and Parkinson's disease. For many of these causes of death that have recently increased, behavior is a less important component than for those causes that have decreased. However, the rising death rates due to Alzheimer's and Parkinson's disease reflect another important trend in health and health care: an increasingly older population.

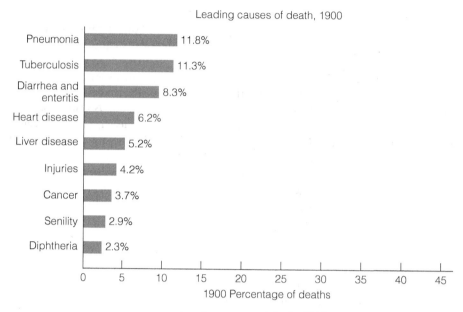

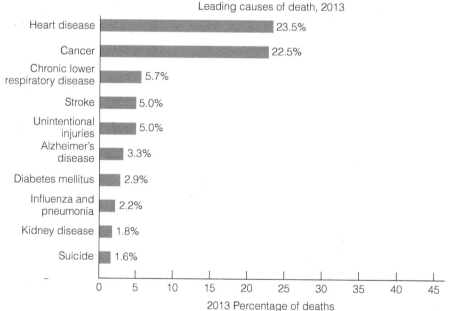

FIGURE 1.1 Leading causes of death, United States, 1900 and 2013.

Source: Healthy people, 2010, 2000, by U.S. Department of Health and Human Services, Washington, DC: U.S. Government Printing Office; "Deaths: Final Data for 2013," 2016, by Xu, J., Murphy, S. L., Kochanek, K. D., & Bastian, B. A., *National Vital Statistics Reports, 64*(2), Table B.

Age Obviously, older people are more likely to die than younger ones, but the causes of death vary among age groups. Thus, the ranking of causes of death for the entire population may not reflect any specific age group and may lead people to misperceive the risk for some ages. For example, cardiovascular disease (which includes heart disease and stroke) and cancer account for over 50% of all deaths in the United States, but they are not the leading cause of death for young people. For individuals between 1 and 44 years of age, unintentional injuries are the leading cause of death, and violent deaths from suicide and homicide rank high on the list as well (National Center for Health Statistics [NCHS], 2016a). Unintentional injuries account for 30% of the deaths in this age group, suicide for almost 12%, and homicide for about 8%. As Figure 1.2 reveals, other causes of death account for much smaller percentages of deaths among adolescents and young adults than unintentional injuries, homicide, and suicide.

For adults 45 to 64 years old, the picture is quite different. Cardiovascular disease and cancer become the leading causes of death. As people age, they become more likely to die, so the causes of death for older people dominate the overall figures for causes of death. However, younger people show very different patterns of mortality.

Ethnicity, Income, and Disease   Question 2 from the quiz inside the front cover asks if the United States is among the top 10 nations in the world in terms of life expectancy. It is not even close; it ranks 34th among all nations (World Health Organization [WHO], 2015c). Within the United States, ethnicity is also a factor in life expectancy, and the leading causes of death also vary among ethnic groups. Table 1.1 shows the ranking of the 10 leading causes of death for four ethnic groups in the United States. No two groups have identical profiles of causes of death, and some causes do not appear on the list for each group, highlighting the influence of ethnicity on mortality.

If African Americans and European Americans in the United States were considered to be different nations, European America would rank higher in life expectancy than African America—34th place and 68th place, respectively (NCHS, 2016; WHO, 2015c). Thus, European Americans have a longer life expectancy than African Americans, but neither should expect to live as long as people in Japan, Canada, Iceland, Australia, the United Kingdom, Italy, France, Hong Kong, Israel, and many other countries.

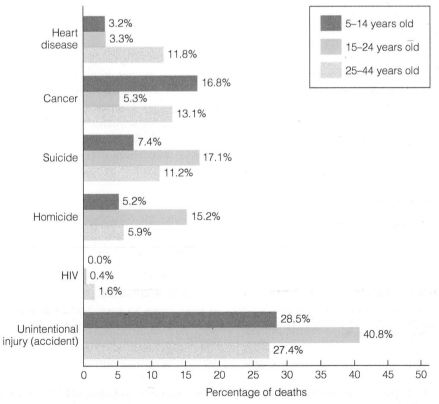

FIGURE 1.2   Leading causes of death among individuals aged 5–14, 15–24, and 25–44, United States, 2013.

Source: "Deaths: Final Data for 2013," 2016, by Xu, J., Murphy, S. L., Kochanek, K. D., & Bastian, B. A., *National Vital Statistics Reports, 64*(2), Table B.

TABLE 1.1   Ten Leading Causes of Death for Four Ethnic Groups in the United States, 2013

	European Americans	Hispanic Americans	African Americans	Asian Americans
Heart disease	1	2	1	2
Cancer	2	1	2	1
Chronic lower respiratory disease	3	7	6	7
Unintentional injuries	4	3	4	4
Stroke	5	4	3	3
Alzheimer's disease	6	8	10	8
Diabetes	7	5	5	5
Pneumonia and influenza	8	9	*	6
Kidney disease	9	10	7	9
Suicide	10	*	*	10
Chronic liver disease	*	6	*	*
Septicemia	*	*	9	*
Homicide	*	*	8	*

*Not among the 10 leading causes of death for this ethnic group.

Source: "Deaths: Leading causes for 2013," 2016, by M. Heron, *National Vital Statistics Reports, 65*(2), Tables D and E.

Hispanics have socioeconomic disadvantages similar to those of African Americans (U.S. Census Bureau [USCB], 2011), including poverty and low educational level. About 10% of European Americans live below the poverty level, whereas 32% of African Americans and 26% of Hispanic Americans do (USCB, 2011). European Americans also have educational advantages: 86% receive high school diplomas, compared with only 81% of African Americans and 59% of Hispanic Americans. These socioeconomic disadvantages translate into health disadvantages (Crimmins, Ki Kim, Alley, Karlamangla, & Seeman, 2007; Smith & Bradshaw, 2006). That is, poverty and low educational level both relate to health problems and lower life expectancy. Thus, some of the ethnic differences in health are due to socioeconomic differences.

Access to health insurance and medical care are not the only factors that make poverty a health risk. Indeed, the health risks associated with poverty begin before birth. Even with the expansion of prenatal care by Medicaid, poor mothers, especially teen mothers, are more likely to deliver low-birth-weight babies, who are more likely than normal-birth-weight infants to die (NCHS, 2016). Also, pregnant women living below the poverty line are more likely than other pregnant women to be physically abused and to deliver babies who suffer the consequences of prenatal child abuse (Zelenko, Lock, Kraemer, & Steiner, 2000).

The association between income level and health is so strong that it appears not only at the poverty level but also at higher income levels. That is, very wealthy people have better health than people who are just, well, wealthy. Why should very wealthy people be healthier than other wealthy people? One possibility comes from the relation of income to educational level, which, in turn, relates to occupation, social class, and ethnicity. The higher the educational level, the less likely people are to engage in unhealthy behaviors such as smoking, eating a high-fat diet, and maintaining a sedentary lifestyle (see Would You Believe ...? box). Another possibility is the perception of social status. People's perception of their social standing may differ from their status as indexed by educational, occupational, and income level, and remarkably, this perception relates to health status more strongly than objective measures (Operario, Adler, & Williams, 2004). Thus, the relationships between health and ethnicity are intertwined with the relationships between health, income, education, and social class.

Changes in Life Expectancy   During the 20th century, life expectancy rose dramatically in the United States

Would You BELIEVE...? College Is Good for Your Health

Would you believe that attending college could be good for your health? You may find that difficult to believe, as college seems to add stress, exposure to alcohol or drugs, and demands that make it difficult to maintain a healthy diet, exercise, and sleep. How could going to college possibly be healthy?

The health benefits of college appear after graduation. People who have been to college have lower death rates than those who have not. This advantage applies to both women and men and to infectious diseases, chronic diseases, and unintentional injuries (NCHS, 2015). Better educated people report fewer daily symptoms and less stress than less educated people (Grzywacz, Almeida, Neupert, & Ettner, 2004).

Even a high school education provides health benefits, but going to college offers much more protection. For example, people with less than a high school education die at a rate of 575 per 100,000; those with a high school degree die at a rate of 509

per 100,000; but people who attend college have a death rate of only 214 per 100,000 (Miniño, Murphy, Xu, & Kochanek, 2011). The benefits of education for health and longevity apply to people around the world. For example, a study of older people in Japan (Fujino et al., 2005) found that low educational level increased the risk of dying. A large-scale study of the Dutch population (Hoeymans, van Lindert, & Westert, 2005) also found that education was related to a wide range of health measures and health-related behaviors.

What factors contribute to this health advantage for people with more education? Part of that advantage may be intelligence, which predicts both health and longevity (Gottfredson & Deary, 2004). In addition, people who are well educated tend to live with and around people with similar education, providing an environment with good health-related knowledge and attitudes (Øystein, 2008). Income and occupation may also contribute (Batty et al., 2008); people who attend

college, especially those who graduate, have better jobs and higher average incomes than those who do not, and thus are more likely to have better access to health care. In addition, educated people are more likely to be informed consumers of health care, gathering information on their diseases and potential treatments. Education is also associated with a variety of habits that contribute to good health and long life. For example, people with a college education are less likely than others to smoke or use illicit drugs (Johnston, O'Malley, Bachman, & Schulenberg, 2007), and they are more likely to eat a low-fat diet and to exercise.

Thus, people who attend college acquire many resources that are reflected in their lower death rate—income potential, health knowledge, more health-conscious spouses and friends, attitudes about the importance of health, and positive health habits. This strong link between education and health is one clear example of how good health is more than simply a matter of biology.

and other industrialized nations. In 1900, life expectancy was 47.3 years, whereas today it is almost 79 years (NCHS, 2016). In other words, infants born today can expect, on average, to live more than a generation longer than their great-great-grandparents born at the beginning of the 20th century.

What accounts for the 30-year increase in life expectancy during the 20th century? Question 3 from the quiz inside the front cover asks if advances in medical care were responsible for this increase. The answer is "False"; other factors have been more important than medical care of sick people. The single most important contributor to the increase in life expectancy is the lowering of infant mortality. When infants die before their first birthday, these deaths lower the population's

average life expectancy much more than do the deaths of middle-aged or older people. As Figure 1.3 shows, infant death rates declined dramatically between 1900 and 1990, but little decrease has occurred since that time.

Prevention of disease also contributes to the recent increase in life expectancy. Widespread vaccination and safer drinking water and milk supplies all reduce infectious disease, which increases life expectancy. A healthier lifestyle also contributes to increased life expectancy, as does more efficient disposal of sewage and better nutrition. In contrast, advances in medical care—such as antibiotics and new surgical technology, efficient paramedic teams, and more skilled intensive care personnel—play a surprisingly minor role in increasing adults' life expectancy.

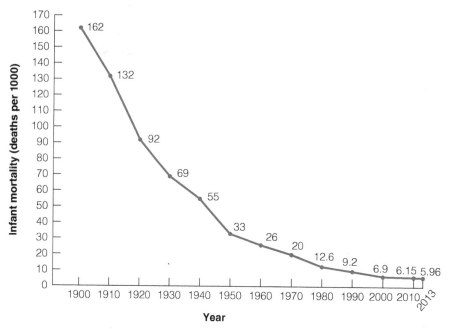

FIGURE 1.3   Decline in infant mortality in the United States, 1900–2013.

Source: Data from *Historical statistics of the United States: Colonial times to 1970,* 1975 by U.S. Bureau of the Census, Washington, DC: U.S. Government Printing Office, p. 60; "Deaths: Final Data for 2013," 2016, by Xu, J., Murphy, S. L., Kochanek, K. D., & Bastian, B. A., *National Vital Statistics Reports, 64*(2), Table B; "Recent Declines in Infant Mortality in the United States, 2005–2011." National Center for Health Statistics, Number 120, 2013.

Escalating Cost of Medical Care

The second major change within the field of health is the escalating cost of medical care. In the United States, medical costs have increased at a much faster rate than inflation, and currently the United States spends the most of all countries on health care. Between 1960 and 2008, medical costs in the United States represented a larger and larger proportion of the gross domestic product (GDP). Since 1995, the increases have slowed, but medical care costs as a percentage of the GDP are over 16% (Organisation for Economic Co-operation and Development [OECD], 2015). Considered on a per person basis, the total yearly cost of health care in the United States increased from $1,067 per person in 1970 to $7,826 in 2013 (NCHS, 2015), a jump of more than 700%!

These costs, of course, have some relationship to increased life expectancy: As people live to middle and old age, they tend to develop chronic diseases that require extended (and often expensive) medical treatment. Nearly half of people in the United States have a chronic condition (Ward, Schiller, & Goodman, 2012),

and they account for 86% of the dollars spent on health care (Gerteis et al., 2014). People with chronic conditions account for 88% of prescriptions written, 72% of physician visits, and 76% of hospital stays. Even though today's aging population is experiencing better health than past generations, their increasing numbers will continue to increase medical costs.

One strategy for curbing mounting medical costs is to limit services, but another approach requires a greater emphasis on the early detection of disease and on changes to a healthier lifestyle and to behaviors that help prevent disease. For example, early detection of high blood pressure, high serum cholesterol, and other precursors of heart disease allow these conditions to be controlled, thereby decreasing the risk of serious disease or death. Screening people for risk is preferable to remedial treatment because chronic diseases are quite difficult to cure and living with chronic disease decreases quality of life. Avoiding disease by adopting a healthy lifestyle is even more preferable to treating diseases or screening for risks. Staying healthy is typically

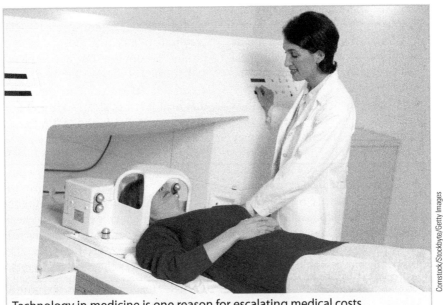

Technology in medicine is one reason for escalating medical costs.

less costly than becoming sick and then getting well. Thus, prevention of disease through a healthy lifestyle, early detection of symptoms, and reduction of health risks are all part of a changing philosophy within the health care field. As you will learn in this book, health psychologists contribute to each of these aims.

What Is Health?

"Once again, the patient as a human being with worries, fears, hopes, and despairs, as an indivisible whole and not merely the bearer of organs—of a diseased liver or stomach—is becoming the legitimate object of medical interest," says Franz Alexander (1950, p. 17), one of the founders of the field of psychosomatic medicine.

What does it mean to be "healthy"? Question 1 from the quiz at the beginning of the book asks if health is merely the absence of disease. But is health more complex? Is health the presence of some positive condition rather than merely the absence of a negative one? Is health simply a state of the physical body, or should health also consider one's beliefs, environment, and behaviors as well?

The **biomedical model** has been the traditional view of Western medicine, which defines health as the absence of disease (Papas, Belar, & Rozensky, 2004). This view conceptualizes disease solely as a biological process that is a result of exposure to a specific **pathogen**,

a disease-causing organism. This view spurred the development of drugs and medical technology oriented toward removing the pathogens and curing disease. The focus is on disease, which is traceable to a specific agent. Removing the pathogen restores health.

The biomedical model of disease is compatible with infectious diseases that were the leading causes of death 100 years ago. Throughout the 20th century, adherence to the biomedical model allowed medicine to conquer or control many of the diseases that once ravaged humanity. However, when chronic illnesses began to replace infectious diseases as leading causes of death, the biomedical model became insufficient (Stone, 1987).

An alternative model of health exists now, one that advocates a more comprehensive approach to medicine. This alternative model is the **biopsychosocial model**, the approach to health that includes biological, psychological, and social influences. This model holds that many diseases result from a combination of factors such as genetics, physiology, social support, personal control, stress, compliance, personality, poverty, ethnic background, and cultural beliefs. We discuss each of these factors in subsequent chapters. For now, it is important to recognize that the biopsychosocial model has at least two advantages over the older biomedical model: First, it incorporates not only biological conditions but also psychological and social factors, and second, it views health as a positive condition. The biopsychosocial model can also account for some surprising findings about who gets sick and who stays healthy (see Would You Believe ...? box). Thus, the biopsychosocial model has not only all of the power of the older biomedical model but also the ability to address problems that the biomedical model has failed to solve.

According to the biopsychosocial view, health is much more than the absence of disease. A person who has no disease condition is not sick, but this person may not be healthy either. A person may have unhealthy lifestyle habits or poor social support, cope poorly with high amounts of stress, or avoid medical care when it is warranted; all of these factors increase risk for future disease. Because health is multidimensional, all aspects of living—biological, psychological, and social—must be considered. This view diverges from the traditional Western conceptualization, but as Table 1.2 shows, other cultures have held different views.

Consistent with this broader view of health, the World Health Organization (WHO) wrote into the preamble of its constitution a modern, Western definition: "Health is a state of complete physical, mental, and social well-being, and not merely the absence of disease or infirmity." This definition clearly affirms that health is a positive state and not just the absence of pathogens. Feeling good is different than not feeling bad, and research in neuroscience has confirmed the difference (Zautra, 2003). The human brain responds in distinctly different patterns to positive feelings and negative feelings. Furthermore, this broader definition of health can account for the importance of preventive behavior in physical health. For example, a healthy person is not merely somebody without current disease or disability but also somebody who behaves in a way that is likely to maintain that state in the future.

Would You BELIEVE...? It Takes More Than a Virus to Give You a Cold

One of the dirtiest jobs an aspiring health psychologist could have is as a research assistant in Sheldon Cohen's laboratory at Carnegie Mellon University. Cohen's assistants sift through study participants' trash in search of used, mucous-filled tissues. When such tissues are found, the assistants unfold them, locate the gooey treasures within, and painstakingly weigh their discoveries. These assistants have good reason to rummage for snot: They want an objective measure of how severely their participants caught the common cold.

Sheldon Cohen and his research team investigate the psychological and social factors that predict the likelihood that a person will succumb to infection. Healthy participants in Cohen's studies receive a virus through a nasal squirt and are then quarantined in a "cold research laboratory"—actually, a hotel room—for 1 week. Participants also answer a number of questionnaires about psychological and social factors such as recent stress, typical positive and negative emotions, and the size and quality of their social networks. Cohen and his team use these questionnaires to predict who gets the cold and who remains healthy.

Cohen's findings expose the inadequacy of the biomedical approach to understanding infection. Despite the fact that everybody in his studies gets exposed to the same pathogen in exactly the same manner, only some participants get sick. Importantly, the people who resist infection share similar psychological and social characteristics. Compared with people who get sick, those who remain healthy are less likely to have dealt with recent stressful experiences (Cohen, Tyrrell, & Smith, 1991), have better sleep habits (Cohen, Doyle, Alper, Janicki-Deverts, & Turner, 2009), typically experience more positive emotion (Cohen, Alper, Doyle, Treanor, & Turner, 2006), are more sociable (Cohen, Doyle, Turner, Alper, & Skoner, 2003), and have more diverse social networks (Cohen, Doyle, Skoner, Rabin, & Gwaltney, 1997).

Thus, it takes more than just exposure to a virus to succumb to a cold or flu bug; exposure to the pathogen interacts with psychological and social factors to produce illness. Only the biopsychosocial model can account for these influences.

TABLE 1.2   Definitions of Health Held by Various Cultures

Culture	Time Period	Health Is
Prehistoric	10,000 BCE	Endangered by spirits that enter the body from outside
Babylonians and Assyrians	1800–700 BCE	Endangered by the gods, who send disease as a punishment
Ancient Hebrews	1000–300 BCE	A gift from God; disease is a punishment from God
Ancient Greeks	500 BCE	A holistic unity of body and spirit
Ancient China	Between 800 and 200 BCE	A state of physical and spiritual harmony with nature
Native Americans	1000 BCE–present	Total harmony with nature and the ability to survive under difficult conditions
Galen in Ancient Rome	130–200 CE	The absence of pathogens, such as bad air or body fluids, that cause disease
Early Christians	300–600 CE	Not as important as disease, which is a sign that one is chosen by God
Descartes in France	1596–1650	A condition of the mechanical body, which is separate from the mind
Western Africans	1600–1800	Harmony achieved through interactions with other people and objects in the world
Virchow in Germany	Late 1800s	Endangered by microscopic organisms that invade cells, producing disease
Freud in Austria	Late 1800s	Influenced by emotions and the mind
World Health Organization	1946	"A state of complete physical, mental, and social well-being"

IN SUMMARY

In the past century, four major trends changed the field of health care. One trend is the changing pattern of disease and death in industrialized nations, including the United States. Chronic diseases now replace infectious diseases as the leading causes of death and disability. These chronic diseases include heart disease, stroke, cancer, emphysema, and adult-onset diabetes, all of which have causes that include individual behavior.

The increase in chronic disease contributed to a second trend: the escalating cost of medical care. Costs for medical care steadily increased from 1970 to 2013. Much of this cost increase is due to a growing elderly population, innovative but expensive medical technology, and inflation.

A third trend is the changing definition of health. Many people continue to view health as the absence of disease, but a growing number of health care professionals view health as a state of positive well-being. To accept this definition of health, one must reconsider the biomedical model that has dominated the health care field.

The fourth trend, the emergence of the biopsychosocial model of health, relates to the changing definition of health. Rather than define disease as simply the presence of pathogens, the biopsychosocial model emphasizes positive health and sees disease, particularly chronic disease, as resulting from the interaction of biological, psychological, and social conditions.

Psychology's Relevance for Health

Although chronic diseases have biological causes, individual behavior and lifestyle contribute to their development. Because behavior is so important for chronic disease, psychology—the science of behavior—is now more relevant to health care than ever before.

It took many years, however, for psychology to gain acceptance by the medical field. In 1911, the American Psychological Association (APA) recommended that psychology be part of the medical school curriculum, but most medical schools did not follow this recommendation. During the 1940s, the medical specialty of psychiatry incorporated the study of psychological factors related to disease into its training, but few psychologists were involved in health research (Matarazzo, 1994). During the 1960s, psychology's role in medicine began to expand with the creation of new medical schools; the number of psychologists who held academic appointments on medical school faculties nearly tripled from 1969 to 1993 (Matarazzo, 1994).

In the past several decades, psychologists have gained greater acceptance by the medical profession (Pingitore, Scheffler, Haley, Seniell, & Schwalm, 2001). In 2002, the American Medical Association (AMA) accepted several new categories for health and behavior that permit psychologists to bill for services to patients with physical diseases. Also, Medicare's Graduate Medical Education program now accepts psychology internships, and the APA worked with the WHO to formulate a diagnostic system for biopsychosocial disorders, the International Classification of Functioning, Disability, and Health (Reed & Scheldeman, 2004). Thus, the role of psychologists in medical settings has expanded beyond traditional mental health problems to include programs to help people stop smoking, eat a healthy diet, exercise, adhere to medical advice, reduce stress, control pain, live with chronic disease, and avoid unintentional injuries.

The Contribution of Psychosomatic Medicine

The biopsychosocial model recognizes that psychological and emotional factors contribute to physical health problems. This notion is not new, as Socrates and Hippocrates proposed similar ideas. Furthermore, Sigmund Freud also proposed that unconscious psychological factors could

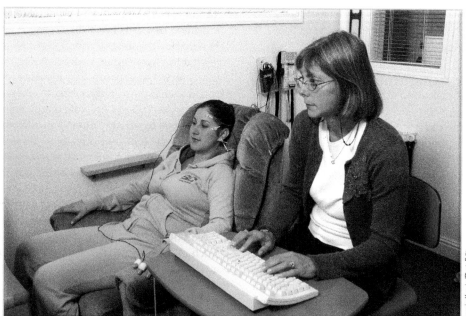

The role of the psychologist in health care settings has expanded beyond traditional mental health problems to include procedures such as biofeedback.

contribute to physical symptoms, but Freud's approach was not based on systematic scientific research.

In 1932, Walter Cannon observed that emotions are accompanied by physiological changes, a discovery that opened up a search to tie emotional causes to illness (Kimball, 1981). Cannon's research demonstrated that emotions can cause physiological changes that are capable of causing disease. From this finding, Helen Flanders Dunbar (1943) developed the notion that habitual responses, which people exhibit as part of their personalities, could relate to specific diseases. In other words, Dunbar hypothesized a relationship between personality type and disease. A little later, Franz Alexander (1950), a onetime follower of Freud, began to see emotional conflicts as a precursor to certain diseases.

These views led others to see a range of specific illnesses as "psychosomatic." These illnesses included disorders such as peptic ulcer, rheumatoid arthritis, hypertension, asthma, hyperthyroidism, and ulcerative colitis. However, the widespread belief at the time in the separation of mind and body—a belief that originated with Descartes (Papas et al., 2004)—led many laypeople to regard these psychosomatic disorders as not being "real" but rather "all in the head." Thus, psychosomatic medicine exerted a mixed impact on the acceptance of psychology within medicine; it benefited by connecting emotional and physical conditions, but it may have harmed by belittling the psychological components of illness. Psychosomatic medicine, however, laid the foundation for the transition to the biopsychosocial model of health and disease (Novack et al., 2007).

The Emergence of Behavioral Medicine

From the psychosomatic medicine movement, two interrelated disciplines emerged: *behavioral medicine* and *health psychology*.

Behavioral medicine is "the interdisciplinary field concerned with the development and integration of behavioral and biomedical science knowledge and techniques relevant to health and illness and the application of this knowledge and these techniques to prevention, diagnosis, treatment and rehabilitation" (Schwartz & Weiss, 1978, p. 250). A key component of this definition is the integration of biomedical science with behavioral sciences, especially psychology. The goals of behavioral medicine are similar to those in other areas of health care: improved prevention, diagnosis, treatment, and rehabilitation. Behavioral medicine, however, attempts to use psychology and the behavioral sciences in conjunction with medicine to achieve these goals. Chapters 3 through 11 cover topics in behavioral medicine.

The Emergence of Health Psychology

At about the same time that behavioral medicine appeared, a task force of the American Psychological Association revealed that few psychologists conducted health research (APA Task Force, 1976). The report envisioned a future in which psychologists would contribute to the enhancement of health and prevention of disease.

In 1978, with the establishment of Division 38 of the American Psychological Association, the field of **health psychology** officially began. Health psychology is the branch of psychology that considers how individual behaviors and lifestyles affect a person's physical health. Health psychology includes psychology's contributions to the enhancement of health, the prevention and treatment of disease, the identification of health risk factors, the improvement of the health care system, and the shaping of public opinion with regard to health. More specifically, it involves the application of psychological principles to physical health areas such as controlling cholesterol, managing stress, alleviating pain, stopping smoking, and moderating other risky behaviors, as well as encouraging regular exercise, medical and dental checkups, and safer behaviors. In addition, health psychology helps identify conditions that affect health, diagnose and treat certain chronic diseases, and modify the behavioral factors involved in physiological and psychological rehabilitation. As such, health psychology interacts with both biology and sociology to produce health- and disease-related outcomes (see Figure 1.4). Note that neither psychology nor sociology contributes directly to outcomes; only biological factors contribute directly to physical health and disease. Thus, the psychological and sociological factors that affect health must "get under the skin" in some way in order to affect biological processes. One of the goals of health psychology is to identify those pathways.

With its promotion of the biopsychosocial model, the field of health psychology continues to grow. One branch of this field, that is, clinical health psychology, continues to gain recognition in providing health care as part of multidisciplinary teams. Health psychology researchers continue to build a knowledge base that will furnish information about the interconnections among psychological, social, and biological factors that relate to health.

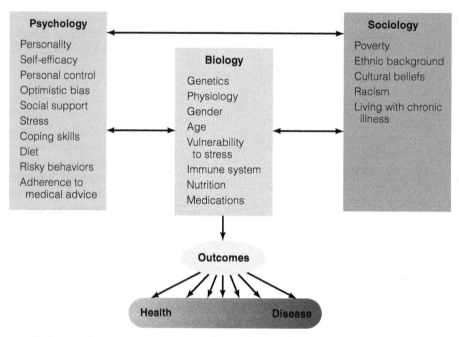

FIGURE 1.4 The biopsychosocial model: Biological, psychological, and sociological factors interact to produce health or disease.

IN SUMMARY

Psychology's involvement in health dates back to the beginning of the 20th century, but at that time, few psychologists were involved in medicine. The psychosomatic medicine movement brought psychological factors into the understanding of disease, and that view gave way to the biopsychosocial approach to health and disease. By the 1970s, psychologists had begun to develop research and treatment aimed at chronic disease and health promotion; this research and treatment led to the founding of two fields, behavioral medicine and health psychology.

Behavioral medicine applies the knowledge and techniques of behavioral research to physical health, including prevention, diagnosis, treatment, and rehabilitation. Health psychology overlaps with behavioral medicine, and the two professions have many common goals. However, behavioral medicine is an interdisciplinary field, whereas health psychology is a specialty within the discipline of psychology. Health psychology strives to enhance health, prevent and treat disease, identify risk factors, improve the health care system, and shape public opinion regarding health issues.

The Profession of Health Psychology

Health psychology now stands as a unique field and profession. Health psychologists have their own associations, publish their research in journals devoted to health psychology (*Health Psychology* and *Annals of Behavioral Medicine,* among others), and acquire training in unique doctoral and postdoctoral programs. In addition, health psychology is recognized within medical schools, schools of public health, universities, and hospitals, and health psychologists work within all of these settings. However, their training occurs within psychology.

The Training of Health Psychologists

Health psychologists are psychologists first and specialists in health second, but the training in health is extensive. People who pursue research in health psychology must learn the topics, theories, and methods of health psychology research. Health psychologists who provide clinical care, known as clinical health psychologists, must learn clinical skills and how to practice as part of a health care team. Some health psychologists also seek out training in medical subspecialties such as neurology, endocrinology, immunology, and epidemiology. This training may occur in a doctoral program (Baum, Perry, & Tarbell, 2004), but many health psychologists also obtain postdoctoral training, with at least 2 years of specialized training in health psychology to follow a PhD or PsyD in psychology (Belar, 1997; Matarazzo, 1987). Practicums and internships in health care settings in hospitals and clinics are common components of training in clinical health psychology (Nicassio, Meyerowitz, & Kerns, 2004).

The Work of Health Psychologists

Health psychologists work in a variety of settings, and their work setting varies according to their specialty. Some health psychologists such as Angela Bryan are primarily researchers, who work in universities or government agencies that conduct research, such as the CDC and the National Institutes of Health. Health psychology research encompasses many topics; it may focus on behaviors related to the development of disease or on evaluation of the effectiveness of new interventions and treatments. Clinical health psychologists are often employed in hospitals, pain clinics, or community clinics. Other settings for clinical health psychologists include health maintenance organizations (HMOs) and private practice.

As Angela Bryan's work shows, health psychologists engage in a variety of activities. Much of their work is collaborative in nature; health psychologists engaged in either research or practice may work with a team of health professionals, including physicians, nurses, physical therapists, and counselors.

The services provided by health psychologists working in clinics and hospitals fit into several categories. One type of service offers alternatives to pharmacological treatment; for example, biofeedback might be an alternative to painkillers for headache patients. Another type of service is providing behavioral interventions to treat physical disorders, such as chronic pain and some gastrointestinal problems, or to improve the rate of patient compliance with medical regimens. Other clinical health psychologists may provide assessments using psychological and neuropsychological tests or provide psychological treatment for patients coping with disease. Those who concentrate on prevention and behavior changes are more likely to be employed in HMOs, school-based prevention programs, or worksite wellness programs.

Like Angela Bryan, many health psychologists engage in both teaching and research. Those who work exclusively in service delivery settings are much less likely to teach and do research and are more likely to spend time providing diagnoses and interventions for people with health problems. Some health psychology students go into allied health profession fields, such as social work, occupational therapy, dietetics, or public health. Those who go into public health often work in academic settings or government agencies and may monitor trends in health issues, or develop and evaluate educational interventions and health awareness campaigns. Health psychologists also contribute to the development and evaluation of wide-scale public health decisions, including taxes and warning labels placed upon healthy products such as cigarettes, and the inclusion of nutrition information on food products and menus. Thus, the health psychologists contribute to the promotion of health in a wide variety of manners.

IN SUMMARY

To maximize their contributions to health care, health psychologists must be both broadly trained in the science of psychology and specifically trained in the knowledge and skills of areas such as neurology, endocrinology, immunology, epidemiology, and other medical subspecialties. Health psychologists work in a variety of settings, including universities, hospitals, clinics, private practice, and HMOs. They typically collaborate with other health care professionals in providing services for physical disorders rather than for traditional areas of mental health care. Research in health psychology is also likely to be a collaborative effort that may include the professions of medicine, epidemiology, nursing, pharmacology, nutrition, and exercise physiology.

Answers

This chapter has addressed three basic questions:

1. **How have views of health changed?**

Views of health are changing, both among health care professionals and among the general public. Several trends have prompted these changes, including (1) the changing pattern of disease and death in the United States from infectious diseases to chronic diseases, (2) the increase in medical costs, (3) the growing acceptance of a view of health that includes not only the absence of disease but also the presence of positive well-being, and (4) the biopsychosocial model of health that departs from the traditional biomedical model and the psychosomatic model by including not only biochemical abnormalities but also psychological and social conditions.

2. **How did psychology become involved in health care?**

Psychology has been involved in health almost from the beginning of the 20th century. During those early years, however, only a few psychologists worked in medical settings, and most were not considered full partners with physicians. Psychosomatic medicine highlighted psychological explanations of certain somatic diseases, emphasizing the role of emotions in the development of disease. By the early 1970s, psychology and other behavioral sciences began to play a role in the prevention and treatment of chronic diseases and in the promotion of positive health, giving rise to two new fields: behavioral medicine and health psychology.

Behavioral medicine is an interdisciplinary field concerned with applying the knowledge and techniques of behavioral science to the maintenance of physical health and to prevention, diagnosis, treatment, and rehabilitation. Behavioral medicine, which is not a branch of psychology, overlaps with health psychology, a division within the field of psychology. Health psychology uses the science of psychology to enhance health, prevent and treat disease, identify risk factors, improve the health care system, and shape public opinion with regard to health.

3. **What type of training do health psychologists receive, and what kinds of work do they do?**

Health psychologists receive doctoral-level training psychology and often receive at least 2 years of postdoctoral work in a specialized area of health psychology.

Health psychologists are employed in a variety of settings, including universities, hospitals, clinics, private practice, and health maintenance organizations. Clinical health psychologists provide services, often as part of a health care team. Health psychologists who are researchers typically collaborate with others, sometimes as part of a multidisciplinary team, to conduct research on behaviors related to the development of disease or to evaluate the effectiveness of new treatments.

Suggested Readings

Baum, A., Perry, N. W., Jr., & Tarbell, S. (2004). The development of psychology as a health science. In R. G. Frank, A. Baum, & J. L. Wallander (Eds.), *Handbook of clinical health psychology* (Vol. 3, pp. 9–28). Washington, DC: American Psychological Association. This recent review of the development of health psychology describes the background and current status of the field of health psychology.

Belar, C. D. (2008). Clinical health psychology: A health care specialty in professional psychology. *Professional Psychology: Research and Practice, 39,* 229–233. Clinical health psychology is the applied branch of health psychology. Cynthia Belar traces the development of this field from the beginning, pointing out the widespread influence of health psychology on research and practice in clinical psychology.

Leventhal, H., Weinman, J., Leventhal, E. A., & Phillips, L. A. (2008). Health psychology: The search for pathways between behavior and health. *Annual Review of Psychology, 59,* 477–505. This article details how psychological theory and research can improve the effectiveness of interventions for managing chronic illness.

CHAPTER 2

Conducting Health Research

CHAPTER OUTLINE

- Real-World Profile of Sylvester Colligan
- *The Placebo in Treatment and Research*
- *Research Methods in Psychology*
- *Research Methods in Epidemiology*
- *Determining Causation*
- *Research Tools*

QUESTIONS

This chapter focuses on five basic questions:

1. What are placebos, and how do they affect research and treatment?

2. How does psychology research contribute to health knowledge?

3. How has epidemiology contributed to health knowledge?

4. How can scientists determine if a behavior causes a disease?

5. How do theory and measurement contribute to health psychology?

☑ Check Your BELIEFS   *About Health Research*

Check the items that are consistent with your beliefs.

☐ 1. Placebo effects can influence physical as well as psychological problems.

☐ 2. Pain patients who expect a medication to relieve their pain often experience a reduction in pain, even after taking a "sugar pill."

☐ 3. Personal testimonials are a good way to decide about treatment effectiveness.

☐ 4. Newspaper and television reports of scientific research give an accurate picture of the importance of the research.

☐ 5. Information from longitudinal studies is generally more informative than information from the study of one person.

☐ 6. All scientific methods yield equally valuable results, so the research method is not important in determining the validity of results.

☐ 7. In determining important health information, studies with non-human subjects can be just as important as those with human participants.

☐ 8. Results from experimental research are more likely than results from observational research to suggest the underlying cause for a disease.

☐ 9. People outside the scientific community conduct valuable research, but scientists try to discount the importance of such research.

☐ 10. Scientific breakthroughs happen every day.

☐ 11. New reports of health research often contradict previous findings, so there is no way to use this information to make good personal decisions about health.

Items 1, 2, 5, and 8 are consistent with sound scientific information, but each of the other items represents a naïve or unrealistic view of research that can make you an uninformed consumer of health research. Information in this chapter will help you become more sophisticated in your evaluation of and expectations for health research.

Real-World Profile of SYLVESTER COLLIGAN

Sylvester Colligan was a 76-year-old man who had been having trouble with his right knee for 5 years (Talbot, 2000). His doctor diagnosed arthritis but had no treatment that would help. However, this physician told Colligan about an experimental study conducted by Dr. J. Bruce Moseley. Colligan talked to Dr. Moseley and reported, "I was very impressed with him, especially when I heard he was the team doctor with the [Houston] Rockets. . . . So, sure, I went ahead and signed up for this new thing he was doing" (Talbot, 2000, p. 36).

The treatment worked. Two years after the surgery, Colligan reported that his knee had not bothered him since the surgery. "It's just like my other knee now. I give a whole lot of credit to Dr. Moseley. Whenever I see him on the TV during a basketball game, I call the wife in and say, "Hey, there's the doctor that fixed my knee!" (Talbot, 2000, p. 36).

Colligan's improvement would not be so surprising, except for one thing: Dr. Moseley did not perform surgery on Colligan. Instead, Dr. Moseley gave Colligan anesthesia, made some cuts around Colligan's knee that *looked* like surgical incisions, and then sent Colligan on his way home.

Why did Sylvester Colligan get better? Was Moseley negligent in performing a fake surgery on Colligan? Surprisingly, many people do not view Moseley's treatment as negligent. Moseley and his colleagues (2002) were conducting a study of the effectiveness of arthroscopic knee surgery. This type of procedure is widely performed but expensive, and Moseley had doubts about its effectiveness (Talbot, 2000). So Moseley decided to perform an experimental study that included a placebo as well as a real arthroscopic surgery. A placebo is an inactive substance or condition that has the appearance of an active treatment and that may cause participants to improve or change because of their belief in the placebo's efficacy.

Moseley suspected that this type of belief and not the surgery was producing improvements, so he designed a study in which half the participants received sham—that is, *fake*—knee surgery. Participants in this condition received anesthesia and surgical lesions to the knee, but no further treatment. The other half of the participants received standard arthroscopic knee surgery. The participants agreed to be in either group, knowing that they might receive sham surgery. The participants, including Colligan, did not know for several years whether they were in the placebo or the arthroscopic surgery group. Moseley discovered, contrary to widespread belief, that arthroscopic knee surgery provided no real benefits beyond a placebo effect. Those who received the sham surgery reported the same level of knee pain and functioning as those who received the real surgical treatment.

Moseley's results suggested that it was patients' beliefs about the surgery, rather than the surgery itself, that provided the benefits. The placebo effect is a fascinating demonstration of the effect of an individual's beliefs on their physical health. However, the placebo effect presents a problem for researchers like Moseley, who want to determine which effects are due to treatment and which are due to beliefs about the treatment.

This chapter looks at the way health psychologists conduct research, emphasizing psychology from the behavioral sciences and epidemiology from the biomedical sciences. These two disciplines share some methods for investigating health-related behaviors, but the two areas also have their own unique contributions to scientific methodology. Before we begin to examine the methods that psychologists and epidemiologists use in their research, let's consider the situation that Colligan experienced—improvement due to the placebo effect.

The Placebo in Treatment and Research

As we described in Chapter 1, health psychology involves the application of psychological principles to the understanding and improvement of physical health. The placebo effect represents one of the clearest examples of the link between people's beliefs and their physical health. Like many people receiving treatment, Colligan benefited from his positive expectations; he improved, even though he received a treatment that technically should not have led to improvement.

Most physicians are aware of the placebo effect, and many may even prescribe placebos when no other effective treatments are available (Tilburt, Emanuel, Kaptchuk, Curlin, & Miller, 2008). However, strong placebo effects can pose a problem for scientists trying to evaluate if a new treatment is effective. Thus, the placebo effect may help individuals who receive treatment but complicate the job of researchers; that is, it can have treatment benefits but research drawbacks.

Treatment and the Placebo

The power of placebo effects was nothing new to Moseley, as the potency of "sugar pills" had been recognized for years. Henry Beecher (1955) observed the effects of placebos on a variety of conditions ranging from headache to the common cold. Beecher concluded that the therapeutic effect of the placebo was substantial—about 35% of patients showed improvement! Hundreds of studies have since examined placebo effects. A recent review of this research confirms that placebos can lead to noticeable improvements in health outcomes, especially in the context of pain and nausea (Hróbjartsson & Gøtzsche, 2010). For example, a meta-analysis of migraine headache prevention (Macedo, Baños, & Farré, 2008) shows a placebo effect of 21%. A more recent review (Cepeda, Berlin, Gao, Wiegand, & Wada, 2012) reveals that anywhere from 7% to 43% of patients in pain improve following administration of a placebo, with the likelihood of improvement largely attributable to the type of pain experienced.

Placebo effects occur in many other health conditions. For example, some researchers (Fournier et al., 2010) argue that the placebo effect is responsible for much of the effectiveness of antidepressant drugs, especially among people with mild to moderate symptoms. Furthermore, the strength of the placebo effect associated with antipsychotic drugs has steadily increased over the past 50 years, suggesting that the effectiveness of these drugs may be in part due to increases in people's beliefs regarding their efficacy (Agid et al., 2013; Rutherford et al., 2014). However, some conditions such as broken bones are not responsive to placebos (Kaptchuk, Eisenberg, & Komaroff, 2002).

The more a placebo resembles an effective treatment, the stronger the placebo effect. Big pills are more

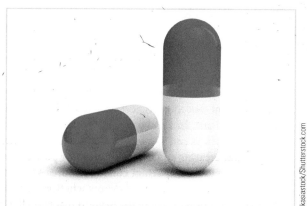

The more a placebo resembles an effective treatment, the stronger the placebo effect. These sugar pills, which look like real pills, are likely to have strong placebo effects.

effective than little ones, and colored pills work better than white tablets. Capsules work better than tablets, and placebos labeled with brand names work better than generics. Two doses provoke a larger placebo response than one dose. An injection is more powerful than a pill, and surgery tends to prompt an even larger placebo response than an injection does. Even cost matters; more expensive placebo pills work better than cheaper pills (Waber, Shiv, Carmon, & Ariely, 2008)!

Both physician and patient expectations also strengthen placebo effects. Physicians who appear positive and hopeful about treatment prompt a stronger response in their patients (Moerman, 2003). Placebo responses also relate to other characteristics of the practitioner, such as his or her reputation, attention, interest, concern, and the confidence he or she projects that a treatment will be effective (Moerman & Jonas, 2002).

Placebos can also produce adverse effects, called the **nocebo effect** (Scott et al., 2008; Turner et al., 1994). Nearly 20% of healthy volunteers given a placebo in a double-blind study experienced some negative effect as a result of the nocebo effect. Sometimes, these negative effects appear as side effects, which show the same symptoms as other drug side effects, such as headaches, nausea and other digestive problems, dry mouth, and sleep disturbances (Amanzio, Corazzini, Vase, & Benedetti, 2009). When participants are led to believe that a treatment might worsen symptoms, the nocebo effect can be as strong as the placebo effect (Petersen et al., 2014). The presence of negative effects demonstrates that the placebo effect is not merely improvement but includes any change resulting from an inert treatment.

How and why do the placebo and nocebo effects occur? Although many people assume that improvements due to placebos are psychological—"It's in people's heads"—research suggests that they have both a physical and psychological basis (Benedetti, 2006; Scott et al., 2008). For example, a placebo analgesic alters levels of brain activity in ways that are consistent with the activity that occurs during pain relief from analgesic drugs (Wager et al., 2004). The nocebo response also activates specific areas of the brain and acts on neurotransmitters, giving additional support to its physical reality (Scott et al., 2008).

Expectancy is a major component of the placebo effect (Finniss & Benedetti, 2005; Stewart-Williams, 2004). People act in ways that they *think* they should. Thus, people who receive treatment without their knowledge do not benefit as much as those who know what to expect (Colloca, Lopiano, Lanotte, & Benedetti, 2004). In addition, culture influences the placebo response. For example, cultures that place greater faith in medical interventions show stronger responses to placebos that resemble a medical intervention (Moerman, 2011). Learning and conditioning are also factors in the placebo response. Through classical and operant conditioning, people associate a treatment with getting better, creating situations in which receiving treatment leads to improvements. Thus, both expectancy and learning contribute to the placebo effect.

In most situations involving medical treatment, patients' improvements may result from a combination of treatment plus the placebo effect (Finniss & Benedetti, 2005). Placebo effects are a tribute to the ability of humans to heal themselves, and practitioners can enlist this ability to help patients become healthier (Ezekiel & Miller, 2001; Walach & Jonas, 2004). Therefore, the placebo effect can be a positive factor in medical and behavioral therapies, as it was for Colligan, whose knee improved as a result of sham surgery. However, the placebo effect makes it difficult to separate the effect of a treatment from the effect of people's *beliefs* about the treatment, so researchers often design studies to try to disentangle these effects, as we will describe.

Research and the Placebo

For researchers to conclude that a treatment is effective, the treatment must show a higher rate of effectiveness than a placebo. This standard calls for researchers to use at least two groups in a study: one that receives the treatment and another that receives a placebo. Both groups must have equal expectations concerning the effectiveness of the treatment. In order to create equal expectancy, not only must the participants be unaware of whether they are receiving a placebo or a treatment but the experimenters who dispense both conditions must also be "blind" as to which group is which. The arrangement in which neither participants nor experimenters know about treatment conditions is called a **double-blind design.** As the Would You Believe . . .? box points out, this design strategy creates ethical dilemmas.

Psychological treatments such as counseling, hypnosis, biofeedback, relaxation training, massage, and a variety of stress and pain management techniques also produce expectancy effects. That is, the placebo effect also applies to research in psychology, but double-blind designs are not easy to perform with these treatments.

Placebo pills can look the same as pills containing an active ingredient, but providers of psychological or behavioral treatments always know when they are providing a sham treatment. In these studies, researchers use a **single-blind design** in which the participants do not know if they are receiving the active or inactive treatment, but the providers are not blind to treatment conditions. In single-blind designs, the control for expectancy is not as complete as in double-blind designs, but creating equal expectancies for participants is usually the more important control feature. Although health researchers often want to know whether a particular treatment provides benefits beyond placebo effects, health researchers also investigate a variety of other questions with a number of other research designs, which we will describe in the next section.

Prescribing Placebos May Be Considered Ethical

Cebocap, a capsule available only by prescription, may be a wonder drug. The ingredients in Cebocap can be remarkably effective in relieving a wide range of health problems, with few serious side effects. Yet, Cebocap is not as widely prescribed as it could be. Surprisingly, many people would be upset to learn that their doctor prescribed them with Cebocap.

Cebocap is a placebo pill made by Forest Pharmaceuticals. Why would a physician prescribe Cebocap, and could it ever be ethical to do so?

Although it is unclear how often physicians prescribe Cebocap, many doctors already report prescribing treatments that they consider to be placebos, such as vitamins or antibiotics for a viral infection (Tilburt et al., 2008). However, nearly three quarters of doctors who admit to prescribing a placebo describe it simply as "Medicine not typically used for your condition but might benefit you" (Tilburt et al., 2008, p. 3). This is truthful and

preserves the active ingredient of placebos: positive expectations. However, critics of this practice argue that the physician is deceiving the patient by withholding the fact that the treatment has no inherent medical benefit.

Could a placebo still be effective if the provider fully informed the patient that the treatment was merely a placebo? A recent study (Kaptchuk et al., 2010) set out to answer this question, by prescribing placebo pills to patients with irritable bowel syndrome (IBS). IBS is a chronic gastrointestinal disorder, characterized by recurrent abdominal pain. With few other effective treatments available for IBS, many view it as ethically permissible to study the effects of placebos on IBS symptoms.

In one experimental condition of this study, researchers told patients to take placebo pills twice daily, describing them as "made of an inert substance, like sugar pills, that have been shown in clinical studies to

produce significant improvement in IBS symptoms through mind-body self-healing processes" (Kaptchuk et al., 2010, p. el5591). Patients in the control condition did not receive any treatment at all. Indeed, the placebo treatment—even when prescribed in this completely transparent manner—led to fewer symptoms, greater improvement, and better quality of life compared with no treatment. Thus, placebos can be both ethically prescribed *and* effective in treatment.

Can placebos be ethically used in research? Typically, clinical researchers do not seek to show that placebos can work. Rather, they seek to show that another treatment performs better than a placebo. Thus, clinical researchers may have to assign patients to an experimental condition that they know does constitute an effective treatment. How do researchers reconcile this ethical difficulty?

Part of the answer to that question lies in the rules governing

(Continued)

research with human participants (American Psychological Association [APA], 2002; World Medical Association, 2004). Providing an ineffective treatment—or any other treatment—may be considered ethical if participants understand the risks fully and still agree to participate in the study. This element of research procedure, known as *informed consent*, stipulates that participants must be informed of factors in the research that may influence their willingness to participate before they consent to participate.

When participants in a clinical trial agree to take part in the study, they receive information about the possibility of getting a placebo rather than a treatment. Those participants who find the chances of receiving a placebo unacceptable may refuse to participate in the study. Colligan, who participated in the study with arthroscopic knee surgery, knew that he might be included in a sham surgery group, and he consented (Talbot, 2000). However, 44% of those interviewed about that study declined to participate (Moseley et al., 2002).

Despite the value of placebo controls in clinical research, some physicians and medical ethicists consider the use of ineffective treatment to be ethically unacceptable because the welfare of patients is not the primary concern. This is a valid concern if a patient-participant receives a placebo instead of the accepted standard of care (Kottow, 2007). These critics contend that control groups should receive the standard treatment rather than a placebo, and that placebo treatment is acceptable only if no treatment exists for the condition. Thus, opinion regarding the ethical acceptability of placebo treatment is divided, with some finding it acceptable and necessary for research and others objecting to the failure to provide an adequate standard of treatment.

IN SUMMARY

A placebo is an inactive substance or condition having the appearance of an active treatment. It may cause participants in an experiment to improve or change behavior because of their belief in the placebo's effectiveness and their prior experiences with receiving effective treatment. Although placebos can have a positive effect from the patient's point of view, they are a problem for the researcher. In general, a placebo's effects are about 35%; its effects on reducing pain may be higher, whereas its effects on other conditions may be lower. Placebos can influence a wide variety of disorders and diseases.

Experimental designs that measure the efficacy of an intervention, such as a drug, typically use a placebo so that people in the control group (who receive the placebo) have the same expectations for success as do people in the experimental group (who receive the active treatment). Drug studies are usually double-blind designs, meaning that neither the participants nor the people administering the drug know who receives the placebo and who receives the active drug. Researchers in psychological treatment studies are often not "blind" concerning the treatment, but participants are, creating a single-blind design for these studies.

Research Methods in Psychology

When you stroll through the breakfast food aisle of your supermarket, do you notice how many cereals boast a high-fiber content? Some cereals are intentionally named to highlight fiber: All Bran, Multi-Bran, Fiber One, Fiber 7. This fascination with fiber may have been at its peak in 1989 when the American television show *Saturday Night Live* aired a mock advertisement for "Colon Blow," a cereal with 30,000 times the fiber content as compared to regular oat bran cereals!

Why were Americans so seemingly obsessed with fiber in the 1980s? One reason for this obsession was the belief that a high-fiber diet could reduce one's risk for cancer, particularly colon cancer. This link between fiber and cancer was first suggested in the early 1970s by Denis Burkitt, a British surgeon who worked in sub-Saharan Africa. Dr. Burkitt observed a very low incidence of colon cancer among native Ugandans. At the time, the Ugandan diet was far different than the typical Western diet. Ugandans ate plenty of fruits, vegetables, raw grains, and nuts but little red meat. Westerners, on the other hand, ate more red meat and fewer vegetables and nuts, and the grains they consumed were typically processed rather than raw. In short, Ugandans had a high-fiber diet, and a low incidence of colon cancer. Dr. Burkitt proposed a seemingly intuitive explanation for this link: Dietary fiber speeds up certain digestive processes, leaving less time for the colon to be exposed to possible carcinogens.

Dr. Burkitt's belief in the benefits of dietary fiber was widely publicized, and led to the marketing of fiber in foods and to decades of research on the possible connection between diet and cancer. In this section, we will review some of this research as a way to illustrate a number of important aspects of health research. Most importantly, we will describe the different types of study designs that health researchers can use to investigate a question. We describe the strengths and weaknesses of these designs, as well as how our confidence in study results can depend on the strength of a research design. Additionally, we will show how health research is a continually evolving pursuit, where old beliefs are often replaced by newer discoveries as researchers acquire and synthesize new evidence.

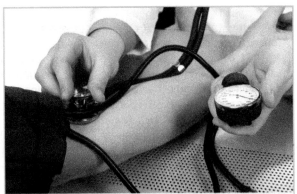

Blood pressure is a risk factor for cardiovascular disease, which means that people with high blood pressure are at increased risk, but not that high blood pressure causes cardiovascular disease.

Correlational Studies

When researchers seek to identify possible factors that predict or are related to a health condition, they use correlational studies. **Correlational studies** are often the first step in the research process, as they yield information about the degree of relationship between two variables. Correlational studies *describe* this relationship and are, therefore, a type of *descriptive research design*. Although scientists cannot use a single descriptive study to determine a causal relationship—such as whether diet *causes* cancer—the degree of relationship between two factors may be exactly what a researcher wants to know.

To assess the degree of relationship between two variables (such as diet and cancer), the researcher measures each of these variables in a group of participants and then calculates the **correlation coefficient** between these measures. The calculation yields a number that varies between −1.00 and +1.00. Positive correlations occur when the two variables increase or decrease together. For example, physical activity and longevity are positively correlated. Negative correlations occur when one of the variables increases as the other decreases, as is the case with the relationship between smoking and longevity. Correlations that are closer to 1.00 (either positive or negative) indicate stronger relationships than do correlations that are closer to 0.00. Small correlations—those less than 0.10—can be *statistically significant* if they are based on a very large number of observations, as in a study with many participants. However, such small correlations, though not

random, offer the researcher very little ability to predict scores on one variable from knowledge of scores on the other variable.

In one of the first examinations of the link between diet and cancer, Armstrong and Doll (1975) utilized a correlational design. These researchers examined the correlation between over 20 countries' average meat consumption and the countries' incidence of colorectal cancer. Indeed, a large and positive correlation of over 0.80 was noted, showing that countries with high meat consumption had significantly higher rates of colon cancer than countries with low meat consumption. However, simply knowing this correlation did not allow the researchers to know whether red meat or some other aspect of diet *caused* cancer. High red meat consumption is generally related to other practices such as low consumption of fiber, fruits, and vegetables, and could be related to environmental factors as well. Thus, this correlational study suggested a link between diet and cancer risk, but could not answer questions of causality directly. Nevertheless, it pointed to a strong association between diet and colon cancer, which fueled the public's interest in consuming foods that might prevent cancer. This finding, together with Dr. Burkitt's highly publicized focus on dietary fiber, led to a widespread public perception of a causal link between fiber intake and colon cancer.

Cross-Sectional and Longitudinal Studies

When health researchers seek to understand how health problems develop over time, they use cross-sectional or longitudinal studies. **Cross-sectional studies** are those conducted at only one point in time, whereas **longitudinal studies** follow participants over an extended period. In a cross-sectional design, the investigator studies a group of people from at least two different age groups to determine the possible differences between the groups on some measure.

Longitudinal studies can yield information that cross-sectional studies cannot because they assess the same people over time, which allows researchers to identify developmental trends and patterns. However, longitudinal studies have one obvious drawback: They take time. Thus, longitudinal studies are costlier than cross-sectional studies and they frequently require a large team of researchers.

Cross-sectional studies have the advantage of speed, but they have a disadvantage as well. Cross-sectional studies compare two or more separate groups of individuals, which make them incapable of revealing information about changes in individuals over a period of time. Cancer incidence increases with age, so a cross-sectional study comparing the cancer rates of young adults to that of older adults would undoubtedly show that older adults have a higher rate of cancer. However, only a longitudinal study, looking at the same people over a long period of time, could confirm that age increases cancer incidence. (In a cross-sectional design, it is always possible that the older adults differed from young adults in some important way other than age, such as exposure to carcinogens).

Due to the time and resources needed to conduct longitudinal research, such studies on the link between diet and cancer did not appear until the late 1990s. For example, one study of over 27,000 Finnish males asked about consumption of fat, meat, fruits, vegetables, calcium, and fiber, and followed the participants for 8 years to track the incidence of colorectal cancer (Pietinen et al., 1999). In this study, colon cancer was linked to some aspects of diet (such as calcium) but was completely unrelated to fiber consumption. Many other longitudinal studies confirmed this lack of relationship. Thus, the results of these longitudinal studies—which provide stronger evidence than the earlier correlational studies—challenged the notion that dietary fiber reduces colon cancer risk.

Experimental Designs

Correlational studies, cross-sectional designs, and longitudinal studies all have important uses in psychology, but none of them can determine causality. Sometimes

psychologists want information on the ability of one variable to cause or directly influence another. Such information requires a well-designed experiment.

An experiment consists of a comparison of at least two groups, often referred to as an **experimental group** and a **control group.** The participants in the experimental group must receive treatment identical to that of participants in the control group except that those in the experimental group receive one level of the **independent variable,** whereas people in the control group receive a different level. The independent variable is the condition of interest, which the experimenter systematically manipulates to observe its influence on a behavior or response—that is, on the **dependent variable.** The manipulation of the independent variable is a critical element of experimental design because this manipulation allows researchers to control the situation by choosing and creating the appropriate levels. In addition, good experimental design requires that experimenters assign participants to the experimental or control group *randomly* to ensure that the groups are equivalent at the beginning of the study.

Often the experimental condition consists of administering a treatment, whereas the control condition consists of withholding that treatment and perhaps presenting some sort of placebo. If the experimental group later shows a different score on the dependent variable than the control group, the independent variable has a cause-and-effect relationship with the dependent variable.

Several large studies have used an experimental design to study the link between diet and cancer (Beresford et al., 2006; Schatzkin et al., 2000). One study randomly assigned nearly 20,000 women to an intervention aimed at reducing fat intake and increasing consumption of fruits, vegetables, and fiber (Beresford et al., 2006). Women randomly assigned to the control group were asked to continue eating as usual. Indeed, women in the experimental group changed their diet as instructed, but they did not show any reduced risk of cancer at an 8-year follow-up compared to the women in the control group. Due to its experimental design, this study provided strong evidence of a lack of a causal relationship between dietary fiber and colon cancer risk.

Figure 2.1 shows a typical experimental design comparing an experimental group with a control group, with counseling as the independent variable and body mass index (BMI) as the dependent variable.

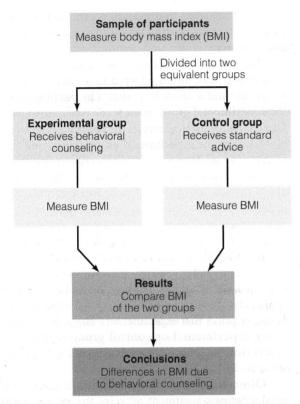

Sample of participants
Measure body mass index (BMI)

Divided into two
equivalent groups

Experimental group
Receives behavioral
counseling

Control group
Receives standard
advice

Measure BMI

Measure BMI

Results
Compare BMI
of the two groups

Conclusions
Differences in BMI due
to behavioral counseling

FIGURE 2.1 Example of an experimental method.

Ex Post Facto Designs

Ethical restrictions or practical limitations prevent researchers from manipulating many variables, such as gender, socioeconomic status, death of a loved one, smoking, or sexual behaviors. This means that experiments are not possible with many such variables, but these limitations do not prevent researchers from studying these variables. When researchers cannot manipulate certain variables in a systematic manner, they sometimes rely on ex post facto designs.

An **ex post facto design,** one of several types of quasi-experimental studies, resembles an experiment in some ways but differs in others. Both types of studies involve contrasting groups to determine differences, but ex post facto designs do not involve the manipulation of independent variables. Instead, researchers choose a variable of interest and select participants who already differ on this variable, called a **subject variable** (or *participant variable*). Both experiments and ex post facto studies involve the measurement of dependent variables. For example, researchers might study the link between meat consumption (subject variable) and cancer risk (dependent variable) by recruiting participants from two community groups: one group being a vegetarian/vegan cooking club and the other being the local chapter of Steak Lovers Anonymous. There is no random assignment in this ex post facto design, but the two groups would certainly differ in red meat consumption.

The comparison group in an ex post facto design is not an equivalent control group, because the participants were assigned to groups on the basis of their food preferences rather than by random assignment. Without random assignment, the groups may potentially differ on variables other than food preferences, such as exercise, alcohol consumption, or smoking. The existence of these other differences means that researchers cannot pinpoint the subject variable as the cause of differences in cancer risk between the groups. However, findings about differences in risk between the two groups can yield useful information, making this type of study a choice for many investigations, particularly when random assignment is difficult or impossible.

IN SUMMARY

Health psychologists use several research methods, including correlational studies, cross-sectional and longitudinal studies, experimental designs, and ex post facto studies. Correlational studies indicate the degree of association between two variables, but they can never show causation. Cross-sectional studies investigate a group of people at one point in time, whereas longitudinal studies follow the participants over an extended period of time. Although longitudinal studies may yield more useful results than cross-sectional studies, they are more time consuming and more expensive. With experimental designs, researchers manipulate the independent variable so that any resulting differences between experimental and control groups can be attributed to their differential exposure to the independent variable. Experimental studies typically include a placebo given to people in a control group so that they will have the same expectations as people in the experimental group. Ex post facto studies are similar to experimental designs in that researchers compare two or more groups and then record group differences in the dependent variable, but differ in that the independent variable is preexisting rather than manipulated.

Research Methods in Epidemiology

The field of health psychology benefits not only from the research methods of psychology but also from medical research—in particular, the research of epidemiologists. **Epidemiology** is a branch of medicine that investigates factors that contribute to health or disease in a particular population (Porta, 2014; Tucker, Phillips, Murphy, & Raczynski, 2004).

With the increase in chronic diseases during the 20th century, epidemiologists make fundamental contributions to health by identifying the risk factors for diseases. A **risk factor** is any characteristic or condition that occurs with greater frequency in people with a disease than in people free from that disease. That is, epidemiologists study those demographic and behavioral factors that relate to heart disease, cancer, and other chronic diseases (Tucker et al., 2004). For example, epidemiology studies were the first to detect a relationship between smoking and heart disease.

Two important concepts in epidemiology are prevalence and incidence. **Prevalence** refers to the proportion of the population that has a particular disease or condition at a specific time; **incidence** measures the frequency of *new cases* during a specified period, usually 1 year (Tucker et al., 2004). With both prevalence and incidence, the number of people in the population at risk is divided into either the number of people with the disorder (prevalence) or the number of new cases in a particular time frame (incidence). The prevalence of a disorder may be quite different from the incidence of that disorder. For example, the prevalence of hypertension is much greater than the incidence because people can live for years after a diagnosis. In a given community, the annual *incidence* of hypertension might be 0.025, meaning that for every 1,000 people of a given age range, ethnic background, and gender, 25 people per year will receive a diagnosis of high blood pressure. But because hypertension is a chronic disorder, the prevalence will accumulate, producing a number much higher than 25 per 1,000. In contrast, for a disease such as influenza with a relatively short duration (due to either the patient's rapid recovery or quick death), the incidence per year will exceed the prevalence at any specific time during that year.

Research in epidemiology uses two broad methods: (1) observational studies and (2) randomized, controlled trials. Each method has its own requirements and yields specific information. Although epidemiologists use some of the same methods and procedures employed by psychologists, their terminology is not always the same. Figure 2.2 lists the broad areas of epidemiological study and shows their approximate counterparts in the field of psychology.

Observational Methods

Epidemiologists use observational methods to estimate the occurrence of a specific disease in a given population. These methods do not show causes of the disease, but researchers can draw inferences about possible factors that relate to the disease. Observational methods are similar to correlational studies in psychology; both show an association between two or more conditions, but neither can be used to demonstrate causation.

Two important types of observational methods are retrospective studies and prospective studies. **Retrospective studies** begin with a group of people already suffering from a particular disease or disorder and then look backward for characteristics or conditions that marked them as being different from people who do not have that problem. This approach is often used in early stages of research because it is relatively quick and inexpensive but can still yield potentially useful information. Indeed, many of the early studies on diet and cancer were retrospective studies in which cancer patients and healthy individuals provided general information about their past patterns of food consumption. Retrospective studies such as these are also referred to as **case–control studies** because cases (people who have a health problem) are compared with controls (people who do not have the problem). Interestingly, many of these early retrospective studies from the 1980s *did* find an association between high-fiber intake and lower incidence of colon cancer (Trock, Lanza, & Greenwald, 1990), no doubt fueling the public's belief in the benefits of dietary fiber. However, one of the major drawbacks of retrospective studies is that they rely on people's recollections of past behavior, which are often inaccurate.

In contrast, **prospective studies** begin with a population of disease-free participants and follow them over a period of time to determine whether a given factor, such as current cigarette smoking, high blood pressure, or obesity, is related to a later health condition, such as heart disease or death. Prospective studies are longitudinal, making them equivalent to longitudinal studies

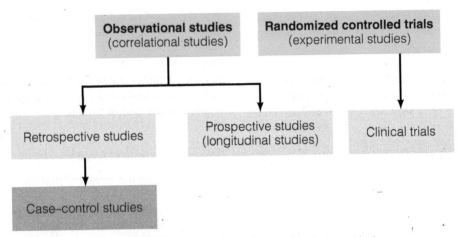

FIGURE 2.2 Research methods in epidemiology, with their psychology counterparts in parentheses.

in psychology: Both provide information about a group of participants over time, and both take a long time to complete. Generally, prospective studies yield stronger evidence than retrospective studies. Prospective studies on diet and colon cancer also led to a different conclusion than retrospective studies. In most prospective studies—which appeared in the 1990s—fiber intake was *not* associated with decreased risk of colon cancer (Pietinen et al., 1999).

Randomized Controlled Trials

A second type of epidemiological research is the randomized controlled trial, which is equivalent to experimental research in psychology. With a randomized controlled trial, researchers randomly assign participants to either a study group or a control group, thus making the two groups equal on all pertinent factors except the variable being studied. (In psychology, this would be called the independent variable.) Researchers must also control variables other than those of primary interest to prevent them from affecting the outcome. A randomized controlled trial, as with the experimental method in psychology, must avoid the problem of self-selection; that is, it must not let participants choose whether to be in the experimental group or the control group, but rather, it must assign them to groups randomly.

A clinical trial is a research design that tests the effects of a new drug or medical treatment. Many clinical trials are randomized controlled trials that feature random assignment and control of other variables, which allow researchers to determine the effectiveness of the new treatment. Epidemiologists often regard randomized, placebo-controlled, double-blind trials as the "gold standard" of research designs (Kertesz, 2003). This design is commonly used to measure the effectiveness of new drugs, as well as psychological and educational interventions. For example, all drugs approved by the U.S. Food and Drug Administration (FDA) must first undergo extensive clinical trials of this nature, demonstrating that the drug is effective and has acceptable levels of side effects or other risks.

When a controlled clinical trial demonstrates the effectiveness of a new drug or intervention, the researchers often publish and publicize the findings so that others can adopt the treatment. In some cases, a controlled trial may fail to demonstrate the effectiveness of a new intervention. When trials fail to show a treatment to be effective, researchers may be less likely to publish the findings. By some estimates, studies that fail to find an intervention as effective are three times less likely to be published (Dwan et al., 2008). Thus, researchers, health care providers, and the public are more likely to learn about research that shows a particular treatment to be effective but less likely to learn about research that shows the same treatment to be ineffective.

Several safeguards are now in place to help ensure that researchers and health care providers can access all available evidence, rather than just the evidence that supports a treatment. For example, major medical journals require that researchers comply with clear guidelines in reporting results of a clinical trial. These guidelines—known as the Consolidated Standards of Reporting Trials (CONSORT) guidelines (Schulz, Altman, Moher, & the CONSORT Group, 2010)—require researchers to register their clinical trial in a registry *prior* to the start of the study. This database allows anybody to locate all clinical trials conducted on a treatment, not simply the trials that found a treatment to be effective.

Meta-Analysis

As we have seen, researchers use a variety of approaches to study behavior and health-related outcomes. Unfortunately, research on the same topic may not yield consistent findings, putting researchers (and everyone else) in the position of wondering which findings are the most valid. Some studies are larger than others, and when it comes to accepting a result, size matters. But sometimes, even large studies furnish results that seem contradictory. However, the statistical technique of meta-analysis allows researchers to evaluate many research studies on the same topic, even if the research methods differed. The results from a meta-analysis include a measure of the overall size of the effect of the variable under study. The ability to offer an estimate of the size of an effect is an advantage. If an effect is statistically significant but small, then people should not be encouraged to change their behavior on the basis of such findings; doing so would provide too few benefits. On the other hand, if an effect is large, then working toward change would be beneficial, even if it is difficult.

Recently, several meta-analyses have synthesized decades of research on diet and colon cancer. In general, dietary fiber shows a weak association, if any, to colon cancer risk (Vargas & Thompson, 2012). However, this does not mean that diet is unimportant. A meta-analysis of 19 case-control and 6 prospective studies show that a diet high in red meat is strongly associated with greater risk of colon cancer (Aune et al., 2013).

Thus, Dr. Burkitt may have been right all along in speculating that the diet of sub-Saharan Africans protected them against colon cancer. But it wasn't the fiber that mattered. It was the absence of red meat. As researchers used stronger designs and larger samples to investigate the link between diet and colon cancer, the evidence began to show that old beliefs about the role of fiber in colon cancer were inaccurate but pointed to the role of red meat instead.

An Example of Epidemiological Research: The Alameda County Study

Epidemiological studies have been crucially important in identifying the role of behavior in health. A famous example of an epidemiological study is the Alameda County Study in California, an ongoing prospective study of a single community to identify health practices that may protect against death and disease. The Alameda County Study was one of the first studies to show how several behaviors decreased people's risk of mortality.

In 1965, epidemiologist Lester Breslow and his colleagues from the Human Population Laboratory of the California State Department of Public Health began a survey of a sample of households in Alameda County (Oakland), California. The researchers sent detailed questionnaires to each resident 20 years of age or older, and nearly 7,000 people returned surveys. Among other questions, these participants answered questions about seven basic health practices: (1) getting 7 or 8 hours of sleep daily, (2) eating breakfast almost every day, (3) rarely eating between meals, (4) drinking alcohol in moderation or not at all, (5) not smoking cigarettes, (6) exercising regularly, and (7) maintaining weight near the prescribed ideal.

At the time of the original survey in 1965, only cigarette smoking had been implicated as a health risk. Evidence that any of the other six practices predicted health or mortality was quite weak. Because several of these practices require some amount of good health, it was necessary to investigate the possibility that original health status might confound subsequent death rates. To control for these possible confounding effects, the Alameda County investigators asked residents about their physical disabilities, acute and chronic illnesses, physical symptoms, and current levels of energy.

A follow-up 5½ years later (Belloc, 1973) revealed that participants who practiced six or seven of the basic health-related behaviors were far less likely to have died than those who practiced zero to three. A 9-year follow-up determined the relationship between mortality and the seven health practices, considered individually as well as in combination (Berkman & Breslow, 1983; Wingard, Berkman, & Brand, 1982). Cigarette smoking, lack of physical activity, and alcohol consumption were strongly related to mortality, whereas obesity and too much or too little sleep were only weakly associated with increased death rates. Skipping breakfast and snacking between meals did not predict mortality.

Moreover, the number of close social relationships also predicted mortality: People with few social contacts were 2½ times more likely to have died than were those with many such contacts (Berkman & Syme, 1979).

The Alameda County Study was the first study to uncover a link between social relationships and mortality. As you will learn in the rest of this book, social relationships and social support are important factors in physical health.

Becoming an Informed Reader of Health-Related Research on the Internet

Not long ago, reports of health research appeared mainly in scientific journals, read primarily by physicians. People typically heard of this research from their physicians. Today, diverse outlets—including television, newspapers, and the Internet—publicize the "latest and greatest" health research. However, with this increased publicity comes an increasing problem: Some of this information may not be trustworthy. The news media are in the business of getting people's attention, so coverage of health information may mislead by focusing on the most sensational findings. And, of course, some commercial advertisements—promoting, for instance, a revolutionary weight loss program or a simple way to stop smoking—may ignore or distort scientific evidence in order to boost sales.

Over 80% of Internet users turn to the Internet for health information (Pew Internet, 2012). The Internet, in particular, presents not only a wealth of useful health information but also some misleading information. How can you judge the worth of health-related information you read or hear? Here are several questions you should ask yourself as you evaluate health information on the Internet.

1. Who runs the website? Any reputable website should clearly state who is responsible for the information. You can often find this information in an "About Us" section of the website. Often,

the website address can also tell you important information. Websites that end in ".gov," ".edu," or ".org" are run by government, educational, or non- for-profit groups. These sites are likely to present unbiased information. In contrast, websites that end in ".com" are run by commercial enterprises and may exist mainly to sell products.

2. What is the purpose of the website? Websites that exist primarily to sell products may not present unbiased information. You should be especially wary of websites that promise "breakthroughs," or try to sell quick, easy, and miraculous cures. Dramatic breakthroughs are rare in science.

3. What is the evidence supporting a claim? Ideally, a website should report information based on studies conducted by trained scientists who are affiliated with universities, research hospitals, or government agencies. Furthermore, websites should include references to these published scientific studies. In contrast, claims supported by testimonials of "satisfied" consumers or from commercial enterprises are less likely to come from scientific research.

4. Is there adequate information available to evaluate the research design of a scientific

study? Findings are more reliable if a study uses a large number of participants. If a study suggests that a factor *causes* a particular health outcome, does it use an experimental design with random assignment? Does it control for placebo effects? If the design is prospective or retrospective, did the researchers adequately control for smoking, diet, exercise, and other possible confounding variables? Lastly, is it clear who the participants in a study were? If a study uses a unique population, then the results may only be applicable to similar individuals.

5. How is the information reviewed before it is posted? Most reputable health information will have somebody with medical or research credentials—such as an MD or a PhD—author or review the material.

6. How current is the information? The date of posting or last review should be clear. Scientific knowledge evolves continually, so the best information is up to date.

You can find many of these tips, and others, on the National Institutes of Health website (www.nih.gov). This website, as well as the Centers for Disease Control and Prevention (www.cdc.gov), is an excellent source for the latest scientific information on a wide variety of health topics.

If some health practices predict greater risk of *mortality,* then a second question concerns how these same factors relate to *morbidity,* or disease. A condition that predicts death need not also predict disease. Many disabilities, chronic illnesses, and illness symptoms do not inevitably lead to death. Therefore, it is important to know whether basic health practices and social contacts predict later physical health. Do health practices merely contribute to survival time, or do they also raise an individual's general level of health?

IN SUMMARY

Epidemiologists conduct research using designs and terminology that differ from those used by psychology researchers. For example, epidemiologists use the concepts of risk factor, prevalence, and incidence. A risk factor is any condition that occurs with greater frequency in people with a disease than it does in people free from that disease. Prevalence refers to the proportion of the population that has a particular disease at a specific time, whereas incidence measures the frequency of new cases of the disease during a specified period of time.

In order to investigate factors that contribute either to health or to the frequency and distribution of a disease, epidemiologists use research methods that are similar to those used by psychologists, but the terminology varies. Observational studies, which are similar to correlational studies, can be either retrospective or prospective. Retrospective studies begin with a group of people already suffering from a disease and then look for characteristics of these people that differ from those of people who do not have the disease; prospective studies are longitudinal designs that follow the forward development of a group of people. Randomized controlled trials are similar to experimental designs in psychology. Clinical trials, a common type of randomized controlled trial, are typically used to determine the effectiveness of new drugs, but they can be used in other controlled studies. The statistical technique of meta-analysis allows researchers to examine a group of studies that have researched the variable of interest and provide an overall estimate of the size of the effect.

Determining Causation

As noted earlier, both prospective and retrospective studies can identify risk factors for a disease, but they do not demonstrate causation. This section looks at the risk factor approach as a means of suggesting causation and then examines evidence that cigarette smoking *causes* disease.

The Risk Factor Approach

The risk factor approach was popularized by the Framingham Heart Study (Levy & Brink, 2005), a large-scale epidemiology investigation that began in 1948 and included more than 5,000 men and women in the town of Framingham, Massachusetts. From its early years and continuing to the present, this study has allowed researchers to identify risk factors for cardiovascular disease (CVD) such as serum cholesterol, gender, high blood pressure, cigarette smoking, and obesity. These risk factors do not necessarily cause CVD, but they relate to it in some way. Obesity, for example, may not be a direct cause of heart disease, but it is generally associated with hypertension, which is strongly associated with CVD. Thus, obesity is a risk factor for CVD.

Two common methods exist for conveying risk: absolute and relative risk. Absolute risk refers to the person's chances of developing a disease or disorder independent of any risk that other people may have for that disease or disorder. These chances tend to be small. For example, a smoker's risk of dying of lung cancer during any one year is about 1 in 1,000. When smokers hear their risk expressed in such terms, they may not recognize the hazards of their behavior (Kertesz, 2003). Other ways of presenting the same information may seem more threatening. For example, a male smoker's risk of getting lung cancer in his *lifetime* is much higher, about 15 in 100 (Crispo et al., 2004).

Relative risk refers to the ratio of the incidence (or prevalence) of a disease in an exposed group to the incidence (or prevalence) of that disease in the unexposed group. The relative risk of the unexposed group is always 1.00. Thus, a relative risk of 1.50 indicates that the exposed group is 50% more likely to develop the disease in question than the unexposed group; a relative risk of 0.70 means that the rate of disease in the exposed group is only 70% of the rate in the unexposed group. Expressed in terms of relative risk, smoking seems much more dangerous. For example, male cigarette smokers have a relative risk of about 23.3 for dying of lung cancer and a relative risk of 14.6 for dying of laryngeal cancer (U.S. Department of Health and Human Services [USDHHS], 2004). This means that, compared with nonsmokers, men who smoke are more than 23 times as likely to die of lung cancer and more than 14 times as likely to die of laryngeal cancer.

The high relative risk for lung cancer among people who have a long history of cigarette smoking may suggest that most smokers will die of lung cancer. However, such is not the case: Most smokers will *not* die of lung cancer. About 39% of male smokers and 40% of female smokers who die of cancer will develop cancer in sites other than the lung (Armour, Woollery, Malarcher, Pechacek, & Husten, 2005). Furthermore, the absolute frequency of death due to heart disease makes a smoker almost as likely to die of heart disease (20% of deaths among smokers) as lung cancer (28% of deaths among smokers). Smokers have a much higher relative risk of dying from lung cancer than CVD, but their *absolute risk* of dying from CVD is much more similar.

Cigarettes and Disease: Is There a Causal Relationship?

In 1994, representatives from all the major tobacco companies came before the Congress House Subcommittee on Health to argue that cigarettes do not cause health problems such as heart disease and lung cancer. The crux of their argument was that no scientific study had ever proven that cigarette smoking causes heart disease or lung cancer in humans. Technically, their contention was correct because only experimental studies can absolutely demonstrate causation, and no such experimental study has ever been (or ever will be) conducted on humans.

During the past 50 years, however, researchers have used nonexperimental studies to establish a link between cigarette smoking and several diseases, especially CVD and lung cancer. Accumulated findings from these studies present an example of how researchers can use nonexperimental studies to make deductions about a causal relationship. In other words, experimental, randomized, placebo-controlled, double-blind studies are not required before scientists can infer a causal link between the independent variable (smoking) and the dependent variables (heart disease and lung cancer). Epidemiologists draw conclusions that a causal relationship exists if certain conditions are met (Susser, 1991; USDHHS, 2004).

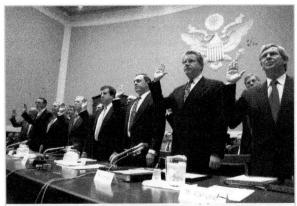

Heads of United States' largest tobacco companies testify before Congress, arguing that no experimental evidence shows that tobacco causes cancer.

The first criterion is that a *dose–response relationship* must exist between a possible cause and changes in the prevalence or incidence of a disease. A **dose–response relationship** is a direct, consistent association between an independent variable, such as a behavior, and a dependent variable, such as a disease; in other words, the higher the dose, the higher the death rate. A body of research evidence (Bhat et al., 2008; Papadopoulos et al., 2011; USDHHS, 1990, 2004) has demonstrated a dose–response relationship between both the number of cigarettes smoked per day and the number of years one has smoked and the subsequent incidence of heart disease, lung cancer, and stroke.

Second, the prevalence or incidence of a *disease should decline with the removal of the possible cause.* Research (USDHHS, 1990, 2004) has consistently demonstrated that quitting cigarette smoking lowers one's risk of CVD and decreases one's risk of lung cancer. People who continue to smoke continue to have increased risks of these diseases. Even laws that ban smoking in the workplace have resulted in decreases in the number of heart attacks attributable to secondhand exposure to cigarette smoke (Hurt et al., 2012).

Third, the *cause must precede the disease.* Cigarette smoking almost always precedes incidence of disease. (We have little evidence that people tend to begin cigarette smoking as a means of coping with heart disease or lung cancer.)

Fourth, a *cause-and-effect relationship between the condition and the disease must be plausible;* that is, it must be consistent with other data, and it must make sense from a biological viewpoint. Although scientists are just beginning to understand the exact

TABLE 2.1 Criteria for Determining Causation Between a Condition and a Disease

1. A dose–response relationship exists between the condition and the disease.
2. Removal of the condition reduces the prevalence or incidence of the disease.
3. The condition precedes the disease.
4. A cause-and-effect relationship between the condition and the disease is physiologically plausible.
5. Relevant research data consistently reveal a relationship between the condition and the disease.
6. The strength of the relationship between the condition and the disease is relatively high.
7. Studies revealing a relationship between the condition and the disease are well designed.

mechanisms responsible for the effect of cigarette smoking on the cardiovascular system and the lungs (USDHHS, 2004), such a physiological connection is plausible.

Fifth, *research findings must be consistent*. For more than 50 years, evidence from ex post facto and correlational studies, as well as from various epidemiological studies, has demonstrated a strong and consistent relationship between cigarette smoking and disease.

Sixth, the *strength of the association between the condition and the disease must be relatively high*. Again, research has revealed that cigarette smokers have at least a twofold risk for CVD and are about 18 times more likely than nonsmokers to die of lung cancer (USDHHS, 2004). Because other studies have found comparable relative risk figures, epidemiologists accept cigarette smoking as a causal agent for both CVD and lung cancer.

The final criterion for inferring causality is the existence of *appropriately designed studies*. Although no experimental designs with human participants have been reported on the relationship between cigarettes and disease, well-designed observational studies can yield the results equivalent to experimental studies (USDHHS, 2004), and a large number of these observational studies consistently reveal a close association between cigarette smoking and both CVD and lung cancer.

Because each of these seven criteria is clearly met by the evidence against smoking, epidemiologists are able to discount the argument of tobacco company representatives that cigarette smoking has not been proven to cause disease. When evidence is as overwhelming as it is in this case, scientists infer a causal link between cigarette smoking and a variety of diseases, including heart disease and lung cancer. Table 2.1 summarizes the criteria for determining causation.

IN SUMMARY

A risk factor is any characteristic or condition that occurs with greater frequency in people with a disease than it does in people free from that disease. Risk may be expressed either in terms of the absolute risk, a person's risk of developing a disease independent of other factors, or the relative risk, the ratio of risk of those exposed to a risk factor compared with those not exposed.

Although the risk factor approach alone cannot determine causation, epidemiologists use several criteria for determining a cause-and-effect relationship between a condition and a disease: (1) A dose–response relationship must exist between the condition and the disease, (2) the removal of the condition must reduce the prevalence or incidence of the disease, (3) the condition must precede the disease, (4) the causal relationship between the condition and the disease must be physiologically plausible, (5) research data must consistently reveal a relationship between the condition and the disease, (6) the strength of the relationship between the condition and the disease must be relatively high, and (7) the relationship between the condition and the disease must be based on well-designed studies. When findings meet all seven of these criteria, scientists can infer a cause-and-effect relationship between an independent variable (such as smoking) and a dependent variable (such as heart disease or lung cancer).

Research Tools

Psychologists frequently rely on two important tools to conduct research: theoretical models and psychometric instruments. Many, but not all, psychology studies use a theoretical model and attempt to test hypotheses suggested by that model. Also, many psychology studies rely on measuring devices to assess behaviors, physiological functions, attitudes, abilities, personality traits, and other variables. This section provides a brief discussion of these two tools.

The Role of Theory in Research

As the scientific study of human behavior, psychology shares the use of scientific methods to investigate natural phenomena with other disciplines. The work of science is not restricted to research methodology; it also involves constructing theoretical models to serve as vehicles for making sense of research findings. Health psychologists have developed a number of models and theories to explain health-related behaviors and conditions, such as stress, pain, smoking, alcohol abuse, and unhealthy eating habits. To the uninitiated, theories may seem impractical and unimportant, but scientists regard them as practical tools that give both direction and meaning to their research.

Scientific theory is "a set of related assumptions that allow scientists to use logical-deductive reasoning to formulate testable hypotheses" (Feist & Feist, 2006, p. 4). Theories and scientific observations have an interactive relationship. A theory gives meaning to observations, and observations, in turn, fit into and alter the theory to explain these observations. Theories, then, are dynamic and become more powerful as they expand to explain more and more relevant observations.

The role of theory in health psychology is basically the same as it is in any other scientific discipline. First, a useful theory should generate research—both descriptive research and hypothesis testing. Descriptive research deals with measurement, labeling, and categorization of observations. Hypothesis testing identifies the conditions that relate to and cause the development of a health condition.

Second, a useful theory should organize and explain the observations derived from research and make them intelligible. Unless research data are organized into some meaningful framework, scientists have no clear direction to follow in their pursuit of further knowledge. A useful theory of the psychosocial factors in obesity, for example, should integrate what researchers know about such factors and allow researchers to frame discerning questions that stimulate further research.

Third, a useful theory should serve as a guide to action, permitting the practitioner to predict behavior

and to implement strategies to change behavior. A practitioner concerned with helping others change health-related behaviors is greatly aided by a theory of behavior change. For instance, a cognitive therapist will follow a cognitive theory of learning to make decisions about how to help clients and will thus focus on changing the thought processes that affect clients' behaviors. Similarly, psychologists with other theoretical orientations rely on their theories to supply them with solutions to the many questions they confront in their practice.

Theories, then, are useful and necessary tools for the development of any scientific discipline. They generate research that leads to more knowledge, organize and explain observations, and help the practitioner (both the researcher and the clinician) handle a variety of daily problems, such as predicting behavior and helping people change unhealthy practices.

The Role of Psychometrics in Research

Health psychologists study a number of phenomena that cannot be described in terms of simple physical measurements, like weight or length. These phenomena include behaviors and conditions such as stress, coping, pain, hostility, eating habits, and personality. To study each of these phenomena, health psychologists must develop new measures that can reliably and validly measure differences between people. Indeed, one of psychology's most important contributions to behavioral medicine and behavioral health is its sophisticated methods of measuring important psychological factors in health.

For any measuring instrument to be useful, it must be both *reliable* (consistent) and *valid* (accurate). The problems of establishing reliability and validity are critical to the development of any measurement scale.

Establishing Reliability   The **reliability** of a measuring instrument is the extent to which it yields consistent results. A reliable ruler, for example, will yield the same measurement across different situations. In health psychology, reliability is most frequently determined by comparing scores on two or more administrations of the same instrument (*test–retest reliability*) or by comparing ratings obtained from two or more judges observing the same phenomenon (*interrater reliability*).

Measuring psychological phenomena is less precise than measuring physical dimensions such as length. Thus, perfect reliability is nearly impossible to come by, and researchers most frequently describe reliability in terms of either correlation coefficients or percentages. The correlation coefficient, which expresses the degree of correspondence between two sets of scores, is the same statistic used in correlational studies. High reliability coefficients (such as 0.80 to 0.90) indicate that participants have obtained nearly the same scores on two administrations of a test. Percentages can express the degree of agreement between the independent ratings of observers. If the agreement between two or more raters is high (such as 85% to 95%), then the instrument should elicit nearly the same ratings from two or more interviewers.

Establishing reliability for the numerous assessment instruments used in health psychology is obviously a formidable task, but it is an essential first step in developing useful measuring devices.

Establishing Validity   A second step in constructing assessment scales is to establish their validity. Validity is the extent to which an instrument measures what it is designed to measure. A valid ruler, for example, will indicate that an object measures 2 centimeters, but only when that object really does measure 2 centimeters. In the context of a psychological measure such as a stress assessment, for example, a valid stress measure should tell you a person is under high stress, but only when that person experiences high stress.

Psychologists determine the validity of a measuring instrument by comparing scores from that instrument with some independent or outside criterion—that is, a standard that exists independently of the instrument being validated. In health psychology, that criterion can be a physiological measure, like a physiological stress response such as elevated blood pressure. A criterion can also be some future event, such as a diagnosis of heart disease or the development of diabetes. An instrument capable of predicting who will receive such a diagnosis and who will remain disease free has *predictive validity*. For example, scales that measure attitudes about body predict the development of eating disorders. For such a scale to demonstrate predictive validity, it must be administered to participants who are currently free of disease. If people who score high on the scale eventually have higher rates of disease than participants with low scores, then the scale can be said to have predictive validity; that is, it differentiates between participants who will remain disease free and those who will become ill.

IN SUMMARY

Two important tools aid the work of scientists: useful theories and accurate measurement. Useful theories (1) generate research, (2) predict and explain research data, and (3) help the practitioner solve a variety of problems. Accurate psychometric instruments are both reliable and valid. *Reliability* is the extent to which an assessment device measures consistently, and *validity* is the extent to which an assessment instrument measures what it is supposed to measure.

Answers

This chapter has addressed five basic questions:

1. **What are placebos, and how do they affect research and treatment?**
A placebo is an inactive substance or condition that has the appearance of an active treatment and that may cause participants to improve or change because of a belief in the placebo's efficacy. In other words, a placebo is any treatment that is effective because patients' expectations based on previous experiences with treatment lead them to believe that it will be effective.

The therapeutic effect of placebos is about 35%, but that rate varies with many conditions, including treatment setting and culture. Placebos, including sham surgery, can be effective in a wide variety of situations, such as decreasing pain, reducing asthma attacks, diminishing anxiety, and decreasing symptoms of Parkinson's disease. Nocebos are placebos that produce adverse effects.

The positive effects of placebos are usually beneficial to patients, but they create problems for researchers attempting to determine the efficacy of a treatment. Experimental designs that measure the effectiveness of a treatment intervention balance that intervention against a placebo so that people in the control (placebo) group have the same expectations as do people in the experimental (treatment intervention) group. Experimental studies frequently use designs in which the participants do not know which treatment condition they are in (*single-blind* design) or in which neither the participants nor the people administering the treatment know who receives the placebo and who receives the treatment intervention (*double-blind* design).

2. How does psychology research contribute to health knowledge?

Psychology has contributed to health knowledge in at least five important ways. First is its long tradition of techniques to change behavior. Second is an emphasis on health rather than disease. Third is the development of reliable and valid measuring instruments. Fourth is the construction of useful theoretical models to explain health-related research. Fifth is various research methods used in psychology. This chapter mostly deals with the fifth contribution.

The variety of research methods used in psychology include (1) correlational studies, (2) cross-sectional studies and longitudinal studies, (3) experimental designs, and (4) ex post facto designs. Correlational studies indicate the degree of association or correlation between two variables, but by themselves, they cannot determine a cause-and-effect relationship. Cross-sectional studies investigate a group of people at one point in time, whereas longitudinal studies follow the participants over an extended period. In general, longitudinal studies are more likely to yield useful and specific results, but they are more time consuming and expensive than cross-sectional studies. With experimental designs, researchers manipulate the independent variable so that any resulting differences in the dependent variable between experimental and control groups can be attributed to their differential exposure to the independent variable. Ex post facto designs are similar to experimental designs in that researchers compare two or more groups and then record group differences on the dependent variable. However, in the ex post facto study, the experimenter merely selects a subject variable on which two or more groups have naturally divided themselves rather than create differences through manipulation.

3. How has epidemiology contributed to health knowledge?

Epidemiology has contributed the concepts of risk factor, prevalence, and incidence. A risk factor is any characteristic or condition that occurs with greater frequency in people with a disease than it does in people free from that disease. Prevalence is the proportion of the population that has a particular disease at a specific time; incidence measures the frequency of new cases of the disease during a specified time.

Many of the research methods used in epidemiology are quite similar to those used in psychology. Epidemiology uses at least three basic kinds of research methodology: (1) observational studies, (2) randomized controlled trials, and (3) natural experiments. Observational studies, which parallel the correlation studies used in psychology, are of two types: retrospective and prospective. Retrospective studies are usually *case–control studies* that begin with a group of people already suffering from a disease (the cases) and then look for characteristics of these people that are different from those of people who do not have that disease (the controls). Prospective studies are longitudinal designs that follow the forward development of a population or sample. Randomized controlled trials are similar to experimental designs in psychology. In these studies, researchers manipulate the independent variable to determine its effect on the dependent variable. Randomized controlled trials are capable of demonstrating cause-and-effect relationships. The most common type of randomized controlled trial is the clinical trial, which is frequently used to measure the efficacy of medications. The statistical technique of meta-analysis allows psychologists and epidemiologists to combine the results of many studies to develop a picture of the size of an effect.

4. How can scientists determine if a behavior causes a disease?

Seven criteria are used for determining a cause-and-effect relationship between a condition and a disease: (1) A dose–response relationship must exist between the condition and the disease, (2) the removal of the condition must reduce the prevalence or incidence of the disease, (3) the condition must precede the disease, (4) the causal relationship between the condition and the disease must be physiologically plausible, (5) research data must consistently reveal a relationship between the condition and the disease, (6) the strength of the relationship between the condition and the disease must be relatively high, and (7) the relationship between the condition and the disease must be based on well-designed studies.

5. **How do theory and measurement contribute to health psychology?**

Theories are important tools used by scientists to (1) generate research, (2) predict and explain research data, and (3) help the practitioner solve a variety of problems. Health psychologists use a variety of measurement instruments to assess behaviors and theoretical concepts. To be useful, these psychometric instruments must be both reliable and valid. Reliability is the extent to which an assessment device measures consistently, and validity is the extent to which an assessment instrument measures what it is supposed to measure.

Suggested Readings

Kertesz, L. (2003). The numbers behind the news. *Healthplan, 44*(5), 10–14, 16, 18. Louise Kertesz offers a thoughtful analysis of the problems of reporting the findings from health research and gives some tips for understanding findings from research studies, including a definition of some of the terminology used in epidemiology research.

Price, D. D., Finniss, D. G., & Benedetti, F. (2008). A comprehensive review of the placebo effect: Recent advances and current thought. *Annual Review of Psychology, 59,* 565–590. This article by one of the leading researchers on the topic of placebo effects describes research on how placebos may work to effect cures.

Russo, E. (2004, August 2). New views on mind–body connection. *The Scientist, 18*(15), 28. This short article describes current research on the placebo and how high-tech methods allow the investigation of brain responses to placebos.

CHAPTER 3

Seeking and Receiving Health Care

CHAPTER OUTLINE

- Real-World Profile of Lance Armstrong
- *Seeking Medical Attention*
- *Seeking Medical Information from Nonmedical Sources*
- *Receiving Medical Care*

QUESTIONS

This chapter focuses on three basic questions:

1. What factors are related to seeking medical attention?

2. Where do people seek medical information?

3. What problems do people encounter in receiving medical care?

☑ Check Your HEALTH RISKS   *Regarding Seeking and Receiving Health Care*

☐ 1. If I feel well, I believe that I am healthy.

☐ 2. I see my dentist twice yearly for regular checkups.

☐ 3. The last time I sought medical care was in a hospital emergency room.

☐ 4. If I had a disease that would be a lot of trouble to manage, I would rather not know about it until I was really sick.

☐ 5. I try not to allow being sick to slow me down.

☐ 6. If I don't understand my physician's recommendations, I ask questions until I understand what I should do.

☐ 7. I think it's better to follow medical advice than to ask questions and cause problems, especially in the hospital.

☐ 8. When facing a stressful medical experience, I think the best strategy is to try not to think about it and hope that it will be over soon.

☐ 9. When I have severe symptoms, I try to find out as much information as possible about my medical condition.

☐ 10. I believe that if people get sick, it is because they were due to get sick, and there was nothing they could have done to prevent their sickness.

☐ 11. In order not to frighten patients faced with a difficult medical procedure, it is best to tell them that they won't be hurt, even if they will.

Items 2, 6, and 9 represent healthy attitudes or behaviors, but each of the other items relates to conditions that may present a risk or lead you to less effective health care. As you read this chapter, you will see the advantages of adopting healthy attitudes or behaviors to make more effective use of the health care system.

Real-World Profile of **LANCE ARMSTRONG**

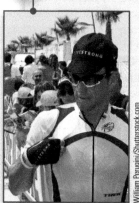

William Perugini/Shutterstock.com

Until 2012, Lance Armstrong was a source of inspiration for millions of people worldwide. He overcame a well-publicized battle with testicular cancer and went on to "win" five Tour de France cycling victories. Armstrong later confessed to using performance-enhancing drugs, his victories were erased, and his reputation instantly tarnished. However, his experience with cancer was what inspired many people, and is what makes his story worth telling here.

For most of his life, Armstrong was never accustomed to being unhealthy or out of shape. However, in 1996, his victory in the Tour DuPont worried some of his fans. Instead of pumping his fists in victory as he crossed the finish line, he looked unusually exhausted. His eyes were bloodshot and his face flushed. Later that year, he dropped out of the Tour de France after only 5 days.

Armstrong later confessed that he did not feel well during that year. He lost energy and suffered from coughs and lower-back pain. When these symptoms appeared, he attributed them to either the flu or a hard training season. He told himself at the time "Suck it up ... you can't afford to be tired" (Jenkins & Armstrong, 2001, "Before and After," paragraph 27).

However, his symptoms did not improve, even after rest. One evening, when he developed a severe headache, Armstrong attributed it to too many margaritas. His vision started to become blurry, but he attributed that to getting older.

Finally, a symptom emerged that he could not ignore: He began coughing up masses of metallic-tasting blood. After the first instance of this symptom, Armstrong called a good friend who happened to be a physician. His friend suggested that Armstrong might only be suffering from a cracked sinus. "Great, so it's no big deal," Armstrong replied, apparently relieved (Jenkins & Armstrong, 2001, "Before and After," paragraph 42).

The next day, Armstrong awoke to find his testicle swollen to the size of an orange. Rather than contact his doctor immediately, Armstrong hopped on his bike for another morning training ride. This time, he could not even manage to sit on the seat. Finally—after his symptoms prevented him doing what he loved most—he set up an appointment with a doctor.

That day, in early October 1996, Armstrong learned that he had Stage 3 testicular cancer. Due to his delays in seeking medical attention, Armstrong's cancer had already spread upwards to his lungs, abdomen, and brain. His doctors gave him only a 40% chance of survival, and he finally sought treatment for his cancer. Later, Armstrong confessed: "My dumb*** just ignored symptoms, obvious glaring symptoms, for a long time and it travelled all the way up" (Gibney, 2013).

Why did it take so long for Armstrong to seek care for his symptoms? His health was critical to his professional success. He was wealthy, could afford medical care, and had access to personal physicians and team doctors. Still, Armstrong resisted seeking medical care. He later wrote, "Of course I should have known that something was wrong with me. But athletes, especially cyclists, are in the business of denial. You deny all the aches and pains because you have to in order to finish the race … You do not give in to pain" (Jenkins & Armstrong, 2001, "Before and After," paragraph 21).

From 1996 to 1998, Lance Armstrong underwent chemotherapy and surgery on both his testicles and brain, and eventually his cancer went into remission. Armstrong is one of the lucky few survivors of advanced-stage cancer. His odds of survival would have surely been better had he sought medical care earlier.

Why do some people, such as Armstrong, seem to behave unwisely on issues of personal health? Why do others seek medical treatment when they are not ill? Psychologists have formulated several models in the attempt to predict and to make sense of behaviors related to health. This chapter looks briefly at some of these models as they relate to health-seeking behavior; Chapter 4 examines theory-driven research about people's adherence to medical advice.

Seeking Medical Attention

How do people know when to seek medical attention? How do they know whether they are ill or not? When Armstrong experienced symptoms that were likely caused by advancing cancer, he tried to ignore them, attributed them to anything but cancer, and consulted friends before making an appointment with a physician. Was Armstrong unusually reluctant to seek medical care, or was his behavior typical? Deciding when formal medical care is necessary is a complex problem, compounded by personal, social, and economic factors.

Before we consider these factors, we should define three terms: *health, disease,* and *illness.* Although the meaning of these concepts may seem obvious, their definitions are elusive. Is health the absence of illness, or is it the attainment of some positive state? In the first chapter, we saw that the World Health Organization (WHO) defines health as positive physical, mental, and social well-being, and not merely as the absence of disease or infirmity. Unfortunately, this definition has little practical value for people trying to make decisions about their state of health or illness, such as Armstrong's decision about whether to seek medical attention for his cancer-related symptoms.

Another difficulty for many people comes from understanding the difference between disease and illness. People often use these terms interchangeably, but most health scientists differentiate the two. Disease refers to the process of physical damage within the body, which can exist even in the absence of a label or diagnosis. Illness, on the other hand, refers to the experience of being sick and having a diagnosis of sickness. People can have a disease and not be ill. For example, people with undiagnosed hypertension, HIV infection, or cancer all have a disease, but they may appear quite healthy and be completely unaware of their disease. Although disease and illness are separate conditions, they often overlap—for example, when a person feels ill and has also received a diagnosis of a specific disease.

People frequently experience physical symptoms, but these symptoms may or may not indicate a disease.

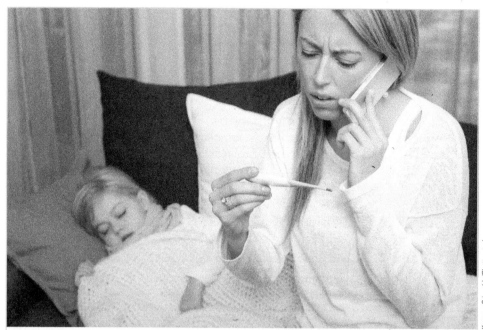

Illness behavior is directed toward determining health status.

Symptoms such as a headache, a painful shoulder, sniffles, or sneezing would probably not prompt a person to seek medical care, but an intense and persistent stomach pain probably would. At what point should a person decide to seek medical care? Errors in both directions are possible. People who decide to go to the doctor when they are not really sick feel foolish, must pay the bill for an office visit, and lose credibility with people who know about the error, including the physician. If they choose not to seek medical care, they may get better, but they may also get worse; trying to ignore their symptoms may make treatment more difficult and seriously endanger their health or increase their risk of death. A prudent action would seem to be to chance the unnecessary visit, but people (for a variety reasons) are often unable or simply reluctant to go to the doctor.

In the United States and other Western countries, people are not "officially" ill until they receive a diagnosis from a physician, making physicians the gatekeepers to further health care. Physicians not only *determine* disease by their diagnoses but also *sanction* it by giving a diagnosis. Hence, the person with symptoms is not the one who officially determines his or her health status.

Dealing with symptoms occurs in two stages, which Stanislav Kasl and Sidney Cobb (1966a, 1966b) called illness behavior and sick role behavior. **Illness behavior** consists of the activities undertaken by people who experience symptoms but who have not yet received a diagnosis. That is, illness behavior occurs *before* diagnosis. People engage in illness behaviors to determine their state of health and to discover suitable remedies. Armstrong was engaging in illness behavior when he sought the opinion of his friend and when he finally made an appointment with a physician. In contrast, **sick role behavior** is the term applied to the behavior of people after a diagnosis, whether from a health care provider or through self-diagnosis. People engage in sick role behavior in order to get well. Armstrong exhibited sick role behavior when he underwent surgery and chemotherapy, kept medical appointments, took a break from cycling, and recovered from his treatments. A *diagnosis*, then, is the event that separates illness behavior from sick role behavior.

Illness Behavior

The goal of illness behavior, which takes place before an official diagnosis, is to determine health status in the presence of symptoms. People routinely experience symptoms that may signal disease, such as chest pain, soreness, or headaches. Symptoms are a critical element in seeking medical care, but the presence of symptoms is not sufficient to prompt a visit to the doctor. Given similar symptoms, some people readily

TABLE 3.1   Factors that Relate to Health Care Seeking

Factor	Findings	Studies
1. Personal factors	Stress, anxiety, and neuroticism all predict greater health care seeking.	Martin & Brantley, 2004; Friedman et al., 2013
2. Gender	Women tend to seek health care more than men.	Galdas et al., 2005; Svendsen et al., 2013.
3. Age	Young adults delay seeking health care, and older adults delay when symptoms appear to be due to aging.	Ryan & Zerwic, 2003.
4. Socioeconomic, ethnic, and cultural factors	People lower in socioeconomic status and ethnic minorities are less likely to seek health care.	Martins et al., 2013.
5. Stigma	People with embarrassing or stigmatized conditions are less likely to seek care.	Barth et al., 2002; Carter-Harris et al., 2014; Wang et al., 2014.
6. Symptom characteristics	Symptoms that are visible, are perceived as severe, interfere with life, and are continuous are more likely to prompt seeking of care.	Unger-Saldaña & Infante-Castañeda, 2011; Quinn, 2005; Irwin et al., 2008.

seek help, others do so reluctantly, and still others do not seek help at all. What determines people's decision to seek professional care?

At least six conditions shape people's response to symptoms (see Table 3.1): (1) personal factors; (2) gender; (3) age; (4) socioeconomic, ethnic, and cultural factors; (5) characteristics of the symptoms; and (6) conceptualization of disease.

Personal Factors   Personal factors include people's way of viewing their own body, their level of stress, and their personality traits. An example comes from people who experience irritable bowel syndrome, an intestinal condition characterized by pain, cramping, constipation, and diarrhea. Stress makes this condition worse. Some people with irritable bowel syndrome seek medical services, whereas many others do not. Interestingly, a person's level of symptoms is *not* the most important reason somebody seeks medical care (Ringström, Abrahamsson, Strid, & Simrén, 2007). Instead, a person typically seeks medical care because of anxiety concerning the condition, coping resources, and level of physical functioning. Those who have adequate resources to cope with the symptoms and feel that the quality of their lives is not too impaired do not seek medical care. These psychological factors are more important than the prominence of symptoms in determining who seeks medical care.

Stress is another personal factor in people's readiness to seek care. People who experience a great deal of stress are more likely to seek health care than those under less stress, even with equal symptoms. Those who experience current or ongoing stress are more likely to seek care when symptoms are ambiguous (Cameron, Leventhal, & Leventhal, 1995; Martin & Brantley, 2004). Ironically, other people are *less* likely to view somebody as having a disease if the person also complains about stress, as others tend to perceive symptoms that coincide with stress as not real. This discounting occurs selectively, with women under high stress judged as less likely to have a physical disease than men in the same circumstances (Chiaramonte & Friend, 2006). This may be particularly true for male physicians who are less likely than female physicians to recommend cardiac testing for women who complain of chest pain (Napoli, Choo, & McGregor, 2014). This tendency to discount symptoms may be a very important factor in the treatment of women who experience symptoms and for the health care providers who hear their reports.

Personality traits also contribute to illness behavior. In a unique and interesting study headed by Sheldon Cohen (Feldman, Cohen, Gwaltney, Doyle, & Skoner, 1999), investigators administered a common cold virus to a group of healthy volunteers to see if participants with different personality traits would report symptoms differently. Participants who scored high on **neuroticism**—that is, those with strong and often negative emotional reactions—generally had high self-reports of illness whether or not objective evidence confirmed their reports. These people also reported more symptoms than other participants, suggesting that people high in the personality trait of neuroticism are more likely to complain of an illness. Not surprisingly, then, people high in the personality trait of neuroticism are more likely to seek medical care than those low in neuroticism (Friedman, Veazie, Chapman, Manning, & Duberstein, 2013).

Gender Differences   In addition to personal factors, gender plays a role in the decision to seek treatment, with women more likely than men to use health care (Galdas, Cheater, & Marshall, 2005). The reasons for this difference are somewhat complex. Women tend to report more body symptoms and distress than men (Koopmans & Lamers, 2007). When asked about their symptoms, men tend to report only life-threatening situations, such as heart disease (Benyamini, Leventhal, & Leventhal, 2000). In contrast, women report not only these symptoms but also non-life-threatening symptoms, such as those from joint disease. Given the same level of symptoms, the female gender role may make it easier for women to seek many sorts of assistance, whereas the male gender role teaches men to act strong and to deny pain and discomfort (as Armstrong did). Indeed, men are more likely than women to delay seeking health care for symptoms that might indicate cancer (Svendsen et al., 2013).

Age   Young adults feel healthy and indestructible, and as such, they show the greatest reluctance to see a health professional. However, as young adults age, they are more likely to seek care for health complaints. Why? As you might imagine, age is inextricably tied to both the development of physical symptoms as well as to people's interpretations of those symptoms.

As people age, they must decide whether their symptoms are due to aging or the result of disease. This distinction is not always easy, as Armstrong incorrectly attributed his blurred vision to the aging process rather than to the cancer that had invaded his brain. In general, people tend to interpret problems with a gradual onset and mild symptoms as resulting from age, whereas they are more ready to see problems with a sudden onset and severe symptoms as being more serious. For example, when older patients with symptoms of acute myocardial infarction can attribute these symptoms to age,

they tend to delay in seeking medical care. One study (Ryan & Zerwic, 2003) looked at patients who failed to realize that a delay in seeking health care could bring about more severe symptoms as well as increased chance of mortality. Compared with younger and middle-aged patients, these older people were more likely to (1) attribute their symptoms to age, (2) experience more severe and lengthy symptoms, (3) attribute their symptoms to some other disorder, and (4) have had previous experience with cardiac problems. Thus, people may be less willing to seek help for symptoms that they view as simply a natural part of aging.

Socioeconomic, Ethnic, and Cultural Factors   People from different cultures and ethnic backgrounds have disparate ways of viewing illness and different patterns of seeking medical care. In the United States, people in higher socioeconomic groups experience fewer symptoms and report a higher level of health than people at lower socioeconomic levels (Matthews & Gallo, 2011; Stone, Krueger, Steptoe, & Harter, 2010). Yet when higher-income people are sick, they are more likely to seek medical care. Nevertheless, poor people are over-represented among the hospitalized, an indication that they are much more likely than middle- and upper-income people to become seriously ill. In addition, people in lower socioeconomic groups tend to wait longer before seeking health care, thus making treatment more difficult and hospitalization more likely. The poor have less access to medical care, have to travel longer to reach health care facilities that will offer them treatment, and must wait longer once they arrive at those facilities. Thus, poor people utilize medical care less than wealthier people; when poor people do utilize medical care, their illnesses are typically more severe.

Ethnic background is another factor in seeking health care, with European Americans being more likely than other groups to report a visit to a physician. Part of the National Health and Nutrition Examination Survey (Harris, 2001) examined some of the reasons behind these ethnic differences, comparing European Americans, African Americans, and Mexican Americans with Type 2 diabetes on access to and use of health care facilities. Ethnic differences appeared in health insurance coverage as well as in common risk factors for diabetes and heart disease. Similarly, ethnic differences in insurance coverage account for ethnic differences in the use of dental health care (Doty & Weech-Maldonado, 2003). However, even in countries where access to health care is not dependent on private health insurance, ethnic minorities tend to show longer delays until diagnosis for cancer-related symptoms (Martins, Hamilton, & Ukoumunne, 2013).

A study from the United Kingdom confirmed the notion that culture and ethnic background—not lack of knowledge—are primarily responsible for differences in seeking medical care. In this study (Adamson, BenShlomo, Chaturvedi, & Donovan, 2003), researchers sent questionnaires to a large, diverse group of participants. Each questionnaire included two clinical vignettes showing (1) people experiencing signs of chest pain and (2) people discovering a lump in their armpit. The experimenters asked each participant to respond to the chest pain and the lump in terms of needing immediate care. Results indicated that respondents who were Black, female, and from lower socioeconomic groups were at least as likely as those who were White, male, and from middle- and upper-class groups to make accurate responses to potential medical problems. That is, poor Black women do not lack information about the potential health hazards of chest pain or a lump in the armpit, but they are more likely to lack the resources to respond quickly to these symptoms. Ethnic minorities are also more likely to experience discrimination in their everyday lives, and those who perceive discrimination are less likely to utilize the health care system (Burgess, Ding, Hargreaves, van Ryn, & Phelan, 2008).

Stigma Some people may neglect to seek help for medical problems because of the stigma associated with a disease. Stigma may occur because a person is embarrassed about the condition itself or because the person is embarrassed about the manner in which he or she may have contracted the condition. Indeed, stigma tends to delay health care seeking for conditions that may be a source of embarrassment, such as incontinence (Wang et al., 2014) or sexually transmitted diseases (Barth et al., 2002). Stigma may also prevent some people, particularly smokers, from seeking care for symptoms related to lung cancer. In one study, people who perceived greater stigma associated with lung cancer waited longer to seek care for initial symptoms of lung cancer (Carter-Harris et al., 2014). Stigma associated with lung cancer may be a particular issue for smokers, as smokers are less likely than nonsmokers to seek help for symptoms that might indicate lung cancer (Smith, Whitaker, Winstanley, & Wardle, 2016), possibly because of fears of negative evaluations from physicians or being blamed for the disease.

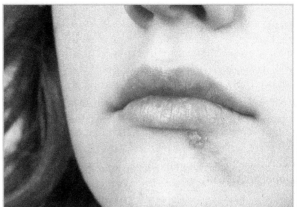
People are more likely to seek care for symptoms that are visible to others.

Symptom Characteristics Symptom characteristics also influence when and how people look for help. Symptoms do not inevitably lead people to seek care, but certain characteristics are important in their response to symptoms. David Mechanic (1978) listed four characteristics of the symptoms that determine people's response to disease.

First is the *visibility of the symptom*—that is, how readily apparent the symptom is to the person and to others. Many of Armstrong's symptoms were not visible to others, including his enlarged testes. In a study of Mexican women who had symptoms of possible breast cancer, those whose symptoms were more visible were more likely to seek medical help (Unger-Saldaña & Infante-Castañeda, 2011). Unfortunately, with many diseases such as breast cancer or testicular cancer, the condition may be worse and treatment options more limited once symptoms become visible.

Mechanic's second symptom characteristic is *perceived severity of the symptom*. According to Mechanic, symptoms seen as severe would be more likely to prompt action than less severe symptoms. Armstrong did not seek immediate medical care partially because he did not see some of his symptoms as serious—he viewed them as the result of the flu or his exhausting training regimen. The perceived severity of the symptom highlights the importance of personal perception and distinguishes between the perceived severity of a symptom and the judgment of severity by medical authorities. Indeed, patients and physicians differ in their perceptions of the severity of a wide variety of symptoms (Peay & Peay, 1998). Symptoms that patients perceive as more serious produce greater concern and a stronger belief that treatment is urgently needed, as a study on women seeking care after experiencing symptoms of heart attack demonstrates (Quinn, 2005). Those women who interpreted their symptoms as indicative of cardiac problems sought care more quickly than women who interpreted their symptoms as some other condition. Thus, perceived severity of symptoms rather than the presence of symptoms is critical in the decision to seek care.

The third symptom characteristic mentioned by Mechanic is the *extent to which the symptom interferes with a person's life*. The more incapacitated the person, the more likely he or she is to seek medical care. Studies on irritable bowel syndrome (Ringström et al., 2007) and overactive bladder (Irwin, Milsom, Kopp, Abrams, & EPIC Study Group, 2008) illustrate this principle; those who seek medical care report a poorer health quality of life than those who do not seek medical care. Armstrong sought attention for his cancer-related symptoms only when they interfered with his ability to ride his bicycle.

Mechanic's fourth hypothesized determinant of illness behavior is the *frequency and persistence of the symptoms*. Conditions that people view as requiring care tend to be those that are both severe and continuous, whereas intermittent symptoms are less likely to generate illness behavior. Severe symptoms—such as coughing up blood, as Armstrong experienced—prompt people to seek help, but even mild symptoms can motivate people to seek help if those symptoms persist.

In Mechanic's description and subsequent research, symptom characteristics alone are not sufficient to prompt illness behavior. However, if symptoms persist or are perceived as severe, people are more likely to evaluate them as indicating a need for care. Thus, people seek care not on the basis of their objective symptoms but rather on the basis of their *interpretation* of their symptoms, highlighting the key role that beliefs and perceptions play in the process of seeking health care.

Conceptualization of Disease   Most people are not experts in physiology or medicine, and are largely unaware of how their body works and how disease develops. People think about diseases in ways that vary substantially from medical explanations. For example, both children (Veldtman et al., 2001) and college students (Nemeroff, 1995) show inaccurate and incomplete understandings of diseases when they describe diseases they have and how they became ill. For example, in one study, college students thought that symptoms of the flu

would be less serious if they contracted the virus from a lover rather than from someone they despised (Nemeroff, 1995)! (A virus is a virus regardless of how you get it.) Thus, people may seek (or not seek) medical care based on their incomplete and sometimes inaccurate beliefs about health and illness.

What are the important ways in which people conceptualize, or think about, diseases? Howard Leventhal and his colleagues (Leventhal, Breland, Mora, & Leventhal, 2010; Leventhal, Leventhal, & Cameron, 2001; Martin & Leventhal, 2004) have looked at five components in the conceptualization process: (1) identity of the disease, (2) time line (the time course of both disease and treatment), (3) cause of the disease, (4) consequences of the disease, and (5) controllability of the disease. Because most people are not medical experts, their beliefs about these components may not always be accurate. Yet, these beliefs have important implications for how people seek care and manage a disease.

The *identity of the disease,* the first component identified by Leventhal and his colleagues, is very important to illness behavior. People who have identified their symptoms as a "heart attack" should (Martin & Leventhal, 2004) and do (Quinn, 2005) react quite differently from those who label the same symptoms as "heartburn." As we have seen, the presence of symptoms is not sufficient to initiate help seeking, but the labeling that occurs in conjunction with symptoms may be critical in a person's either seeking help or ignoring symptoms.

Labels provide a framework within which people can recognize and interpret symptoms. In one study, Leventhal and his team gave young adults a blood pressure test and randomly assigned them to receive one of two results: high blood pressure or normal blood pressure (Baumann, Cameron, Zimmerman, & Leventhal, 1989). Compared with the young adults who received results labeled as normal blood pressure, those who received results labeled as high blood pressure were more likely to subsequently report other symptoms related to hypertension. In other words, the label made them report other symptoms consistent with their diagnosis.

People experience less emotional arousal when they find a label that indicates a minor problem (heartburn rather than heart attack). Initially, they will probably adopt the least serious label that fits their symptoms. For example, Armstrong interpreted headaches as hangovers and blurred vision as a normal part of aging. Armstrong—as well as his physician friend—also preferred to interpret his blood-expelling coughs as a sinus problem rather than something more severe. To a large extent, a label carries with it some prediction about the symptoms and time course of the disease, so if the symptoms and time course do not correspond to the expectation implied by the label, the person has to relabel the symptoms. When a swollen testicle became another prominent symptom, Armstrong quickly realized that he had more than merely a sinus problem. Thus, the tendency to interpret symptoms as indicating minor rather than major problems is the source of many optimistic self-diagnoses, of which Armstrong's is an example.

The second component in conceptualizing an illness is the *time line*. Even though a diagnosis usually implies the time course of a disease, people's understanding of the time involved is not necessarily accurate. People with a chronic disorder often view their disease as acute and of short duration. For example, patients with heart disease (a chronic disorder) may see their disease as "heartburn," an acute disorder (Martin & Leventhal, 2004). With most acute diseases, patients can expect a temporary disorder with a quick onset of symptoms, followed by treatment, a remission of symptoms, and then a cure. In fact, people who conceptualize their illness as an acute disorder tend to manage their symptoms better (Horne et al., 2004). Unfortunately, this scenario does not fit the majority of diseases, such as heart disease and diabetes, which are chronic and persist over a lifetime. In a study of adults with diabetes, those who conceptualized their illness as acute rather than chronic managed their illness worse, likely because they took medications only when acute symptoms were present (Mann, Ponieman, Leventhal, & Halm, 2009). However, conceptualizing a chronic disease as time limited may provide patients with some psychological comfort; patients who conceptualize their cancer as chronic report greater distress than those who view the disease as an acute illness (Rabin, Leventhal, & Goodin, 2004).

The third component in conceptualizing an illness is the *determination of cause*. For the most part, determining causality is more a facet of the sick role than of illness behavior because it usually occurs after a diagnosis has been made. But the attribution of causality for symptoms is an important factor in illness behavior. For example, if a person can attribute the pain in his hand to a blow received the day before, he will not have to consider the possibility of bone cancer as the cause of the pain.

Attribution of causality, however, is often faulty. People may attribute a cold to "germs" or to the weather, and they may see cancer as caused by microwave ovens or by the will of God. These conceptualizations have important implications for illness behavior. People are less likely to seek professional treatment for conditions they consider as having emotional or spiritual causes. Culture may also play a role in attributions of causes for diseases. Cultural differences appeared in a study that compared Britons' and Taiwanese beliefs about heart disease: Britons were more likely to see heart disease as caused by lifestyle choices, whereas Taiwanese were more likely to see heart disease as caused by worry and stress (Lin, Furze, Spilsbury, & Lewin, 2009). It is reasonable to expect that someone who views heart disease as due to lifestyle will manage the illness differently than someone who views it as due to stress. Therefore, people's conceptualizations of disease causality can influence their behavior.

The *consequences of a disease* are the fourth component in Leventhal's description of illness. Even though the consequences of a disease are implied by the diagnosis, an incorrect understanding of the consequences can have a profound effect on illness behavior. Many people view a diagnosis of cancer as a death sentence. Some neglect health care because they believe themselves to be in a hopeless situation. Women who find a lump in their breast sometimes delay making an appointment with a doctor, not because they fail to recognize this symptom of cancer but because they fear the possible consequences—surgery and possibly the loss of a breast, chemotherapy, radiation, or some combination of these consequences.

The *controllability* of a disease refers to people's belief that they can control the course of their illness by controlling the treatment or the disease. People who believe that their behaviors will not change the course of a disease are more distressed by their illness and less likely to seek treatment than those who believe that treatment will be effective (Evans & Norman, 2009; Hagger & Orbell, 2003). However, people who are able to control the symptoms of their disease without medical consultation will be less likely to seek professional medical care (Ringström et al., 2007).

In sum, the five beliefs in Leventhal's model predict several important outcomes, including distress, seeking of health care, and disease management. Can changing these beliefs improve health outcomes? A recent study of asthma sufferers suggests that these components can be useful targets for intervention

(Petrie, Perry, Broadbent, & Weinman, 2011). In this study, researchers sent some asthma patients periodic text messages that accurately informed the patients of the identity, time line, cause, consequences, and controllability of asthma. Compared with a control group, patients who received the text message intervention reported more accurate beliefs about their asthma, as well as much better management of their condition. Thus, the five beliefs in Leventhal's model are useful to understand why some people behave not only in unhealthy ways but also as targets for intervention to improve self-management.

The Sick Role

Kasl and Cobb (1966b) defined sick role behavior as the activities engaged in by people who believe themselves ill, for the purpose of getting well. In other words, sick role behavior occurs after a person receives a diagnosis. Alexander Segall (1997) expanded this concept, proposing that the sick role concept includes three rights or privileges and three duties or responsibilities. The privileges are (1) the right to make decisions concerning health-related issues, (2) the right to be exempt from normal duties, and (3) the right to become dependent on others for assistance. The three responsibilities are (1) the duty to maintain health along with the responsibility to get well, (2) the duty to perform routine health care management, and (3) the duty to use a range of health care resources.

Segall's formulation of rights and duties is an ideal—not a realistic—conception of sick role behavior in the United States. The first right—to make decisions concerning health-related issues—does not extend to children and many people living in poverty (Bailis, Segall, Mahon, Chipperfield, & Dunn, 2001). The second feature of the sick role is the exemption of the sick person from normal duties. Sick people are usually not expected to go to work, attend school, go to meetings, cook meals, clean house, care for children, do homework, or mow the lawn. However, meeting these expectations is not always possible. Many sick people neither stay home nor go to the hospital but continue to go to work. People who feel in danger of losing their jobs are more likely to go to work when they are sick (Bloor, 2005), but so do those who experience good working relationships with their colleagues and are dedicated to their jobs (Biron, Brun, Ivers, & Cooper, 2006). Similarly, the third privilege—to be dependent on others—is more of an ideal than a reflection of reality. For example,

sick mothers often must continue to be responsible for their children.

Segall's three duties of sick people all fall under the single obligation to do whatever is necessary to get well. However, the goal of getting well applies more to acute than to chronic diseases. People with chronic diseases will never be completely well. This situation presents a conflict for many people with a chronic disease, who have difficulty accepting their condition as one of continuing disability; instead, they erroneously believe that their disease is a temporary state.

IN SUMMARY

No easy distinction exists between health and illness. The WHO sees health as more than the absence of disease; rather, health is the attainment of positive physical, mental, and social well-being. Curiously, the distinction between disease and illness is clearer. Disease refers to the process of physical damage within the body, whether or not the person is aware of this damage. Illness, on the other hand, refers to the experience of being sick; people can feel sick but have no identifiable disease.

At least six factors determine how people respond to illness symptoms: (1) personal factors, such as the way people look upon their own body, their stress, and their personality; (2) gender—women are more likely than men to seek professional care; (3) age—older people attribute many ailments to their age; (4) ethnic and cultural factors—people who cannot afford medical care are more likely than affluent people to become ill but less likely to seek health care; (5) stigma—people often delay seeking care for conditions that are shameful or embarrassing; (6) characteristics of the symptoms—symptoms that interfere with daily activities as well as visible, severe, and frequent symptoms are most likely to prompt medical attention; and (7) people's conceptualization of disease.

People tend to incorporate five components into their concept of disease: (1) the identity of the disease, (2) the time line of the disease, (3) the cause of the disease, (4) the consequences of the disease, and (5) the controllability of the disease. If a patient receives a diagnosis of a disease, the diagnosis implies its time course and its consequences. However, people who know the name of their disease do not always have an accurate concept of its time course and consequence and may wrongly see a chronic disease as having a short time course. People want to know the cause of their illness and to understand how they can control it, but beliefs that an illness is uncontrollable may lead people to neglect treatment.

After receiving a diagnosis, people engage in sick role behavior in order to get well. People who are sick should be relieved from normal responsibilities and should have the obligation of trying to get well. However, these rights and duties are difficult and often impossible to fulfill.

Seeking Medical Information from Nonmedical Sources

After people notice symptoms that they perceive as being a potential problem, they must decide whether and how to seek help. People's first step in seeking health care, however, is often not to seek help from a doctor. Instead, people often turn to two more easily accessible sources—their lay referral network and the Internet.

Lay Referral Network

When Armstrong finally decided to seek advice about his symptoms, he did not immediately go to a specialist. Instead, he consulted his friends, one of whom happened to be a physician. Armstrong's friends were part of his lay referral network, a network of family and friends who offer information and advice before any official medical treatment is sought (Friedson, 1961; Suls, Martin, & Leventhal, 1997). Like Armstrong, most people who seek health care do so as a result of prior conversations with friends and family about symptoms (Cornford & Cornford, 1999). For example, in the study of irritable bowel syndrome (Ringström et al., 2007), about half of those who did not seek medical care sought alternative care or the advice of someone with the same condition. Thus, most people sought help but not necessarily from a physician.

The lay referral network can help a person understand the meaning of symptoms, such as what its label, cause, and cure might be. A lay referral network can also prime a person's perception of symptoms. A woman with chest pain, for example, would react quite differently if her family had a history of heart attacks compared with a history of heartburn. In some cases, people in the lay referral network might advise *against* seeking medical care, particularly if they can recommend simple home remedies or recommend complementary and alternative treatments (see Chapter 8 for a review of complementary and alternative therapies). Thus, people's social networks are often a first source of information and advice on health matters but may not always encourage people to seek traditional medical care (Dimsdale et al., 1979).

The Internet

In recent years, the Internet has become an additional source of information for people who seek information and help with symptoms. Indeed, a majority of Internet users in the United States report using the Internet to search for health information for themselves (Atkinson, Saperstein, & Pleis, 2009) or for other people (Sadasivam et al., 2013). Women and those with higher education are more likely than others to use the Internet for this purpose (McCully, Don, & Updegraff, 2013; Powell, Inglis, Ronnie, & Large, 2011). In fact, public health researchers can use sudden increases in the number of Internet searches about specific disease symptoms to reliably identify outbreaks of infectious diseases in near real time (Ginsberg et al., 2009)!

The Internet is a common source of health information because it satisfies a number of motivations, such as to seek a greater understanding of a health issue, get a second opinion, seek reassurance, and overcome difficulties in getting health information through other sources (Amante et al., 2015; Powell et al., 2011). However, increased access to the Internet opens a vast source of medical information *and* misinformation to the public (Wald, Dube, & Anthony, 2007) (see "Would You Believe …?" box). One of the challenges that Internet users face is how to distinguish trustworthy websites from those that are simply trying to sell health products. Many people use Wikipedia as a primary source of health information (Laurent & Vickers, 2009), despite the fact that the information on Wikipedia may not be as accurate as other sources. Excellent and credible sources of health information include the Center for Advancing Health website (www.cfah.org) and the National Institutes of Health website (health.nih.gov). Chapter 2 also includes helpful tips on how to identify valid health information on the Internet.

Patients who go to the web for information become more active in their health care, but this knowledge may

Would You BELIEVE...?   There Is Controversy about Childhood Vaccinations

In 1980, prior to widespread vaccination for measles, the contagious virus killed approximately 2.6 million people each year. Following widespread vaccination, measles-related deaths have declined to the point that few people in developed countries don't even know what measles is. However, measles-related deaths still occur in regions where vaccination rates are low. In fact, measles remains the leading cause of vaccine-preventable death among children worldwide.

Why, then, is vaccination for measles such an emotionally charged and controversial issue for many people? Why do many parents feel it is safer to not immunize their children? How did this controversy arise, and why might it continue?

The controversy began in 1998, when Andrew Wakefield published a study about 12 children who experienced the sudden onset of gastrointestinal problems and autism-related symptoms (Wakefield et al., 1998, later retracted). Parents or doctors of 8 of those 12 children stated that the symptoms started soon after the child received the measles, mumps, and rubella (MMR) vaccination.

Children typically receive the first dose of an MMR vaccination in their first 2 years of life. This is also the time when parents or doctors usually begin to notice symptoms of autism in children. Thus, it is expected that some parents would observe symptoms of autism develop around the same time as an MMR vaccination. If some parents notice this *correlation*, it may be easy for them to conclude that the vaccination *caused* autism.

Did the MMR vaccine cause autism among 8 of the 12 children in Wakefield's study? Wakefield's study raised this question, but it was a small study of a dozen children, and after investigation, serious questions about the validity of Wakefield's data were raised and the study was retracted. Spurred by the controversy of Wakefield's paper, nearly a dozen large epidemiological studies have tackled this question, including one that examined over 500,000 children (Madsen et al., 2002). None of these later studies found *any* evidence that children who receive an MMR vaccination show higher risk for autism than those who do not. If Wakefield's study of 12 children detected a valid association between vaccination and autism, then surely a study of half a million children should find the same association as well. But it, and many other studies, did not.

Why, then, do questions about the safety of vaccinations persist? Several explanations exist. First, some of most outspoken anti-vaccination critics are celebrities with a high degree of media exposure, such as actors Jim Carrey and Jenny McCarthy (whose own son was diagnosed with autism). Second, the exact cause of autism is unknown, and no cure currently exists. When medical research offers few answers, people often look to nonmedical sources, the Internet, and social media for answers.

The Internet and social media can be sources of both information and misinformation. One study found that *less than half* of the websites that resulted from a Google search of "Is there a link between MMR and autism?" provided scientifically accurate answers to the question (Scullard, Peacock, & Davies, 2010). Social media sites—such as Facebook or blogs—offer emotional accounts of personal experiences with vaccinations or autism, which most often focus on perceived harms of vaccines (Betsch et al., 2012). Decades of research in the field of persuasion show that personal stories and narratives are more engaging and powerful—regardless of accuracy—than drier, more scientifically based information. Thus, for a parent searching for information about MMR vaccination, the Internet and other media outlets may be powerful sources of misinformation. Furthermore, people tend to seek out information that confirms—rather than disconfirms—their beliefs, making people resistant to new information that contradicts their views.

This misinformation may lead many parents to forego vaccination for their children. When vaccination rates decrease, the public is at increased risk for contracting measles. In fact, for a highly contagious virus such as measles, 90–95% of a population needs to be vaccinated in order for the population to avoid exposure to the disease. Even small decreases in vaccination rates can lead to outbreaks of a disease, as occurred in 2015 when nearly 150 visitors to an amusement park in California contracted measles. This outbreak was likely due to a single person who contracted measles overseas and unknowingly transmitted it to others who were not vaccinated.

Thus, the controversy over childhood vaccinations highlights many key issues in seeking out medical information, including the persuasive power of anecdotal information over results from large-scale studies, people's need to find answers when few are available, as well as the difficulty that people often have in changing firmly held views in the face of new information.

decrease physicians' authority and change the nature of the physician–patient relationship. When patients bring information to the physician that the physician views as accurate and relevant, then the relationship can benefit (Murray et al., 2003). However, when the patient brings information that is not accurate or relevant, it can deteriorate the relationship and challenge the physician's authority. Many patients are reluctant to bring up Internet health information with their providers out of fear of challenging the provider (Imes et al., 2008). Thus, the Internet is an important source of health information, and patients who do not have access to accurate and relevant information may not be in as good position to be effective users of the medical system (Hall & Schneider, 2008).

Receiving Medical Care

Most people have experience in receiving medical care. In some situations, this experience may be satisfying; in other situations, people face challenges in receiving medical care. These problems include having only limited access to medical care, choosing the right practitioner, and being in the hospital.

Limited Access to Medical Care

The cost of medical care prevents many people from receiving proper treatment and care. This limited access to medical care is more restricted in the United States than in other industrialized nations (Weitz, 2010). Many countries have developed national health insurance or other plans for universal coverage, but the United States has typically resisted this strategy. Hospitalization and complex medical treatments are so expensive that most people cannot afford these services. This situation has led to the rise and development of health insurance, which people may purchase as individuals but more often obtain as part of workplace groups that offer coverage to their members.

Individual insurance tends to be expensive and to offer less coverage, especially for people with health problems, but these individuals may be able to get some insurance as part of a workplace group. Thus, employment is an important factor in access to medical care in the United States. People who are unemployed or whose jobs do not offer the benefit of health insurance are often uninsured, a situation describing about 11% of people in the United States (NCHS, 2016a). However, even people with insurance may face barriers to receiving care; their policies often fail to cover services such as dental care,

mental health services, and eyeglasses, forcing people to pay these expenses out of their own pockets or forego these services. For insured people who experience a catastrophic illness, coverage may be inadequate for many expenses, creating enormous medical costs. Indeed, medical costs are the underlying cause for over 60% of all personal bankruptcies in the United States (Himmelstein, Thorne, Warren, & Woolhandler, 2009).

The problem of providing medical care for those who cannot afford to pay for these services was a concern throughout the 20th century in the United States (Weitz, 2010). In response to these concerns, the U.S. Congress created two programs in 1965—Medicare and Medicaid. Medicare pays hospital expenses for most Americans over the age of 65, and thus few people in this age group are without hospitalization insurance. Medicare also offers medical insurance that those who participate may purchase for a monthly fee, but many expenses are not covered, such as routine dental care. Medicaid provides health care based on low income and physical problems, such as disability or pregnancy. These restrictions make many poor people ineligible; only about half of people living in poverty receive coverage through Medicaid (NCHS, 2016a). Children may be eligible for health insurance, even if their parents are not, through the State Children's Health Insurance Program.

People with low incomes struggle to obtain insurance coverage, but even those with insurance may face barriers such as finding a provider who will accept their plan and the out-of-pocket cost of services (Carrillo et al., 2011; DeVoe et al., 2007). The uninsured face more restrictions. These people are less likely to have a regular physician, more likely to have a chronic health problem, and less likely to seek medical care because of the cost (Finkelstein et al., 2011; Pauly & Pagán, 2007). This reluctance has consequences for the management of their diseases. People with chronic diseases and without health insurance have poorly controlled conditions, difficulty in obtaining medications, more health crises, and higher risk of mortality than people with insurance (McWilliams, 2009). In addition, a high proportion of people without insurance may create a spillover effect in which those with insurance experience higher costs and poorer quality of care. Thus, health insurance is an important issue in the access to medical care and plays a role in choosing a practitioner.

Choosing a Practitioner

As part of their attempts to get well, sick people usually consult a health care practitioner. Beginning during the

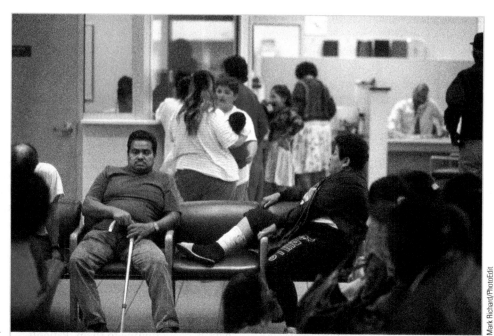

Cost and accessibility of services present barriers to obtaining health care.

19th century, physicians became the dominant medical providers (Weitz, 2010). Most middle-class and wealthy people in industrialized nations seek the services of a physician. Toward the end of the 20th century, however, medical dominance began to decline, and other types of health care providers' popularity rose. For example, midwives, nurses, pharmacists, physical therapists, psychologists, osteopaths, chiropractors, dentists, nutritionists, and herbal healers all provide various types of health care.

Some of these sources of health care are considered "alternative" because they provide alternatives to conventional medical care. Almost a third of U.S. residents who seek conventional health care also use some form of alternative health care, and nearly everyone (96%) who uses alternative health care also uses conventional health care (Weitz, 2010). Some people who consult practitioners such as herbal healers do so because these healers are part of a cultural tradition, such as *curanderos* in Latin American culture. However, the recent growth of alternative medicine has come mainly from well-educated people who are dissatisfied with standard medical care and who hold attitudes that are compatible with the alternative care they seek (Weitz, 2010). Well-educated people are more likely to turn to alternative medicine because they are better able to pay for this care, which is less likely to be covered by insurance than conventional care.

People without health insurance are less likely to have a regular health care provider than are those with insurance (Pauly & Pagán, 2007). People who do not have health insurance may receive care from convenient care clinics or hospital emergency rooms, even for chronic conditions. Convenient care clinics offer basic health care, primarily by physicians' assistants and nurse practitioners (Hanson-Turton, Ryan, Miller, Counts, & Nash, 2007). Seeking care through the emergency room may result in people receiving care only after their condition meets the definition of an emergency. Thus, these patients are sicker than they might have been if they had easier access to care. In addition, seeking care from emergency rooms is more expensive and overburdens these facilities, decreasing their ability to provide care to those with acute conditions.

Practitioner–Patient Interaction   The interaction between a patient and practitioner is an important consideration in receiving medical care. Practitioners who are successful in forming a working alliance with their patients are more likely to have patients who are satisfied (Fuertes et al., 2007). A satisfying patient–practitioner relationship offers important practical benefits: Satisfied patients are more likely to follow medical advice (Fuertes et al., 2007), more likely to continue to use medical services and obtain checkups, and less likely to file complaints against their practitioners (Stelfox, Gandhi, Orav, & Gustafson, 2005). Important factors in building successful practitioner–patient alliances include verbal communication and the practitioner's personal characteristics.

Verbal Communication   Poor verbal communication is perhaps the most crucial factor in practitioner-patient interaction (Cutting Edge Information, 2004). In fact, patients are significantly less likely to follow a practitioner's medical advice when the practitioner communicates poorly (Ratanawongsa et al., 2013; Zolnierek & DiMatteo, 2009). Communication problems may arise when physicians ask patients to report on their symptoms but fail to listen to patients' concerns, interrupting their stories within seconds (Galland, 2006). What constitutes a concern for the patient may not be essential to the diagnostic process, and the practitioner may simply be trying to elicit information relevant to making a diagnosis. However, patients may misinterpret the physician's behavior as a lack of personal concern or as overlooking what patients consider important symptoms. After practitioners have made a diagnosis, they typically tell patients about that diagnosis. If the diagnosis is minor, patients may be relieved and not highly motivated to adhere to (or even listen to) any instructions that may follow. If the verdict is serious, patients may become anxious or frightened, and these feelings may then interfere with their concentration on subsequent medical advice. The patient–practitioner interaction is especially important at this juncture: When patients do not receive information that they have requested, they feel less satisfied with their physician and are less likely to comply with the advice they receive (Bell, Kravitz, Thom, Krupat, & Azari, 2002). However, when patients believe that physicians understand their reasons for seeking treatment and that both agree about treatment, they are more likely to comply with medical advice (Kerse et al., 2004).

For a variety of reasons, physicians and patients frequently do not speak the same language. First, physicians operate in familiar territory. They know the subject matter, are comfortable with the physical surroundings, and are ordinarily calm and relaxed with procedures that have become routine to them. Patients, in contrast, are often unfamiliar with medical terminology (Castro, Wilson, Wang, & Schillinger, 2007); distracted by the strange environment; and distressed by anxiety, fear, or pain

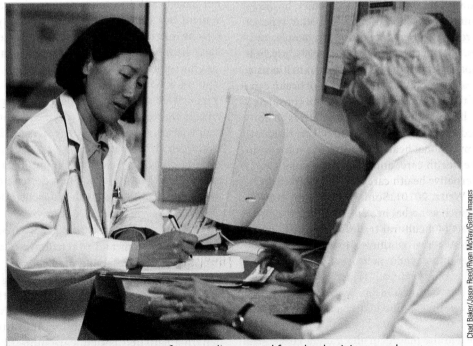

Communication is important for compliance, and female physicians tend to encourage interaction and communication.

Chad Baker/Jason Reed/Ryan McVay/Getty Images

(Charlee, Goldsmith, Chambers, & Haynes, 1996). In some cases, practitioners and patients do not speak the same language—literally. Differences in native language present a major barrier to communication (Blanchard & Lurie, 2004; Flores, 2006). Even with interpreters, substantial miscommunication may occur (Rosenberg, Leanza, & Seller, 2007). As a result, patients either fail to understand or to remember significant portions of the information their doctors give them.

The Practitioner's Personal Characteristics   A second aspect of the practitioner–patient interaction is the perceived personal characteristics of the physician. When people have the freedom to choose their practitioners, they value technical competence (Bendapudi, Berry, Frey, Parish, & Rayburn, 2006). However, because most patients lack medical training of their own, patients have difficulty judging the technical competence of practitioners. Instead, they often base their judgments of technical quality on a practitioner's personal characteristics. Behaviors that differentiate practitioners whom patients rate as providing excellent treatment include being confident, thorough, personable, humane, forthright, respectful, and empathetic. Female physicians are more likely to show these behaviors than male physicians. Two meta-analyses covering nearly 35 years of research (Hall, Blanch-Hartigan, & Roter, 2011; Roter & Hall, 2004) showed that female physicians were more patient centered, spent 10% more time with patients, employed more partnership behaviors, were more positive in their communication, engaged in more psychosocial counseling, asked more questions, used more emotionally focused talk, and were evaluated more highly by patients than male physicians. Moreover, the patients of female physicians were more likely to disclose more information about their medical symptoms as well as their psychological concerns. This research suggests that when choosing a physician, a person may wish to consider the physician's gender.

Indeed, people are more likely to follow the advice of doctors they see as warm, caring, friendly, and interested in the welfare of patients (DiNicola & DiMatteo, 1984). Alternatively, when patients believe that physicians look down on them or treat them with disrespect, patients are less likely to follow physicians' advice or keep medical appointments (Blanchard & Lurie, 2004). In fact, poor communication between the physician and patient may have a particularly detrimental effect on adherence when the physician and patient come from different ethnic backgrounds (Schoenthaler, Allegrante, Chaplin, & Ogedegbe, 2012).

Being in the Hospital

In serious cases, seeking health care may result in hospitalization. Over the past 30 years, hospitals and the experience of being in the hospital have both changed. First, many types of surgery and tests that were formerly handled through hospitalization are now performed on an outpatient basis. Second, hospital stays have become shorter. Third, an expanding array of technology is available for diagnosis and treatment. Fourth, patients feel increasingly free to voice their concerns to their physician (Bell, Kravitz, Thom, Krupat, & Azari, 2001). As a result of these changes, people who are not severely ill are not likely to be hospitalized, and people who are admitted to a hospital are more severely ill than those admitted 30 years ago.

Ironically, although managed care has helped control costs through shorter hospital stays, it has not always been in the interest of the patient. Technological medicine has become more prominent in patient care, and personal treatment by the hospital staff has become less so. These factors can combine to make hospitalization a stressful experience (Weitz, 2010). In addition, understaffing and the challenges of monitoring complex technology and medication regimens have created an alarming number of medical mistakes (see Would You Believe …? box).

The Hospital Patient Role   Part of the sick role is to be a patient, and being a patient means conforming to the rules of a hospital and complying with medical advice. When a person enters the hospital as a patient, that person becomes part of a complex institution and assumes a role within that institution. That role includes some difficult aspects: being treated as a "nonperson," tolerating lack of information, and losing control of daily activities. Patients find incidents such as waits, delays, and communication problems with staff distressing, and such incidents decrease patients' satisfaction (Weingart et al., 2006).

When people are hospitalized, all but their illness becomes invisible, and their status is reduced to that of a "nonperson." Not only are patients' identities ignored, but their comments and questions may also be overlooked. Hospital procedure focuses on the technical aspects of medical care; it usually ignores patients' emotional needs and leaves them less satisfied with their treatment than patients who are treated as persons, listened to, and informed about their condition (Boudreaux & O'Hea, 2004; Clever, Jin, Levinson, & Meltzer, 2008).

Would You BELIEVE...?   Hospitals May Be a Leading Cause of Death

Would you believe that receiving medical care, especially in an American hospital, can be fatal? Newspaper headlines have painted an alarming picture of the dangers of receiving health care, based on a series of studies. In 1999, a study from the Institute of Medicine made headlines with its findings that at least 44,000—and perhaps as many as 98,000—people die in U.S. hospitals every year as a result of medical errors (Kohn, Corrigan, & Donaldson, 1999). Later reports found even higher numbers of medical mistakes (HealthGrades, 2011; Zhan & Miller, 2003). Although the United States does not recognize medical error as a cause of death, the *Washington Post* (Weiss, 1999) calculated that medical errors are the fifth leading cause of death in the United States.

Unfortunately, medical errors aren't the only cause of unnecessary deaths of patients in U.S. hospitals. Medication, too, can be fatal. An Institute of Medicine study (Aspden, Wolcott, Bootman, & Cronenwett, 2007) estimated that hospitalized patients experience an average of one medication error per patient per day of hospitalization, resulting in morbidity, mortality, and increased cost of hospitalization. A meta-analysis of studies on adverse drug reactions (Lazarou, Pomeranz, & Corey, 1998) found that, even when prescribed and taken properly, prescription drugs account for between 76,000 and 137,000 deaths each year. This analysis included patients admitted to a hospital for an adverse drug reaction as well as those already in the hospital who suffered a fatal drug reaction. This meta-analysis also estimated the total number of toxic drug reactions among hospitalized patients at more than 2 million. Despite widespread publicity and growing concern, little improvement seems to have occurred during the past 15 years. The medical profession has achieved only limited progress toward solving the problem of medical errors (Leape & Berwick, 2005), and a recent study (HealthGrades, 2011) indicated that medical errors in hospitals have not decreased.

One barrier to correcting the situation comes from the climate of silence and blame that surrounds errors—health care professionals do not want to admit to errors or report colleagues who have made errors because of the blame involved. Rather than silence and blame, Lucian Leape (Leape & Berwick, 2005) suggested that hospitals should be eager to seek information about errors and that analysis should focus on the systems that allow errors rather than the people who make errors.

Interventions may be able to reduce the incidence of medical errors (Woodward et al., 2010). These include patient-focused interventions, such as encouraging patients to state their name to physicians and asking physicians whether they washed their hands. In addition, institutional interventions may also reduce medical errors, such as reducing the number of hours in a typical physician's or nurse's shift and implementing computer systems to better detect potential medication errors. The practice of medicine will never be free of errors, but creating systems that make errors more difficult to commit will improve patient safety and cut hospitalization costs.

The lack of information that patients experience comes from hospital routine rather than from an attempt to keep information from patients. Most physicians believe that patients should receive full information about their conditions. However, an open exchange of information between patient and practitioner is difficult to achieve in the hospital, where physicians spend only a brief amount of time talking to patients. In addition, information may be unavailable because patients are undergoing diagnostic tests. The hospital staff may not explain the purpose or results of diagnostic testing, leaving the patient without information and filled with anxiety.

Hospitalized patients are expected to conform submissively to the rules of the hospital and the orders of their doctor, thus relinquishing much control over their lives. People tend to manifest heightened physiological responses and to react on a physical level to uncontrollable stimulation more strongly than they do when they can exert some control over their condition. Lack of control can decrease people's capacity to concentrate and can increase their tendency to report physical symptoms.

For the efficiency of the organization, uniform treatment and conformity to hospital routine are desirable, even though they deprive patients of information and control. Hospitals have no insidious plot to deprive patients of their freedom, but this occurs when hospitals impose their routine on patients. Restoring control to patients in any significant way would further

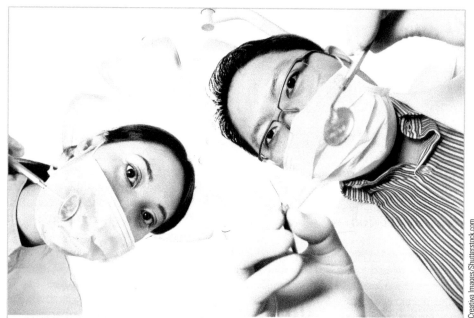

Increased use of technology, lack of information, and lack of control contribute to the stress of hospitalization.

complicate an already complex organization, but the restoration of small types of control may be effective. For example, most hospitals now allow patients some choice of foods and provide TV remote controls to give patients the power to select a program to watch (or not watch). These aspects of control are small but possibly important, as we discuss in Chapter 5 (Langer & Rodin, 1976; Rodin & Langer, 1977).

Children and Hospitalization   Few children pass through childhood without some injury, disease, or condition that requires hospitalization, and the hospitalization experience can be a source of stress and anxiety—separation from parents, an unfamiliar environment, diagnostic tests, administration of anesthesia, immunization "shots," surgery, and postoperative pain. Pediatric hospitals often offer some type of preparation program for children. Training children to cope with their fear of treatment presents special problems to health psychologists. Providing children and parents with information about hospital procedures and equipment can be an effective way to decrease anxiety.

Contrary to what many parents may think, reassuring a child is not an effective way to reduce fear in either the child or the parent. In a study with 4- to

6-year-old children who were about to receive preschool immunization shots, researchers (Manimala, Blount, & Cohen, 2000) paired each child with her or his parent and then randomly assigned each dyad to either a distraction group or a reassurance group. Researchers asked the parents of children in the distraction group to distract their child's attention away from the immunization procedure but asked parents of children in the reassurance group to reduce their child's anxiety by reassuring them that they had nothing to fear. Results strongly favored the distraction group, with three times as many children in the reassurance group requiring physical restraint. Also, children in the reassurance group showed much more verbal fear than did the other children. An interesting adjunct to these findings involved the training received by parents prior to the immunization process. Those who received training on how to reassure their child expressed a high level of confidence that they could calm their child. Then, after immunization, the reassuring parents not only had problems helping their children but they also rated themselves as being much more distressed than did the other parents. In turn, parents' distress increases the child's anxiety (Wolff et al., 2009). Reassurance, it seems, does not reduce stress for either the parent or the child.

Another strategy for helping children is modeling—that is, seeing another child cope successfully with a similar stressful procedure. A combination of modeling with a cognitive behavioral intervention and self-talk reduced distress for children who were receiving painful treatments for leukemia (Jay, Elliott, Woody, & Siegel, 1991). Indeed, this intervention was more successful than a drug treatment that included the tranquilizer Valium. A review of interventions for children (Mitchell, Johnston, & Keppel, 2004) indicated that multicomponent programs were generally more effective than single-component programs; providing information and teaching coping skills are both important for children and their parents when faced with hospitalization.

Cost, not effectiveness, is the main problem with intervention strategies to reduce children's distress resulting from hospitalization for specific medical procedures. The trend is toward cost cutting, and all interventions add to medical care costs. Some of these interventions may be cost effective if they reduce the need for additional care or decrease other expenses.

IN SUMMARY

The expense of medical care has led to restricted access for most U.S. residents. People who have medical insurance receive better care and have more choices about their care than people without insurance. Concerns about medical costs led to the creation of two U.S. government programs: Medicare, which pays for hospitalization for those over age 65, and Medicaid, which pays for care for poor people who are aged, blind, disabled, pregnant, or the parents of a dependent child.

Physicians are primary sources of medical care, but alternative sources have become more popular over the past two decades. People without medical insurance often have limitations in securing a regular medical care practitioner. Patients' satisfaction with their providers is an important factor in seeking medical care, as well as adherence to medical advice. Physicians who listen to their patients and are perceived as personable, confident, and empathetic are those who are most likely to be rated as excellent physicians. Female physicians tend to exhibit these characteristics more than male physicians.

Hospitalized patients often experience added stress as a result of being in the hospital. They are typically regarded as "nonpersons," receive inadequate information concerning their illness, and experience some loss of control over their lives. They are expected to conform to hospital routine and to comply with frequent requests of the hospital staff.

Hospitalized children and their parents experience special problems and may receive special training to help them deal with hospitalization. Several types of interventions, including modeling and cognitive behavioral programs, are effective in helping children and their parents cope with this difficult situation.

Answers

This chapter has addressed three basic questions:

1. **What factors are related to seeking medical attention?**

   How people determine their health status when they don't feel well depends not only on social, ethnic, and demographic factors but also on the characteristics of their symptoms and their concept of illness. In deciding whether they are ill, people consider at least four characteristics of their symptoms: (1) the obvious visibility of the symptoms, (2) the perceived severity of the illness, (3) the degree to which the symptoms interfere with their lives, and (4) the frequency and persistence of the symptoms. Once people are diagnosed as sick, they adopt the sick role that involves relief from normal social and occupational responsibilities and the duty to try to get better.

2. **Where do people seek medical information?**

   Prior to seeking medical care and information from the health care system, people often turn to other people and the Internet. The lay referral network is people's family and friends, who often help interpret the meaning of symptoms as well as suggest possible causes and cures. In recent years, the Internet is a common source of health information, although the quality of health information on the Internet varies widely. When patients find accurate and relevant health information, it can benefit the patient–practitioner relationship. However, not all patients have access to health information through the Internet or are wary of bringing up such information with their providers.

3. What problems do people encounter in receiving medical care?

People encounter problems in paying for medical care, and those without insurance often have limited access to health care. The U.S. government's creation of Medicare and Medicaid has helped people over 65 and some poor people with access to health care, but many people have problems finding a regular practitioner and receiving optimal health care.

Physicians may not have a lot of time to devote to a patient, which may create communication problems that reduce patients' satisfaction.

Communication problems include using medical language that is unfamiliar to the patient, as well as focusing on determining and describing a diagnosis rather than allowing the patients to fully describe their concerns.

Although hospital stays are shorter than they were 30 years ago, being in the hospital is a difficult experience for both adults and children. As a hospital patient, a person must conform to hospital procedures and policies, which include being treated as a "nonperson," tolerating lack of information, and losing control of daily activities. Children who are hospitalized are placed in an unfamiliar environment, may be separated from parents, and may undergo surgery or other painful medical procedures. Interventions that help children and parents manage this stressful experience may ease the distress, but cost is a factor that limits the availability of these services.

Suggested Readings

Leventhal, H., Breland, J. Y., Mora, P. A., & Leventhal, E. A. (2010). Lay representations of illness and treatment: A framework for action. In A. Steptoe (Ed.), *Handbook of behavioral medicine: Methods and applications* (pp. 137–154). New York: Springer. This chapter not only discusses the importance of people's conceptualizations of illness in terms of both health seeking and disease management but also outlines ways in which illness conceptualizations may be used as targets for intervention.

Martin, R., & Leventhal, H. (2004). Symptom perception and health care–seeking behavior. In J. M. Raczynski & L. C. Leviton (Eds.), *Handbook of clinical health psychology* (Vol. 2, pp. 299–328). Washington, DC: American Psychological Association. This chapter explores the situations and perceptions that underlie seeking health care, including the difficulty of interpreting symptoms and the theories that attempt to explain this behavior.

Weitz, R. (2010). *The sociology of health, illness, and health care: A critical approach* (5th ed.). Belmont, CA: Cengage. Weitz critically reviews the health care situation in the United States in this medical sociology book. Chapters 10, 11, and 12 provide a description of health care settings and professions, including many alternatives to traditional health care.

CHAPTER **4**

Adhering to Healthy Behavior

CHAPTER OUTLINE

QUESTIONS

This chapter focuses on six basic questions:

1. What is adherence, how is it measured, and how frequently does it occur?

2. What factors predict adherence?

3. What are continuum theories of health behavior, and how do they explain adherence?

4. What are stage theories of health behavior, and how do they explain adherence?

5. What is the intention–behavior gap, and what factors predict whether intentions are translated into behavior?

6. How can adherence be improved?

57

☑ Check Your **HEALTH RISKS**   *Regarding Adhering to Healthy Behavior*

☐ 1. I believe physical activity is important, but every time I try to exercise I can never keep it up for very long.

☐ 2. If my prescription medicine doesn't seem to be working, I will continue taking it.

☐ 3. I do not need to engage in any planning to change my health habits, as my good intentions always carry me through.

☐ 4. I won't have a prescription filled if it costs too much.

☐ 5. I see my dentist twice a year whether or not I have a problem.

☐ 6. I'm a smoker who knows that smoking can cause heart disease and lung cancer, but I believe that other smokers are much more likely to get these diseases than I am.

☐ 7. I am a woman who doesn't worry about breast cancer because I don't have any symptoms.

☐ 8. I am a man who doesn't worry about testicular cancer because I don't have any symptoms.

☐ 9. People have advised me to stop smoking, but I have never been able to quit.

☐ 10. I frequently forget to take my medication.

☐ 11. When I set a goal to improve my health, I plan out the specific ways and specific situations in which I can act to achieve the goal.

☐ 12. The last time I was sick, the doctor gave me advice that I didn't completely understand, but I was too embarrassed to say so.

Items 2, 5, and 11 represent good adherence beliefs and habits, but each of the other items represents a risk factor for being able to adhere to medical advice. Although it may be nearly impossible to adhere to all good health recommendations (such as not smoking, eating a healthy diet, exercising, and having regular dental and medical checkups), you can improve your health by adhering to sound medical advice. As you read this chapter, you will learn more about the health benefits of adherence, as well as the beliefs and techniques that can improve adherence.

Real-World Profile of **RAJIV KUMAR**

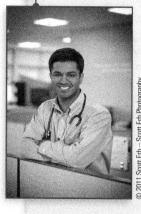

© 2011 Scott Erb – Scott Erb Photography

In 2005, Rajiv Kumar was a medical student at Brown University in Rhode Island. Soon into his medical training, he noticed that every patient he worked with seemed to struggle with making healthy changes to their behavior, such as eating healthier or increasing physical activity. The only help that physicians seemed to provide was to simply tell patients to join a gym or go on a diet. This well-intentioned advice rarely seemed enough to get patients to make lasting changes to their behavior.

Based on these experiences, Kumar decided to drop out of medical school. But rather than giving up on his goal of making people healthier, he used one of his observations as a source of inspiration: "I noticed that all of the patients who succeeded told us that they had social support from family and friends."

Kumar teamed up with one of his fellow medical students to develop a comprehensive program that harnessed the power of social support to get people to succeed at their diet and physical activity goals. Kumar secured a small amount of money to start his endeavor and emailed every person he knew in Rhode Island to sign up for his program, which became known as ShapeUp Rhode Island.

The initial ShapeUp program was a 16-week program that helped people form "teams" of friends and work colleagues who all shared the same goal of improving their lifestyle. An online platform allowed people to set goals, track their progress, receive reminders, and, most importantly, share and compare results with other team members. In addition, teams could compete against each other. Kumar called it "a Facebook for health."

The program seemed to work remarkably. Over 2,000 people signed up for the program, with 80% of them completing it and losing about 8 pounds on average. These results generated the interest of many local businesses that were interested in including the program as part of their workplace wellness initiatives. This allowed the program to expand.

A recent study demonstrated what Kumar suspected all along: The social aspect of the ShapeUp program was a major component of its success. The more the ShapeUp participants felt there was social support—and social pressure—to succeed at their plans, the better they did (Leahey, Kumar, Weinberg, & Wing, 2012).

As of 2016, over 800 companies provide the ShapeUp program to their employees, with over 2 million participants. Kumar, who eventually re-enrolled in medical school and earned his medical degree in 2011, is working to develop a similar program for children and adolescents. Now, many other online physical activity programs such as FitBit, DietBet, and Daily Challenge, all include some aspect of social influence to help people achieve their health goals.

Issues in Adherence

Why was Rajiv Kumar's ShapeUp program effective in encouraging people to improve their diet and physical activity? What did the ShapeUp program provide to participants that brief advice from a physician typically does not?

For medical advice to benefit a patient's health, two requirements must be met. First, the advice must be valid. Second, the patient must follow this advice. Both conditions are essential. Ill-founded advice that patients strictly follow may produce new health problems, such as when parents follow inaccurate advice to not have children vaccinated for common health problems (see Chapter 3 box on "There Is Controversy about Childhood Vaccinations"). On the other hand, excellent advice is worthless if patients have difficulty following it. As many as 125,000 people in the United States may die each year because they fail to adhere to medical advice, especially by failing to take prescribed medications (Cutting Edge Information, 2004). As two meta-analyses show, adhering to a medical regimen makes a large difference in improvement (DiMatteo, Giordani, Lepper, & Croghan, 2002; Simpson et al., 2006).

Kumar developed his program to increase people's social support and, as you will learn in this chapter, social support is one factor that helps people adhere to medical advice. There are other elements of the ShapeUp program that also contributed to its success, and we will also describe these factors in this chapter. In addition, we will present some of the major theories that attempt to explain why some people adhere to recommendations for healthy behavior, but others often have difficulty.

What Is Adherence?

What does it mean to be adherent? We define adherence as a person's ability and willingness to follow recommended health practices. R. Brian Haynes (1979) suggested a broader definition of the term, defining adherence as "the extent to which a person's behavior (in terms of taking medications, following diets, or executing lifestyle changes) coincides with medical or health advice" (pp. 1–2). This definition expands the concept of adherence beyond merely taking medications to include maintaining healthy lifestyle practices, such as eating properly, getting sufficient exercise, avoiding undue stress, abstaining from smoking cigarettes, and not abusing alcohol. In addition, adherence includes making and keeping periodic medical and dental appointments, using seatbelts, and engaging in other behaviors that are consistent with the best health advice available. Adherence is a complex concept, with people being adherent in one situation and nonadherent in another (Ogedegbe, Schoenthaler, & Fernandez, 2007).

How Is Adherence Measured?

How do researchers know the percentage of patients who fail to adhere to practitioners' recommendations? What methods do they use to identify those who fail to adhere? The answer to the first question is that adherence rates are not known with certainty, but researchers use techniques that yield a great deal of information about nonadherence. At least six basic methods of measuring patient adherence are available: (1) ask the practitioner, (2) ask the patient, (3) ask other people, (4) monitor medication usage, (5) examine biochemical evidence, and (6) use a combination of these procedures.

The first of these methods, asking the practitioner, is usually the poorest choice. Physicians generally overestimate their patients' adherence rates, and even when their guesses are not overly optimistic, they are usually wrong (Miller et al., 2002). In general, practitioners' accuracy is only slightly better than chance, as practitioners may rely on cues such as age, race, and weight to make inferences about adherence (Huizinga et al., 2010; Lutfey & Ketcham, 2005; Parker et al., 2007).

Asking patients themselves is a slightly more valid procedure, but it is fraught with many problems. Self-reports are inaccurate for at least two reasons. First, patients tend to report behaviors that make them appear more adherent than they actually are. Second, they may simply not know their own rate of adherence, as people do not typically pay close attention to their health-related behaviors. Interviews are more prone to these types of errors than asking patients to keep records or diaries of their behavior (Garber, 2004). Because self-report measures have questionable validity, researchers often supplement them with other methods (Parker et al., 2007).

Another method is to ask hospital personnel and family members to monitor the patient, but this procedure also has at least two problems. First, constant observation may be physically impossible, especially with regard to behaviors such as diet, smoking, and alcohol consumption (observing risky sexual behavior raises clear ethical issues as well!). Second, persistent monitoring creates an artificial situation and frequently results in higher rates of adherence than would otherwise occur. This outcome is desirable, of course, but as a means of assessing adherence, it contains a built-in error that makes observation by others inaccurate.

A fourth method of assessing adherence is to objectively monitor a person's behavior. This may occur by monitoring a patient's medicine usage, such as counting pills or assessing whether patients obtain prescriptions or refills (Balkrishnan & Jayawant, 2007). These procedures seem to be more objective because very few errors are likely to be made in counting the number of pills absent from a bottle or the number of patients who have their prescriptions filled. Even if the required number of pills are gone or the prescriptions filled, however, the patient may not have taken the medication or may have taken it in a manner other than the one prescribed.

The development of electronic technology makes possible more sophisticated methods to monitor adherence. Researchers can assess physical activity by using devices that record physical movement or by sending surveys to people's mobile phones that ask about physical activity in the past 30 minutes (Dunton, Liao, Intille, Spruijt-Metz, & Pentz, 2011). Researchers can ask patients to send photographs of pill capsules from mobile phones to verify the time when they take their medications (Galloway, Coyle, Guillén, Flower, & Mendelson, 2011). Other methods such as the Medication Event Monitoring System (MEMS) include a microprocessor in a pill cap that records the date and time of every bottle opening and closing, thus yielding a record of usage (assuming that opening the bottle equates to using the medication). In addition, this system includes an Internet link that uploads the data stored in the device so that researchers can monitor adherence on a daily or weekly basis. Not surprisingly, assessment by MEMS does not show high consistency with self-reports of medication usage (Balkrishnan & Jayawant, 2007; Shi et al., 2010), but assessment by MEMS is likely to be more valid. In a study of HIV-positive children in Uganda who were prescribed antiretroviral medications to control their condition, adherence measured by MEMS predicted biochemical measures of viral load over a 1-year period, but adherence measured by self-report did not (Haberer et al., 2012).

Examination of biochemical evidence is a fifth method of measuring adherence. This procedure looks at biochemical evidence, such as analysis of blood or urine samples that reflect adherence, to determine whether a patient behaved in an adherent fashion. For example, researchers can measure the progression of HIV infection with assessments of viral load, a biochemical measure of the amount of HIV in the blood; adherence to HIV medication relates to changes in HIV viral load. Researchers can assess proper management of diabetes by a blood test that gauges the amount of glucose in the blood over a period of months. However, problems can arise with the use of biochemical evidence as a means of assessing adherence because individuals vary in their biochemical response to drugs. In addition, this approach requires frequent medical monitoring that may be intrusive and expensive.

Finally, clinicians can use a combination of these methods to assess adherence. Several studies (Haberer et al., 2012; Velligan et al., 2007) used a variety of methods to assess adherence, including interviewing patients, counting pills, electronic monitoring, and measuring biochemical evidence, as well as a combination of all these methods. The results indicate good agreement among pill counts, electronic monitoring, and measuring biochemical evidence but poor agreement between these objective measures and patients' or clinicians' reports. A weakness of using multiple methods of measuring adherence is the cost, but it is an important strategy when researchers need the most accurate evidence to measure adherence.

How Frequent Is Nonadherence?

How common are failures of adherence? Kumar's experience as a medical student suggested that nonadherence among his patients was common. However, the answer to this question depends in part on how adherence is defined, the nature of the illness under consideration, the demographic features of the population, and the methods used to assess adherence. When interest in these questions developed in the late 1970s, David Sackett and John C. Snow (1979) reviewed more than 500 studies that dealt with the frequency of adherence. Sackett and Snow found higher rates for patients' keeping appointments when patients initiated the appointments (75%) than when appointments were scheduled for them (50%). As expected, adherence rates were higher when treatment was meant to cure rather than to prevent a disease. However, adherence was lower for medication taken for a chronic condition over a long period; adherence was around 50% for either prevention or cure.

More recent reviews confirm the problem of nonadherence, estimating nonadherence to medication regimens at nearly 25% (DiMatteo, 2004b). Adherence rates tend to be higher in more recent studies than in older ones, but many of the factors identified in Sackett and Snow's (1979) review continued to be significant predictors of adherence. Medication treatments yielded higher adherence rates than recommendations for exercise, diet, or other types of health-related behavior change. However, DiMatteo's analysis revealed that not all chronic conditions yielded equally low adherence rates. Some chronic conditions, such as HIV, arthritis, gastrointestinal disorders, and cancer, showed high adherences rates, whereas diabetes and pulmonary disease showed lower adherence. Nevertheless, failure to adhere to medical advice is a widespread problem, with one prominent review stating that finding "effective ways to help people *follow* medical treatments could have far larger effects on health than any treatment itself" (Haynes, Ackloo, Sahota, McDonald & Yao, 2008, p. 20).

What Are the Barriers to Adherence?

One category of reasons for nonadherence includes all those problems inherent in hearing and heeding physicians' advice. Patients may have financial or practical problems in making and keeping appointments and in filling, taking, and refilling prescriptions. Patients may reject the prescribed regimen as being too difficult, time consuming, expensive, or not adequately effective. Or they may just forget. Patients tend to pick and choose among the elements of the regimen their practitioners offer, treating this information as advice rather than orders (Vermeire, Hearnshaw, Van Royen, & Denekens, 2001). These patients may stop taking their medication because adherence is too much trouble or does not fit into the routine of their daily lives.

Patients may stop taking medication or changing other behaviors when their symptoms disappear. Paradoxically, others stop because they fail to feel better or begin to feel worse, leading them to believe that the medication is useless. Still others, in squirrel-like fashion, save a few pills for the next time they get sick.

Some patients may make irrational choices about adherence because they have an **optimistic bias**—a belief that they will be spared the negative consequences of nonadherence that afflict other people (Weinstein, 1980, 2001). Other patients may be nonadherent because prescription labels are too difficult to read. Visual handicaps that are common among older patients form one barrier. However, even college students may find prescription labels difficult to understand; fewer than half of college students were able to correctly understand prescription labels that had been randomly selected from a pharmacist's records (Mustard & Harris, 1989).

Another set of reasons for high rates of nonadherence is that the current definition of adherence demands lifestyle choices that are difficult to attain. At the beginning of the 20th century, when the leading causes of death and disease were infectious diseases, adherence was simpler. Patients were adherent when they followed the doctor's advice with regard to medication, rest, and so on. Adherence is no longer a matter of taking the proper pills and following short-term advice. The three leading causes of death in the United States—cardiovascular disease, cancer, and chronic obstructive lung disease—are all affected by unhealthy lifestyle choices such as smoking cigarettes, abusing alcohol, not eating properly, and not exercising regularly. In addition, of course, people now must also make and keep medical and dental

TABLE 4.1 Reasons Why Patients May Not Adhere to Medical Advice

"It's too much trouble."

"The medication was too expensive, so I took fewer pills to make them last."

"The medication didn't work very well. I was still sick, so I stopped taking it."

"The medication worked after only 1 week, so I stopped taking it."

"I won't get sick. God will save me."

"I'll start the diet tomorrow."

"I'll never be able to stick to that diet plan."

"I'm too embarrassed to go to the gym."

"I don't have the time in my schedule to exercise."

"A cancer screening test will be too painful and uncomfortable."

"The medication makes me sick."

"I feel fine. I don't see any reason to take something to prevent illness."

"Healthy foods take too long to prepare."

"I don't like my doctor. He looks down on people without insurance."

"I didn't understand my doctor's instructions and was too embarrassed to ask her to repeat them."

"I don't like the taste of nicotine chewing gum."

"I didn't understand the directions on the label."

appointments, listen with understanding to the advice of health care providers, and, finally, follow that advice. These conditions present a complex array of requirements that are difficult for anyone to fulfill completely. Table 4.1 summarizes some of the reasons patients give for not adhering to medical advice.

IN SUMMARY

Adherence is the extent to which a person is able and willing to follow medical and health advice. In order for people to profit from adherence, first, the advice must be valid, and second, patients must follow that advice. Inability or unwillingness to adhere to health-related behaviors increases people's chances of serious health problems or even death.

Researchers can assess adherence in at least six ways: (1) ask the physician, (2) ask the patient, (3) ask other people, (4) monitor medical usage, (5) examine biochemical evidence, and (6) use a combination of these procedures. No one of these procedures is both reliable and valid. However, with the exception of clinician judgment, most have some validity and usefulness. When accuracy is crucial, using two or more of these methods yields greater accuracy than reliance on a single technique.

The frequency of nonadherence depends on the nature of the illness. People are more likely to adhere to a medication regimen than to a diet plan or exercise program. The average rate of nonadherence is slightly less than 25%. To understand and improve adherence, health psychologists seek to understand the barriers that keep people from adhering, including the difficulty of altering lifestyles of long duration, inadequate practitioner–patient communications, and erroneous beliefs as to what advice patients should follow.

What Factors Predict Adherence?

Who adheres and who does not? The factors that predict adherence include personal characteristics and environmental factors that are difficult or impossible to change, such as age or socioeconomic factors. The factors also include specific health beliefs that are more easily modifiable. In this section, we consider the first set of factors, which include severity of the disease; treatment characteristics, including side effects and complexity of the treatment; personal characteristics, such as age, gender, and personality; and environmental factors such as social support, income, and cultural norms (see Table 4.2). Later in this chapter, we will present major theories of adherence that identify specific beliefs and behavioral strategies that are more easily modifiable through intervention.

Severity of the Disease

At the start of this chapter, Kumar was disheartened by his observations that many patients had difficulties following doctor's recommendations. Even when people should be highly motivated to adhere—such as when they have a severe, potentially crippling, or life-threatening illness—they often do not adhere. In general, people with a serious disease are no more likely than

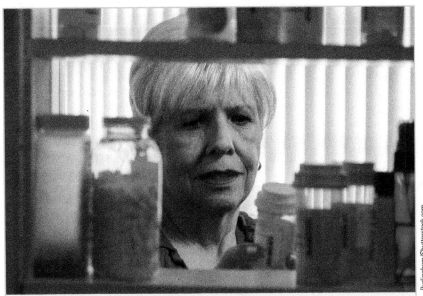

More complex treatments tend to lower compliance rates.

Researchers observe this relationship between number of doses and adherence across a variety of chronic medical conditions, including diabetes, hypertension, and HIV (Ingersoll & Cohen, 2008; Pollack, Chastek, Williams, & Moran, 2010). For example, people who need to take one pill per day adhere fairly well (as high as 90%), and increasing the dosage to two per day produces little decrease (Claxton, Cramer, & Pierce, 2001). When people must take four doses per day, however, adherence plummets to below 40%; this may be due to people having difficulty fitting medications into daily routines. For example, pills prescribed once a day can be cued to routine activities, such as waking up; those prescribed twice a day can be cued to early morning and late night; and those prescribed three times a day can be cued to meals. Schedules calling for patients to take medication four or more times a day, or to take two or more medications a day, create difficulties and lower adherence rates. Other aspects of a medical regimen can contribute to complexity, such as the need to cut pills in half prior to taking them. In a study of nearly 100,000 patients of Type 2 diabetes, patients who were prescribed the most complex regimen—in terms of both the need to split pills as well as the number of doses per day—showed the lowest rates of adherence (Pollack et al., 2010).

people with a less serious problem to adhere to medical advice (DiMatteo, 2004b). What matters in predicting adherence is not the objective severity of a patient's disease but, rather, the patient's *perception* of the severity of the disease (DiMatteo, Haskard, & Williams, 2007). That is, the objective severity of a disease is less closely related to adherence to treatment or prevention regimens than the threat that people perceive from a disease.

Treatment Characteristics

Characteristics of the treatment, such as side effects of a prescribed medication and the complexity of the treatment, also present potential problems for adherence.

Side Effects of the Medication Research with diabetes medications (Mann, Ponieman, Leventhal, & Halm, 2009) and the complex regimen of HIV medication (Applebaum, Richardson, Brady, Brief, & Keane, 2009; Herrmann et al., 2008) shows that those who experience or have concerns about severe side effects are less likely to take their medications than those who do not have such concerns.

Complexity of the Treatment Are people less likely to adhere as treatment procedures become increasingly complex? In general, the greater the number of doses or variety of medications people must take, the greater the likelihood that they will not take pills as prescribed (Piette, Heisler, Horne, & Caleb Alexander, 2006).

Personal Factors

Who is most adherent, women or men? The young or the old? Are there certain personality patterns that predict adherence? In general, demographic factors such as age and gender show some relationship to adherence, but each of these factors alone is too small to be a good predictor of who will adhere and who will not (DiMatteo, 2004b). Personality was one of the first factors considered in relation to adherence, but other personal factors such as emotional factors and personal beliefs appear more important in understanding adherence.

Age The relationship between age and adherence is not simple. Assessing adherence among children is difficult because the person whose adherence is important is actually the parent and not the child (De Civita & Dobkin, 2005). As children grow into adolescents, they become more responsible for adhering to medical regimens, and this situation continues throughout adulthood. However, older people may face situations that make adherence difficult, such as memory problems, poor health, and regimens that include many medications (Gans & McPhillips, 2003). These developmental issues contribute to a complex relationship between age and adherence. One study (Thomas et al., 1995) found a curvilinear relationship between age and adherence to colorectal cancer screening. That is, those who adhered best were around 70 years old, with older and younger participants adhering least. Those who are 70 years old may not be the best at adhering to all medical advice, but this result suggests that both older and younger adults, plus children and adolescents, experience more problems with adherence. Other research confirms the problems with these age groups.

Even with caregivers to assist them, children with asthma (Penza-Clyve, Mansell & McQuaid, 2004), diabetes (Cramer, 2004), and HIV infection (Farley et al., 2004) often fail to adhere to their medical regimens. As they grow into adolescence and exert more control over their own health care, adherence problems become even more prominent (DiMatteo, 2004b). Several studies (Miller & Drotar, 2003; Olsen & Sutton, 1998) show that as diabetic children become adolescents, their adherence to recommended exercise and insulin regimens decreases, and conflicts with parents over diabetes management increase. Young adults with these diseases also experience adherence problems (Ellis et al., 2007; Herrmann et al., 2008). Thus, age shows a small but complex relationship with adherence.

Gender   Overall, researchers find few differences in the adherence rates of women and men, but some differences exist in following specific recommendations. In general, men and women are about equal in adhering to taking medication (Andersson, Melander, Svensson, Lind, & Nilsson, 2005; Chapman, Petrilla, Benner, Schwartz, & Tang, 2008), controlling diabetes (Hartz et al., 2006), or keeping an appointment for a medical test (Sola-Vera et al., 2008). However, women are less adherent than men in taking medications to lower cholesterol, but this may be due to the higher prevalence of heart disease among men (Mann, Woodward, Muntner, Falzon, & Kronish, 2010). Women may be better at adhering to healthy diets, such as sodium-restricted diets (Chung et al., 2006) and diets with lots of fruits and vegetables (Emanuel, McCully, Gallagher, & Updegraff, 2012; Thompson et al., 2011). Aside from these differences, men and women have similar levels of adherence (DiMatteo, 2004b).

Personality Patterns   When the problem of nonadherence became obvious, researchers initially considered the concept of a nonadherent personality. According to this concept, people with certain personality patterns would have low adherence rates. If this concept is accurate, then the same people should be nonadherent in a variety of situations. However, most evidence does not support this notion. Nonadherence is often specific to the situation (Lutz, Silbret, & Olshan, 1983), and adherence to one treatment program is typically unrelated to adherence to others (Ogedegbe, Schoenthaler, & Fernandez, 2007). However, there may be a few "clusters" of nonadherent behaviors that occur together. For example, people who smoke tobacco often tend to overuse alcohol and be physically inactive (deRuiter et al., 2014; Morris, D'Este, Sargent-Cox, & Anstey, 2016). Thus, the evidence suggests that nonadherence is not a global personality trait but is specific to a given situation (Haynes, 2001).

Emotional Factors   People who experience stress and emotional problems also have difficulties with adherence. Stressful life events often interfere with efforts to be physically active (Stults-Kolehmainen & Sinha, 2014). Similarly, HIV-positive individuals who report high levels of stress are often less adherent to taking antiretroviral medication (Bottonari, Roberts, Ciesla, & Hewitt, 2005; Leserman, Ironson, O'Cleirigh, Fordiani, & Balbin, 2008).

Do anxiety and depression reduce adherence rates? Whereas anxiety has only a small relationship with adherence, depression has a major influence on adherence (DiMatteo, Lepper, & Croghan, 2000). The risk of nonadherence is three times greater in depressed patients than in those who are not depressed. More recent studies show that depression relates to lower adherence among people managing chronic illnesses, such as diabetes and HIV (Gonzalez et al., 2008; Katon et al., 2010; Sin & DiMatteo, 2014). Given that coping with a chronic illness can increase risk for depression (Nouwen et al., 2010), the link between depression, chronic illness, and adherence is an important public health concern (Moussavi et al., 2007).

Emotional factors clearly present risks, but do some personality characteristics relate to better adherence and improved health? Patients who express optimism and positive states of mind have better physical health (Chida & Steptoe, 2008; Pressman & Cohen, 2005; Rasmussen, Scheier, & Greenhouse, 2009) and are more likely to adhere to their medical regimens (Gonzalez et al., 2004). Furthermore, the trait of **conscientiousness**, one of the factors in the five factor model of personality (McCrae & Costa, 2003), shows a reliable relationship to adherence and improved health (Bogg & Roberts, 2013). For example, conscientiousness predicts adherence to an overall healthy lifestyle (Takahashi, Edmonds, Jackson, & Roberts, 2013). Conscientiousness also relates to slower progression of HIV infection (O'Cleirigh, Ironson, Weiss, & Costa, 2007) and greater medication adherence (Hill & Roberts, 2011; Molloy, O'Carroll, & Ferguson, 2014). Thus, emotional factors and personality traits may present either a risk or an advantage for adherence.

Environmental Factors

Although some personal factors are important for adherence, environmental factors exert an even larger influence. Included in this group of environmental factors are economic factors, social support, and cultural norms.

Economic Factors   Of all the demographic factors examined by Robin DiMatteo (2004b), socioeconomic factors such as education and income were the most strongly related to adherence. People with greater income and education tend to be more adherent. Two meta-analyses show that it is income rather than education that relates more strongly to adherence (DiMatteo, 2004b; Falagas, Zarkadoulia, Pliatsika, & Panos, 2008). Difference in income may also explain some ethnic differences in adherence. For example, Hispanic American children and adolescents have a lower rate of adherence to a diabetes regimen, but this difference disappears after controlling for income differences (Gallegos-Macias, Macias, Kaufman, Skipper, & Kalishman, 2003). Thus, economic factors show a relationship to health; one avenue is through access to health care, and another is through the ability to pay for treatments.

In the United States, people without insurance experience difficulties in obtaining access to health care and in follow-up care such as filling prescriptions (Gans & McPhillips, 2003). Many of the people who experience cost concerns have chronic diseases, which often require daily medications over long periods of time (Piette et al., 2006). In a study of Medicare beneficiaries over age 65 (Gellad, Haas, & Safran, 2007), cost concerns predicted nonadherence, and such concerns were more common for African Americans and Hispanic Americans than for European Americans. In another study, people who had been admitted to the hospital for heart disease were more likely to adhere to their medications to reduce cholesterol level during the next year if their insurance plan paid more of the cost of the prescription (Ye, Gross, Schommer, Cline, & St. Peter, 2007). Therefore, how much people must pay for their treatment affects not only access to medical care but also the likelihood that they will adhere to the treatment regimen. These limitations and concerns about costs affect older people and those from ethnic minorities more often than others.

Social Support   Social support is a broad concept that refers to both tangible and intangible help a person receives from family members and from friends. A social support network is important for dealing with a chronic disease and for adhering to the required medical regimen (Kyngäs, 2004). Social support networks for adolescents include parents, peers (both those with and without similar conditions), people at school or work, health care providers, and even pets. In addition, adolescents use technology such as cell phones and computers to contact others and obtain support.

The level of social support one receives from friends and family is a strong predictor of adherence. In general, people who are isolated from others are likely to be nonadherent; those who enjoy many close interpersonal relationships are more likely to follow medical advice. A review of 50 years of research (DiMatteo, 2004a) confirmed the importance of social support for adherence.

Researchers can analyze social support in terms of the variety and function of relationships that people have, as well as the types of support that people receive from these relationships (DiMatteo, 2004a). For example, living with someone is a significant contributor to adherence; people who are married and those who live with families are more adherent than those who live alone. However, simply living with someone is not sufficient—family conflict and partner stress may lead to reductions in adherence (Molloy, Perkins-Porras, Strike, & Steptoe, 2008). Thus, the living situation itself is not the important factor; rather, the support a person receives is the critical issue (DiMatteo, 2004a).

In the ShapeUp program described at the start of the chapter, a participant's teammates could provide social support in a number of ways, by either offering useful tips or by providing encouragement for success. Social support may consist of either practical or emotional support. Practical support includes reminders, helpful advice, and physical assistance in adhering. Emotional support includes nurturance, empathy, and encouragement. In studies of both patients recovering from heart problems (Molloy, Perkins-Porras, Bhattacharyya, Strike, & Steptoe, 2008) and adolescents with diabetes (Ellis et al., 2007), practical support was a more important determinant of adherence than emotional support. Thus, social support is an important factor in adherence, and those who lack a support network have more trouble adhering to medical advice.

Cultural Norms Cultural beliefs and norms have a powerful effect not only on rates of adherence but also on what constitutes adherence. For example, if one's family or tribal traditions include strong beliefs in the efficacy of tribal healers, then the individual's adherence to modern medical recommendations might be low. A study of diabetic and hypertensive patients in Zimbabwe (Zyazema, 1984) found a large number of people who were not adhering to their recommended therapies. As might be expected, many of these patients believed in traditional healers and had little faith in Western medical procedures. Thus, the extent to which people accept a medical practice has a large impact on adherence to that practice, resulting in poorer adherence for individuals who are less acculturated to Western medicine, such as immigrants or people who retain strong ties to another culture (Barron, Hunter, Mayo, & Willoughby, 2004).

Failures to adhere to Western, technological medicine do not necessarily indicate a failure to adhere to some other medical tradition. People who maintain a cultural tradition may also retain its healers. For example, a study of Native Americans (Novins, Beals, Moore, Spicer, & Manson, 2004) revealed that many sick people sought the services of traditional healers, sometimes in combination with biomedical services. This strategy of combining treatments might be considered nonadherent by both types of healers.

People who accept a different healing tradition should not necessarily be considered nonadherent when their illness calls for a complex biomedical regimen. Native Hawaiians have a poor record of adherence (Kaʻopua & Mueller, 2004), partly because their cultural beliefs are more holistic and spiritual, and their traditions emphasize family support and cohesion. These

cultural values are not compatible with those that form the basis of Western medicine. Thus, Native Hawaiians have more trouble than other ethnic groups in Hawaii in adhering to medical regimens to control diabetes and risks for heart disease. The health-related beliefs of Native Hawaiians with heart failure lead them to prefer native healers over physicians (Kaholokula, Saito, Mau, Latimer, & Seto, 2008). However, no differences appear in their rates of adherence to the complex regimen of antiretroviral therapy that helps to control HIV infection, and their cultural value of family support may be a positive factor (Kaʻopua & Mueller, 2004).

Cultural beliefs can also increase adherence. For example, older Japanese patients are typically more adherent than similar patients from the United States or Europe (Chia, Schlenk, & Dunbar-Jacob, 2006). The Japanese health care system provides care for all citizens through a variety of services, which creates trust in the health care system. This trust extends to physicians; Japanese patients accept their physicians' authority, preferring to allow physicians to make health care decisions rather than make those decisions themselves. Consistent with this attitude, patients tend to respect the advice they receive from physicians and to follow their orders carefully.

Culture and ethnicity also influence adherence through the treatment that people from different cultures and ethnic groups receive when seeking medical care. Physicians and other health care providers may be influenced by their patients' ethnic background and socioeconomic status, and this influence can affect patient adherence. Physicians tend to have stereotypical and negative attitudes toward African American and low- and middle-income patients (Dovidio et al., 2008; van Ryn & Burke, 2000), including pessimistic beliefs about their rates of adherence. Perceived discrimination and disrespect may contribute to ethnic differences in following physicians' recommendations and keeping appointments (Blanchard & Lurie, 2004). African Americans (14.1%), Asian Americans (20.2%), and Hispanic Americans (19.4%) reported that they felt discriminated against or treated with a lack of respect by a physician from whom they had received care within the past 2 years. In contrast, only about 9% of European American patients felt that they had been treated with disrespect by their physician. In this study, patients' perception of disrespect predicted lower adherence and more missed medical appointments.

These findings have important implications for physicians and other health care providers whose

TABLE 4.2   Factors that Predict Adherence

Factors	Findings	Studies
1. Severity of the disease	People adhere more when they perceive a disease as severe.	DiMatteo et al., 2007
2. Treatment characteristics	People adhere less to treatments that are complex and produce unpleasant side effects.	Applebaum et al., 2009; Ingersoll & Cohen, 2008; Pollack et al., 2010.
3. Age	Complex relationship exists between age and adherence, with younger and older adults adhering less than middle-aged adults.	Thomas et al., 1995
4. Personal factors	Stress and depression predict poorer adherence; conscientiousness predicts better adherence.	Stults-Kolehmainen & Sinha, 2014; DiMatteo et al., 2000; Bogg & Roberts, 2013.
5. Economic factors	People with lower income generally show poorer adherence.	DiMatteo, 2004a; Falagas et al., 2008.
6. Social support	People adhere better when they have strong social support.	DiMatteo, 2004b.
7. Culture	People adhere more to modern medicine when their cultural beliefs support a reliance and trust in modern medicine.	Zyazema, 1984; Kaholokula et al., 2008; Chia et al., 2006.

clientele consists largely of people from different cultural backgrounds. In addition, these findings highlight the importance of interactions between patient and practitioner in adhering to medical advice.

Interaction of Factors

Researchers have identified dozens of factors, each of which shows some relation to adherence. However, many of these factors account for a very small amount of the variation in adhering to medical advice. To gain a fuller understanding of adherence, researchers must study the mutual influence of factors that affect adherence. For example, patients' beliefs about the disease are related to adherence, but those beliefs are affected by interactions with physicians, another factor that has been identified as influential for adherence. Thus, many of the factors described earlier are not independent of one another. Many of the factors identified as being related to adherence overlap with and influence other factors in complex ways. Therefore, both researchers and practitioners must understand the complex interplay of factors that affect adherence. Furthermore, many of the factors we have discussed so far are not modifiable. Health psychologists are not only interested

in understanding adherence but also in *improving* adherence. In the next section, we focus on theories of adherence that identify these potentially modifiable factors, how they might interact with each other, and suggest specific ways to improve adherence.

IN SUMMARY

Several conditions predict poor adherence: (1) side effects of the medication, (2) long and complicated treatment regimens, (3) personal factors such as old or young age, (4) emotional factors such as conscientiousness and emotional problems such as stress and depression, (5) economic barriers to obtaining treatment or paying for prescriptions, (6) lack of social support, and (7) patients' cultural beliefs that the medical regimen is ineffective. Researchers and practitioners need to understand that the factors identified as influencing adherence interact in complex ways. However, many of these factors may not be easy to change; thus, researchers develop theories of health behavior that identify factors that may be easier to modify.

Why and How Do People Adhere to Healthy Behaviors?

In order to intervene to improve people's adherence, it is critical to identify the potentially modifiable factors that predict adherence. To do this, health psychologists develop theories to understand *why* people make the health decisions they do and *how* they successfully adhere to medical advice. In Chapter 2, we said that useful theories (1) generate research, (2) organize and explain observations, and (3) guide the practitioner in predicting behavior. Theories that successfully identify why people adhere or do not adhere are also useful for practitioners in designing interventions to improve adherence. As you will see in this section, theories of adherence develop over time, as researchers notice the weaknesses of existing theories and propose newer models that account for these weaknesses. Furthermore, theories of health behavior can be classified into two general types: continuum theories and stage theories, each with different assumptions.

Continuum Theories of Health Behavior

Continuum theories were the first class of theories developed to understand health behavior and include the health belief model (Becker & Rosenstock, 1984), self-efficacy theory (Bandura, 1986, 1997, 2001), the theory of planned behavior (Ajzen, 1985, 1991), and behavioral theory. **Continuum theories** are a name given to theories that seek to explain adherence with a single set of factors that should apply equally to all people regardless of their existing levels or motivations for adhering. In other words, continuum theories take a "one size fits all" approach. Stage theories, which we will describe later in this chapter, take a different approach to explaining adherence, by first classifying people into different stages of behavior change and then identifying the unique variables that predict adherence among people in different stages.

The Health Belief Model In the 1950s, tuberculosis was a major health problem. The United States Public Health Service initiated a free tuberculosis health-screening program. Mobile units went to convenient neighborhood locations and provided screening X-rays free of charge. Yet, very few people took advantage of the screening program. Why?

Geoffrey Hochbaum (1958) and his colleagues developed the health belief model to answer this question. Several versions of the health belief model exist; the one that has attracted the most attention is that of Marshall Becker and Irwin Rosenstock (Becker & Rosenstock, 1984).

The model developed by Becker and Rosenstock assumes that beliefs are important contributors to health behavior. This model includes four beliefs that should combine to predict health-related behaviors: (1) perceived *susceptibility* to disease or disability, (2) perceived *severity* of the disease or disability, (3) perceived *benefits* of health-enhancing behaviors, and (4) perceived *barriers* to health-enhancing behaviors, including financial costs.

Consider how these factors might motivate a smoker to quit. First, a smoker should believe that smoking increases the likelihood of some disease such as lung cancer or heart disease. Second, the person should believe that such diseases are, indeed, serious. If a person does not believe that smoking leads to diseases or that the diseases are not life-threatening, then there would be little motivation to quit. Third, a person needs to believe that there are obvious benefits to quitting smoking, such as reducing the likelihood of future disease. Lastly, a person needs to believe that there are few barriers to quitting; in other words, that quitting smoking would be a relatively painless process. However, smokers often perceive many barriers to quitting, including few other options for managing stress or lack of support from others (Twyman, Bonevski, Paul, & Bryant, 2014). Thus, a smoking cessation intervention based on the health belief model would seek to educate people on susceptibility to smoking-related diseases, the severity of those diseases, the benefits of quitting, and ways to deal with perceived barriers.

Although the health belief model corresponds with common sense in many ways, common sense does not always predict adherence to health-related behaviors. While some interventions based on the health belief model have been successful at promoting adherence to relatively simple and infrequent behaviors such as mammography screening (Aiken et al., 1994), the health belief model does not predict adherence very well, especially to ongoing, lifestyle behaviors such as smoking cessation. Of the health belief model's four factors, perceived benefits and barriers are the best predictors of behavior, whereas perceived susceptibility and severity are generally weak predictors of behavior (Carpenter, 2010). Similarly, the factors in the health belief model may be more predictive for some groups than for other

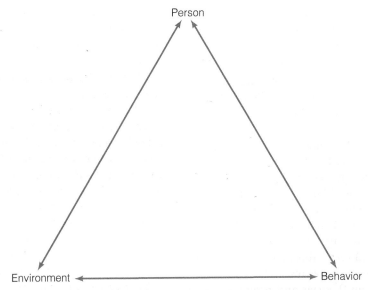

FIGURE 4.1   Bandura's concept of reciprocal determinism. Human functioning is a product of the interaction of behavior, environment, and person variables, especially self-efficacy and other cognitive processes.

Source: Adapted from "The self system in reciprocal determinism," by A. Bandura, 1979, *American Psychologist, 33*, p. 345.

groups. For example, susceptibility and severity more strongly predict vaccination for African Americans and European Americans than for Hispanic Americans. For Hispanic Americans, barriers more strongly predict vaccination than the other factors (Chen, Fox, Cantrell, Stockdale, & Kagawa-Singer, 2007). These ethnic differences point to the importance of other factors omitted by the health belief model.

Some critics (Armitage & Conner, 2000) argue that the health belief model emphasizes motivational factors too heavily and behavioral factors too little, and thus can never be a completely adequate model of health behavior. One of the biggest limitations of the health belief model, however, is its omission of beliefs about a person's control over a health behavior.

Self-Efficacy Theory   Albert Bandura (1986, 1997, 2001) proposed a social cognitive theory that assumes that humans have some capacity to exercise limited control over their lives. That is, they use their cognitive processes to pursue goals they view as important and achievable. Bandura suggests that human action results from an interaction of behavior, environment, and person factors, especially people's beliefs. Bandura

(1986, 2001) referred to this interactive triadic model as **reciprocal determinism**. The concept of reciprocal determinism can be illustrated by a triangle, with behavior, environment, and person factors occupying the three corners of the triangle and each having some influence on the other two (see Figure 4.1).

An important component of the person factor is **self-efficacy**, defined by Bandura (2001) as "people's beliefs in their capability to exercise some measure of control over their own functioning and over environmental events" (p. 10). Self-efficacy is a situation-specific rather than a global concept; that is, it refers to people's confidence that they can perform necessary behaviors to produce desired outcomes in a *particular* situation, such as fighting off a temptation to smoke. Bandura (1986) suggested that self-efficacy can be acquired, enhanced, or decreased in one of four ways: (1) performance, or enacting a behavior such as successfully resisting cigarette cravings; (2) vicarious experience, or seeing another person with similar skills perform a behavior; (3) verbal persuasion, or listening to the encouraging words of a trusted person; and (4) physiological arousal states, such as feelings of anxiety or stress, which ordinarily *decrease* self-efficacy.

According to self-efficacy theory, people's beliefs concerning their ability to initiate difficult behaviors (such as quitting smoking) predict their likelihood of accomplishing those behaviors. People who think they can do something will try and persist at it; people who do not believe they can do something will not try or will give up quickly. Also important in self-efficacy theory are **outcome expectations**, which are people's beliefs that those behaviors will produce valuable outcomes, such as lower risk for heart problems. According to Bandura's theory, the combination of self-efficacy and outcome expectations plays an important role in predicting behavior. To successfully adhere to a health behavior, people must believe that the behavior will bring about a valuable outcome and that they have the ability to successfully carry out the behavior.

Indeed, self-efficacy theory predicts adherence to a variety of health recommendations, including relapse in a smoking cessation program, maintenance of an exercise regimen, adherence to diabetes management, and adherence to HIV medication regimens. For example, a study on self-efficacy and smoking relapse (Shiffman et al., 2000) found that, after an initial lapse, smokers with high self-efficacy tended to remain abstinent, whereas those with waning self-efficacy were likely to relapse. Self-efficacy was the best predictor of completing versus dropping out of an exercise rehabilitation program (Guillot, Kilpatrick, Hebert, & Hollander, 2004) and adhering to an exercise program for cardiac rehabilitation (Schwarzer, Luszczynska, Ziegelmann, Scholz, & Lippke, 2008). One team of researchers (Iannotti et al., 2006) studied diabetes management among adolescents and found self-efficacy to predict better self-management and optimal blood sugar levels. Research with a group of women with AIDS (Ironson et al., 2005) and women and men with HIV/AIDS (Simoni, Frick, & Huang, 2006) found that self-efficacy related to adherence to taking medications as prescribed and to physical indicators of decreased disease severity. Thus, self-efficacy predicts good adherence and good medical outcomes. For this reason, self-efficacy is now incorporated into nearly all health behavior models. However, one limitation of self-efficacy theory is that it focuses chiefly on self-efficacy as a predictor of behavior but omits other factors that also supply a person with motivation for adherence, such as social pressure.

The Theory of Planned Behavior   Like self-efficacy theory, the theory of planned behavior assumes that people act in ways that help them achieve important goals.

The *theory of planned behavior* (Ajzen, 1985, 1991), one of the most commonly used theories of health behavior, assumes that people are generally reasonable and make systematic use of information when deciding how to behave; they think about the outcome of their actions before making a decision to engage in a particular behavior. They can also choose not to act, if they believe that an action would move them away from their goal.

According to the theory of planned behavior, the immediate determinant of behavior is the *intention* to act or not to act. Intentions, in turn, are shaped by three factors. The first is a personal evaluation of the behavior—that is, one's *attitude toward the behavior*. One's attitude toward the behavior arises from beliefs that the behavior will lead to positively or negatively valued outcomes. The second factor is one's *perception of how much control* exists over one's behavior (Ajzen, 1985, 1991). Perceived behavioral control is the ease or difficulty one has in achieving desired behavioral outcomes, which reflects both past behaviors and perceived ability to overcome obstacles. This belief in perceived behavioral control is very similar to Bandura's concept of self-efficacy. The more resources and opportunities people believe they have, the stronger their beliefs that they can control their behavior.

The third factor is one's perception of the social pressure to perform or not perform the action—that is, one's *subjective norm*. The focus on subjective norms is a unique aspect of the theory of planned behavior. A person's subjective norm is shaped by both his or her belief that other people encourage the behavior, as well as his or her motivation to adhere to the wishes of others. The ShapeUp program described at the start of this chapter sought to increase participants' subjective

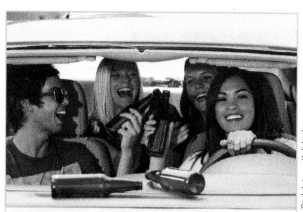

Young adults' perception of social norms can influence their behavior.

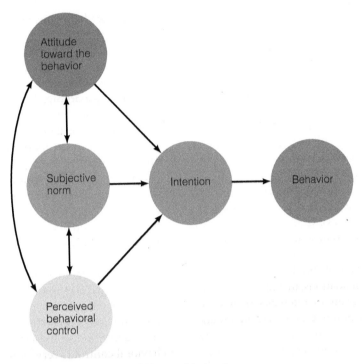

FIGURE 4.2   Theory of planned behavior.

Source: Reprinted from *Organizational Behavior and Human Decision Processes*, 50, I. Ajzen, "The Theory of Planned Behavior," p. 182.

norm for physical activity and healthy eating by ensuring that friends and co-workers believed that participants should exercise and eat better. Furthermore, by encouraging friendly competition among participants, the ShapeUp program made participants more motivated to live up to the expectations of fellow teammates! Indeed, two of the best predictors of weight loss in the ShapeUp program were whether other people in one's own team successfully lost weight and one's own perception of strong social influence to lose weight (Leahey et al., 2012) (see also Would You Believe ...? box).

Figure 4.2 shows that we can predict a person's behavior from knowledge of a person's (1) attitude toward the behavior, (2) subjective norm, and (3) perceived behavioral control. All three components interact to shape the person's intention to behave.

One strength of the theory of planned behavior is that it identifies beliefs that shape behavior. For example, American men consume less fruits and vegetables than American women. This gender difference relates directly to gender differences in components of the theory of planned behavior: Men have less favorable attitudes toward and perceive less control over their ability

to eat fruits and vegetables than women do (Emanuel et al., 2012). A study on the topic of premarital sex among Korean university students (Cha, Doswell, Kim, Charron-Prochownik, & Patrick, 2007) also highlights this theory's strengths and weaknesses. In this study, subjective norms were significant predictors for both male and female students. However, perceived behavioral control was a factor only for male students because virginity may be a more deliberate choice for Korean men but not for women (Cha et al., 2007). For females, attitudes were more strongly predictive. Thus, the theory of planned behavior was a good model to explain this behavior, but more so for male students. Similarly, a study of fruit and vegetable consumption found that norms were significant predictors of intentions for African American participants but not for European American participants (Blanchard et al., 2009), suggesting that cultural differences exist in how much people are motivated by the expectations of close friends and family.

Despite these limitations, the theory of planned behavior has been useful in guiding the development of Internet-based interventions for a variety of health behaviors (Webb, Joseph, Yardley, & Michie, 2010).

A recent meta-analysis of over 200 studies found that the theory of planned behavior was most successful at predicting physical activity and dietary behaviors (McEachan, Conner, Taylor, & Lawton, 2011). In contrast, the theory of planned behavior was less successful at predicting risk-taking behaviors such as speeding, smoking, and alcohol and drug use, as well as screening, safe sex, and abstinence behaviors. What could account for these differences across types of behavior? For the most part, physical activity and diet represent ongoing, planned, individual choices that the theory of planned behavior was designed to predict. On the other hand, intentions and perceived behavioral control were less likely to predict risk-taking and sexual behaviors because these behaviors are likely to be reactions to specific situations rather than planned choices. Across nearly all behaviors, subjective norms were the weakest predictor of behavior, with two exceptions. Subjective norms more strongly predicted behavior for adolescents compared with adults, and subjective norms more strongly predicted risk-taking behaviors than other behaviors. Thus, subjective norms may be especially important in understanding risk-taking behavior among adolescents, a point we will return to later in this chapter.

Behavioral Theory   When people begin to engage in a health behavior, behavioral principles may strengthen or extinguish those behaviors. The *behavioral model* of adherence employs the principles of operant conditioning proposed by B. F. Skinner (1953). The key to operant conditioning is the immediate *reinforcement* of any response that moves the organism (person) toward the target behavior—in this case, following medical recommendations. Skinner found that reinforcement, either positive or negative, strengthens the behavior it follows. With **positive reinforcement**, a positively valued stimulus is added to the situation, thus increasing the probability that the behavior will recur. An example of positive reinforcement of adherent behavior would be a monetary payment contingent on a patient's keeping a doctor's appointment. With **negative reinforcement**, behavior is strengthened by the removal of an unpleasant or negatively valued stimulus. An example of negative reinforcement would be taking medication to stop your spouse from nagging you about taking your medication.

Punishment also changes behavior by decreasing the chances that a behavior will be repeated, but psychologists seldom use it to modify nonadherent behaviors. The effects of positive and negative reinforcers

are quite predictable: They both strengthen behavior. However, the effects of punishment are limited and sometimes difficult to predict. At best, punishment will inhibit or suppress a behavior, and it can condition strong negative feelings toward any persons or environmental conditions associated with it. Punishment, including threats of harm, is seldom useful in improving a person's adherence to medical advice.

The behavioral model also predicts that adherence will be difficult, because learned behaviors form patterns or habits that often resist change. When a person must make changes in habitual behavior patterns to take medication, change diet or physical activity, or take blood glucose readings several times a day, the individual often has trouble accommodating a new routine. People need help in establishing such changes, and advocates of the behavioral model also use cues, rewards, and contingency contracts to reinforce adherent behaviors. Cues include written reminders of appointments, telephone calls from the practitioner's office, and a variety of self-reminders; the ShapeUp online program periodically reminded participants of their health goals. Rewards for adherence can be extrinsic (money and compliments) or intrinsic (feeling healthier); the ShapeUp online program included numerous rewards, including the opportunity for praise or encouragement from team members, or the possibility of beating another team in a competition. Contingency contracts can be verbal, but they are more often written agreements between practitioner and patient. In other cases, people can form contracts through online services like DietBet, where they place a bet with friends and earn money back only if they meet their goal. Most adherence models recognize the importance of such incentives and contracts in improving adherence, but research also shows that adherence often drops after incentives are taken away (DeFulio & Silverman, 2012; Mantzari et al., 2015; Mitchell et al., 2013). However, behavioral techniques may be useful in helping people initiate new behaviors, with the hopes that they will eventually translate into habits.

Critique of Continuum Theories   In Chapter 2, we suggested that a useful theory should (1) generate significant research, (2) organize and explain observations, and (3) help the practitioner predict and change behaviors. How well do continuum theories meet these three criteria?

First, substantial amounts of research apply continuum theories to understanding adherence. The health belief model has prompted the most research, but a body of evidence exists for all these models.

Second, do these models organize and explain health-related behaviors? In general, all these models do better than chance in explaining and predicting behavior. However, the health belief model and the theory of planned behavior address motivation, attitudes, and intentions, but not actual behavior or behavior change (Schwarzer, 2008). Thus, they are only moderately successful in predicting adherence. The theory of planned behavior, however, does a better job than the health belief model and self-efficacy theory in recognizing the social and environmental pressures that influence behavior, in the form of subjective norms.

Another type of challenge comes from the necessity of relying on instruments to assess the various components of the models because such measures are not yet consistent and accurate. The health belief model, for example, might predict health-seeking behavior more accurately if valid measurements existed for each of its components. If a person feels susceptible to a disease, perceives his or her symptoms to be severe, believes that treatment will be effective, and sees few barriers to treatment, then logically that person should seek health care. But each of these four factors is difficult to assess reliably and validly.

Finally, do continuum theories allow practitioners to predict and change behavior? One strength of continuum theories is that they identify several beliefs that should motivate *anyone* to change his or her behaviors. Thus, continuum theories have guided the development of "one size fits all" interventions that target these beliefs. Despite these strengths, continuum theories also leave out important psychological factors that predict behavior, such as self-identity and anticipated emotions (Rise, Sheeran, & Hukkelberg, 2010; Rivis, Sheeran, & Armitage, 2009). For example, people who simply think about the regret they might experience if they do not enroll in an organ donation program are more likely to enroll than people who think about all of the beliefs in the theory of planned behavior combined (O'Carroll, Dryden, Hamilton-Barclay, & Ferguson, 2011).

Lastly, health habits are often very ingrained behaviors and are difficult to change. Indeed, people's past behavior is often a better predictor of their future behavior than any of the beliefs identified in many continuum theories (Ogden, 2003; Sutton, McVey, & Glanz, 1999). Changing people's beliefs about a health behavior may provide motivation, but people often need more concrete steps and skills to translate intention into behavior change (Bryan, Fisher, & Fisher, 2002).

IN SUMMARY

The health belief model includes the concepts of perceived severity of the disease, personal susceptibility, and perceived benefits of and barriers to health-enhancing behaviors. The health belief model has only limited success in predicting health-related behaviors.

Self-efficacy theory emphasizes people's beliefs about their ability to control their own health behaviors. Self-efficacy is one of the most important predictors of health behavior, particularly for behaviors that are relatively difficult to adhere to.

Ajzen's theory of planned behavior focuses on intentional behavior, with the predictors of intentions being attitudes, perceived behavioral control, and subjective norms. Perceived behavioral control and intentions tend to be the strongest predictors of adherence. Subjective norms also predict behavior, and have the strongest influence among adolescents and for risk-taking behaviors.

Behavioral theory focuses on reinforcement and habits that must be changed. When a person's attempts to change behavior are met with rewards, it is more likely that those changes will persist. Rewards can be extrinsic (money and compliments) or intrinsic (feeling healthier). Behavioral theory also recognizes the importance of cues and contracts in improving adherence.

Stage Theories of Health Behavior

Stage theories include the transtheoretical model (Prochaska, DiClemente, & Norcross, 1992; Prochaska, Norcross, & DiClemente, 1994), and the health action process approach (Schwarzer, 2008). These models of health behavior differ in several important ways from continuum models. Most importantly, stage models propose that people pass through discrete stages as they attempt to change their behavior. In this way, stage models seem to better describe the *processes* by which people change their behavior than continuum models. Stage models also suggest that different variables will be important depending on what stage a person is in. In this way, stage models differ from continuum models, as people in different stages should benefit from different types of interventions. As you will learn in this section of this chapter, interventions based on stage theories typically tailor information to the specific stage that a person is in, rather than employ a "one size fits all" approach.

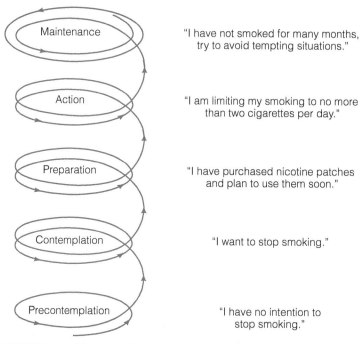

"I have not smoked for many months, try to avoid tempting situations."

"I am limiting my smoking to no more than two cigarettes per day."

"I have purchased nicotine patches and plan to use them soon."

"I want to stop smoking."

"I have no intention to stop smoking."

FIGURE 4.3 The transtheoretical model and stages of changing from smoking to stopping smoking.

The Transtheoretical Model The most well-known stage model is the *transtheoretical model* because it cuts across and borrows from other theoretical models; the *stages-of-change model* is another name for this theory. The transtheoretical model, developed by James Prochaska, Carlo DiClemente, and John Norcross (1992, 1994), assumes that people progress as well as regress through five spiraling stages in making changes in behavior: precontemplation, contemplation, preparation, action, and maintenance. A smoker's progression through these five stages of change in stopping smoking is illustrated in Figure 4.3.

During the *precontemplation stage,* the person has no intention of stopping smoking. In the *contemplation stage,* the person is aware of the problem and has thoughts about quitting, but has not yet made an effort to change. The *preparation stage* includes both thoughts (such as intending to quit within the next month) and action (such as learning about effective quitting techniques or telling others about intentions). During the *action stage,* the person makes overt changes in behavior, such as stopping smoking or using nicotine replacement therapy. In the *maintenance stage,* the person tries to sustain the changes previously made and attempts to resist temptation to relapse back into old habits.

Prochaska and his associates maintain that a person moves from one stage to another in a spiral rather than a linear fashion and argue that this model captures the time factor of behavior change better than other models (Velicer & Prochaska, 2008). Relapses propel people back into a previous stage, or perhaps all the way back to the contemplation or precontemplation stages. From that point, the person may progress several times through the stages until completing behavioral change successfully. Thus, relapses are to be expected and can serve as learning experiences that help a person recycle upward through the various stages.

Prochaska and colleagues (1992, 1994) suggested that people in different stages require different types of assistance to make changes successfully. For example, people in the contemplation and preparation stages should benefit from techniques that raise their awareness of a health problem. In contrast, people in the action and maintenance stages should benefit from strategies that directly address behaviors. Put simply, people in the precontemplation stage need to learn *why* they should change, whereas people in the contemplation and action stages need to learn *how* to change. People in the maintenance stage need help or information oriented toward preserving their changes.

Research tends to support these contentions. For example, a longitudinal study of adopting a low-fat diet (Armitage, Sheeran, Conner, & Arden, 2004) revealed that people's attitudes and behavior fall into the various stages of the transtheoretical model, and individuals both progress through the stages and regress into earlier stages, much as the model predicts. Furthermore, the interventions that moved people from one stage to another varied by stage. Unfortunately, these researchers found that moving people from the preparation to the action stage was more difficult than other transitions. Thus, the transitions from one stage to another may not be equally easy to influence.

Does the transtheoretical model apply equally to different problem behaviors? A meta-analysis of 47 studies (Rosen, 2000) attempted to answer this question by looking at the model across several health-related issues, including smoking, substance abuse, exercise, diet, and psychotherapy. The results showed that the transtheoretical model worked best for understanding smoking cessation compared with many other health behaviors. For example, in the case of smoking cessation, cognitive processes were more frequently used in deciding to quit, whereas behavioral techniques were more effective when a person was in the process of quitting. However, other reviews of stage-matched interventions for smoking cessation have shown that stage-matched interventions are just as effective as interventions that provide the same information to all people regardless of stage (Cahill, Lancaster, & Green, 2010). Compared with its success in understanding smoking cessation, the transtheoretical model has not been as successful in predicting adherence to other

behaviors such as special diets, exercise, or condom use (Bogart & Delahanty, 2004).

The lack of success of stage-matched interventions based on the transtheoretical model may be due to problems with how researchers classify people into stages. For example, the five stages in the transtheoretical model may not represent distinctly different stages (Herzog, 2008). For this reason, some have suggested that stage models with fewer stages may be more accurate and useful (Armitage, 2009). The health action process approach is such a simplified stage model.

The Health Action Process Approach   Schwarzer's (2008) *health action process approach* is a recent model that incorporates some of the most important aspects of both continuum theories and stage theories. The health action process approach can be viewed as a simplified stage model, with two general stages. In the first stage, called the **motivational phase**, a person forms the intention to either adopt a preventive measure or to change a risk behavior. During the motivational phase, three beliefs are necessary for an intention to form. First, people must perceive a personal risk. Second, people must have favorable outcome expectations. Third, people must have a sense of self-efficacy. In the motivational phase, Schwarzer refers to *action self-efficacy*—or the confidence in one's ability to make the change—as being the important belief. Thus, in many ways the motivational phase of the health action process approach resembles many of the continuum models (as shown in Figure 4.4).

However, simply intending to change a behavior is rarely enough to produce lasting change, as anyone who has failed at a New Year's resolution knows. In the second

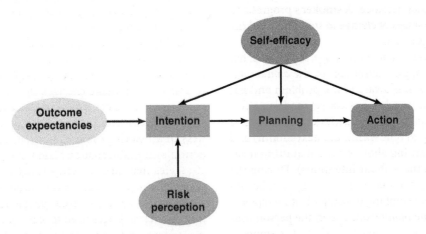

FIGURE 4.4   The health action process approach.

Source: Adapted by permission of Ralf Schwarzer.

stage, called the **volitional phase**, a person attempts to make the change to his or her behavior, as well as persist in those changes over time. During the volitional phase, a different set of beliefs and strategies become important. For example, planning is crucial during the volitional phase. To lose weight, a person must make detailed plans for what foods to eat, what foods to buy, and where and when to exercise. However, many people who wish to change their behavior may not realize the importance of planning until they have already failed at their goals.

A large web-based study of German adults (Parschau et al., 2012) reveals the importance of planning in promoting physical activity. Among adults who intended to exercise but had not yet started, those who engaged in more planning were more likely to be physically active 3 weeks later. However, among the adults who had no intention to exercise, planning had little influence; this finding illustrates the stage-specific role that planning plays in adherence. Planning not only includes detailing the "what, where, and when" but also planning for how to cope with anticipated setbacks. For example, what will a person do if he or she misses an exercise session, or experiences pain when exercising? People who anticipate and plan for such setbacks tend to be more successful in pursuing their health goals (Craciun, Schüz, Lippke, & Schwarzer, 2012; Evers, Klusmann, Ziegelmann, Schwarzer, & Heuser, 2011; Reuter et al., 2010).

Although the health action process approach is not yet studied as widely as other models, many studies support its propositions. Compared with the health belief model and the theory of planned behavior, the health action process approach does a better job of predicting young adults' intentions to resist unhealthy dieting and to perform breast self-exams (Garcia & Mann, 2003).

Critique of Stage Theories   How well do stage theories organize and explain observations? Of the stage theories, the transtheoretical model is the most complex. It proposes five stages, as well as 10 different processes that could potentially move people from stage to stage. As some have noted (Armitage, 2009; Herzog, 2008), this degree of complexity may be unnecessary, as more complex stage models may not explain behavior any better than simpler stage models such as the health action process approach.

Do stage theories help a practitioner predict and change behavior? One of the strengths of stage models is that they recognize the benefit of tailoring interventions to a person's stage of behavior change. For example, people who choose to participate in the ShapeUp program are those in the action or maintenance stage (transtheoretical model) or the volitional stage (health action process approach), as they are acting on their intentions to change their behavior. Many of the behavioral techniques used by the ShapeUp program, such as reminder cues and self-monitoring, are useful for people in those stages of the behavior change process.

Regarding the transtheoretical model, the evidence is mixed for whether stage-matched interventions are more effective than non-stage-matched interventions. Regarding the health action process approach, there is accumulating evidence for the effectiveness of stage-matched interventions based on the health action process approach for promoting physical activity (Lippke, Schwarzer, Ziegelmann, Scholz, & Schüz, 2010; Lippke, Ziegelmann, & Schwarzer, 2004) and oral health (Schüz, Sniehotta, & Schwarzer, 2007). At this point, most studies of stage models use cross-sectional designs, which make it difficult to observe how an individual changes over time. With all stage models, more longitudinal research is needed to evaluate their validity (Ogden, 2003).

Health psychologists who seek to build valid models for health-related behaviors face challenges. One challenge is that health behavior is often determined by factors other than an individual's beliefs or perceptions. Among such factors are poor interpersonal relationships that keep people away from the health care system and public policies (including laws) that affect health behaviors. In addition, certain health-related behaviors, such as cigarette smoking and dental care, can develop into habits that become so automatic that they are largely outside the personal decision-making process. All of these factors present challenges for researchers to create theories of health behavior that account for all of this variability while also keeping the models as simple and parsimonious as possible.

Most of the models postulate some type of barrier or obstacle to seeking health care, and an almost unlimited number of barriers are possible. Often these barriers are beyond the life experience of researchers. For example, barriers for affluent European Americans may be quite different from those faced by poor Hispanic Americans, Africans living in sub-Saharan Africa, or Hmong immigrants in Canada; thus, the health belief model and the theory of planned behavior may not apply equally to all ethnic and socioeconomic groups (Poss, 2000). Models for health-seeking behavior tend to emphasize the importance of direct and personal control of behavioral choices. Little allowance is made for barriers such as racism and poverty.

IN SUMMARY

Stage models of health behavior classify people into different stages of adherence and suggest that progression through each stage is predicted by different sets of variables. Prochaska's transtheoretical model assumes that people spiral through five stages as they make changes in behavior: precontemplation, contemplation, preparation, action, and maintenance. Relapse should be expected, but after relapse, people can move forward again through the various stages.

Schwarzer's health action process approach proposes only two general stages: the motivational phase and the volitional phase. Planning and specific forms of self-efficacy are thought to be important factors for helping people translate intentions into lasting behavior change.

Stage models suggest that interventions should use a tailored, stage-matched approach, by only addressing the variables relevant in the person's current stage. Thus, the effectiveness of stage-matched interventions depends in part on how well practitioners can classify people into discrete stages. One criticism of the transtheoretical model is that the five stages do not represent discrete stages, and people in different stages may be more similar to each other than the theory suggests. This may explain why there is only mixed support for stage-matched interventions based on the transtheoretical model.

The Intention–Behavior Gap

Stage models acknowledge what many of us already know from our own experiences—that even our best intentions do not always translate into behavior. This "intention–behavior gap" (Sheeran, 2002) is exemplified by people who intend to behave healthily but do not. In this section, we describe models and strategies that help understanding the reasons for this intention–behavior gap, as well as ways to help bridge this gap.

Behavioral Willingness

In some situations, strong social pressures are capable of thwarting the best of intentions. A person may enter into a potential sexual encounter with every intention of using a condom or embark on a night out on the town

with the intent of resisting binge drinking. At some point in the evening, however, the person may forget these intentions altogether. **Behavioral willingness** refers to a person's motivation *at a given moment* to engage in a risky behavior (Gibbons, Gerrard, Blanton, & Russell, 1998). Behavioral willingness reflects more of a *reaction* to a situation than a deliberate, planned choice. This concept of behavioral willingness has been helpful in understanding a number of adolescent risk-taking behaviors, such as smoking, alcohol use, and lack of safe sex practices (Andrews, Hampson, Barckley, Gerrard, & Gibbons, 2008; Gibbons et al., 1998). In these studies, intention and willingness relate to each other, showing that people with stronger intentions tend to report less of a willingness to engage in risky behaviors "in the moment." However, behavioral willingness is a unique predictor of actual behavior. That is, if you take two people with equally strong intentions to

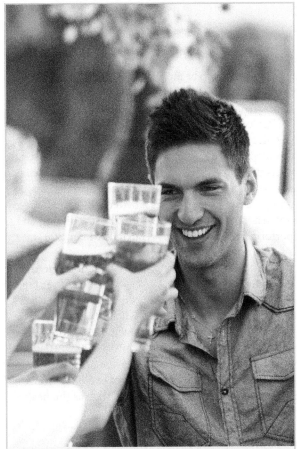

People may intend to avoid risky behaviors, but strong social pressures often make them willing to engage in them.

iStockphoto.com/Ajkkafe

avoid risky behaviors, the person with the greater willingness will be the one whose intentions will ultimately fall short.

What drives people's willingness to engage in risky behaviors? Many times, people's concern about their social image is what leads to the willingness to engage in risky behavior. When people have positive images of others who engage in risky behaviors, they are more likely to report a willingness to engage in those behaviors (Gibbons et al., 1998). In turn, that willingness can break down the best of intentions.

Implementational Intentions

As emphasized in the health action process approach, planning is an important factor in translating intention into action. A growing body of research shows that short and simple planning exercises can help people adhere to medical advice. **Implementational intentions** are specific plans that people can make that identify not only *what* they intend to do but also *where*, *when*, and *how*. In essence, implementational intentions connect a situation with the goal that the person

Would You BELIEVE...? Both Real and Online Social Networks Can Influence Health

How much do our social networks influence our health behaviors? While it's tempting to think of a person's health as mainly a reflection of his or her personal preferences, behavior is also strongly related to a person's social network: both real and online. What kind of people tend to influence our behaviors the most, and what kind of people do we look toward for inspiration and influence?

Using a rich longitudinal dataset from the Framingham Heart Study, Nicholas Christakis examined the influence of our real social networks on health behaviors by tracking how health behaviors such as smoking and obesity spread through social networks over a period of three decades. The study collected health information from over 5,000 adults as well as 8 to 10 of their closest family members, friends, and co-workers. Christakis found that a person's chances of becoming obese or quitting smoking were significantly predicted by what occurred in one's immediate social network. For example, if a person's spouse became obese or quit smoking, that person's chances of also becoming obese or quitting smoking increased by nearly 60% (Christakis & Fowler, 2007, 2008)!

Clearly, spouses had a strong influence on a person's health, but siblings, friends, and even co-workers also had a noticeable influence on people's health. Thus, a person's health was closely tied to the health of those around them, either for better (smoking cessation) or for worse (obesity).

Could our online social networks also influence health? In a series of clever studies, Damon Centola examined how health behaviors could spread through an online social network. Centola teamed up with a fitness-promoting website, where upon registration, users would be assigned a number of "neighbors" who were also users of the site. Users could also choose to "friend" new neighbors or "unfriend" existing neighbors from their network. How did people select who to add or remove from their network? Interestingly, Centola found that users overwhelmingly chose to add neighbors who were *similar* to them—especially in terms of age, gender, and body mass index (BMI)—and to drop neighbors who were dissimilar (Centola & van de Rijt, 2015). In short, people didn't choose to associate with people who might have been fitter or more "aspirational." Rather, they

chose to associate with people like themselves.

Could this tendency toward *homophily* (associating with people who are similar) have a detrimental influence on people who are not fit? To test this idea, Centola (2011) set up a fitness social network site where a user's neighbors were either assigned randomly or assigned so that they were similar in age, gender, and BMI to the user. Centola then had one neighbor in everyone's network make mention of a new diet plan, and Centola tracked how interest in the diet spread through the networks. Not surprisingly, interest in the diet spread more rapidly in the homophilic networks than in the random networks. In other words, a network had greater influence if the people in the networks were similar to each other. More importantly, it didn't matter if a user was less fit and therefore surrounded by friends who were also less fit. The interest in the diet plan spread as rapidly among "fit" networks as it did among "less fit" networks. Thus, these results suggest that online social networks can have positive influences on health, even among people who may have the greatest health risks.

wants to achieve. For example, someone who wants to exercise more could form an implementational intention of "I will run 30 minutes immediately after work on Tuesday evening." In this way, implementational intentions go beyond the intention of "I plan to exercise more." Over time, it is thought that forming implementational intentions can help make people's pursuit of their goals more automatic.

Indeed, simple implementational intentions exercises are effective in helping people to adhere to a wide variety of health behaviors. These include one-time behaviors such as cervical cancer screening (Sheeran & Orbell, 2000) and breast self-exam (Orbell, Hodgkins, & Sheeran, 1997). Implementational intentions also make it more likely that people engage in behaviors that require action over time, such as taking vitamin supplements and medications (Brown, Sheeran, & Rueber, 2009; Sheeran & Orbell, 1999), eating healthily (Armitage, 2004; Verplanken & Faes, 1999), and resisting binge drinking (Murgraff, White, & Phillips, 1996). A meta-analysis of over 20 studies on physical activity confirmed the usefulness of implementational intentions in promoting adherence (Bélanger-Gravel, Godin, & Amireault, 2011).

Why do implementation intentions work? One reason is that they make people less likely to forget their intentions. For example, in a study of cervical cancer screening, 74% of participants scheduled their appointment on the very date they had specified in their implementation intention exercise (Sheeran & Orbell, 2000). Thus, implementational intentions can help turn "intenders" into "actors."

IN SUMMARY

Many people fail to adhere because their intentions do not translate into behavior. For some people, this may occur because of *behavioral willingness*, which represents a person's willingness to engage in risky behaviors at a given moment. Behavioral willingness can put people at risk of nonadherence when strong social pressures exist. People may also not adhere because they do not plan adequately. *Implementational intentions* represent specific plans that link a situation with the enactment of a behavior and can boost adherence to a variety of health behaviors.

Improving Adherence

In this chapter, we have surveyed several issues related to adherence, including theoretical models that might explain or predict adherence, techniques for measuring adherence, the frequency of adherence, and factors that relate to adherence. This information, along with knowledge of why some people fail to adhere, can help answer an important question of this chapter: How can adherence be improved?

Methods for improving adherence can generally be divided into (1) educational and (2) behavioral strategies. Educational procedures are those that impart information, sometimes in an emotion-arousing manner designed to frighten the nonadherent patient into becoming adherent. Included with educational strategies are procedures such as health education messages, individual patient counseling with various professional health care providers, programmed instruction, lectures, demonstrations, and individual counseling accompanied by written instructions. Haynes (1976) reported that strategies that relied on education and threats of disastrous consequences for nonadherence were only marginally effective in bringing about a meaningful change in patients' behaviors; more recent reviews (Harrington, Noble, & Newman, 2004; Schroeder, Fahey, & Ebrahim, 2007) come to similar conclusions. Educational methods may increase patients' knowledge, but behavioral approaches offer a more effective way of enhancing adherence. People, it seems, do not misbehave because they do not know better but because adherent behavior, for a variety of reasons, is less appealing or difficult to enact.

Behavioral strategies focus more directly on changing the behaviors involved in compliance. They include a wide variety of techniques, such as notifying patients of upcoming appointments, simplifying medical schedules, providing cues to prompt taking medication, monitoring and rewarding patients' compliant behaviors, and shaping people toward self-monitoring and self-care. Behavioral techniques are typically more effective than educational strategies in improving patient adherence, particularly for people who know *why* they should change their behavior but may not know *how*. Indeed, one reason why the ShapeUp program may have been so successful is that it included a number of behavioral strategies, such as reminders and self-monitoring of physical activity. Self-monitoring is known to be one of the most powerful techniques to improve one's diet and physical activity (Michie et al., 2009).

Adherence researchers Robin DiMatteo and Dante DiNicola (1982) recommended four categories of behavioral strategies for improving adherence, and their categories are still a valid way to approach the topic. First, various *prompts* can be used to remind patients to initiate health-enhancing behaviors. These prompts may be cued by regular events in the patient's life, such as taking medication before each meal, or they may take the form of telephone calls from a clinic to remind the person to keep an appointment or to refill a prescription. Another type of prompt comes in the form of reminder packaging, which presents information about the date or time that the medication should be taken on the packaging for the medication (Heneghan, Glasziou, & Perera, 2007). In addition, electronic technology such as text messaging or smartphone apps can be useful in providing prompts.

A second behavioral strategy proposed by DiMatteo and DiNicola is *tailoring the regimen,* which involves fitting the treatment to habits and routines in the patient's daily life. For example, pill organizers work toward this goal by making medication more compatible with the person's life, and some drug companies are creating medication packaging, called compliance packaging, that is similar to pill organizers in providing a tailored regimen (Gans & McPhillips, 2003). Another approach that fits within this category is simplifying the medication schedule; a review of adherence studies (Schroeder et al., 2007) indicated that this approach was among the most successful in increasing adherence.

Another way to tailor the regimen involves assessing important characteristics of the patient—such as personality or stages of change—and orienting change-related messages to these characteristics (Gans & McPhillips, 2003; Sherman, Updegraff, & Mann, 2008). For example, a person in the contemplation stage is aware of the problem but has not yet decided to adopt a behavior (see Figure 4.2). This person might benefit from an intervention that includes information or counseling, whereas a person in the maintenance stage would not. Instead, people in the maintenance stage might benefit from monitoring devices or prompts that remind them to take their medication or to exercise. Applying this approach to the problem of preventing the complications that accompany heart disease, a group of researchers (Turpin et al., 2004) concluded that tailoring adherence programs to patients' previous levels of adherence is critical; patients who are mostly adherent differ from those who are partially adherent or nonadherent. These successes suggest that different stages of readiness to change require different types of assistance to achieve adherence.

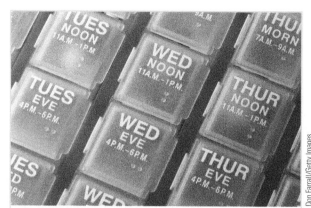

Finding effective prompts helps patients fit medication into their schedules.

A similar way to tailor the regimen involves helping clients resolve the problems that prevent them from changing their behavior. **Motivational interviewing** is a therapeutic approach that originated within substance abuse treatment (Miller & Rollnick, 2002) but has been applied to many other health-related behaviors, including medication adherence, physical activity, diet, and diabetes management (Martins & McNeil, 2009). This technique attempts to change a client's motivation and prepares the client to enact changes in behavior. The procedure includes an interview in which the practitioner attempts to show empathy with the client's situation; discusses and clarifies the client's goals and contrasts them with the client's current, unacceptable behavior; and helps the client formulate ways to change behavior. Reviews indicate that the technique is effective, particularly for motivating people to stop smoking (Lai, Cahill, Qin, & Tang, 2010; Lundahl & Burke, 2009; Martins & McNeil, 2009).

Third, DiMatteo and DiNicola suggested a *graduated regimen implementation* that reinforces successive approximations to the desired behavior. Such shaping procedures would be appropriate for exercise, diet, and possibly smoking cessation programs but not for taking medications.

The final behavioral strategy listed by DiMatteo and DiNicola is a *contingency contract* (or behavioral contract)—an agreement, usually written, between patients and health care professionals that provides for some kind of reward to patients contingent on their achieving compliance. These contracts may also involve penalties for noncompliance (Gans & McPhillips, 2003). Contingency contracts are most effective when they are enacted at the beginning of therapy and when the provisions are negotiated and agreed upon by patients and providers. Even with these provisions, contracts have not been demonstrated to boost adherence by a great deal (Bosch-Capblanch, Abba, Prictor, & Garner, 2007), and any beneficial effects on adherence are likely to dissipate after the contract is complete (Mantzari et al., 2015).

Despite these suggestions, many health care providers put little effort into improving adherence, and adherence rates have improved little over the past 50 years (DiMatteo, 2004a). Evidence indicates that clear instructions about taking medications are the best strategy to boost adherence for short-term regimens (Haynes, McDonald, & Garg, 2002); the instructions work better if they are both verbal and in writing (Johnson, Sandford, & Tyndall, 2007). For long-term regimens, many strategies show some effectiveness, but none offer dramatic improvement (Haynes et al., 2008). Furthermore, the interventions that demonstrate greater effectiveness tend to be complex and costly.

Therefore, adherence remains a costly problem, both in terms of the cost in lives and ill health of failures and in terms of the added costs of even marginally effective interventions. Despite these challenges, addressing the issue of nonadherence is an ongoing task in the field of health psychology.

IN SUMMARY

Effective programs to improve compliance rates frequently include cues to signal the time for taking medication, clearly written instructions, simplified medication regimens, prescriptions tailored to the patient's daily schedule, and rewards for compliant behavior. Despite these effective strategies, the problem of nonadherence remains a major challenge for the health psychologist.

 # Becoming Healthier

You can improve your health by following sound health-related advice. Here are some things you can do to make adherence pay off.

1. Adopt an overall healthy lifestyle—one that includes not smoking, using alcohol in moderation or not at all, eating a diet high in fiber and low in saturated fats, getting an optimum amount of regular physical activity, and incorporating safety into your life. Procedures for adopting each of these health habits are discussed in *Becoming Healthier* boxes in Chapters 12 through 15.

2. Establish a working alliance with your physician that is based on cooperation, not obedience. You and your doctor are the two most important people involved in your health, and the two of you should cooperate in designing your health practices.

3. Another important person interested in your health is your spouse, parent, friend, or sibling. Enlist the support of a significant person or persons in your life. High levels of social support improve one's rate of adherence.

4. Before visiting a health care provider, jot down some questions you would like to have answered; ask the questions and write down the answers during the visit. If you receive a prescription, ask the doctor about possible side effects—you don't want an unanticipated unpleasant side effect to be an excuse to stop taking the medication. Also, be sure you know how long you must take the medication—some chronic diseases require a lifetime of treatment.

5. If your physician gives you complex medical information that you don't comprehend, ask for clarification in language that you can understand. Enlist the cooperation of your pharmacist,

who can be another valuable health care provider.

6. Remember that some recommendations such as beginning a regular exercise program should be adopted gradually. If you do too much the first day, you won't feel like exercising again the next day.

7. Find a practitioner who understands and appreciates your cultural beliefs, ethnic background, language, and religious beliefs.

8. Make specific plans for when and how you will act to achieve your goals. Research on implementational intentions shows that simple planning exercises are effective in helping people adhere.

9. Reward yourself for following your good health practices. If you faithfully followed your diet for a day or a week, do something nice for yourself!

Answers

This chapter addresses six basic questions:

1. **What is adherence, how is it measured, and how frequently does it occur?**

Adherence is the extent to which a person's behavior coincides with appropriate medical and health advice. For people to profit from medical advice, first, the advice must be accurate and, second, patients must follow the advice. When people do not adhere to sound health behaviors, they may risk serious health problems or even death. As many as 125,000 people in the United States die each year because of adherence failures.

Researchers can measure adherence in at least six ways: (1) ask the practitioner, (2) ask the patient, (3) ask other people, (4) monitor use of medicine, (5) examine biochemical evidence, and (6) use a combination of these procedures. Of these, physician judgment is the least valid, but each of the others also has serious flaws; a combination of procedures provides the best assessment.

These different methods of assessment complicate the determination of the frequency of nonadherence. However, an analysis of more than 500 studies revealed that the average rate of nonadherence is around 25%, with people on medication regimens more adherent than those who must change health-related behaviors.

2. **What factors predict adherence?**

The severity of a disease does not predict adherence, but unpleasant or painful side effects of medication do lower adherence. Some personal factors relate to adherence, but a nonadherent personality does not exist. Age shows a curvilinear relationship, with older adults and children and adolescents experiencing problems in adhering to medication regimens, but gender shows little overall effect. Emotional factors such as stress, anxiety, and depression lower adherence, but conscientiousness improves adherence. Personal beliefs are a significant factor, with beliefs in a regimen's ineffectiveness lowering adherence and self-efficacy beliefs increasing adherence.

A person's life situation also affects adherence. Lower income endangers adherence; people are not able to pay for treatment or medications. Higher income levels and greater social support generally increase adherence. Individuals with a cultural background that fails to accept Western medicine are less likely to adhere. Ethnicity may also affect the treatment that patients receive from practitioners, and people who feel discriminated against adhere at lower rates. No one factor accounts for adherence, so researchers must consider a combination of factors.

3. **What are continuum theories of health behavior, and how do they explain adherence?**

Continuum theories of health behavior identify variables that should predict the likelihood a person will adhere to a healthy behavior. Continuum theories propose that the variables should predict adherence in the same manner for all individuals.

The health belief model focuses on people's beliefs in perceived susceptibility to a health problem, perceived severity of the problem, perceived benefits of adhering to a behavior, and perceived barriers to adherence. Self-efficacy theory focuses on beliefs about people's confidence that they can control adherence, as well as their beliefs that adherence will bring about good outcomes. The theory of planned behavior focuses on people's attitudes toward a behavior, their beliefs about subjective norms, and their perceived behavioral control as predictors of intentions. Behavioral theory explains adherence in terms of reinforcement and habits that must be changed. Rewards and reinforcements can help a person to initiate a behavior, as well as maintain it over time. Behavioral theory also recognizes the importance of cues and contracts in improving adherence.

Continuum theories generate a large amount of research across a wide variety of behaviors and are typically successful at predicting people's motivations to adhere to health behaviors. However, they neglect behavioral factors, so they are often better at predicting people's motivations and intentions than they are at predicting behavior.

4. **What are stage theories of health behavior, and how do they explain adherence?**

Stage theories propose that people progress through discrete stages in the process of changing their behavior, and that different variables will be important depending on what stage a person is in. The transtheoretical model proposes that people progress in spiral fashion through five stages in making changes in behavior—precontemplation, contemplation, preparation, action, and maintenance. People in the earlier stages of contemplation and preparation are thought to benefit more from techniques that raise their awareness of a health problem, such as education or motivational interviewing. In contrast, people in the later stages of action and maintenance should benefit most from strategies that directly address behaviors.

The health action process approach proposes two stages: a motivational phase and a volitional phase. Perceived susceptibility, self-efficacy, and outcome expectations are the important factors in the motivational phase. Planning and self-efficacy are the important factors in the volitional phase.

The success of stage theories in predicting and changing behavior rests on having accurate and valid methods of assessing a person's stage of behavior change. All theories—continuum and stage theories—are useful for understanding adherence but limited by their omission of various social, economic, ethnic, and other demographic factors that also affect people's health behavior.

5. **What is the intention–behavior gap, and what factors predict whether intentions are translated into behavior?**

The intention–behavior gap refers to the fact that intentions are imperfect predictors of adherence. Behavioral willingness refers to a person's motivation at a given moment to engage in a risky behavior and is driven largely by social pressures in a specific situation. Poor planning can also explain why intentions are not always translated into behavior. Implementational intentions are effective planning exercises that help people identify the specific situations in which they will perform a specific behavior.

6. **How can adherence be improved?**

Methods for improving adherence can generally be divided into educational and behavioral strategies. Educational methods may increase patients' knowledge, but behavioral approaches are better at enhancing adherence. Strategies for enhancing adherence fall into four approaches: (1) providing prompts, (2) tailoring the regimen, (3) implementing the regimen gradually, and (4) making a contingency contract. Effective programs frequently include clearly written as well as clear verbal instructions, simple medication schedules, follow-up calls for missed appointments, prescriptions tailored to the patient's daily schedule, rewards for compliant behavior, and cues to signal the time for taking medication.

Suggested Readings

Bogart, L. M., & Delahanty, D. L. (2004). Psychosocial models. In T. J. Boll, R. G. Frank, A. Baum, & J. L. Wallander (Eds.), *Handbook of clinical health psychology: Vol. 3: Models and perspectives in health psychology* (pp. 201–248). Washington, DC: American Psychological Association. This review of models of health-related behaviors critically examines the health belief model and theories of reasoned action and planned behavior. The review is oriented around an evaluation of how well these models predict important health behaviors, including condom use, exercise, smoking, and dieting.

DiMatteo, M. R. (2004). Variations in patients' adherence to medical recommendations: A quantitative review of 50 years of research. *Medical Care, 42,* 200–209. DiMatteo analyzes more than 500 studies published over a span of 50 years to determine factors that relate to failures in adherence. Her concise summary of these results reveals the relative contribution of demographic factors as well as illness characteristics.

Schwarzer, R. (2008). Modeling health behavior change: How to predict and modify the adoption and maintenance of health behaviors. *Applied Psychology: An International Review, 57,* 1–29. This review outlines the health action process approach, and its application to understanding both the adoption and the maintenance of several health behaviors, such as physical activity, breast self-examination, seat belt use, dietary change, and dental flossing.

will work out.

CHAPTER 5

Defining, Measuring, and Managing Stress

CHAPTER OUTLINE

QUESTIONS

This chapter focuses on six basic questions:

1. What is the physiology of stress?

2. What theories explain stress?

3. What sources produce stress?

4. How is stress measured?

5. What factors influence coping, and what strategies are effective?

6. What behavioral techniques are effective for stress management?

☑ Check Your **HEALTH RISKS** *Life Events Scale for Students*

Has this stressful event happened to you at any time during the last 4 months? If it has, please check the box next to it. If it has not, leave it blank.

- ☐ Death of a parent (100)
- ☐ Death of your best or very good friend (91)
- ☐ Time in jail (80)
- ☐ Pregnancy, either yourself or being the father (78)
- ☐ Major car accident (car wrecked, people injured) (77)
- ☐ Major personal injury or illness (75)
- ☐ Break-up of parent's marriage/divorce (70)
- ☐ Getting kicked out of college (68)
- ☐ Major change of health in close family member (68)
- ☐ Break-up with boy/girlfriend (65)
- ☐ Major and/or chronic financial problems (63)
- ☐ Parent losing a job (57)
- ☐ Losing a good friend (57)
- ☐ Failing a number of courses (56)
- ☐ Seeking psychological or psychiatric consultation (56)

- ☐ Seriously thinking about dropping out of college (55)
- ☐ Failing a course (53)
- ☐ Major argument with boy/girlfriend (53)
- ☐ Major argument with parents (48)
- ☐ Sex difficulties with boy/girlfriend (48)
- ☐ Beginning an undergraduate program at university (47)
- ☐ Moving away from home (46)
- ☐ Moving out of town with parents (44)
- ☐ Change of job (43)
- ☐ Minor car accident (42)
- ☐ Switch in program within same college or university (37)
- ☐ Getting an unjustified low grade on a test (36)
- ☐ Establishing new steady relationship with partner (35)
- ☐ Minor financial problems (32)
- ☐ Losing a part-time job (31)
- ☐ Vacation with parents (27)

- ☐ Finding a part-time job (25)
- ☐ Family get-togethers (25)
- ☐ Minor violation of the law (e.g., speeding ticket) (24)
- ☐ Getting your own car (21)
- ☐ Vacation alone/with friends (16)

For all of the items you checked, add up the numbers in parentheses next to the items. Healthy undergraduate students, on average, have total scores around 190. Clearly, college students experience stress in their lives. However, as scores increase, so do people's risk of health problems. For example, people with scores of 300 and higher have a very high risk of a serious health change within 2 years. This chapter explores why stressful life events such as those listed in this checklist can worsen physical health.

Source: Reprinted from *Personality and Individual Differences*, Vol. 20, Issue 6. Clements, K., & Turpin, G., The life events scale for students: Validation for use with British Samples, 747–751, 1996.

Real-World Profile of **HOPE SOLO**

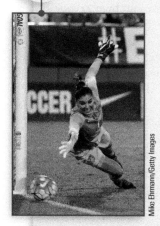

Mike Ehrmann/Getty Images

What is the most stressful position in professional sports? Ask this question to any sports fan, you will likely hear one of three positions: a football placekicker, a hockey goaltender, or a soccer goaltender. In all of these positions, the success of an entire team rests on the ability of a single person to perform in the most intense of situations. A successful kick or block is what the team and fans expect. But a missed kick or an allowed goal can be devastating.

Hope Solo, regarded as one of the top female soccer goalkeepers in the world, is no stranger to stress. In her 13-year professional career, she has continually moved, playing for teams in Pennsylvania, Missouri, Washington, Florida, Sweden, and France. She earned two Olympic gold medals and a World Cup gold medal. She currently holds the U.S. record for most career "clean sheets"—that is, the most games played in which the opposing team could not score a goal against her. Despite her successes, she has also responded to stress in ways that have caused her problems.

Hope's experiences with stress began early in life. Hope's father, a war veteran and ex-con man, taught her how to play soccer at the age of 5, but soon left her family and spent time homeless on the streets of Seattle. When Hope was 7, her father took her and her brother on what seemed to be a vacation but was actually an attempted kidnapping. Hope's father was rarely around during her childhood and adolescence.

Hope focused her attention on soccer throughout high school and college. While playing for the University of Washington, she rekindled her relationship with her father and the two became very close. Her father would attend every home game she played, and Hope would bring him food and talk with him for hours. Hope, a self-described loner, said that her father was "the only one who really knew me" (Hass, 2012). During Hope's time in college, her father was named as a suspect in a brutal murder case. Both Hope and her father maintained his innocence for years, and the experience angered Hope. Although the charge against Hope's father was later shown to be false, Hope's father died of a heart attack just months prior to her first appearance in the 2007 FIFA Women's World Cup.

At the start of every match that Hope played in the 2007 Women's World Cup, she spread ashes of her father in the goal area she protected. However, Hope's coach chose not to play her in a critical semifinal match against the Brazilian team, which angered her. Hope publicly criticized the decision, upsetting her coach, team, and the soccer community. As a result of her outburst, Solo was dropped from playing in the rest of the World Cup matches that year.

S tress is a reality of life. The causes of stress are widespread and include major life-changing events such as death of a loved one, unemployment, and disasters such as the terrorist attacks of September 11, 2001, Hurricane Katrina, and the 2011 tsunami in Japan that left over 300,000 people displaced from their homes and villages. Seemingly minor hassles such as relationship breakups and transportation problems can be ongoing sources of stress. Even people who are expert in handling some kinds of stress, such as Hope Solo, may find other forms of stress difficult. This chapter looks at what stress is, how it can be measured, some of the effective and ineffective strategies that people use to cope, and some behavioral management techniques that can help people cope more effectively. Chapter 6 examines the question of whether stress can cause illness and even death. In this chapter, we first look at the physiological bases of stress.

The Nervous System and the Physiology of Stress

Stress is a psychological experience that easily gets "under the skin" to influence how our bodies function. To understand the physiological effects of stress, we must first understand several aspects of the nervous and endocrine system.

The effects of stress on the body result from our nervous system's responses to our environment. The human nervous system contains billions of individual cells called **neurons**, which function electrochemically. Within each neuron, electrically charged ions hold the potential for an electrical discharge. The discharge of this potential produces a small electrical current, which travels the length of the neuron. The electrical charge leads to the release of chemicals called **neurotransmitters** that are manufactured within each neuron and stored in vesicles at the ends of the neurons. The released neurotransmitters diffuse across the **synaptic cleft**, the space between neurons. Thus, neurotransmitters are the primary ways that neurons communicate with each other.

Billions of neurons make up the nervous system, which is organized in a hierarchy with major divisions and subdivisions. The two major divisions of the nervous system are the **central nervous system (CNS)** and the **peripheral nervous system (PNS)**. The CNS consists of the brain and the spinal cord. The PNS consists of all other neurons, which extend from the spinal cord to all other parts of the body. Figure 5.1 illustrates these divisions and subdivisions of the nervous system.

The Peripheral Nervous System

The PNS, that part of the nervous system lying outside the brain and spinal cord, is divided into two parts:

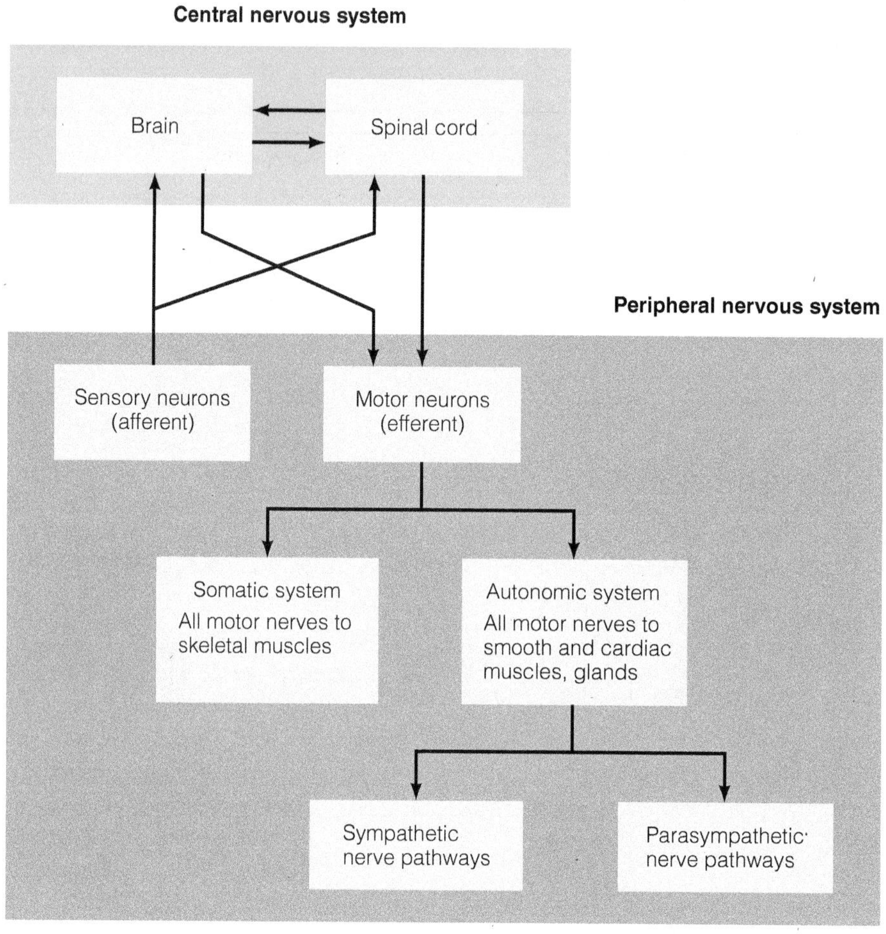

Central nervous system

Peripheral nervous system

FIGURE 5.1 Divisions of the human nervous system.

the **somatic nervous system** and the **autonomic nervous system** (ANS). The somatic nervous system primarily serves the skin and the voluntary muscles. The ANS primarily serves internal organs and is therefore important in understanding responses to stress.

The ANS allows for a variety of responses through its two divisions: the **sympathetic nervous system** and the **parasympathetic nervous system**. These two subdivisions differ anatomically as well as functionally. They, along with their target organs, appear in Figure 5.2.

The sympathetic division of the ANS mobilizes the body's resources in emergency, stressful, and emotional situations. The reactions include an increase in the rate and strength of heart contractions, increase in rate of breathing, constriction of blood vessels in the skin, a decrease of gastrointestinal activity, stimulation of the sweat glands, and dilation of the pupils in the eyes. Many of these physiological changes serve

to direct the flow of blood and oxygen to the skeletal muscles, enabling the organism to mount a quick motor response to a potentially threatening event.

The parasympathetic division of the ANS, on the other hand, promotes relaxation, digestion, and normal growth functions. The parasympathetic nervous system is active under normal, nonstressful conditions. The parasympathetic and sympathetic nervous systems serve the same target organs, but they tend to function reciprocally, with the activation of one increasing as the other decreases. For example, the activation of the sympathetic division reduces the secretion of saliva, producing the sensation of a dry mouth. The activation of the parasympathetic division promotes secretion of saliva.

Neurons in the ANS are activated by neurotransmitters, principally **acetylcholine** and **norepinephrine**. These neurotransmitters have complex effects; each has different effects in different organ systems because

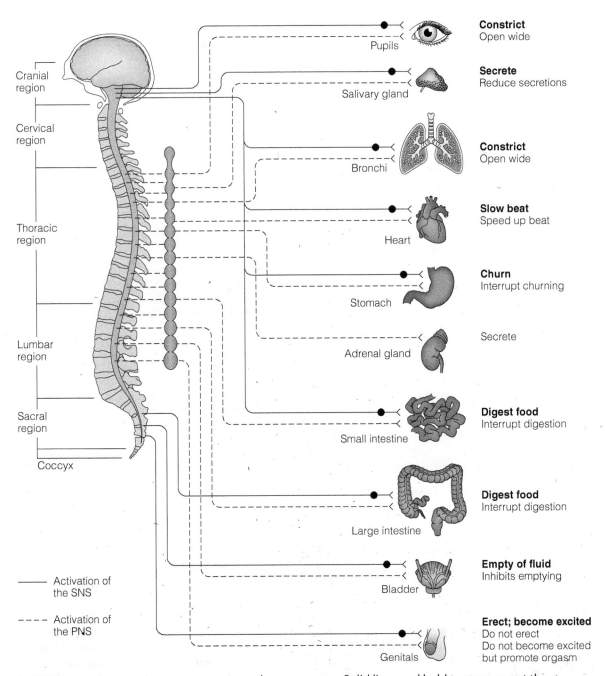

FIGURE 5.2 Autonomic nervous system and target organs. Solid lines and bold type represent the parasympathetic system, whereas dashed lines and lighter type represent the sympathetic system.

the organs contain different neurochemical receptors. In addition, the balance between these two main neurotransmitters, as well as their absolute quantity, is important. Therefore, these two major ANS neurotransmitters can produce a wide variety of responses. Norepinephrine, as we will describe shortly, plays a number of important roles in the stress response.

The Neuroendocrine System

The **endocrine system** consists of ductless glands distributed throughout the body (see Figure 5.3). The **neuroendocrine system** consists of those endocrine glands that are controlled by and interact with the nervous system. Glands of the endocrine

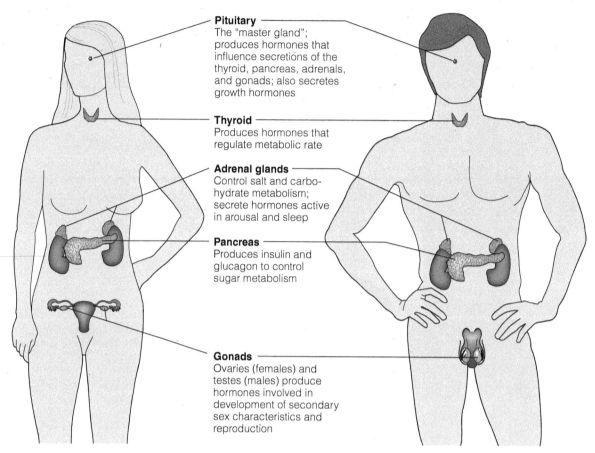

Pituitary
The "master gland"; produces hormones that influence secretions of the thyroid, pancreas, adrenals, and gonads; also secretes growth hormones

Thyroid
Produces hormones that regulate metabolic rate

Adrenal glands
Control salt and carbo-hydrate metabolism; secrete hormones active in arousal and sleep

Pancreas
Produces insulin and glucagon to control sugar metabolism

Gonads
Ovaries (females) and testes (males) produce hormones involved in development of secondary sex characteristics and reproduction

FIGURE 5.3 Some important endocrine glands.

and neuroendocrine systems secrete chemicals known as **hormones**, which move into the bloodstream to be carried to different parts of the body. Specialized receptors on target tissues or organs allow hormones to have specific effects, even though the hormones circulate throughout the body. At the target, hormones may have a direct effect, or they may cause the secretion of another hormone.

The endocrine and nervous systems work closely together because they have several similarities, but they also differ in important ways. Both systems share, synthesize, and release chemicals. In the nervous system, these chemicals are called neurotransmitters; in the endocrine system, they are called hormones. The activation of neurons is usually rapid, and the effect is short term; the endocrine system responds more slowly, and its action persists longer. In the nervous system, neurotransmitters are released by the stimulation of neural impulses, flow across the synaptic cleft, and are immediately either reabsorbed or inactivated. In the

endocrine system, hormones are synthesized by the endocrine cells, are released into the blood, reach their targets in minutes or even hours, and exert prolonged effects. The endocrine and nervous systems both have communication and control functions, and both work toward integrated, adaptive behaviors. The two systems are related in function and interact in neuroendocrine responses.

The Pituitary Gland   The **pituitary gland** is located in the brain and is an excellent example of the intricate relationship between the nervous and endocrine systems. The pituitary is connected to the hypothalamus, a structure in the forebrain, and is sometimes referred to as the "master gland" because it produces a number of hormones that affect other glands and prompt the production of yet other hormones.

Of the seven hormones produced by the anterior portion of the pituitary gland, **adrenocorticotropic hormone (ACTH)** plays an essential role in the stress response. When stimulated by the hypothalamus, the pituitary releases ACTH, which in turn acts on the adrenal glands.

The Adrenal Glands   The adrenal glands are endocrine glands located on top of each kidney. Each gland is composed of an outer covering, the adrenal cortex, and an inner part, the adrenal medulla. Both secrete hormones that are important in the response to stress. The adrenocortical response occurs when ACTH from the pituitary stimulates the adrenal cortex to release glucocorticoids, one type of hormone. Cortisol, the most important of these hormones, exerts a wide range of effects on major organs in the body (Kemeny, 2003).

This hormone is so closely associated with stress that the level of cortisol circulating in the blood can be used as an index of stress. Its peak levels appear 20 to 40 minutes after a stressor, allowing time for measurement of this stress hormone. Cortisol can also be assessed in the saliva and urine.

The **adrenomedullary response** occurs when the sympathetic nervous system activates the adrenal medulla. This action prompts secretion of **catecholamines**, a class of chemicals containing norepinephrine and **epinephrine**. Norepinephrine is both a hormone and a neurotransmitter and is produced in many places in the body besides the adrenal medulla. Figure 5.4 shows this adrenomedullary response.

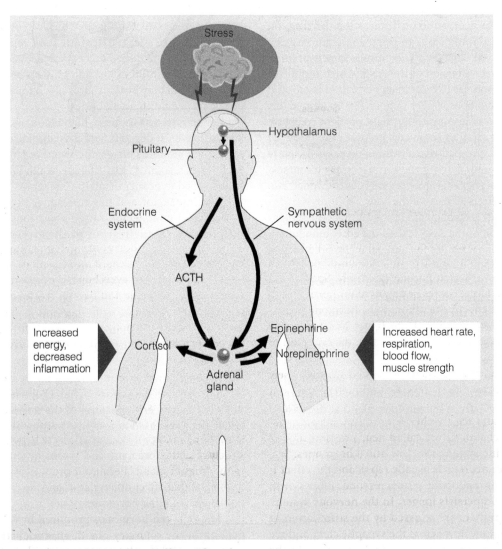

FIGURE 5.4 Physiological effects of stress.

On the other hand, epinephrine (sometimes referred to as adrenaline) is produced exclusively in the adrenal medulla. It is so closely and uniquely associated with the adrenomedullary stress response that it is sometimes used as an index of stress. The amount of epinephrine secreted can be determined by assaying a person's urine, thus measuring stress by tapping into the physiology of the stress response. Like other hormones, epinephrine and norepinephrine circulate through the bloodstream, so their action is both slower and more prolonged than the action of neurotransmitters.

Physiology of the Stress Response

Each of these physiological reactions to stress begins with the perception of some kind of stress or threat, whether it be an unfair accusation or insult, a job demand, or, perhaps as in Solo's case, an opposing team rushing toward her goal. That *perception* results in activation of the sympathetic division of the ANS, which mobilizes the body's resources to react in emotional, stressful, and emergency situations. Walter Cannon (1932) termed this configuration of responses the "fight or flight" reaction because this array of responses prepares the body for either option. Sympathetic activation prepares the body for intense motor activity, the sort necessary for attack, defense, or escape. This mobilization occurs through two routes and affects all parts of the body.

One route is through direct activation of the sympathetic division of the ANS (called the adrenomedullary system), which activates the adrenal medulla to secrete epinephrine and norepinephrine (Kemeny, 2003). The effects occur throughout the body, affecting the cardiovascular, digestive, and respiratory systems. The other route is through the **hypothalamic-pituitary-adrenal (HPA) axis**, which involves all of these structures. The action begins with perception of a threatening situation, which prompts action in the hypothalamus. The hypothalamic response is the release of corticotropin-releasing hormone, which stimulates the anterior pituitary (the part of the pituitary gland at the base of the brain) to secrete ACTH. This hormone stimulates the adrenal cortex to secrete glucocorticoids, including cortisol. The secretion of cortisol mobilizes the body's energy resources, raising the level of blood sugar to provide energy for the cells. Cortisol also has an anti-inflammatory effect, giving the body a natural defense against swelling from injuries that might be sustained during a fight or a flight. Figure 5.4 shows these two routes of activation.

Together, these physiological reactions to stress prepare the body for a variety of responses that allow adaptation to a threatening situation. **Allostasis** is a term that refers to the body's maintenance of an appropriate level of activation under changing circumstances (McEwen, 2005). Activation of the sympathetic nervous system is the body's attempt to meet the needs of the situation during emergencies. At its optimum in maintaining allostasis, the ANS adapts smoothly, adjusting to normal demands by parasympathetic activation and rapidly mobilizing resources for threatening or stressful situations by sympathetic activation. Not all sympathetic activation leads to health problems, however: Short-term activation of the sympathetic nervous system by physical activity, for example, confers a number of health benefits. Prolonged sympathetic activation, however, creates *allostatic load,* which can overcome the body's ability to adapt. **Allostatic load** represents the "wear and tear" that the body experiences as a result of prolonged activation of physiological stress responses. Allostatic load may be the source of a number of health problems, including weak or dysregulated cortisol production in response to stress, high blood pressure, insulin resistance, fat deposits, and even decline in cognitive abilities over time (Juster, McEwen, & Lupien, 2010; McEwen & Gianaros, 2010). These health problems will be described in greater detail in Chapter 6.

Shelley Taylor and her colleagues (Taylor, 2002, 2006; Taylor et al., 2000) raised objections to the traditional conceptualization of the stress response, questioning the basic notion that people's behavioral responses to stress are necessarily fight-or-flight. These theorists contended that concentrating on men has biased research and theory on stress responses, as fight-or-flight is a more valid description of behavioral responses for men than for women. Although they acknowledge that men's and women's nervous system responses to stress are virtually identical, they argue that women exhibit neuroendocrine responses to stress that differ from men's reactions. They propose that these differences may arise because of the hormone oxytocin, which is released in response to some stressors and linked to a number of social activities such as bonding and affiliation. The effects of oxytocin are especially influenced by estrogen, an interaction that may lay the biological foundation for gender differences in behavioral responses to stress. Taylor and her colleagues propose that women's behavioral responses to stress are better characterized as "tend and befriend" than "fight or flight." That is, women tend to respond to stressful situations with nurturing responses and by seeking and giving social support, rather than by either fighting or fleeing. Indeed, one of the largest gender differences in coping with stress relates to social support seeking: Women seek out the company and comfort of others when stressed more than men (Taylor et al., 2000), and also provide better support when stressed than men (Bodenmann et al., 2015).

Taylor and her colleagues argued that this pattern of responses arose in women during human evolutionary history. Although some researchers criticized this evolutionary explanation (Geary & Flinn, 2002), recent human research is consistent with the tend-and-befriend view (Taylor, 2006). For example, the patterns of hormone secretion during competition differ for women and men (Kivlinghan, Granger, & Booth, 2005). Furthermore, among women, relationship problems correlate with greater levels of oxytocin in the blood (Taylor et al., 2006; Taylor, Saphire-Bernstein, & Seeman, 2010), confirming a gender difference in responses to stress.

IN SUMMARY

The physiology of the stress response is complex. When a person perceives stress, the sympathetic division of the ANS rouses the person from a resting state in two ways: by stimulating the sympathetic nervous system and by producing hormones. The ANS activation is rapid, as is all neural transmission, whereas the action of the neuroendocrine system is slower but longer lasting. The pituitary releases ACTH, which in turn affects the adrenal cortex. Glucocorticoid release prepares the body to resist the stress and even to cope with injury by the release of cortisol. Together the two systems form the physiological basis for allostasis, adaptive responses under conditions of change.

An understanding of the physiology of stress does not completely clarify the meaning of stress. Several models, described next, attempt to better define and explain stress.

Theories of Stress

If you ask people you know whether they are stressed, it is unlikely anyone will ask you what you mean. People seem to know what stress is without having to define it.

However, for researchers, *stress* has no simple definition (McEwen, 2005). Indeed, stress has been defined in three different ways: as a stimulus, as a response, and as an interaction. When some people talk about stress, they are referring to an environmental *stimulus,* as in "I have a high-stress job." Others consider stress a physical *response,* as in "My heart races when I feel a lot of stress." Still others consider stress to result from the *interaction* between environmental stimuli and the person, as in "I feel stressed when I have to make financial decisions at work, but other types of decisions do not stress me."

These three views of stress also appear in different theories of stress. The view of stress as an external event was the first approach taken by stress researchers, the most prominent of whom was Hans Selye. During the course of his research, Selye changed to a more physical response-based view of stress. The most influential view of stress among psychologists is the interactionist approach, proposed by Richard Lazarus, which focuses on stress as a product of both the person and the environment. The next two sections discuss the views of Selye and Lazarus.

Selye's View

Beginning in the 1930s and continuing until his death in 1982, Selye (1956, 1976, 1982) made a strong case for the relationship between stress and physical illness and brought this issue to the public's attention. Selye first conceptualized stress as a stimulus and focused his attention on the environmental conditions that produce stress. In the 1950s, he shifted his focus to stress as a response that the organism makes. To distinguish the two, Selye started using the term *stressor* to refer to the stimulus and *stress* to mean the response.

Selye's contributions to stress research included a model for how the body defends itself in stressful situations. According to Selye's model, stress was a nonspecific response, that is, a wide variety of stressors could prompt the stress response but the response would always be the same.

The General Adaptation Syndrome   Selye coined the term general adaptation syndrome (GAS) to refer to the body's generalized attempt to defend itself against a stressor. This syndrome is divided into three stages, the first of which is the **alarm reaction**. During alarm, the body's defenses against a stressor are mobilized through activation of the sympathetic nervous system. Adrenaline (epinephrine) is released, heart rate and blood pressure increase, respiration becomes faster, blood is diverted away from the internal organs toward the skeletal muscles, sweat glands are activated, and the gastrointestinal system decreases its activity.

Selye called the second phase of the GAS the **resistance stage.** In this stage, the organism adapts to the stressor. How long this stage lasts depends on the severity of the stressor and the adaptive capacity of the organism. If the organism can adapt, the resistance stage will continue for a long time. During this stage, the person gives the outward appearance of normality, but physiologically the body's internal functioning is not normal. Continuing stress will cause continued neurological and hormonal changes. Selye believed that these demands take a toll, setting the stage for what he described as *diseases of adaptation*—diseases related to continued, persistent stress. Figure 5.5 illustrates these stages and the point in the process at which diseases develop.

Among the diseases Selye considered to be the result of prolonged resistance to stress are peptic ulcers and ulcerative colitis, hypertension and cardiovascular disease, hyperthyroidism, and bronchial asthma. In addition, Selye hypothesized that resistance to stress would cause changes in the immune system, making infection more likely.

The capacity to resist stress is finite, and the final stage of the GAS is the **exhaustion stage.** At the end, the organism's ability to resist is depleted, and a breakdown results. This stage is characterized by activation of the parasympathetic division of the ANS. Under normal circumstances, parasympathetic activation keeps the body functioning in a balanced state. In the exhaustion stage, however, the parasympathetic system functions abnormally, causing a person to become exhausted. Selye believed that exhaustion frequently results in depression and sometimes even death.

Evaluation of Selye's View Selye's early concept of stress as a stimulus and his later concentration on the physical aspects of stress influenced stress research. The stimulus-based view of stress prompted researchers to investigate the various environmental conditions that cause people to experience stress and also led to the construction of stress inventories, such as the Life Events Scale for Students that introduces this chapter.

However, Selye's view of the physiology of stress is probably too simplistic (McEwen, 2005). He considered the stress response to all events to be similar, a view that research does not support. He also believed that the physiological responses to stress were oriented toward

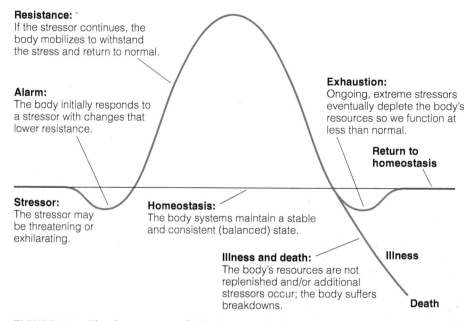

FIGURE 5.5 The three stages of Selye's general adaptation syndrome—alarm, resistance, exhaustion—and their consequences.

Source: An invitation to health (7th ed., p. 40) by D. Hales, 1997, Pacific Grove, CA: Brooks/Cole. From HALES, *Invitation to Health*, 7E. © 1997 Cengage Learning.

maintaining functioning within a narrow range of the optimal level. The concepts of *allostasis* and *allostatic load,* which emphasize the processes of adaptation and change rather than narrow regulation, now replace Selye's view. Allostatic load occurs when many changes are required by presence of chronic stressors. Thus, allostatic load can become overload, resulting in damage and disease. This view of stress is similar to Selye's but shows subtle differences that are more compatible with modern research.

The major criticism of Selye's view is that it ignores the situational and psychological factors that contribute to stress. These factors include the emotional component and a person's interpretation of stressful events (Mason, 1971, 1975), which makes Selye's view of stress incomplete in the view of most psychologists. Although Selye's view has had great influence on the popular conception of stress, an alternative model formulated by psychologist Richard Lazarus is more widely accepted among today's psychologists.

Lazarus's View

In Lazarus's view, the interpretation of stressful events is more important than the events themselves. Neither the environmental event nor the person's response defines stress; rather, the individual's *perception* of the psychological situation is the critical factor. For example, a job promotion may represent an opportunity and challenge for one person but a significant source of stress for another person. Tending a soccer goal in the midst of a World Cup match might be a challenge for Solo, but a panic-inducing event for almost anyone else.

Psychological Factors   Lazarus's emphasis on interpretation and perception differs from that of Selye. This emphasis arose from another difference: Lazarus worked largely with humans rather than nonhuman animals. The ability of people to think about and evaluate future events makes them vulnerable to psychological stressors in ways that other animals are not. People feel stressed about situations that would probably not concern an animal, such as employment, finances, public speaking, bad hair days, deadlines, and upcoming exams in psychology classes. Humans encounter stresses because they have high-level cognitive abilities that other animals lack.

According to Lazarus (1984, 1993), the effect that stress has on a person is based more on that person's feelings of threat, vulnerability, and ability to cope than on the stressful event itself. For example, losing a job

may be extremely stressful for someone who has no money saved or who believes that finding another job will be difficult. But for someone who hated the job, has money saved, and believes finding a new job will be easy, the experience may cause little stress. These examples highlight Lazarus's view that a life event is not what produces stress; rather, it is one's view of the situation that causes an event to become stressful.

Lazarus and Susan Folkman defined psychological stress as a "particular relationship between the person and the environment that is appraised by the person as taxing or exceeding his or her resources and endangering his or her well-being" (1984, p. 19). This definition makes several important points. First, it emphasizes Lazarus and Folkman's interactional or *transactional* view of stress, holding that stress refers to a relationship between person and environment. Second, this definition emphasizes the key role of a person's appraisal of the psychological situation. Third, the definition holds that stress arises when a person appraises a situation as threatening, challenging, or harmful.

Appraisal   According to Lazarus and Folkman (1984), people make three kinds of appraisals of situations: primary appraisal, secondary appraisal, and reappraisal. **Primary appraisal** is not necessarily first in importance, but it is first in time. When people first encounter an event, such as an offer of a job promotion, they appraise the offer in terms of its effect on their well-being. They may view the event as irrelevant, benign-positive, or stressful. Irrelevant events are those that have no implications for a person's well-being, such as a snowstorm in another state. Benign-positive events are those that are appraised as having good implications. A stressful event means that the event is appraised as being harmful, threatening, or challenging. Lazarus (1993) defined *harm* as damage that has already been done, such as an illness or injury; *threat* as the anticipation of harm; and *challenge* as a person's confidence in overcoming difficult demands. Research indicates that the perception of threat or challenge makes a difference for performance; perception of challenge leads to better performance than perception of threat (Moore, Vine, Wilson, & Friedman, 2012).

After their initial appraisal of an event, people form an impression of their ability to control or cope with harm, threat, or challenge, an impression called **secondary appraisal.** People typically ask three questions in making secondary appraisals. The first is "What options are available to me?" The second is

"What is the likelihood that I can successfully apply the necessary strategies to reduce this stress?" The third is "Will this procedure work—that is, will it alleviate my stress?" Each of these secondary appraisals can also influence the degree of stress experienced. Naturally, having a number of options available that you feel you can use to reduce harm or threat will make the event less stressful.

The third type of appraisal is **reappraisal**. Appraisals change constantly as new information becomes available. Reappraisal does not always result in more stress; sometimes it decreases stress. For example, a person could reappraise the stress of a breakup with a boyfriend or girlfriend as an opportunity to spend time with other friends, which could make the experience less stressful.

Coping   An important ingredient in Lazarus's theory of stress is the ability or inability to cope with a stressful situation. Lazarus and Folkman defined coping as "constantly changing cognitive and behavioral efforts to manage specific external and/or internal demands that are appraised as taxing or exceeding the resources of the person" (1984, p. 141). This definition spells out several important features of coping. First, coping is a process, constantly changing as one's efforts are evaluated as more or less successful. Second, coping is not automatic; it is a learned pattern of responding to stressful situations. Third, coping requires effort. People need not be completely aware of their coping response, and the outcome may or may not be successful, but effort must have been expended. Fourth, coping is an effort to *manage* the situation; control and mastery are not necessary. For example, most of us make an effort to manage our physical environment by striving for a comfortable air temperature. Thus, we cope with our environment even though complete mastery of the climate is impossible. How well people are able to cope depends on the resources they have available and the strategies they use. We will discuss effective coping strategies later in this chapter.

IN SUMMARY

Two leading theories of stress are those of Selye and Lazarus. Selye, the first researcher to look closely at stress, first saw stress as a stimulus but later viewed it as a response. Whenever animals (including humans) encounter a threatening stimulus, they mobilize themselves in a generalized attempt to adapt to that stimulus. This mobilization, called the general adaptation syndrome, has three stages—alarm, resistance, and exhaustion—and the potential for trauma or illness exists at all three stages.

In contrast, Lazarus held a cognitively oriented, transactional view of stress and coping. Stressful encounters are dynamic and complex, constantly changing and unfolding, so that the outcomes of one stressful event alter subsequent appraisals of new events. Individual differences in coping strategies and in the appraisal of stressful events are crucial to a person's experience of stress; therefore, the likelihood of developing any stress-related disorder varies with the individual.

Sources of Stress

Stress can flow from myriad sources: cataclysmic events with natural or human causes, changes in an individual's life history, and ongoing hassles of daily life. In organizing sources of stress, we follow the model set forth by Lazarus and Judith Cohen (1977), but as these two researchers emphasized, an individual's perception of a stressful event is more crucial than the event itself.

Cataclysmic Events

Lazarus and Cohen defined cataclysmic events as "sudden, unique, and powerful single life-events requiring major adaptive responses from population groups sharing the experience" (1997, p. 91). A number of cataclysmic events, both intentional and unintentional, strike unpredictably in areas around the world. Unintentional major events include natural disasters such as hurricanes, typhoons, fires, tornadoes, floods, earthquakes, and other cataclysmic events that kill large numbers of people and create stress, grief, and fear among survivors. Mass shootings and acts of terrorism are examples of intentional cataclysmic events.

Occasionally, stressful events are so powerful that they affect nearly the entire globe, such as the great earthquake and tsunami that devastated large parts of Japan in March 2011, the tsunami in the Indian Ocean in December 2004, and Hurricane Katrina and its aftermath, which destroyed New Orleans and other cities on the Gulf of Mexico in August 2005. The physical damage of these natural events was astronomical. More than 200,000 people were killed or missing and countless others left injured, sick, and homeless. Survivors of

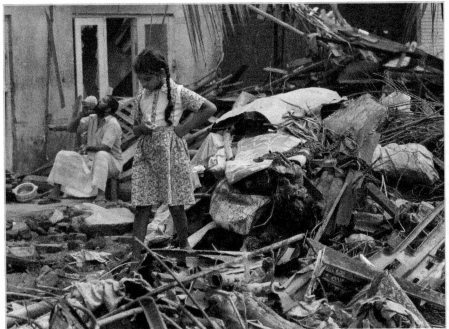

Paula Bronstein/Getty Images

Cataclysmic events require major adaptive responses from large groups of people.

the Indian Ocean tsunami (Dewaraja & Kawa-mura, 2006) and residents in the New Orleans area (Weems et al., 2007) experienced symptoms of depression and **posttraumatic stress disorder (PTSD)**. However, several factors moderated or exacerbated these symptoms, such as their feelings of support from others, discrimination, and their proximity to the destruction.

Natural disasters can be devastating to huge numbers of people, but they cannot be blamed on any single person or group of persons. In contrast, the 1995 bombing of the Murrah Federal Building in Oklahoma City and the attack on the World Trade Center and the Pentagon on September 11, 2001, were all *intentional* acts. Each was sudden, unique, and powerful, and each required adaptive responses from large numbers of people. Television and the media brought the aftermath of these cataclysmic events into millions of homes, resulting in multitudes of people having similar stress-related experiences.

Several factors contribute to how much stress an event creates, including physical proximity to the event, time elapsed since the event, and the intention of the perpetrators. The September 11 attack on the World Trade Center included all three factors for those living in New York City, creating lingering trauma for

people close to the site (Hasin, Keyes, Hat-zenbuehler, Aharonovich, & Alderson, 2007). For those not in New York City, stress associated with the attacks began to dissipate within weeks (Schlenger et al., 2002), but other evidence suggests that some people continued to experience negative psychological and physical health effects several years later (Holman et al., 2008; Richman, Cloninger, & Rospenda, 2008; Updegraff, Silver, & Holman, 2008). The intentional nature of the attacks added to the stress, making these violent events more traumatic than natural disasters.

In summary, cataclysmic events can be either intentional or unintentional, with different effects on stress. Such events strike suddenly, without warning, and people who survive them as well as those who help with the aftermath often see their experience as life altering. Despite the power of cataclysmic events to affect people, researchers have focused more attention on life events as sources of stress (Richman et al., 2008).

Life Events

Major life events—such as experiencing the death of a spouse or parent, getting a divorce, being fired from your job, or moving to a different country—are major sources of stress, but minor life events can also be stressful. Some of the items on the Life Events Scale for Students at the beginning of this chapter are life events, and the popular Holmes and Rahe (1967) Social Readjustment Rating Scale described later in this chapter also consists of life events. Indeed, many of the stressors that Solo faced such as frequent moves and the death of her father are life events that are generally viewed as major sources of stress. Troubles with the law, such as what Solo's father faced, can also be highly stressful.

Life events differ from cataclysmic events in three important ways. Life events and life event scales emphasize the importance of *change*. When events require people to make some sort of change or readjustment, they feel stressed. Positive events such as getting married, becoming a parent, and starting a new job all require some adjustment, but negative events such as losing a job, the death of a family member, or being a victim of a violent crime also require adaptation. Unlike cataclysmic events that affect huge numbers of people, stressful life events affect a few people or perhaps only one. Divorce that happens to you can be more profound in changing your life than an earthquake in a far-off location that affects thousands.

Life events usually evolve more slowly than cataclysmic events. Divorce does not happen in a single day, and being dismissed from a job is ordinarily preceded by a period of conflict. Crime victimization, however, is often sudden and unexpected. All of these life events produce stress, and subsequent problems are common. For example, divorce may decrease stress between the divorcing partners (Amato & Hohmann-Marriott, 2007) but more often creates short-term and sometimes long-term problems for both the adults and their children (Michael, Torres, & Seeman, 2007). When losing a job results in long-term unemployment, this situation creates a cascade of stressors, including financial problems and family conflict (Howe, Levy, & Caplan, 2004; Song, Foo, Uy, & Sun, 2011). Being the victim of a violent crime "transforms people into victims and changes their lives forever" (Koss, 1990, p. 374). Crime victims tend to lose their sense of invulnerability, and their risk of PTSD increases (Koss, Bailey, Yuan, Herrera, & Lichter, 2003). This risk applies to a variety of types of victimization, and studies have established the risk of PTSD for both children (Sebre et al., 2004) and adults. Even exposure to community violence increases risks for children (Rosario, Salzinger, Feldman, & Ng-Mak, 2008).

Daily Hassles

Unlike life events that call for people to make adjustments in their lives, daily hassles are part of everyday life. Living in poverty, fearing crime, arguing with one's spouse, balancing work with family life, living in crowded and polluted conditions, and fighting a long daily commute to work are examples of daily hassles. The stress brought on by daily hassles can originate from both the physical and the psychosocial environment.

Daily Hassles and the Physical Environment

Noise, pollution, crowding, fear of crime, and personal alienation are often a part of urban life. Although these environmental sources of stress may be more concentrated in urban settings, rural life can also be noisy, polluted, hot, cold, humid, or even crowded, with many people living together in a one- or two-room dwelling. Nonetheless, the crowding, noise, pollution, fear of crime, and personal alienation more typical of urban living combine to produce what Eric Graig (1993) termed **urban press**. The results from one study (Christenfeld, Glynn, Phillips, & Shrira, 1999) suggested that the combined sources of stress affecting residents of New York City are factors in that city's higher heart attack death rate. Living in a polluted, noisy, and crowded environment creates chronic daily hassles that not only make life unpleasant but may also affect behavior and performance (Evans & Stecker, 2004) and pose a risk to health (Schell & Denham, 2003). Access to a garden or park can diminish this stress; individuals whose living situations include access to such "green spaces" report lower stress (Nielsen & Hansen, 2007) and better self-reported health (van Dillen, de Vries, Groenewegen, & Spreeuwenberg, 2011).

Noise is a type of pollution because it can be a noxious, unwanted stimulus that intrudes into a person's environment, but it is quite difficult to define in any objective way. One person's music is another person's noise. The importance of subjective attitude toward noise is illustrated by a study (Nivison & Endresen, 1993) that asked residents living beside a busy street about their health, sleep, anxiety level, and attitude toward noise. The level of noise was not a factor, but the residents' subjective view of noise showed a strong relationship to the number of their health complaints. Similarly, workers who are more sensitive to noise (Waye et al., 2002) show a higher cortisol level and rate low-frequency noises as more annoying than workers who are less sensitive.

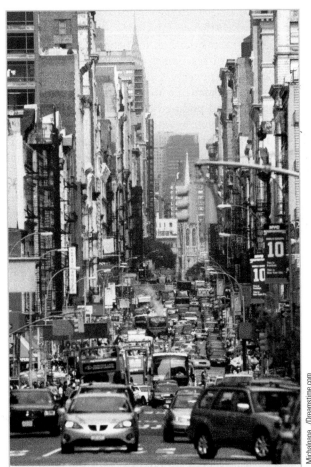

Crowding, noise, and pollution increase the stress of urban life.

Michalnapa.../Dreamstime.com

Another source of hassles is *crowding*. A series of classic experiments with rats living in crowded conditions (Calhoun, 1956, 1962) showed that crowding produced changes in social and sexual behavior that included increases in territoriality, aggression, and infant mortality and decreases in levels of social integration. More recent work confirms that in primates too, crowding is associated with increases in physiological stress responses (Dettmer, Novak, Meyer, & Suomi, 2014; Pearson, Reeder, & Judge, 2015). These results suggest that crowding is a source of stress that affects behavior, but studies with humans are complicated by several factors, including a definition of crowding.

A distinction between the concepts of population density and crowding helps in understanding the effects of crowding on humans. In 1972, Daniel Stokols defined **population density** as a *physical* condition in which a large population occupies a limited space. **Crowding**, however, is a *psychological* condition that arises from a person's perception of the high-density environment in which that person is confined. Thus, density is necessary for crowding but does not automatically produce the feeling of being crowded. Being in a packed subway train may not make you feel crowded if you have an empty seat next to you, but being stuck sitting between two strangers would increase your feelings of crowding and your physiological stress response. Indeed, this is what researchers found in a study of train commuters (Evans & Wener, 2007). The distinction between density and crowding means that personal perceptions, such as a feeling of control, are critical in the definition of crowding. Crowding in both neighborhoods and residences plays a role in how stressed a person will be (Regoeczi, 2003).

Pollution, noise, and crowding often co-occur in "the environment of poverty" (Ulrich, 2002, p. 16). The environment of poverty may also include violence or the threat of violence and discrimination. On a daily basis, wealthier people experience fewer stressors than poor people (Grzywacz et al., 2004), but even wealthy people are not exempt. The threat of violence and fear of crime are a part of the stress of modern life. Some evidence suggests that community violence is especially stressful for children and adolescents (Ozer, 2005; Rosario et al., 2008). Children who grow up in an environment of poverty experience greater chronic stress and allostatic load, which may contribute to health problems later in life (Matthews, Gallo, & Taylor, 2010). For example, children growing up in lower socioeconomic status households perceive greater threat and family chaos, which are linked to greater cortisol production as they age (Chen, Cohen, & Miller, 2010).

In the United States, poverty is more common among ethnic minorities than among European Americans (U.S. Census Bureau [USCB], 2015), and discrimination is another type of daily hassle that is often associated with the environment of poverty. However, discrimination is part of the psychosocial environment.

Daily Hassles and the Psychosocial Environment

People's psychosocial environment can be fertile ground for creating daily hassles. These stressors originate in the everyday social environment from sources such as community, workplace, and family interactions.

Discrimination is a stressor that occurs with alarming regularity in a variety of social situations in

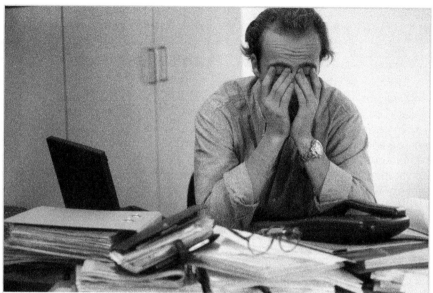

David De Lossy/Getty Images

High job demands can produce stress, especially when combined with low levels of control.

the community and workplace for African Americans in the United States (Landrine & Klonoff, 1996), but other ethnic groups (Edwards & Romero, 2008), women, and gay and bisexual individuals (Huebner & Davis, 2007) also face discrimination. Unfair treatment creates both disadvantage for the individuals discriminated against and a stigma that is stressful (Major & O'Brien, 2005). Discrimination is a source of stress that may increase the risk for cardiovascular disease (Troxel, Matthews, Bromberger, & Sutton-Tyrrell, 2003). A meta-analysis of over 100 studies confirmed this link between perceived discrimination and both mental and physical health problems (Pascoe & Richman, 2009). Discrimination is associated with both increased physiological stress responses, as well as maladaptive health behaviors that people use to cope with discrimination.

Discrimination is not the only stressor that occurs in the workplace—some jobs are more stressful than others. Contrary to some people's assumption, business executives who must make many decisions every day have *less* job-related stress than their employees who merely carry out those decisions. Most executives have jobs in which the demands are high but so is their level of control, and lack of control is more stressful than the burden of making decisions. Lower-level occupations are actually more stressful than executive jobs (Wamala,

Mittleman, Horsten, Schenck-Gustafsson, & Orth-Gomér, 2000). Using stress-related illness as a criterion, the jobs of construction worker, secretary, laboratory technician, waiter or waitress, machine operator, farmworker, and painter are among the most stressful. These jobs all share a high level of demand combined with a low level of control, status, and compensation. Stress can even be influenced by whether people find their work engaging or not. People who are engaged and committed to their work environment have lower cortisol production during the workweek compared with those with little engagement in their work (Harter & Stone, 2012). Brief vacations from work may help relieve work-related stress, but this relief does not last as long as people may hope (see Would You Believe ...? box).

Stress from trying to balance the roles of worker and family member affects men as well as women. Half of all workers are married to someone who is also employed, creating multiple roles for both women and men (Moen & Yu, 2000). Problems may arise from work stress spilling over into the family or from family conflicts intruding into the workplace (Ilies et al., 2007; Schieman, Milkie, & Glavin, 2009). The differences in men's and women's roles and expectations within the family mean that family and work conflicts influence women and men in different ways. Women often encounter stress because of the increased burden of doing the work associated

Would You BELIEVE...?   Vacations Relieve Work Stress ... But Not for Long

Summer vacation. Spring break. Winter holiday. Every year, Americans spend millions of dollars on vacations from work and school. Vacations take people away from work and also provide opportunities for fun, travel, and relaxation. But do vacations serve as an effective long-term "intervention" for alleviating work-related stress?

A number of studies attempt to answer this question, and a review of this research yields some surprising results (de Bloom et al., 2009). People experience less stress during a vacation than they did prior to a vacation, which we expect. Furthermore, in the days following a vacation, people report substantially less stress than they did prior to the vacation. In some cases, vacations may even offer relief from physical health symptoms.

However, this "vacation effect" tends to disappear quickly. Typically, any stress reduction effects of a vacation disappear within 3 to 4 weeks (de Bloom et al., 2009; Kuhnel & Sonnentag, 2011). One study showed the effect to fade within a single week (de Bloom et al., 2010). This decrease may occur because a person's return to work leaves him or her needing to work extra hours or overtime to "catch up," which increases stress.

Certainly, these findings do not suggest that people should avoid vacations altogether. Instead, they suggest that vacations should not be the only way to cope with work- or school-related stress. People can more effectively manage stress by using proven techniques, such as those described at the end of this chapter.

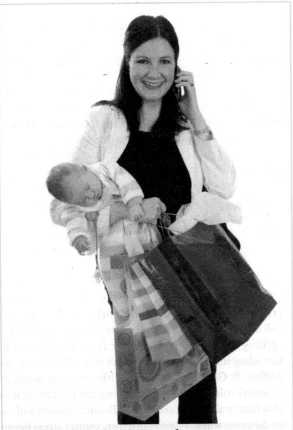

Multiple roles can be a source of stress.

with their multiple roles as employee, wife, and mother, but overall, these multiple roles offer health benefits (Barnett & Hyde, 2001; Schnittker, 2007).

The positive or negative effects of work and family roles depend on the resources people have available. Partner and family support affects both men and women, but its absence more strongly affects women's health (Walen & Lachman, 2000). Women with children and no partner are especially burdened and, therefore, stressed (Livermore & Powers, 2006). Thus, filling multiple obligations is not necessarily stressful for women, but low control and poor support for multiple roles can produce stress for both men and women. Despite the possibilities for conflict and stress, families are a major source of social support, a resource that is important for coping with stress.

IN SUMMARY

Stress has a number of sources, which can be classified according to the magnitude of the event: cataclysmic events, life events, and daily hassles. Cataclysmic events include natural disasters such as floods and earthquakes and intentional violence such as terrorist attacks.

Life events are events that produce changes in people's lives that require adaptation. Life events may be either negative or positive. Negative life events such as divorce, death of a family member, or crime victimization can produce severe and long-lasting stress.

Daily hassles are everyday events that create repetitive, chronic distress. Some hassles arise from the physical environment; others come from the psychosocial environment. Stress from pollution, noise, crowding, and violence combine in urban settings with commuting hassles to create a situation described as *urban press*. Each of these sources of stress may also be considered individually. Noise and crowding are annoyances, but there is some evidence that even low levels of these stressors can prompt stress responses, which suggests that long-term exposure may have negative health consequences. The combination of community stressors such as crowding, noise, and threat of violence is common in poor neighborhoods, creating an environment of poverty.

Daily hassles in the psychosocial environment occur within the situations of the everyday social environment, including community, workplace, and family. Within the community, racism and sexism produce stress for the targets of these types of discrimination. Within the workplace, jobs with high demands and little control create stress, and poor support adds to the stress. Within the family, relationships such as spouse and parent present possibilities for conflict and stress as well as support. In addition, the conflict between family and work demands is a source of stress for many people.

Measurement of Stress

Given the nearly endless sources of stress that exist in modern life, how do researchers measure stress? The measurement of stress is an important part of a health psychologist's job, as researchers need to first measure stress in order to understand the effect of stress on health. This section discusses some of the more widely used methods and addresses the problems involved in determining their reliability and validity.

Methods of Measurement

Researchers have used a variety of approaches to measure stress, but most fall into two broad categories: physiological measures and self-reports (Monroe, 2008).

Physiological measures directly assess aspects of the body's physical stress response. Self-reports measure either life events or daily hassles that a person experiences. Both approaches hold some potential for investigating the effects of stress on illness and health.

Physiological Measures Physiological measures of stress include blood pressure, heart rate, galvanic skin response, respiration rate, and increased secretion of stress hormones such as cortisol and epinephrine. These physiological measures provide researchers with a window into the activation of the body's sympathetic nervous system and HPA axis.

Another common approach to the physiological measurement of stress is through its association with the release of hormones. Epinephrine and norepinephrine, for example, can be measured in either blood or urine samples and can provide an index of stress (Eller, Netterstrøm, & Hansen, 2006; Krantz, Forsman, & Lundberg, 2004). The levels of these hormones circulating in the blood decrease within a few minutes after the stressful experience, so measurement must be quick to capture the changes. The levels of hormones persist longer in the urine, but factors other than stress contribute to urinary levels of these hormones. The stress hormone cortisol persists for at least 20 minutes, and measurement of salivary cortisol provides an index of the changes in this hormone. A newer method assesses the cortisol in human hair, which represents the body's cortisol production over the preceding 6 months (Kirschbaum, Tietze, Skoluda, & Dettenborn, 2009).

The advantage of these physiological measures of stress is that they are direct, highly reliable, and easily quantified. A disadvantage is that the mechanical and electrical hardware and clinical settings that are frequently used may themselves produce stress. Thus, this approach to measuring stress is useful but not the most widely used method. Self-report measures are far more common.

Life Events Scales Since the late 1950s and early 1960s, researchers have developed a number of self-report instruments to measure stress. The earliest and best known of these self-report procedures is the Social Readjustment Rating Scale (SRRS), developed by Thomas H. Holmes and Richard Rahe in 1967. The scale is simply a list of 43 life events arranged in rank order from most to least stressful. Each event carries an assigned value, ranging from 100 points for death of a spouse to 11 points for minor violations of the law. Respondents check the items they experienced during a recent period, usually the previous 6 to 24 months. Adding each item's point value and totaling scores yields a stress score for each person. These scores can then be correlated with future events, such as incidence of illness, to determine the relationship between this measure of stress and the occurrence of physical illness.

Other stress inventories exist, including the Life Events Scale for Students (Clements & Turpin, 1996), the assessment that appears as Check Your Health Risks at the beginning of this chapter. College students who check more stress situations tend to use health services more than students who check fewer events.

The Perceived Stress Scale (PSS) (Cohen, Kamarck, & Mermelstein, 1983) emphasizes *perception* of events rather than the events themselves. The PSS is a 14-item scale that attempts to measure the degree to which people appraise events in the past month as being "unpredictable, uncontrollable, and overloading" (Cohen et al., 1983, p. 387). The scale assesses three components of stress: (1) daily hassles, (2) major events, and (3) changes in coping resources. Researchers use the PSS in a variety of situations, such as measuring prenatal stress in expectant mothers (Nast et al., 2013), determining the effectiveness of a relaxation program for elementary teachers (Nassiri, 2005), and predicting burnout among college athletic coaches (Tashman, Tenenbaum, & Eklund, 2010). Its brevity combined with good reliability and validity has led to use of this scale in a variety of research projects.

Everyday Hassles Scales   Lazarus and his associates pioneered an approach to stress measurement that looks at daily hassles rather than life events. Daily hassles are "experiences and conditions of daily living that have been appraised as salient and harmful or threatening to the endorser's well-being" (Lazarus, 1984, p. 376). Recall from the discussion of theories of stress that Lazarus views stress as a transactional, dynamic complex shaped by people's *appraisal* of the environmental situation and their *perceived capabilities to cope* with this situation. Consistent with this view, Lazarus and his associates insisted that self-report scales must be able to assess subjective elements such as personal appraisal, beliefs, goals, and commitments (Lazarus, 2000; Lazarus, DeLongis, Folkman, & Gruen, 1985).

The original Hassles Scale (Kanner, Coyne, Schaefer, & Lazarus, 1981) consists of 117 items about annoying, irritating, or frustrating situations in which people may *feel* hassled. These include concerns about weight, home maintenance, crime, and having too many things to do. People also rate the degree to which each item produced stress. The Hassles Scale only modestly correlates with life events, which suggests that these two types of stress are not the same thing. Furthermore, the Hassles Scale can be more accurate predictor of psychological health than life events scales (Lazarus, 1984). A shorter Hassles Scale, developed by the same research team (DeLongis, Folkman, & Lazarus, 1988), is a better predictor than the Social Readjustment Rating Scale of both the frequency and intensity of headaches (Fernandez & Sheffield, 1996) and episodes of inflammatory bowel disease (Searle & Bennett, 2001). Thus, everyday hassles can have more of an influence on health than the more serious life events measured by the Social Readjustment Rating Scale.

The measurement of everyday hassles also extends to specific situations. For example, the Urban Hassles Index (Miller & Townsend, 2005) measures stressors that commonly affect adolescents in urban environments, and the Family Daily Hassles Inventory (Rollins & Garrison, 2002) targets daily stressors commonly experienced by parents. Thus, researchers have a variety of self-report stress measures to choose from, depending on their purposes and specific populations of study.

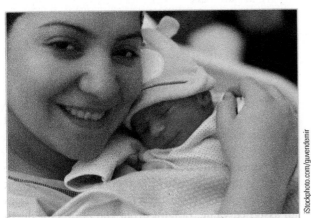

iStockphoto.com/guvendemir

Life events scales also include positive events because such events also require adjustment.

IN SUMMARY

Researchers and clinicians measure stress by several methods, including physiological and biochemical measures and self-reports of stressful events. The most popular life events scale is the Social Readjustment Rating Scale, which emphasizes change in life events. Despite its popularity, the SRRS is a modest predictor of subsequent illness. Lazarus and his associates pioneered the measurement of stress as daily hassles and uplifts. These inventories emphasize the perceived severity and importance of daily events. In general, the revised Hassles and Uplifts Scale is more accurate than the SRRS in predicting future illness.

Coping with Stress

People constantly attempt to manage the problems and stresses of their lives, and most of these attempts fit into the category of coping. However, the term **coping** is usually applied to strategies that individuals use to manage the distressing problems and emotions in their lives. Coping is an active topic of research: thousands of studies have explored the personal and situational characteristics that affect coping efforts, as well as the effectiveness of various coping strategies.

Personal Resources That Influence Coping

Lazarus and Folkman (1984) suggested a number of personal resources that could help people manage the demands of a stressful situation, including good health, optimistic beliefs, socioeconomic resources, social skills, and social support. Although research supports the importance of each of these resources, the most important personal resources for coping with stress are social support, a sense of personal control, and optimistic beliefs.

Social Support **Social support** refers to a variety of material and emotional supports a person receives from others. The related concepts of **social contacts** and **social network** are sometimes used interchangeably; both refer to the number and types of people with whom one associates. The opposite of social contacts is **social isolation,** which refers to an absence of specific, meaningful interpersonal relations. People with a high level of social support ordinarily have a broad social network and many social contacts; socially isolated people have neither. Solo, who lost her father in 2007 and who did not feel close with many of her teammates in that year's Women's World Cup, probably had low levels of social support during portions of her career.

The Alameda County Study (Berkman & Syme, 1979) was the first to establish a strong link between social support and longevity. This study indicated that lack of social support was as strongly linked to mortality as cigarette smoking and a sedentary lifestyle. Subsequent research confirms the importance of social support. A recent meta-analysis of nearly 150 studies shows that people with strong social ties have substantially lower mortality rates than those with weak social ties (Holt-Lunstad, Smith, & Layton, 2010). Furthermore, as Figure 5.6 shows, the association between social support and longevity is nearly as strong as the benefits of refraining from smoking, and stronger than the benefits of consuming little or no alcohol, maintaining a healthy weight, exercising, and taking medication for hypertension. Thus, the benefits of social support are strong and robust. (But, how often has your physician recommended that you improve your social relationships in order to stay healthy?)

Social support may influence stress in several ways. For example, stressed individuals may benefit from a support network with members who encourage them to adopt healthier habits, such as stopping smoking, beginning an exercise program, or keeping doctor's appointments. Social support may also help people gain confidence in their ability to handle stressful situations; thus, when they experience stress, they may appraise the stressor as less threatening than do people who have fewer coping resources (Wills, 1998). Another possibility is that social support may alter the physiological responses to stress (DeVries, Glasper, & Detillion, 2003; Kiecolt-Glaser & Newton, 2001). This view, referred to as the *stress-buffering hypothesis,* suggests that social support lessens or eliminates the harmful effects of stress and therefore protects against disease and death. A large epidemiological survey of over 30,000 Americans supports this view (Moak & Agrawal, 2010). For adults who experienced little life stress, social support was not strongly related to their feelings of distress or overall physical health. For those who experienced more life stress, higher levels of social support related to less depression and anxiety and greater self-reported physical health.

The positive effects of social support for health are well established (Martin & Brantley, 2004), but some individuals benefit more than others. For example, marriage (or at least happy marriage) would seem to provide excellent social support for both partners, but the benefits of marriage are not equal for women and men—being married benefits men's health more than women's (Kiecolt-Glaser & Newton, 2001). The reason

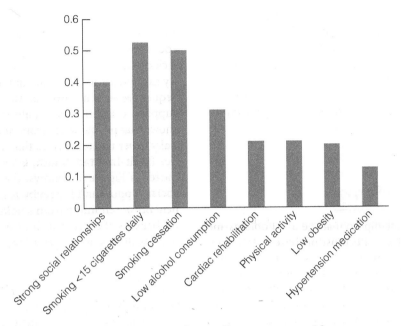

FIGURE 5.6 Odds of decreased mortality across several factors associated with mortality, including social support.

Source: From "Social relationships and mortality risk: A meta-analytic review," by J. Holt-Lunstad, T. B. Smith, & J. B. Layton, 2010, *PLoS Med, 7*(7), e1000316.

for men's advantage is not clear, but one possibility is that women's role as caregivers puts them in the position of providing more care than they receive. Providing companionship is a positive factor for the caregiver as well as the recipient, but providing help comes at a cost to the helper (Strazdins & Broom, 2007). This situation may describe women's more than men's caregiving role, and thus the gender difference.

Social support is a significant factor in predicting both the development of disease and the course of chronic disease (Martin & Brantley, 2004). Surprisingly, the stress-buffering benefits of social support are not limited to support provided by humans (see Would You Believe ...? box). Furthermore, the benefits of social support are entwined with another factor that influences coping: perceptions of personal control.

Personal Control A second factor that affects people's ability to cope with stressful life events is a feeling of **personal control**—that is, confidence that they have some control over the events that shape their lives. Both classic and current research confirm the benefits of a sense of control. One classic approach is Julian Rotter's (1966) concept of locus of control, a continuum that captures the extent to which people believe they are in

control of the important events in their lives. According to Rotter, people who believe that they control their own lives have an *internal locus of control*, whereas those who believe that luck, fate, or the acts of others determine their lives score high on *external locus of control*. The value of an internal locus of control appeared in a study of people with chronic illness (Livneh, Lott, & Antonak, 2004); those who had adapted well showed a higher sense of control than those who had adapted poorly.

Ellen Langer and Judith Rodin (1976), who studied older nursing home residents, reported another classic example of the effects of personal control. This research project encouraged some residents to assume more responsibility for and control over their daily lives, whereas others had decisions made for them. The areas of control were fairly minor, such as rearranging furniture, choosing when and with whom to visit in the home, and deciding what leisure activities to pursue. In addition, residents were offered a small growing plant, which they were free to accept or reject and to care for as they wished. A comparison group of residents received information that emphasized the responsibility of the nursing staff, and each of them also received a live plant. Although equal in most other ways, the amount of control made a substantial difference in health. Residents in the responsibility-induced group were happier, more active, and more alert, with a higher level of general well-being. In just 3 weeks, most of the comparison group (71%) had become more debilitated, whereas nearly all the responsibility-induced group (93%) showed some overall mental and physical improvement. In an 18-month follow-up (Rodin & Langer, 1977), residents in the original responsibility-induced group retained their advantage, and their mortality rate was lower than that of the comparison group.

How do perceptions of control influence health? While there may be many ways in which control buffers stress, one route may be through reductions in potentially harmful physiological responses. A meta-analysis of over 200 studies examined the characteristics of laboratory stress tasks that led to the greatest production of the stress hormone cortisol (Dickerson & Kemeny, 2004). Stress tasks that offered participants very little control—such as completing impossible tasks, performing under extreme time pressures, or exposure to uncontrollable loud noises—led to the largest increases in cortisol production and the longest times to recovery.

These results suggest that people who frequently face situations that offer little control may be most likely to suffer the long-term health consequences of prolonged HPA activation.

These studies suggest that lack of control may impair health, and even a minimal amount of control can be beneficial to health. However, the benefits of control may be bound to Western cultures that emphasize individual autonomy and effort. In a comparison of stress and coping among people from Japan and Great Britain (O'Connor & Shimizu, 2002), the Japanese participants reported a lower sense of personal control, but only the British reported that loss of control produced stress. Thus, the benefits of personal control may be restricted to people in Western societies. However, the universal occurrence of stress means that strategies for coping with stress occur in all societies.

Optimism   In times of uncertainty, do you usually expect the best? Do you expect more good things to happen to you than bad? If you answered yes to these two questions, you are probably high in the trait of optimism.

Would You BELIEVE...? Pets May Be Better Support Providers Than People

Sometimes, the best social support may not come from a friend, but instead from "man's best friend." But can pets—such as dogs and cats—really help people cope with stress and improve health?

Nearly 40% of households in the United States own a dog or a cat (Humane Society of the United States, 2011). Pets provide companionship and affection, and, in some cases, force their owners to be more physically active. It may be no surprise that among survivors of heart attacks, dog owners are over *8 times* more likely to be alive 1 year after their heart attack than those who do not own a dog (Friedmann & Thomas, 1995).

Can pets also dampen people's physiological responses to stress? In one study, researchers asked adults to perform a series of difficult and painful laboratory stress-tasks—including mental arithmetic—while measuring their cardiovascular stress responses (Allen, Blascovich, & Mendes, 2002). Some participants did the tasks alone; some did the tasks in front of a close friend or spouse; others did the tasks in front of a pet dog or cat.

The results are striking. The presence of a pet led to the lowest stress response of all. Surprisingly, the presence of a spouse or friend led to the greatest stress response! Pets, it seems, provide comfort and support, without the possibility of criticism or evaluation. Friends and spouses provide support, too, but they are also more likely to notice someone's poor math skills. In this situation, the support of a trusted pet provides all

the benefits of social support without any apparent costs.

Pet support may be especially helpful for people who are sensitive to criticism. For example, a recent study of children with insecure attachment styles shows that those who performed a stressful lab task in the presence of a dog produced significantly lower salivary cortisol than children who completed the task in front of a friendly human (Beetz et al., 2011).

Thus, pets are an excellent source of unconditional social support. Humorist Dave Barry might have said it best: "You can say any foolish thing to a dog, and the dog will give you a look that says, 'My God, you're right! I never would've thought of that!'"

Psychologists define optimism simply: **Optimists are people who expect good things to happen to them,** whereas pessimists are people who generally expect bad things. Of course, lay conceptualizations of these traits view optimists as cheery and upbeat and pessimists as "doom-and-gloom." But to psychologists, the defining feature of optimism is not positive mood, but rather a person's general *belief* that good things will happen. This belief substantially influences both mental and physical health, as well as how people cope with stress.

Optimists experience less emotional distress than pessimists, as shown in studies of students beginning college (Aspinwall & Taylor, 1992), cancer patients (Carver et al., 1993), coronary bypass surgery patients (Fitzgerald et al., 1993), and Alzheimer's caregivers (Shifren & Hooker, 1995). Even more striking are findings that show that optimistic beliefs predict physical health and mortality. For example, a study of nearly 100,000 women found that optimistic women were 30% less likely to die from cardiovascular problems at an 8-year follow-up, compared to their pessimistic peers (Tindle et al., 2009). The physical health benefits of optimism are not limited to cardiovascular health, as a meta-analysis of over 80 studies of a variety of health conditions showed that optimists have better physical health than pessimists (Rasmussen, Scheier, & Greenhouse, 2009).

There are several reasons why the personal resource of optimism may confer health benefits. First, optimists are likely to have stronger social support networks than pessimists (MacLeod & Conway, 2005). Due to their positive expectations, optimists may be more likely than pessimists to invest time and energy into building social relationships (Brissette et al., 2002). Also, optimistic people are usually more likable than pessimistic people, so they may find it easier to develop a social network.

Second, the positive moods associated with optimism may speed the recovery of cardiovascular responses to stress (Fredrickson & Levenson, 1998). Optimists and others who experience frequent positive moods may, then, experience less cumulative wear and tear on their bodies and, possibly, improved immune functioning (Marsland, Pressman, & Cohen, 2007).

Lastly, when people feel confident that good things are likely to happen, they are more likely to persist in pursuing important goals in the face of stress and setbacks. Pessimists, when confronted with problems, tend to retreat from their woes. In other words, optimists deal with stress differently than pessimists. In fact, one of the key differences between optimists and pessimists is in the coping strategies they use.

Personal Coping Strategies

Psychologists have categorized coping strategies in many ways, but Folkman and Lazarus's (1980) conceptualization of coping strategies as emotion focused or problem focused is the most influential. **Problem-focused coping** is aimed at changing the source of the stress, whereas **emotion-focused coping** is oriented toward managing the emotions that accompany the perception of stress. Both approaches can be effective in making the stressed individual feel better, but the two approaches may not be equally effective in managing the stressful situation.

As shown in Table 5.1, several different strategies fall within the emotion-focused and problem-focused categories. For example, taking action to try to get rid of the problem is a problem-focused strategy, but seeking the company of friends or family for comfort and reassurance is an emotion-focused strategy. If an upcoming

TABLE 5.1   Examples of Problem-Focused and Emotion-Focused Coping Strategies

Problem-Focused Coping	Emotion-Focused Coping
Studying for upcoming exam	Writing in a journal
Developing a budget to save money	Exercising
Talking to a friend to solve a conflict	Watching a comedy
Asking boss for extra time to complete a project	Praying, meditating
Trying to get back together with a partner who dumped you	Drinking alcohol or drugs
	Denial

exam is a source of stress, making (and following) a schedule for studying is a problem-focused strategy. Calling up a friend and complaining about the test or going out to a movie might help manage the distress, but these strategies are almost certainly not effective for dealing with the upcoming test. The problem-focused strategy sounds like a better choice in this case, but emotion-focused coping can be effective in some situations (Folkman & Moskowitz, 2004). When stress is unavoidable, finding a way to feel better may be the best option. For example, if you were dumped by someone who has no intention of getting back together with you, then it may be better to manage your feelings instead of trying to win the person back.

However, certain specific coping strategies may be unhealthy. A meta-analysis of the effects of coping strategies on psychological and physical health (Penley, Tomaka, & Wiebe, 2002) showed that problem-focused coping generally contributed to good health, whereas emotion-focused coping strategies contributed to poorer health. In particular, those who used the emotion-focused strategies of eating more, drinking, sleeping, or using drugs, reported poorer health. Several recent meta-analyses have confirmed this general pattern of findings—problem-focused coping is better than emotion-focused coping in dealing with chronic stress such as discrimination (Pascoe & Richman, 2009), HIV infection (Moskowitz, Hult, Bussolari, & Acree, 2009), and diabetes (Duangdao & Roesch, 2008).

People are more likely to use problem-focused coping when they appraise a situation as controllable. Among people coping with cancer, those who appraise their situation as a challenge are more likely to use problem-focused coping; those who appraise their situation as harm or loss are more likely to use avoidance coping (Franks & Roesch, 2006). Optimists are more likely than pessimists to employ problem-focused strategies, less likely to use avoidance strategies, and also more likely to adjust their coping strategies to meet the specific demands of the situation (Nes & Segerstrom, 2006). Thus, the "wise" use of coping strategies explains why optimists adjust better to stress than pessimists.

Additional categories of coping strategies exist (Folkman & Moskowitz, 2004). These include *social coping*, such as seeking support from others, and *meaning-focused coping*, in which the person concentrates on deriving meaning from the stressful experience. For example, people who experience a trauma such as loss of a loved one or a diagnosis of a serious disease often attempt to understand the personal (and often spiritual) meaning within the situation. People who take this approach often succeed (Folkman & Moskowitz, 2000) and in doing so often experience better psychological adjustment (Helgeson, Reynolds, & Tomich, 2006; Updegraff, Silver, & Holman, 2008).

Culture exerts a powerful influence on coping, and gender also shows some effects. One might imagine that people who live in cultures that emphasize social harmony would be more likely to use social coping strategies, but such is not the case (Kim, Sherman, & Taylor, 2008). Indeed, Asian Americans are *less* likely than European Americans to seek social support when coping with stress, largely because of the motivation to maintain harmony with others (Wang, Shih, Hu, Louie, & Lau, 2010). However, another study (Lincoln, Chatters, & Taylor, 2003) found that African Americans were more likely than European Americans to seek social support from their families. Some studies find cross-cultural similarities in coping strategies, and those studies tend to study people in similar situations. For example, a study of adolescents in seven European nations (Gelhaar et al., 2007) found similarities among coping strategies for adolescents in all of the nations, especially in job-related situations.

Females tend to use social coping strategies more than men (Tamres, Janicki, & Helgeson, 2002). Aside from this difference, research on gender differences in coping tends to find small differences between women's and men's coping strategies when studying individuals in similar situations (Adams, Aranda, Kemp, & Takagi, 2002; Ronan, Dreer, Dollard, & Ronan, 2004; Sigmon, Stanton, & Snyder, 1995). However, the stressors that men and women face may differ due to gender roles, resulting in gender differences in coping strategies. For example, in one study that found gender differences in coping, women experienced more family-related stressors but men experienced more finance and work-related stressors (Matud, 2004). Because gender roles vary among cultures, gender and culture may interact to create different situational demands for coping by men and women in various cultures.

IN SUMMARY

Personal resources and a variety of coping strategies allow people to cope with stress in order to avoid or minimize distress. Social support, defined as the emotional quality of one's social contacts, is inversely related to disease and death. In general, people with high levels of social support experience health advantages and lower mortality. People with adequate social support probably receive more encouragement and advice regarding good health practices and may react less strongly to stress, which may buffer them against the harmful effects of stress more than people who are socially isolated.

Adequate feelings of personal control also seem to enable people to cope better with stress and illness. People who believe that their lives are controlled by fate or outside forces have greater difficulty changing health-related behaviors than do those who believe that the locus of control resides with themselves. The classic studies of nursing home residents demonstrated that when people are allowed to assume even small amounts of personal control and responsibility, they seem to live longer and healthier lives.

Coping strategies are classified in many ways, but the distinction between problem-focused coping, which is oriented toward solving the problem, and emotion-focused coping, which is oriented toward managing distress associated with stress, is useful. In addition, meaning-focused coping helps people find underlying meaning in negative experiences. In general, problem-focused coping is more effective than other types, but all types of coping strategies may be effective in some situations. The key to successful coping is flexibility, leading to the use of an appropriate strategy for the situation.

Behavioral Interventions for Managing Stress

In addition to studying stress, psychologists develop techniques that teach people how to manage stress. These include relaxation training, cognitive behavioral therapy, emotional disclosure, and mindfulness.

Relaxation Training

Relaxation training is perhaps the simplest and easiest to use of all psychological interventions, and relaxation may be the key ingredient in other types of therapeutic interventions for managing stress.

What Is Relaxation Training? · During the 1930s, Edmond Jacobson (1938) discussed a type of relaxation he called *progressive muscle relaxation*. With this procedure, patients first receive the explanation that their present tension is mostly a physical state resulting from tense muscles. While reclining in a comfortable chair, often with eyes closed and with no distracting lights or sounds, patients first breathe deeply and exhale slowly. After this, the series of deep muscle relaxation exercises begins, a process described in the Becoming Healthier box. Once patients learn the relaxation technique, they may practice independently or with prerecorded audio-tapes at home. Length of relaxation training programs varies, but 6 to 8 weeks and about 10 sessions with an instructor are usually sufficient to allow patients to easily and independently enter a state of deep relaxation (Blanchard & Andrasik, 1985).

Autogenics training is another approach to relaxation. Pioneered by Johannes Schultz during the 1920s and 1930s in Germany, the technique was refined by Wolfgang Luthe (Naylor & Marshall, 2007). Autogenics training consists of a series of exercises designed to reduce muscle tension, change the way people think, and change the content of people's thoughts. The process begins with a mental check of the body and proceeds with suggestions for relaxation and warmth throughout the body. Advocates contend that practicing autogenics for 10 minutes at least twice a day reduces stress and thus improves health.

How Effective Is Relaxation Training?   Like other psychological interventions, relaxation is effective only if it proves more powerful than a control situation, or placebo. Relaxation techniques generally meet this criterion (Jacobs, 2001). Indeed, relaxation may be an essential part of other interventions such as biofeedback and hypnotic treatment (see Chapter 8).

Relaxation training was a component in a successful stress management program for college students (Iglesias et al., 2005), and children were able to learn and to benefit from relaxation training (Lohaus & Klein-Hessling, 2003). Both progressive muscle relaxation and autogenic training are components in effective treatment programs for stress-related disorders such as depression, anxiety, hypertension, and insomnia (Stetter & Kupper, 2002; McCallie, Blum, & Hood, 2006). Techniques also help reduce hormonal stress responses following breast cancer surgery (Phillips et al., 2011) and promote faster healing following gallbladder surgery (Broadbent et al., 2012). Table 5.2 summarizes the effectiveness of relaxation techniques for stress-related problems.

Becoming Healthier

Progressive muscle relaxation is a technique that you may be able to use to cope with stress and pain. Although some people may need the help of a trained therapist to master this approach, others are able to train themselves. To learn progressive muscle relaxation, recline in a comfortable chair in a room with no distractions. You may wish to remove your shoes and either dim the lights or close your eyes to enhance relaxation. Next, breathe deeply and exhale slowly. Repeat this deep breathing exercise several times until you begin to feel your body becoming more and more relaxed.

The next step is to select a muscle group (for example, your left hand) and deliberately tense that group of muscles. If you begin with your hand, make a fist and squeeze the fingers into your hand as hard as you can. Hold that tension for about 10 seconds and then slowly release the tension, concentrating on the relaxing, soothing sensations in your hand as the tension gradually drains away. Once the left hand is relaxed, shift to the right hand and repeat the procedure, while keeping your left hand as relaxed as possible. After both hands are relaxed, go through the same tensing and relaxing

sequence progressively with other muscle groups, including the arms, shoulders, neck, mouth, tongue, forehead, eyes, toes, feet, calves, thighs, back, and stomach. Then repeat the deep breathing exercises until you achieve a complete feeling of relaxation. Focus on the enjoyable sensation of relaxation, restricting your attention to the pleasant internal events and away from irritating external sources of pain or stress. You will probably need to practice this procedure several times to learn to quickly place your body into a state of deep relaxation.

TABLE 5.2 Effectiveness of Relaxation Techniques

Problems	Findings	Studies
1. Stress management for college students	Relaxation is a component in successful stress management.	Iglesias et al., 2005
2. Depression, anxiety, hypertension, and insomnia	Autogenics and progressive muscle relaxation are effective components in programs to manage these disorders.	McCallie et al., 2006; Stetter & Kupper, 2002
3. Laboratory stress	Progressive muscle relaxation produces changes in heart rate, skin conductance, and skin temperature in children.	Lohaus & Klein-Hessling, 2003
4. Stress following surgery for breast cancer	Relaxation training is an important component of a stress management program that lowered women's cortisol levels over a 12-month period.	Phillips et al., 2011
5. Recovery following gallbladder surgery	Relaxation training leads to lower perceived stress and faster wound healing.	Broadbent et al., 2012

Cognitive Behavioral Therapy

Health psychologists use the same types of interventions for managing stress that they use for other behavior problems, including *cognitive behavioral therapy*. This approach is a combination of *behavior modification*, which arose from the laboratory research on operant conditioning, and *cognitive therapy*, which can be traced to research on mental processes. Cognitive behavioral therapy is more effective than any other approach for stress management.

What Is Cognitive Behavioral Therapy? Cognitive behavioral therapy (CBT) is a type of therapy that aims to develop beliefs, attitudes, thoughts, and skills to make positive changes in behavior. Like cognitive therapy, CBT assumes that thoughts and feelings are the basis of behavior, so CBT begins with changing attitudes. Like behavior modification, CBT focuses on modifying environmental contingencies and building skills to change observable behavior.

An example of CBT for stress management is the stress inoculation program developed by Donald Meichenbaum and Roy Cameron (1983; Meichenbaum, 2007). The procedure works in a manner analogous to vaccination. By introducing a weakened dose of a pathogen (in this case, the pathogen is stress), the therapist attempts to build some immunity against high levels of stress. Stress inoculation includes three stages: conceptualization, skills acquisition and rehearsal, and follow-through or application. The *conceptualization* stage is a cognitive intervention in which the therapist works with clients to identify and clarify their problems. During this overtly educational stage, patients learn about stress inoculation and how this technique can reduce their stress. The *skills acquisition and rehearsal* stage involves both educational and behavioral components to enhance patients' repertoire of coping skills. At this time, patients learn and practice new ways of coping with stress. One of the goals of this stage is to improve self-instruction by changing cognitions, a process that includes monitoring one's internal monologue—that is, self-talk. During the *application and follow-through* stage, patients put into practice the cognitive changes they have achieved in the two previous stages.

Another CBT approach to stress is cognitive behavioral stress management (CBSM; Antoni, Ironson, & Schneiderman, 2007), a 10-week group intervention that shares many features with stress inoculation training. CBSM also works toward changing cognitions concerning stress, enlarging clients' repertoire of coping skills, and guiding clients to apply these skills in effective ways. Other researchers use variations of CBT to investigate the effectiveness of this approach to stress management.

How Effective Is Cognitive Behavioral Therapy?

Research on the efficacy of CBT indicates that it is effective for both prevention and management of stress and stress-related disorders. Furthermore, CBT is effective with a wide variety of clients, and is one of the most effective techniques for reducing stress among college students (Regehr, Glancy, & Pitts, 2013).

An early meta-analysis (Saunders, Driskell, Johnston, & Sales, 1996) of nearly 40 studies found that stress inoculation training decreased anxiety and raised performance under stress. Stress inoculation training is effective for a range of stressors. For example, one program (Sheehy & Horan, 2004) tested the benefits of stress inoculation training for first-year law students to determine if the training helped these students alleviate some of their anxiety and stress. The program succeeded in meeting those goals and also raised grades.

Stress inoculation can also be effective in helping victims of trauma manage their severe distress (Cahill & Foa, 2007). For example, stress inoculation is helpful for crime victims who experience PTSD (Hembree & Foa, 2003). Researchers adapted stress inoculation therapy for use on the Internet (Litz, Williams, Wang, Bryant, & Engel, 2004), making it available to a larger number of people.

Other varieties of cognitive behavioral therapy are effective for stress management, including CBSM. This intervention may even help counteract the negative effects of stress by moderating the increased cortisol production that accompanies the stress response (Antoni et al., 2009; Gaab, Sonderegger, Scherrer, & Ehlert, 2007), an accomplishment that few techniques have achieved (see Chapter 6). One recent study showed that a prenatal CBSM intervention reduced cortisol production of both mothers *and* their infants (Urizar & Muñoz, 2011). However, these effects may not include dramatic improvement in immune functioning. A meta-analysis of cognitive behavioral interventions for people who are HIV positive (Crepaz et al., 2008) revealed significant positive effects for reductions in stress, depression, anxiety, and anger, but immune functioning was less improved. Like stress inoculation programs, cognitive behavioral interventions are also adapted for use on the Internet (Benight, Ruzek, & Waldrep, 2008).

CBSM also helps those with substance abuse problems manage stress-induced cravings, which could give a boost to substance abuse treatment (Back, Gentilin, & Brady, 2007). Cognitive behavioral therapy is also an effective intervention for PTSD (Bisson & Andrew, 2007), chronic back pain (Hoffman, Papas, Chatkoff, & Kerns, 2007), and chronic fatigue syndrome (Lopez et al., 2011). Cognitive behavioral techniques are used in workplace stress management, and this approach has demonstrated consistently larger effects than other programs (Richardson & Rothstein, 2008). Furthermore, cognitive behavioral stress techniques can help students improve their performance; a cognitive behavioral stress intervention improved students' motivations and scores on standardized exams (Keogh, Bond, & Flaxman, 2006).

In summary, many studies show that cognitive behavioral therapy interventions are effective for stress management for people with a variety of stress-related problems. Table 5.3 summarizes the effectiveness of cognitive behavioral therapy for stress-related problems.

Emotional Disclosure

In 2015, following a period in which she faced legal and personal problems, Solo began to deal with her stress by starting a blog: in her words, a way to "process and share my experiences." Could emotional disclosure, such as writing a blog, help people such as Solo cope with stress? Indeed, research by James Pennebaker and colleagues (Pennebaker, Barger, & Tiebout, 1989) shows that emotional self-disclosure improves both psychological and physical health. Subsequent research has

extended the positive effects of emotional disclosure to a variety of people and settings.

What Is Emotional Disclosure? Emotional **disclosure** is a therapeutic technique in which people express their strong emotions by talking or writing about negative events that precipitated those emotions. For centuries, confession of sinful deeds has been part of personal healing in many religious rituals. During the late 19th century, Joseph Breuer and Sigmund Freud (1895/1955) recognized the value of the "talking cure," and **catharsis**—the verbal expression of emotions—became an important part of psychotherapy. Pennebaker took the notion of catharsis beyond Breuer and Freud, by demonstrating the health benefits of talking or writing about traumatic life events.

The general pattern of Pennebaker's research is to ask people to write or talk about traumatic events for 15 to 20 minutes, three or four times a week. Emotional disclosure should be distinguished from emotional expression, which refers to emotional outbursts

TABLE 5.3   Effectiveness of Cognitive Behavioral Therapy

Problems	Findings	Studies
1. Performance anxiety	Inoculation training reduces performance anxiety and boosts performance under stress.	Saunders et al., 1996
2. Stress of law school	Stress inoculation training decreases stress and increases grades.	Sheehy & Horan, 2004
3. Posttraumatic stress disorder	Inoculation procedures lessen negative effects of posttraumatic stress disorder.	Cahill & Foa, 2007; Hembree & Foa, 2003; Litz et al., 2004
4. Hormonal stress responses	Cognitive behavioral stress management moderates cortisol production during stress response.	Antoni et al., 2009; Gaab et al., 2007; Urizar & Muñoz, 2011
5. Stress, anxiety, depression in people with HIV	Cognitive behavioral therapy improves these symptoms of HIV.	Crepaz et al., 2008
6. Stress-related cravings	Cognitive behavioral stress management decreased cravings.	Back et al., 2007
7. Psychological and physical health symptoms	Cognitive behavioral therapy is an effective treatment.	Bisson & Andrew, 2007; Hoffman et al., 2007; Lopez et al., 2011
8. Workplace stress	Cognitive behavioral therapy is effective.	Richardson & Rothstein, 2008
9. School-related stress	Cognitive behavioral therapy boosts motivation and test performance.	Keogh et al., 2006

or emotional venting, such as crying, laughing, yelling, or throwing objects. Emotional disclosure, in contrast, involves the transfer of emotions into language and thus requires a measure of self-reflection. Emotional outbursts are often unhealthy and may add more stress to an already unpleasant situation.

In one of their early studies on emotional disclosure, Pennebaker and colleagues (Pennebaker et al., 1989) asked survivors of the Holocaust to talk for 1 to 2 hours about their war experiences. Those survivors who disclosed the most personally traumatic experiences had better subsequent health than survivors who expressed less painful experiences. Since then, Pennebaker and his colleagues have investigated other forms of emotional disclosure, such as asking people to talk into a tape recorder, write their thoughts privately, or speak to a therapist about highly stressful events. With each of these techniques, the key ingredient is language—emotions must be expressed through language.

The physical and psychological changes in people who use emotional disclosure are typically compared with those of a control group, who are asked to write or talk about superficial events. This relatively simple procedure is responsible for physiological changes such as fewer physician visits, improved immune functioning, and lower rates of asthma, arthritis, cancer, and heart disease. In addition, disclosure has produced psychological and behavioral changes, such as fewer depressive symptoms before taking graduate school entrance exams and better performance on those exams (Frattaroli, Thomas, & Lyubomirsky, 2011).

How Effective Is Emotional Disclosure? A substantial number of studies by Pennebaker's team and other researchers demonstrate the effectiveness of disclosure in reducing a variety of illnesses. A review of 146 studies of emotional disclosure found a positive effect on most psychological outcomes and some physical health outcomes (Frattaroli, 2006). This review also identified a number of factors that make emotional disclosure more effective. One of these factors is the amount of stress in a person's life: People who experience more stress benefit from emotional disclosure more than those who experience less stress. Other factors that make emotional disclosure more effective include writing in private, writing for more than 15 minutes, and writing about a stressful event not previously shared with other people. Importantly, the effectiveness of emotional disclosure does not differ based on gender, age, or ethnicity (Frattaroli, 2006).

A notable example of the effect of emotional disclosure on physical health includes an early study that showed that students who disclosed feelings about entering college had fewer illnesses than those who wrote about superficial topics (Pennebaker, Colder, & Sharp, 1990). Despite its emotional basis, a meta-analysis of studies on emotional disclosure (Frisina, Borod, & Lepore, 2004) concluded that this approach is more effective in helping people with physical than psychological problems. Emotional disclosure can reduce symptoms in patients with asthma and arthritis (Smyth, Stone, Hurewitz, & Kaell, 1999) and buffer some of the problems associated with breast cancer among women who perceive low levels of social support (Low, Stanton, Bower, & Gyllenhammer, 2010).

Must the emotional disclosure focus on trauma? Some evidence indicates that when people focus on finding some positive aspect of a traumatic experience, they may accrue even more benefits than when they focus on the negative aspects of the experience. In one

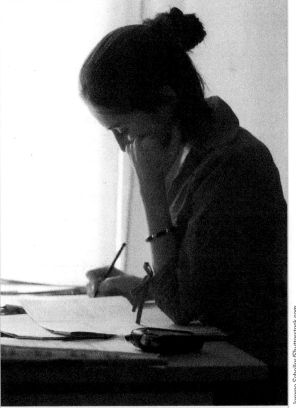

Writing about traumatic or highly stressful events produces physical as well as emotional benefits.

study, when participants were led to a less negative interpretation of a traumatic event, they experienced greater benefits than did those whose negative interpretations were validated (Lepore, Fernandez-Berrocal, Ragan, & Ramos, 2004). Other research suggests that when writing about a stressful situation, developing a plan for dealing with the situation (Lestideau & Lavallee, 2007) or focusing on positive aspects of the stressor (Lu & Stanton, 2010) boosts the benefits of expressive writing. These findings extend Pennebaker's research on disclosure by suggesting that people who concentrate on the positive aspects of a traumatic experience or develop a plan to deal with the stressful situation can receive health benefits equal or superior to those who simply write about a traumatic life event.

Pennebaker's research adds an effective and easily accessible tool to the arsenal of strategies for managing stress. Indeed, benefits can occur through a program of writing by e-mail (Sheese, Brown, & Graziano, 2004) or through an Internet-based intervention (Possemato, Ouimette, & Geller, 2010). See Table 5.4 for a summary of the effectiveness of self-disclosure through writing or talking.

Mindfulness

While a graduate student in molecular biology at Massachusetts Institute of Technology, Jon Kabat-Zinn chanced upon small talk given by a Zen missionary on the topic of meditation. The missionary described his experience in a Zen monastery: primitive, no heat, and freezing cold in the winter. However, within several months at the monastery, the missionary observed that his chronic ulcers began to subside and never returned again.

What does meditation provide that could cause a stress-related ailment such as chronic ulcers to subside, especially under seemingly unpleasant living conditions? Dr. Kabat-Zinn dedicated his career to investigating this question, and for the next three decades spearheaded a movement to examine the possible mental health and physical health benefits of mindfulness meditation.

TABLE 5.4   Effectiveness of Emotional Disclosure

Problems	Findings	Studies
1. General health problems	Holocaust survivors who talked most about 'their experience had fewer health problems 14 months later.	Pennebaker et al., 1989
2. Performance on graduate entrance exams (GRE, LSAT, MCAT)	Written disclosure about upcoming exam improved performance.	Frattaroli et al., 2011
3. Emotional and physical symptoms	Disclosure associated with better psychological and physical health outcomes.	Frisina et al., 2004; Frattaroli, 2006
4. Anxiety about entering college	Students who disclosed had fewer illnesses.	Pennebaker et al., 1990
5. Asthma, rheumatoid arthritis, and living with cancer	Keeping a journal of stressful events reduces symptoms and improves functioning.	Smyth et al., 1999
6. Emotional and physical symptoms of breast cancer	Disclosure associated with less distress among women with low social support.	Low et al., 2010
7. Emotional and physical symptoms	Focusing on positive aspects of situation produced greater benefits.	Lepore et al., 2004; Lu & Stanton, 2010
8. Emotional and physical symptoms	Focusing on developing a plan produced greater benefits than focusing only on emotions.	Lestideau & Levallee, 2007
9. Problems in mental and physical health	E-mail and Internet intervention about traumatic events showed benefits.	Sheese et al., 2004; Possemato et al., 2010

What Is Mindfulness?   Although there are many definitions of mindfulness, most Western views of mindfulness define it as a quality of consciousness or awareness that comes about through intentionally focusing one's attention on the present moment in a nonjudgmental and accepting manner (Kabat-Zinn, 1994). Kabat-Zinn developed an 8-week mindfulness-based stress reduction program that taught people mindfulness skills through exercises such as focusing attention on one's immediate breathing, thoughts, bodily sensations, sounds, and everyday activities. For most people, attending to one's present environment and sensations is not a typical response to stress; people have a natural tendency to respond to stress with preoccupation on one's past or ongoing troubles and their effects on their future. Mindfulness meditation aims to take this preoccupation with past- and future-directed thoughts and emotions, and redirect it toward their immediate situation.

How Effective Is Mindfulness?   Reviews of this literature indeed suggest that mindfulness-based stress reduction interventions can decrease stress, depression, and anxiety in breast cancer patients (Cramer, Lauche, Paul, & Dobos, 2012; Zainal, Booth, & Huppert, 2013), increase acceptance of pain in patients with low back pain (Cramer, Haller, Lauche, & Dobos, 2012), decrease distress and possibly improve disease progression among people living with HIV (Riley & Kalichman, 2015). While the benefits of mindfulness are most pronounced when looking at outcomes such as self-reported stress, depression, and anxiety, the effects of mindfulness may also extend to physical health outcomes as well. For example, a mindfulness-based stress reduction intervention was associated with better outcomes in terms of immune measures, stress hormones, and blood pressure in cancer patients (Carlson, Speca, Faris, & Patel, 2007), as well as reduced blood pressure among adults at risk for hypertension (Hughes et al., 2013). Furthermore, the effects of mindfulness-based stress reduction interventions on mental health seem to be due to their ability to improve mindfulness, reduce worry, and reduce people's tendency to dwell on stressful experiences (Gu, Strauss, Bond, & Cavanagh, 2015). Although most mindfulness-based stress reduction interventions last 8 weeks, some research shows that even

participating in fewer sessions can also lead to similar benefits (Carmody & Baer, 2009; Hofmann, Sawyer, Witt, & Oh, 2010).

IN SUMMARY

Health psychologists help people cope with stress by using relaxation training, cognitive behavioral therapy, emotional disclosure, and mindfulness. Relaxation techniques include progressive muscle relaxation and autogenics training. Relaxation approaches have some success in helping patients manage stress and anxiety and are generally more effective than a placebo.

Cognitive behavioral therapy draws upon operant conditioning and behavior modification as well as cognitive therapy, which strives to change behavior through changing attitudes and beliefs. Cognitive behavioral therapists attempt to get patients to think differently about their stress experiences and teach strategies that lead to more effective self-management.

Stress inoculation and CBSM are types of cognitive behavioral therapy interventions. Stress inoculation introduces low levels of stress and then teaches skills for coping and application of those skills. Stress inoculation and CBSM are successful interventions for preventing stress and in treating a wide variety of stress problems, including anxiety and depression in people with HIV, stress cravings in people with substance use disorders, PTSD, workplace stress, and school-related stress.

Emotional disclosure calls for patients to disclose strong negative emotions, most often through writing. People using this technique write about traumatic life events for 15 to 20 minutes, three or four times a week. Emotional disclosure generally enhances health, relieves anxiety, and reduces visits to health care providers, and may reduce the symptoms of asthma, rheumatoid arthritis, and cancer.

Mindfulness-based stress reduction interventions foster a nonjudgmental focus and attention on the present moment. Mindfulness interventions can decrease stress, depression, anxiety, and may also improve physiological measures such as blood pressure as well.

Answers

This chapter has addressed six basic questions:

1. **What is the physiology of stress?**

   The nervous system plays a central role in the physiology of stress. When a person perceives stress, the sympathetic division of the autonomic nervous system stimulates the adrenal medulla, producing catecholamines and arousing the person from a resting state. The perception of stress also prompts a second route of response through the pituitary gland, which releases adrenocorticotropic hormone. This hormone, in turn, affects the adrenal cortex, which produces glucocorticoids. These hormones prepare the body to resist stress.

2. **What theories explain stress?**

   Hans Selye and Richard Lazarus both proposed theories of stress. During his career, Selye defined stress first as a stimulus and then as a response. Whenever the body encounters a disruptive stimulus, it mobilizes itself in a generalized attempt to adapt to that stimulus. Selye called this mobilization the general adaptation syndrome. The GAS has three stages—alarm, resistance, and exhaustion—and the potential for trauma or illness exists at all three stages. Lazarus insisted that a person's perception of a situation is the most significant component of stress. To Lazarus, stress depends on one's appraisal of an event rather than on the event itself. Whether or not stress produces illness is closely tied to one's vulnerability as well as to one's perceived ability to cope with the situation.

3. **How has stress been measured?**

   Several methods exist for assessing stress, including physiological and biochemical measures and self-reports of stressful events. Most life events scales are patterned after Holmes and Rahe's Social Readjustment Rating Scale. Some of these instruments include only undesirable events, but the SRRS and other self-report inventories are based on the premise that any major change is stressful. Lazarus and his associates pioneered scales that measure daily hassles and uplifts. These scales, which generally have better validity than the SRRS, emphasize the severity of the event as perceived by the person.

   Physiological and biochemical measures have the advantage of good reliability, whereas self-report inventories pose more problems in demonstrating reliability and validity. Although most self-report inventories have acceptable reliability, their ability to predict illness remains to be established. For these stress inventories to predict illness, two conditions must be met: First, they must be valid measures of stress; second, stress must be related to illness. Chapter 6 takes up the question of whether stress causes illness.

4. **What sources produce stress?**

   Sources of stress can be categorized as cataclysmic events, life events, and daily hassles. Cataclysmic events include sudden, unexpected events that produce major demands for adaptation. Such events include natural disasters such as earthquakes and hurricanes and intentional events such as terrorist attacks. Posttraumatic stress disorder is a possibility in the aftermath of such events.

   Life events such as divorce, criminal victimization, or death of a family member also produce major life changes and require adaptation, but life events are usually not as sudden and dramatic as cataclysmic events. Daily hassles are even smaller and more common, but produce distress. Such daily events may arise from the community, as with noise, crowding, and pollution; from workplace conditions, such as work with high demands and little control; or from conflicts in relationships.

5. **What factors influence coping, and what strategies are effective?**

   Factors that influence coping include social support, personal control, and personal hardiness. Social support, defined as the emotional quality of one's social contacts, is important to a person's ability to cope and to one's health. People with social support receive more encouragement and advice to seek medical care, and social support may provide a buffer against the physical effects of stress. Second, people's beliefs that they have control over the events of their life seem to have a positive impact on health. Even a sense of control over small matters may improve health and prolong life. The factor of personal hardiness includes components of commitment, control, and interpreting events as challenges rather than as stressors.

People use a variety of strategies to cope with stress, all of which may be successful. Problem-focused coping is often a better choice than emotion-focused efforts because problem-focused coping can change the source of the problem, eliminating the stress-producing situation. Emotion-focused coping is oriented toward managing the distress that accompanies stress. Research indicates that most people use a variety of coping strategies, often in combination, and this flexibility is important for effective coping.

6. **What behavioral techniques are effective for stress management?**

Four types of interventions are available to health psychologists in helping people cope with stress. First, relaxation training can help people cope with a variety of stress problems. Second, cognitive behavioral therapy—including stress inoculation and cognitive behavioral stress management—is effective in reducing both stress and stress-related disorders such as posttraumatic stress disorder. Third, emotional disclosure—including writing about traumatic events—can help people recover from traumatic experiences and experience better psychological and physical health. Fourth, mindfulness-based stress reduction interventions can help reduce stress, depression, and anxiety.

Suggested Readings

Kemeny, M. E. (2003). The psychobiology of stress. *Current Directions in Psychological Science, 12,* 124–129. This concise review furnishes a summary of the physiology of stress, how stress can "get under the skin" to influence disease, and some psychosocial factors that moderate this process.

Lazarus, R. S., & Folkman, S. (1984). *Stress, appraisal, and coping.* New York: Springer. In this classic book, Richard Lazarus and Susan Folkman present a comprehensive treatment of Lazarus's views of stress, cognitive appraisal, and coping. This book also discusses the relevant literature up to that time.

McEwen, B. S. (2005). Stressed or stressed out: What is the difference? *Journal of Psychiatry and Neuroscience, 30,* 315–318. This brief, readable article summarizes the evolution of the concept of stress, including Selye's work and changes to that framework.

Monroe, S. M. (2008). Modern approaches to conceptualizing and measuring human life stress. *Annual Review of Clinical Psychology, 4,* 33–52. This readable review describes many of the issues in defining and measuring stress in humans, as well as understanding pathways by which life stress may influence physical health.

CHAPTER 6

Understanding Stress, Immunity, and Disease

CHAPTER OUTLINE

- Real-World Profile of Big City Taxi Drivers
- *Physiology of the Immune System*
- *Psychoneuroimmunology*
- *Does Stress Cause Disease?*

QUESTIONS

This chapter focuses on three basic questions:

1. How does the immune system function?
2. How does the field of psychoneuroimmunology relate behavior to disease?
3. Does stress cause disease?

Real-World Profile of **BIG CITY TAXI DRIVERS**

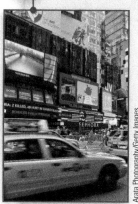

One of the most stressful occupations is driving a taxi cab, particularly in a bustling metropolis such as New York City. Taxi drivers often earn little money, work 60 to 70 hours per week, and face steep competition from other drivers and increasing job insecurity. In addition to navigating hectic traffic under intense time pressures, taxi drivers deal with impatient customers, poor weather and road conditions, unsuspecting pedestrians and cyclists, and the need to pack in as many customers in each day as possible. Taxi drivers who are ethnic minorities may also experience discrimination as a result of both their race and occupation. Taxi drivers also face homicide risks far higher than those in most other occupations.

"You never know who's getting in your cab, so you have to be constantly vigilant and expect trouble at any time," says Kathy Pavlofsky, a taxi driver from Berkeley, California (Kloberdanz, 2016).

The health risks of being a cab driver extend beyond assault and homicide. Taxi drivers are at increased risk for obesity and diabetes, due to a largely sedentary occupation and frequent reliance on a fast-food diet. The small compartment of a taxicab and the continual exposure to strangers also put cab drivers at high risk of exposure to airborne viruses.

The stress of the job can also increase risk for long-term health problems. A survey by the New York Taxi Worker's Alliance found that more than 20% of drivers have cardiovascular disease or cancer. By other estimates, more than 60% of taxi drivers have high blood pressure.

For example, Rafael Arias, a New York City taxi driver for 17 years, developed a buildup of blood in his brain that, without treatment, could have developed into a stroke. His doctor noted stress as a likely cause of the problem.

Emotional problems may also be common among people in high stress occupations such as taxi drivers. "Many of them need to see a psychiatrist," says Maria Ramos, an activist who recognized the stress-related problems of New York City cab drivers and created a city-wide program called the Taxi/Limousine Drivers Health Initiative to help alleviate the health problems the group faces (Camhi, 2012). Ramos received a Community Health Leaders Award from the Robert Wood Johnson Foundation for recognizing and addressing the health needs of drivers such as Arias.

In this chapter, you will learn how stress—such as that faced by taxi drivers and others in highly stressful occupations—can increase one's risk for a variety of health problem, as well as the biological pathways by which stress can influence disease.

Arata Photography/Getty Images

This chapter reviews the evidence relating to stress as a possible cause of disease. In Chapter 5, you learned that stress can influence health-related behaviors, which can increase risk for disease or death. If stress, a psychological factor, can also influence physical disease *directly*, some mechanism must exist to allow this interaction. In this chapter, we will examine how stress can increase risk for health problems through biological processes. We begin with a discussion of the immune system, which protects the body against stress-related diseases and provides one mechanism for stress to cause disease.

Physiology of the Immune System

At any given moment, you are surrounded by microorganisms such as bacteria, viruses, and fungi. Some of these microorganisms are harmless, but others can endanger your health. The immune system consists of tissues, organs, and processes that protect the body from invasion by such foreign microorganisms. In addition, the immune system performs housekeeping functions by removing worn-out or damaged cells and patrolling for mutant cells. Once the immune system locates these invaders and renegades, it activates processes to eliminate them. Thus, a well-functioning immune system plays a crucial role in maintaining health.

Organs of the Immune System

The immune system is spread throughout the body in the form of the lymphatic system. The tissue of the lymphatic system is lymph; it consists of the tissue components of blood other than red cells and platelets. In the process of vascular circulation, fluid and *leukocytes* (white blood cells) leak from the capillaries, escaping the circulatory system. Body cells also secrete white blood cells. This tissue fluid is referred to as lymph when it enters the lymph vessels, which circulate lymph and eventually return it to the bloodstream.

Lymph circulates by entering the lymphatic system and then reentering the bloodstream rather than staying exclusively in the lymphatic system. The structure of the lymphatic system (see Figure 6.1) roughly parallels the circulatory system for blood. In its circulation, all lymph travels through at least one lymph node. The lymph nodes are round or oval capsules spaced throughout the lymphatic system that help clean lymph of cellular debris, bacteria, and even dust that has entered the body.

Lymphocytes are a type of white blood cell found in lymph. There are several types of lymphocytes, the most fully understood of which are T-lymphocytes, or T-cells; B-lymphocytes, or B-cells; and natural killer (NK) cells. Lymphocytes originate in the bone marrow, but they mature and differentiate in other structures of the immune system. In addition to lymphocytes, two other types of leukocytes are granulocytes and monocytes/macrophages. These leukocytes have roles in the nonspecific and specific immune system responses (discussed in detail later).

The thymus, which has endocrine functions, secretes a hormone called thymosin, which is involved in the maturation and differentiation of the T-cells. Interestingly, the thymus is largest during infancy and childhood and then atrophies during adulthood. Its function is not entirely understood, but the thymus is clearly important in the immune system because its removal impairs immune function. Its atrophy also suggests that the immune system's production of T-cells is more efficient during childhood and that aging is related to lowered immune efficiency (Briones, 2007). The tonsils are masses of lymphatic tissue located in the throat. Their function seems to be similar to that of the

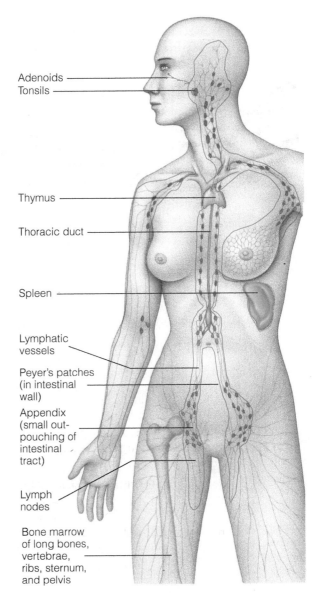

Adenoids
Tonsils
Thymus
Thoracic duct
Spleen
Lymphatic vessels
Peyer's patches (in intestinal wall)
Appendix (small out-pouching of intestinal tract)
Lymph nodes
Bone marrow of long bones, vertebrae, ribs, sternum, and pelvis

FIGURE 6.1   Lymphatic system.

Source: Introduction to microbiology (p. 407), by J. L. Ingraham & C. A. Ingraham. From INGRAHAM/INGRAHAM, *Introduction to Microbiology*, 1E. © 1995 Cengage Learning.

lymph nodes: trapping and killing invading cells and particles. The spleen, an organ near the stomach in the abdominal cavity, is one site where lymphocytes mature. In addition, it serves as a holding station for lymphocytes as well as a disposal site for worn-out blood cells.

Thus, the organs of the immune system produce, store, and circulate lymph throughout the rest of the body. The surveillance and protection that the immune system offers is not limited to the lymph nodes. Rather, it takes place in other tissues of the body that contain lymphocytes. To protect the entire body, immune function must occur in all parts of the body.

Function of the Immune System

The immune system's function is to defend against foreign substances that the body encounters. The immune system must be extraordinarily effective to prevent 100% of the invading bacteria, viruses, and fungi from damaging our bodies. Few other body functions must operate at 100% efficiency, but when this system performs at some lesser capacity, the person (or animal) becomes vulnerable.

Invading organisms can enter the body in many ways, and the immune system has methods to combat each mode of entry. In general, there are two ways the immune system fights invading foreign substances: general (nonspecific) and specific responses. Both may be involved in fighting an invader.

Nonspecific Immune System Responses   To enter the body, foreign substances must first pass the skin and mucous membranes. Thus, these organs and tissues are the body's first line of defense against the outside world. Foreign substances that are able to pass these barriers face two general (nonspecific) mechanisms. One is **phagocytosis**, the attacking of foreign particles by cells of the immune system. Two types of leukocytes perform this function. **Granulocytes** contain granules filled with chemicals. When these cells come into contact with invaders, they release their chemicals, which attack the invaders. **Macrophages** perform a variety of immune functions, including scavenging for worn-out cells and debris, initiating specific immune responses, and secreting a variety of chemicals that break down the cell membranes of invaders. Thus, phagocytosis involves several mechanisms that can quickly result in the destruction of invading bacteria, viruses, and fungi. However, some invaders escape this nonspecific action.

A second type of nonspecific immune system response is **inflammation**, which works to restore tissues that have been damaged by invaders. When an injury occurs, blood vessels in the area of injury dilate, increasing blood flow to the tissues and causing the warmth and redness that accompany inflammation. The damaged cells release enzymes that help destroy invading microorganisms; these enzymes can also aid in their own digestion, should the cells die. Both granulocytes and macrophages migrate to the site of injury

to battle the invaders. Finally, tissue repair begins. Figure 6.2 illustrates the process of inflammation.

Specific Immune Systems Responses   Specific immune responses are specific to one invader, such as a certain virus or bacteria. Two types of lymphocytes, T-cells and B-cells, carry out specific immune responses. When a lymphocyte encounters a foreign substance for the first time, both the general response and a specific response occur. Invading microorganisms are killed and eaten by macrophages, which present fragments of these invaders to T-cells that have moved to the area of inflammation. This contact sensitizes the T-cells, and they acquire specific receptors on their surfaces that enable them to recognize the invader. An army of *cytotoxic T-cells* forms through this process, and it soon mobilizes a direct attack on the invaders. This process is referred to as *cell-mediated immunity* because it occurs at the level of the body cells rather than in the bloodstream. Cell-mediated immunity is especially effective against fungi, viruses that have already entered the cells, parasites, and mutations of body cells.

The other variety of lymphocyte, the B-cell, mobilizes an indirect attack on invading microorganisms. With the help of one variety of T-cell (the *helper T-cell*), B-cells differentiate into **plasma cells** and secrete **antibodies**. Each antibody is manufactured in response to a specific invader. Foreign substances that provoke antibody manufacture are called **antigens** (for antibody generator). Antibodies circulate, find their antigens, bind to them, and mark them for later destruction. Figure 6.3 shows the differentiation of T-cells and B-cells.

The specific reactions of the immune system constitute the *primary immune response*. Figure 6.4 shows the development of the primary immune response and depicts how subsequent exposure activates the *secondary immune response*. During initial exposure to an invader, some of the sensitized T-cells and B-cells replicate and, rather than go into action, are held in reserve. These *memory lymphocytes* form the basis for a rapid immune response on second exposure to the same invader. Memory lymphocytes can persist for years but will not be activated unless the antigen invader reappears. If it does, then the memory lymphocytes initiate the same sort of direct and indirect attacks that occurred at the first exposure, but much more rapidly. This specifically tailored rapid response to foreign microorganisms that occurs with repeated exposure is what most people consider **immunity**.

This system of immune response through B-cell recognition of antigens and their manufacture of

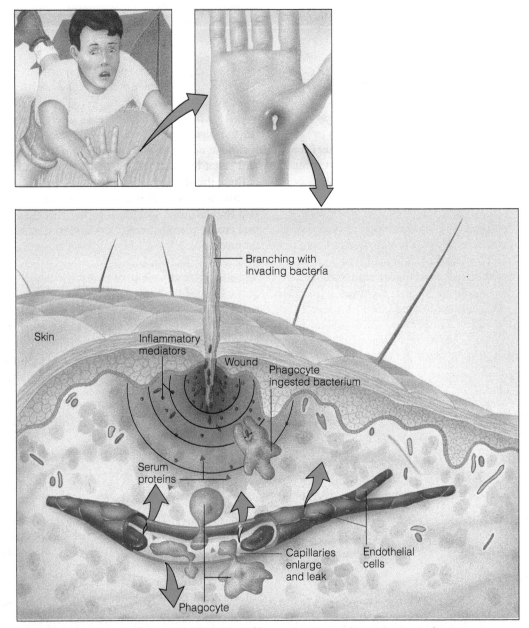

FIGURE 6.2   Acute inflammation is initiated by a stimulus such as injury or infection. Inflammatory mediators, produced at the site of the stimulus, cause blood vessels to dilate and increase their permeability; they also attract phagocytes to the site of inflammation and activate them.

Source: Introduction to microbiology (p. 386), by J. L. Ingraham & C. A. Ingraham. From INGRAHAM/INGRAHAM, *Introduction to Microbiology*, 1E. © 1995 Cengage Learning.

antibodies is called **humoral immunity** because it happens in the bloodstream. The process is especially effective in fighting viruses that have already entered the cells, parasites, and mutations of body cells.

Creating Immunity   One widely used method to induce immunity is **vaccination.** In vaccination, a weakened form of a virus or bacterium is introduced into the body, stimulating the production of antibodies.

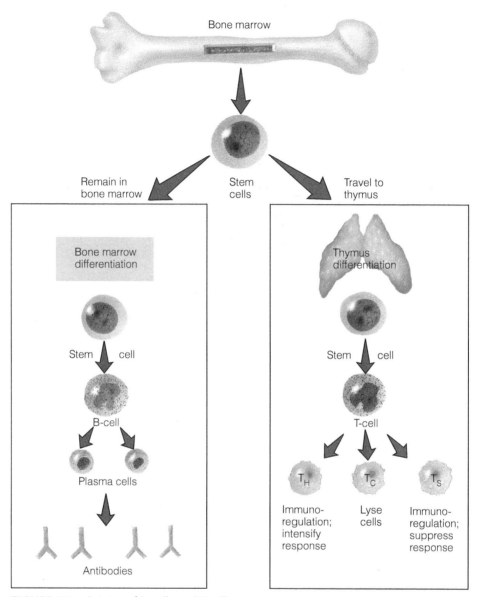

FIGURE 6.3 Origins of B-cells and T-cells.

Source: Introduction to microbiology (p. 406), by J. L. Ingraham & C. A. Ingraham. From INGRAHAM/INGRAHAM, *Introduction to Microbiology*, 1E. © 1995 Cengage Learning.

These antibodies then confer immunity for an extended period. Smallpox, which once killed thousands of people each year, was eradicated through the use of vaccination. As a result, people are no longer vaccinated against this disease.

Other vaccines exist for a variety of diseases. They are especially useful in the prevention of viral infections. However, immunity must be created for each specific virus, and thousands of viruses exist. Even viral diseases that produce similar symptoms, such as the common cold, may be caused by many different viruses. Therefore, immunity for colds would require many vaccinations, and such a process has not yet proven practical.

Immune System Disorders

Immune deficiency, an inadequate immune response, may occur for several reasons. For example, it is a side

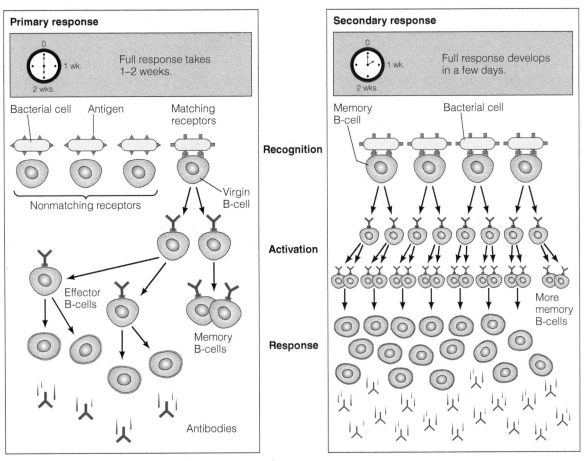

FIGURE 6.4   Primary and secondary immune pathways.

Source: Introduction to microbiology (p. 414), by J. L. Ingraham & C. A. Ingraham. From INGRAHAM/INGRAHAM, *Introduction to Microbiology*, 1E. © 1995 Cengage Learning.

effect of most chemotherapy drugs used to treat cancer. Immune deficiency also occurs naturally. Although the immune system is not fully functional at birth, infants are protected by antibodies they receive from their mothers through the placenta, and infants who breast-feed receive antibodies from their mothers' milk. These antibodies offer protection until the infant's own immune system develops during the first months of life.

In rare cases, the immune system fails to develop, leaving the child without immune protection. Physicians can try to boost immune function, but the well-publicized "children in plastic bubbles" still possess immune deficiency. Exposure to any virus or bacterium can be fatal to these children. They are sealed into sterile quarters to isolate them from the microorganisms that are part of the normal world.

A much more common type of immune deficiency is **acquired immune deficiency syndrome (AIDS)**.

This disease is caused by a virus, the human immuno-deficiency virus (HIV), which destroys the T-cells and macrophages in the immune system. People infected with HIV may progress to AIDS and become vulnerable to a wide range of bacterial, viral, and malignant diseases. HIV is contagious, but not easily transmitted from person to person. The highest concentrations of the virus are found in blood and in semen. Blood transfusions from an infected person, injection with a contaminated needle, sexual intercourse, and transmission during the birth process are the most common routes of infection. Treatment consists of controlling the proliferation of the virus through antiviral drugs and management of the diseases that develop as a result of immune deficiency. As of 2016, a combination of antiviral drugs is capable of slowing the progress of HIV infection, but no treatment is yet capable of eliminating HIV from an infected person.

Allergies are another immune system disorder. An allergic response is an abnormal reaction to a foreign substance that normally elicits little or no immune reaction. A wide range of substances can cause allergic reactions, and the severity of the reactions also varies widely. Some allergic reactions may be life threatening, whereas others may cause annoyances such as runny noses. Some allergies are treated by introducing regular, small doses of the allergen to desensitize the person and to diminish or alleviate the allergic response. Sometimes, for reasons not well understood, the immune system may attack its own body. This situation occurs with **autoimmune diseases**. Recall that a function of the immune system is to recognize foreign invaders and mark them for destruction. In autoimmune diseases, the immune system loses the ability to distinguish the body from an invader, and it mounts the same vicious attack against itself that it would against an intruder. Lupus erythematosus, rheumatoid arthritis, and multiple sclerosis are autoimmune diseases.

IN SUMMARY

If stress can cause disease directly, it can do so only by affecting biological processes (see Figure 1.4). One likely candidate for this interaction is the immune system, which is made up of tissues, organs, and processes that protect the body from invasion by foreign material such as bacteria, viruses, and fungi. The immune system also protects the body by eliminating damaged cells. Immune system responses can be either nonspecific or specific. The nonspecific response is capable of attacking any invader, whereas specific responses attack one particular invader. Immune system problems can stem from several sources, including organ transplants, allergies, drugs used for cancer chemotherapy, and immune deficiency. The HIV damages the immune system, creating a deficiency that leaves the person vulnerable to a variety of infectious and malignant diseases.

Psychoneuroimmunology

The previous section described the function of the immune system as well as its tissues, structure, and disorders. Physiologists have traditionally taken a similar approach, studying the immune system as separate from and independent of other body systems. About 30 years ago, however, accumulating evidence suggested that the immune system interacts with the central nervous system (CNS) and the endocrine system. This evidence shows that psychological and social factors can affect the CNS, endocrine system, and immune system. In addition, immune function can affect neural function, providing the potential for the immune system to alter behavior and thought (Maier, 2003). This recognition led to the founding and rapid growth of the field of **psychoneuroimmunology** (PNI), a multidisciplinary field that focuses on the interactions among behavior, the nervous system, the endocrine system, and the immune system.

History of Psychoneuroimmunology

In the early 1900s, Ivan Pavlov discovered that dogs could be trained to salivate at the sound of a bell. Pavlov showed that, through the process of classical conditioning, environmental events could become automatic triggers of basic physiological processes. Could classical conditioning also influence the functioning of physiological processes as seemingly "invisible" as the immune system?

In 1975, Robert Ader and Nicholas Cohen published a study that investigated this simple question. In doing so, Ader and Cohen showed how the nervous system, the immune system, and behavior could interact—a discovery that essentially created the field of PNI. Ader and Cohen's approach was straightforward and similar to Pavlov's approach: They paired a conditioned stimulus (CS) with an unconditioned stimulus (UCS), to see whether the conditioned stimulus alone would later produce a conditioned response (CR). However, the difference was that Ader and Cohen's conditioned stimulus was a saccharin and water solution that rats drank, and the unconditioned stimulus was the administration of a drug that suppresses the immune system. During the conditioning process, the rats were allowed to drink the saccharin solution and then were injected with the immunosuppressive drug. Much like Pavlov's dogs, the rats quickly associated the two stimuli, such that the rats later showed immune suppression when they were given *only* the saccharine solution! In this groundbreaking study, Ader and Cohen demonstrated that the immune system was subject to the same type of associative learning as other body systems.

Until Ader and Cohen's 1975 report, most physiologists believed that the immune system and the nervous system did not interact, and their results were not immediately accepted (Fleshner & Laudenslager, 2004). After many replications of their findings, physiologists now accept that the immune system and other body systems exchange information in a variety of ways. One mechanism is through cytokines, chemical messengers secreted by cells in the immune system (Blalock & Smith, 2007; Maier & Watkins, 2003). One type of cytokine is known as **proinflammatory cytokine** because it promotes inflammation. These cytokines, which include several types of *interleukins,* may underlie a number of states, including feelings associated with sickness, depression, and social withdrawal (Eisenberger, Inagaki, Mashal, & Irwin, 2010; Irwin, 2008; Kelley et al., 2003). This is one example of how the functioning of the immune system may influence psychological states.

The developing knowledge of the connections between the immune and nervous systems spurred researchers to explore the physical mechanisms by which interactions occur. Psychologists began using measures of immune function to test the effects of behavior on the immune system. During the 1980s, the AIDS epidemic focused public attention and research funding on how behavior influences the immune system and therefore health. As a result of this attention, some of the clearest evidence of the role of psychological factors in immune functioning comes from studies of people coping with HIV infection (Chida & Vedhara, 2009). However, researchers in the field of psychoneuroimmunology use a variety of populations and methods to examine the links between psychological factors and the functioning of the immune system (see Would You Believe ...? box).

Research in Psychoneuroimmunology

Research in psychoneuroimmunology aims to develop an understanding of the role of behavior in changes in the immune system and the development of disease. To reach this goal, researchers must establish a connection between psychological factors and changes in immune function and also demonstrate a relationship between this impaired immune function and changes

Would You BELIEVE...?   Pictures of Disease Are Enough to Activate the Immune System

The ability of the immune system to mount an effective attack against a biological invader is amazing in both its complexity and effectiveness. However, the immune system may have evolved to respond to more than simply pathogens that already entered the body. The immune system may mount defenses against pathogens that the brain *anticipates may soon enter the body.*

Canadian researchers (Schaller, Miller, Gervais, Yager, & Chen, 2010) presented a series of photographs to college student participants. Some participants saw pictures of infectious diseases—such as pox, skin lesions, and sneezing. These pictures were stimuli that were expected to activate an immune response. Participants in a control group saw pictures of guns, which were threatening stimuli but were not expected to activate an immune response. Indeed, participants who viewed the pictures of infectious diseases produced significantly more proinflammatory cytokines than participants who viewed the pictures of guns.

An Australian research team (Stevenson, Hodgson, Oaten, Barouei, & Case, 2011) found similar results when they had participants view images intended to induce a feeling of disgust, such as a dead animal, dirty toilet, and a cockroach on a pizza. Compared with participants who viewed neutral or threatening (but not disgusting) images, participants viewing the disgusting images produced greater quantities of the proinflammatory cytokine TNF-a.

Why might such disgusting images stimulate the immune system? While he exact reason is unknown, some researchers suggest the responses may be rooted in evolution. Organisms that mount an immune response when exposed to stimuli that are associated with pathogens may have less likelihood of succumbing to infection when those pathogens eventually enter the body (Schaller et al., 2010). However, such a response may be ineffectual—or even costly—in contexts where disgusting stimuli are not typically followed by exposure to pathogens, for example, when watching a particularly gory horror film.

Taken together, these findings highlight the fascinating links between the brain and the immune system. Pass the popcorn!

in health status. Ideally, research should include all three components—psychological factors such as stress, immune system malfunction, and development of disease—to establish the connection between stress and disease (Forlenza & Baum, 2004). This task is difficult for several reasons.

One reason for the difficulty is the less-than-perfect relationship between immune system malfunction and disease. Not all people with impaired immune systems become ill (Segerstrom & Miller, 2004). Disease is a function of both the immune system's competence and the person's exposure to pathogens, the agents that produce illness. The best approach in PNI comes from longitudinal studies that follow people for a period of time after they (1) experience stress that (2) prompts a decline in immunocompetence and then (3) assess changes in their health status. Few studies included all three components, and most such studies are restricted to nonhuman animals. However, one such study followed older adults who were responsible for providing care to a spouse with dementia (Kiecolt-Glaser, Dura, Speicher, Trask, & Glaser, 1991). Compared to non-caregiving controls, the caregivers showed poorer functioning in several measures of immune status. Furthermore, the caregivers reported more days of infectious illness. The poorer immune functioning was particularly apparent in the caregivers who had low levels of social support.

The majority of research in PNI focuses on the relationship between various stressors and altered immune system function. Most studies measure the immune system's function by testing blood samples rather than by testing immune function in people's bodies (Coe & Laudenslager, 2007; Segerstrom & Miller, 2004). Some research concentrates on the relationship between altered immune system function and the development of disease or spread of cancer (Cohen, 2005; Reiche, Nunes, & Morimoto, 2004), but such studies are in the minority. Furthermore, the types of stressors, the species of animals, and the facet of immune system function studied varied, resulting in a variety of findings (Forlenza & Baum, 2004).

Some researchers manipulate short-term stressors such as electric shock, loud noises, or complex cognitive tasks in a laboratory situation; others use naturally occurring stress in people's lives to test the effect of stress on immune system function. Laboratory studies allow researchers to investigate the physical changes that accompany stress, and such studies show correlations between sympathetic nervous system activation and immune responses (Glaser, 2005; Irwin, 2008). This research suggests that sympathetic activation may be a pathway through which stress can affect the immune system. The effect is initially positive, mobilizing resources, but continued stress activates physiological processes that can be damaging.

The naturally occurring stress of medical school exams provides another opportunity to study the relationship between stress and immune function in students (Kiecolt-Glaser, Malarkey, Cacioppo, & Glaser, 1994). A series of studies showed differences in immunocompetence, measured by numbers of natural killer cells, percentages of T-cells, and percentages of total lymphocytes. Indeed, medical students show more symptoms of infectious disease immediately before and after exams. More recent research (Chandrashekara et al., 2007) confirms that anxious students taking exams experience a lowering of immune function, which demonstrates that the effect on immune function is specific to the situation and to the students' psychological state.

Exam stress is typically a short-term stress, but chronic stress has even more severe effects on immune competence. Relationship conflict predicts immune system suppression for couples that experience marital conflict (Kiecolt-Glaser & Newton, 2001). Indeed, marriage is important in immune function and to a wide range of health outcomes (Graham, Christian, & Kiecolt-Glaser, 2006). For example, effects of marital conflict may include poorer response to immunization and slower wound healing (Ebrecht et al., 2004), and lack of partner support may play a role in increased stress during pregnancy, which raises health risk (Coussons-Read, Okun, & Nettles, 2007). However, marital conflict may not always lead to poorer immune response. Partners who deal with conflict with productive communication patterns have immune responses that are less dysregulated by episodes of marital conflict (Graham et al., 2009).

Other chronic stressors also suppress immune function. For example, people who are caregivers for someone with Alzheimer's disease experience chronic stress (see Chapter 11 for more about the disease and the stress of caregiving). Alzheimer's caregivers experience poorer psychological and physical health, longer healing times for wounds, and lowered immune function (Damjanovic et al., 2007; Kiecolt-Glaser, 1999; Kiecolt-Glaser, Marucha, Malarkey, Mercado, & Glaser, 1995). Furthermore, the death of the Alzheimer's patient fails to improve the stressed caregivers' psychological health or immune system functioning (Robinson-Whelen, Tada, MacCallum, McGuire, & Kiecolt-Glaser, 2001). Both caregivers and former caregivers were more depressed and showed lowered immune system functioning, suggesting that this stress continues even after the caregiving is over.

The results of meta-analyses of 30 years of studies on stress and immunity (Segerstrom & Miller, 2004) show a clear relationship between stress and decreased immune function, especially for chronic sources of stress. The stressors that exert the most chronic effects have the most global influence on the immune system. Refugees, the unemployed, taxi drivers, and those who live in high-crime neighborhoods experience the type of chronic, uncontrollable stress that has the most widespread negative effect on the immune system. Short-term stress may produce changes that are adaptive, such as mobilizing hormone production, but chronic stress exerts effects on many types of immune system response that weaken immune system effectiveness.

Some of the PNI research that most clearly demonstrates the three-way link among stress, immune function, and disease uses stressed rats as subjects, injecting material that provokes an immune system response and observing the resulting changes in immune function and disease (Bowers, Bilbo, Dhabhar, & Nelson, 2008). Some research with human participants also demonstrates the link among stress, immune function, and disease (Cohen, 2005; Kiecolt-Glaser, McGuire, Robles, & Glaser, 2002). For example, healing time after receiving a standardized wound varies, depending on whether the wound occurs during vacation or during exams. Students under exam stress show a decline in a specific immune function related to wound healing; the same students took 40% longer to heal during exams than they did during vacation. Thus, both human and animal research demonstrate that stress can affect immune function and disease processes.

If behavioral and social factors can decrease immune system function, is it possible to *boost* immunocompetence through changes in behavior? Would such an increase enhance health? Researchers have designed interventions aimed at increasing the effectiveness of the immune system—such as hypnosis, relaxation, and stress management—but a meta-analysis of these studies (Miller & Cohen, 2001) indicated only modest effects. Similarly, a meta-analysis of cognitive behavioral interventions for HIV-positive men (Crepaz et al., 2008) showed significant effects for improvements in anxiety, stress, and depression but limited changes

in immune system function. However, a 10-week cognitive behavioral stress management intervention for women under treatment for breast cancer led to some improvements in immune measures over a 6-month period (Antoni et al., 2009). Cancer treatment weakens the immune system, so even small improvements may be an advantage for these individuals.

Physical Mechanisms of Influence

How does stress influence the functioning of the immune system? The effects of stress can occur through at least three routes—through the peripheral nervous system, through the secretion of hormones, and through behaviors that affect their immune system negatively, such as missing sleep, drinking alcohol, or smoking (Segerstrom & Miller, 2004).

The peripheral nervous system provides connections to immune system organs such as the thymus, spleen, and lymph nodes. The brain can also communicate with the immune system through the production of *releasing factors,* hormones that stimulate endocrine glands to secrete hormones. These hormones travel through the bloodstream and affect target organs, such as the adrenal glands. (Chapter 5 included a description of these systems and the endocrine component of the stress response.) T-cells and B-cells have receptors for the glucocorticoid stress hormones.

When the sympathetic nervous system is activated, the adrenal glands release several hormones. The adrenal medulla releases epinephrine and norepinephrine, and the adrenal cortex releases cortisol. The modulation of immunity by epinephrine and norepinephrine seems to come about through the autonomic nervous system (Dougall & Baum, 2001).

The release of cortisol from the adrenal cortex results from the release of adrenocorticotropic hormone (ACTH) by the pituitary in the brain. Another brain structure, the hypothalamus, stimulates the pituitary to release ACTH. Elevated cortisol is associated with a number of physical and emotional distress conditions (Dickerson & Kemeny, 2004), and it exerts an anti-inflammatory effect. Cortisol and the glucocorticoids tend to depress immune responses, phagocytosis, and macrophage activation. The nervous system can influence the immune system either through the sympathetic nervous system or through neuroendocrine response to stress.

Communication also occurs in the other direction: The immune system can signal the nervous system by way of cytokines, chemicals secreted by immune system cells (Irwin, 2008; Maier, 2003). Cytokines communicate with the brain, probably by way of the peripheral nervous system. This interconnection makes possible bidirectional interactions of immune and nervous systems and may even enable effects on behavior such as fatigue and depression, which are common symptoms of sickness. Michael Irwin (2008) emphasized the many possibilities for communication between the nervous and immune systems and how behavioral responses are the key to activating processes that influence the immune system. The interrelationship between the nervous system and the immune system makes it possible for each to influence the other to produce the symptoms associated with stress and disease.

Stress may also "get under the skin" by altering health-related behaviors (Segerstrom & Miller, 2004). For example, people under stress may smoke more cigarettes, drink more alcohol, use illicit drugs, and get less sleep. As described at the start of this chapter, the highly stressful lives of taxi drivers may leave little opportunity for physical activity or proper diet. Each of these behaviors increases risk for a variety of diseases and may influence the immune system in negative ways.

IN SUMMARY

Psychoneuroimmunology research demonstrates that various functions of the immune system respond to both short-term and long-term psychological stress. Researchers are making progress toward linking psychological factors, immune system function, and disease, but few studies have included all three elements.

Some research is successful in linking immune system changes to changes in health status; this link is necessary to complete the chain between psychological factors and disease. In addition to establishing links between psychological factors and immune system changes, researchers attempt to specify the physical mechanisms through which these changes occur. Possible mechanisms include direct connections between nervous and immune systems and an indirect connection through the neuroendocrine system. Chemical messengers called cytokines also allow for communication between immune and nervous system and possible effects on behavior. In addition, stress may prompt people to change their behaviors, adopting less healthy habits that are risk factors for disease.

Does Stress Cause Disease?

Many factors cause disease, and stress may be one of those factors. When considering the link between stress and disease, remember that most people who experience substantial stress do *not* develop a disease. Furthermore, in contrast to other risk factors—such as having high cholesterol levels, smoking cigarettes, or drinking alcohol—the risks conferred by life events are usually temporary. Yet, even temporary stress affects some people more than others.

Why does stress affect some people, apparently causing them to get sick, and leave others unaffected? The diathesis–stress model offers a possible answer to this question.

The Diathesis–Stress Model

The **diathesis–stress model** suggests that some individuals are vulnerable to stress-related diseases because either genetic weakness or biochemical imbalance inherently predisposes them to those diseases. The diathesis–stress model has a long history in psychology, particularly in explaining the development of psychological disorders. During the 1960s and 1970s, the concept was used as an explanation for the development of psychophysiological disorders (Levi, 1974) as well as schizophrenic episodes, depression, and anxiety disorders (Zubin & Spring, 1977).

Applied to either psychological or physiological disorders, the diathesis–stress model holds that some people are predisposed to react maladaptively to environmental stressors. This predisposition (diathesis) is usually thought to be inherited through biochemical or organ system weakness, but some theorists (Zubin & Spring, 1977) also consider learned patterns of thought and behavior as components of vulnerability. Whether inherited or learned, the vulnerability is relatively permanent. What varies over time is the presence of environmental stressors, which may account for the waxing and waning of illnesses.

Thus, the diathesis–stress model assumes that two factors are necessary to produce disease. First, the person must have a relatively permanent predisposition to the disease, and second, that person must experience some sort of stress. Diathetic individuals respond pathologically to the same stressful conditions with which most people are able to cope. For people with a strong predisposition to a disease, even a mild environmental stressor may be sufficient to produce an illness episode. For example, a study of symptom stress and depression (Schroeder, 2004) revealed that surgical patients with low coping competence were vulnerable to developing depression in the months following their surgery, whereas patients with better coping skills were less vulnerable to depression. Abuse or maltreatment during childhood may create another source of vulnerability to physical and psychological disorders. As adults, these individuals show increased vulnerability to schizophrenia (Rosenberg, Lu, Mueser, Jankowski, & Cournos, 2007), anxiety and depression (Stein, Schork, & Gelernter, 2008), posttraumatic stress disorder (Storr, Lalongo, Anthony, & Breslau, 2007), and infectious disease (Cohen, 2005). A person's social environment may also create a diathesis; stressful life events can increase suicide risk among adults, but especially for those who also report high levels of loneliness (Chang, Sanna, Hirsch, & Jeglic, 2010). Therefore, personal and psychosocial factors have the power to create vulnerabilities to disorders.

The diathesis–stress model may explain why life event scales (see Chapter 5) are so inconsistent in predicting illness. The number of points accumulated on the Holmes and Rahe Social Readjustment Rating Scale or the number of items checked on the Life Events Scale for Students is only a weak predictor of illness. The diathesis–stress model holds that a person's diathesis (vulnerability) must be considered along with stressful life events in predicting who will get sick and who will stay well; it allows for a great deal of individual variability in who gets sick and who stays well under conditions of stress (Marsland, Bachen, Cohen, & Manuck, 2001).

In this section, we review the evidence concerning the link between stress and several diseases, including headache, infectious disease, cardiovascular disease, diabetes mellitus, premature birth, asthma, and rheumatoid arthritis. In addition, stress shows some relationship to psychological disorders such as depression and anxiety disorders.

Stress and Disease

What is the evidence linking stress to disease? Which diseases have been implicated? What physiological mechanism might mediate the connection between stress and disease?

Hans Selye's concept of stress (see Chapter 5) included suppression of the immune response, and a growing body of evidence now supports this hypothesis through interactions among the nervous, endocrine, and immune systems (Kemeny & Schedlowski, 2007). These interactions are similar to the responses hypothesized by Selye and provide strong evidence that stress could be involved in a variety of physical ailments. Figure 6.5 shows some possible effects.

Several possibilities exist for pathways through which stress could produce disease (Segerstrom & Miller, 2004). Direct influence could occur through the effects of stress on the nervous, endocrine, and immune systems. Because any or all of these systems can create disease, sufficient physiological foundations exist to provide a link between stress and disease. In addition, indirect effects could occur through changes in health practices that increase risks; that is, stress tends to be related to increases in drinking, smoking, drug use, and sleep problems, all of which can increase the risk for disease.

Stress may also accelerate the normal aging process by shortening the length of telomeres. A telomere is a region of repetitive nucleotide sequences that appears at each end of a chromosome. Telomeres serve as a protective cap that prevents a chromosome from deterioration, much in the same way that the tip of a shoelace prevents it from fraying apart. Each time a cell divides and a chromosome replicates, however, the length of the telomere shortens. When telomeres shorten to a certain point, affected cells undergo senescence; that is, they lose the ability to replicate normally. Senescence is a normal part of the aging process, and for this reason, telomere length can be a useful measure of cellular aging.

Importantly, recent research shows that the experience of life stress—both early life stress as well as recent chronic stress—is associated with accelerated shortening of telomeres (Mathur et al., 2016; Verhoeven, van Oppen et al., 2015). Long working hours, lower socioeconomic status, and childhood trauma all have been linked to shorter telomere length. In one study of healthy mothers, those who reported the highest levels of stress had shorter telomeres than those with the lowest levels of stress, a difference corresponding to what would be expected from 10 years of normal aging (Epel et al., 2004)! Longitudinal research shows that other psychological states such as anxiety, depression, and PTSD predict shortened telomere length over time (Shalev et al., 2014). Even having ambivalent social relationships—that is, having many social relationships that you feel neither particularly positive or negative about—is associated with shorter telomeres, particularly among women (Uchino et al., 2012).

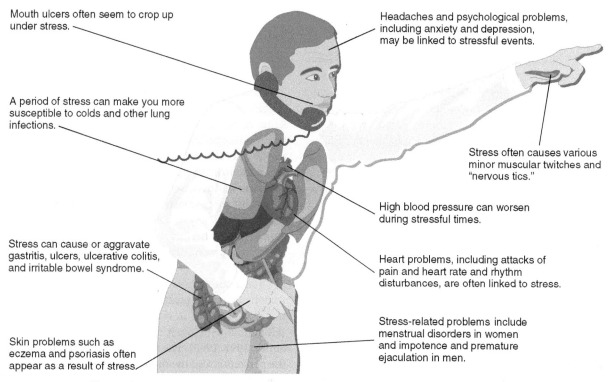

Mouth ulcers often seem to crop up under stress.

Headaches and psychological problems, including anxiety and depression, may be linked to stressful events.

A period of stress can make you more susceptible to colds and other lung infections.

Stress often causes various minor muscular twitches and "nervous tics."

High blood pressure can worsen during stressful times.

Stress can cause or aggravate gastritis, ulcers, ulcerative colitis, and irritable bowel syndrome.

Heart problems, including attacks of pain and heart rate and rhythm disturbances, are often linked to stress.

Stress-related problems include menstrual disorders in women and impotence and premature ejaculation in men.

Skin problems such as eczema and psoriasis often appear as a result of stress.

FIGURE 6.5   Effects of long-term stress.

Source: *An invitation to health* (7th ed., p. 58), by D. Hales, 1997, Pacific Grove, CA: Brooks/Cole. From HALES, *Invitation to Health*, 7E. © 1997 Cengage Learning.

While the exact mechanisms by which stress or other psychosocial states contribute to the shortening of telomere remains unclear, the release of glucocorticoids by the HPA axis during stress may result in oxidative damage to DNA and the shortening of telomeres (Epel et al., 2004; von Zglinicki, 2002). It is unknown at this point, however, whether the effect of stress on telomere length increases a person's chances of succumbing to specific diseases. Shortened telomeres may contribute to the susceptibility to infection (Cohen et al., 2013a), and in one study, the shortened telomere length partially explained the link between low childhood socioeconomic status and adult risk of infection (Cohen et al., 2013b). Shortened telomere length has also been associated with the development of cancer (Günes & Rudolph, 2013), but life stress appears to have a small, if any, relationship to the risk of developing cancer (Chida, Hamer, Wardle, & Steptoe, 2008; Heikkilä et al., 2013). Investigations into the potential role of stress in accelerating cellular aging remains an active and exciting area of research, and highlights the multiple ways in which stress could influence disease.

Headaches   Headaches are a common problem; more than 99% of people will experience headaches at some time in their lives (Smetana, 2000). For most people, headaches are an uncomfortable occurrence, but others experience serious, chronic pain. Headache can signal serious medical conditions, but most often the pain associated with the headache is the problem. This source of pain is a major cause of disability (D'Amico et al., 2011). The majority of people who seek medical assistance for headaches experience the same sorts of headaches as those who do not; the difference stems from the frequency and severity of the headaches or from personal factors involved in seeking assistance.

Although more than 100 types of headaches may exist, distinguishing among them is controversial, and the underlying causes for the most common types remain unclear (Andrasik, 2001). Nevertheless, diagnostic criteria have been devised for several types of headaches. The most frequent type is *tension headache,* usually associated with increased muscle tension in the head and neck region. Tension is also a factor in migraine headaches, which are believed to originate in neurons in the brain stem (Silberstein, 2004). Migraines are associated with throbbing pain localized in one side of the head.

Stress is a factor in headaches; people with either tension or vascular headaches name stress as one of the leading precipitating factors (Deniz, Aygül, Koçak, Orhan, & Kaya, 2004; Spierings, Ranke, & Honkoop, 2001). However, a comparison of people with daily headaches and those with infrequent headaches found no difference in stress as measured either by life events or by hassles (Barton-Donovan & Blanchard, 2005), and a study comparing traumatic life events for headache patients found no difference from a comparison group (de Leeuw, Schmidt, & Carlson, 2005). The type of stress that people associate with headaches tends not to be traumatic life events but, rather, daily hassles. Students with chronic or frequent headaches reported more hassles than did students with infrequent headaches (Bottos & Dewey, 2004).

Nash and Thebarge (2006) discussed the ways through which stress might influence headaches. First, stress may be a predisposing factor that influences the development of headaches. Second, stress may act to transform a person who experiences occasional headaches into one who has chronic headaches. Third, stress may worsen headache episodes, magnifying the pain. These routes allow for several possibilities through which stress can contribute to the development of a headache and to chronic headaches. Furthermore, stress may decrease the quality of life for those with headaches.

Infectious Disease   Are people who are under stress more likely than nonstressed individuals to develop infectious diseases such as the common cold? Research suggests that the answer is yes. An early study (Stone, Reed, & Neale, 1987) followed married couples who kept diaries on their own and their spouse's desirable and undesirable daily life experiences. Results indicated that participants who experienced a decline in desirable events or an increase in undesirable events developed somewhat more infectious diseases (colds or flu) 3 and 4 days later. The association was not strong, but this study was the first prospective design to show a relationship between daily life experiences and subsequent disease.

Later studies used a more direct approach, intentionally exposing healthy volunteers with cold viruses to see who would develop a cold and who would not (Cohen, 2005; Cohen et al., 1998; Cohen, Tyrrell, & Smith, 1991, 1993). The results indicated that the higher the person's stress, the more likely it was that the person would become ill.

Cohen and his colleagues (1998) also used the same inoculation procedure to see what types of stressors increase susceptibility to a cold virus. They found that duration of a stressful life event was more important than severity. Acute severe stress of less

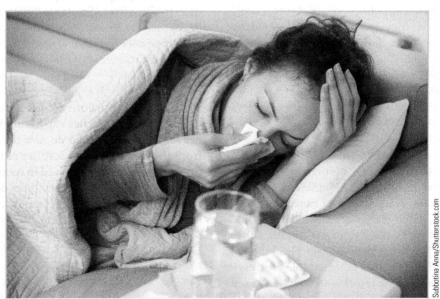

Research has shown that stress can influence development of infectious disease.

Subbotina Anna/Shutterstock.com

than 1 month did not lead to the development of colds, but severe chronic stress (more than 1 month) led to a substantial increase in colds. Later research showed that susceptibility varied from individual to individual (Marsland, Bachen, Cohen, Rabin, & Manuck, 2002); people who are sociable and agreeable develop fewer colds than others after exposure to a cold virus (Cohen, Doyle, Turner, Alper, & Skoner, 2003). A naturalistic study of stress and colds (Takkouche, Regueira, & Gestal-Otero, 2001) showed that high levels of stress were related to increases in infection. People in the upper 25% of perceived stress were about twice as likely as those in the lowest 25% to get a cold, which suggests that stress may be a significant predictor of developing infectious disease.

Stress may also influence the extent to which vaccinations provide protection against infectious disease. Vaccinations, as you recall, stimulate the immune system to produce antibodies against specific viruses. People under substantial stress—such as caregivers—show weakened antibody production following flu vaccination compared with people under less life stress (Pedersen, Zachariae, & Bovbjerg, 2009). This relationship between stress and weakened response to vaccination suggests it is as apparent among younger adults as it is among older adults. Thus, vaccinations may be less effective in protecting against infectious disease among people who experience stress.

Stress may also affect the progression of infectious disease. Reviews of psychosocial factors in HIV infection (Cole et al., 2001; Kopnisky, Stoff, & Rausch, 2004) explored the effect of stress on HIV infection; they concluded that stress affects both the progression of HIV infection and the infected person's immune response to antiviral drug treatment. HIV is not the only infectious disease that stresses influences. The herpes simplex virus (HSV) is transmitted through contact with the skin of an infected person and can cause blisters on the mouth, lips, or genitals. Often, these physical symptoms are not present in the infected person but only appear during periodic active outbreaks of HSV. Stress predicts these symptomatic outbreaks of HSV symptoms (Chida & Mao, 2009; Strachan et al., 2011). For example, in a study of women with a sexually transmitted form of HSV, researchers found that experiences of psychosocial distress predicted the onset of genital lesions 5 days later (Strachan et al., 2011). Stress also plays a role in other bacterial, viral, and fungal infections, including pneumonia, hepatitis, and recurrent urinary tract infections (Levenson & Schneider, 2007). Thus, stress is a

significant factor in susceptibility, severity, and progression of infection.

Cardiovascular Disease Cardiovascular disease (CVD) has a number of behavioral risk factors, some of which are related to stress. Chapter 9 examines these behavioral risk factors in more detail; in this section we look only at stress as a contributor to CVD. People who have had heart attacks named stress as the cause of their disorder (Cameron, Petrie, Ellis, Buick, & Weinman, 2005), but the relationship is less direct than they imagine. Two lines of research relate stress to CVD: studies that evaluate stress as a precipitating factor in heart attack or stroke and studies that investigate stress as a cause in the development of CVD.

Evidence for the role of stress as a precipitating factor for heart attack or stroke in people with CVD is clear; stress increases the risks. Stress can serve as a trigger for heart attacks for people with coronary heart disease (Kop, 2003; Sheps, 2007). A large cross-cultural study called the INTERHEART Study compared more than 15,000 people who had experienced a heart attack with almost as many who had not, attempting to identify significant risk factors that held across cultures and continents (Yusuf et al., 2004). This study identified a set of psychological stressors that showed a significant relationship to heart attack, including workplace and home stress, financial problems, major life events in the past year, depression, and external locus of control (Rosengren et al., 2004). These stress factors related to heart attack and made a substantial contribution to the risk within each population. The individuals who experienced heart attacks may have had long-standing CVD, but stress may also contribute to the development of this disease. However, even positive stress may create a risk for cardiovascular problems (see Would You Believe ...? box).

The role of stress in the development of heart disease is indirect but may occur through several routes, including hormone release as a response to stress or as a result of the immune system response (Matthews, 2005). For example, job-related stress (Smith, Roman, Dollard, Winefield, & Siegrist, 2005) and other situations with high demands and low control (Kamarck, Muldoon, Shiffman, & Sutton-Tyrrell, 2007) are implicated in heart disease. One possible route for this effect is through the action of the immune system, which reacts by releasing cytokines, which promote inflammation. This inflammation is a factor in the development of coronary artery disease (Steptoe, Hamer, & Chida,

Would You BELIEVE...?   Being a Sports Fan May Be a Danger to Your Health

Would you believe that being a sports fan may endanger your health? A week or so before the 2015 Super Bowl, stories appeared in the media suggesting that watching this sports event might present a risk for heart attack. This risk did not stem from the pizza, chips, and beer from Super Bowl parties, but from the emotional stress and excitement of the game.

The warnings were not based on research on the dangers of American football but, rather, on the increase in cardiovascular events during the World Cup Soccer championship held in Germany in 2006 (Wilbert-Lampen et al., 2008). Researchers compared the frequency of cardiac events such as heart attack and cardiac arrhythmia during the month of the World Cup championship with the month before and after the playoffs and found an elevated rate during the playoffs. The incidence of such cardiac events was three times higher for men and almost twice as high for women on days when the German team played compared with days during the comparison period. The risk was greatest during the 2 hours after the beginning of a match, suggesting that fans truly had their "hearts in the game."

As you'd expect, winning or losing matters. Fans of losing teams have the greater chances of being admitted to a hospital for cardiovascular problems, compared to fans of winning teams. But watching your team win a game doesn't get you off the hook: The thrill of cheering on a victory also increases chances of cardiovascular problems (Olsen, Elliott, Frampton, & Bradley, 2015). Some evidence suggests that this heightened risk is attributable to stress-induced inflammatory responses (Wilbert-Lampen et al., 2010), and the risk is greatest for people who already have cardiovascular problems. So, before sitting down to watch the next big championship game, you may want to consult with your doctor first.

2007). The action of stress hormones such as the corticoids also affects the development of diseased arteries, exacerbating artery damage and making the development of arterial plaque more likely. These stress-related responses apply to any source of stress, forming an indirect route to heart disease.

Hypertension   Although high blood pressure would seem to be the result of stress, no simple relationship exists between stress and blood pressure. Situational factors such as noise can elevate blood pressure, but most studies show that blood pressure returns to normal when the situational stimulus is removed. However, a longitudinal study of blood pressure (Stewart, Janicki, & Kamarck, 2006) showed that the time to return to normal blood pressure after a psychological stressor predicted hypertension over 3 years. This response is similar to reactivity.

Reactivity   The idea that some people react more strongly to stress than others is another possibility for the link between stress and CVD. This response, called *reactivity*, may play a role in the development of CVD if the response is relatively stable within an individual and prompted by events that occur frequently in the individual's life. Many life events can prompt stress responses that include cardiac reactions.

One study showed that reactivity relates to incidence of stroke (Everson et al., 2001). Men with higher systolic blood pressure reactivity were at greater risk for stroke than men with less blood pressure reactivity. The higher rate of CVD for African Americans than for European Americans leads researchers to examine differences in reactivity between these two ethnic groups, as well as the stressors that prompt such reaction. Many African Americans experience a continuous struggle to cope with a variety of stressors that relate to their ethnicity, and this struggle constitutes the type of long-term stressor that poses health threats (Bennett et al., 2004). Beginning during childhood and continuing into adolescence, African Americans show greater reactivity than European Americans (Murphy, Stoney, Alpert, & Walker, 1995); these differences appeared among children as young as 6 (Treiber et al., 1993). In addition, African American children with a family history of CVD showed significantly greater reactivity than any other group of children in the study.

Research on the experience of discrimination shows that racist provocations produce reactivity. A study comparing the reactions of African American and European American women (Lepore et al., 2006) showed that African American women who evaluated a stressful situation as racist showed stronger cardiac

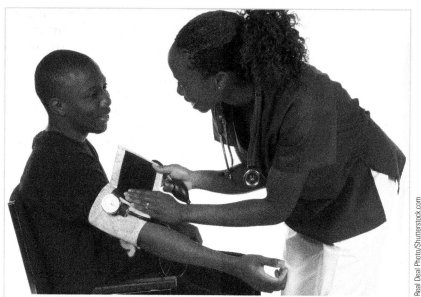

Beginning during childhood, African Americans show higher cardiac reactivity than other ethnic groups, which may relate to their higher levels of cardiovascular disease.

reactions than women who did not identify the stress as racist. Both European American and African American men who viewed a racist film clip experienced a greater increase in blood pressure than they did while viewing emotionally neutral films (Fang & Myers, 2001). Differences exist in reactivity for African Americans and Caribbean Americans, with both showing higher reactivity than European Americans (Arthur, Katkin, & Mezzacappa, 2004). However, Asian Americans showed lower reactivity than European Americans to a laboratory stressor (Shen, Stroud, & Niaura, 2004). This result is consistent with a lower rate of CVD among Asian Americans.

Ulcers   At one time, stress was widely accepted as the cause of ulcers, but during the 1980s, two Australian researchers, Barry Marshall and J. Robin Warren, proposed that ulcers were the result of a bacterial infection rather than stress (Okuda & Nakazawa, 2004). At the time, their hypothesis seemed unlikely because most physiologists and physicians believed that bacteria could not live in the stomach environment with its extreme acidity. Marshall had trouble obtaining funding to research the possibility of a bacterial basis for ulcers.

With no funding for his research and the belief that he was correct, Marshall took matters into his own hands: He infected himself with the bacterium to demonstrate its gastric effects. He developed severe gastritis and took antibiotics to cure himself, providing further evidence that this bacterium has gastric effects. A clinical trial later supported Marshall's hypothesis: Stomach ulcers were less likely to return in patients who received antibiotics compared with patients who received an acid suppressant (Alper, 1993). These findings demonstrated the role that bacterial infection plays in ulcer development. However, the psychological component has not disappeared from explanations for the development and reoccurrence of ulcers because *H. pylori* infection does not seem to account for all ulcers (Levenstein, 2000; Watanabe et al., 2002). This infection is very common and related to a variety of gastric problems, yet most infected people do not develop ulcers (Weiner & Shapiro, 2001). Thus, *H. pylori* infection may create a vulnerability to ulcers, which stress or other psychosocial conditions then precipitate. For example, smoking, heavy drinking, caffeine consumption, and use of nonsteroidal anti-inflammatory drugs all relate to ulcer formation. Stress may be a factor in any of these behaviors, providing an indirect link between stress and ulcer formation in infected individuals. In addition, the hormones and altered immune function associated with the experience of chronic stress may be a more direct link. Therefore, behavioral factors play a role in the development of ulcers, but so does *H. pylori* infection, creating a complex interaction of factors in the formation of ulcers.

Other Physical Disorders   Besides headache, infectious disease, CVD, and ulcers, stress is linked to several other physical disorders, including diabetes, premature delivery for pregnant women, asthma, and rheumatoid arthritis.

Diabetes mellitus is a chronic disease that is also related to stress. Two kinds of diabetes mellitus are Type 1, or insulin-dependent, and Type 2, or non-insulin-dependent. Type 1 diabetes usually begins in childhood and requires insulin injections for its control. Type 2 diabetes usually appears during adulthood and can most often be controlled by dietary changes. (The lifestyle adjustments and behavioral management required by diabetes mellitus are discussed in Chapter 11.)

Stress may contribute to the *development* of both types of diabetes. First, stress may contribute directly to the development of insulin-dependent diabetes through the disruption of the immune system, possibly during infancy (Sepa, Wahlberg, Vaarala, Frodi, & Ludvigsson, 2005). Immune system measures at age 1 year indicated that those infants who had experienced higher family stress showed more indications of antibodies consistent with diabetes. Second, a recent epidemiological study of over 55,000 Japanese adults showed that greater perceived stress increased the risk of developing Type 2 diabetes at a 10-year follow-up (Kato, Noda, Inoue, Kadowaki, & Tsugane, 2009). Stress may contribute to the development of Type 2 through its effect on cytokines that initiate an inflammatory process that affects insulin metabolism and produces insulin resistance (Black, 2003; Tsiotra & Tsigos, 2006). Third, stress may contribute to Type 2 through its possible effects on obesity. Research on stress and Type 2 diabetics shows that stress can be a triggering factor and thus play a role in the age at which people develop Type 2 diabetes.

In addition, stress may affect the *management* of diabetes mellitus through its direct effects on blood glucose (Riazi, Pickup, & Bradley, 2004) and through the indirect route of hindering people's adherence with controlling glucose levels (Farrell, Hains, Davies, Smith, & Parton, 2004). Indeed, adherence, discussed in Chapter 4, is a major problem for this disorder.

Stress during pregnancy is the topic of research for both human and nonhuman subjects (Kofman, 2002). Research with nonhuman subjects conclusively demonstrates that stressful environments relate to lower birth weight and developmental delays, and that infants of stressed mothers show higher reactivity to stress. Research with human participants cannot experimentally manipulate such stressors, so the results are not as conclusive, but studies on stress during pregnancy reveal a tendency for stress to make preterm deliveries more likely and to result in babies with lower birth weights (Dunkel-Schetter, 2011). Both factors contribute to a number of problems for the infants. The importance of type and timing of stress remains unclear, but there is some indication that chronic stress may be more damaging than acute stress and that stress late in pregnancy is riskier than earlier stress.

Asthma is a respiratory disorder characterized by difficulty in breathing due to reversible airway obstruction, airway inflammation, and increase in airway responsiveness to a variety of stimuli (Cohn, Elias, & Chupp, 2004). The prevalence and mortality rate of asthma is increasing for both European American and African American women, men, and children, but asthma disproportionately affects poor African Americans living in urban environments (Gold & Wright, 2005).

Because inflammation is an essential part of asthma, researchers hypothesize that the proinflammatory cytokines play a fundamental (possibly a causal) role in the development of this disease (Wills-Karp, 2004). The link between stress and the immune system presents the possibility that stress plays a role in the development of this disorder, but stress is also involved in asthma attacks (Chen & Miller, 2007).

Physical stimuli such as smoke can trigger an attack, but stressors, such as emotional events and pain, can also stimulate an asthma attack (Gustafson, Meadows-Oliver, & Banasiak, 2008). Both acute and chronic stress increase the risk of asthma attacks in children with asthma; a population-based study in South Korea (Oh, Kim, Yoo, Kim, & Kim, 2004) found that people who reported more stress were more likely to experience more severe problems with their asthma. Children living in inner-city neighborhoods with parents who have mental problems are at sharply heightened risk (Weil et al., 1999). Even in a laboratory setting, the influence of chronic stress on asthma is evident: Children of low socioeconomic status show greater asthma symptoms following an acute stress task than children of high socioeconomic status (Chen, Strunk, Bacharier, Chan, & Miller, 2010). Thus, stress is a significant factor in triggering asthma attacks.

Rheumatoid arthritis, a chronic inflammatory disease of the joints, may also be related to stress. Although the cause is unknown, rheumatoid arthritis is believed to be an autoimmune disorder in which a person's own immune system attacks itself (Ligier & Sternberg, 2001). The attack produces inflammation and damage to the tissue lining of the joints, resulting in pain and loss of flexibility and mobility. Stress is hypothesized to be a factor in the development of autoimmune diseases through the production of stress hormones and cytokines (Stojanovich & Marisavljevich, 2008).

Stress can make arthritis worse by increasing sensitivity to pain, reducing coping efforts, and possibly affecting the process of inflammation itself. Although it is unclear whether people with rheumatoid arthritis have different cortisol responses to stress than healthy people, there is evidence of greater immune dysregulation among arthritis patients (Davis et al., 2008; de Brouwer et al., 2010). These findings suggest a role for stress in this disease. For example, people with rheumatoid arthritis reported more pain on workdays that were stressful (Fifield et al., 2004). Other factors are important for the development of rheumatoid arthritis, but the stress that results from rheumatoid arthritis brings about negative changes in people's lives and requires extensive coping efforts.

Stress and Psychological Disorders

Stress can put people in a bad mood. For some people, these emotional responses of stress are short lived. For other people, stress may lead to persistent emotional difficulties that can qualify as psychological disorders. Therefore, the study of stress as a factor in psychological disorders parallels other research about stress and disease by adopting the diathesis–stress model. This research concentrates not only on the sources of stress that relate to psychological disorders but also on the factors that create vulnerability.

Mood changes can also lead to changes in immune function. Changes in immune functioning may underlie several psychological disorders (Dantzer, O'Connor, Freund, Johnson, & Kelley, 2008; Harrison, Olver, Norman, & Nathan, 2002). As you will learn, the relationship between stress and psychological disorders may be mediated through processes similar to those involved in other diseases—through the immune system.

Depression There is clear evidence that stress contributes to the development of depressive symptoms. Much of the research that focuses on this relationship attempts to answer two questions. First, what factors

make some people more vulnerable to depression? Second, what physical mechanisms translate stress into depression? A large body of research attempts to identify the factors that make some people particularly vulnerable to depression.

Ineffective coping may be one source of vulnerability to depression. People who can cope effectively are able to avoid depression, even with many stressful events in their lives. As you will recall from Chapter 5, Richard Lazarus and his colleagues (Kanner et al., 1981; Lazarus & DeLongis, 1983; Lazarus & Folkman, 1984) regarded stress as the combination of an environmental stimulus with the person's appraisal, vulnerability, and perceived coping strength. According to this theory, people become ill not only because they have had too many stressful experiences but also because they evaluate these experiences as threatening or damaging, because they are physically or socially vulnerable at the time, or because they lack the ability to cope with the stressful event.

Another proposal for vulnerability to depression is the "kindling" hypothesis (Monroe & Harkness, 2005). This view holds that major life stress provides a "kindling" experience that may prompt the development of depression. This experience then sensitizes people to depression, and future experiences of stress need not be major to prompt recurrences of depression (Stroud, Davila, Hammen, & Vrshek-Schallhorn, 2011). A meta-analysis of studies on this topic (Stroud, Davila, & Moyer, 2008) showed some support, especially for the hypothesis of stress predicting first episodes of depression.

A negative outlook or the tendency to dwell on problems may exacerbate stress, making people more likely to think in ways that increase depression (Ciesla & Roberts, 2007; Gonzalez, Nolen-Hoeksema, & Treynor, 2003). Rumination—the tendency to dwell on negative thoughts—is one factor implicated in depression. For example, a longitudinal study of Japanese university students (Ito, Takenaka, Tomita, & Agari, 2006) demonstrated that rumination predicted depression. Thus, the tendency to dwell on negative thoughts is one type of vulnerability for depression. Consistent with the diathesis–stress view, more positive ways of thinking or less stress would result in lower risk for depression.

Genetic vulnerability is another type of risk factor for depression. In a longitudinal study of Swedish twins (Kendler, Gatz, Gardner, & Pedersen, 2007), stress was a significant factor in depression, but only under some circumstances. Stress was more likely to predict earlier

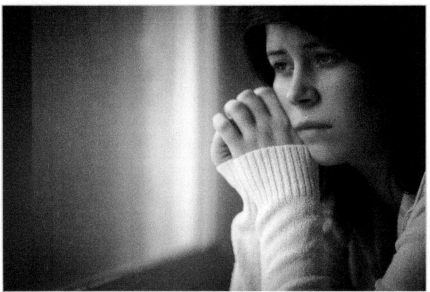

Stress can make people more vulnerable to depression.

compared with later episodes of depression, consistent with the kindling hypothesis. Importantly, stress was also more likely to predict depression for people with low rather than high genetic risk. Another longitudinal study (Caspi et al., 2003) demonstrated the interaction between genes and environment in the development of depression. Individuals who inherited a particular version of a gene pair that is involved with the neurotransmitter serotonin developed depression and suicidal thoughts significantly more frequently than did individuals with a different version of this gene pair, but only when the vulnerable individuals experienced stressful life events. These studies suggest that genes furnish the basis for a vulnerability that interacts with stressful life events to precipitate depression.

Some types of stressful situations produce greater risks for depression than other events. For example, chronic workplace stress is linked to the development of depression, especially for people with low decision-making authority (Blackmore et al., 2007), as is living in a neighborhood where crime and drug use are common (Cutrona et al., 2005). Illness is another type of stress that shows a relationship to depression. Experiencing health problems produces stress both for the sick person and for caregivers. Heart disease (Guck, Kavan, Elsasser, & Barone, 2001), cancer (Spiegel & Giese-Davis, 2003), AIDS (Cruess et al., 2003), and Alzheimer's disease (Dorenlot, Harboun, Bige, Henrard, & Ankri, 2005) are all tied to increased incidence of depression. The relationship between stress and this variety of diseases occurs through the immune system.

Depression that meets the diagnostic criteria for clinical depression (American Psychiatric Association, 2013) is also associated with immune function, with stronger relationships found among older and hospitalized patients. In addition, the more severe the depression, the greater the alteration of immune function. A meta-analysis of depression and immune function (Zorrilla et al., 2001) indicated that depression related to many facets of immune system function, including reduced T-cells and decreased activity of natural killer cells. This link between depression and reduced immune functioning is apparent among women receiving treatment for breast cancer, for whom a healthy immune system is critical in defending against infection (Sephton et al., 2009).

This link between depression and reduced immune functioning may develop when prolonged stress disrupts regulation of the immune system through the action of proinflammatory cytokines (Robles, Glaser, & Kiecolt-Glaser, 2005). The release of proinflammatory cytokines by the immune system (Anisman, Merali, Poulter, & Hayley, 2005; Dantzer et al., 2008) sends a signal to the nervous system, which may generate fatigue, feelings of listlessness, and a loss of feelings of pleasure. Cytokine production increases when people are depressed, and people undergoing treatments that increase the production of certain cytokines also experience symptoms of depression. Thus, several lines of evidence support the role of cytokines in depression. Indeed, the brain may even interpret cytokines as stressors (Anisman et al., 2005), which interact with environmental stressors to increase risk for depression.

Anxiety Disorders   Anxiety disorders include a variety of fears and phobias, often leading to avoidance behaviors. Included in this category are conditions such as panic attacks, **agoraphobia**, generalized anxiety, obsessive-compulsive disorders, and posttraumatic stress disorder (American Psychiatric Association, 2013). This section looks at stress as a possible contributor to anxiety states.

One anxiety disorder that, by definition, is related to stress is **posttraumatic stress disorder (PTSD)**. The *Diagnostic and Statistical Manual of Mental Disorders* (5th ed.; American Psychiatric Association, 2013) defines PTSD as "the development of characteristic symptoms following exposure to one or more traumatic events" (p. 274). PTSD can also stem from experiencing threats to one's physical integrity; witnessing another person's serious injury, death, or threatened physical integrity; and learning about death of or injury to family members or friends. The traumatic events often include military combat, but sexual assault, physical attack, robbery, mugging, and other personal violent assaults can also trigger PTSD.

Symptoms of PTSD include recurrent and intrusive memories of the traumatic event, recurrent distressing dreams that replay the event, and extreme psychological and physiological distress. Events that resemble or symbolize the original traumatic event, as well as anniversaries of that event, may also trigger symptoms. People with PTSD attempt to avoid thoughts, feelings, or conversations about the event and to avoid any person or place that might trigger acute distress. Lifetime prevalence of PTSD in the general population of the United States is around 7% (Kessler et al., 2005).

However, most people who experience traumatic events do not develop PTSD (McNally, 2003), and researchers have sought to identify the risk factors for PTSD. Initially, PTSD was viewed primarily as a response to combat stress. Now, many types of experiences are considered potential risks for PTSD. People who are the victims of crime (Scarpa, Haden, & Hurley, 2006), terrorist attacks (Gabriel et al., 2007), domestic violence or sexual abuse (Pimlott-Kubiak & Cortina,

2003), and natural disasters (Dewaraja & Kawamura, 2006; Norris, Byrne, Diaz, & Kaniasty, 2001) are vulnerable. Personal factors and life circumstances also show a relationship to the development of PTSD (McNally, 2003), such as prior emotional problems, but poor social support and reactions to the traumatic event are more important in predicting who will develop PTSD (Ozer, Best, Lipsey, & Weiss, 2003).

The list of experiences that make people vulnerable to PTSD includes more events experienced by women than by men, and women are more likely to show symptoms of PTSD (Pimlott-Kubiak & Cortina, 2003). Hispanic Americans also seem more vulnerable to PTSD than other ethnic groups (Pole, Best, Metzler, & Marmar, 2005). The disorder is not limited to adults; children and adolescents who are the victims of violence or who observe violence are at increased risk (Griffing et al., 2006). PTSD increases the risk for medical disorders; its effects on the immune system may be the underlying reason. PTSD produces long-lasting suppression of the immune system and an increase in proinflammatory cytokines (Pace & Heim, 2011).

The relationship between stress and other anxiety disorders is less clear, perhaps because of the overlap between anxiety and depression (Suls & Bunde, 2005). Disentangling symptoms of negative affect presents problems for researchers. However, a study conducted in China (Shen et al., 2003) found that people with generalized anxiety disorder reported more stressful life events than did people with no psychological disorder. Furthermore, those with anxiety disorder showed lower levels of some immune system functioning. Thus, stress may play a role in anxiety disorders, and again the route may be through an effect on the immune system.

IN SUMMARY

Much evidence points to a relationship between stress and disease, but the relationship between stressful life events or daily hassles and disease is indirect and complex. The diathesis–stress model is the major framework for understanding the relationship between stress and development of disease. The diathesis–stress model hypothesizes that without some vulnerability, stress does not produce disease; much of the research on stress and various diseases is consistent with this model. Stress plays a role in the development of several physical disorders, including headache and infectious disease. The evidence for a relationship between stress and heart disease is complex. Stress is not directly responsible for hypertension, but some individuals show higher cardiac reactivity to stress, which may contribute to the development of CVD. Experiences of discrimination are also a factor in reactivity. Stress also plays an indirect and minor role in the development of ulcers. Other diseases have a more direct relationship with stress, including diabetes, asthma, and rheumatoid arthritis, as well as some premature deliveries; the influence of stress on the immune system and the involvement of cytokines may underlie all these relationships.

Depression is related to the experience of stressful life events in people who are vulnerable, but not in others. The source of this vulnerability may be genetic, but experiences and attitudes may also contribute to increased vulnerability, especially the experience of abuse or maltreatment during childhood. PTSD, by definition, is related to stress, but most people who experience trauma do not develop this disorder. Thus, vulnerability is also a factor for the effect of stress on the development of anxiety disorders.

 # Becoming Healthier

Stress may erode people's good intentions to maintain a healthy lifestyle. Stress may underlie people's decisions to eat an unhealthy diet, smoke, drink, use drugs, miss sleep, or avoid exercise. According to Dianne Tice and her colleagues (Tice, Bratslavsky, & Baumeister, 2001), distressed people tend to behave more impulsively. These researchers showed that when distressed, people do things oriented toward making them feel better, and some of those things are health threatening, such as eating high-fat and high-sugar snacks. Stress is also the rationalization that some people use to smoke (or not quit), have a few drinks, or use drugs.

Some of these indulgences may make people feel better temporarily, but others are poor choices. Maintaining a healthy lifestyle is a better choice. People feel better when they eat a healthy diet, engage in physical exercise, have positive interactions with friends or family, and get enough sleep. Indeed, these steps may be good for your immune system. Social isolation decreases immune function (Hawkley & Cacioppo, 2003), but social support improves its function (Miyazaki et al., 2003), as does getting enough sleep (Lange, Dimitrov, & Born, 2011). So, when you are feeling a lot of stress, try to withstand the temptation to indulge in unhealthy behaviors. Instead, prepare to treat yourself with healthy indulgences, such as time with friends or family, more (rather than less) sleep, or participation in sports or other physical activity.

Answers

This chapter has addressed three basic questions:

1. **How does the immune system function?**

   The immune system consists of tissues, organs, and processes that protect the body from invasion by foreign material such as bacteria, viruses, and fungi. The immune system marshals both a nonspecific response capable of attacking any invader and a specific response tailored to specific invaders. The immune system can also be a source of problems when it is deficient (as in HIV infection) or when it is too active (as in allergies and autoimmune diseases).

2. **How does the field of psychoneuroimmunology relate behavior to disease?**

   The field of psychoneuroimmunology relates behavior to illness by finding relationships among behavior, the central nervous system, the immune system, and the endocrine system. Psychological factors can depress immune function, and some research has linked these factors with immune system depression and severity of physiological symptoms.

3. Does stress cause disease?

Research indicates that stress and illness are related, but as the diathesis–stress model holds, individuals must have some vulnerability for stress to cause disease. Stress is a moderate risk factor for headache and infectious disease. The role of stress in heart disease is complex; reactivity to stress may be involved in hypertension and the development of cardiovascular disease. Most ulcers can be traced to a bacterial infection rather than stress. The experience of stress is one of the many factors that contributes to psychological and mood disorders, but the route through which stress influences the development of these disorders may also be through the immune system.

Suggested Readings

Cohen, S. (2005). Keynote presentation at the eighth International Congress of Behavioral Medicine. *International Journal of Behavioral Medicine, 12*(3), 123–131. Shelton Cohen summarizes his fascinating research on stress and vulnerability to infectious disease.

Irwin, M. R. (2008). Human psychoneuroimmunology: 20 years of discovery. *Brain, Behavior and Immunity, 22,* 129–139. This recent review of the area of psychoneuroimmunology presents an overview of the immune system and the research on the links among psychosocial factors, immune system response, and the development of disease in humans.

Robles, T. F., Glaser, R., & Kiecolt-Glaser, J. K. (2005). Out of balance: A new look at chronic stress, depression, and immunity. *Current Directions in Psychological Science, 14,* 111–115. This short article looks at chronic stress and hypothesizes its relationship to depression through the immune system.

CHAPTER 7

Understanding and Managing Pain

CHAPTER OUTLINE

QUESTIONS

This chapter focuses on five basic questions:

1. How does the nervous system register pain?
2. What is the meaning of pain?
3. What types of pain present the biggest problems?
4. How can pain be measured?
5. What techniques are effective for pain management?

☑ Check Your **EXPERIENCES** *Regarding Your Most Recent Episode of Pain*

Nearly everybody experiences pain, but people experience pain in many different ways. The following questions allow you to understand the role pain plays in your life. To complete the exercise, think of the most significant pain that you have experienced within the past month, or if you have chronic pain, make your ratings with that pain problem in mind.

1. How long did your pain persist? _____ hours and _____ minutes

2. If this pain is chronic, how often does it occur?
   ☐ Less than once a month
   ☐ Once a month
   ☐ Two or three times a month
   ☐ About once a week
   ☐ Two or three times a week
   ☐ Daily
   ☐ Throughout most of every day

3. What did you do to alleviate your pain? (Check all that apply.)
   ☐ Took a prescription drug
   ☐ Tried to relax
   ☐ Did something to distract myself from the pain
   ☐ Took an over-the-counter drug
   ☐ Tried to ignore the pain

4. Place a mark on the line below to indicate how serious your pain was.

   Not at all   Unbearable

   | 0 | 10 | 20 | 30 | 40 | 50 | 60 | 70 | 80 | 90 | 100 |

5. Place a mark on the line below to indicate how much this pain interfered with your daily routine.

   Not at all   Completely disrupted

   | 0 | 10 | 20 | 30 | 40 | 50 | 60 | 70 | 80 | 90 | 100 |

6. During your pain, what did people around you do? (Check all that apply.)
   ☐ Gave me a lot of sympathy
   ☐ Did my work for me
   ☐ Complained when I could not fulfill my normal responsibilities
   ☐ Ignored me
   ☐ Relieved me of my normal responsibilities

Completing this assessment will show you something about your own pain experience. Some of the items on this assessment are similar to those on some of the standardized pain scales described in "The Measurement of Pain" later in the chapter.

Real-World Profile of **ARON RALSTON**

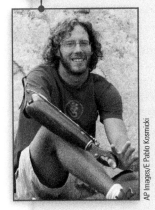

AP Images/E Pablo Kosmicki

"I smiled as I cut off my arm. I was grateful to be free."—Aron Ralston, 27 years old.

In April 2003, Aron Ralston was hiking alone in a remote area of Utah when an 800-pound boulder dislodged and pinned his right arm against a canyon wall. Ralston had not told anybody about his hiking plans, nor did he have a mobile phone with him. With no way to move the boulder, Ralston was stranded. After 5 days of trying to free his arm from the boulder, Ralston reached a grim realization: He could save his life only if he amputated his arm. With no food or water and little chance of rescue, this was his only option for survival.

To amputate his arm, Ralston first used the weight of his body to snap the bones in his forearm. He then used a small, dull pocketknife to cut his flesh, muscles, and tendons. Ralston, an experienced outdoorsman, then used his teeth and his other arm to tighten a tourniquet around the stump to stop the profuse blood loss. After freeing himself from the boulder, Ralston hiked several more hours until he was eventually rescued.

Did Ralston experience pain? Certainly he did. "I wanted to be free. I wanted to be with my family . . . So it was a case of whatever it took. It was going to hurt. I knew that," Ralston said in a later interview. "The pain was irrelevant" (Rollings, 2011).

The complex interplay between the brain and the body is no more apparent than it is in the study of pain. You might think that a life without pain would be wonderful. However, pain plays a necessary and basic role in survival; pain is the body's way of calling attention to injury.

People with the rare genetic disorder called *congenital insensitivity to pain* are not able to feel pain. Because of this condition, these people must be carefully monitored. They often experience serious injuries without any awareness, such as broken bones, bitten tongues, cuts, burns, eye damage, and infections. Many people with this disorder die at a relatively young age, due to health problems that could have been treated if they were only able to heed the warning signs that pain provides.

In other cases, such as with people suffering from chronic pain, pain may exist for no clear reason. In the more extreme cases of phantom limb pain, people experience pain in parts of the body that do not exist! However, for most people, pain is an unpleasant and uncomfortable experience to be avoided whenever possible. Can people's beliefs about pain—such as Aron Ralston's belief that enduring excruciating pain was his only hope for survival—influence their experience of pain? In this chapter, we explore these many mysteries of pain. To understand these mysteries, we must first examine how the nervous system registers pain.

Pain and the Nervous System

All sensory information, including pain, begins with sense receptors on or near the surface of the body. These receptors change physical energy—such as light, sound, heat, and pressure—into neural impulses. We can feel pain through any of our senses, but most of what we think of as pain originates as stimulation to the skin and muscles.

Neural impulses that originate in the skin and muscles are part of the peripheral nervous system (PNS); you will recall from Chapter 5 that all neurons outside the brain and spinal cord (the central nervous system, or CNS) are part of the PNS. Neural impulses that originate in the PNS travel toward the spinal cord and brain. Therefore, it is possible to trace the path of neural impulses from the receptors to the brain. Tracing this path is a way to understand the physiology of pain.

The Somatosensory System

The **somatosensory system** conveys sensory information from the body to the brain. All the PNS neurons from the skin's surface and muscles are part of the somatic nervous system. For example, a neural impulse that originates in the right index finger travels through the somatic nervous system to the spinal cord. The interpretation of this information in the brain results in a person's perception of sensations about his or her body and its movements. The somatosensory system consists of several senses, including touch, light and deep pressure, cold, warmth, tickling, movement, and body position.

Afferent Neurons   Afferent neurons are one of three types of neurons—*afferent, efferent,* and *interneurons.* **Afferent (sensory) neurons** relay information from the sense organs toward the brain. **Efferent (motor) neurons** result in the movement of muscles or the stimulation of organs or glands; **interneurons** connect sensory to motor neurons. The sense organs contain afferent neurons, called **primary afferents**, with specialized receptors that convert physical energy into neural impulses, which travel to the spinal cord and then to the brain, where that information is processed and interpreted.

Involvement in Pain   **Nociception** refers to the stimulation of sensory nerve cells that may lead to the perception of pain. The skin is the largest of the sense organs, and receptors in the skin and organs—called **nociceptors**—are capable of responding to various types of stimulation that may cause tissue damage, such as heat, cold, crushing, cutting, and burning.

Some neurons that convey sensory information (including nociception) are covered with **myelin**, a fatty substance that acts as insulation. Myelinated afferent neurons, called **A fibers**, conduct neural impulses faster than unmyelinated **C fibers** do. In addition, neurons differ in size, and larger ones conduct impulses faster than smaller ones. Two types of A fibers are important in pain perception: the large **A-beta fibers** and the smaller **A-delta fibers**. The large, myelinated A-beta fibers conduct impulses more than 100 times faster than small, unmyelinated C fibers (Melzack, 1973). C fibers are much more common; more than 60% of all sensory afferents are C fibers (Melzack & Wall, 1982). A-beta fibers fire with little stimulation, whereas C fibers require more stimulation to fire. Thus, these different types of fibers respond to different stimulation (Slugg, Meyer, & Campbell, 2000). Stimulation of A-delta fibers produces "fast" pain that is sharp or pricking, whereas stimulation of C fibers often results in a slower developing sensation of burning or dull aching (Chapman, Nakamura, & Flores, 1999).

The Spinal Cord

Protected by the vertebrae, the spinal cord is the avenue through which sensory information travels toward the brain and motor information comes from the brain. The spinal cord also produces the spinal reflexes. Damage to the spinal cord may interrupt the flow of sensory information, motor messages, or both, creating permanent impairment but leaving spinal reflexes intact. However, the most important role of the spinal cord is to provide a pathway for ascending sensory information and descending motor messages.

The afferent fibers group together after leaving the skin and this grouping forms a *nerve.* Nerves may be entirely afferent, entirely efferent, or a mixture of both. Just outside the spinal cord, each nerve bundle divides into two branches (see Figure 7.1). The sensory tracts, which funnel information toward the brain, enter the dorsal (toward the back) side of the spinal cord. The motor tracts, which come from the brain, exit the ventral (toward the stomach) side of the cord. On each side of the spinal cord, the dorsal root swells into a dorsal root ganglion, which contains the cell bodies of the primary afferent neurons. The neuron fibers extend into the **dorsal horns** of the spinal cord.

The dorsal horns contain several layers, or **laminae**. In general, the larger fibers penetrate more deeply into the laminae than the smaller fibers do (Melzack & Wall, 1982). The cells in lamina 1 and especially those in lamina 2 receive information from the small A-delta and C fibers; these two laminae form the **substantia gelatinosa**. In their gate control theory of pain, described later in this chapter, Ronald Melzack and Peter Wall (1965) hypothesized that the substantia gelatinosa modulates sensory input information, and subsequent research shows that they were correct (Chapman et al., 1999). Other laminae also receive projections from A and C fibers, as well as fibers descending from the brain and fibers from other laminae. These connections allow for elaborate interactions between sensory input from the body and the central processing of neural information in the brain.

The Brain

The **thalamus** receives information from afferent neurons in the spinal cord. After making connections in the thalamus, the information travels to other parts of

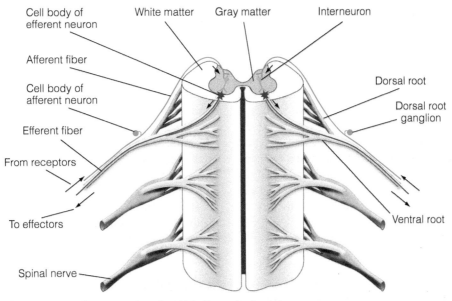

FIGURE 7.1   Cross-section through the spinal cord.

Source: Human physiology: From cells to systems (4th ed.), by L. Sherwood, 2001, p. 164. From SHERWOOD, *Human Physiology*, 4E. © 2001 Cengage Learning.

the brain, including the **somatosensory cortex** in the cerebral cortex. The primary somatosensory cortex receives information from the thalamus that allows the entire surface of the skin to be mapped onto the somatosensory cortex. However, not all areas of the skin are equally represented. Figure 7.2 shows the area of the primary somatosensory cortex allotted to various regions of the body. Areas that are particularly rich in receptors occupy more of the somatosensory cortex than those areas that are poorer in receptors. For example, even though the back has more skin, the hands have more receptors, and therefore more area of the brain is devoted to interpreting the information from receptors in the hand. This abundance of receptors also means that the hands are more sensitive; hands are capable of sensing stimuli that the back cannot.

A person's ability to localize pain on the skin's surface is more precise than it is for internal organs. Internal stimulation can also give rise to sensations, including pain, but the brain does not map the viscera in the same way that it maps the skin, so localizing internal sensation is much less precise. Intense stimulation of internal organs can result in the spread of neural stimulation to the pathways serving skin senses, creating the perception of visceral pain as originating on the skin's surface. This type of pain is called **referred pain**, when pain is experienced in a part of the body other than the

site where the pain stimulus originates. For example, a person who feels pain in the upper arm may not associate this sensation with the heart, even though a heart attack can cause this kind of pain.

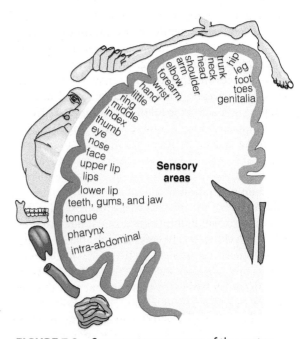

FIGURE 7.2   Somatosensory areas of the cortex.

The development of positron emission tomography (PET) and functional magnetic resonance imaging (fMRI) allows researchers to study what happens in the brain when people experience pain. These techniques confirm that brain activity occurs when nociceptors are activated, but they paint a complex picture of how pain activates the brain (Apkarian, Bushnell, Treede, & Zubieta, 2005). Studies of brain responses to specific pain stimuli show activation in not only many areas of the brain, including the primary and secondary somatosensory cortices, but also the anterior cingulate cortex, the thalamus, and even the cerebellum in the lower part of the brain (Buffington, Hanlon, & McKeown, 2005; Davis, 2000). Adding to the complexity, an emotional reaction usually accompanies the experience of pain, and brain imaging studies indicate activation in areas of the brain associated with emotion when people experience pain (Eisenberger, Gable, & Lieberman, 2007; see Would You Believe . . .? box). Thus, brain imaging studies using PET and fMRI do not reveal a "pain center" in the brain. Rather, these studies show that the experience of pain produces a variety of activation in the brain, ranging from the lower brain to several centers in the forebrain.

Neurotransmitters and Pain

Neurotransmitters are chemicals that are synthesized and stored in neurons. The electrical action potential

Would You BELIEVE...? Emotional and Physical Pain Are Mainly the Same in the Brain

Social rejection is painful. People use phrases such as "emotionally scarred," "slap in the face," "deeply hurt," or "crushed" to describe experiences of social rejection (MacDonald & Leary, 2005). This is as true for English speakers as it is for native speakers of German, Hebrew, Armenian, Cantonese, and Inuktitut.

It may not be a coincidence that people think about social pain in a similar manner to physical pain. Using functional magnetic resonance imaging, Naomi Eisenberger and her colleagues (Eisenberger & Lieberman, 2004; Eisenberger, Lieberman, & Williams, 2003) examined the brain activity of people whose feelings were "hurt" and found that the human brain reacts in similar ways to emotional and physical pain. The participants in this study experienced a virtual-reality, ball-tossing game called "Cyberball" while an fMRI scanner imaged their brains. During the game, the researchers excluded the participants from continuing the game by what participants believed were decisions of two other players.

This exclusion represented social rejection, the type of situation in which people's feelings get hurt.

Eisenberger and her colleagues (2003) found that both the anterior cingulate cortex and the right ventral prefrontal cortex became more active during the experience of social exclusion. Importantly, these two regions of the brain also become more active when people experience *physical* pain. Furthermore, the level of activation in the anterior cingulate cortex correlated with the participants' ratings of distress. A subsequent study showed that social rejection triggers the release of endogenous opioid painkillers in the brain, just as experiences of physical pain do (Hsu et al., 2013). Thus, the experience of social exclusion affects brain activity in a way that is quite similar to the experience of physical pain, suggesting that the two types of pain are similar in the brain.

If social and physical pain lead to similar patterns of brain activation, could a pill that relieves physical pain also relieve social pain?

Acetaminophen—known by the brand name Tylenol—is a pain reliever that acts on the central nervous system. Nathan DeWall and colleagues (DeWall et al., 2010) examined whether acetaminophen would reduce people's reports of social pain. These researchers randomly assigned young adults to take either acetaminophen or a placebo pill daily for 3 weeks. Participants who took the acetaminophen pill reported less social pain over those 3 weeks—such as feeling hurt by being teased—than participants who took the placebo pill! In a follow-up fMRI study, these researchers additionally showed that participants who took acetaminophen prior to being socially excluded during a game of "Cyberball" showed less activity in the anterior cingulate cortex than participants who took a placebo pill.

Thus, there may be many similarities between social pain and physical pain. Will your doctor soon be prescribing two Tylenol as a remedy for both headache *and* heartache?

causes the release of neurotransmitters from neurons, which carries neural impulses across the synaptic cleft, the space between neurons. After flowing across the synaptic cleft, neurotransmitters act on other neurons by occupying specialized receptor sites. Each fits a specialized receptor site in the same way that a key fits into a lock; without the proper fit, the neurotransmitter will not affect the neuron. Sufficient amounts of neurotransmitters prompt the formation of an action potential in the stimulated neuron. Many different neurotransmitters exist, and each one is capable of causing an action.

In the 1970s, researchers (Pert & Snyder, 1973; Snyder, 1977) demonstrated that the neurochemistry of the brain plays a role in the perception of pain. This realization came about through an examination of how drugs affect the brain to alter pain perception. Receptors in the brain are sensitive to opiate drugs, which are painkillers such as morphine and codeine that are derived from opium in the poppy plant. This discovery explained how opiates reduce pain—these drugs fit into brain receptors, modulate neuron activity, and alter pain perception.

The discovery of opiate receptors in the brain raised another question: Why does the brain respond to the resin of the opium poppy? In general, the brain is selective about the types of molecules that it allows to enter; only substances similar to naturally occurring neurochemicals can enter the brain. This reasoning led to the search for and identification of naturally occurring chemicals in the brain that affect pain perception. These neurochemicals have properties similar to those of the opiate drugs (Goldstein, 1976; Hughes, 1975). This discovery prompted a flurry of research that identified more opiate-like neurochemicals, including the **endorphins,** the *enkephalins,* and *dynorphin.* These neurochemicals seem to be one of the brain's mechanisms for modulating pain. Stress, suggestion, and electrical stimulation of the brain can all trigger the release of these endorphins (Turk, 2001). Thus, opiate drugs such as morphine may be effective at relieving pain because the brain contains its own system for pain relief, which the opiates stimulate!

Neurochemicals also seem to be involved in producing pain. The neurotransmitters *glutamate* and *substance P,* as well as the chemicals *bradykinin* and *prostaglandins,* sensitize or excite the neurons that relay pain messages (Sherwood, 2001). Glutamate and substance P act in the spinal cord to increase neural firings related to pain. Bradykinin and prostaglandins are substances released by tissue damage; they prolong the experience of pain by continuing to stimulate the nociceptors.

In addition, proteins produced by the immune system, *proinflammatory cytokines,* also influence pain (Watkins et al., 2007; Watkins & Maier, 2003, 2005). Infection and inflammation prompt the immune system to release these cytokines, which signal the nervous system and produce a range of responses associated with sickness, including decreased activity, increased fatigue, and increased pain sensitivity. Indeed, these cytokines may intensify chronic pain, by sensitizing the structures in the dorsal horn of the spinal cord that modulate the sensory message from the primary afferents (Watkins et al., 2007). Thus, the action of neurotransmitters and other chemicals produced by the body is complex, with the potential to both increase and decrease the experience of pain.

The Modulation of Pain

The **periaqueductal gray,** a structure near the center of the midbrain, is involved in modulating pain. When it is stimulated, neural activity spreads downward to the spinal cord, and pain relief occurs (Goffaux, Redmond, Rainville, & Marchand, 2007; Sherwood, 2001). Neurons in the periaqueductal gray run down into the reticular formation and the **medulla,** a structure in the lower part of the brain that is also involved in pain perception (Fairhurst, Weich, Dunckley, & Tracey, 2007). These neurons descend into the spinal cord and make connections with neurons in the substantia gelatinosa. The result is that the dorsal horn neurons cannot carry pain information to the thalamus.

The inhibition of transmission also involves some familiar neurotransmitters. Endorphins in the periaqueductal gray initiate activity in this descending inhibitory system. Figure 7.3 illustrates this type of modulation. The substantia gelatinosa contains synapses that use enkephalin as a transmitter. Indeed, neurons that contain enkephalin seem to be concentrated in the same parts of the brain that contain substance P, the transmitter that activates pain messages (McLean, Skirboll, & Pert, 1985).

These elaborate physical and chemical systems are the body's way of modulating the neural impulses of pain. The value of pain is obvious. Pain after injury is adaptive, furnishing a reminder of injury and discouraging activity that adds to the damage. In some situations, however, pain modulation is also adaptive. When people or other animals are fighting or fleeing, the ability to ignore pain can be an advantage. Thus, the nervous system has complex systems that allow not only for the perception but also for the modulation of pain.

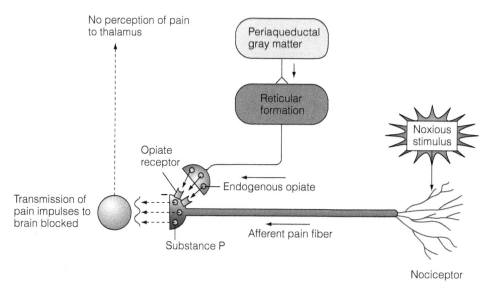

FIGURE 7.3   Descending pathways from the periaqueductal gray prompt the release of endogenous opiates (endorphins) that block the transmission of pain impulses to the brain.

Source: Human physiology: From cells to systems (4th ed.), by L. Sherwood, 2001, p. 181. From SHERWOOD, *Human Physiology*, 4E. © 2001 Cengage Learning.

IN SUMMARY

The activation of receptors in the skin results in neural impulses that move along afferent pathways to the spinal cord by way of the dorsal root. In the spinal cord, the afferent impulses continue to the thalamus in the brain. The primary somatosensory cortex includes a map of the skin, with more of the cortex devoted to areas of the body richer in skin receptors. The A-delta and C fibers are involved in pain, with A-delta fibers relaying pain messages quickly and C fibers sending pain messages more slowly.

The brain and spinal cord also contain mechanisms for modulating sensory input and thereby affecting the perception of pain. One mechanism is through the naturally occurring neurochemicals that relieve pain and mimic the action of opiate drugs, which exist in many places in the central and peripheral nervous systems. The second mechanism is a system of descending control through the periaqueductal gray and the medulla. This system affects the activity of the spinal cord and provides a descending modulation of activity in the spinal cord.

The Meaning of Pain

Until about 100 years ago, people thought that pain was a direct consequence of physical injury, and the extent of tissue damage determined the intensity of pain. Near the end of the 19th century, C. A. Strong changed this very simplistic view. Strong (1895) hypothesized that pain was due to two factors: the sensation and the person's reaction to that sensation. In this view, psychological factors and physical causes were of equal importance. This attention to psychological factors signaled the beginning of a new definition, an altered view of the experience, and new theories of pain.

Definition of Pain

Pain is an almost universal experience. Only those rare people with congenital insensitivity to pain escape the experience of pain. Nevertheless, pain is remarkably difficult to define. Some experts (Covington, 2000) concentrate on the physiology that underlies the perception of pain, whereas others (Wall, 2000) emphasize the subjective nature of pain. These different views reflect the multidimensional nature of pain, which the International Association for the Study of Pain (IASP) has incorporated into its definition. The IASP

Subcommittee on Taxonomy (1979, p. 250) defined pain as "an unpleasant sensory and emotional experience associated with actual or potential tissue damage, or described in terms of such damage." Most pain researchers and clinicians continue to agree with this definition.

Another way to understand the meaning of pain is to view it in terms of three stages: acute, chronic, and prechronic (Keefe, 1982). **Acute pain** is the type of pain that most people experience when injured; it includes pains from cuts, burns, childbirth, surgery, dental work, and other injuries. Its duration is normally brief. This type of pain is ordinarily adaptive; it signals the person to avoid further injury. In contrast, **chronic pain** endures over months or even years. This type of pain may be due to a chronic condition such as rheumatoid arthritis, or it may be the result of an injury that persists beyond the time of healing (Turk & Melzack, 2001). Chronic pain frequently exists in the absence of any identifiable tissue damage. It is not adaptive but, rather, can be debilitating and demoralizing and often leads to feelings of helplessness and hopelessness. Chronic pain never has a biological benefit.

Perhaps the most crucial stage of pain is the **prechronic pain** stage, which comes between the acute and the chronic stages. This period is critical because the person either overcomes the pain at this time or develops the feelings of fear and helplessness that can lead to chronic pain. These three stages do not exhaust all possibilities of pain. Several other types of pain exist, the most common of which is **chronic recurrent pain**, or pain marked by alternating episodes of intense pain and no pain. A common example of chronic recurrent pain is headache pain.

The Experience of Pain

The experience of pain is individual and subjective, but situational and cultural factors influence that experience. Henry Beecher, an anesthesiologist, was one of the first researchers to identify the situational influences on the experience of pain. Beecher (1946) observed soldiers wounded at the Anzio beachhead during World War II. Beecher noted that, despite their serious battle injuries, many of these men reported very little pain. What made the experience of pain different in this situation? These men had been removed from the battlefront and thus from the threat of death or further injury, in the same way that Ralston's amputation of his own arm led to his rescue. Under these conditions, the wounded soldiers were in a cheerful, optimistic state of mind. In contrast, civilian patients with comparable injuries experienced much more pain and requested more pain-killing drugs than the soldiers (Beecher, 1956). These findings prompted Beecher (1956) to conclude that "the intensity of suffering is largely determined by what the pain means to the patient" (p. 1609) and that "the extent of wound bears only a slight relationship, if any (often none at all), to the pain experienced" (p. 1612). Finally, Beecher (1957) described pain as a two-dimensional experience consisting of both a sensory stimulus and an emotional component. Other pain researchers came to accept Beecher's view of pain as *both* a psychological and physical phenomenon.

Battle wounds are an extreme example of sudden injury, but people who experience injuries that are more mundane also report variable amounts of pain. For example, most—but not all—people admitted to an emergency room for treatment of injury report pain (Wall, 2000). Pain is more common among people with injuries such as broken bones, sprains, and stabs than among people with injuries to the skin. Indeed, 53% of those with cuts, burns, or scrapes report that they feel no pain for at least some time after their injury, whereas only 28% of those with deep tissue injury fail to feel immediate pain. These individual variations of pain contrast with people who have been tortured, all of whom feel pain, even though their injuries may not be as serious as those of people reporting to an emergency room. People who believe that a stimulus will be harmful experience more pain than those who have different beliefs about the situation (Arntz & Claassens, 2004; Harvie et al., 2015). The threat, intent to inflict pain, and lack of control give torture a very different meaning from unintentional injury and thus produce a different pain experience. These variations in pain perception suggest either individual differences, a cultural component for variations in pain-related behaviors, or some combination of these factors.

Individual Differences in the Experience of Pain

Individual factors and personal experience make a difference in the experience of pain. People learn to associate stimuli related to a painful experience with the pain and thus develop classically conditioned responses to the associated stimuli (Sanders, 2006). For example, many people dislike the smell of hospitals or become anxious when they hear the dentist's drill because they have had experiences associating these stimuli with pain.

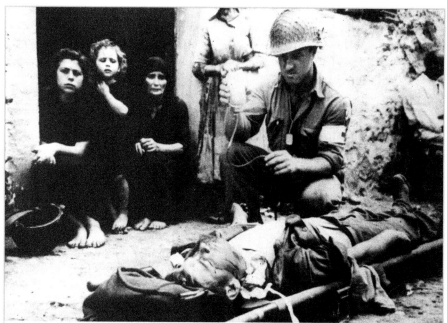

The experience of pain varies with the situation. Wounded soldiers removed from the front lines may feel little pain despite extreme injuries.

Popperfoto/Getty Images

Operant conditioning may also play an important role in pain by providing a means for acute pain to develop into chronic pain. Pioneering pain researcher John J. Bonica (1990) believed that being rewarded for pain behaviors is a key factor that transforms acute pain into chronic pain. According to Bonica, people who receive attention, sympathy, relief from normal responsibilities, and disability compensation for their injuries and pain behaviors are more likely to develop chronic pain than are people who have similar injury but receive fewer rewards. Consistent with Bonica's hypotheses, headache patients report more pain behaviors and greater pain intensity when their spouses or significant others respond to pain complaints with seemingly helpful responses, such as taking over chores, turning on the television, or encouraging the patient to rest (Pence, Thorn, Jensen, & Romano, 2008).

Despite people's belief in a "pain-resistant" personality, no such thing exists. Some people such as Ralston endure pain with little or no complaint, but nevertheless, they perceive discomfort. They display no sign of their pain because of situational factors, cultural sanctions against the display of emotion, or some combination of these two factors. For example, some Native American, African, and South Pacific island cultures have initiation rituals that involve the silent endurance of pain. These rituals may include body piercing, cutting, tattooing, burning, or beating. To show signs of pain would result in failure, so individuals are motivated to hide their pain. Individuals may withstand these injuries with no visible sign of distress yet react with an obvious display of pain behavior to an unintentional injury in a situation outside the ritual (Wall, 2000). These variations in expressions of pain suggest cultural variations in pain behaviors rather than the existence of a pain-resistant personality.

If a pain-resistant personality does not exist, could there be evidence for a *pain-prone* personality? Research does not support the concept of a pain-prone personality either (Turk, 2001). However, people who are anxious, worried, and have a negative outlook tend to experience heightened sensitivity to pain (Janssen, 2002). Fear may be part of this negative outlook; individuals who experience a heightened fear of pain also experience more pain (Leeuw et al., 2007). In addition, people with severe chronic pain are much more likely than others to suffer from some type of psychopathology, such as anxiety disorders or depression (McWilliams, Goodwin, & Cox, 2004; Williams, Jacka, Pasco, Dodd, & Berk, 2006). However, the direction of the cause and effect is not always clear (Gatchel & Epker, 1999). Patients suffering from chronic pain are more likely to be depressed, to abuse alcohol and other drugs, and to suffer from personality disorders. Some chronic pain patients develop these disorders as a result of their chronic pain, but others have some form of psychopathology prior to the beginning of their pain. Thus, individual differences exist in the experience of pain, but cultural and situational factors are more important.

Cultural Variations in Pain Perception   Large culture differences exist in pain sensitivity and the expression of pain behaviors. In addition, cultural background and social context affect the experience (Cleland, Palmer, & Venzke, 2005) and treatment (Cintron & Morrison, 2006) of pain. These differences come from varying meanings that different cultures attach to pain and from stereotypes associated with various cultural groups.

Cultural expectations for pain are apparent in the pain that women experience during childbirth (Callister, 2003; Streltzer, 1997). Some cultures hold birth as a dangerous and painful process, and women in these cultures reflect these expectations by experiencing great pain. Other cultures expect quiet acceptance during the experience of giving birth, and women in those cultures tend not to show much evidence of pain. When questioned about their apparent lack of pain, however, these women reported that they felt pain but that their culture did not expect women to show pain under these circumstances, so they did not (Wall, 2000).

Since the 1950s, studies have compared pain expression for people from various ethnic backgrounds (Ondeck, 2003; Streltzer, 1997). Some studies have shown differences and others have not, but the studies tend to suffer from the criticism of stereotyping. For example, a stereotype exists of Italians as people who show a lot of emotion. Consistent with this stereotype, studies have found that Italian Americans express more distress and demand more pain medication than "Yankees" (Americans of Anglo-Saxon descent who have lived in the United States for generations), who have a reputation for stoically ignoring pain (Rollman, 1998). These variations in pain behaviors among different cultures may reflect behavioral differences in learning and modeling, differences in sensitivity to pain, or some combination of these factors.

Laboratory studies confirm differences between African Americans and European Americans in sensitivity to painful stimuli. African Americans and Hispanic Americans show higher sensitivity to pain than

European Americans (Rahim-Williams et al., 2007). These sensitivities carry over to clinical pain (Edwards, Fillingim, & Keefe, 2001) and chronic pain (Riley et al., 2002); African Americans report higher levels of both. These differences may be due to racial and ethnic differences in endogenous pain modulation as well as differences in coping strategies (Anderson, Green, & Payne, 2009).

Greater sensitivity to pain is doubly unfortunate for African Americans because physicians are more likely to underestimate their pain (Staton et al., 2007) and to prescribe less analgesia than they do for European Americans as outpatients, in hospitals, and in nursing homes, despite similar complaints about pain (Cintron & Morrison, 2006). Hispanics receive similar treatment—less analgesia in many types of medical settings. This discrimination in treatment is a source of needless pain for patients from these ethnic groups.

Gender Differences in Pain Perception   Another common stereotype about pain perception is that women are more sensitive to pain than men (Robinson et al., 2003), and this belief has some research support. Women report pain more readily than men (Fillingim, King, Ribeiro-Dasilva, Rahim-Williams, & Riley, 2009). Women also experience disabilities and pain-related conditions more often than men (Croft, Blyth, & van der Windt, 2010; Henderson, Gandevia, & Macefield, 2008). However, in laboratory studies in which men and women are exposed to the same pain stimulus, women tend to report lower thresholds for only certain kinds of pain, such as heat, cold, and pressure pain, but not for pain caused by the restriction of blood flow (Racine et al., 2012).

One explanation for these gender differences involves gender roles and socialization. A study of Swedish 9-, 12-, and 15-year-olds (Sundblad, Saartok, & Engström, 2007) showed more frequent reports of pain from girls than boys, and a decrease in pain reports for older boys but an increase among older girls. These changes are consistent with adoption of the male and female gender role; boys may learn to deny pain, whereas girls learn that reporting pain is consistent with their gender role. Consistent with this view, men who identify more highly with the male gender role are less likely than other men and less likely than women to report pain in a laboratory experiment (Pool, Schwegler, Theodore, & Fuchs, 2007).

Another explanation for gender differences posits that women may be more vulnerable than men to developing certain pain conditions. Some chronic pain syndromes occur only or mostly in women, such as chronic fatigue syndrome, endometriosis, and fibromyalgia (Fillingim et al., 2009). Sex hormones and gender differences in coping strategies may also contribute to gender differences in sensitivity to musculoskeletal pain (Institute of Medicine, 2011; Picavet, 2010).

However, other research fails to find dramatic differences between men and women. A study on women and men who had dental surgery (Averbuch & Katzper, 2000) reported that more women than men described their pain as severe but found very small differences between pain reports for men and women and no difference in their responses to analgesic drugs. A similar study with adolescents (Logan & Rose, 2004) showed similar results: Girls reported more pain but used no more analgesics than boys. Another study (Kim et al., 2004) found that women reported pain more readily than men in a laboratory situation but showed similar responses to pain associated with oral surgery. One reason why women may report more pain than men could be due to women's higher anxiety and threat related to their experiences of pain, which may be an important factor in gender differences in pain perception (Racine et al., 2012).

Theories of Pain

How people experience pain is the subject of a number of theories. Of the several models of pain, two capture the divergent ways of conceptualizing pain: the specificity theory and the gate control theory.

Specificity Theory   Specificity theory explains pain by hypothesizing that specific pain fibers and pain pathways exist, making the experience of pain virtually equal to the amount of tissue damage or injury (Craig, 2003). The view that pain is the result of transmission of pain signals from the body to a "pain center" in the brain originated with Descartes, who in the 1600s proposed that the body works mechanically (DeLeo, 2006). Descartes hypothesized that the mind works by a different set of principles, and body and mind interact in only a limited way. Descartes's view influenced not only the development of a science of physiology and medicine but also the view that pain is a physical experience largely uninfluenced by psychological factors (Melzack, 1993).

Working under the assumption that pain was the transmission of one type of sensory information, researchers tried to determine which type of receptor conveyed what type of sensory information (Melzack, 1973). For example, they tried to determine which type of receptor relayed information about heat, cold, and other types of pain. The attempt failed, as researchers found that some parts of the body (such as the cornea of the eye) contain only one type of receptor, yet those areas feel a full range of sensations. Specificity does exist in the different types of sensory receptors and nerve fibers, such as light touch, pressure, itching, pricking, warmth, and cold (Craig, 2003). Yet, each of these sensations can become painful when intense, so any simple version of specificity theory is not valid.

The Gate Control Theory   In 1965, Melzack and Wall formulated a new theory of pain, which suggests that pain is *not* the result of a linear process that begins with sensory stimulation of pain pathways and ends with the experience of pain. Rather, pain perception is subject to a number of modulations that can influence the experience of pain. These modulations begin in the spinal cord.

Melzack and Wall hypothesized that structures in the spinal cord act as a gate for the sensory input that the brain interprets as pain. Melzack and Wall's theory is thus known as the **gate control theory** (see Figure 7.4). It has a basis in physiology but explains both sensory and psychological aspects of pain perception.

Melzack and Wall (1965, 1982, 1988) pointed out that the nervous system is never at rest; the patterns of neural activation constantly change. When sensory information from the body reaches the dorsal horns of the spinal cord, that neural impulse enters a system that is already active, much like a car entering a highway from an on-ramp. The existing activity in the spinal cord and brain—like varying levels of traffic on a highway—influences the fate of incoming sensory information, sometimes amplifying and sometimes decreasing the incoming neural signals. The gate control theory hypothesizes that these complex modulations in the spinal cord and in the brain are critical factors in the perception of pain.

According to the gate control theory, neural mechanisms in the spinal cord act like a gate that can either increase (open the gate) or decrease (close the gate) the flow of neural impulses. If there is a lot of activity already occurring on the brain and spinal cord, the gate could close to prevent further traffic. However, if there is little activity in the brain and spinal cord, the gate could open to allow for more traffic. Figure 7.4 shows the results of opening and closing the gate. With the gate open, impulses flow through the spinal cord toward the brain, neural messages reach the brain, and the

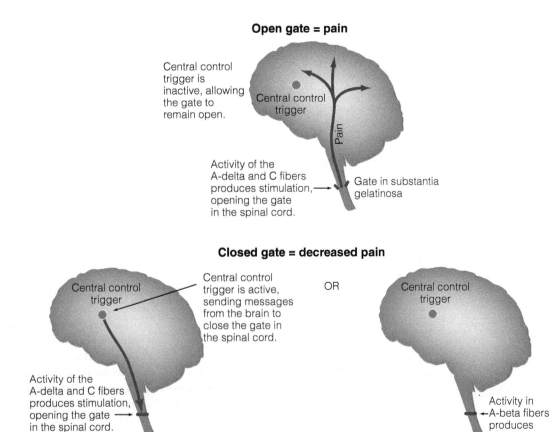

FIGURE 7.4   Gate control theory of pain.

person feels pain. With the gate closed, impulses do not ascend through the spinal cord, messages do not reach the brain, and the person does not feel pain. Moreover, sensory input is subject to modulation, depending on the activity of the large A-beta fibers, the small A-delta fibers, and the small C fibers that enter the spinal cord and synapse in the dorsal horns.

The dorsal horns of the spinal cord are composed of several layers (laminae). As described earlier, two of these laminae make up the substantia gelatinosa, which is the hypothesized location of the gate (Melzack & Wall, 1965). Both the small A-delta and C fibers and the large A-beta fibers travel through the substantia gelatinosa, which also receives projections from other laminae (Melzack & Wall, 1982, 1988). This arrangement of neurons provides the physiological basis for the modulation of incoming sensory impulses.

Melzack and Wall (1982) proposed that activity in the small A-delta and C fibers causes prolonged activity in the spinal cord. This type of activity would promote sensitivity, which increases sensitivity to pain. Activity of these small fibers would thus open the gate. On the other hand, activity of the large A-beta fibers produces an initial burst of activity in the spinal cord, followed by inhibition. Activity of these fibers closes the gate. Subsequent research does not confirm this feature of the gate control theory in a clear way, however (Turk, 2001). Activity of A-delta and C fibers seems to relate to the experience of pain, but under conditions of inflammation, increased activity of A-beta fibers can increase rather than decrease pain.

The gate may be closed by activity in the spinal cord, as well as by messages that descend from the brain. Melzack and Wall (1965, 1982, 1988) proposed the concept of a **central control trigger** consisting of nerve impulses that descend from the brain and influence the gating mechanism. They hypothesized that this system consists of large neurons that conduct impulses rapidly.

These impulses from the brain, which cognitive processes can influence, affect the opening and closing of the gate in the spinal cord. That is, Melzack and Wall proposed that the experience of pain is influenced by beliefs and prior experience, and they also hypothesized a physiological mechanism that can account for such factors in pain perception. As we discussed, the periaqueductal gray matter furnishes descending controls (Mason, 2005), which is consistent with this aspect of the gate control theory.

According to the gate control theory, then, pain has not only sensory components but also motivational and emotional components. This aspect of the theory revolutionized conceptualizations of pain (Melzack, 2008). The gate control theory explains the influence of cognitive aspects of pain and allows for learning and experience to affect the experience of pain. Anxiety, worry, depression, and focusing on an injury can increase pain by affecting the central control trigger, thus opening the gate. Distraction, relaxation, and positive emotions can cause the gate to close, thereby decreasing pain. The gate control theory is not specific about how these experiences affect pain, but recent experimental research confirms that factors such as mood indeed influence the extent of pain-related activity in the CNS. A team of Japanese researchers experimentally induced participants to experience either a sad, neutral, or positive mood. Following the mood induction, all participants experienced moderately painful electric shocks. Participants in a sad mood showed greater activity in brain regions associated with pain than participants in a neutral or positive mood (Yoshino et al., 2010). Thus, a person's emotional state modulated the amount of pain-related activity in the brain.

Many personal experiences with pain are consistent with the gate control theory. When you accidentally hit your finger with a hammer, many of the small fibers are activated, opening the gate. An emotional reaction accompanies your perception of acute pain. You may then grasp your injured finger and rub it. According to the gate control theory, rubbing stimulates the large fibers that close the gate, thus blocking stimulation from the small fibers and decreasing pain.

The gate control theory also explains how injuries can go virtually unnoticed. If sensory input enters into a heavily activated nervous system, then the stimulation may not be perceived as pain. A tennis player may sprain an ankle during a game but not notice the acute pain because of excitement and concentration on the game. After the game is finished, however, the player may notice the pain because the nervous system functions at a different level of activation and the gate opens more easily.

Although it is not universally accepted, the gate control theory is the most influential theory of pain (Sufka & Price, 2002). This theory allows for the complexities of pain experiences. Melzack and Wall proposed the gate control theory before the discovery of the body's own opiates or of the descending control mechanisms through the periaqueductal gray and the medulla, both of which offer supporting evidence. The gate control theory has been and continues to be successful in spurring research and generating interest in the psychological and perceptual factors involved in pain.

More recently, Melzack (1993, 2005) proposed an extension to the gate control theory called the *neuromatrix theory,* which places a stronger emphasis on the brain's role in pain perception. He hypothesized a network of brain neurons that he called the neuromatrix, "a large, widespread network of neurons that consists of loops between the thalamus and cortex as well as between the cortex and limbic system" (Melzack, 2005, p. 86). Normally, the neuromatrix processes incoming sensory information including pain, but the neuromatrix acts even in the absence of sensory input, producing phantom limb sensations (phantom limb sensations are an unusual form of pain that we describe in the next section). Melzack's neuromatrix theory extends gate control theory but maintains that pain perception is part of a complex process affected not only by sensory input but also by activity of the nervous system and by experience and expectation.

IN SUMMARY

Although the extent of damage is important in the pain experience, personal perception is also important. Pain can be acute, prechronic, or chronic, depending on the length of time that the pain has persisted. Acute pain is usually adaptive and lasts for less than 6 months. Chronic pain continues beyond the time of healing, often in the absence of detectable tissue damage. Prechronic pain occurs between acute and chronic pain. All of these stages of pain appear in pain syndromes, such as headache pain, low back pain, arthritic pain, cancer pain, and phantom limb pain.

Several models seek to explain pain, but specificity theory does not capture the complexity of the pain experience. The gate control theory is the most influential model of pain. This theory holds that mechanisms in the spinal cord and the brain can increase or diminish pain. Since its formulation, increased knowledge of the physiology of the brain and spinal cord has supported this theory. The neuromatrix theory extends the gate control theory by hypothesizing the existence of a set of neurons in the brain that maintain a pattern of activity that defines the self and yet also responds to expectations and to incoming signals such as pain.

Pain Syndromes

Acute pain is both a blessing and a burden. The blessing comes from the signals it sends about injury and the reminders it conveys to avoid further injury and allow healing. The burden is that it hurts.

Chronic pain, in contrast, serves no clear purpose—it signals no injury and causes people to live in misery. More than 30% of the population of the United States (Institute of Medicine, 2011) and almost 20% of those in Europe (Corasaniti, Amantea, Russo, & Bagetta, 2006) experience chronic or intermittent persistent pain. Nearly 10% of Americans report not just some chronic pain, but a *lot* of it (Nahin, 2015). Indeed, chronic pain accounts for more than 80% of visits to doctors (Gatchel, Peng, Peters, Fuchs, & Turk, 2007). Chronic pain often results in poor sleep, and poor sleep intensifies pain, creating a cycle that may prolong suffering (Schuh-Hofer et al., 2013). Unfortunately, the prevalence of chronic pain in the United States is likely to rise in the upcoming decades due to an aging population and increases in the prevalence of obesity (Croft et al., 2010). In fact, one aim of the United States 2010 Patient Protection and Affordable Care Act is to "increase the recognition of pain as a significant public health problem in the United States."

Chronic pain is categorized according to **syndrome**, symptoms that occur together and characterize a condition. Headache and low back pain are the two most frequently treated pain syndromes, but people also seek treatment for several other common pain syndromes.

Headache Pain

Headache pain is the most common of all types of pain, with more than 99% of people experiencing headache at some time during their lives (Smetana, 2000) and

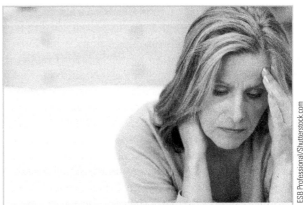

Headache is the most common of all types of pain—more than 99% of people have experienced a headache.

16% of people reporting severe headaches in the last 3 months (CDC and NCHS, 2010d). Until the 1980s, no reliable classification of headache pain was available to researchers and therapists. Then in 1988, the Headache Classification Committee of the International Headache Society (IHS) published a classification system that standardized definitions of various headache pains (Olesen, 1988). Although the IHS identifies many different kinds of headache, the three primary pain syndromes are migraine, tension, and cluster headaches.

Migraine headaches represent recurrent attacks of pain that vary widely in intensity, frequency, and duration. Originally conceptualized as originating in the blood vessels in the head, migraine headaches are now believed to involve not only blood vessels but also a complex cascade of reactions that include neurons in the brain stem (Corasaniti et al., 2006) and to have a genetic component (Bigal & Lipton, 2008a). The underlying cause and the exact mechanism for producing pain remain controversial. Migraine attacks often occur with loss of appetite, nausea, vomiting, and exaggerated sensitivity to light and sound. Migraine headaches often involve sensory, motor, or mood disturbances. Migraines also exist in two varieties: those with aura and those without aura. Migraines with aura have identifiable sensory disturbances that precede the headache pain; migraines without aura have a sudden onset and an intense throbbing, usually (but not always) restricted to one side of the head. Brain imaging studies indicate that these two varieties of migraine affect the brain in somewhat different ways (Sánchez del Rio & Alvarez Linera, 2004).

The epidemiology of migraine headaches includes gender differences and variations in prevalence around the world. Women are two to three times more likely than men to have migraine headaches, with rates in the United States of 6% to 9% for men and 17% to 18% for women (Lipton et al., 2007; Victor, Hu, Campbell, Buse, & Lipton, 2010). Rates for non-Western countries are lower. For example, between 3% and 7% of people in Africa report migraines (Haimanot, 2002). However, the experience of migraine is similar; men and women who have chronic migraines have similar experiences of symptoms, frequency, and severity (Marcus, 2001). Most migraine patients experience their first headache before age 30 and some before the age of 10. However, the period for the greatest frequency of migraines is between ages 30 and 50 (Morillo et al., 2005). Few patients have a first migraine after age 40, but people who have migraines continue to do so, often throughout their lives.

Tension headaches are muscular in origin, accompanied by sustained contractions of the muscles of the neck, shoulders, scalp, and face, but current explanations (Fumal & Schoenen, 2008) also include mechanisms within the CNS. Tension headaches have a gradual onset; sensations of tightness; constriction or pressure; highly variable intensity, frequency, and duration; and a dull, steady ache on both sides of the head. Nearly 40% of the U.S. population experiences tension headaches (Schwartz, Stewart, Simon, & Lipton, 1998), and people with this pain syndrome reported lost workdays and decreased effectiveness at work, home, and school because of their pain.

A third type of headache is the **cluster headache**, a severe headache that occurs in daily or nearly daily clusters (Favier, Haan, & Ferrari, 2005). Some symptoms are similar to those of migraine, including severe pain and vomiting, but cluster headaches are much briefer, rarely lasting longer than 2 hours (Smetana, 2000). The headache occurs on one side of the head, and often the eye on the other side becomes bloodshot and waters. In addition, cluster headaches are more common in men than in women, by a ratio of 2:1 (Bigal & Lipton, 2008b). Most people who have cluster headaches experience episodes of headache, with weeks, months, or years of no headache (Favier et al., 2005). Cluster headaches are even more mysterious than other types of headaches, with no clear understanding of risk factors.

Low Back Pain

As many as 80% of people in the United States experience low back pain at some time, making the problem extensive but not necessarily serious. Most injuries are not permanent, and most people recover (Leeuw et al., 2007). Those who do not recover quickly have a poor prognosis and are likely to develop chronic pain problems. Health care expenditures for these people total more than $90 billion a year in the United States (Luo, 2004). The incidence of low back pain shows some variation for countries around the world (European Vertebral Osteoporosis Study Group, 2004), but this condition produces direct expenses, such as medical care, and indirect costs, such as lost workdays and disability, affecting people in countries around the world (Dagenais, Caro, & Haldeman, 2008).

Infections, degenerative diseases, and malignancies can all cause low back pain. However, the most frequent cause of low back pain is probably injury or stress resulting in musculoskeletal, ligament, and neurological problems in the lower back (Chou et al., 2007). Pregnancy is also a cause of low back pain, with nearly 90% of pregnant women suffering from the syndrome (Hayes et al., 2000). Aging is yet another factor in back pain, because the fluid content and elasticity of the intervertebral disks decrease as one grows older, and arthritis and osteoporosis become more likely. However, fewer than 20% of back pain patients have a definite identification of the physical cause of their pain (Chou et al., 2007).

Stress and psychological factors most likely play a role not only in back pain but also in all types of chronic pain. Making the transition from the prechronic stage to chronic pain is a complex process, and physiological and psychological processes accompany this progression. Some researchers (Baliki, Geha, Apkarian, & Chialvo, 2008; Corasaniti et al., 2006) focus on physical changes in the nervous system that occur when pain becomes chronic. Other researchers (Leeuw et al., 2007; Sanders, 2006) emphasize psychological factors such as fear, anxiety, depression, a history of trauma and abuse, and reinforcement experiences, all of which are more common among chronic pain patients. However, most chronic pain researchers recognize the role that both physical and psychological factors play in causing and maintaining chronic pain.

Arthritis Pain

Rheumatoid arthritis is an autoimmune disorder characterized by swelling and inflammation of the joints as well as destruction of cartilage, bone, and tendons. These changes alter the joint, producing direct pain, and the changes in joint structure lead to

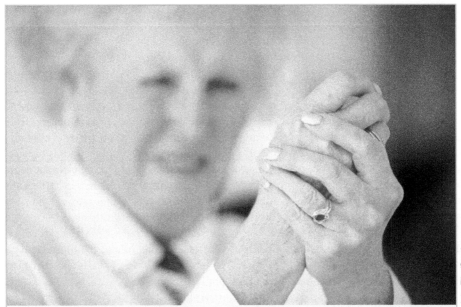

Arthritis is a source of pain and disability for more than 20 million Americans.

Arthur Tilley/Getty Images

changes in movement, which may result in additional pain through this indirect route (Dillard, 2002). Rheumatoid arthritis can occur at any age, even during adolescence and young adulthood, but it is most prevalent among people 40 to 70 years old. Women are more than twice as likely as men to develop this disease (Theis, Helmick, & Hootman, 2007). The symptoms of rheumatoid arthritis are extremely variable. Some people experience a steady worsening of symptoms, but most people face alternating remission and intensification of symptoms. Rheumatoid arthritis interferes with work, family life, recreational activities, and sexuality (Pouchot, Le Parc, Queffelec, Sichère, & Flinois, 2007).

Osteoarthritis is a progressive inflammation of the joints that produces degeneration of cartilage and bone (Goldring & Goldring, 2007); it affects mostly older people. Osteoarthritis causes a dull ache in the joint area, which worsens with movement; the resulting lack of movement increases joint problems and pain. Osteoarthritis is the most common form of arthritis, which is one of the primary causes of disability in older people, affecting about 50% of those over 70 (Keefe et al., 2002). Older women make up a disproportionate number of those affected. As joints stiffen and pain increases, people with arthritis begin to have difficulties engaging in enjoyable activities and even basic self-care. They often experience feelings of helplessness, depression, and anxiety, which exacerbate their pain.

Fibromyalgia is a chronic pain condition characterized by tender points throughout the body. This disorder also has symptoms of fatigue, headache, cognitive difficulties, anxiety, and sleep disturbances (Chakrabarty & Zoorob, 2007). Although fibromyalgia is not arthritis (Endresen, 2007), some symptoms are common to both, as is a diminished quality of life (Birtane, Uzunca, Tastekin, & Tuna, 2007).

Cancer Pain

More than 13 million people in the United States have a cancer diagnosis (Mariotto, Yabroff, Shao, Feuer, & Brown, 2011). Cancer can produce pain in two ways: through its growth and progression and through the various treatments to control its growth. Pain is present in 44% of all cancer cases and in 64% or more of advanced cases (Institute of Medicine, 2011). Some cancers are much more likely than others to produce pain. Head, neck, and cervical cancer patients experience more pain than leukemia patients (Anderson, Syrjala, & Cleeland, 2001). In addition, treatments for cancer may also produce pain; surgery, chemotherapy, and radiation therapy all produce painful effects. Thus, either the disease or its treatment creates pain for most cancer patients. However, many cancer patients do not get adequate relief from pain. A review of 26 international studies showed that across countries, almost half of cancer patients' pain was untreated (Deandrea, Montanari, Moja, & Apolone, 2008).

Phantom Limb Pain

Just as injury can occur without producing pain, pain can occur in the absence of injury. One such type of pain is **phantom limb pain**, the experience of chronic pain in a part of the body that is missing! Amputation removes the nerves that produce the impulses leading to the experience of pain, but not the sensations. Most amputees experience some sensations from the amputated limb, and many of these sensations are painful (Czerniecki & Ehde, 2003).

Until the 1970s, phantom pain was believed to be rare, with less than 1% of amputees experiencing a painful phantom limb, but more recent research has indicated that the percentage may be as high as 80% (Ephraim, Wegener, MacKenzie, Dillingham, & Pezzin, 2005). The sensations often start soon after surgery as a tingling and then develop into other sensations that resemble actual feelings in the missing limb, including pain. Nor are the sensations of phantom pain limited to limbs. Women who have undergone breast removal also perceive sensations from the amputated breast, and people who have had teeth pulled sometimes continue to experience feelings from those teeth.

Amputees sometimes feel that a phantom limb is of abnormal size or in an uncomfortable position (Melzack & Wall, 1982). Phantom limbs can also produce painful feelings of cramping, shooting, burning, or crushing. These pains vary from mild and infrequent to severe and continuous. Early research suggested that the severity and frequency of the pain decrease over time (Melzack & Wall, 1988); however, subsequent research suggests that phantom pain remains over time (Ephraim et al., 2005). In fact, nearly 75% of amputees who lost a limb over 10 years earlier still report phantom pains (Ephraim et al., 2005). Pain is more likely to occur in the missing limb when the person experienced a great deal of pain before the amputation (Hanley et al., 2007).

The underlying cause of phantom limb pain is the subject of heated controversy (Melzack, 1992; Woodhouse, 2005). Because surgery rarely relieves the pain, some authorities suggest that phantom limb pain has an emotional basis. Melzack (1992) argued that phantom limb sensations arise because of the activation of a characteristic pattern of neural activity in the brain, which he called a *neuromatrix*. This neuromatrix pattern continues to operate, even if the neurons in the PNS do not furnish input to the brain.

Melzack believed that this pattern of brain activity is the basis for phantom limb sensations, which may include pain, and recent research is consistent with his theory (Woodhouse, 2005). Brain imaging technology allows researchers to investigate patterns of brain activation, and such studies show that the brain is capable of reorganization after injury, producing changes in the nervous system. Such changes are observed in the somatosensory and motor cortex of amputees (Flor, Nikolajsen, & Staehelin Jensen, 2006; Karl, Mühlnickel, Kurth, & Flor, 2004), which is consistent with Melzack's concept of the neuromatrix and its role in phantom limb pain. Therefore, phantom limb pain may arise from changes that occur in both peripheral and central nervous systems after removal of the limb. Rather than compensate for the loss, the nervous system makes changes that are maladaptive, creating the perception of pain in a body part that no longer exists.

IN SUMMARY

Acute pain may result from hundreds of different types of injuries and diseases, but chronic pain exists as a limited number of syndromes. A few of these syndromes account for the majority of people who suffer from chronic pain. Headache is the most common type of pain, but only some people experience chronic problems with migraine, tension, or cluster headaches. Most people's experience of low back pain is acute, but for some people the pain becomes chronic and debilitating. Arthritis is a degenerative disease that affects the joints, producing chronic pain. Rheumatoid arthritis is an autoimmune disease that may affect people of any age; osteoarthritis is the result of progressive inflammation of the joints that affects mostly older people. Fibromyalgia is a chronic pain condition characterized by pain throughout the body, sleep disturbances, fatigue, and anxiety. Pain is not an inevitable consequence of cancer, but most people with cancer experience pain either as a result of the progression of the disease or from the various treatments for cancer. One of the most puzzling pain syndromes is phantom limb pain, which represents pain that occurs in a missing body part. A majority of people with amputations experience this pain syndrome.

The Measurement of Pain

"I have been told to 'suck it up'; I have been asked if I was having trouble at home; I have been accused of being a 'druggy.' I have also found some practitioners who could 'read the tea leaves,' so to speak and TELL ME how much pain I must be in, based on my physical exam."—A person with chronic pain (Institute of Medicine, 2011, p. 59).

Pain, at its core, is a subjective experience. No doctor or other outside observer can know how much pain a patient experiences. The subjective nature of pain presents a great challenge to researchers and clinicians who seek to understand and treat pain. How can clinicians and researchers assess pain most accurately? Are there reliable and valid ways of assessing pain, other than asking a person to tell you?

Asking physicians (Marquié et al., 2003; Staton et al., 2007) or nurses (Wilson & McSherry, 2006) to rate their patients' pain is not a valid approach because these professionals tend to underestimate patients' pain. Asking people to rate their own pain on a scale would seem reliable and valid. Who knows better than patients themselves how much pain they are feeling? However, some pain experts (Turk & Melzack, 2001) have questioned both the reliability and the validity of this procedure, stating that people do not reliably remember how they rated an earlier pain. For this reason, pain researchers have developed a number of techniques for measuring pain, including (1) self-report ratings, (2) behavioral assessments, and (3) physiological measures.

Self-Reports

Self-report pain assessments ask people to evaluate and make ratings of their pain on simple rating scales, standardized pain inventories, or standardized personality tests.

Rating Scales   Simple rating scales are an important part of the pain measurement toolbox. For example, patients may rate the intensity of their pain on a scale from 0 to 10 (or 0 to 100), with 10 being the most excruciating pain possible and 0 being the complete absence of pain. Such numeric ratings showed advantages over other types of self-reports in a comparison of several approaches to pain assessment (Gagliese, Weizblit, Ellis, & Chan, 2005).

A similar technique is the Visual Analog Scale (VAS), which is simply a line anchored on the left by a phrase such as "no pain" and on the right by a phrase such as "worst pain imaginable." Both the VAS and numerical rating scales are easy to use. For some pain patients, the VAS is superior to word descriptors of pain (Rosier, Iadarola, & Coghill, 2002) and numerical ratings (Bigatti & Cronan, 2002). Visual analog scales have been criticized as sometimes being confusing to patients not accustomed to quantifying their experience (Burckhardt & Jones, 2003b) and difficult for those who cannot comprehend the instructions, such as older people with dementia or young children (Feldt, 2007). Another rating scale is the face scales, consisting of 8 to 10 drawings of faces expressing emotions from intense joy to intense pain; patients merely indicate which illustration best fits their level of pain (Jensen & Karoly, 2001). This type of rating is effective with both children and older adults (Benaim et al., 2007). A limitation of each of these rating scales is that they measure only the intensity of pain; they do not tap into patients' verbal description of their pain, such as whether is it sharp or dull. Despite this limitation, this approach to pain assessment may be the simplest and most effective for many patients.

Pain Questionnaires   Melzack (1975, p. 278) contended that describing pain on a single dimension was "like specifying the visual world only in terms of light flux without regard to pattern, color, texture, and the many other dimensions of visual experience." Rating scales make no distinction, for example, among pains that are pounding, shooting, stabbing, or hot.

To rectify some of these weaknesses, Melzack (1975) developed the McGill Pain Questionnaire (MPQ), an inventory that provides a subjective report of pain and categorizes it in three dimensions: sensory, affective, and evaluative. *Sensory* qualities of pain are its temporal, spatial, pressure, and thermal properties; *affective* qualities are the fear, tension, and autonomic properties that are part of the pain experience; and *evaluative* qualities are the words that describe the subjective overall intensity of the pain experience.

The MPQ has four parts that assess these three dimensions of pain. Part 1 consists of front and back drawings of the human body. Patients mark on these drawings indicating the areas where they feel pain. Part 2 consists of 20 sets of words describing pain, and patients draw a circle around the one word in each set that most accurately describes their pain. These adjectives appear from least to most painful—for example, *nagging, nauseating, agonizing, dreadful,* and *torturing.*

Part 3 asks how the patient's pain has changed with time. Part 4 measures the intensity of pain on a 5-point scale from *mild* to *excruciating*. This fourth part yields a Present Pain Intensity (PPI) score.

The MPQ is the most frequently used pain questionnaire (Piotrowski, 1998, 2007), and a short form of the McGill Pain Questionnaire (Melzack, 1987) preserves the multidimensional assessment and correlates highly with scores on the standard MPQ (Burckhardt & Jones, 2003a). Clinicians use the MPQ to assess pain relief in a variety of treatment programs and in multiple pain syndromes (Melzack & Katz, 2001). The MPQ also exists in 26 different languages (Costa, Maher, McAuley, & Costa, 2009). The short form is growing in use and demonstrates a high degree of reliability (Grafton, Foster, & Wright, 2005). In addition, a computerized, touch-screen administration of this test exists, which shows a high degree of consistency with the paper-and-pencil version (Cook et al., 2004).

The Multidimensional Pain Inventory (MPI), also known as the West Haven–Yale Multidimensional Pain Inventory (WHYMPI), is another assessment tool specifically designed for pain patients (Kerns, Turk, & Rudy, 1985). The 52-item MPI is divided into three sections. The first rates characteristics of the pain, interference with patients' lives and functioning, and patients' moods. The second section rates patients' perceptions of the responses of significant others, and the third measures how often patients engage in each of the 30 different daily activities. Using this inventory allowed researchers (Kerns et al., 1985) to develop 12 different scales that capture various important dimensions of the lives of pain patients.

Standardized Psychological Tests   In addition to the specialized pain inventories, clinicians and researchers also use a variety of standardized psychological tests in assessing pain. The most frequently used of these tests is the MMPI-2 (Arbisi & Seime, 2006). The MMPI measures clinical diagnoses such as depression, paranoia, schizophrenia, and other psychopathologies. Research from the early 1950s (Hanvik, 1951) found that different types of pain patients could be differentiated on several MMPI scales, and more recent research (Arbisi & Seime, 2006) confirms the use of the MMPI for such assessment. One of the major advantages of using the MMPI-2 for pain assessment is its ability to detect patients who are being dishonest about their experience of pain (Bianchini, Etherton, Greve, Heinly, & Meyers, 2008).

Researchers also use the Beck Depression Inventory (Beck, Ward, Mendelson, Mock, & Erbaugh, 1961) and the Symptom Checklist–90 (Derogatis, 1977) to measure pain. The Beck Depression Inventory is a short self-report questionnaire that assesses depression; the Symptom Checklist–90 measures symptoms related to various types of behavioral problems. People with chronic pain often experience negative moods, so the relationship between scores on psychological tests and pain is not surprising. However, factor analyses of the Beck Depression Inventory with pain patients (Morley, de C. Williams, & Black, 2002; Poole, Branwell, & Murphy, 2006) indicate that pain patients present a different profile than depressed people with no chronic pain. Specifically, chronic pain patients are less likely to endorse negative beliefs about the self than depressed people but are more likely to report behavioral and emotional symptoms of depression. Like the MMPI-2, the Symptom Checklist–90 (McGuire & Shores, 2001) is also able to differentiate pain patients from those instructed to fake pain symptoms. Thus, these standardized psychological tests may have something to offer in the assessment of pain, including the ability to identify people who may be exaggerating symptoms of pain.

Behavioral Assessments

A second major approach to pain measurement is observation of patients' behavior. Influential researcher Wilbert Fordyce (1974) noted that people in pain often groan, grimace, rub, sigh, limp, miss work, remain in bed, or engage in other behaviors that signify to observers that they may be suffering from pain, including lowered levels of activity, use of pain medication, body posture, and facial expressions. Behavioral observation began as an informal way to assess pain; Fordyce (1976) trained spouses to record pain behaviors, working to obtain a list of between 5 and 10 behaviors that indicate pain for each individual.

Health care professionals tend to underestimate patients' pain (Staton et al., 2007; Wilson & McSherry, 2006) and require extensive training to overcome their bias (Keefe & Smith, 2002; Rapoff, 2003). Another way for health care professionals to assess pain is through the development of behavioral observation into a standardized assessment strategy (Keefe & Smith, 2002). During an observational protocol, pain patients perform a series of tasks while a trained observer records their body movements and facial expressions, noting signs of pain. For example, patients with low back pain

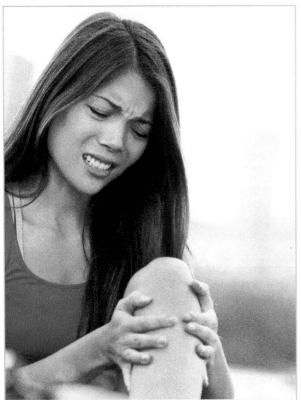

Facial expressions provide a behavioral measure of pain.

may be asked to sit, stand, walk, and recline during a 1- to 2-minute observation. The session may be videotaped to allow other observers to rate pain-related behaviors such as limping and grimacing. This strategy for collecting information yields data about pain behaviors, and analyses confirm that these data are reliable and valid indicators of pain (Keefe & Smith, 2002).

Behavioral observation is especially useful in assessing the pain of people who have difficulty furnishing self-reports—children, the cognitively impaired, and some elderly patients. This approach includes assessments of children's pain (von Baeyer & Spagrud, 2007) and a coding system that allows observers to assess the pain of infants by observing five facial movements and two hand actions (Holsti & Grunau, 2007). Many older patients can report on their pain, but some cannot, and behavioral observation of facial expressions allows an assessment of this difficult group (Clark, Jones, & Pennington, 2004; Lints-Martindale, Hadjistavropoulos, Barber, & Gibson, 2007).

Physiological Measures

A third approach to pain assessment is the use of physiological measures (Gatchel, 2005). Electromyography (EMG), which measures the level of muscle tension, is one of these physiological techniques. The notion behind this approach is that pain increases muscle tension. Attaching the measuring electrodes to the surface of the skin provides an easy way to measure muscle tension, but questions have arisen over the validity of this measurement as a pain indicator. For example, Herta Flor (2001) reported little consistency between self-reports of pain and EMG levels. A meta-analysis of EMG assessment of low back pain (Geisser et al., 2005) indicated that EMG was useful in discriminating those with versus those without low back pain, but EMG alone was not an adequate assessment.

Researchers have also attempted to assess pain through several autonomic indices, including involuntary processes such as hyperventilation, blood flow in the temporal artery, heart rate, hand surface temperature, finger pulse volume, and skin conductance level. Heart rate predicts perceptions of pain, but only for men (Loggia, Juneau, & Bushnell, 2011; Tousignant-Laflamme, Rainville, & Marchand, 2005). In experimental tasks, changes in skin conductance levels correlate with changes in the intensity of a pain stimulus and changes in pain perceptions; however, this method is not well suited for assessing differences between people in clinical pain reports (Loggia et al., 2011). Researchers and clinicians primarily use these physiological assessments with patients who cannot furnish self-reports but more often use behavioral observation of pain-related behaviors for these groups.

IN SUMMARY

Pain measurement techniques fall into three general categories: (1) self-reports, (2) behavioral observation, and (3) physiological measures. Self-reports include rating scales, pain questionnaires such as the MPQ and the MPI, and standardized objective tests such as the Minnesota Multiphasic Personality Inventory and the Beck Depression Inventory. Clinicians who treat pain patients often use a combination of assessments, relying most often on self-report inventories. Behavioral assessments of pain began as informal observation but have evolved into standardized ratings by trained clinicians that are especially useful for individuals, such as young children and people with dementia, who cannot complete self-reports. Physiological measures include muscle tension and autonomic indices such as heart rate, but these approaches are not as reliable or valid as self-reports or behavioral observation.

Managing Pain

Pain presents complex problems for management. Treatment for acute pain is usually straightforward because the source of the pain is clear. However, helping people with chronic pain is a challenge because this type of pain exists without obvious tissue damage. Some people achieve relief through medical treatments, and others experience improvement through behavioral management of their pain.

Medical Approaches to Managing Pain

Drugs are the main medical strategy for treating acute pain. Although drugs are also a choice for some chronic pain syndromes, this strategy carries greater risks. Chronic pain that has not responded to drugs may be treated by surgery, which also presents risks.

Drugs   **Analgesic drugs** relieve pain without causing loss of consciousness. Hundreds of different analgesic drugs are available, but almost all fall into two major groups: the opiates and the nonnarcotic analgesics (Julien, Advokat, & Comaty, 2010). Both types exist naturally as derivatives of plants, and both have many synthetic variations. Of the two, the opium type is more powerful and has a longer history of use, dating back at least 5,000 years (Melzack & Wall, 1982).

Contemporary **opiate painkillers** include substances such as morphine, codeine, oxycodone, and hydrocodone (an active ingredient in the drug known as Vicodin). The use of these painkillers is limited by prescription from a physician, because use can lead to the development of both tolerance and dependence. **Tolerance** is the body's decreased responsiveness to a drug. When tolerance occurs, larger and larger doses of a drug are required to bring about the same effect. **Dependence** occurs when the drug's removal produces withdrawal symptoms. Because opiates produce both tolerance and dependence, they are potentially dangerous and subject to abuse.

How realistic are the fears of drug abuse as a consequence of opiate prescription? Do patients become addicted while recovering from surgery? What about the dangers to patients with terminal illnesses? According to one study (Porter & Jick, 1980), the risk of addiction is less than 1%. During the late 1990s, prescriptions for opiate analgesics increased dramatically, and publicity about an epidemic of analgesic abuse fueled the fear that increased prescriptions for these drugs were leading to widespread addiction. Despite increases in opiate use and abuse, the number of chronic pain patients who develop an addiction to opiate pain medications is less than 4% of the number who are prescribed them (Fishbain, Cole, Lewis, Rosomoff, & Rosomoff, 2008). To date, the best predictor of opiate painkiller abuse is personal history of illegal drug and alcohol use; people who misuse these substances are more likely to also misuse opiate painkillers (Turk, Swanson, & Gatchel, 2008).

Between 1997 and 2007, the use of opiate analgesic drugs increased over 600% (Paulozzi et al., 2012). Since 1999, the number of opioid-related deaths quadrupled as well (CDC, 2016a). Much of this increase was for the drugs oxycodone and hydrocodone. Both are opiates with a potential for abuse, which increased during the time when prescriptions increased. Wariness about abuse of these drugs affects both physicians, who are reluctant to prescribe them (Breuer, Fleishman, Cruciani, & Portenoy, 2011), and many patients, who are reluctant to take sufficient doses to obtain relief (Lewis, Combs, & Trafton, 2010). This reluctance applies to all opiate drugs, even for cancer pain (Reid, Gooberman-Hill, & Hanks, 2008). Thus, people with either acute or chronic pain frequently fail to receive sufficient relief.

The advantages of opiate drugs outweigh their dangers for some people in some situations; no other type of drug produces more complete pain relief. However, their potential for abuse and their side effects make them more suitable for treating acute pain than for managing chronic pain, as there is limited evidence supporting their long-term use for chronic pain (Manchikanti et al., 2011). The opiate drugs remain an essential part of pain management for the most severe, acute injuries, for recovery from surgery, and for terminal illnesses.

One procedure that has overcome the undermedication problem is a system of self-paced administration. Patients can activate a pump attached to their intravenous lines and deliver a dose of medication whenever they wish, within well-defined limits. Such systems began to appear in the late 1970s and have since gained wide acceptance because patients tend to use less medication, obtain better pain relief (Sri Vengadesh, Sistla, & Smile, 2005), and experience higher satisfaction (Gan, Gordon, Bolge, & Allen, 2007). Because an intravenous line is necessary for this system of drug delivery, it is most commonly used to control pain following surgery. However, a patient-controlled transdermal delivery system is also available (D'Arcy, 2005). This system allows people to self-administer analgesia through a device about the size of a credit card that adheres to their upper arm. These types of self-administered analgesics help prevent undermedication.

Whereas undermedication may be a problem for cancer pain patients, overmedication is often a problem for patients suffering from low back pain. One team of investigators (Von Korff, Barlow, Cherkin, & Deyo, 1994) grouped primary care physicians according to their low, moderate, or high frequency of prescribing pain medication and bed rest for back pain patients. A 1- and 2-year follow-up found that back pain patients who took less medication and remained active did just as well as those who were told to take more medication and to rest. Another study (Rhee, Taitel, Walker, & Lau, 2007) found that back pain patients who took opiate drugs experienced more frequent health problems such as hypertension, anxiety, depression, and arthritis; in addition, they were more likely to make a visit to a hospital emergency room. Both studies indicated that treatment for these patients was more costly than for patients who took other approaches to managing back pain. Thus, low back pain patients who use pain medication have poorer outcomes, more health problems, and higher costs than those who do not. Unfortunately, opiate prescriptions for low back pain appear to be increasing rather than decreasing in frequency (Mafi, McCarthy, Davis, & Landon, 2013).

The **nonnarcotic analgesics** include a variety of nonsteroidal anti-inflammatory drugs (NSAIDs) as well as acetaminophen. Aspirin, ibuprofen, and naproxen sodium appear to block the synthesis of prostaglandins (Julien et al., 2010), a class of chemicals released by damaged tissue and involved in inflammation. The presence of these chemicals sensitizes neurons and increases pain. These drugs act at the site of injury instead of crossing into the brain, but they change neurochemical activity in the nervous system and affect pain perception. As a result of their mechanism of action, NSAIDs do not alter pain perception when no injury is present—for example, in laboratory situations with people who receive experimental pain stimuli.

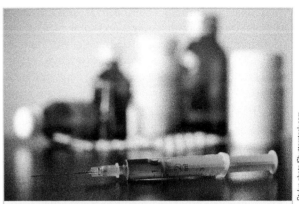

Drugs offer effective treatment for acute pain but are not a good choice to treat chronic pain.

Aspirin and other NSAIDs have many uses in pain relief, including for minor cuts and scratches as well as more severe injuries such as broken bones. But pain that occurs without inflammation is not so readily relieved by NSAIDs. In addition, NSAIDs can irritate and damage the stomach lining, even producing ulcers (Huang, Sridhar, & Hunt, 2002). Aspirin's side effects include the alteration of blood clotting time, and aspirin and other NSAIDs are toxic in large doses, causing damage to the liver and kidneys.

A new type of NSAID, the Cox-2 inhibitor, affects prostaglandins but has lower gastric toxicity. After the approval and heavy marketing of these drugs, their sales skyrocketed, especially among people with arthritis. However, the discovery of increased heart attack risk led to the withdrawal of two Cox-2 inhibitors from the market in the United States and increased caution in the use of this type of NSAID (Shi & Klotz, 2008).

Acetaminophen, another nonnarcotic analgesic, is not one of the NSAIDs. Under brand names such as Tylenol, acetaminophen has become a widely used painkiller. It has few anti-inflammatory properties but has a pain-relieving capability similar to that of aspirin, though somewhat weaker. Acetaminophen does not have the gastric side effects of aspirin, so people who cannot tolerate aspirin find it a good substitute. However, acetaminophen is not harmless. Large quantities of acetaminophen can be fatal, and even nonlethal doses can do serious damage to the liver, especially when combined with alcohol (Julien et al., 2010).

Analgesic drugs are not the only drugs that affect pain. Antidepressant drugs and drugs used to treat seizures also influence pain perception, and these drugs can be used to treat some types of pain

(Maizels & McCarberg, 2005). Antidepressants can be useful in treating low back pain, and some types of anticonvulsant medication can help people with migraine headaches. In addition, other drugs exist that have some ability to prevent migraine headaches (Peres, Mercante, Tanuri, & Nunes, 2006) and to reduce the inflammation that is a damaging part of rheumatoid arthritis (Iagnocco et al., 2008). Similar developments for other chronic pain syndromes would change the lives of millions of people. Unfortunately, even the variety of drugs and strategies for their use are not adequate for many people with chronic pain. Those individuals may consider surgery or other treatments to attain relief.

Surgery   Another traditional medical treatment for pain is surgery, which aims to repair the source of the pain or alter the nervous system to alleviate the pain. Low back surgery is the most common surgical approach to pain, but surgery is not an option that physicians recommend until other, less invasive possibilities have failed (van Zundert & van Kleef, 2005).

Surgery can also alter nerves that transmit pain (van Zundert & van Kleef, 2005). This procedure may use heat, cold, or radiofrequency stimulation to change neural transmission and control pain. Complete destruction of nerves is not typically the aim because it can lead to loss of all sensation, which may be more distressing than pain. Another tactic for altering pain through changing nerve transmission involves stimulation of nerves through implanted wires that stimulate rather than damage nerves. Surgery is required for this approach, which involves implanting devices that can deliver electrical stimulation to either the spinal cord or the brain. Activation of the system produces pain relief by activating neurons and by releasing neurotransmitters that block pain. This process does not destroy neural tissue.

Spinal stimulation is a promising technique for controlling back pain (De Andrés & Van Buyten, 2006), but a related type of stimulation, **transcutaneous electrical nerve stimulation** (TENS), has proven to be less effective. The TENS system typically consists of electrodes that attach to the skin and are connected to a unit that supplies electrical stimulation. Despite some promising early indications of success, TENS has demonstrated only limited effectiveness in controlling pain (Claydon, Chesterton, Barlas, & Sim, 2011).

Surgery has at least two drawbacks as a treatment for pain. First, it does not always repair damaged tissue, and second, it does not provide all patients with sufficient pain relief. Even those for whom surgery is initially successful may experience a return of pain. That is, surgery is not a successful treatment for many people with chronic back pain (Ehrlich, 2003). Thus, this approach is an expensive but unreliable approach to controlling this pain syndrome (Turk & McCarberg, 2005). Also, surgery has its own potential dangers and possibilities for complications, which lead many pain patients to behavioral approaches for managing their pain.

Behavioral Techniques for Managing Pain

Psychologists have been prominent in devising therapies that teach people how to manage pain, and several behavioral techniques have proven effective with a variety of pain syndromes. These techniques include relaxation training, behavioral therapy, cognitive therapy, and cognitive behavioral therapy. Some authorities consider these techniques to be part of mind–body medicine and thus part of alternative medicine (covered in Chapter 8). Psychologists see these techniques as part of psychology.

Relaxation Training   Relaxation is one approach to managing pain and may be the key ingredient in other types of pain management. *Progressive muscle relaxation* consists of sitting in a comfortable chair with no distractions and then systematic tensing and relaxing of muscle groups throughout the body (Jacobson, 1938). After learning the procedure, people can practice this relaxation technique independently.

Relaxation techniques have been used successfully to treat pain problems such as tension and migraine headache (Fumal & Schoenen, 2008; Penzien, Rains, & Andrasik, 2002), rheumatoid arthritis (McCallie et al., 2006), and low back pain (Henschke et al., 2010). A National Institutes of Health Technology (NIHT) panel evaluated the evidence for progressive muscle relaxation and gave this technique its highest rating in controlling pain (Lebovits, 2007). However, relaxation training typically functions as part of a multicomponent program (Astin, 2004).

Table 7.1 summarizes the effectiveness of relaxation techniques.

Behavioral Therapy   The most prominent behavioral therapy is *behavior modification,* which arose from the laboratory research on operant conditioning. **Behavior modification** is the process of shaping behavior

TABLE 7.1 Effectiveness of Relaxation Techniques

Problems	Findings	Studies
1. Tension and migraine headaches	Relaxation helps in managing headache.	Fumal & Schoenen, 2008; Penzien et al., 2002
2. Rheumatoid arthritis	Progressive muscle relaxation is an effective component in programs to manage these disorders.	McCallie et al., 2006
3. Low back pain	Relaxation is effective in programs to treat low back pain.	Henschke et al., 2010
4. Variety of chronic pain conditions	Progressive muscle relaxation is effective according to an NIHT review.	Lebovits, 2007

through the application of operant conditioning principles. The goal of behavior modification is to shape *behavior,* not to alleviate *feelings* or *sensations* of pain. People in pain usually communicate their discomfort to others through their behavior—they complain, moan, sigh, limp, rub, grimace, and miss work.

Wilbert E. Fordyce (1974) was among the first to emphasize the role of operant conditioning in the perpetuation of pain behaviors. He recognized the *reward* value of increased attention and sympathy, financial compensation, and other **positive reinforcers** that frequently follow pain behaviors. These conditions create what pain expert Frank Andrasik (2003) called pain traps, situations that push people who experience pain toward developing and maintaining chronic pain. The situations that create chronic pain include attention from family, relief from normal responsibilities, compensation from employers, and medications that people receive from physicians. These reinforcers make it difficult to get better (Newton-John, 2013).

Behavior modification works against these pain traps, identifying the reinforcers and training people in the patient's environment to use praise and attention to reinforce more desirable behaviors and to withhold reinforcement when the patient exhibits less desired pain behaviors. In other words, the groans and complaints are now ignored, whereas efforts toward greater physical activity and other positive behaviors are reinforced. Objective outcomes indicate progress, such as the amount of medication taken, absences from work, time in bed or off one's feet, number of pain complaints, physical activity, range of motion, and length of sitting tolerance. The strength of the operant conditioning technique is its ability to increase levels of physical activity and decrease the use of medication—two important targets in any pain treatment regimen (Roelofs, Boissevain, Peters, de Jong, & Vlaeyen, 2002). In addition, this behavioral approach can decrease pain intensity, reduce disability, and improve quality of life (Gatzounis, Schrooten, Crombez, & Vlaeyan, 2012). The behavior modification approach does not address the cognitions that underlie and contribute to behaviors, but cognitive therapy focuses on these cognitions.

Cognitive therapy is based on the principle that people's beliefs, personal standards, and feelings of self-efficacy strongly affect their behavior (Bandura, 1986, 2001; Beck, 1976; Ellis, 1962). Cognitive therapies concentrate on techniques designed to change cognitions, assuming that behavior will change when a person alters his or her cognitions. Albert Ellis (1962) argued that thoughts, especially irrational thoughts, are the root of behavior problems. He focused on the tendency to "catastrophize," which escalates an unpleasant situation into something worse. Examples of pain-related catastrophizing might include "This pain will never get better," "I can't go on any longer," or "There is nothing I can do to stop this pain."

The experience of pain can easily turn into a catastrophe, and any exaggeration of feelings of pain can lead to maladaptive behaviors and further exacerbation of irrational beliefs. The tendency to catastrophize is associated with the magnification of pain, both acute (Pavlin, Sullivan, Freund, & Roesen, 2005) and chronic (Karoly & Ruehlman, 2007).

Once irrational cognitions have been identified, the therapist actively attacks these beliefs, with the goal of eliminating or changing them into more rational beliefs. For example, cognitive therapy for pain addresses the tendency to catastrophize, leading people to abandon the belief that their pain is unbearable and will never stop (Thorn & Kuhajda, 2006). Cognitive therapists address these cognitions and work with patients to change them. Rather than concentrate exclusively on thoughts, however, most cognitive therapists working with pain patients address changes in both cognitions and behavior. That is, they practice cognitive behavioral therapy.

Cognitive behavioral therapy (CBT) is a type of therapy that aims to develop beliefs, attitudes, thoughts, and skills to make positive changes in behavior. Like cognitive therapy, CBT assumes that thoughts and feelings are the basis of behavior, so CBT begins with changing attitudes. Like behavior modification, CBT focuses on modifying environmental contingencies and building skills to change observable behavior.

One approach to CBT for pain management is the pain inoculation program designed by Dennis Turk and Donald Meichenbaum (Meichenbaum & Turk, 1976; Turk, 1978, 2001), which is similar to stress inoculation explained in Chapter 5. Pain inoculation includes a cognitive stage, the *reconceptualization* stage, during which patients learn to accept the importance of psychological factors for at least some of their pain and often receive an explanation of the gate control theory of pain. The second stage—*acquisition and rehearsal of skills*—includes learning relaxation and controlled breathing skills. The final, or *follow-through,* phase of treatment includes instructions to spouses and other family members to ignore patients' pain behaviors and to reinforce healthy behaviors such as greater levels of physical activity, decreased use of medication, fewer visits to the pain clinic, or an increased number of days at work. With the help of their therapists, patients construct a posttreatment plan for coping with future pain; and finally, they apply their coping skills to everyday situations outside the pain clinic. A study of laboratory-induced pain (Milling, Levine, & Meunier, 2003) indicated that inoculation training was as effective as hypnosis in helping participants control pain. A study of athletes recovering from knee injury (Ross & Berger, 1996) also found that pain inoculation procedures were effective.

Other CBT programs have demonstrated their effectiveness for a wide variety of pain syndromes. CBT includes strategies for addressing the harmful cognitions that are common among chronic pain patients, such as fear and catastrophizing (Leeuw et al., 2007; Thorn et al., 2007) and a behavioral component to help pain patients behave in ways that are compatible

with health rather than illness. Evaluations of CBT for low back pain (Hoffman, Papas, Chatkoff, & Kerns, 2007) indicate its effectiveness for this pain syndrome, and studies of CBT with headache patients (Martin, Forsyth, & Reece, 2007; Nash, Park, Walker, Gordon, & Nicholson, 2004; Thorn et al., 2007) have also demonstrated its benefits. Fibromyalgia patients benefited more from CBT than from a drug treatment (García, Simón, Durán, Canceller, & Aneiros, 2006), and CBT proved beneficial for people with rheumatoid arthritis (Astin, 2004; Sharpe et al., 2001) as well as cancer and AIDS pain (Breibart & Payne, 2001).

Recently, researchers evaluated a form of CBT for pain management called **acceptance and commitment therapy (ACT)**. ACT encourages pain patients to increase acceptance of their pain, while focusing their attention on other goals and activities that they value. This form of therapy may be especially helpful for chronic pain patients, as attempting to directly control pain may lead to distress and disability (McCracken, Eccleston, & Bell, 2005). A recent meta-analysis of 10 studies of chronic pain patients found that ACT led to significant reduction in pain intensity and improvements in physical functioning compared with a comparison group (Hann & McCracken, 2014). Thus, ACT may be another good alternative to traditional CBT for the management of chronic pain. ACT's focus on acceptance of pain is also a focus of mindfulness-based interventions for chronic pain.

As described in Chapter 5, **mindfulness** is a quality of consciousness or awareness that comes about through intentionally focusing one's attention on the present moment in a nonjudgmental and accepting manner (Kabat-Zinn, 1994). In the context of chronic pain, a mindfulness-based intervention aims to increase a person's awareness and acceptance of all sensations—even those of pain and physical discomfort—and the emotions that accompany those sensations. Although it may seem odd that deliberately encouraging a person to focus attention on pain could be effective in reducing it, recent evidence suggests that mindfulness works in helping chronic pain patients. One large randomized trial compared CBT, mindfulness, and usual care in adults with chronic low back pain (Cherkin et al., 2016). Both the mindfulness and the cognitive behavioral interventions led to clinically significant reductions in pain in over 40% of the patients, compared to only 25% of the patients in the usual care condition. There may be several reasons why mindfulness appears to help people manage pain. First, mindfulness can help reduce depression and anxiety, and as discussed earlier in this chapter, anxiety increases people's perception of pain. Perhaps more importantly, mindfulness seeks to reduce people's tendency to catastrophize about pain. In a mindfulness-based intervention, people are encouraged to do frequent "body scans" in which they not only pay close attention to the sensations in all parts of their body but are also instructed to attend to them without jumping to judgment about how severe, crippling, or debilitating any pain sensations might be. Such a non-judgmental approach to attending to pain may make a person realize that their pain occurs less frequently than they typically believe, notice situations that tend to increase or decrease the pain, and also help them refrain from judgments such as "This pain will never go away."

Several studies show that mindfulness reduces pain by reducing this tendency toward catastrophizing (Cassidy, Atherton, Robertson, Walsh, & Gillett, 2012; Garland et al., 2011). Given the promise and relatively low cost of mindfulness-based interventions for chronic pain, some authorities suggest that such non-pharmacological interventions could be an effective first step in treatment for chronic pain patients (Dowell et al., 2016).

In summary, these studies show that behavior modification, CBT, and mindfulness can be effective interventions for pain management for people with a variety of pain syndromes. These techniques are among the most effective types of pain management strategies. Table 7.2 summarizes the effectiveness of these therapies and the problems they can treat.

TABLE 7.2   Effectiveness of Behavioral, Cognitive, and Cognitive Behavioral Therapy and Mindfulness

Problems	Findings	Studies
1. Increase in pain behaviors	Verbal reinforcement increases pain behaviors.	Jolliffe & Nicholas, 2004
2. Chronic low back pain	Operant conditioning increases physical activity and lowers medication usage; behavior modification and CBT can also be effective.	Roelofs et al., 2002; Smeets et al., 2009
3. Pain intensity	Behavior modification decreases pain intensity.	Sanders, 2006
4. Catastrophizing the experience of pain	Catastrophizing intensifies acute and chronic pain.	Karoly & Ruehlman, 2007; Pavlin et al., 2005; Thorn & Kuhajda, 2006
5. Laboratory-induced pain	Inoculation training was as effective as hypnosis for pain.	Milling et al., 2003
6. Athletes with knee pain	Pain inoculation reduces pain.	Ross & Berger, 1996
7. Low back pain	CBT was evaluated as effective in a meta-analysis and in a systematic review.	Hoffman et al., 2007
8. Headache pain and prevention	CBT is effective in both management and prevention.	Martin et al., 2007; Nash et al., 2004; Thorn et al., 2007
9. Fibromyalgia	CBT is more effective than drug treatment.	García et al., 2006
10. Rheumatoid arthritis	CBT can relieve some pain.	Astin, 2004; Sharpe et al., 2001
11. Cancer and AIDS pain	CBT helps people cope.	Breibart & Payne, 2000
12. Chronic pain	ACT is effective in reducing pain intensity in two meta-analyses.	Hann & McCracken, 2014; Veehof et al., 2010
13. Low back pain	Mindfulness and CBT are equally effective at reducing pain and improving physical functioning.	Cherkin et al., 2016

IN SUMMARY

A variety of medical treatments for pain are effective but also have limitations. Analgesic drugs offer pain relief for acute pain and can be of use for chronic pain. These drugs include opiates and nonnarcotic drugs. Opiates are effective in managing severe pain, but their tolerance and dependence properties pose problems for use by chronic pain patients, making health care professionals and patients reluctant to use effective doses. Nonnarcotic drugs such as aspirin, nonsteroidal anti-inflammatory drugs, and acetaminophen are effective in managing mild to moderate acute pain and have some uses in managing chronic pain.

Surgery can alter either peripheral nerves or the CNS. Surgical procedures are often a last resort in controlling chronic pain, and procedures that involve destruction of nerve pathways are often unsuccessful. Procedures that allow for stimulation of the spinal cord show more promise in pain management, but transcutaneous electrical nerve stimulation is not an effective method.

Health psychologists help people cope with stress and chronic pain by using relaxation training, behavioral therapy, cognitive therapy, and CBT. Relaxation techniques such as progressive muscle relaxation have demonstrated some success in helping patients manage headache pain, postoperative pain, and low back pain. Behavior modification can be effective in helping pain patients become more active and decrease their dependence on medication, but this approach does not address the negative emotions and suffering that accompany pain. Cognitive therapy addresses feelings and thus helps in reducing the catastrophizing that exacerbates pain. Combined with the behavioral components of operant conditioning, CBT has demonstrated greater effectiveness than other therapies.

CBT includes pain inoculation therapy, but other combinations of changes in cognitions concerning pain and behavioral strategies for changing pain-related behavior also fit within this category. These approaches have been successful in treating low back pain, headache pain, rheumatoid arthritis pain, fibromyalgia, and the pain that accompanies cancer and AIDS.

Answers

This chapter has addressed five basic questions:

1. **How does the nervous system register pain?**
   Receptors near the skin's surface react to stimulation, and the nerve impulses from this stimulation relay the message to the spinal cord. The spinal cord includes laminae (layers) that modulate the sensory message and relay it toward the brain. The somatosensory cortex in the brain receives and interprets sensory input. Neurochemicals and the periaqueductal gray can also modulate the information and change the perception of pain.

2. **What is the meaning of pain?**
   Pain is difficult to define, but it can be classified as acute (resulting from specific injury and lasting less than 6 months), chronic (continuing beyond the time of healing), or prechronic (the critical stage between acute and chronic). The personal experience of pain is affected by situational and cultural factors as well as individual variation and learning history. The meaning of pain can also be understood through theories. The leading model is the gate control theory of pain, which takes both physical and psychological factors into account in the experience of pain.

3. **What types of pain present the biggest problems?**
   Pain syndromes are a common way of classifying chronic pain according to symptoms. These syndromes include headache pain, low back pain, arthritic pain, cancer pain, and phantom limb pain; the first two are the most common sources of chronic pain and lead to the most time lost from work or school.

4. **How can pain be measured?**
   Pain can be measured physiologically by assessing muscle tension or autonomic arousal, but these measurements do not have high validity. Observations of pain-related behaviors (such as limping,

grimacing, or complaining) have some reliability and validity. Self-reports are the most common approach to pain measurement; they include rating scales, pain questionnaires, and standardized psychological tests.

5. What techniques are effective for pain management?

The techniques that health psychologists use in helping people cope with pain include relaxation training and behavioral techniques. Relaxation training can help people cope with pain problems such as headache and low back pain. Behavioral approaches include behavior modification, which guides people to behave in ways compatible with health rather than pain. Cognitive therapy concentrates on thoughts, guiding pain patients to minimize catastrophizing and fear. Cognitive behavioral therapy combines strategies to change cognitions with behavioral application, which is an especially effective approach for pain control.

Suggested Readings

Baar, K. (2008, March/April). Pain, pain, go away. *Psychology Today, 41*(2), 56–57. This very brief article provides a summary of psychological factors in pain and the treatments psychologists have used successfully to help people manage pain.

Gatchel, R., Haggard, R., Thomas, C., & Howard, K. J. (2012). Biopsychosocial approaches to understanding chronic pain and disability. In R. J. Moore (Ed.), *Handbook of pain and palliative care* (pp. 1–16). New York: Springer. This chapter walks the reader through the development of major theories of pain, discusses how acute pain can turn into chronic pain, and presents issues in the assessment and management of chronic pain.

Kabat-Zinn, J. (2010). Mindfulness meditation for pain relief: Guided practices for reclaiming your body and your life (audio recording). SoundsTrue. This audio recording by Dr. Kabat-Zinn, one of the leading figures in mindfulness research and practice, provides an overview of mindfulness and several approaches for using it as a way to reduce suffering that accompanies experiences of chronic pain.

Wall, P. (2000). *Pain: The science of suffering.* New York: Columbia University Press. Peter Wall, one of the originators of the gate control theory of pain, tells about his extensive experience in trying to understand this phenomenon. He provides a nontechnical examination of the experience of pain, considering the cultural and individual factors that contribute.

CHAPTER 8

Considering Alternative Approaches

CHAPTER OUTLINE

QUESTIONS

This chapter focuses on six questions:

1. What are some alternatives to conventional medicine?

2. What products and diets count as alternative medicine?

3. What manipulative practices fall within alternative practices?

4. What is mind–body medicine?

5. Who uses complementary and alternative medicine?

6. What are the effective uses and limitations of alternative treatments?

☑ Check Your **HEALTH CARE PREFERENCES**

Check the items that are consistent with your beliefs.

☐ 1. When I am in pain, I go to the medicine cabinet to find something to alleviate my pain.

☐ 2. I believe that herbal treatments can be as effective as drugs in treating pain.

☐ 3. Drug companies should develop a pill to help people deal with stress.

☐ 4. Stress and pain arise from sources outside the person.

☐ 5. If my pain did not respond to medical treatment, I would be willing to try some alternative approach such as hypnosis or acupuncture.

☐ 6. Too many people take drugs to help them cope with their problems.

☐ 7. I would prefer some alternative to medical treatments for stress and pain problems.

☐ 8. Stress and pain come from an interaction of the person and the situation.

☐ 9. Chiropractic care offers no real benefits.

☐ 10. Alternative treatments cannot be as effective as conventional medical treatments.

☐ 11. Alternative treatments are safer than conventional medical approaches.

☐ 12. I believe that a combination of alternative and conventional medical treatments offers the best approach for pain management.

If you agreed with items 1, 3, 4, 9, and 10, then you probably have a strong belief in conventional medical approaches to treatment, including treatments for stress and pain problems. If you agreed with items 2, 5, 6, 7, 8, 11, and 12, then you show some beliefs that are compatible with alternative and behavioral treatments.

This chapter examines alternative treatments, describes alternative approaches to managing stress and pain, and reviews evidence about the effectiveness of these approaches.

Real-World Profile of **NORMAN COUSINS**

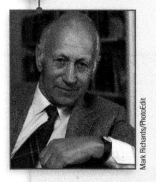

Mark Richards/PhotoEdit

In 1964 Norman Cousins was editor of the influential magazine *Saturday Review* when he was stricken by ankylosing spondylitis, a degenerative, inflammatory disease that affects the connective tissue in the spine. His physician told Cousins that his chances of recovery were 1 in 500 (Cousins, 1979). The treatment involved hospitalization and large doses of anti-inflammatory drugs; Cousins checked into the hospital and began taking the drugs. However, he decided that he could not remain a passive observer in his health care. Furthermore, he began to question the effectiveness of hospital routine, hospital food, seemingly endless tests, and high doses of drugs. Cousins left the hospital.

Cousins continued treatment, but instead of a hospital room, he chose a nice hotel. Rather than drugs, Cousins prescribed himself a healthy diet, large doses of vitamin C, an optimistic attitude, and a regimen of laughter from episodes of *Candid Camera* and old Marx brothers' movies. His physician was skeptical but agreed to this unusual course of treatment, and to his surprise, Cousins began to improve; eventually, he made a complete recovery. Cousins reported his experience in an article published in 1976 in the *New England Journal of Medicine*, which became the first chapter of his 1979 book, *Anatomy of an Illness as Perceived by the Patient*.

Cousins became a vocal advocate for the power that lies within people to heal themselves. He argued for the necessity of broadening medicine to focus on the patient and including psychological factors in the healing process. By accepting the position of Adjunct Professor of Medical Humanities at the University of California at Los Angeles, Cousins was able to work within conventional medicine to advocate for alternatives. He spoke and wrote about the possibilities for the healing power of positive emotions until his death in 1990. Cousins helped move medical care from one dominated by the biomedical model based on the concept of pathogens as the underlying cause of disease to a biopsychosocial model that includes social, cultural, and psychological factors.

The biopsychosocial model is an expansion of the biomedical view, but other conceptualizations of illness differ so much from mainstream medicine that they fall into another category. **Alternative medicine** is the term applied to this group of diverse medical and health care systems, practices, and products that are not currently considered part of conventional medicine (National Center for Complementary and Integrative Health [NCCIH], 2008/2015). Alternatives to conventional medicine come from systems of medicine that arose in different cultures, such as traditional Chinese medicine; from practices that are not yet accepted in mainstream medicine, such as yoga and massage therapy; and from products that are not yet recognized as having medicinal value, such as glucosamine or melatonin.

People may use these practices and products as alternatives to conventional medicine—for example, when a person seeks acupuncture or massage therapy for back pain rather than take an analgesic drug. However, people usually combine alternative with conventional treatments (Clarke, Black, Stussman, Barnes, & Nahin, 2015). In such circumstances, the term **complementary medicine** applies—for example, when a person uses both massage and analgesic drugs to control pain. The group of systems, practices, and products is often termed *complementary and alternative medicine (CAM)*. However, the ideal situation for many practitioners and patients would be a mixture of both conventional and alternative approaches, which constitutes **integrative medicine** (or *integrative health*). We will return to this goal later but will first examine the systems that originated many alternative approaches.

Alternative Medical Systems

The classification of procedures and products as complementary or alternative depends not only on cultural context but also on time period. In the United States 150 years ago, surgery was an alternative treatment not well accepted by established medicine (Weitz, 2010). As surgical techniques improved and evidence began to accumulate that surgery was the best treatment for some conditions, it became part of conventional medicine. More recently, the value of whole-grain diets made the transition from alternative medicine to mainstream medical recommendation when evidence about the health value of high-fiber diets began to accumulate (Hufford, 2003). Some of the techniques now classified as CAM will, with research and time, become part of conventional medicine.

Making the transition from CAM to conventional medicine requires demonstration of the effectiveness of the procedure or substance through scientific research (Berman & Straus, 2004; Committee on the Use of Complementary and Alternative Medicine, 2005). To assist this process, the U.S. Congress created an agency that became the National Center for Complementary and Alternative Medicine, and then in 2014, the National Center for Complementary and Integrative Health. Beginning in 1992, this agency has sponsored research on CAM in an attempt to determine which approaches are effective for what conditions, as well as who uses CAM and for what conditions. Before considering the findings on CAM approaches for managing stress, pain, and other conditions, we will review some of the major CAM approaches and techniques.

The health care most people receive in North America, Europe, and other places around the world comes from physicians, surgeons, nurses, and pharmacists who represent the biomedical system of medicine. Various alternative systems have arisen at different times and places; some have evolved during the same time frame as Western conventional medicine (NCCIH, 2008/2015). Each of these alternative systems includes a complete theory of disease (and possibly of health as well) and a description of what constitutes appropriate medical practice. In the United States, over 20% of people have used a treatment based on at least one of these systems (Clarke et al., 2015).

Traditional Chinese Medicine

Traditional Chinese medicine (TCM) originated in China at least 2,000 years ago (Xutian, Zhang, & Louise, 2009) and remains a major treatment approach in Asian countries. The system of TCM holds that a vital force, called *qi* (pronounced "chee" and sometimes written *chi*), animates the body. Qi flows through channels in the body called *meridians,* which connect parts of the body to each other and to the universe as a whole. Keeping the qi in balance is important to maintaining and restoring health. If the qi is blocked or becomes stagnant, health impairment and disease can develop.

The body exists in a balance between two opposing energies or forces, *yin* and *yang* (Xutian et al., 2009). Yin represents cold, passive, and slow energy, whereas yang is hot, active, and rapid. The two always operate together—achieving a balance between the two is essential for health; attaining harmony is ideal. Imbalances may occur through physical, emotional, or environmental events, and thus TCM takes a holistic approach to diagnosis and treatment. Practitioners have a variety of techniques to help individuals revitalize and unblock qi, bring yin and yang into balance, and restore health. These techniques include acupuncture, massage, herbal preparations, diet, and exercise.

Acupuncture became the first component of TCM to gain widespread publicity in the West in 1971, when *New York Times* journalist James Reston experienced and reported on the acupuncture treatment he received in China (Harrington, 2008). Reston had accompanied Secretary of State Henry Kissinger to China as Kissinger worked toward a meeting between Chinese leader Mao Tse-tung and U.S. President Richard Nixon, who wanted to establish diplomatic relations with China. Reston's story about the success of acupuncture in controlling his postoperative pain captured the interest of many people and led the way toward acupuncture becoming well known as a treatment in alternative medicine. Acupuncture holds an important place in the system of TCM.

Acupuncture consists of inserting needles into specific points on the skin and stimulating the needles continuously (NCCIH, 2007/2016a). The stimulation can be accomplished electrically or by twirling the needles. About 1.5% of people in the United States reported that they have used acupuncture (Clarke et al., 2015).

Acupressure is a manipulative technique that involves the application of pressure rather than needles to the points used in acupuncture. In the system of TCM, acupuncture and acupressure help to unblock the flow of qi and thus restore health. Another strategy for stimulating or subduing qi is a massage technique called *tui na*. TCM holds that this process regulates the nervous system, boosts immune function, and helps flush wastes out of the system.

The Chinese *Materia Medica* is a reference guide to the use of herbs and herbal preparations in treatment. Herbs such as ginseng and ginger are common, but many other plant, mineral, and even animal preparations are part of herbal remedies. The ingredients are ground into a powder and either made into tea or formed into pills.

Diet and exercise are also part of TCM. Rather than aim for a diet with a balance of carbohydrates, protein, and fats, recommendations in TCM strive to remedy imbalances in yin and yang by eating certain foods and avoiding others (Xutian et al., 2009). The exercise with therapeutic properties is *qi gong*, which consists of a series of movements and breathing techniques that help with the circulation of qi.

The practices of acupuncture and qi gong as well as products such as herbal preparations are used as

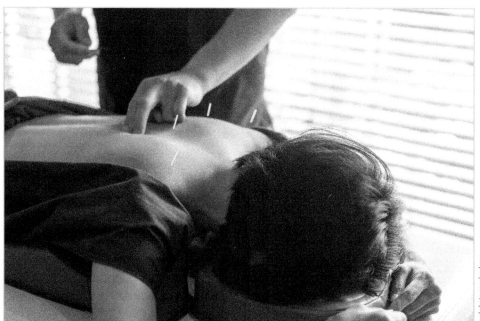

Acupuncture originated within traditional Chinese medicine and has become a popular alternative treatment.

alternative treatments for specific problems in many cultures. However, TCM consists of an integrated theory of health and practice of medicine. Ayurveda is another system of medicine that emphasizes balance.

Ayurvedic Medicine

Ayurveda, or Ayurvedic medicine, is an ancient system that arose in India; the first written texts appeared more than 2,000 years ago (NCCIH, 2005/2015). The term originated in two Sanskrit words, the combination of which means "science of life." The goal of Ayurvedic medicine is to integrate and balance the body, mind, and spirit. These three elements are believed to be an extension of the relationship among all things in the universe. Humans are born in a state of balance, but events can disrupt this balance. When these elements are out of balance, health is endangered; bringing them back into balance restores health.

Ayurvedic practitioners diagnose patients through examinations that include observation of physical characteristics as well as questions about lifestyle and behavior (NCCIH, 2005/2015). Formulating a treatment plan may require consultation with family members as well as the patient. The goals of treatment are to eliminate impurities and to increase harmony and balance, which are achieved through changes to exercise and diet. These changes may include yoga exercises and special diets or fasting to eliminate impurities in the body. Massage to vital points on the body is also part of Ayurvedic medicine, which provides pain relief and improves circulation. The use of herbs, medicated oils, spices, and minerals is extensive, yielding more than 5,000 products. Patients may also receive directions to change behaviors to reduce worry and increase harmony in their lives; yoga practice may be part of this element. Less than 1% of people in the United States have sought Ayurvedic treatment, making it much less common than TCM (Clarke et al., 2015). However, 9.5% of adults and 3.1% of children (Black et al., 2015) in the United States have practiced yoga. Table 8.1 presents elements of TCM and Ayurvedic medicine, which show the similarities in underlying philosophy and differences in terminology of these two systems.

Other alternative medical systems include *naturopathy* and *homeopathy*; both arose during the 19th century in Europe and came to North America. Each became prominent and then faded from popularity with the rise of conventional medicine. In the United States, homeopathic treatment is more common (2.2%) than naturopathic treatment (0.5%; Clarke et al., 2015), which means that neither system experiences widespread use.

TABLE 8.1   Elements of Traditional Chinese and Ayurvedic Medicine

Traditional Chinese Medicine	Ayurvedic Medicine
Basic Philosophy	
Life force (qi/chi) flows through the body along meridians and must be balanced to maintain health.	Health is achieved by a balance of body, mind, and spirit.
Origin of Disease	
There is blockage of the flow of qi.	Life circumstances and events can produce impurities and imbalances among body, mind, and spirit.
Treatments	
Exercise, including qi gong and tai chi	Exercise, including yoga
Changes to diet to balance the forces of yin and yang by eating certain foods and avoiding others	Changes to diet, including fasting or special diets
Acupuncture or acupressure to relieve pain	Massage to relieve pain and improve circulation
Tui na massage to regulate the nervous system, increase immune function, and eliminate wastes	
Preparations with herbs	Preparations with herbs, oils, spices, or minerals

IN SUMMARY

Alternative medicine consists of a group of health care systems, practices, and products that are not currently part of conventional medicine but that people use rather than (alternative medicine) or along with conventional treatments (complementary medicine).

Alternative health care systems include TCM, Ayurvedic medicine, naturopathy, and homeopathy. TCM and Ayurvedic medicine are ancient; naturopathy and homeopathy arose in the 19th century. Each of these systems presents a theory of health and disease as well as practices for diagnosis and treatment.

TCM holds that the body contains a vital energy called qi; keeping this energy in balance is essential to health. Techniques such as acupuncture and acupressure, herbal remedies, massage (called *tui na*), and the energy-channeling practices of qi gong and tai chi are aimed at achieving this balance. Ayurvedic medicine accepts the notion of vital energy and holds that the integration of body, mind, and spirit is essential to health. Diet and herbal preparations are part of Ayurvedic medicine and so is exercise, including yoga.

Naturopathy and homeopathy were prominent treatments 100 years ago in the United States, but their popularity declined and has not rebounded.

Alternative Products and Diets

The practice of supplementing the diet to improve health is ancient, originating in many cultures and variations dating back thousands of years. Currently, millions of people take vitamin and mineral supplements to preserve their health and to promote wellness, often at the suggestion of a physician or other conventional health practitioner. Thus, that practice falls within the category of conventional treatment, but some natural products are classified as alternative treatments. In the United States, the Food and Drug Administration regulates natural products as food rather than as drugs; such products are sold without restriction, without evaluations of effectiveness, but with evaluations of safety (NCCAM, 2009/2014).

The category of natural products includes a variety of supplements, probiotics and functional foods. Natural product supplements include omega-3 fatty acid supplements as a method of reducing the risks of cardiovascular disease, echinacea as a treatment for colds and flu, glucosamine for osteoarthritis, melatonin to promote sleep, and many others. *Probiotics* consist of live microorganisms that occur naturally in the digestive tract that people take to enhance digestion or to remedy digestive problems. The most common example of a probiotic is yogurt cultured with live bacteria. People also try to maintain or enhance their health by supplementing their diets with a wide variety of herbs, amino acids, extracts, special foods, and other natural products. *Functional foods* are components of a normal diet that have biologically active components, such as soy, chocolate, cranberries, and other foods containing antioxidants.

Sales of dietary supplements amount to billions of dollars each year in the United States, and supplements are among the most widely used types of alternative medicine. Table 8.2 presents the frequency of use of supplements for adults and children in the United States.

Diet is an important factor in health, and some people follow specific diet plans as a way to improve their health (rather than—or in addition to—losing weight). Such diets include vegetarian, macrobiotic, Atkins, Ornish, and Zone diets.

All vegetarian diets restrict meat and fish and focus on vegetables, fruits, grains, legumes, seeds, and plant-based oils. However, varieties of vegetarian diets include lactovegetarian, which allows dairy products, ovolacto vegetarian, which allows dairy products and eggs, and vegan diets, which allow neither dairy nor egg products. Diets that restrict meat and meat products tend to be lower in fat and higher in fiber than other diets, which make them beneficial for people with health problems such as high cholesterol levels. The American Heart Association and the American Cancer Society have recommended limiting meat consumption for health reasons. All three varieties of vegetarian diets are capable of furnishing adequate nutrition for people in all stages of development, but vegetarians must plan their meals carefully to assure that they receive adequate protein, calcium, and other nutrients that are plentiful in meat (Phillips, 2005). Those who follow very restrictive vegetarian diets such as a *macrobiotic diet* must be more careful than other vegetarians to obtain adequate nutrients. This vegetarian diet plan is not only largely vegetarian but also restricts food choices to grains, cereals, cooked vegetables, and an occasional, limited amount of fruit and fish.

The Atkins, Pritikin, Ornish, and Zone diets vary in terms of the amount of carbohydrates and fats allowed

TABLE 8.2   Most Frequently Used CAM Products

Product or Diet	Percentage of Adults Who Used This Approach	Percentage of Children (<18 years) Who Used This Approach
Nonvitamin/nonmineral supplement	17.7	4.9
Fish oil	7.8	—
Glucosamine or chondroitin	2.6	—
Probiotics	1.6	—
Melatonin	1.3	—
Echinacea	0.9	—
Diet-based therapies	3.0	0.7

Sources: Data from "Use of complementary health approaches among children aged 4–17 years in the United States: National Health Interview Survey, 2007–2012" by L. I. Black, T. C. Clarke, P. M. Barnes, B. J. Stussman, R. L. Nahin, 2015, *National Health Statistics Reports,* no. 78, Hyattsville, MD: National Center for Health Statistics; and "Trends in the use of complementary health approaches among adults: United States, 2002–2012" by T. C. Clarke, L. I. Black, B. J. Stussman, P. M. Barnes, & R. L. Nahin, 2015, *National Health Statistics Reports,* no. 79, Hyattsville, MD: National Center for Health Statistics.

and also vary in their overall goals (Gardner et al., 2007). For example, the Atkins diet program limits carbohydrates but not fat or calories, whereas the Ornish program strives to limit fat intake to 10% of calories, which makes this diet almost entirely vegetarian, difficult to follow, and thus rarely followed (Clarke et al., 2015). Special diets to promote health are not a common practice; most people who follow a restrictive diet have the goal of losing weight. As Table 8.2 shows, only 3% of people in the United States follow one of these special diets, a number that has decreased over the past 10 years (Clarke et al., 2015).

IN SUMMARY

Alternative products include dietary supplements; specialized diets are an alternative procedure. People are more likely to supplement their diets with a wide variety of vitamins, minerals, and natural products such as herbs, amino acids, extracts, and special foods to improve health or to treat specific conditions. This approach has become the most commonly used alternative medicine in the United States. Some special diets have the goal of lowering cholesterol levels, such as the Ornish, South Beach, or Zone diets; other diets have the goal of improving health, such as vegetarian and macrobiotic diets. Following a special diet is less common (3%) than using a dietary supplement (17.7%).

Manipulative Practices

Manipulative practices consist of practices oriented toward symptom relief or treatment of disease conditions. The most common are chiropractic treatment and massage. Chiropractic focuses on spinal alignment and the joints, using adjustment techniques to bring the spine back into alignment. Massage is also a manipulation technique, but massage focuses on the soft tissue. Several different types of massage exist, but many share the underlying premise that this type of manipulation helps the body to heal itself.

Chiropractic Treatment

Daniel David Palmer founded chiropractic in 1895 (NCCIH, 2007/2012). Palmer believed that manipulation of the spine was the key not only to curing illness but also to preventing it. That focus forms the basis for chiropractic care—performing adjustments to the spine and joints to correct misalignments that underlie health problems. Chiropractic adjustments involve applying pressure with the hands or with a machine that forces a joint to move beyond its passive range of motion. Chiropractors may also use heat, ice, and electric stimulation as part of treatment; they may also prescribe exercise for rehabilitation, dietary changes, or dietary supplements. With these problems corrected, the body can heal itself.

Palmer founded the first chiropractic school in 1896, and chiropractic began to spread in the United

States during the early 20th century (Pettman, 2007). Students are accepted into schools of chiropractic training after completing at least 90 hours in undergraduate college courses, focusing on science (NCCIH, 2007/2012). Chiropractic training requires an additional 4 years of study in one of the schools accredited by the Council of Chiropractic Education. The program involves coursework and patient care. All 50 states of the United States license chiropractors after they finish their course of study and undergo board examinations.

Almost from the beginning of chiropractic, physicians attacked the practice, initiating prosecutions against chiropractors for practicing medicine without a license (Pettman, 2007). The American Medical Association waged a bitter battle against chiropractic throughout the mid-20th century, but the chiropractors prevailed. Chiropractic is in the process of becoming integrated into conventional medicine; for example, requests by athletes for chiropractic treatment have encouraged its integration into sport medicine (Theberge, 2008). Chiropractic treatment is also available for clients served through the U.S. Department of Defense and the Department of Veterans Affairs, either through Veteran's Hospitals or through contracts with private providers (U.S. Department of Veterans Affairs, n.d.). Indeed, chiropractic treatment has become so well accepted that many insurance plans pay for these services. Back, neck, and headache pain are the most common condition that prompt people to seek chiropractic treatment (NCCIH, 2007/2012). Table 8.3 shows the frequency of seeking chiropractic care in the United States for children as well as adults; the percentage is somewhat higher for Canadian adults, where 11% used chiropractic within the year before the survey (Park, 2005).

Massage

Chiropractic manipulation focuses on the spine and joints, but massage manipulates soft tissue to produce health benefits. Considered a luxury a few years ago, massage is now recognized as an alternative therapy used to control stress and pain. This approach dates back thousands of years and arose in many cultures (Moyer, Rounds, & Hannum, 2004). Records of massage date back to 2000 BCE., and early healers such as Hippocrates and Galen wrote about its benefits. Table 8.3 presents the percentage of adults and children in the United States who have used massage for health benefits.

Several different types of therapeutic massage exist. Although Per Henrik Ling is often credited, it was Johann Mezger who developed the massage techniques during the 19th century that became known as Swedish massage (Pettman, 2007). This type of massage achieves relaxation by using light strokes in one direction combined with kneading muscles using deeper pressure in the opposite direction (NCCIH, 2006/2015a). Originally part of physical therapy and rehabilitation, massage is now a therapy for stress, anxiety, and various types of pain management.

Other types of massage come from other systems of medicine, including TCM, Ayurveda, and naturopathy. Acupressure and *tui na* are both manipulative techniques originating in TCM (Xue, Zhang, Greenwood, Lin, & Story, 2010). Acupressure involves the application of pressure to meridians on the body, with the goal of unblocking the flow of qi. *Shiatsu massage* is the Japanese counterpart of acupressure. *Tui na* is another approach from TCM for allowing the qi to flow freely throughout the body. It may involve pushing the qi along specific meridians using one finger or thumb, which is also similar to shiatsu massage. The rationale for Ayurvedic

TABLE 8.3   Most Frequently Used Manipulative Practices

Manipulative Practices	Percentage of Adults Who Used This Approach	Percentage of Children (<18 years) Who Used This Approach
Chiropractic manipulation	8.4	3.3
Massage	6.9	0.7

Source: Data from "Use of complementary health approaches among children aged 4–17 years in the United States: National Health Interview Survey, 2007–2012" by L. I. Black, T. C. Clarke, P. M. Barnes, B. J. Stussman, R. L. Nahin, 2015, *National Health Statistics Reports,* no. 78, Hyattsville, MD: National Center for Health Statistics; and "Trends in the use of complementary health approaches among adults: United States, 2002–2012" by T. C. Clarke, L. I. Black, B. J. Stussman, P. M. Barnes, & R. L. Nahin, 2015, *National Health Statistics Reports,* no. 79, Hyattsville, MD: National Center for Health Statistics.

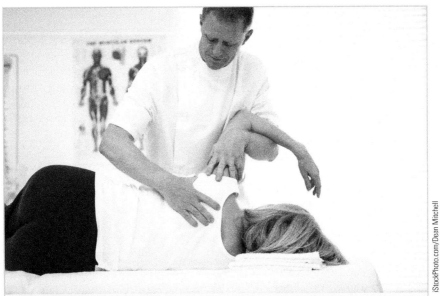

Manipulating the spinal cord or muscles can be effective in helping to relieve pain.

massage holds that manipulating specific points on the body will channel healing energy within the body. Its practice often involves medicinal oils to decrease friction and to help with the healing. Thus, the practice of massage is common in CAM, arising from several systems and used as an independent healing practice.

IN SUMMARY

Manipulative practices include chiropractic treatments and massage. Chiropractic focuses on spinal alignment and the joints, using adjustment techniques to bring the spine back into alignment. Massage is also a manipulation technique, but massage focuses on the soft tissue. Several different types of massage exist, but many share the underlying premise that this type of manipulation helps the body to heal itself.

Mind–Body Medicine

Mind–body medicine   It is the term applied to a variety of techniques based on the notion that the brain, mind, body, and behavior interact in complex ways and that

emotional, mental, social, and behavioral factors exert important effects on health (NCCIH, 2008/2015). Some of these techniques are associated with psychology and some with conventional medicine, but all share the notion that mind and body represent a holistic system of dynamic interactions. Norman Cousins, whose story began this chapter, was an enthusiastic proponent of this view. However, this conception is not recent; it forms the basis for TCM, Ayurvedic medicine, and many other systems of traditional and folk medicine. This notion was also prominent in Europe until the 17th century, when French philosopher René Descartes proposed that the mind and the body work according to different principles. Descartes' pronouncement promoted the view that the body functions according to mechanistic principles, which was important in the development of Western medicine but discounted the importance of the mind in physical health.

Those who accept mind–body medicine seek to understand the interaction of mind and body and its relationship to health. Some of the techniques of mind–body medicine come from those systems that propose a holistic view, such as TCM and Ayurvedic medicine. However, the techniques include not only meditation, tai chi, qi gong, and yoga, which arose within those systems of medicine but also guided imagery, hypnosis, and biofeedback. A component that is common to most

TABLE 8.4   Most Frequently Used CAM Therapies

Mind–Body Approaches	Percentage of Adults Who Used This Approach	Percentage of Children (<18 years) Who Used This Approach
Deep breathing	10.9	2.7
Meditation	8.0	1.6
Guided imagery	1.7	0.4
Yoga	9.5	3.1
Tai chi	1.1	0.2
Qi gong	0.3	0.1
Biofeedback	0.1	<0.1
Hypnosis	0.1	—

Source: Data from "Use of complementary health approaches among children aged 4–17 years in the United States: National Health Interview Survey, 2007–2012" by L. I. Black, T. C. Clarke, P. M. Barnes, B. J. Stussman, R. L. Nahin, 2015, *National Health Statistics Reports,* no. 78, Hyattsville, MD: National Center for Health Statistics; and "Trends in the use of complementary health approaches among adults: United States, 2002–2012" by T. C. Clarke, L. I. Black, B. J. Stussman, P. M. Barnes, & R. L. Nahin, 2015, *National Health Statistics Reports,* no. 79, Hyattsville, MD: National Center for Health Statistics.

of these practices is deep, controlled breathing, but many people in the United States use deep-breathing exercises alone rather than as a part of other mind–body techniques (Clarke et al., 2015). Table 8.4 shows the frequency of this and other mind–body practices among adults and children in the United States.

Meditation and Yoga

Most approaches to meditation originated in Asia as part of religious practices, but the mind–body approaches to meditation typically have no religious connotations (NCCIH, 2007/2016b). Many variations of meditation exist, but all involve a quiet location, a specific posture, a focus of attention, and an open attitude. Table 8.4 shows the use of meditation among adults and children in the United States. The two most prominent types of meditation are transcendental meditation and mindfulness meditation.

Transcendental Meditation   Transcendental meditation originated in the Vedic tradition in India. Participants who practice this type of meditation usually sit with eyes closed and muscles relaxed. They then focus attention on their breathing and silently repeat a sound, such as "om" or any other personally meaningful word or phrase, with each breath for about 20 minutes. Repetition of the single word is intended to prevent distracting thoughts and to sustain muscle relaxation. Meditation requires a conscious motivation to focus

attention on a single thought or image along with effort not to be distracted by other thoughts.

Mindfulness Meditation   Mindfulness meditation has roots in ancient Buddhist practice (Bodhi, 2011) but has been adapted as a modern stress reduction practice. In mindfulness meditation, people usually sit in a relaxed, upright posture and focus on any thoughts or sensations as they occur, trying to enhance their own awareness of their perceptions and thought processes in a nonjudgmental way (Kabat-Zinn, 1993). If unpleasant thoughts or sensations occur, meditators are encouraged not to ignore them, but to let them pass and to concentrate on the breath. By noting thoughts objectively, without censoring or editing them, people can gain insight into how they see the world and what motivates them.

Mindfulness meditation has been adapted into a program of mindfulness-based stress reduction (Kabat-Zinn, 1993). This procedure involves an 8-week course of training, which typically occurs for at least 2 hours per day and may also include an intensive retreat to develop meditation skills. Mindfulness-based stress reduction is useful in a wide variety of settings to help people control anxiety and manage chronic disease and pain conditions. Systematic review and meta-analysis (Goyal et al., 2014) indicated that this approach showed a moderate-sized effect in helping people manage anxiety, depression, and pain.

Becoming Healthier

One technique that helps people manage and minimize pain is guided imagery. This technique involves creating an image and being guided (or guiding yourself) through it. The process can be helpful in dealing with both chronic pain and acute pain, such as medical or dental procedures. Those who are not experienced at guided imagery will benefit from having a recorded version of the guided imagery instructions.

To practice guided imagery, choose a quiet place where you will not be disturbed and where you will be comfortable. Prepare for the experience by placing the recording where you can turn it on, seating yourself in a comfortable chair, and taking a few deep breaths. Turn on the player, close your eyes, and follow the instructions you have recorded.

The instructions should include a description of a special place, one that you either imagine or have experienced, where you feel safe and at peace. Tailor the place to fit with your life and experiences—one person's magic place may not be so attractive to another person, so think about what will be appealing to you. Many people enjoy a beach scene, but others like woods, fields, or special rooms. The goal is to imagine somewhere that you will feel relaxed and at peace.

Put instructions on your recording concerning this place and its description. Spend time in this place and experience it in detail. Pay attention to the sights and sounds, but do not neglect the smells and skin senses associated with the place. Spend time imagining each of these

sensory experiences, and include instructions to yourself about the feelings. You should feel relaxed and peaceful as you go through this scene. Linger over the details and aim to allow yourself to become completely absorbed in the experience.

Include some instructions for relaxed breathing in your tour of your special place. Your goal is to achieve peace and relaxation that will replace the anxiety and pain that you have felt. As you repeat the guided imagery exercise, you may want to revise the recorded instructions to include more details. The recording should include at least 10 minutes of guided instructions, and your experience and practice may lead you to lengthen it. Eventually, you will not need the recording, and you will be able to use this technique wherever you go.

Guided Imagery   Guided imagery shares some elements with meditation but also has important differences. In guided imagery, people conjure up a calm, peaceful image, such as the repetitive rhythmic roar of an ocean or the quiet beauty of an outdoor scene. They then concentrate on that image for the duration of a situation, often one that is painful or anxiety provoking. The assumption underlying guided imagery is that a person cannot concentrate on more than one thing at a time. Therefore, imagining an especially powerful or peaceful scene will divert attention from the painful experience (see Becoming Healthier box). Table 8.4 shows how uncommon guided imagery practice is.

Yoga   Yoga has its origins in ancient India (refer back to Table 8.1) but is now part of mind–body practice (NCCIH, 2008/2013). It includes physical postures, breathing, and meditation, and its goal is to balance body, mind, and spirit. Of the various schools of yoga, Hatha yoga is the most common in the United States and Europe. The many postures of yoga furnish ways to move

and concentrate energy in the body. This concentration of attention on the body permits people to ignore other situations and problems and to live in their bodies in the moment. The controlled breathing fosters relaxation. Table 8.4 shows that yoga is among the more common mind–body practices among both adults and children.

Qi Gong and Tai Chi

TCM includes movement-based approaches to unblock qi and improve health. The basic technique is *qi gong* (also written *qigong, chi gung,* and *chi gong*), which consists of a series of exercises or movements intended to concentrate and balance the body's vital energy (Sancier & Holman, 2004). Its practice promotes relaxation and provides exercise. Tai chi or *tai chi chuan* originated as one of the martial arts but evolved into a set of movements used for therapeutic benefits (Gallagher, 2003).

Qi Gong   Qi gong involves the practice or cultivation (gong) of the qi (energy) by postures and simple movements that channel vital energy and restore balance in the body. It is one of the basic practices of TCM (Twicken, 2011). One way to view qi gong is as "the manipulation of the regulation of the body, breath, and mind into an integrative whole, with the breath as the key regulator practice to make this happen" (Shinnick, 2006, p. 351). These postures and movements may be practiced individually or integrated into a sequence, called a *form*. Within TCM, the practice of qi gong increases health and decreases the need for treatments such as acupuncture and herbal remedies.

Although qi gong fits within the philosophy of TCM, its practice has been adapted to be compatible with Western medicine, under the name *medical qi gong* (He, 2005; Twicken, 2011). Researchers have investigated the physical existence of qi, with claims that the practice of qi gong creates measurable changes in thermal and electrical energy (Shinnick, 2006). The practice of medical qi gong seeks to prevent disease, promote long life, and treat specific disease conditions such as hypertension, diabetes, and heart disease as well as stress and pain. Table 8.4 shows that the rate of qi gong practice is low in the United States.

Tai Chi Tai chi (or *tai chi chuan*) is one category of qi gong form, which has evolved from a martial art with a

long but disputed history. Some advocates trace its history back thousands of years, whereas others point to a history of only several hundred years (Kurland, 2000). The key figures in its development are also the subject of debate, but a commonly cited story involves a Shaolin monk who noticed the struggle between a snake and a crane and adapted their movements to a form of defense. Over time, the practice of tai chi became increasingly popular as a way to promote health, spreading throughout China and around the world. As one of the practices of TCM, tai chi cultivates balance between the yin and yang energies and thus promotes health.

Tai chi involves slow, gentle movements that shift the weight while the person maintains an upright yet relaxed posture and controlled breathing (NCCIH, 2006/2015b). One movement flows into another, and those who practice tai chi strive to maintain a steady rate of movement while coordinating the breath with the movements, creating a "moving meditation." The history of tai chi includes the development of many different styles, originally perpetuated within families. Currently, the Yang style is the most common in China and among those who practice tai chi as alternative medicine. All of the variations in styles include a set of movements connected together into a sequence, called

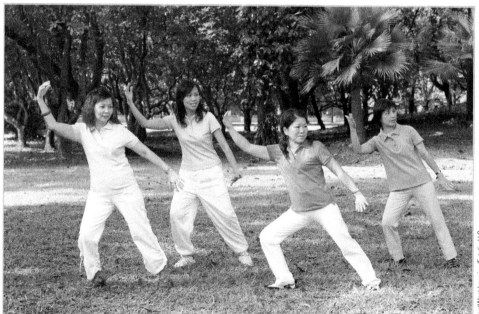

Tai chi chuan is a movement-based technique that produces physical and psychological benefits.

EastWest Imaging/Fotolia LLC

a form. Tai chi provides moderate intensity aerobic exercise equivalent to brisk walking and a low-impact form of exercise that is appropriate for a wide variety of individuals (Taylor-Piliae, Haskell, Waters, & Froelicher, 2006). As Table 8.4 shows, tai chi is more widely practiced in the United States than qi gong.

Biofeedback

Until the 1960s, most people in the Western world assumed that it was impossible to consciously control physiological processes such as heart rate, the secretion of digestive juices, and the constriction of blood vessels. These biological functions do not require conscious attention for their regulation, and conscious attempts at regulation seem to have little effect. Then, during the late 1960s, a number of researchers began to explore the possibility of controlling biological processes traditionally believed to be beyond conscious control. Their efforts culminated in the development of **biofeedback,** the process of providing feedback information about the status of biological systems. Early experiments indicated that biofeedback made possible the control of some otherwise automatic functions. In 1969, Neal E. Miller reported a series of experiments in which he and his colleagues altered the levels of animals' visceral response through reinforcement. Some subjects received rewards for raising their heart rate and others for lowering it. Within a few hours, significant differences in heart rate appeared. After other investigators demonstrated that biofeedback could be used with humans (Brown, 1970; Kamiya, 1969), interest in this procedure became widespread.

In biofeedback, electronic instruments measure biological responses, and the status of those responses becomes immediately available to the person using the machines. By using biofeedback, a person gains information about changes in biological responses as those responses are taking place. This immediate feedback allows the person to alter physiological responses that are otherwise almost impossible to control voluntarily.

Many types of biofeedback exist; few are common in clinical use, but electromyography and thermal biofeedback are more common than other types. **Electromyograph (EMG) biofeedback** reflects the activity of the skeletal muscles by measuring the electrical discharge in muscle fibers. The measurement is taken by attaching electrodes to the surface of the skin over the muscles to be monitored. The level of electrical activity reflects the degree of tension or relaxation of the muscles. The machine responds with a signal that varies according to that muscle activity. Biofeedback can be used to increase muscle tension in rehabilitation or to decrease muscle tension in stress management. The most common use of EMG biofeedback among CAM users is in the control of low back pain and headaches; however, EMG biofeedback is becoming more widely recognized as being useful in rehabilitation (Giggins, Persson, & Caulfield, 2013).

Thermal biofeedback, which may also be used to help people cope with stress and pain, is based on the principle that skin temperature varies in relation to levels of stress. Stress tends to constrict blood vessels, whereas relaxation opens them. Therefore, cool surface skin temperature may indicate stress and tension; warm skin temperature suggests calm and relaxation. Thermal biofeedback involves placing a **thermistor**—a temperature-sensitive resistor—on the skin's surface. The thermistor signals changes in skin temperature, thereby furnishing the information that allows control. The feedback signal, as with EMG biofeedback, may be auditory, visual, or both. As Table 8.4 shows, children rarely receive biofeedback, and the practice is not common among adults.

Hypnotic Treatment

Although trancelike conditions are probably older than human history, modern hypnosis is usually traced to the last part of the 18th century, when Austrian physician Franz Anton Mesmer conducted elaborate demonstrations in Paris. Although Mesmer's work was attacked, modifications of his technique, known as *mesmerism,* soon spread to other parts of the world. By the 1830s, mesmerism was being used by some surgeons as an anesthetic during major operations (Hilgard & Hilgard, 1994).

With the discovery of chemical anesthetics, the popularity of hypnosis waned, but during the late 19th century, many European physicians, including Sigmund Freud, employed hypnotic procedures in the treatment of mental illness. Since the beginning of the 20th century, the popularity of hypnosis as a medical and psychological tool has continued to wax and wane. Its present position is still somewhat controversial, but a significant number of practitioners within medicine and psychology are using hypnotherapy to treat health-related problems, especially pain. As Table 8.4 shows, the technique remains in limited use.

Not only is the use of hypnotic processes still controversial but the precise nature of hypnosis is also debatable. Some authorities, such as Joseph Barber (1996) and Ernest Hilgard (1978), regarded hypnosis as an altered *state* of consciousness in which a person's stream of consciousness is divided or dissociated. Barber argued that hypnotic analgesia works through a process of negative hallucination—not perceiving something that one would ordinarily perceive. To Hilgard, the process of **induction**—that is, being placed into a hypnotic state—is central to the hypnotic process. After induction, the responsive person enters a state of divided or dissociated consciousness that is essentially different from the normal state. This altered state of consciousness allows people to respond to suggestion and to control physiological processes that they cannot control in the normal state of consciousness.

The alternative view of hypnosis holds that it is a more generalized *trait,* or a relatively permanent characteristic of some people who respond well to suggestion (T. X. Barber, 1984, 2000). Those who hold this view reject the basic conception that hypnosis is altered consciousness. Rather, they argue that hypnosis is nothing more than relaxation, induction is not necessary, and suggestive procedures can be just as effective without entering a trancelike state.

Research has not resolved this controversy. Brain imaging studies (De Benedittis, 2003; Rainville & Price, 2003) tend to support the view that hypnosis is an altered state of consciousness. However, in a study comparing hypnotic to nonhypnotic suggestion (Milling, Kirsch, Allen, & Reutenauer, 2005), both types were comparably effective. That is, expectancy and suggestion led to a reduction of pain whether participants were hypnotized or not.

Physiology and Mind–Body Medicine

A growing body of research validates the extent to which mind–body medicine lives up to its name; that is, these behavioral techniques affect a variety of biological processes. For example, brain imaging studies have helped clarify what happens when a person relaxes and meditates. Attention and executive function monitoring are altered in meditation (Manna et al., 2010), and different meditation techniques prompt different patterns of brain activation. Other research has explored what brain changes accompany meditation, suggesting that practicing meditation may have the capability to delay or even reverse some of the brain changes that occur through aging (Luders, 2013).

Research into the nature of mindfulness training (Jha, Krompinger, & Baime, 2007) suggests that it improves attention processes by altering the subcomponents of attention such as orienting attention and alerting attention. In mindfulness meditation, the prefrontal cortex and anterior cingulate cortex show higher levels of activation, and long-term experience with meditation prompts changes in brain structures involved in attention (Chiesa & Serretti, 2010). Additional research (Hölzel et al., 2011) confirmed that mindfulness meditation works by altering brain function.

Another physiological effect of mindfulness-based stress reduction involves improved function in several immune system components (Rosenkranz et al., 2013). A meta-analysis (Morgan, Irwin, Chung, & Wang, 2014) confirmed the ability of mind–body techniques to modulate immune system function. Evidence also exists that qi gong training produces changes in the function of the immune system (Lee, Kim, & Ryu, 2005). These physiological effects specify routes through which meditation and qi gong might improve health.

IN SUMMARY

Mind–body medicine is a term applied to a variety of techniques that people use to improve their health or treat health problems, including meditation, guided imagery, yoga, qi gong, tai chi, biofeedback, and hypnosis. Transcendental meditation directs people to focus on a single thought or sound to achieve relaxation, whereas mindfulness meditation encourages practitioners to focus on the moment, becoming mindful of the details of their current experience. Guided imagery encourages people to create a pleasant scene to achieve relaxation and anxiety relief. Yoga uses physical postures, breathing, and meditation, with the goal of balancing body, mind, and spirit. The movement-based practices of qi gong and tai chi originated in TCM. Qi gong and tai chi involve postures and movements intended to direct and balance the body's vital energy.

Biofeedback is the process of providing feedback information about the status of biological systems with the goal of controlling them. Many types of biofeedback exist, but learning to control muscle tension through electromyograph biofeedback and skin temperature through thermal biofeedback have the widest clinical applications. Hypnotic treatment is controversial, with some authorities arguing that it represents an altered state of consciousness that boosts relaxation and suggestibility, whereas others contend that it is a trait of some individuals. In either case, relaxation and suggestibility both have the potential to improve health.

Mind–body medicine also has the power to alter physiology. Meditation, mindfulness meditation, and qi gong have all shown the power to alter physiological processes. These beneficial changes include altering brain function for more effective cognitive processing, slowing brain changes that accompany aging, and boosting some components of immune efficiency.

Who Uses Complementary and Alternative Medicine?

People use techniques from CAM to enhance health, prevent disease, and manage health problems. Many of the techniques from CAM are applicable and widely used in managing anxiety, stress, and pain. Indeed, a great deal of the research funded by the U.S. National Center for Complementary and Integrative Health is oriented toward assessing the effectiveness of these approaches for these conditions.

The number of people who find CAM techniques appealing has grown, and research has also tracked that growth. A comparison of CAM use in 2002, 2007, and 2012 in the United States (Black et al., 2015; Clarke et al., 2015) showed increases between 2002 and 2007 for many categories and continued increases in 2012 for a few. The number of people who use natural products such as omege-3 fatty acid supplements, glucosamine, and echinacea remained the most popular CAM over the three assessments. Increases also appeared between 2002 and 2007 for the use of deep-breathing exercises, meditation, yoga, massage, and chiropractic care. Between 2007 and 2012, few increases occurred. However, the practice of yoga, which increased to 9.5%, was an exception.

People not only use a variety of CAM techniques but they also use the techniques for a variety of reasons. However, pain is a prominent problem that brings adults (Zhang et al., 2015) and children (Black et al., 2015) to use CAM. The situation suggests that CAM users tend to have conditions that are painful, a suggestion confirmed by other analyses (Ayers & Kronenfeld, 2011; Wells, Phillips, Schachter, & McCarthy, 2010).

In addition, the pain has often not been addressed through conventional medicine (Freedman, 2011), leading these patients to seek alternative care in addition to conventional treatment. Indeed, most people who use CAM combine the techniques with conventional treatments rather than abandoning conventional treatments. This pattern is similar to CAM use in Europe (Rössler et al., 2007), Canada (Foltz et al., 2005), and Israel (Shmueli, Igudin, & Shuval, 2011).

Culture, Ethnicity, and Gender

The use of CAM varies among countries to some extent. In a population study in Australia, 68.9% of people (Xue, Zhang, Lin, Da Costa, & Story, 2007) and over 70% of Australian women (Bowe, Adams, Liu, & Sibbritt, 2015) reported using some form of CAM, indicating a substantially higher level of use than in the United States. The Australian government has integrated CAM into health care delivery to a greater extent than in most other English-speaking countries (Baer, 2008), so high prevalence is reasonable.

In Europe, the percentage of users varies by country. Some countries are similar to the United States, whereas others use CAM as frequently as Australians do (di Sarsina, 2007). The types of treatments and demographics of users are similar among these three geographic areas. Nutritional supplements, massage therapy, meditation, chiropractic treatments, yoga, and acupuncture are among the most popular CAM therapies (Xue et al., 2007).

Within Europe, the availability of CAM varies. In some countries, such as Sweden, the availability is limited; the Swedish health service does not consider offering CAM treatments because of insufficient evidence of their effectiveness (di Sarsina, 2007). In other countries, such as Germany and the United Kingdom, CAM is integrated into medical practice; physicians receive training in CAM and refer patients to CAM practitioners. In countries in which CAM is integrated into the health services, users tend to come from a wider variety of socioeconomic backgrounds than in countries such as the United States, where most CAM users must pay out-of-pocket for such treatment (Romeyke & Stummer, 2015).

In the United States and Canada, CAM use varies with ethnicity in complex ways (Park, 2013). The variations do not correspond to stereotypes that link CAM with ethnic minorities and immigrants (Keith, Kronenfeld, Rivers, & Liang, 2005; Roth &

Kobayashi, 2008): Non-Hispanic European Americans are more likely than African Americans or Hispanic Americans to use CAM (Clarke et al., 2015). Indeed, recent immigrants are *less* likely to use CAM than immigrants who have been in the United States for years (Su, Li, & Pagán, 2008). A similar finding emerged from a study of Asian Americans (Hsiao, Wong, et al., 2006) and Asians in Canada (Roth & Kobayashi, 2008). However, Asian Americans used CAM at higher rates than non-Hispanic European Americans, and Asians in Canada use CAM more frequently than the Canadian population in general. Chinese Americans' usage of CAM tended to correspond to their culture: Chinese Americans were more likely than other Asian Americans to use herbal products (Hsiao, Wong, et al., 2006) and to seek acupuncture treatment (Burke, Upchurch, Dye, & Chyu, 2006). Similar patterns apply to countries around the world: Acupuncture is more common in Japan, Singapore, Australia, and Canada than in Saudi Arabia, Israel, or Denmark (Cooper, Harris, Relton, & Thomas, 2013). In Canada, use of CAM is related to how strongly users identified with Asian culture (Roth & Kobayashi, 2008).

In all ethnic groups and in various countries, individuals who seek CAM tend to be female, in the upper-income brackets, and well-educated. In the United States, well-educated European American women are more likely than others to use CAM (Zhang et al., 2015). Even among children who use CAM, girls from upper-income families are more common than others (Groenewald, Beals-Erickson, Ralston-Wilson, Rabbitts, & Palermo, 2016). Education is also a factor, and one study (Burke, Nahin, & Stussman, 2015) pointed to a lack of health knowledge as a factor that prevents people from using CAM. The willingness of women to use CAM may relate to health concerns but also to personal beliefs (Furnham, 2007). The importance of personal beliefs and the compatibility of CAM with one's beliefs may explain the motivation of some people to seek alternative treatments, whereas others do not.

Motivations for Seeking Alternative Treatment

Although culture, ethnicity, and gender each shows a relationship to CAM use, other factors are probably more important. One of those important factors is acceptance of the underlying values of CAM. Research findings suggest that people use CAM when the techniques are compatible with their personal worldviews and concerns about health (Astin, 1998). For example,

young men who expressed strong beliefs in science were less likely to use CAM than other people (Furnham, 2007). People who have less faith in conventional medicine and stronger beliefs in the role of attitude and emotion in health are more likely to try CAM. Thus, openness to different worldviews, acceptance of the value in holistic treatment, and belief in the contribution of biopsychosocial factors to health are more typical of CAM users than of those who stay with conventional treatments exclusively.

A person's current health status is also an important predictor of CAM usage. People tend to seek alternative treatments when conventional medicine has not offered relief for their conditions. Those who use CAM may not be dissatisfied with conventional medicine (Astin, 1998); people tend to add alternative treatments to the conventional ones they are using rather than replace conventional treatments with alternative ones. Research on a representative sample of U.S. residents (Nerurkar, Yeh, Davis, Birdee, & Phillips, 2011) found the combination of chronic health problems and a persistence of those problems related to the willingness of physicians to refer these patients to CAM practitioners. The findings from this study and an older study (Freedman, 2011) suggest that unresponsive chronic conditions make people more willing to seek alternative treatments. Reasonably enough, people who are unwell and continue to experience distressing symptoms are motivated to find some effective treatment, including alternative medicine. For example, people who received treatment for cancer were substantially more likely to use CAM than those who had not been treated for cancer (Mao, Palmer, Healy, Desai, & Amsterdam, 2011). One analysis (Ayers & Kronenfeld, 2011) indicated that the experience of pain was the best predictor of who had used CAM, which is also true for children who use CAM (Groenewald et al., 2016). However, one survey of CAM users (Nguyen, Davis, Kaptchuk, & Phillips, 2011) indicated that they were more likely than nonusers to rate their health as excellent and to say that their health had improved over the previous year. This combination of findings suggests that CAM users may fall into one group who seek alternative treatments due to some health problem and another who strive to maintain or better their health through CAM.

Within both conventional and alternative medicine lie concerns about effectiveness and safety for the various products and practices that fall within CAM. What is the evidence of success for these alternative approaches?

IN SUMMARY

Most people who use CAM use it as a complementary rather than an alternative treatment. People in the United States and other countries use a great variety of CAM products and practices, including natural products, deep-breathing exercises, massage, meditation, chiropractic treatments, and yoga. People in Australia and some European countries use CAM more often than people in the United States, but the assortment of techniques is similar. Ethnicity is a factor in CAM use in the United States, but ethnic stereotypes of recent immigrants' using traditional remedies is incorrect. CAM usage is associated with being female, European American, well-educated, and in a high-income bracket. This combination of demographic characteristics also applies to CAM use in Canada, Australia, and some European countries.

People are motivated to use CAM if their worldviews are compatible with the philosophies that underlie CAM—accepting a biopsychosocial view of health rather than a biomedical view. Health status is also a motivation for seeking CAM; people who have health problems that have not responded to conventional treatments may be motivated to seek CAM.

How Effective Are Alternative Treatments?

Alternative treatments are classified as *alternative* because insufficient evidence exists for their effectiveness. However, a great deal of controversy exists concerning fair evaluation of alternative medicine. Advocates of conventional medicine contend that evidence is weak concerning the effectiveness of alternative treatments and that the dangers remain unevaluated (Berman & Straus, 2004; Wahlberg, 2007). According to this view, the only acceptable method of establishing effectiveness is the randomized controlled trial in which participants are assigned randomly to a treatment group or a placebo control group in a double-blind design; neither practitioner nor participants know to which treatment condition participants belong.

Using the randomized controlled method of conducting experiments allows researchers to minimize the influence of bias and expectation. Both of these factors are important in evaluating treatment studies (as discussed in Chapter 2). People who have expectations concerning CAM will bring this bias into treatment, which may affect the outcome. For example, a study on acupuncture (Linde et al., 2007) assessed participants' attitudes about the effectiveness of acupuncture at the beginning of the study. The results indicated that those who expressed belief that acupuncture was an effective treatment experienced greater pain relief from an 8-week course of treatment than did those who had lower expectations for success. Although expectations for success boost treatment effectiveness, these expectations are a placebo response rather than a response to the treatment. Thus, those who advocate for randomized placebo-controlled trials have a valid point: This design represents a stringent criterion for evidence of effectiveness.

Unfortunately, many alternative treatments do not lend themselves to placebo control and blinding as easily as drug treatments do. For example, most people who receive a massage, practice meditation, or learn biofeedback training cannot be blind to their treatment, nor can practitioners of massage, biofeedback, or yoga be unaware of the treatment they deliver. Thus, fewer options exist for controlling for expectation in CAM than in research on conventional medicine. When studies lack random assignment, placebo control, and "blinding," advocates of conventional medicine judge these studies to be of lesser quality and thus less convincing. By these standards, CAM is inadequate; the standards that advocates of conventional medicine believe to be essential cannot be met. Regardless of the number of studies with positive results, treatments that have few randomized controlled trials will always yield judgments of insufficient evidence to make conclusions of effectiveness in systematic reviews.

Disputing the standard of randomized controlled trials is one strategy that CAM advocates have used to argue that CAM is the target of inappropriate judgments (Clark-Grill, 2007; Schneider & Perle, 2012), and others (Wider & Boddy, 2009) have warned that conducting systematic reviews on CAM treatments requires extra care to achieve a fair evaluation.

Another type of objection has come from the argument that conventional medicine has not met the standards that its defenders have required of CAM. Kenneth Pelletier (2002) argued that many of the treatments used in conventional medicine have not submitted this standard of evidence. Rather, much of the practice of conventional medicine has not come to be accepted through evidence from randomized controlled trials. Instead, many of the standard treatments in medicine and surgery have evolved through clinical practice and observation of what works rather than through experimental evidence of effectiveness. Indeed, the concept of evidence-based medicine is relatively recent. This standard is being applied to CAM more stringently than to treatments within conventional medicine.

Despite these barriers, CAM researchers strive to conduct research that demonstrates effectiveness and safety; this route allows for greater acceptability of CAM treatments (Shannon, Weil, & Kaplan, 2011). What does the evidence say about alternative treatments? Which approaches have demonstrated that they are effective, and for what conditions?

Alternative Treatments for Anxiety, Stress, and Depression

Many CAM modalities have targeted anxiety, stress, and depression, and some have demonstrated their effectiveness. Meditation is an obvious choice for these conditions, and the research evidence confirms its effectiveness.

A systematic review of meditation for stress and stress-related health problems (Goyal et al., 2014) indicated benefits large enough to have clinical significance. In addition, similar evaluations of specific meditation techniques offer support for their effectiveness. For example, meta-analyses and systematic reviews of mindfulness-based stress reduction (Chisea & Serretti, 2010; Grossman, Niemann, Schmidt, & Walach, 2004; Ivanovski & Malhi, 2007) and mindfulness-based cognitive therapy (Fjorback, Arendt, Ørnbøl, Fink, & Walach, 2011) have found positive results. Mindfulness-based approaches seem to be effective for a wide variety of people for anxiety, stress-related problems, and prevention of relapse into depression. The analyses also indicated that mindfulness meditation can help not only people with stress-related and anxiety disorders but also people without clinical problems who are seeking better ways to manage the stresses in their lives. Those who practiced the technique more also received greater benefits, indicating a dose–response relationship (Carmody & Baer, 2008).

Studies on transcendental meditation have also been the focus of a systematic review (Krisanaprakornkit, Krisanaprakornkit, Piyavhatkul, & Laopaiboon, 2006), which indicated that this type of meditation is similar to other relaxation modalities in helping people with anxiety disorders. A systematic review of

yoga (Chong, Tsunaka, Tsang, Chan, & Cheung, 2011) showed that yoga also constitutes an effective approach to stress management. Thus, the majority of evidence indicates that meditation and programs that include meditation are effective treatment for managing anxiety and depression.

The movement-based practices of qi gong and tai chi also show stress-reducing effects. A number of physiological measurements indicate that the practice of qi gong reduces stress (Sancier & Holman, 2004) and affects the nervous system in ways that reduce the stress response and improve several chronic illnesses (Ng & Tsang, 2009). A study of older Chinese immigrants at risk for cardiovascular disease showed improvements in mood and stress after practicing tai chi for 12 weeks (Taylor-Piliae et al., 2006). A systematic review of tai chi practice (Wang, Bannuru, et al., 2010) indicated a wide range of benefits including relief from anxiety, stress, and depression. A systematic review of qi gong practice (Wang et al., 2014) revealed benefits in reducing anxiety and stress.

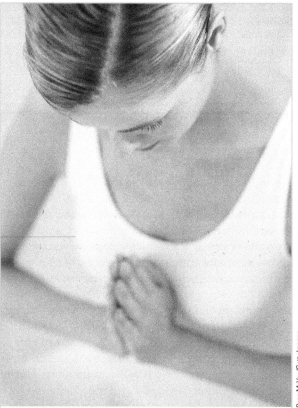

Meditation can help people cope with depression and a variety of stress-related problems.

Acupuncture also holds some promise in treating depression. In systematic reviews (Leo & Ligot, 2007; Smith, Hay, & MacPherson, 2010), evaluating the effectiveness of acupuncture for depression was difficult, but results indicated that responses to acupuncture treatment were comparable to the use of antidepressant drugs in relieving symptoms of depression. The possibility also exists that combining acupuncture treatment with medication will lead to a boost in effectiveness (Smith et al., 2010). Yoga has also been a successful complementary treatment for depressed people who did not experience a complete response to antidepressant drugs (Shapiro, Cook, et al., 2007). Another effective alternative treatment for depression is the herbal remedy Saint-John's wort. A meta-analysis of randomized controlled trials indicated that an extract of this herb alleviates mild to moderate clinical depression, with effectiveness similar to that of antidepressant drugs, but with fewer side effects (Linde, Berner, & Kriston, 2008).

Therefore, a variety of alternative medicine approaches have demonstrated effectiveness in treating anxiety, stress, and depression. Table 8.5 summarizes the evidence for alternative treatments for anxiety, stress, and depression.

Alternative Treatments for Pain

As Chapter 7 presents, chronic pain presents problems for those who experience it and for those who attempt to treat it. Conventional medicine often fails to control pain adequately, which motivates many people to seek alternative treatments (Ayers & Kronenfeld, 2011; Wells et al., 2010). A variety of alternative treatments have been applied to the problem of pain, but the CAM techniques that are successful in managing pain vary somewhat from those that are effective in managing anxiety, stress, and depression.

Meditation and the related technique of guided imagery received a strong endorsement from a National Institutes of Health Technology panel review, which concluded that these interventions were effective in managing chronic pain (Lebovits, 2007). More recent research (Grant, Courtemanche, Duerden, Duncan, & Rainville, 2010) has determined that experienced meditators' pain sensitivity decreases, including detectable brain changes that underlie this benefit. A test of mindfulness-based stress reduction, which consists of mindfulness-based meditation and yoga, demonstrated effectiveness in managing low back pain, both after an 8-week training and at a 1-year follow-up (Cherkin et al., 2016).

Guided imagery has also been described as a best practice for the pain associated with pregnancy and childbirth (Naparstek, 2007). This technique is also effective in managing headaches (Tsao & Zeltzer, 2005) and for reducing postoperative pain in children (Huth, Broome, & Good, 2004) and in older people (Antall & Kresevic, 2004).

Techniques derived from TCM can also be useful in pain control, including tai chi, qi gong, and acupuncture. Tai chi demonstrated its effectiveness in helping adults with tension headache manage their pain (Abbott, Hui, Hays, Li, & Pan, 2007). A systematic review of studies of qi gong (Lee, Pittler, & Ernst, 2007a) found encouraging evidence regarding its effectiveness in treating chronic pain. Randomized controlled trials showed that qi gong (Haak & Scott, 2008) and tai chi (Wang, Schmid, et al., 2010) provided relief from pain and improvement in quality of life for people with fibromyalgia.

Acupuncture is better established as a pain treatment than either tai chi or qi gong. A study of the brain changes in connection with acupuncture (Napadow et al., 2007) revealed that participants who received acupuncture, compared with those who received sham acupuncture, showed changes in brain activity that were consistent with decreases in pain perception. Acupuncture also produces complex reactions in the somatosensory system and alters the neurochemistry of the central nervous system, which is likely related to its analgesic effects (Manni, Albanesi, Guaragna, Barbaro Paparo, & Aloe, 2010).

Reviews of the effectiveness of acupuncture for a variety of pain conditions have indicated that acupuncture has demonstrated positive effects for some pain conditions but not for others. For example, the evidence about benefits of acupuncture is persuasive for success in treating neck pain (Trinh, Graham, Irnich, Cameron, & Forget, 2016) and more successful for neck pain than shoulder or elbow pain (Dhanani, Caruso, & Carinci, 2011). Acupuncture is also more effective in treating tension-type headache pain than migraine headache pain (Linde et al., 2016). The evidence for acupuncture as a treatment for decreasing arthritis knee pain has become more positive as more studies have been conducted and methodology has improved.

Back pain is a common and challenging pain problem, and acupuncture has demonstrated some effectiveness in dealing with this pain syndrome. A meta-analysis of acupuncture for low back pain (Manheimer, White, Berman, Forys, & Ernst, 2005) indicated that this treatment is more effective for

TABLE 8.5 Effectiveness of Alternative Treatments for Anxiety, Stress, and Depression

Problems	Findings	Type of Assessment	Studies
1. Anxiety and stress	Mindfulness-based stress reduction is effective.	Systematic review	Chiesa & Serretti, 2010; Goyal et al., 2014; Grossman et al., 2004
2. Anxiety and stress	Qi gong decreases anxiety and stress.	Systematic review	Wang et al., 2014
3. Relapse into depression	Mindfulness-based cognitive therapy is effective.	Systematic review	Fjorback et al., 2011; Goyal et al., 2014
4. Anxiety disorders and depression	Mindfulness meditation is effective.	Systematic review	Goyal et al., 2014, Ivanovski & Malhi, 2007
5. Stress	Mindfulness-based stress reduction is more effective if practiced more frequently.	Pretest–posttest design	Carmody & Baer, 2008
6. Anxiety disorders	Transcendental meditation is comparable to relaxation training.	Systematic review	Krisanaprakornkit et al., 2006
7. Anxiety and stress management	Yoga is effective.	Systematic review	Chong et al., 2011
8. Stress	Qi gong reduces physiological indicators of stress.	Case study	Sancier & Holman, 2004
9. Altering the stress response	Qi gong alters the stress response in ways that are beneficial to several chronic health conditions in older people.	Systematic review	Ng & Tsang, 2009
10. Stress and negative mood	Tai chi practice improves stress and mood among older Chinese immigrants.	Quasi-experimental, longitudinal study	Taylor-Piliae et al., 2006
11. Anxiety, stress, and depression	Tai chi practice improves these conditions.	Systematic review	Wang, Bannuru, et al., 2010
12. Depression	Acupuncture showed effectiveness comparable to antidepressant drugs.	Systematic reviews	Leo & Ligot, 2007; Smith, Hay, & MacPherson, 2010
13. Depression	Yoga is a successful complementary treatment for people taking antidepressants.	Systematic review	Shapiro, Berkman, et al., 2007
14. Depression	Saint-John's wort is as effective as antidepressant drugs and produces fewer side effects.	Systematic review	Linde et al., 2008

short-term relief of chronic back pain than sham acupuncture or no treatment. In a systematic review that considered all types of treatment for back pain (Keller, Hayden, Bombardier, & van Tulder, 2007), acupuncture was among the most effective treatments, although none of the treatments revealed a high degree of effectiveness. This result may point to an answer to some of the confusion concerning the effectiveness of acupuncture (Johnson, 2006): When compared with other treatments, acupuncture may fail to show advantages.

Would You BELIEVE...?   Humans Are Not the Only Ones Who Benefit from Acupuncture

Nonhuman animals are common in medical research, and the growing research base to establish the effectiveness of acupuncture uses animals as substitutes for humans. However, acupuncture also occurs in veterinary care. Whereas rats are the most common species in creating animal models in research, horses, dogs, cats, and other animals receive acupuncture for the same pain problems that prompt humans to seek it. Another similarity in veterinary acupuncture is the combination of this alternative treatment with conventional veterinary care; that is, nonhuman animals receive acupuncture along with and not a substitute for conventional veterinary care (Boldt, 2016).

However, some differences exist that pose challenges for the veterinary use of acupuncture. One challenge is determining when a horse or dog might need treatment; they can't tell anyone when their back hurts. However, sensitivity to touch and differences in behavior provide cues (Boldt, 2016). An additional challenge is mapping animals' bodies to locate equivalent sites to human acupuncture points (Alfaro, 2014). TCM has mapped these points for horses, but other species receive veterinary acupuncture.

For example, people seek acupuncture for their companion animals, and the reasons are similar to humans' reasons for seeking CAM for themselves: back, neck, and arthritis pain (Woods, Burke, & Rodzon, 2011). People who sought acupuncture for their dogs or cats also tended to fit the same demographics as people who seek such care for themselves: well-educated, upper-income range, and more women than men. The pet owners were more likely than the average person to have experience with acupuncture (over 50%) and to believe in its effectiveness. Similar to the results from studies on humans, acupuncture is also effective for nonhuman animals in producing relief of back and neck pain, arthritis pain, surgical and postsurgical pain, and postsurgical nausea and vomiting (Boldt, 2016).

When compared to no treatment, the effects may be small. However, none of the available treatment for this condition is very effective. Therefore, acupuncture may be at least as effective a treatment as any for low back pain. A systematic review and meta-analysis (Furlan et al., 2012) confirmed the effectiveness of acupuncture for low back pain, but the review also showed that other CAM modalities were equally effective, including massage and spinal manipulation.

A large-scale research project (Witt, Brinkhaus, Reinhold, & Willich, 2006) examined the benefits of integrating acupuncture into standard medical care for chronic pain. Low back pain, osteoarthritis of the hip and knee, neck pain, and headache were among the types of pain included in treatment. The study found that acupuncture was effective in addition to the benefit obtained from standard medical care. That is, in addition to providing benefits as an alternative treatment, acupuncture was an effective complementary therapy for a variety of pain syndromes. This benefit is not confined to human patients, as the Would You Believe...? box describes.

Massage is another treatment for pain, and a review of massage for all types of chronic pain except cancer pain (Tsao, 2007) indicated varying degrees of effectiveness for different pain syndromes. The strongest evidence of effectiveness came from studies on low back pain (Furlan, Imamura, Dryden, & Irvin, 2008), whereas the evidence for shoulder and headache pain was more modest (Tsao, 2007). A later study (Cherkin et al., 2011) confirmed the benefits for low back pain, and another study (Sherman, Cherkin, Hawkes, Miglioretti, & Deyo, 2009) showed benefits for massage in relieving neck pain. Because of a lack of high-quality studies, a review of massage for musculoskeletal pain (Lewis & Johnson, 2006) failed to reach conclusions concerning effectiveness.

Chiropractic manipulation has also been the subject of systematic review. This type of CAM is most often used for back and neck pain, but a recent review found only small benefits (Rubenstein, van Middlekoop, Assendelft, de Boer, & van Tulder, 2011). However, a review of studies on spinal manipulation for musculoskeletal pain (Perram, 2006) indicated that chiropractic treatment was superior to conventional medical treatment for this type of pain. However, chiropractic manipulation did not appear to be effective in treating tension headaches (Lenssinck et al., 2004), but another review (Haas, Spegman, Peterson, Aickin, & Vavrek, 2010) indicated benefits of spinal manipulation for neck-related headaches.

Early research on the effectiveness of biofeedback (Blanchard et al., 1990) looked promising: Thermal biofeedback with relaxation showed positive results as a treatment for migraine and tension headaches. Later research has painted a less optimistic picture; biofeedback demonstrated no greater effects than relaxation training in preventing migraine headaches (Stewart, 2004). A meta-analysis of biofeedback studies in the treatment of migraine (Nestoriuc & Martin, 2007) indicated a medium-sized effect, but no such benefit appeared in an assessment of treatment effectiveness for tension-type headache (Verhagen, Damen, Berger, Passchier, & Koes, 2009) or for low back pain (Roelofs, Boissevain, Peters, de Jong, & Vlaeyen, 2002). The added expense associated with providing biofeedback is a drawback for this CAM. On balance, then, biofeedback shows more limited benefits than do some other CAM treatments for pain management.

Hypnotic treatment also has some applications in controlling pain, and the list of pains that are responsive to hypnotic procedures is extensive. A meta-analysis (Montgomery, DuHamel, & Redd, 2000) showed that hypnotic suggestion is equally effective in reducing both experimental pain induced in the laboratory and clinical pain that people experience in the world for about 75% of participants. Research exploring brain activity during hypnosis showed that hypnosis altered the brain response to painful stimulation in areas that underlie both the sensory and emotional responses to pain (Röder, Michal, Overbeck, van de Ven, & Linden, 2007). Indeed, the effectiveness of hypnosis in managing pain may be its power to change the fear that often accompanies pain (De Benedittis, 2003).

Hypnosis is not equally effective with all types of clinical pain; it is more effective in controlling acute pain than in managing chronic pain (Patterson & Jensen, 2003). Hypnosis is most effective in helping people manage pain associated with invasive medical procedures, postoperative recovery, and burns. For example, research shows that hypnosis was effective in reducing the need for preoperative medication in children (Calipel, Lucaspolomeni, Wodey, & Ecoffey, 2005), in stabilizing the pain of invasive surgical procedures, and in reducing surgery patients' need for analgesic drugs (Lang et al., 2000). Hypnosis is especially effective in relieving gastrointestinal pain in children (Kröner-Herwig, 2009) and appears very effective in

managing pain associated with childbirth (Landolt & Milling, 2011). Burns are notoriously difficult to treat because they involve severe pain and suffering. An early review of the effectiveness of hypnosis in treating the pain associated with burns (Van der Does & Van Dyck, 1989) examined 28 studies that used hypnosis with burn patients and found consistent evidence of its benefits. Evidence of those benefits continues to accrue, and David Patterson (2010) has argued that hypnosis has shown such convincing results that it should no longer be considered alternative medicine.

Although hypnotic treatment is effective with many types of acute pain, chronic pain is a more difficult management issue, and hypnosis is not as successful with chronic pain such as headache and low back pain as it is with acute pain (Patterson & Jensen, 2003). Hypnosis is also more effective with some people than with others. Individual differences in susceptibility to hypnosis are a factor in the analgesic effects of hypnosis—highly suggestible people may receive substantial analgesic benefits from this technique, whereas others receive limited benefits. Thus, hypnosis can be very effective with some people for some pain problems.

Table 8.6 summarizes the effectiveness of CAM treatments for pain. Although the studies on pain management using CAM could benefit from better design, evaluations of the results indicate that several of these techniques work for a variety of pain problems. Conventional medicine has not been very successful for many patients in managing chronic pain, and the conventional treatments tend to have many side effects, a criticism that is uncommon for CAM and thus an additional benefit.

Fewer side effects are not the only additional benefit to CAM use; a study of participants in several CAM clinical trials for pain (Hsu, BlueSpruce, Sherman, & Cherkin, 2010) identified a range of benefits that occurred in addition to the goals of the trial, including positive changes in emotion, ability to cope, health, and well-being. Thus, CAM treatments have few of the risks of conventional medicine and may have some benefits not assessed in most studies of effectiveness.

Alternative Treatments for Other Conditions

Although anxiety, stress, depression, and pain are the most common problems for which people use CAM, some products and procedures have been found effective for other conditions. Both the products and

TABLE 8.6   Effectiveness of Alternative Therapies for Pain

Problems	Findings	Type of Assessment	Studies
1. Chronic pain	Meditation is effective.	Panel review, NIH Technology	Lebovits, 2007
2. Pain associated with pregnancy and childbirth	Guided imagery is the best practice for this type of pain.	Narrative review	Naparstek, 2007
	Hypnosis is effective for managing labor and delivery pain.	Methodological review	Landolt & Milling, 2011
3. Headache pain	Guided imagery is effective in managing headache pain.	Narrative review	Tsao & Zeltzer, 2005
	Acupuncture is effective for tension headache.	Systematic review	Linde et al., 2016
4. Postoperative pain in children	Guided imagery reduces postoperative pain.	Experimental study	Huth et al., 2004
5. Postoperative pain in older people	Guided imagery reduces postoperative pain.	Experimental study	Antall & Kresevic, 2004
6. Tension headache pain in adults	Tai chi was effective in a randomized controlled trial.	Randomized controlled trial	Abbott et al., 2007
7. Chronic pain	Qi gong was evaluated as promising in a systematic review.	Systematic review	Lee et al., 2007a
8. Fibromyalgia	Qi gong provided pain relief and lowered distress in a randomized controlled trial.	Randomized controlled trial	Haak & Scott, 2008
	Tai chi provided pain relief and improved quality of life.	Randomized controlled trial	Wang, Schmid, et al., 2010
9. Low back pain	Mindfulness-based stress reduction is effective both after training and at 1-year follow-up.	Randomized controlled trial	Cherkin et al., 2016
10. Low back pain	Acupuncture is as or more effective than other approaches.	Review of systematic reviews	Keller et al., 2007; Manheimer et al., 2005
11. Low back pain	Acupuncture, massage, and spinal manipulation were all more effective than placebo.	Systematic review	Furlan et al., 2012
12. Low back pain, osteoarthritis, neck pain, and headache	Acupuncture was effective as a complementary treatment.	Randomized controlled trial	Witt et al., 2006
13. Low back pain, shoulder pain, and headache pain	Massage was effective for low back pain and modestly effective for shoulder and headache pain.	Review of meta-analyses and other reviews	Tsao, 2007
14. Low back pain	Massage can be effective for pain relief.	Randomized controlled trial	Cherkin et al., 2011

TABLE 8.6   *(Continued)*

Problems	Findings	Type of Assessment	Studies
15. Neck pain	Acupuncture is effective.	Systematic review	Trihn et al., 2016
	Massage can be effective.	Randomized trial	Sherman et al., 2009
16. Musculoskeletal pain	Massage studies are too limited to allow conclusions of effectiveness.	Systematic review	Lewis & Johnson, 2006
17. Back and neck pain	Chiropractic manipulation has only small benefits.	Systematic review	Rubenstein et al., 2011
18. Musculoskeletal pain	Chiropractic manipulation was more effective than conventional medical treatment.	Systematic review	Perram, 2006
19. Tension headache	Chiropractic manipulation was not found effective.	Systematic review	Lenssinck et al., 2004
20. Neck-related headaches	Spinal manipulation showed benefits.	Randomized controlled trial	Haas et al., 2010
21. Migraine and tension headache	Thermal biofeedback plus relaxation produced a significant reduction in headache activity.	Randomized controlled trial	Blanchard et al., 1990
22. Migraine headache prevention	Thermal biofeedback is comparable to other preventive treatments.	Meta-analysis	Stewart, 2004
23. Migraine headache treatment	Biofeedback produced a medium-sized effect.	Systematic review	Nestoriuc & Martin, 2007
24. Tension headache treatment	Biofeedback produced no benefit.	Qualitative review	Verhagen et al., 2009
25. Low back pain	EMG biofeedback was not effective.	Narrative review	Roelofs et al., 2002
26. Experimental and clinical pain	Hypnotic suggestion is effective for clinical and experimental pain.	Meta-analysis	Montgomery et al., 2000
27. Fear and anxiety associated with pain	Hypnosis is especially effective.	Narrative review	De Benedittis, 2003
28. Clinical pain	Hypnosis is more effective in controlling acute than in managing chronic pain.	Narrative review of randomized controlled trials	Patterson & Jensen, 2003
29. Preoperative distress	Hypnosis reduces preoperative distress better than medication.	Experimental design	Calipel et al., 2005
30. Surgery pain	Self-hypnosis decreases postoperative pain and reduces need for drugs.	Randomized trial	Lang et al., 2000
31. Gastrointestinal pain in children	Hypnosis is especially effective.	Review of systematic reviews	Kröner-Herwig, 2009
32. Burn pain	Hypnosis is a valuable component in treating severe burn pain.	Narrative review	Patterson, 2010; Van der Does & Van Dyck, 1989

procedures and the conditions for which they are effective vary widely; CAM has been used to achieve more rapid healing, to lower blood pressure, and to improve balance. For example, use of aloe vera speeds burn wound healing significantly (Maenthaisong, Chaiyakunapruk, Niruntraporn, & Kongkaew, 2007). Although biofeedback is not as effective as other CAM for stress and pain, thermal biofeedback is effective in the management of **Raynaud's disease,** a disorder that involves painful constriction of peripheral blood vessels in the hands and feet (Karavidas, Tsai, Yucha, McGrady, & Lehrer, 2006). In addition, biofeedback has demonstrated its usefulness in the rehabilitation of motor abilities (Giggins et al., 2013), including after stroke (Langhorne, Coupar, & Pollock, 2009). Hypnosis was found to be effective in controlling nausea and vomiting associated with chemotherapy in children (Richardson et al., 2007). The practice of transcendental meditation received a positive evaluation in controlling risk factors such as high blood pressure and some of the physiological changes that underlie cardiovascular disease and thus may offer protection (Horowitz, 2010). Yoga may help not only to control some of the risks for Type 2 diabetes (Innes & Vincent, 2007) but also to prevent cardiovascular complications in diabetics. A mindfulness-based meditation program was successful with male and female prisoners in improving mood and decreasing hostility (Samuelson, Carmody, Kabat-Zinn, & Bratt, 2007). This assortment of effective treatments represents many different complementary and alternative interventions, but some systems of alternative medicine have yielded successful treatments for a number of problems.

TCM includes acupuncture, qi gong, and tai chi, all of which produce a wide range of effective treatments and other health benefits. For example, acupuncture (Ezzo, Streitberger, & Schneider, 2006) has been found to be effective in controlling nausea and vomiting associated with postoperative symptoms. Also, a systematic review showed that acupuncture was effective in treating insomnia (H. Y. Chen et al., 2007). Tai chi and qi gong produce improvements in blood pressure and other cardiovascular measures compared to a nonexercise intervention and benefits comparable to other exercise interventions (Jahnke, Larkey, Rogers, & Etnier, 2010). Qi gong practice, however, was not superior to drug treatment for blood pressure treatment (Guo, Zhou, Nishimura, Teramukai, & Fukushima, 2008) but appeared to be as effective as drug treatment in managing the risk factors for diabetes such as oral glucose tolerance and blood glucose (Xin, Miller, & Brown, 2007).

Qi gong and the related practice of tai chi seem to have the ability to improve immune system function, which would give these practices the potential for many health benefits. Compared with healthy control participants who did not practice qi gong or tai chi, the immune system response of those who practiced qi gong was enhanced in ways that would resolve inflammation more rapidly (Li, Li, Garcia, Johnson, & Feng, 2005). Older adults who practiced qi gong or tai chi showed an enhanced immune system response to influenza immunization (Yang et al., 2007). Indeed, the immune response was sufficiently strong to produce positive health consequences before immunization. In a randomized controlled trial (Irwin, Pike, Cole, & Oxman, 2003), older adults who practiced tai chi exhibited an enhanced immune response to the herpes zoster (shingles) virus, even before they received the immunization for this virus. Thus, the practice of qi gong and tai chi seems to confer some immune system benefits that have been researched most extensively with older people but may apply to all.

The most common applications of tai chi have been among older people to improve balance and flexibility and to decrease falls. A large body of evidence, including systematic reviews, leads to the conclusion that these practices are successful in reducing fear of falling, improving balance, and reducing fall rates (Jahnke et al., 2010; Leung, Chan, Tsang, Tsang, & Jones, 2011). Qi gong and tai chi are also beneficial to bone density, which is an important underlying factor in falls among older people (Jahnke et al., 2010). Calcium and vitamin D supplements, another CAM treatment, are also effective in helping people over age 50 retain bone minerals (Tang, Eslick, Nowson, Smith, & Bensoussan, 2007).

Reasoning that the benefits of tai chi for balance and flexibility might apply to individuals with multiple sclerosis and rheumatoid arthritis, researchers have tested those benefits. A systematic review of the research on rheumatoid arthritis (Lee, Pittler, & Ernst, 2007b) found some positive effects for disability, quality of life, and mood but not enough clear evidence to recommend this practice. Two studies have assessed the benefits of tai chi for people with multiple sclerosis (Burschka, Keune, Oy, Oschmann, & Kuhn, 2014; Mills, Allen, & Morgan, 2000), both indicating substantial benefits for balance and mobility.

Thus, CAM interventions are effective for a variety of problems. The most persuasive evidence comes from mind–body medicine and TCM, but an assortment of products and procedures have demonstrated their effectiveness in randomized controlled trials, in meta-analyses, and in systematic reviews. Table 8.7 summarizes these treatments. Despite some impressive evidence for effectiveness, treatments within CAM also have limitations.

Limitations of Alternative Therapies

All forms of therapy have limitations, including CAM. One of the primary limitations is the reason any technique is considered *alternative*: the lack of information on its effectiveness. As we have seen, this deficit may be due to the sparseness of research rather than a lack of effectiveness. The growing interest in CAM and the funding for research through the U.S. National Center for Complementary and Integrative Health have worked toward solving this problem, revealing that some products and procedures are effective, whereas others are not. Both conventional and alternative treatments are limited by their success for some conditions and not others. However, specific CAM techniques have limitations and even dangers.

Herbal remedies and botanicals are part of many CAM systems, including Ayurvedic medicine, TCM, naturopathy, and homeopathy. These types of natural products are the most commonly used CAM approaches in the United States (Black et al., 2015; Clarke et al., 2015). Like drug treatments, natural products such as herbal and botanical products carry risks of adverse reactions and interactions with over-the-counter and prescription drugs (Firenzuoli & Gori, 2007; Lake, 2009). Unlike drugs, the U. S. government classifies herbal remedies, dietary supplements, and other natural products as food, so these products receive evaluations only for safety and not for effectiveness. People often consider natural herbs and botanicals to be safe and even if not effective, then at least harmless. Such is not always the case. Sometimes, evidence of dangers accumulates only after these products have been available for some time. Natural products may interact with each other or with prescription or over-the-counter medications, and many people who use natural products fail to inform their physicians of their CAM usage (Lake, 2009).

Massage has many benefits but is not suitable for people with problems related to joints, weakened bones, damaged nerves, a tumor, an open wound, or infection, or for people with bleeding disorders or those who are taking blood thinning agents (NCCIH, 2006/2015a). Serious complications such as spinal disc herniation, tissue damage, and neurological damage are possible, but serious injury is very rare (Yin, Wu, Litscher, & Xu, 2014). Chiropractic treatment may do harm when applied to individuals with broken bones or infection, and treatment may produce headache or other discomfort (NCCIH, 2007/2012).

Acupuncture and acupressure do not work for everyone. Some people do not respond, some types of manipulation of the needles are more effective than others, and some needle placements work better than others (Martindale, 2001). Needles should be sterile and inserted properly; improper insertion and needles that are not sterile can cause damage and infection (Yamashita & Tsukayama, 2008). However, incidents involving these dangers occur rarely (Xu et al., 2013). Tai chi and qi gong are generally safe, but people with severe osteoporosis, sprains, fractures, or joint problems should exercise caution or modify the positions (NCCIH, 2006/2015b). Meditation carries few health risks (NCCIH, 2007/2016b). Indeed, compared with the prevalence of medical errors made by conventional practitioners (Makary & Daniel, 2016), the risks from these alternative practices are small.

However, people should exercise caution in using any CAM treatment as an alternative to conventional medical care. People who trust alternative approaches and mistrust conventional medicine may fail to seek treatment that could be more effective. For example, yoga may help to control some of the risks for Type 2 diabetes (Innes & Vincent, 2007), but for most people, yoga will not be sufficient to control diabetes. The majority of people who use CAM recognize the limitations of these therapies and use them as additions to conventional medical care. However, many people who use some CAM modality fail to tell their conventional medical practitioner that they are using an alternative as a well as conventional treatment (Lake, 2009). This failure may present risks due to interactions between the two treatments.

Another limitation for CAM is its accessibility. Not everyone who is interested in CAM may be able to find or to afford CAM treatment. Many CAM treatments are limited by the number of qualified practitioners and by their geographic location. For example, acupuncture use increased dramatically between 1997 and 2007 (Nahin, Barnes, Stussman, & Bloom, 2009) and continued to increase between 2007 and 2012 (Clarke et al., 2015).

TABLE 8.7   Effectiveness of Alternative Treatments for Other Conditions

Problems	Findings	Method of Assessment	Studies
1. Burn healing	Aloe vera speeds healing.	Systematic review	Maenthaisong et al., 2007
2. Raynaud's disease	Thermal biofeedback is an effective treatment.	Narrative review	Karavidas et al., 2006
3. Rehabilitation of motor abilities after injury or stroke	EMG biofeedback is effective.	Systematic review	Langhorne et al., 2009
4. Nausea and vomiting associated with chemotherapy	Hypnosis is effective in controlling these symptoms.	Systematic review	Richardson et al., 2007
5. Physical reactions related to cardiovascular disease	Transcendental meditation shows beneficial effects.	Narrative review	Horowitz, 2010
6. Risks for Type 2 diabetes	Yoga is effective in controlling risks and in decreasing CVD complications.	Systematic review	Innes & Vincent, 2007
7. Hostility	Mindfulness meditation is effective in moderating hostility among prisoners.	Pretest–posttest design	Samuelson et al., 2007
8. Postoperative nausea and vomiting	Acupuncture is effective.	Systematic review	Ezzo et al., 2006
9. Insomnia	Acupuncture is effective.	Systematic review	H. Y. Chen et al., 2007
10. High blood pressure and other responses related to cardiovascular disease	Tai chi and qi gong produce improvements. Qi gong practice lowered blood pressure, but not as much as drugs.	Review of randomized controlled trials Meta-analysis	Jahnke et al., 2010 Guo et al., 2008
11. Risk factors for diabetes	Qi gong was effective in lowering risk.	Qualitative review	Xin et al., 2007
12. Immune system function	Qi gong and tai chi enhanced immune system response to influenza vaccination in older adults.	Controlled experiment	Yang et al., 2007
13. Immune system function	Tai chi practice enhanced older adults' immune system response to herpes zoster before and after immunization.	Randomized controlled experiment	Irwin et al., 2003
14. Fear of falling, balance, and falls	Tai chi and qi gong practice decreased fear of falling, increased balance, and decreased falls among older adults.	Review of randomized controlled trials	Jahnke et al., 2010; Leung et al., 2011
15. Osteoporosis	Calcium and vitamin D supplements slowed bone mineral loss in people over age 50.	Meta-analysis	Tang et al., 2007
16. Rheumatoid arthritis	Tai chi showed some positive effects but not clear enough evidence for a recommendation.	Systematic review	Lee et al., 2007b
17. Multiple sclerosis	Tai chi practice improved balance.	Controlled experiments	Burschka et al., 2014; Mills et al., 2000

However, accessibility may remain a problem that limits its use (Burke & Upchurch, 2006). People who used alternative medicine products or procedures are not reimbursed often for the products they purchase or the services they receive (Burke & Upchurch, 2006). The failure to include CAM services in insurance reimbursement is typical in the United States and represents huge out-of-pocket expenditures to CAM users—an estimated $27 billion (Nahin et al., 2009). One way to remove this barrier is to increase the presence of alternative treatments in conventional medical settings. This is the focus of integrative medicine.

Integrative Medicine

Integrating conventional and alternative medicine is what Norman Cousins, whose story began this chapter, envisioned for health care and treatment. Cousins's experience with a debilitating disease and cure through a very unorthodox treatment prompted him to work toward changes to conventional medicine. As Cousins said,

> It becomes necessary therefore to create a balanced perspective, one that recognizes that attitudes such as a strong will to live, high purpose, a capacity for festivity, and a reasonable degree of confidence are not an alternative to competent medical attention, but a way of enhancing the environment of treatment. The wise physician favors a spirit of responsible participation by the patients in a total strategy of medical care. (UCLA Cousins Center for Psychoneuroimmunology, 2011, paragraph 1)

This approach is what most people attempt when they choose techniques and products from conventional and alternative medicine, but most people work toward this combination on their own rather than within the medical care system. However, this integration is the ideal for many individuals and for a growing number of practitioners in the United States and most other high-income countries. This integration offers benefits but also faces barriers.

Currently, many people who use CAM do so without the guidance of their physician (Nerurkar et al., 2011) and often without informing their physician (Lake, 2009). These people may feel reluctant to discuss their use of alternative treatment with a conventional practitioner because of the skepticism within conventional medicine about CAM (Frank, Ratanawongsa, & Carrera, 2010). This skepticism makes physicians reluctant to refer patients to practitioners of alternative

treatments and even hesitant to enter into collaborative relationships. Integrative medicine requires conventional and alternative medicine practitioners to accept the effectiveness of both approaches and to form a working relationship focused on the patient's health. Both the acceptance and the cooperation present challenges.

Practitioners who follow the biomedical model have basic differences from those who hold a biopsychosocial model, which affects the way that each views health and treatment (Lake, 2007). For example, the assumptions of TCM, chiropractic, and homeopathy have been difficult for many physicians trained in Western medicine to accept (Shere-Wolfe, Tilburt, D'Adamo, & Chesney, 2013). Some conventional practitioners are vehemently opposed (Freedman, 2011), but others are more open, especially to techniques that are beginning to accumulate research support for effectiveness. Practitioners whose training has not included alternative treatments are more resistant than those who have training in CAM (Hsiao, Ryan, et al., 2006). Students in a variety of professional schools of health care have a great interest in CAM (Chow, Liou, & Heffron, 2016; Song, John, & Dobs, 2007). An increasing number of medical schools include CAM departments and curricula (Frank et al., 2010), but the philosophy of practice and treatment methods and strategies differ (Shannon, Weil, & Kaplan, 2011). In 2009, the U.S. Institute of Medicine sponsored a conference titled "Summit on Integrative Medicine and the Health of the Public" (Ullman, 2010). Those who attended expressed hopes for an integration of conventional and alternative approaches to health and treatment, but they also acknowledged that this integration would require large changes in the medical delivery system.

Integration of care is more common in some areas of practice than others, such as pain treatment, cancer care, and mental health problems. In pain clinics, pain is the problem, and treatment is oriented toward managing it and not the condition that originally caused it. Such a clinic often include health care professionals from several specialties (Dillard, 2002), including (1) a physician trained in neurology, anesthesia, rehabilitation, or psychiatry; (2) a physical rehabilitation expert; (3) a psychiatrist or psychologist; and (4) a chiropractor, massage therapist, or acupuncturist (or all three). Integrative oncology also involves treatment by a team of providers. In addition to conventional treatments for cancer such as chemotherapy, radiation, and surgery, patients may participate in interventions aimed at pain control, stress management, nutrition, and physical activity. Stress management, healthy diet, and exercise represent changes that improve the quality of life for most people, but these lifestyle changes may also affect the progression of cancer (Boyd, 2007).

Several studies have researched integrated medicine programs to explore how the integration worked as well as the benefits and barriers for staff. One such program is available at the famous Mayo Clinic in Minnesota (Pang et al., 2015), where referrals to CAM increased between 2007 and 2010. The most common referrals to CAM practitioners were consistent with the practice of integrative medicine—pain management and stress management. Another study focused on another common setting for integrative medicine—cancer treatment centers. The practitioners in these centers in Germany and the United States (Mittring, Pérard, & Witt, 2013) had developed similar views, regardless of their background in conventional or alternative medicine, which included an emphasis on evidence-based treatment centered on a holistic approach to treating each patient. Conventional practitioners reported no difficulties in accepting alternative approaches but voiced problems with the additional time that the patient-centered, holistic approach created for scheduling and waiting times.

Such an integrated approach could apply to the treatment of many chronic diseases. The growing consumer interest in CAM has led an increasing number of patients to expect that their conventional medicine practitioners will be knowledgeable concerning CAM and willing to refer to them CAM practitioners (Ben-Arye, Frenkel, Klein, & Schraf, 2008). Despite a history of resistance, conventional medicine practitioners also have an increasing interest in CAM and a willingness to provide some alternative procedures or refer patients to CAM practitioners (Shere-Wolfe et al., 2013). Thus, the goal to attain the "best of both worlds" by combining conventional medicine with effective treatments from alternative medicine through a cooperation of the practitioners seems to have started.

IN SUMMARY

For alternative treatments to be accepted by conventional medicine, research evidence must confirm their effectiveness. The standard for this evidence is controversial. Should CAM be held to the standard of effectiveness as demonstrated by randomized controlled trials? Some in conventional medicine say so, but some in alternative medicine argue that most treatments in conventional medicine fail to meet this criterion. Nonetheless, evidence is accruing concerning effectiveness for CAM.

Both transcendental meditation and mindfulness meditation have demonstrated effectiveness for anxiety. Mindfulness-based stress reduction and the movement-based practices of qi gong and tai chi are effective in managing stress. Acupuncture and yoga show some promise of reducing depression, and the herbal remedy Saint-John's wort reduces depression.

Guided imagery is an effective intervention in helping people manage several types of pain. Techniques from TCM have been successful in pain management, including qi gong, tai chi, and acupuncture. Qi gong and tai chi may be good choices for people with chronic pain problems, including headache and fibromyalgia. Acupuncture can be effective for easing low back and neck pain as well as pain from osteoarthritis. Research also indicates that massage is effective for low back pain, neck pain, musculoskeletal pain, and headache; chiropractic manipulation also helps the same set of pain syndromes. However, biofeedback is not as effective as other CAM treatments; biofeedback is similar to relaxation in managing migraine headaches but shows few benefits for treating other types of pain. Hypnosis is effective for a variety of types of pain but is more effective for acute pain such as postsurgical and burn pain than for chronic pain.

Techniques from CAM are also effective for a variety of other conditions, including speeding burn healing (aloe vera), treating insomnia (acupuncture), controlling nausea and vomiting (hypnosis and acupuncture), managing Raynaud's disease (thermal biofeedback), increasing motor movement after stroke (EMG biofeedback), and lowering risk for cardiovascular disease (meditation and qi gong) and diabetes (qi gong). Research has indicated that the practice of qi gong and tai chi can alter the immune system in beneficial ways, and tai chi improves balance and flexibility and decreases both fear of falling and number of falls in older adults.

Like all treatments, CAM has limitations and even dangers. Some herbal remedies and botanical products may be toxic or may interact with each other or with over-the-counter or prescription drugs. Individuals with some conditions should avoid some treatments; for example, people with weakened bones should be cautious in seeking massage or chiropractic treatment. Another limitation for CAM is its accessibility, in terms of both availability and cost of treatments.

Integrative medicine is the integration of alternative and conventional medicine, which should provide the best of both approaches. The challenges for achieving such integration include melding the two discrepant traditions and training practitioners who will refer patients to each other when appropriate. The movement toward integrative medicine and integrative health is gaining popularity in many countries throughout the world. Two areas in which integrative medicine is advancing most rapidly are pain management and cancer treatment.

Answers

This chapter has addressed six basic questions:

1. **What medical systems represent alternatives to conventional medicine?**

The alternative medical systems include TCM, Ayurvedic medicine, naturopathy, and homeopathy. TCM and Ayurvedic medicine are ancient; naturopathy and homeopathy arose in the 19th century and gained popularity in the early 20th century. Each of these systems presents a theory of health and disease as well as practices for diagnosis and treatment. All of the alternative systems share the concept of vital energy and the notion that bringing the mind and body together is important to health.

2. **What products and diets count as alternative medicine?**

Alternative products include dietary supplements, including nonvitamin products such as echinacea, glucosamine, omega-3 fatty acids, and a variety of herbs, extracts, and special foods that may be taken as curatives or preventatives. Diets such as the Atkins, Ornish, Zone, and various vegetarian diets may be undertaken to maintain or enhance health or to control risk factors for disease.

3. **What manipulative practices fall within alternative practices?**

Manipulative techniques include chiropractic and massage; chiropractic manipulation focuses on adjusting the spine and joints, whereas massage manipulates soft tissue. Chiropractic treatment has grown in popularity, and increasing research has demonstrated its effectiveness for dealing with several types of chronic pain. Massage has also increased in popularity as a therapeutic intervention to manage both pain and stress.

4. **What is mind–body medicine?**

Mind–body medicine is the term applied to a variety of techniques that are based on the notion that the brain, mind, body, and behavior interact in complex ways and that emotional, mental, social, and behavioral factors exert important effects on health. According to mind–body medicine, overlooking psychological factors will lead to an incomplete form of health treatment and lose the power that can come from enlisting mind and emotions in treatment. Included within mind–body medicine are meditation, guided imagery, yoga, qi gong, tai chi, biofeedback, and hypnosis.

5. **Who uses complementary and alternative medicine?**

Countries vary in CAM usage, and within countries, some demographic factors predict CAM use. Australia, Canada, and some European countries show higher percentages of the population seeking CAM treatments than in the United States. Within the United States, ethnicity shows some relationship to CAM use, with European American, well-educated, and upper-income individuals using CAM more often than others. In all countries, women are more likely than men to use CAM. Personal attitudes of acceptance of the underlying philosophy of CAM also predict use, as does health status—people who have a persistent health problem that conventional medicine has not helped are more likely to seek alternative treatment.

6. **What are the effective uses and limitations of alternative treatments?**

A variety of techniques are available to help people manage anxiety, stress, depression, pain, and other problems, and an increasing body of research indicates that some alternative treatments are effective in managing these problems. Both transcendental and mindfulness meditation are effective in managing anxiety; mindfulness-based stress reduction helps in coping with stress. No one alternative technique is effective for all pain situations, but several are effective for some type of pain. Manipulation techniques such as massage and chiropractic treatment and mind–body techniques such as acupuncture seem to be as effective as any treatment for the difficult problem of chronic low back pain. The movement-based approaches of qi gong and tai chi show promise of helping to manage headaches and fibromyalgia and also influence the immune system in beneficial ways. However, their primary therapeutic use is to help older people maintain balance and flexibility. Hypnosis also has benefits for pain control, but these benefits apply more to acute pain than to chronic pain.

Limitations to CAM come from limited research on its effectiveness, but that situation is changing. Other limitations are similar to those of treatments in conventional medicine—hazards for some individuals using some treatments and drug interactions arising from the use of herbal treatments or dietary supplements. Availability and cost of treatments are other limitations of CAM, but the growing interest in integrating CAM and conventional treatments holds the promise of greater access and more effective delivery of complementary treatments.

Suggested Readings

Freedman, D. H. (2011). The triumph of new-age medicine. *The Atlantic, 308*(1), 90–100. This article in a popular magazine explores integrative medicine, interviewing advocates and detractors of alternative approaches to treatment. Through this evaluation, Freedman provides a critique of the current level of medical care in the United States.

Harrington, A. (2008). *The cure within: A history of mind–body medicine*. New York: Norton. Harrington's book takes a social and historical perspective on the status of alternative medicine, weaving together a wide collection of information concerning the interaction between mind and body.

Lake, J. (2007). Philosophical problems in medicine and psychiatry, part II. *Integrative Medicine: A Clinician's Journal, 6*(3), 44–47. This brief article takes a historical and philosophical perspective in explaining the underlying differences in assumptions and worldviews between advocates of conventional and alternative medicine and how these differences present barriers to integrating the two types of medical care.

Shannon, S., Weil, A., & Kaplan, B. J. (2011). Medical decision making in integrative medicine: Safety, efficacy, and patient preference. *Alternative & Complementary Therapies, 17*(2), 84–91. This thoughtful critique of both conventional and alternative medicine details safety and effectiveness concerns that should be used in all types of medicine.

CHAPTER 9

Behavioral Factors in Cardiovascular Disease

CHAPTER OUTLINE

QUESTIONS

This chapter focuses on four basic questions:

1. What are the structures, functions, and disorders of the cardiovascular system?

2. What are the risk factors for cardiovascular disease?

3. How does lifestyle relate to cardiovascular health?

4. What behaviors allow people to lower their cardiovascular risks?

☑ Check Your **HEALTH RISKS**   *Regarding Cardiovascular Disease*

Question	Point
Age	
Are you a man 55 years or older OR woman 65 years or older?	2 if Yes
Smoking	
I never smoked	0
I am a former smoker (last smoked more than 12 months ago)	2
I smoke 1–5 cigarettes per day	2
I smoke 6–10 cigarettes per day	4
I smoke 11–15 cigarettes per day	6
I smoke 16–20 cigarettes per day	7
I smoke more than 20 cigarettes per day	11
Over the past 12 months, what has been your typical exposure to other people's tobacco smoke?	
Secondhand smoke	
Less than 1 hour of exposure per week	0
One or more hours of secondhand smoke exposure per week	2
Other health conditions	
Do you have diabetes mellitus?	6 if Yes
Do you have high blood pressure?	5 if Yes
Have either or both of your biological parents had a heart attack?	4 if Yes
Waist-to-hip ratio	
Less than 0.873	0
Between 0.873 and 0.963	2
Greater than 0.964	4
Psychosocial factors	
How often have you felt work or home life stress in the last year?	
Never or some periods	0
Several periods of stress or permanent stress	3
During the past 12 months, was there ever a time when you felt sad, blue, or depressed for weeks or more in a row?	3 if Yes
Dietary factors	
Do you eat salty food or snacks one or more times a day?	1 if Yes
Do you eat deep fried foods or snacks or fast foods three or more times a week?	1 if Yes
Do you eat fruit one or more times daily?	1 if No
Do you eat vegetables one or more times daily?	1 if No
Do you eat meat and/or poultry two or more times daily?	2 if Yes
Physical activity	
I am mainly sedentary or perform mild exercise (requiring minimal effort)	2
I perform moderate or strenuous physical activity in my leisure time	0

Source: "Estimating modifiable coronary heart disease risk globally in multiple regions of the world: The INTERHEART modifiable risk score" by C. McGorrian et al. (2011), *European Heart Journal, 32,* Supplementary Table 2.

This checklist supplies you with your INTERHEART Modifiable Risk Score. The score derives from research on over 30,000 people from 52 different countries and represents the most recent method for calculating heart attack risk. If you score below 9, congratulations: You are at lowest risk for heart attack. If you score above 15, you are at highest risk for heart attack; however, most of these factors are under your control. In this chapter, you will learn why each of these factors increases risk for cardiovascular problems, and how you can decrease your risk.

Real-World Profile of **PRESIDENT BILL CLINTON**

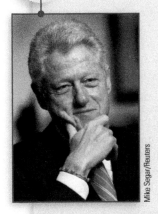

Mike Segar/Reuters

In early September 2004, former President Bill Clinton went to the hospital because he experienced chest pains and shortness of breath (King & Henry, 2004). Soon after, he learned that his coronary arteries were blocked, which led to coronary bypass surgery. Had Clinton not obtained treatment, his chances of a heart attack would have been substantial. Like many people, Clinton did not experience any major symptoms beforehand, so he considered himself fortunate to have a warning of coronary problems. His diagnosis and treatment were opportunities to avoid a heart attack and to gain additional years of healthy life.

Clinton also speculated about the underlying cause of his heart problems. He had a history of heart disease in his family and, because of this, tried to jog regularly and get regular check-ups with his doctors. But, he was also fond of high-fat fast food. Clinton's unhealthy diet during his White House years was "legendary" (Templeton, 2008). Clinton also had a history of high blood pressure and high cholesterol.

Clinton looked healthy, but despite the appearance of health, his coronary arteries were seriously blocked—one more than 90% (Associated Press, 2004). Clinton recovered from his quadruple coronary bypass surgery, but additional surgery was required 6 months later to remove scar tissue (Matthews, 2005). Clinton's experience turned him into an advocate for prevention of heart disease (Clinton, 2005). He joined with the American Heart Association to begin an initiative to combat childhood obesity, including urging fast-food restaurants to provide healthier menu choices for children.

n this chapter, we examine the behavioral risks for cardiovascular disease—the most frequent cause of death in the United States and other industrialized nations—and look at Bill Clinton's risk from both inherent and behavioral factors. But first, we describe the cardiovascular system. What is it, and what are methods of measuring how well it functions?

The Cardiovascular System

The **cardiovascular system** consists of the heart, arteries, and veins. The heart is a muscle that, by contracting and relaxing, pumps blood throughout the body. The heart is, essentially, the center of a rapid-transit system that carries oxygen to body cells and removes carbon dioxide and other wastes from cells. Under healthy conditions, the cardiovascular, respiratory, and digestive systems are integrated: The digestive system produces nutrients and the respiratory system furnishes oxygen, both of which circulate through the blood to various parts of the body. In addition, the endocrine system affects the cardiovascular system by stimulating or depressing the rate of cardiovascular activity. Although we will view the cardiovascular system in isolation in this chapter, it does not function that way.

The blood's route through the body appears in Figure 9.1. The entire circuit takes about 20 seconds when the body is at rest, but exertion speeds the process. Blood travels from the right ventricle of the heart to the lungs, where hemoglobin (one of the components of blood) saturates it with oxygen. From the lungs, oxygenated blood travels back to the left atrium of the heart, then to the left ventricle, and finally out to the rest of the body. The **arteries** carry the oxygenated blood branch into vessels of smaller and smaller diameter, called **arterioles**, and finally terminate in tiny **capillaries** that connect arteries and **veins**. Oxygen diffuses out to body cells, and carbon dioxide and other chemical wastes pass into the blood so they can be disposed of. Blood that has been stripped of its oxygen returns to the heart by way of the system of veins, beginning with the tiny **venules** and ending with the two large veins that empty into the right atrium, the upper right chamber of the heart.

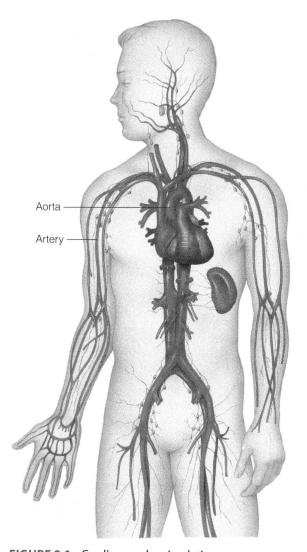

Aorta

Artery

FIGURE 9.1   Cardiovascular circulation.

Source: Introduction to microbiology (p. 671), by J. L. Ingraham & C. A. Ingraham. From INGRAHAM/ INGRAHAM, *Introduction to Microbiology,* 1E.

This section briefly considers the functioning of the cardiovascular system, concentrating on the physiology underlying **cardiovascular disease (CVD)**, a general term that includes coronary artery disease, coronary heart disease, and stroke.

The Coronary Arteries

The coronary arteries supply blood to the heart muscle, the **myocardium**. The two principal coronary arteries branch off from the aorta (see Figure 9.2), the main artery that carries oxygenated blood from the heart. Left and right coronary arteries divide into smaller branches, providing the blood supply to the myocardium.

With each beat, the heart makes a slight twisting motion, which moves the coronary arteries. The coronary arteries, therefore, receive a great deal of strain as part of their normal function. This movement of the heart has been hypothesized to almost inevitably cause injury to the coronary arteries (Friedman & Rosenman, 1974). The damage can heal in two different ways. The preferable route involves the formation of small amounts of scar tissue and results in no serious problem. The second route involves the formation of **atheromatous plaques**, deposits composed of cholesterol and other lipids (fats), connective tissue, and muscle tissue. The plaques grow and calcify into a hard, bony substance that thickens the arterial walls (Kharbanda & MacAllister, 2005). This process also involves inflammation (Abi-Saleh, Iskandar, Elgharib, & Cohen, 2008). The formation of plaques and the resulting occlusion of the arteries are called **atherosclerosis**, shown in Figure 9.3.

A related but different problem is **arteriosclerosis**, or the loss of elasticity of the arteries. The beating of the heart pushes blood through the arteries with great force, and arterial elasticity allows adaptation to this pressure. Loss of elasticity tends to make the cardiovascular system less capable of tolerating increases in cardiac blood volume. Hence, a potential danger exists during strenuous exercise for people with arteriosclerosis.

The formation of arterial plaques (atherosclerosis) and the "hardening" of the arteries (arteriosclerosis) often occur together. Both can affect any artery in the cardiovascular system, but when the coronary arteries are affected, the heart's oxygen supply may be threatened.

Coronary Artery Disease

Coronary artery disease (CAD) refers to damage to the coronary arteries, typically through the processes of atherosclerosis and arteriosclerosis. No clear visible outward symptoms accompany the buildup of plaques in the coronary arteries, as Bill Clinton discovered. CAD can develop while a person remains totally unaware of its progress. In CAD, the plaques narrow the arteries and restrict the supply of blood to the myocardium. Deposits of plaque may also rupture and form blood clots that can obstruct an artery. If such an obstruction deprives the heart of oxygen, the heart will not function properly. Restriction of blood flow is called **ischemia**.

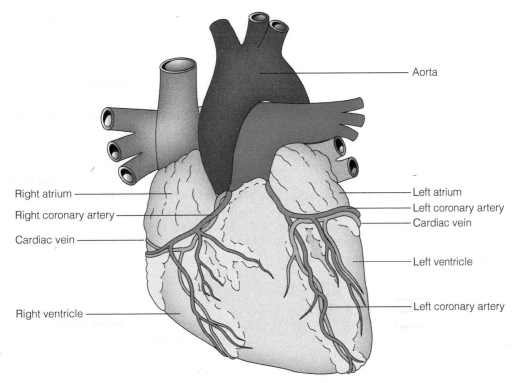

FIGURE 9.2 Heart (myocardium) with coronary arteries and veins.

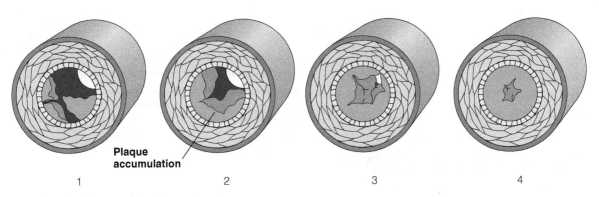

FIGURE 9.3 Progressive atherosclerosis.

Bill Clinton's symptoms of chest pain and shortness of breath were likely due to ischemia.

Coronary heart disease (CHD) refers to any damage to the myocardium as a result of insufficient blood supply. Clinton had coronary artery disease, but the disease had not damaged his heart when he experienced symptoms and sought treatment. Thus, Clinton did not yet have coronary heart disease.

Complete blockage of either coronary artery shuts off the blood flow and thus the oxygen supply to the myocardium. Like other tissue, the myocardium cannot survive without oxygen; therefore, coronary blockage results in the death of myocardial tissue, an infarction. **Myocardial infarction** is the medical term for the condition commonly referred to as a heart attack. During myocardial infarction, the damage may be so extensive as to completely disrupt the heartbeat. In less severe cases, heart contractions may become less effective. The signals for a myocardial infarction include a feeling of weakness or dizziness combined with nausea, cold sweating, difficulty in breathing, and a sensation of crushing or squeezing pain in the chest, arms, shoulders, jaw, or back. Rapid loss of consciousness or death may occur, but the victim sometimes remains quite alert throughout the experience. The severity of symptoms depends on the extent of damage to the heart muscle.

In those people who survive a myocardial infarction (more than half do), the damaged portion of the myocardium will not regrow or repair itself. Instead, scar tissue forms at the infarcted area. Scar tissue does not have the elasticity and function of healthy tissue, so a heart attack lessens the capacity of the heart to pump blood efficiently. A myocardial infarction can limit the type and vigor of activities that a person can safely do, prompting some lifestyle changes. The coronary artery disease that caused a first attack can cause another, but future infarctions are not a certainty.

The process of **cardiac rehabilitation** may involve psychologists, who help cardiac patients adjust their lifestyle to minimize risk factors and lessen the chances of future attacks. Because heart disease is the most frequent cause of death in the United States, preventing heart attacks and furnishing cardiac rehabilitation are major tasks for the health care system.

A less serious result of restriction of the blood supply to the myocardium is **angina pectoris**, a disorder with symptoms of crushing pain in the chest and difficulty in breathing—the symptoms Bill Clinton experienced. Angina is usually precipitated by exercise or stress because these conditions increase demand on the heart. Clinton had experienced such symptoms during exercise and was not distressed, but when he had difficulty in breathing and tightness across the chest during his normal activities, he sought medical attention (Clinton, 2005). With oxygen restriction, the reserve capacity of the cardiovascular system is reduced, and heart disease becomes evident. The uncomfortable symptoms of angina rarely last more than a few minutes, but angina is a sign of obstruction in the coronary arteries.

Former President Clinton's symptoms led to a diagnosis of CAD, and his treatment was bypass surgery, one of the common treatments for this disorder. This procedure replaces the blocked portion of the coronary artery (or arteries) with grafts of healthy sections of the coronary arteries (see Figure 9.4). Bypass surgery is expensive, carries some risk of death, and may not extend the patient's life significantly, but it is generally

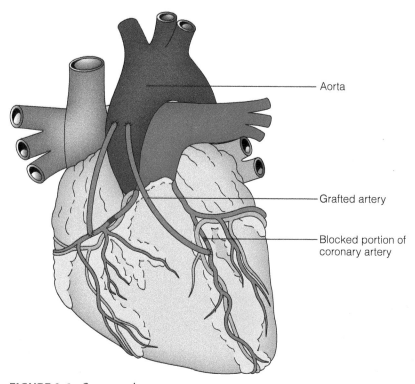

Aorta

Grafted artery

Blocked portion of coronary artery

FIGURE 9.4   Coronary bypass.

successful in relieving angina and improving quality of life, as it has been for Clinton.

Stroke

Atherosclerosis and arteriosclerosis can also affect the arteries that serve the head and neck, thereby restricting the blood supply to the brain. That is, the same disease process that causes CAD and CHD may affect the brain. Any obstruction in the arteries of the brain will restrict or completely stop the flow of blood to the area of the brain served by that portion of the system. Oxygen deprivation causes the death of brain tissue within 3 to 5 minutes. This damage to the

brain resulting from lack of oxygen is called a **stroke**, the fifth most frequent cause of death in the United States. But strokes have other causes as well—for example, a bubble of air (air embolism) or an infection that impedes blood flow in the brain. In addition, the weakening of artery walls associated with arteriosclerosis may lead to an *aneurysm*, a sac formed by the ballooning of a weakened artery wall. Aneurysms may burst, causing a *hemorrhagic stroke* or death (see Figure 9.5).

A stroke damages neurons in the brain, and these neurons have no capacity to replace themselves. Most commonly, some of the neurons devoted to a particular function (such as speech production) are lost,

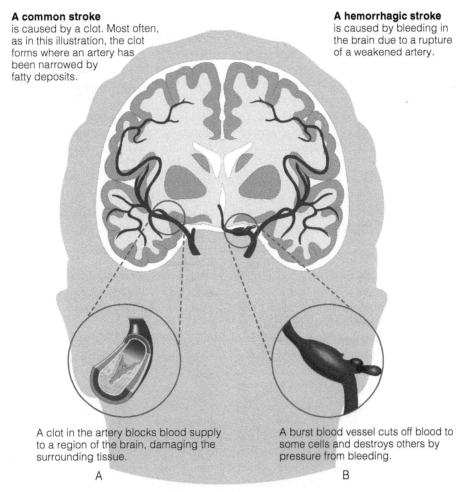

A common stroke is caused by a clot. Most often, as in this illustration, the clot forms where an artery has been narrowed by fatty deposits.

A hemorrhagic stroke is caused by bleeding in the brain due to a rupture of a weakened artery.

A clot in the artery blocks blood supply to a region of the brain, damaging the surrounding tissue.

A burst blood vessel cuts off blood to some cells and destroys others by pressure from bleeding.

A

B

FIGURE 9.5   There are two types of strokes: Common strokes are caused by blockage of an artery; hemorrhagic strokes are caused by the bursting of an artery in the brain.

Source: An invitation to health (7th ed., p. 379), by D. Hales, 1997, Pacific Grove, CA: Brooks/Cole. From HALES, *Invitation to Health*, 7E.

impairing brain function. The extent of the loss is related to the amount of damage to the area; more extensive damage results in greater impairment. Damage may be so extensive—or in such a critical area—as to bring about immediate death or damage may be so slight as to go unnoticed.

Blood Pressure

When the heart pumps blood, the force must be substantial to power circulation for an entire cycle through the body and back to the heart. In a healthy cardiovascular system, the pressure in the arteries is not a problem because arteries are quite elastic. In a cardiovascular system diseased by atherosclerosis and arteriosclerosis, however, the pressure of the blood in the arteries can produce serious consequences. The narrowing of the arteries that occurs in atherosclerosis and the loss of elasticity that characterizes arteriosclerosis both tend to raise blood pressure. In addition, these disease processes make the cardiovascular system less capable of adapting to the demands of heavy exercise and stress.

Blood pressure measurements are usually expressed by two numbers. The first number represents **systolic pressure**, the pressure generated by the heart's contraction. The second number represents **diastolic pressure**, or the pressure experienced between contractions, reflecting the elasticity of the vessel walls. Both numbers are expressed in millimeters (mm) of mercury (Hg) because original measurements of blood pressure were obtained by determining how high mercury would rise in a glass column by the pressure of blood in circulation.

Blood pressure elevates through several mechanisms. Some elevations in blood pressure are normal and even adaptive. Temporary activation of the sympathetic nervous system, for example, increases heart rate and also causes constriction of the blood vessels, both of which raise blood pressure. Other elevations in blood pressure, however, are neither normal nor adaptive—they are symptoms of CVD.

Millions of people in the United States have **hypertension**—that is, abnormally high blood pressure. This "silent" illness is the single best predictor of both heart attack and stroke, but it can also cause eye damage and kidney failure (see Figure 9.6). **Essential hypertension** refers to a chronic elevation of blood pressure, which has both genetic and environmental causes (Staessen, Wang, Bianchi, & Birkenhager, 2003). This condition affects *one-third* of people in the United States and other developed countries, for a total of about 76 million in the United States and 1 billion worldwide (Roger et al.,

2012; U.S. Department of Health and Human Services [USDHHS], 2003). It is strongly related to aging but also to factors such as African American ancestry, weight, sodium intake, tobacco use, and lack of exercise.

Table 9.1 shows the ranges for normal blood pressure, prehypertension, and Stage 1 and Stage 2 hypertension. Despite beliefs to the contrary, hypertension does not have easily discernible symptoms, so people with hypertension can have dangerously elevated blood pressure and remain completely unaware of their vulnerability to heart attack and stroke.

In younger individuals, high diastolic pressure is most strongly related to cardiovascular risk, but in older individuals, elevated systolic pressure is a better predictor (Staessen et al., 2003). Each 20-mm-Hg increase in systolic blood pressure doubles the risk of CVD (Roger et al., 2012). Systolic pressure that exceeds 200 mm Hg presents a danger of rupture in the arterial walls (Berne & Levy, 2000). Diastolic hypertension tends to result in vascular damage that may injure organs served by the affected vessels, most commonly the kidneys, liver, pancreas, brain, and retina.

Because the underlying cause of essential hypertension is complex and not fully understood, no treatment exists that will remedy its basic cause. Treatment tends to be oriented toward drugs or changes in behavior and lifestyle that can lower blood pressure (USDHHS, 2003). Because part of the treatment of hypertension involves behavioral changes, health psychologists play an important role in encouraging behaviors such as controlling weight, maintaining a regular exercise program, and restricting sodium intake. Adherence to these behaviors is important for controlling blood pressure. Unfortunately, adherence to medications is notoriously poor for patients with hypertension.

IN SUMMARY

The cardiovascular system consists of the heart and blood vessels. The heart pumps blood, which circulates throughout the body, supplying oxygen and removing waste products. The coronary arteries supply blood to the heart itself, and when atherosclerosis affects these arteries, coronary artery disease occurs. In this disease process, plaques form within the arteries, restricting the blood supply to the heart muscle. The restriction can cause angina pectoris, with symptoms of chest pain and difficulty in breathing. Blocked coronary arteries can

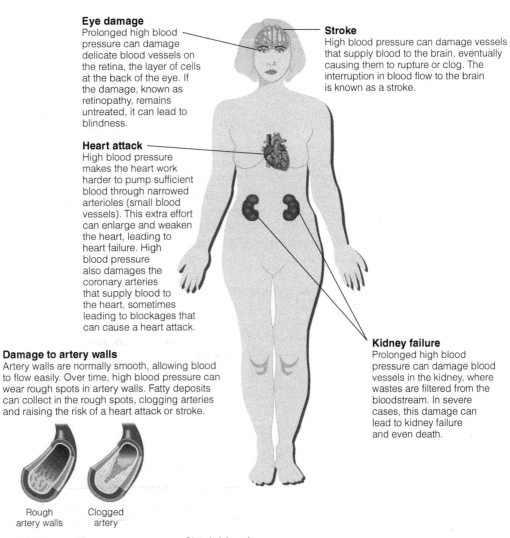

Eye damage
Prolonged high blood pressure can damage delicate blood vessels on the retina, the layer of cells at the back of the eye. If the damage, known as retinopathy, remains untreated, it can lead to blindness.

Stroke
High blood pressure can damage vessels that supply blood to the brain, eventually causing them to rupture or clog. The interruption in blood flow to the brain is known as a stroke.

Heart attack
High blood pressure makes the heart work harder to pump sufficient blood through narrowed arterioles (small blood vessels). This extra effort can enlarge and weaken the heart, leading to heart failure. High blood pressure also damages the coronary arteries that supply blood to the heart, sometimes leading to blockages that can cause a heart attack.

Kidney failure
Prolonged high blood pressure can damage blood vessels in the kidney, where wastes are filtered from the bloodstream. In severe cases, this damage can lead to kidney failure and even death.

Damage to artery walls
Artery walls are normally smooth, allowing blood to flow easily. Over time, high blood pressure can wear rough spots in artery walls. Fatty deposits can collect in the rough spots, clogging arteries and raising the risk of a heart attack or stroke.

Rough artery walls

Clogged artery

FIGURE 9.6   The consequences of high blood pressure.

Source: An invitation to health (7th ed., p. 370), by D. Hales, 1997, Pacific Grove, CA: Brooks/Cole. From HALES, *Invitation to Health,* 7E.

TABLE 9.1   Ranges of Blood Pressure (Expressed in mm of Hg)

	Systolic		Diastolic
Normal	<120	and	<80
Prehypertension	120–139	or	80–89
Stage 1 hypertension	140–159	or	90–99
Stage 2 hypertension	≥160	or	≥100

Source: Adapted from *The seventh report of the joint national committee on prevention, detection, evaluation and treatment of high blood pressure* (NIH Publication No. 03-5233), 2003, by U.S. Department of Health and Human Services (USDHHS). Washington, DC: Author. Table 1.

also lead to a myocardial infarction (heart attack). When the oxygen supply to the brain is disrupted, stroke occurs. Stroke can affect any part of the brain and can vary in severity from minor to fatal. Hypertension—high blood pressure—is a predictor of both heart attack and stroke. Both behavioral and medical treatments can lower hypertension as well as other risk factors for CVD.

The Changing Rates of Cardiovascular Disease

The current mortality rate from CVD for people in the United States is lower than it was in 1920. However, between 1920 and 2002, the death rates changed dramatically. Figure 9.7 reveals a sharp rise in CVD deaths from 1920 until the 1950s and 1960s, followed by a decline that continues to the present day. Currently, nearly 30% of all deaths in the United States are from CVD (NCHS, 2016a, 2016b).

In 1920, the rate of deaths due to heart disease was similar for women and men. Overall, the rates of death from CVD remain similar, but the pattern of deaths began to differ when CVD rates began to rise. During the middle of the 20th century, men died from CVD at younger ages than women, creating a gender gap in heart disease.

Reasons for the Decline in Death Rates

The decline in cardiac mortality in the United States is due largely to two causes: improved emergency coronary care and changes in risk factors for CVD (Ford et al., 2007; Wise, 2000). Beginning in the 1960s, many people in the United States began to change their lifestyle. They began to smoke less, be more aware of their blood pressure, control serum cholesterol, watch their weight, and follow a regular exercise program.

Publicity from two monumental research studies prompted these lifestyle changes. The first was the Framingham Heart Study that began to issue reports during the 1960s, implicating cigarette smoking, high cholesterol, hypertension, a sedentary lifestyle, and obesity as risk factors in CVD (Levy & Brink, 2005). The second study was the highly publicized 1964 Surgeon General's report (U.S. Public Health Service [USPHS], 1964), which found

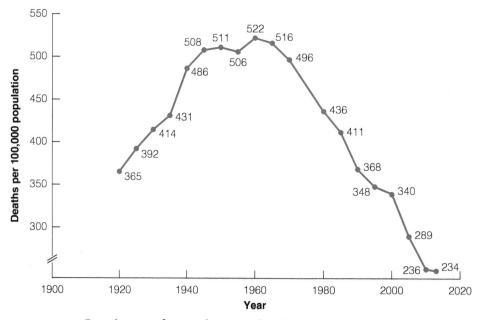

FIGURE 9.7 Death rates for cardiovascular disease per 100,000 population, United States, 1920–2013.

Source: U.S. Public Health Service, *Vital Statistics of the United States,* annual, Vol. I and Vol. II (1900–1970); U.S. National Center for Health Statistics, *Vital Statistics of the United States,* annual (1971–2001); *National Vital Statistics Report,* monthly (2002–2005). Retrieved August 21, 2008, from http://www.infoplease.com/ipa/A0922292.html; *National Vital Statistics Report* (2016). Retrieved July 20, 2016, from http://www.cdc.gov/nchs/data/nvsr/nvsr64/nvsr64_02.pdf

a strong association between cigarette smoking and heart disease. Many people became aware of these studies and began to alter their way of living.

Although these lifestyle changes closely parallel declining heart disease death rates, they offer no proof of a causal link between behavior changes and the drop in cardiovascular mortality. During this same period, medical care and technology continued to improve, and many cardiac patients who in earlier years would have died were saved by better and faster treatment. Which factor—lifestyle changes or better medical care—contributed more to the declining death rate from heart disease? The answer is both. About 47% of the decline in CHD was due to improvements in treatment and 44% to changes in risk factors (Ford et al., 2007). Thus, the declining rate of death from heart disease is due about as much to changes in behavior and lifestyle as it is to improved medical care.

Heart Disease Throughout the World

Heart disease is the leading cause of death, not only in the United States but also worldwide. The total number of deaths from heart disease and stroke accounts for about 30% of all deaths (Mackay & Mensah, 2004). The United States is only one of many high-income Western countries that have seen lifestyle changes and dramatic reductions in cardiovascular deaths among its population (World Health Organization [WHO], 2008b).

In Finland, CVD rates fell more than 70% from the 1970s through the 1990s (Puska, 2002; Puska, Vartiainen, Tuomilehto, Salomaa, & Nissinen, 1998). Part of this decrease was the result of a countrywide effort to change risk factors. That effort began with a community intervention that targeted an area of Finland with particularly high rates of CVD and attempted to change diet, hypertension, and smoking. This lowering of risk factors was largely responsible for the majority of the reduction (Laatikainen et al., 2005).

In contrast, during decades when rates of CVD were dropping in many countries, rates of heart disease were increasing in countries that were once part of the Soviet Union (Weidner, 2000; Weidner & Cain, 2003). This epidemic affected middle-aged men more than other groups, and the gender gap in heart disease is larger in Russia and other former Soviet republics than in most all other countries. The risk of premature death from heart disease is four times greater for a Russian man than for one in the United States. In some countries in Eastern Europe, coronary heart disease

accounts for 80% of deaths; the average life expectancy has decreased and is not expected to increase in the near future. The reasons for this plague of heart disease are not completely understood, but lack of social support, and high levels of stress, smoking, and alcohol abuse are common, and these psychosocial and behavioral differences may underlie the increased rates of CVD (Weidner & Cain, 2003). Fortunately, in the last decade, rates of mortality due to CVD are beginning to drop in many of the countries of the former Soviet Union (Nichols, Townsend, Scarborough, & Rayner, 2014).

Heart disease and stroke are also leading causes of death in developing and underdeveloped countries, where an increase in heart disease and stroke continues (WHO, 2008b). As tobacco smoking, obesity, physical activity, and dietary patterns in these countries become more like those of developed nations, CVD will increase in developing nations. Thus, the worldwide burden of CVD is immense.

IN SUMMARY

Since the mid-1960s, deaths from coronary artery disease and stroke have steadily declined in the United States and most (but not all) other high-income nations. Although some of that decline is a result of better and faster coronary care, lifestyle changes account for 50% or more of this decrease. In low-income countries around the world, the opposite has occurred: Smoking and obesity have increased and physical activity has decreased. These habits have increased risks for CVD, which will grow in these countries in the coming years.

Risk Factors in Cardiovascular Disease

Research links several risk factors to the development of CVD. In Chapter 2, we defined a *risk factor* as any characteristic or condition that occurs with greater frequency in people with a disease than in people free from that disease. The risk factor approach does not identify the cause of a disease. Nor does it allow a precise prediction of who will succumb to disease and who will remain healthy. The risk factor approach simply yields information concerning which conditions are associated—directly or indirectly—with a particular disease or disorder.

The risk factor approach to predicting heart disease began with the Framingham Heart Study in 1948, an investigation of more than 5,000 people in the town of Framingham, Massachusetts (Levy & Brink, 2005). The study was a prospective design; thus, all participants were free of heart disease at the beginning of the study. The original plan was to follow these people for 20 years to study heart disease and the factors related to its development. The results proved so valuable that the study has continued now for more than 50 years and includes both children and grandchildren of the original participants.

At the time of their discovery, medicine had not considered many typical American lifestyle behaviors to be particularly dangerous (Levy & Brink, 2005). Prompted by the growing epidemic of heart disease in the 1950s, the Framingham study revealed that these risk factors are reliably related to the development of heart disease and stroke.

Several large-scale studies followed the Framingham study. These include the Nurses' Health Study, a long-term epidemiological study of women's health that confirms the link between several risk factors and women's risk for CVD (Oh, Hu, Manson, Stampfer, & Willett, 2005). The largest study of cardiovascular health to date is the 52-country INTERHEART Study (Yusuf et al., 2004), which matched over 15,000 people who experienced a heart attack with nearly 15,000 similar people who had not. This case–control study examined a host of other potential risk factors and the extent to which risk factors for CVD are similar across countries. Thus, much of our knowledge about the risk factors for major cardiovascular problems comes from the Framingham, Nurses' Health, and INTERHEART studies.

Cardiovascular risk factors include those that are inherent, those that arise from physiological conditions, those that arise from behavior, and a variety of psychosocial factors.

Inherent Risk Factors

Inherent risk factors result from genetic or physical conditions that cannot be readily modified. Although inherent risk factors cannot be changed, people with these risk factors are not necessarily destined to develop CVD. Identifying people with inherent risk factors enables these high-risk individuals to minimize their overall risk profile by controlling the things that they can, such as hypertension, smoking, and diet. Inherent risk factors for CVD include advancing age, family history, gender, and ethnic background.

Advancing Age   Advancing age is the primary risk factor for CVD as well as for cancer and many other diseases. As people become older, their risk for cardiovascular death rises sharply. Figure 9.8 shows that for every 10-year increase in age, both men and women more than double their chances of dying of CVD. For example, men 85 and older are about 2.7 times as likely to die of CVD as men between the ages of 75 and 84, and women 85 and older are about 3.7 times as likely as women 75 to 84 to die from CVD.

Family History   Family history is also an inherent risk factor for CVD. People with a history of CVD in their family are more likely to die of heart disease than those with no such history. Similarly, people with a parent who has suffered a heart attack are more likely to suffer a heart attack themselves (Chow et al., 2011). Bill Clinton mentioned his family history as a factor that put him at risk for CVD. This familial risk is likely to occur through the action of many genes and their interactions with environmental factors in people's lives (Doevendans, Van der Smagt, Loh, De Jonge, & Touw, 2003). Like other inherent risk factors, genes cannot be altered through lifestyle changes, but people with a family history of heart disease can lower their risk by changing their lifestyle.

Gender   Although gender is an inherent risk factor, many behaviors and social conditions are related to gender. Thus, the differing risk for women and men may or may not be inherent.

In 1920, the rate of deaths due to heart disease was similar for women and men. Overall, the rates of death from CVD remain similar, but the pattern of deaths began to differ when CVD rates began to rise. During the middle of the 20th century, men died from CVD at younger ages than women, creating a gender gap in heart disease.

As Figure 9.8 shows, this gender gap continues to exist. Men have a higher rate of death from CVD than women, and this discrepancy shows most prominently during the middle-age years. After that age, the percentage of women's deaths due to CVD increases sharply, and a larger number of older women than older men die of CVD; nonetheless, the rate of death from CVD remains higher for men.

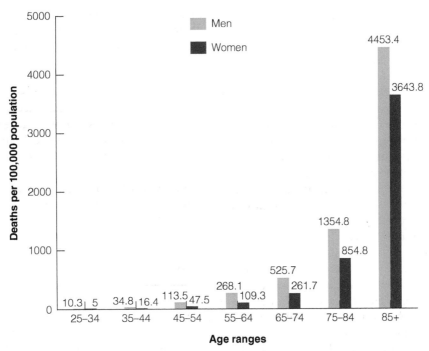

FIGURE 9.8   Mortality rates for diseases of the heart by age and gender, United States, 2014.

Source: Health United States, 2015, by National Center for Health Statistics, 2016, Hyattsville, MD: U.S. Table 23. Retrieved July 20, 2016, from http://www.cdc.gov/nchs/data/hus/hus15.pdf

What factors explain this gender gap? Both physiology and lifestyle contribute (Pilote et al., 2007). Before menopause, women experience a lower rate of CVD than men. At one time, estrogen was believed to furnish protection, but the failure to produce any benefit in a large-scale hormone replacement trial engendered doubt (Writing Group for the Women's Health Initiative Investigators, 2002). A more recent focus is on androgens, including the possibility that these hormones may involve both protections and risks for both men and women (Ng, 2007).

However, lifestyle is responsible for much of the gender gap in heart disease. Across the world, men tend to experience a heart attack at an earlier age than women do, and this difference is explained by men's higher rates of unhealthy lifestyle factors during their younger years (Anand et al., 2008). Furthermore, the gender gap is particularly large in some countries. Russia has the widest gender gap in life expectancy in the world—women can expect to outlive men by an average of 12 years—and most of the discrepancy comes from higher rates of CVD among men (CIA, 2016). Russian men's health habits include more smoking and drinking, and

they show poorer coping skills for dealing with stress. In other countries, such as Iceland, the gender difference in CVD rate is small (Weidner, 2000). The fact that gender differences in CVD mortality are much greater in some countries than in others suggests that behavioral factors, rather than inherent biological differences, explain the CVD mortality discrepancy between men and women.

Ethnic Background   A fourth inherent risk for CVD is ethnic background. In the United States, African Americans have more than a 30% greater risk for cardiovascular death than European Americans, but Native Americans, Asian Americans, and Hispanic Americans have lower rates (CDC/NCHS, 2010d). The increased risk for African Americans may be related to social, economic, or behavioral factors rather than to any biological basis, because the INTERHEART Study (Yusuf et al., 2004) indicated that the risk factors for heart disease are the same for people in countries around the world. Thus, ethnic differences in heart disease are likely due to ethnic differences in levels of known risk factors.

African Americans follow that pattern: They have higher levels of risk factors for heart disease than European Americans, Hispanics, Asians, and Native Americans. The strongest risk for African Americans is high blood pressure (Jones et al., 2002), but psychosocial risks such as low income and low educational level also have a major impact (Karlamangla et al., 2005; Pilote et al., 2007). The higher rates of cardiovascular death among African Americans may be due to their higher rate of hypertension. Their higher rate of hypertension may be partly due to greater cardiac reactivity, as a possible result of ongoing experiences of racial discrimination. Even threats of discrimination can raise blood pressure in African Americans (Blascovich, Spencer, Quinn, & Steele, 2001). The tendency to react to stress and threats of stress with increased cardiac reactivity may arise from years of racial discrimination, discrimination most likely to be experienced by dark-skinned people. For example, Elizabeth Klonoff and Hope Landrine (2000) found that dark-skinned African Americans were 11 times more likely than light-skinned African Americans to experience frequent racial discrimination. Thus, racial discrimination seems to be a factor in the increased blood pressure levels among African Americans, but these responses are classified as psychosocial risks that relate to ethnicity rather than as a risk that is inherent in ethnic differences.

Physiological Conditions

A second category of risk factors in CVD includes the physiological conditions of hypertension, serum cholesterol level, problems in glucose metabolism, and inflammation.

Hypertension   Other than advancing age, hypertension is the single most important risk factor for CVD, yet millions of people with high blood pressure are not aware of their vulnerability. Unlike most disorders, hypertension produces no overt symptoms, and dangerously elevated blood pressure levels commonly occur with no signals or symptoms.

The Framingham Heart Study provided the first solid evidence of the risks of hypertension. More recently, the 52-country INTERHEART Study confirmed the strong link between hypertension and cardiovascular problems across age, gender, ethnicity, and country of residence (Yusuf et al., 2004). As a U.S. government report stated, "The risk between BP and risk of CVD events is continuous, consistent, and independent of other risk factors. The higher the BP, the greater the chance of heart attack, heart failure, stroke, and kidney disease" (USDHHS, 2003, p. 2).

Serum Cholesterol Level   A second physiological condition related to CVD is high serum cholesterol level. Cholesterol is a waxy, fat-like substance that is essential for human life as a component of cell membranes. *Serum* or *blood cholesterol* is the level of cholesterol circulating through the bloodstream; this level is related (but not perfectly related) to *dietary cholesterol*, or the amount of cholesterol in one's food. Dietary cholesterol comes from animal fats and oils but not from vegetables or vegetable products. Although cholesterol is essential for life, too much may contribute to the process of developing CVD.

After a person eats cholesterol, the bloodstream transports it as part of the process of digestion. A measurement of the amount of cholesterol carried in the serum (the liquid, cell-free part of the blood) is typically expressed in milligrams (mg) of cholesterol per deciliters (dl) of serum. Thus, a cholesterol reading of 210 means 210 mg of cholesterol per deciliter of blood serum.

However, total cholesterol in the bloodstream is not the best predictor of CVD. Cholesterol circulates in the blood in several forms of **lipoproteins**, which can be distinguished by analyzing their density and function. **Low-density lipoprotein** (LDL) carries cholesterol from the liver to the cells of the body, whereas **high-density lipoprotein** (HDL) carries cholesterol from the tissues back to the liver. The Framingham researchers found that LDL was positively related to CVD, whereas HDL was negatively related. Subsequent research supports this relationship. High-density lipoprotein actually seems to offer some protection against CVD, whereas LDL seems to promote atherosclerosis. For these reasons, LDL is sometimes referred to as "bad cholesterol" and HDL as "good cholesterol." Indeed, women's higher levels of HDL may be a partial explanation for the gender gap in heart disease (Pilote et al., 2007).

Total cholesterol (TC) is determined by adding the values for HDL, LDL, and 20% of very low-density lipoprotein (VLDL), also called **triglycerides**. A low ratio of total cholesterol to HDL is more desirable than a high ratio. A ratio of less than 4.5 to 1 is healthier than a ratio of 6.0 to 1; that is, people whose HDL level is about 20% to 22% of total cholesterol have a reduced risk of CVD. Most authorities now believe that a favorable balance

TABLE 9.2   Desirable Ranges for Serum Cholesterol, Along with Examples of Favorable and Risky Profiles

Cholesterol Component	Desirable Range	Good Profile	Risky Profile
HDL cholesterol	>60 mg/dl	70	40
LDL cholesterol	<130 mg/dl	60	180
Triglycerides	<200 mg/dl	150	250
	(20% of VLDL)	30 (= 150 × 0.20)	50 (= 250 × 0.20)
Total cholesterol	<200 mg/dl	70 + 60 + 30 = 160	40 + 180 + 50 = 270
Cholesterol/HDL ratio	<4.00	160/70 = 2.28	270/40 = 6.75

of total cholesterol to HDL is more critical than total cholesterol in avoiding CVD, and much recent research has focused on lowering LDL via dietary changes or pharmaceuticals known as *statins* (Grundy et al., 2004). Table 9.2 presents the desirable ranges for total cholesterol and each of the subfractions, along with a desirable and an undesirable profile.

Research on cholesterol suggests several conclusions. First, cholesterol intake and blood cholesterol are related. Second, the relationship between dietary intake of cholesterol and blood cholesterol relates strongly to habitual diet—that is, eating habits maintained over many years. Lowering blood cholesterol level by changing diet is possible, but the process is neither quick nor easy. Third, the ratio of total cholesterol to HDL is probably more important than total cholesterol alone, but lowering LDL is an important goal.

Problems in Glucose Metabolism   A third physiological risk factor for CVD comes from problems with glucose metabolism. The most obvious of such problems is diabetes, a condition in which glucose cannot be taken into the cells because of problems in producing or using insulin. When this situation occurs, glucose remains in the blood at abnormally high levels. People who have juvenile onset (Type 1) diabetes are more likely to develop CVD, and longer-duration problems with glucose metabolism increase the risk (Pambianco, Costacou, & Orchard, 2007). Type 2 diabetes also elevates the risk of CVD (Sobel & Schneider, 2005). (We discuss the risks of diabetes more fully in Chapter 11.)

Many people have problems with glucose metabolism that do not qualify as diabetes but may still create CVD risk. One study (Khaw et al., 2004) showed that people who have problems in glucose metabolism (but

not diabetes) had greater risks for CVD development or death than those with normal glucose metabolism. Such problems in glucose metabolism constitute one of the factors in the *metabolic syndrome*, a collection of factors proposed to elevate the risk for CVD (Johnson & Weinstock, 2006). Other components of metabolic syndrome include excess abdominal fat, elevated blood pressure, and problems with the levels of two components of cholesterol. People with metabolic syndrome are twice as likely to experience cardiovascular health problems as those without the syndrome (Mottillo et al., 2010). In a study testing the components of the metabolic syndrome (Anderson et al., 2004), problems in insulin metabolism were more strongly related to arterial damage than the other components.

Inflammation   As unlikely as it may sound, atherosclerosis results in part from the body's natural inflammatory response. As you learned in Chapter 6, inflammation is a nonspecific immune response. When a tissue is damaged, white blood cells (such as granulocytes and macrophages) migrate to the site of the injury and defend against potential invaders by engulfing them through the process of phagocytosis. When an artery is injured or infected, these white blood cells migrate toward and accumulate on the artery wall. When a person's diet is high in cholesterol, the "diet" of these white blood cells is likewise high in cholesterol. Arterial plaques—the precursors to atherosclerosis—are simply accumulations of cholesterol-filled white blood cells. Inflammation influences not only the development of plaques but also their stability, making them more likely to rupture and cause a heart attack or stroke (Abi-Saleh et al., 2008).

Because chronic inflammation may raise the risk for the development of atherosclerosis (Pilote et al.,

2007), factors that produce chronic inflammation may also increase risk for CVD. Stress and depression are two factors that may contribute to inflammation (Miller & Blackwell, 2006) and are two known risk factors for CVD. Indeed, inflammatory processes account for some, but not all, of the association between depression and increased risk of cardiovascular mortality (Kop et al., 2010). Metabolic syndrome may also be related to inflammation (Vlachopoulos, Rokkas, Ioakeimidis, & Stefanadis, 2007), suggesting that these conditions interact or have some common pathways for causing damage to the cardiovascular system.

Similarly, any factor that reduces inflammation may reduce risk for CVD. For example, aspirin—an anti-inflammatory pain reliever—lowers the risk of heart attack. Thus, the findings about the risks from inflammation explain why taking aspirin lowers the risk of heart attack, and the findings about stress and depression suggest that other behavioral factors may present risks as well as ways to protect against CVD. These findings also help explain why taking care of your teeth and gums may also keep your heart healthy (see Would You Believe … ? box).

Behavioral Factors

Behavioral factors constitute a third risk category for CVD; the most important of these lifestyle factors are smoking, diet, and physical activity. For example, women who do not smoke, eat a diet high in fiber and low in saturated fat, are not overweight, and are physically active have an 80% lower risk for coronary heart disease than other people (Stampfer, Hu, Manson, Rimm, & Willett, 2000)! Each of these behaviors—smoking, food choice, weight maintenance, and physical activity—is related to CVD.

Smoking   Cigarette smoking is the leading behavioral risk factor for cardiovascular death in the United States, and a major contributor to deaths throughout the world (American Cancer Society, 2012; USDHHS, 2010c). In the United States, cardiovascular deaths due to smoking have begun to decline (Rodu & Cole, 2007). For example, between 1987 and 2002, deaths attributable to smoking declined 41% in men and 30% in women. However, such a decline has not occurred in all parts of the world—smoking continues at higher rates in many other countries than in the United States. Smoking accounts for about 35% of the risk for heart attack worldwide (Yusuf

et al., 2004), which translates into more than a million deaths per year.

People who currently smoke are three times more likely to suffer a heart attack than people who never smoked (Teo et al., 2006). Fortunately, quitting smoking does reduce the risk of heart attack: within 3 years of quitting, former smokers are only twice as likely to suffer a heart attack as those who never smoke (Teo et al., 2006). However, the risks of past smoking do not disappear completely, as a small risk for heart attack persists even 20 years after a person quits. Even when tobacco is not inhaled, it still presents risks, as chewing tobacco also increases the risk of heart attack. Passive smoking—or "secondhand" smoking—is not as dangerous as personal tobacco use, but exposure to environmental tobacco smoke raises the risk for CVD by about 15% (Kaur, Cohen, Dolor, Coffman, & Bastian, 2004). Thus, tobacco contributes to increased risk for cardiovascular problems in a number of ways.

Weight and Diet   Obesity and diet also increase risk for CVD. Although the dangers of obesity seem obvious, the evaluation of obesity as an independent risk for CVD is difficult. The main problem is that obesity is related to other risks, such as blood pressure, Type 2 diabetes, total cholesterol, LDL, and triglycerides (Ashton, Nanchahal, & Wood, 2001). A high degree of abdominal fat is a risk factor for heart attack in men (Smith, et al., 2005), in women (Iribarren, Darbinian, Lo, Fireman, & Go, 2006), and in people worldwide (Yusuf et al., 2005).

The dietary choices that people make may either increase or decrease their chances of developing CVD, depending on the foods they eat. Results from two large-scale studies—the Framingham Study (Levy & Brink, 2005) and the INTERHEART Study (Iqbal et al., 2008)—show that diets heavy in saturated fats are positively related to CVD and risk of heart attack. These high-fat foods have an obvious link to serum cholesterol levels, but other nutrients may also affect CVD risks.

For example, sodium intake contributes to high blood pressure (one of the major risks for CVD; Stamler et al., 2003), and some individuals seem to be more sensitive to the effects of sodium intake than others (Brooks, Haywood, & Johnson, 2005). Potassium intake, however, seems to decrease the risk, which brings up the question: Can diet serve as protection against CVD? A growing body of results indicates that some diets, and perhaps even some foods, offer protective effects.

Would You BELIEVE...?   Chocolate May Help Prevent Heart Disease

Would you believe that chocolate—rather than being bad for you—may contain chemicals that help prevent coronary artery disease? One of the dietary components that seems to offer some protection against artery damage is a class of chemicals called *flavonoids*, which are derived primarily from fruits and vegetables (Engler & Engler, 2006). Several subcategories of flavonoids exist, each with slightly different properties. The subcategory that contains chocolate is the flavonols, which also occur in tea, red wine, grapes, and blackberries. However, all of the subcategories have been linked to health benefits, including growing evidence of the advantages of chocolate.

Not all chocolate contains the same amount of flavonoids, and thus some types of chocolate may offer more protection than others (Engler & Engler, 2006). The processing of the cacao bean, from which chocolate is made, affects the flavonoid content. Dark chocolate contains two to three times more flavonoids than milk chocolate or Dutch chocolate.

Flavonoids exert their health benefits by reducing oxidation, making them one type of antioxidant. The benefits may occur through effects on the lining of arteries (Engler & Engler, 2006). Flavonoids may be especially effective in protecting arteries against the harmful effects of low-density cholesterol and increase vascular dilation. If flavonoids protect arteries, that mechanism would explain the connection between flavonol intake and lower rates of coronary heart disease mortality (Huxley & Neil, 2003). However, chocolate consumption has also shown cardiovascular benefits in lowering blood pressure and decreasing inflammation, both of which lower risk factors for CVD (Engler & Engler, 2006). This body of research indicates that chocolate consumption may protect against heart disease in a variety of ways.

Chocolate is not the only food that is rich in flavonols. High concentrations of this micronutrient also occur in green and black tea, grapes, red wine, cherries, apples, blackberries, and raspberries. Thus, chocolate may not offer unique health benefits, but legions of chocoholics would testify that its taste is unique. These devotees are overjoyed that a food that was once considered a sin may now offer salvation from heart disease.

Over more than two decades, researchers showed that diets high in fruits and vegetables predict lower CVD risks. The INTERHEART Study, for example, found that people who ate a diet high in fruits and vegetables had a lower risk of heart attack (Iqbal et al., 2008). One analysis of worldwide consumption of fruits and vegetables (Lock, Pomerleau, Causer, Altmann, & McKee, 2005) concluded that if these levels increased to a minimal acceptable level, the rate of heart disease could be reduced by 31% and stroke by 19%.

A diet high in fish seems to offer some protection against heart disease and stroke (Iso et al., 2001; Torpy, 2006); the protective component is *omega-3 fatty acids*. Fish such as tuna, salmon, mackerel, and other high-fat fish and shellfish are high in this nutrient, but research on the benefits of fish has yielded mixed results. Not all fish meals offer the same protection (Mozaffarian et al., 2005). For example, baked or broiled fish was more beneficial than fried fish in decreasing the risk of stroke in older adults. The American Heart Association recommends at least two servings of fish per week (Smith & Sahyoun, 2005) based on this evidence. That advantage is balanced against the high level of mercury in some fish, which also presents risks.

Do certain vitamins or other micronutrients protect against CVD? People who eat diets high in antioxidants such as vitamin E, beta carotene or lycopene, selenium, and riboflavin show a number of health advantages, including lower levels of CVD (Stanner, Hughes, Kelly, & Buttriss, 2004). These antioxidants protect LDL from oxidation and thus from its potentially damaging effects on the cardiovascular system. However, research findings do not show that taking supplements of these nutrients is as effective as eating a diet that contains the nutrients in high levels. Such a diet may include some surprising choices (see Would You Believe …? box).

Physical Activity   Across the world, two factors consistently predict higher risk of heart attack: owning a car and owning a television (Held et al., 2012). These two factors have one thing in common: they both reduce physical activity. The benefits of physical activity in lowering cardiovascular risk are clear and "irrefutable" (Warburton, Nicol, & Bredin, 2006, p. 801; see Chapter 15

Would You BELIEVE...? Nearly All the Risk for Stroke Is Due to Modifiable Factors

In the United States, nearly 1 million people suffer a stroke each year, and strokes are the fifth leading cause of death. Despite its prevalence and its role as a leading cause of mortality, would you believe that people's risk for stroke is due almost entirely to *modifiable* factors?

An international team of researchers examined the medical records of 6,000 men and women from across the world (O'Donnell et al., 2010). The researchers utilized a case-control method, where 3,000 of the participants had been admitted to a hospital for a first stroke, and the other 3,000 participants had not experienced a stroke. The researchers compared the two groups to identify the extent to which a number of risk factors predicted the likelihood of stroke.

The researchers found that 10 risk factors were associated with 90% of their population's risk of stroke! The factors that contributed to risk most strongly were hypertension, lack of physical activity, high cholesterol, and poor diet; these four factors alone accounted for 80% of the population's stroke risk. Other significant factors were obesity, smoking, alcohol intake, and stress. You will notice that many of these factors are the same factors that contribute to cardiovascular disease more generally. However, the role of modifiable, behavioral risk factors in disease is perhaps no more apparent than it is in the case of stroke risk.

for a review of this evidence). Unfortunately, people's jobs have become less physically strenuous, and many individuals do not engage in physical activity in their leisure time, creating large numbers of sedentary people in many industrialized societies.

The risks of inactivity apply to the entire life span. In the United States, children have become less physically active, and their sedentary lifestyle has contributed to their increasing obesity and growing risk for CVD (Wang, 2004). At the other end of the age spectrum, women over age 65 showed better health and lower CVD risks when they voluntarily engaged in exercise (Simonsick, Guralnik, Volpato, Balfour, & Fried, 2005). Sedentary lifestyle also contributes to the metabolic syndrome, the pattern of CVD risks that include overweight, abdominal fat, and blood glucose metabolism problems (Ekelund et al., 2005). Thus, physical inactivity is an important behavioral risk factor for CVD.

Psychosocial Factors

A number of psychosocial factors relate to heart disease (Smith & Ruiz, 2002). These factors are education, income, marital status, social support, stress, anxiety, depression, cynical hostility, and anger.

Educational Level and Income Low socioeconomic status—often assessed by low educational level and low income—are risk factors for CVD. For example, in the INTERHEART Study, low socioeconomic status

emerged as a risk factor for heart attack (Rosengren et al., 2009). In particular, low education placed people at increased risk for heart attack. In many countries, educational levels are related to ethnicity, but studies in the United States (Yan et al., 2006), Netherlands (Bos, Kunst, Garssen, & Mackenbach, 2005), and Israel (Manor, Eisenbach, Friedlander, & Kark, 2004) examined educational level within ethnic groups. The results showed that, independent of ethnicity, low educational level increased risk for CVD.

What factors link low levels of education to high levels of heart disease? One possibility is that people with low education practice fewer protective health behaviors than those with higher educational levels; they eat a less healthy diet, smoke, and lead more sedentary lives (Laaksonen et al., 2008). Indeed, in the INTERHEART Study, much of the influence of socioeconomic factors such as education on cardiovascular risk was explained by the modifiable lifestyle factors of smoking, physical activity, diet, and obesity (Rosengren et al., 2009).

Income level is another risk factor for CVD; people with lower incomes have higher rates of heart disease than people in the higher income brackets. A report from China (Yu et al., 2000) showed that socioeconomic level—defined as education, occupation, income, and marital status—related to cardiovascular risk factors such as blood pressure, body mass index, and cigarette smoking. This finding is not isolated—many studies show links between socioeconomic status and health, mortality, and CVD. A cross-national study (Kim, Kawachi, Hoorn, & Ezzati, 2008) revealed that in societies with a large discrepancy in income levels, individuals in the lower part of the income distribution had higher risk factors for CVD. The effect may occur through income level or social status; evidence exists for both. Income level relates to longevity in the form of a gradient, with higher income predicting longer life (Krantz & McCeney, 2002). Social rank and status have a variety of cardiovascular effects in many species, including humans (Sapolsky, 2004). In addition, research suggests that these socioeconomic cardiovascular risks begin to accumulate during adolescence or even childhood (Karlamangla et al., 2005). Thus, educational level, income, and social status all show effects on the cardiovascular system and on diseases of this system.

Social Support and Marriage   Prospective studies confirm that lacking social support is also a risk for CVD (Krantz & McCeney, 2002). This conclusion is consistent with the wide body of research discussed in Chapter 5 that shows the value of social support and the problems that can arise from its absence. Indeed, loneliness during childhood, adolescence, and young adulthood relates to CVD risk factors (Caspi, Harrington, Moffitt, Milne, & Poulton, 2006), and these effects may become more serious with aging (Hawkley & Cacioppo, 2007). For example, older people who had experienced a heart attack were more likely to have another, fatal heart attack if they lived alone (Schmaltz et al., 2007).

Lack of social support may be a factor even more important in the progression of CVD. Studies that measured the progression of blockage of the coronary arteries in women (Wang, Mittleman, & Orth-Gomér, 2005; Wang et al., 2007) found that support at home and at work affected the progression of coronary artery blockage; high stress in either area predicted progressive blockage, whereas satisfactory support in both led to regression of arterial plaques. Another study showed that the number of people in a person's social network related to coronary mortality; CAD patients with only one to three people in their social network were nearly 2½ times more likely to die of coronary artery disease than patients with four or more close friends (Brummett et al., 2001). Older men who were more socially involved were less likely to die of CVD than those who were more isolated (Ramsay et al., 2008).

Marriage should provide social support, and in general, married people are at decreased risk for

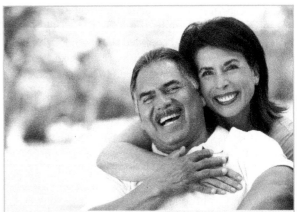

Marriage appears to provide protection against cardiovascular disease.

cardiovascular health problems (Empana et al., 2008; Hu et al., 2012). For example, two large population studies—one in France (Empana et al., 2008) and another in China (Hu et al., 2012)—both found that married individuals were less likely to suffer a heart attack than people who were not married. However, the quality of the marital relationship may be a factor. In a 10-year follow-up, married men were almost half as likely to die as unmarried men (Eaker, Sullivan, Kelly-Hayes, D'Agostino, & Benjamin, 2007). For women, the benefits depended on marital communication and quality, with poor communication increasing heart disease risk. Another study (Holt-Lunstad, Birmingham, & Jones, 2008) focused specifically on marriage and also found that marital quality was important; marriage was not beneficial if the individual was dissatisfied with the relationship. However, happily married people received greater benefits in the form of lower blood pressure than single people, even those with a supportive social network.

Spouses (and other sources of social support) may reduce the risk of cardiovascular mortality by providing encouragement for compliance with a healthy lifestyle or a medical regimen or by urging a person to seek medical care (Williams et al., 1992). Sources of social support are usually friends, family, spouses, and even pets (Allen, 2003). Support may also affect CVD through its influence on the experience of stress and depression.

Stress, Anxiety, and Depression   Stress, anxiety, and depression relate to CVD, but they also relate to each other (Suls & Bunde, 2005). This overlap makes independent assessment of each component difficult.

However, a great deal of evidence implicates these factors in CVD. For example, the INTERHEART Study (Rosengren et al., 2004) revealed that people who had heart attacks also experienced more work and financial stress and more life events than their matched controls. In a large, prospective study of young adults in the United States, increases in work-related stress led to greater incidence of hypertension 8 years later (Markovitz, Matthews, Whooley, Lewis, & Greenlund, 2004).

Anxiety and depression also increase risk for CVD; the evidence for the risks from depression is especially strong. Even after controlling for other risk factors such as smoking and cholesterol, anxiety (Shen et al., 2008) and depression (Goldston & Baillie, 2008; Whang et al., 2009) predict the development of CVD. The risks of depression and anxiety apply not only to the development of CVD but also to its progression, as depression in the year following a heart attack predicts subsequent risk of cardiovascular mortality (Bekke-Hansen, Trockel, Burg, & Taylor, 2012). However, the evidence is stronger for these two negative emotions in the development of CVD (Suls & Bunde, 2005). Indeed, evidence for the beginning of artery damage appeared in a study of depressed adolescents (Tomfohr, Martin, & Miller, 2008), which is consistent with the long-term damage that accompanies CVD. More evidence about the harm of negative emotions has come from the study of hostility and anger.

Hostility and Anger   Researchers have also found that some types of hostility and anger are risk factors for CVD. Much of this research grew out of work on the Type A behavior pattern, originally proposed by cardiologists Meyer Friedman and Ray Rosenman (1974; Rosenman et al., 1975), physicians who specialized in heart disease. Friedman and Rosenman may have gotten their inspiration for studying the Type A behavior pattern from a rather unusual source: an upholsterer. On numerous occasions, Friedman and Rosenman paid an upholsterer to repair the fabric on the seats in their waiting room. One day the upholsterer commented that only the cardiology patients wore out the seats so quickly, with a pattern that suggested they were habitually sitting on the edges of their seats. Years later, Meyer Friedman reported that this was the first time he remembered anybody making a connection between people's behavior patterns and their risk for CVD (Sapolsky, 1997).

Friedman and Rosenman described people with the Type A behavior pattern as hostile, competitive, concerned with numbers and the acquisition of objects, and possessed of an exaggerated sense of time urgency. During the early years of its history, the Type A behavior pattern demonstrated promise as a predictor of heart disease, but later researchers were unable to affirm a consistent link between the global Type A behavior pattern and incidence of heart disease. This situation led investigators to consider the possibility that some component of the pattern—rather than the entire pattern— might be a predictor.

Hostility appeared to be the component of Type A that was risky. In 1989, Redford Williams suggested that cynical hostility is especially harmful to cardiovascular health. He contended that people who mistrust others, think the worst of humanity, and interact with others with cynical hostility are harming themselves and their hearts. Furthermore, he suggested that people who use *anger* as a response to interpersonal problems have an elevated risk for heart disease.

Hostility early in life does predict cardiovascular health later in life. In one long-term prospective study, young adults who scored high in hostility had higher levels of coronary calcification—a precursor of atherosclerosis—at a 10-year follow-up than young adults low in hostility (Iribarren et al., 2000). Higher levels of hostility also predicted greater incidence of hypertension at a 15-year follow-up (Yan et al., 2003). In addition to increasing risk for these two precursors to CVD, a recent review of over 20 longitudinal studies confirmed hostility as a significant predictor of subsequent CVD (Chida & Steptoe, 2009). The cardiovascular health of men, in particular, relates to both hostility as well as another related emotion: anger.

Anger and hostility may seem the same, but they have important differences. Anger is an unpleasant *emotion* accompanied by physiological arousal, whereas hostility is a negative *attitude* toward others (Suls & Bunde, 2005). The *experience* of anger is probably unavoidable and may not present much of a risk. However, the manner in which a person deals with anger may be a factor in the development of CVD. People may express their anger, including yelling back when someone yells at them, raising their voice when arguing, and throwing temper tantrums. Alternatively, people may suppress their anger, holding in their feelings. Some evidence suggests that either strategy may pose problems.

Anger and Cardiovascular Reactivity   One way that the expression of anger might relate to coronary heart

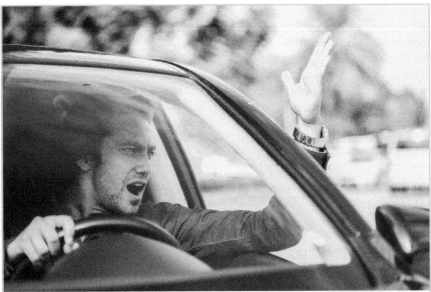

Hostility and expressed anger are risk factors for cardiovascular disease.

lstockphoto.com/seb_ra

disease is through **cardiovascular reactivity (CVR)**, typically defined as increases in blood pressure and heart rate due to frustration, harassment, or any laboratory stress task. Most past research on CVR used laboratory methods in which researchers presented participants with various situations intended to arouse anger and monitored their physiological responses, often using a variety of cardiac measurements such as blood pressure and heart rate. Sometimes, the measurements also included the persistence of such cardiac responses.

In one study using such a procedure (Suarez, Saab, Llabre, Kuhn, & Zimmerman, 2004), African American men showed a stronger blood pressure response than did European American men or women from either ethnic group. This result suggests that the higher prevalence of hypertension among African American men may relate to their tendency to higher reactivity. Another reactivity study (Merritt, Bennett, Williams, Sollers, & Thayer, 2004) focused on educational level and anger-coping strategies among African American men and found that low educational level and a high-effort style of coping are associated with higher blood pressure reactivity. For African Americans, the experiences of racism constitute a source of anger, and one study (Clark, 2003) connected the perception of racism with blood pressure reactivity. This type of reactivity difference also appeared in a study comparing African American and European American women (Lepore

et al., 2006). Thus, reactivity may relate to hypertension among African Americans.

Suppressed Anger   If expressing anger can undermine cardiac health for some people, then would it be better to suppress anger? Results from early studies (Dembroski, MacDougall, Williams, Haney, & Blumenthal, 1985; MacDougall, Dembroski, Dimsdale, & Hackett, 1985) and more recent findings (Harburg, Julius, Kaciroti, Gleiberman, & Schork, 2003; Jorgensen & Kolodziej, 2007) suggest that suppressing anger may be more toxic than forcefully expressing anger. One version of suppressed emotion is rumination—repeated negative thoughts about an incident—which tends to increase negative feelings and depression (Hogan & Linden, 2004). Thus, people who suppress their anger but "stew" over their feelings may be using a coping style that puts them in danger. However, expressing anger (and other negative emotions) in a forceful way may act as triggers for those with CVD, precipitating a heart attack or stroke (Suls & Bunde, 2005).

So when it comes to expressing anger, are you "Damned if you do, damned if you don't" (Dorr, Brosschot, Sollers, & Thayer, 2007, p. 125)? How can people handle anger situations? Aron Siegman (1994) suggested that people learn to recognize their anger but to express it calmly and rationally, in a way that will be likely to resolve rather than escalate a conflict. Indeed, the manner in which a person expresses anger may affect cardiovascular health. People who discuss anger in a way that seeks to resolve a situation have better cardiovascular health, particular among men (Davidson & Mostofsky, 2010). In contrast, people who justify their anger by blaming other people have greater long-term incidence of cardiovascular health problems (Davidson & Mostofsky, 2010). Thus, it may not be just the anger that increases risk for cardiovascular problems, but also the additional stress caused by alienating others with hostile expressions of anger.

It may not be surprising, then, that anger combines with the negative emotions that accompany anxiety and depression to present greater risk for the development of CVD (Bleil, Gianaros, Jennings, Flory, & Manuck, 2008; Suls & Bunde, 2005). In addition, cynical hostility and anger relate to each other and may interact with other risk factors such as high blood pressure to increase a person's risk for heart disease. Figure 9.9 shows the evolution of the Type A behavior pattern to hostility, to anger, to the expression or suppression of anger, and finally to negative emotionality.

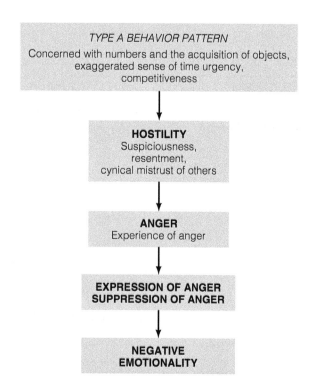

Note: **BOLDFACE** denotes components suggested by research to be the strongest link to heart disease.

FIGURE 9.9 Evolution from the Type A behavior pattern to negative emotionality.

IN SUMMARY

Although the causes of CVD are not fully understood, an accumulating body of evidence points to certain risk factors. These factors include inherent risks such as advancing age, family history of heart disease, gender, and ethnic background. Other risk factors include physiological conditions such as hypertension, problems in glucose metabolism, and high serum cholesterol levels. Other than age, hypertension is the best predictor of coronary artery disease, and a higher blood pressure equals higher risk for heart disease. Total cholesterol level is also related to coronary artery disease, but the *ratio* of total cholesterol to high-density lipoprotein is a more critical risk factor.

Behaviors such as smoking and unwise eating also relate to heart disease. Cigarette smoking is associated with increased risk for heart disease worldwide. Stopping smoking reduces risks, but deciding to never start smoking is the best choice for maintaining cardiovascular health. Eating foods high in saturated fat may lead to obesity, which is a risk for CVD. Also, consuming low levels of fruits and vegetables add to one's risk of heart disease.

Psychosocial risk factors related to coronary artery disease include low educational and income levels; low levels of social support and marital satisfaction; and high levels of stress, anxiety, and depression. The anger and hostility components descended from the Type A behavior pattern are independent risk factors for heart disease. Both the violent expression and the suppression of anger may contribute to CHD disease. Expressing anger in a soft, calm voice is a better coping strategy than violently expressing anger or timidly holding it in.

Reducing Cardiovascular Risks

Psychology's main contribution to cardiovascular health involves changing unhealthy behaviors before these behaviors lead to heart disease. In addition, psychologists may help people who have been diagnosed with heart disease; that is, they often help cardiac rehabilitation patients adhere to an exercise program, a medical regimen, a healthy diet, and smoking cessation.

Before Diagnosis: Preventing First Heart Attacks

What can people do to lower their risks for CVD? Ideally, people should prevent CVD by modifying risk factors before the disease process causes damage. A longitudinal study by Jerry Stamler and his colleagues (1999) indicated that prevention is possible—maintaining a low level of risk factors protects against CVD. This study examined young adult and middle-aged men and women in five large cohorts to see if a low-risk profile would reduce both CVD and other causes of mortality. After dividing the participants into risk groups and screening for as long as 57 years, results indicated that low-risk participants had lower rates of death not only from CHD and stroke but also from all causes. Thus, young and middle-aged men and women who can modify CVD risks to attain low-risk profiles will also lower their risk for all-cause mortality and can expect to live 6 to 10 years longer.

The factors examined by Stamler et al. (1999) included smoking, cholesterol levels, and blood pressure—three major risk factors for CVD. However, the importance of maintaining a healthy lifestyle may begin as early as childhood (Beilin & Huang, 2008), when dietary and physical activity patterns are often established, and definitely continues during adolescence, when most smokers begin their habit. Keeping risk factors low can pay substantial dividends in later years (Matthews, Kuller, Chang, & Edmundowicz, 2007). After people acquire high risks from behavioral factors such as smoking and unwise eating, managing those risks is more difficult. As psychologists are frequently concerned with changing behavior, many of their techniques can be helpful in modifying behaviors that place people at risk for developing CVD.

The most serious behavioral risk factor is cigarette smoking, a behavior that also contributes to many other disorders, especially lung cancer. For this reason, all of Chapter 12 is devoted to a discussion of tobacco use. Although hypertension and serum cholesterol are not behaviors, both can change indirectly through changes in behavior, making these factors candidates for intervention (Linden, 2000).

Before people cooperate with programs to change their behavior, they must perceive that these behaviors place them in jeopardy, which is often a problem for people who have no symptoms of CVD. These individuals may recognize established risk factors in calculating their personal risk, but they often display what Neil Weinstein (1984) called an optimistic bias in assessing their risk. That is, people—particularly young adults—believe they will not develop the problems that other people with similar risk profiles will develop. These thoughts place such individuals in the precontemplation or contemplation stage, according to the transtheoretical model, when they are not ready to make changes (Prochaska et al., 1992, 1994; see Chapter 4 for more on this model). The technique of motivational interviewing, for example, challenges people's beliefs with the goal of moving people toward making positive change; this technique was part of a successful program to increase fruit and vegetable consumption (Resnicow et al., 2001). Thus, moving people to the point of making changes in their health habits is a major challenge for health psychologists involved in cardiovascular health.

Reducing Hypertension   Lowering high blood pressure into the normal range is often a difficult task because a number of physiological mechanisms act to keep blood pressure at a set point (Osborn, 2005). Despite the difficulty, interventions aim to increase people's adherence to behaviors that can, over time, reduce hypertension. One such behavior is the regular use of antihypertensive drugs that require a physician's prescription. The goal is typically to lower blood pressure to 130/80 mmHg or lower (USDHHS, 2003). Because hypertension presents no unpleasant symptoms and the medications may cause side effects, many patients are reluctant to follow this regimen. (The factors affecting adherence to this and other medical regimens are discussed in Chapter 4.)

Several behaviors relate to both the development and the treatment of hypertension, and these behaviors are also targets of interventions. Obesity correlates with hypertension, and many obese people who lose weight lower their blood pressure into the normal range (Moore et al., 2005). Thus, losing weight is part of blood pressure control. (We discuss strategies for losing weight in Chapter 15.) Hypertensive individuals also typically receive recommendations to restrict sodium intake and make dietary changes (Bhatt, Luqman-Arafath, & Guleria, 2007). The Dietary Approach to Stop Hypertension (DASH) originated as a plan to control hypertension; it includes a diet high in fruits, vegetables, whole grains, and low-fat dairy products as well as other lifestyle changes. Table 9.3 shows a daily menu that adheres to the DASH diet, with both regular and low-sodium options. Not only is the DASH diet

TABLE 9.3   Sample Daily Menu from the DASH Plan, with Regular and Low-Sodium Options

2,300 mg Menu	Sodium	Substitution to Reduce Sodium to 1,500 mg	Sodium
Breakfast			
¾ cup bran flakes cereal	220	¾ cup shredded wheat cereal	1
1 medium banana	1		
1 cup low-fat milk	107		
1 slice whole wheat bread	149		
1 tsp margarine	26	1 tsp unsalted margarine	0
1 cup orange juice	5		
Lunch			
¾ cup chicken salad	179	Remove salt from recipe	120
2 slices whole wheat bread	299		
1 tbsp Dijon mustard	373	1 tbsp regular mustard	175
Salad			
½ cup cucumber slices	1		
½ cup tomato wedges	5		
1 tbsp sunflower seeds	0		
1 tsp Italian dressing, low calorie	43		
½ cup fruit cocktail, juice pack	5		
Dinner			
3 oz roast beef	35		
2 tbsp fat-free gravy	165		
1 cup green beans	12		
1 small baked potato	14		
1 tbsp sour cream, fat free	21		
1 tbsp reduced-fat cheddar cheese	67	1 tbsp reduced-fat cheddar cheese, low sodium	1
1 small whole wheat roll	148		
1 tsp margarine	26	1 tsp unsalted margarine	0
1 small apple	1		
1 cup low-fat milk	107		
Snacks			
⅓ cup unsalted almonds	0		
¼ cup raisins	4		
½ cup fruit yogurt, fat free, no added sugar	86		

Source: Adapted from *Your guide to lowering your blood pressure with DASH* (NIH Publication No. 06-4082), 2006, by U.S. Department of Health and Human Services (USDHHS). Washington, DC: Author.

effective in lowering blood pressure but also decreases the risk for stroke and CHD in women (Fung et al., 2008). A regular physical activity program is also effective in controlling hypertension, especially in people who have been sedentary (Murphy, Nevill, Murtagh, & Holder, 2007). (We discuss exercise in Chapter 15.) Other techniques for reducing blood pressure include stress management, meditation, and relaxation training, and we discuss these interventions in Chapters 5 and 8. Thus, a program to control hypertension may have both drug and behavioral components.

Lowering Serum Cholesterol   Interventions aimed at lowering cholesterol levels can include drugs, dietary changes, increased physical activity, or a combination of these components. Eating a diet low in saturated fat and high in fruits and vegetables and maintaining a program of regular physical activity are good strategies for preventing high cholesterol levels, and dietary and exercise interventions are key components in managing high cholesterol levels (USDHHS, 2003). However, once a person develops high cholesterol levels, a prudent diet and physical activity are not likely to lower cholesterol to an acceptable level. Thus, many people with high cholesterol cannot achieve substantially lower cholesterol levels through diet and exercise.

Physicians may prescribe cholesterol-lowering drugs such as the statin drugs to patients with high total cholesterol levels or high LDL levels (Grundy, 2007). These drugs act by blocking an enzyme that the liver needs to manufacture cholesterol. They are especially effective in lowering LDL cholesterol and can reduce risks and improve survival of people at risk for CVD (Brugts et al., 2009; Cholesterol Treatment Trialists' [CTT] Collaboration, 2010). Despite their effectiveness, these drugs require a prescription, cost money, and have side effects.

The recommendations for cholesterol lowering are complex. First, relying on drugs to lower cholesterol without behavioral changes is not a good strategy. Behavioral interventions can help both men and women adhere to a regular exercise program as well as a low-fat diet. Such adherence can lower LDL and improve the ratio of total cholesterol to HDL. If lifestyle changes do not lower cholesterol, then drugs are an option, but not before, especially for people with low levels of risk. Second, the ratio of total cholesterol to HDL is more important than total cholesterol. Statins tend to lower LDL rather than raise HDL, but these drugs lower cholesterol and incidence of heart attacks and stroke,

making them a good choice for people with very high or resistant cholesterol levels (Cheng, Lauder, Chu-Pak, & Kumana, 2004). Third, people with multiple risks for CVD, such as hypertension, diabetes, or smoking, should consider the task of lowering cholesterol as more urgent than those with fewer risks (Grundy, 2007).

Modifying Psychosocial Risk Factors   Earlier, we discussed research that links psychosocial factors such as stress, anxiety, depression, and anger with CVD. The evidence for these risks is sufficiently compelling for some authorities to call for the development of *behavioral cardiology* (Rozanski, Blumenthal, Davidson, Saab, & Kubzansky, 2005), urging cardiologists to screen for psychological risks and to recommend psychological interventions to decrease anxiety and depression and to manage stress and anger. Consistent with this concept, research on people who received angioplasty (Helgeson, 2003) indicated that those who had a more positive outlook about themselves and their future were less likely to experience a recurrence of CVD. These results are good news for former president Bill Clinton, whose optimistic outlook was evident even before his cardiac surgery (King & Henry, 2004).

Anger and negative emotions are also a target of intervention, and clinical health psychologists recommend a variety of strategies for coping with hostility, anger, and depression. To reduce the toxic element in anger, perpetually angry people can learn to become aware of cues from others that typically provoke angry responses. They can also remove themselves from provocative situations before they become angry, or they can do something else. In interpersonal encounters, angry people can use self-talk as a reminder that the situation will not last forever. Humor is another potentially effective means of coping with anger (Godfrey, 2004), but it may present its own risks. Sarcastic or hostile humor can incite additional anger, but silliness or mock exaggerations often defuse potentially volatile situations. Relaxation techniques can also be effective strategies for dealing with anger. These techniques can include progressive relaxation, deep-breathing exercises, tension reduction training, relaxing to the slow repetition of the word "relax," and relaxation imagery, in which the person imagines a peaceful scene. Finally, angry people can lower their blood pressure by constructively discussing their feelings with other people (Davidson, MacGregor, Stuhr, Dixon, & MacLean, 2000).

Discussing feelings with a therapist may also benefit people who are depressed, but physicians may not always

Becoming Healthier

1. Learn about your family risk for heart disease. Although you cannot change this risk factor, knowing that you are at high risk can motivate you to change some modifiable risk factors.

2. Have your blood pressure checked. If it is in the normal range, you can keep it that way by exercising, controlling your weight, and moderating alcohol consumption. Also try some of the relaxation techniques discussed in Chapter 8. If your blood pressure is above the normal range (even a little), consult a physician.

3. Know your cholesterol level, but be sure to ask for a complete profile, one that includes measures of both HDL and LDL as well as the ratio of total cholesterol to HDL.

4. If you are a smoker but have failed at prior attempts to quit, keep trying. Many smokers make multiple attempts before quitting successfully.

5. Keep a food diary for at least 1 week. Note the amount of saturated fat as well as fruits and vegetables you eat and the approximate number of calories consumed per day. A heart-healthy diet is low in saturated fat and includes five servings of fruits and vegetables per day.

6. If you are persistently angry and react to anger-arousing events with loud, sudden explosions of anger or if you "stew" over such events, try to change your reactions by expressing your frustrations in a soft, quiet voice.

recognize this problem. Thus, screening for depression among people at risk for CVD is an urgent need (Goldston & Baillie, 2008). Depression is also common among people who experience a heart attack or other CVD event. These individuals may be more willing to undertake changes to avoid another heart attack or stroke.

After Diagnosis: Rehabilitating Cardiac Patients

After people experience a heart attack, angina, or other symptoms of CVD, they sometimes receive a referral to a cardiac rehabilitation program to change their lifestyle and lower risk for a subsequent (and possibly even more serious) event. In addition to survival, the goals of cardiac rehabilitation programs are to help patients deal with psychological reactions to their diagnosis, to return to normal activities as soon as possible, and to change to a healthier lifestyle.

Patients recovering from heart disease, as well as their spouses, often experience a variety of psychological reactions that include depression, anxiety, anger, fear, guilt, and interpersonal conflict. For cardiac patients, the most common psychological reaction to a myocardial infarction is *depression*, which decreases adherence to medication and lifestyle changes (Kronish et al., 2006) and increases the risk of death to 3.5 times that for non-depressed cardiac patients (Guck et al., 2001).

Treating depression among cardiac patients is an important, but difficult problem. Two large-scale interventions sought to treat depression among cardiac patients, through the use of antidepressant medications (Glassman, Bigger, & Gaffney, 2009) or cognitive behavioral therapy (Berkman et al., 2003). Although these trials have some success in treating depression, the antidepressant intervention did not improve survival. The cognitive behavioral intervention improved survival among European American men, but not among ethnic minority men or among women (Schneiderman et al., 2004).

Another common psychological reaction related to depression is *anxiety*. A follow-up study of cardiac rehabilitation patients (Michie, O'Connor, Bath, Giles, & Earll, 2005) showed that those who completed the rehabilitation program continued to make progress not only in lowering their physiological risks but also in lowering their levels of anxiety and depression and increasing their feelings of control. One common source of anxiety among heart patients and their spouses is the resumption of sexual activity. The probable source of this anxiety is concern about the elevation of heart rate during sex, especially during orgasm. However, sexual activity poses little threat to cardiac patients. Also, male CAD patients who take Viagra do not have an elevated risk of subsequent heart problems, but this drug may interact in dangerous ways with drugs for hypertension that such patients may be taking (Jackson, 2004).

Cardiac rehabilitation programs usually include components to help patients stop smoking, eat a low-fat and low-cholesterol diet, control weight, moderate alcohol intake, learn to manage stress and hostility, and adhere to a prescribed medication regimen. Also, cardiac patients frequently participate in a graduated or structured exercise program in which they gradually increase their level of physical activity. In other words, the same lifestyle recommendations for avoiding a first cardiovascular event also apply to survivors of myocardial infarction, coronary artery bypass graft surgery, and stroke. In addition, cardiac patients are often encouraged to join a social support group, participate in health education programs, and allow support from their primary caregiver. Some research (Clark, Whelan, Barbour, & MacIntyre, 2005) indicated that cardiac patients rated such social support and being with others who shared the same problem as the most valuable aspects of the program.

Dean Ornish and his colleagues (1998) devised a comprehensive cardiac rehabilitation program with diet, stress management, smoking cessation, and physical activity components in an effort to *reverse* heart patients' coronary artery damage. Although similar to the interventions that attempt to alter risk factors, this program was more comprehensive and imposed more stringent modifications, especially with regard to diet. The Ornish program recommends that cardiac patients reduce their consumption of fat to only 10% of their total caloric intake, which necessitates a careful vegetarian diet with no added fats from oils, eggs, butter, or nuts. An evaluation of the program included a control group that received a typical cardiac rehabilitation program along with the experimental group of participants on the Ornish program.

Early research on the benefits of the program painted a slightly more optimistic picture of its benefits than later research. After 1 year of the program, Ornish and his colleagues (1990) found that 82% of patients in the treatment group showed a regression of plaques in the coronary arteries. After 5 years, this program produced less artery blockage and fewer coronary events. Although a later study (Aldana et al., 2007) failed to confirm the reversal of arterial plaque, it did show that patients on the Ornish program decreased their risk factors to a greater extent than those in a standard cardiac rehabilitation program and decreased their symptoms of angina substantially. The benefits in decreasing angina also appeared in another study (Frattaroli, Weidner, Merritt-Worden, Frenda, & Ornish, 2008),

and other research confirms that dietary change can reverse arterial plaque (Shai et al., 2010). The main disadvantage of a program such as the Ornish plan is the difficulty of following such a stringent diet (Dansinger, Gleason, Griffith, Selker, & Schaefer, 2005). At the advice of Dr. Ornish, Bill Clinton followed a very stringent diet following his surgery; it improved several of his risk factors, but even Clinton had difficulty following all of the recommendations.

Adherence is a major problem with cardiac rehabilitation programs in general. Less than half of cardiac patients complete their rehabilitation regimen (Taylor, Wilson, & Sharp, 2011). One factor that may influence adherence involves the physician, rather than the patient: Many cardiologists fail to endorse rehabilitation programs, which affects their patients' willingness to participate. Many patients also cite difficulties in finding time for and traveling to a clinic for rehabilitation. However, the same factors that predict the development of CVD also predict failure to adhere to rehabilitation: depression, being a smoker, being overweight, and having a high cardiovascular risk profile (Taylor et al., 2011). Thus, the patients who are most in need of intervention may be least likely to adhere. When used as intended, many different rehabilitation programs are effective, including brief interventions (Fernandez et al., 2007) and at-home rehabilitation programs (Dalal, Zawada, Jolly, Moxham, & Taylor, 2010).

A meta-analysis of studies on the effectiveness of two components of cardiac rehabilitation programs (Dusseldrop, van Elderen, Maes, Meulman, & Kraaj, 1999) found that heart disease patients who followed a health education and stress management program had a 34% reduction in cardiac mortality and a 29% reduction in recurrence of a heart attack. Exercise-based cardiac rehabilitation programs are also effective in reducing cardiac mortality and heart attack recurrence (Lawler, Filion, & Eisenberg, 2011). Exercise may present some risks for cardiac patients, but the benefits far outweigh the risks. For example, a graded exercise program can enhance patients' self-efficacy for increasing levels of activity (Cheng & Boey, 2002) as well as increase self-esteem and physical mobility (Ng & Tam, 2000). After a diagnosis of heart problems, exercise programs have three main goals (Thompson, 2001). First, exercise can maintain or improve functional capacity; second, it can enhance a person's quality of life; and third, it can help prevent recurrent heart attacks. Thus, cardiac rehabilitation programs are an effective but underused strategy.

IN SUMMARY

Health psychologists contribute to reducing risks for a first cardiovascular incident as well as to rehabilitating people who have already been diagnosed with CVD. Many of the risks for CVD relate to behaviors, such as smoking, diet, physical activity, and management of negative emotions. Combinations of lifestyle change and drugs are effective in lowering hypertension and cholesterol level, two important risks for CVD. In addition, health psychologists can help people modify negative emotions such as anxiety, depression, and anger, all of which are risks for CVD and often occur in patients after heart attacks. Health psychologists also strive to keep cardiac patients in rehabilitation and boost their levels of physical activity.

Answers

This chapter has addressed four basic questions:

1. What are the structures, functions, and disorders of the cardiovascular system?

The cardiovascular system includes the heart and blood vessels (veins, venules, arteries, arterioles, and capillaries). The heart pumps blood throughout the body, delivering oxygen and removing wastes from body cells. Disorders of the cardiovascular system include (1) coronary artery disease, which occurs when the arteries that supply blood to the heart become clogged with plaque and restrict the blood supply to the heart muscle; (2) myocardial infarction (heart attack), which is caused by blockage of coronary arteries; (3) angina pectoris, which is a nonfatal disorder with symptoms of chest pain and difficulty in breathing; (4) stroke, which occurs when the oxygen supply to the brain is disrupted; and (5) hypertension (high blood pressure), which is a silent disorder but a good predictor of both heart attack and stroke. Heart attack and stroke account for more than 30% of deaths in the United States.

2. What are the risk factors for cardiovascular disease?

Beginning with the Framingham study, researchers identified a number of cardiovascular risk factors. These factors include (1) inherent risk, (2) physiological risks, (3) behavioral and lifestyle risks, and (4) psychosocial risks. Inherent risk factors, such as advancing age, family history, gender, and ethnicity, are not modifiable, but people with inherent risk can alter their other risks to lower their chances of developing heart disease.

The two primary physiological risk factors are hypertension and high cholesterol, and diet can play a role in controlling each of these. Behavioral factors in CVD include smoking, a diet high in saturated fat and low in fiber and antioxidant vitamins, and low physical activity level. Psychosocial risks include low educational and income levels; lack of social support; and persistently high levels of stress, anxiety, and depression. In addition, hostility and both loud, violent expressions of anger and suppression of anger elevate risk slightly.

3. How does lifestyle relate to cardiovascular health?

Lifestyle factors such as cigarette smoking, unwise eating, and a sedentary lifestyle all predict cardiovascular health. During the past three decades, deaths from heart disease have steadily decreased in the United States; perhaps as much as 50% of that drop is a result of changes in behavior and lifestyle. During this same time period, millions of people have quit smoking, altered their diet to control weight and cholesterol, and begun an exercise program.

4. What behaviors allow people to lower their cardiovascular risks?

Both before and after a diagnosis of heart disease, people can use a variety of approaches to reduce their risks for CVD. Drugs, sodium restriction, and weight loss all can control hypertension. Also, drugs, diet, and exercise can lower cholesterol levels. Lowering the ratio of total cholesterol to HDL is probably a better idea, but the statin type of cholesterol-lowering drugs tends to lower LDL, which can also be beneficial. Also, people can learn to manage stress more effectively, enter therapy to improve depression, and learn to manage anger to avoid loud, quick outbursts and to express their frustrations in a soft, slow manner.

Suggested Readings

Holt-Lunstad, J., Birmingham, W., & Jones, B. Q. (2008). Is there something unique about marriage? The relative impact of marital status, relationship quality, and network social support on ambulatory blood pressure and mental health. *Annals of Behavioral Medicine, 35,* 239–244. This journal article gives a technical analysis of social support, considering the notion that good marriages provide the best type of support.

Levy, D., & Brink, S. (2005). *A change of heart: How the Framingham Heart Study helped unravel the mysteries of cardiovascular disease.* New York, NY: Knopf. This report on the Framingham Heart Study includes not only the fascinating history of this project but also the major findings from the study and tips for maintaining heart health.

Miller, G. E., & Blackwell, E. (2006). Turning up the heat: Inflammation as a mechanism linking chronic stress, depression, and heart disease. *Current Directions in Psychological Science, 15,* 269–272. This brief article reviews the concept of inflammation and its risks while attempting to build a model that integrates stress and depression into an explanation for the development of heart disease.

Yusuf, S., Hawken, S., Ôunpuu, S., Dans, T., Avezum, A., Lanas, F., ... INTERHEART Study Investigators (2004). Effect of potentially modifiable risk factors associated with myocardial infarction in 52 countries (the INTERHEART Study): Case-control study. *Lancet, 364,* 937–952. The INTERHEART Study identified nine factors that predicted most of the variance in heart attack deaths in countries throughout the world. This report details the study and presents the relative contributions of each of the nine.

Behavioral Factors in Cancer

CHAPTER OUTLINE

QUESTIONS

This chapter focuses on five basic questions:

1. What is cancer?
2. Are cancer death rates increasing or decreasing?
3. What are the inherent and environmental risk factors for cancer?
4. What are the behavioral risk factors for cancer?
5. How can cancer patients be helped in coping with their disease?

☑ Check Your **HEALTH RISKS**   *Regarding Cancer*

☐ 1. Someone in my immediate family (a parent, sibling, aunt, uncle, or grandparent) developed cancer before age 50.

☐ 2. I am African American.

☐ 3. I have never had a job where I was exposed to radiation or hazardous chemicals.

☐ 4. I have never been a cigarette smoker.

☐ 5. I am a former smoker who quit during the past 5 years.

☐ 6. I have used tobacco products other than cigarettes (such as chewing tobacco, a pipe, or cigars).

☐ 7. My diet is low in fat.

☐ 8. My diet includes lots of smoked, salt-cured, or pickled foods.

☐ 9. I rarely eat fruits or vegetables.

☐ 10. My diet is high in fiber.

☐ 11. I have light-colored skin, but I like to get at least one nice tan every year.

☐ 12. I have had more than 15 sexual partners during my life.

☐ 13. I have never had unprotected sex with a partner who was at high risk for HIV infection.

☐ 14. I am a woman over age 30 who has not given birth to a child.

☐ 15. I have at least two alcoholic drinks every day.

☐ 16. I exercise on a regular basis.

Each of these topics is either a known risk factor for some type of cancer or has the potential to protect against it. Items 3, 4, 7, 10, 13, and 16 describe situations that may offer some protection against cancer. If you checked none or only a few of these items and a large number of the remaining items, your risk for some type of cancer is higher than people who checked different items. Behaviors related to smoking and diet (items 4–10) place you at a greater risk than other behaviors, such as item 15 (alcohol).

Real-World Profile of **STEVE JOBS**

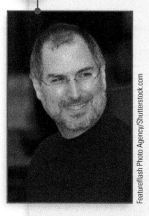

Featureflash Photo Agency/Shutterstock.com

In 2003, Steve Jobs and his company Apple were revolutionizing the technology world. The iPod, unveiled a year and a half earlier, changed how the world listened to music. Jobs and his team started developing the iPhone and the iPad, two products that would similarly revolutionize the mobile phone and computer industries. Steve Jobs—a charismatic, perfectionistic, and demanding workaholic—had already appeared on the cover of *Time* magazine four times. Apple's worth steadily mounted.

In this same year, during a CT scan to look for kidney stones, Steve's doctors noticed something unexpected on his pancreas. The diagnosis soon became islet cell neuroendocrine pancreatic cancer, a rare form of one of the deadliest of cancers. With a low survival rate for conventional treatments, people diagnosed with pancreatic cancer often try alternative therapies. Steve initially refused his doctors' suggestions for surgery, saying, "I really didn't want them to open up my body" (Isaacson, 2011, "Cancer," paragraph 6).

Jobs first tried a variety of alternative treatments, including a vegan diet, acupuncture, herbal remedies, and even a psychic. After delaying standard medical treatment for 9 months, Steve finally relented to surgery. By then, the cancer had already spread to other parts of his body. Steve then sought the most advanced treatments for his condition, which included radiation therapy and a liver transplant. The treatments and transplant took a physical toll with Steve becoming increasingly gaunt.

In August 2011, he resigned from Apple for health reasons. Two months later, Steve Jobs died of respiratory failure due to complications arising from advanced pancreatic cancer.

Steve Jobs' battle with cancer lasted a total of 8 years, far longer than his initial prognosis. Steve's wealth afforded him the best medical treatments, which may have extended his life. However, he later came to regret his decision to delay initial surgery. Why did Steve initially reject treatment for his cancer? What issues did Steve likely cope with in his battle against cancer? Was Steve's "fighting spirit" something that helped him live for so long after his diagnosis? We will explore these questions in this chapter, but first, we need to define what cancer is.

What Is Cancer?

Cancer is a group of diseases characterized by the presence of new cells that grow and spread beyond control. During the 19th century, the great physiologist Johannes Muller discovered that tumors, like other tissues, consisted of cells and were not formless collections of material. However, their growth seemed unrestrained by the mechanisms that control other body cells.

The finding that tumors consist of cells did not shed light on what causes their growth. During the 19th century, the leading theory of cancer was that a parasite or infectious agent caused the disorder, but researchers could find no such agent. Because of this failure, the mutation theory arose, holding that cancer originates because of a change in the cell—a mutation. The cell continues to grow and reproduce in its mutated form, and the result is a tumor.

Cancer is not unique to humans; all animals get cancer, as do plants. Indeed, any cell that is capable of division can transform into a cancer cell. In addition to the diverse *causes* of cancer, many different *types* exist. However, different cancers share certain characteristics, the most common of which is the presence of **neoplastic** tissue cells, which have nearly unlimited growth that robs the host of nutrients and that yields no compensatory beneficial effects. All true cancers share this characteristic of neoplastic growth.

Neoplastic cells may be **benign** or **malignant**, although the distinction is not always easy to determine. Both types consist of altered cells that reproduce true to their altered type. However, benign growths tend to remain localized, whereas malignant tumors tend to spread and establish secondary colonies. The tendency for benign tumors to remain localized usually makes them less threatening than malignant tumors, but not all benign tumors are harmless. Malignant tumors are much more dangerous because they invade and destroy surrounding tissue and may also move, or **metastasize**, through blood or lymph and thus spread to other sites in the body.

The most dangerous characteristic of tumor cells is their autonomy—that is, their ability to grow without regard to the needs of other body cells and without being subject to the restraints of growth that govern other cells. This unrestrained tumor growth makes cancer capable of overwhelming its host, damaging other organs or physiological processes, or using nutrients essential for body functions. The tumor then becomes a parasite on its host, gaining priority over other body cells.

Malignant growths fall into four main groups: carcinomas, sarcomas, leukemias, and lymphomas. **Carcinomas** are cancers of the epithelial tissue, cells that line the outer and inner surfaces of the body, such as skin, stomach lining, and mucous membranes. **Sarcomas** are cancers that arise from cells in connective tissue, such as bone, muscles, and cartilage. **Leukemias** are cancers that originate in the blood or blood-forming cells, such as stem cells in the bone marrow. These three types of cancers—carcinomas, sarcomas, and leukemias—account for more than 95% of malignancies. The fourth type of cancer is **lymphoma**, a cancer of the lymphatic system, which is one of the rarer types of cancer.

Although some people may have a genetic predisposition to cancer, people almost never inherit the disease. Behavior and lifestyle are primary contributors to cancer, making it possible for the rates of cancer to change over relatively short periods.

The Changing Rates of Cancer Deaths

For the first time on record, the death rate from cancer in the United States declined during the 1990s. This trend ended a century-long increase in cancer deaths that peaked in 1993, when cancer mortality was more than three times higher than in 1900. Figure 10.1 shows an increase in total cancer death rates in the United States from 1900 to 1990 and then a gradual decline. The decrease is significant—more than 22% for men and more than 15% for women since 1990 (Siegel, Naishadham, & Jemal, 2012).

Why did cancer death rates drop? At least two explanations are possible. First, the decline might be

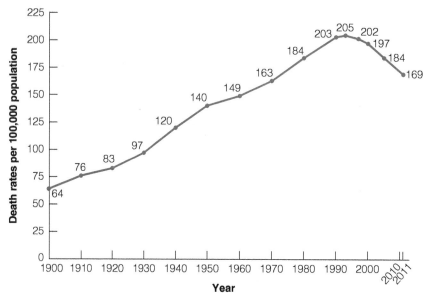

FIGURE 10.1   Death rates from cancer per 100,000 population, United States, 1900–2011.

Source: Data from Historical statistics of the United States: Colonial times to 1970, Part 1 (p. 68) by U.S. Bureau of the Census, 1975, Washington, DC: U.S. Government Printing Office; *Statistical abstract of the United States, 2008* (127th edition), by U.S. Census Bureau, (2007). Washington, DC: U.S. Government Printing Office; Cancer statistics, 2008, by A. Jemal et al., 2008, CA: *Cancer Journal for Clinicians, 58,* 71–96. Siegel, R. L., Miller, K. D., & Jemal, A. (2015). Cancer statistics, 2015. CA: *a cancer journal for clinicians,* 65(1), 5-29.

due to improved treatment that prolongs the life of cancer patients. We can test the validity of this explanation by examining the difference between cancer incidence and cancer deaths. If incidence remained the same or even increased while deaths declined, then better treatment would account for the drop in cancer deaths. However, the evidence does not support this hypothesis, as both cancer incidence and cancer deaths declined during the 1990s (Siegel et al., 2012). Some of that decrease is attributable to the lower incidence of certain cancers, such as lung cancer in men, and some of it is due to improved early detection and treatment, such as the decline in deaths from prostate and breast cancer. Thus, better treatment regimens play a role in the recent decrease in cancer rates, but people are developing cancer less often than they did over a decade ago. In the United States, for example, people are smoking much less and eating a healthier diet than they did 40 years ago. Because lifestyle factors such as smoking, diet, and physical inactivity account for about two-thirds of all cancer deaths in the United States (American Cancer Society [ACS], 2012), improvements in these areas should result in lower rates of cancer.

Cancers with Decreasing Death Rates

Cancer of the lungs, breast, prostate, and colon/rectum account for about half of all cancer deaths in the United States, and mortality rates for each of these sites are currently declining.

Lung cancer accounts for about 14% of all cancer cases, but 28% of all cancer deaths—figures that reveal the deadliness of lung cancer. Between 1990 and 2008, mortality due to lung cancer in the United States declined for men but not for women (ACS, 2012; see Figures 10.2 and 10.3). Figure 10.2 shows that lung cancer mortality for women rose dramatically from 1965 to 1995, but since that time death rates have been almost level. In Europe, this pattern is somewhat similar, with lung cancer mortality for men declining since 1990; however, lung cancer mortality for women continues to rise (Ferlay, Parkin, & Steliarova-Foucher, 2010). Because cigarette smoking is the primary cause of lung cancer deaths, the current decline in women's smoking rates in the United States should eventually effect a decrease in lung cancer mortality for women.

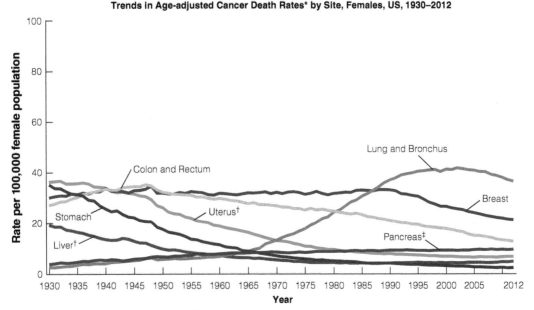

Trends in Age-adjusted Cancer Death Rates* by Site, Females, US, 1930–2012

*Per 100,000, age adjusted to the 2000 US standard population.
†Uterus refers to uterine cervix and uterine corpus combined.
‡ Mortality rates for pancreatic and liver cancers are increasing.

NOTE: Due to changes in ICD coding, numerator information has changed over time. Rates for cancers of the liver, lung and bronchus, and colon and rectum are affected by these coding changes.

SOURCE: US Mortality Volumes 1930 to 1959, US Mortality Data 1960 to 2012, National Center for Health Statistics, Centers for Disease Control and Prevention.

©2016, American Cancer Society, Inc., Surveillance Research

FIGURE 10.2   Cancer death rates for selected sites, women, United States, 1930–2012.

Source: The American Cancer Society. *Cancer Facts and Figures 2016.* Atlanta: American Cancer Society, Inc.

Other than prostate cancer, *breast cancer* has the highest incidence (but not death rate) of any cancer in the United States, accounting for about 29% of cancer cases among women. Men also develop breast cancer, but women account for 99% of all new cases. The incidence of female breast cancer increased from 1980 to 2001 but then began to decline. One factor that may be involved in this decline is the decrease in the number of postmenopausal women using hormone replacement therapy, some types of which were linked to breast cancer (Siegel et al., 2012). The decline in the breast cancer death rate is due mainly to improvements in early detection and treatment.

Prostate cancer has the highest incidence of cancer among men in the United States, but again, it does not have the highest mortality rate—about twice as many men die each year from lung cancer as from prostate cancer. In 2012, the number of men diagnosed with prostate cancer was higher than the number of women diagnosed with breast cancer (Siegel et al., 2012).

As with breast cancer incidence, new cases of prostate cancer increased sharply during the 1980s when prostate-specific antigen (PSA) screening was first introduced. From 2000 to 2012, however, the number of new cases—about 29% of all cancer cases in men—declined significantly.

Colorectal cancer is the second leading cause of cancer deaths in the United States and other developed countries, exceeded only by lung cancer. However, in the United States, both the incidence and the mortality rates of colorectal cancer are decreasing. Incidence and mortality rates vary widely by ethnic background, with African Americans more likely to receive a diagnosis of and die from colorectal cancer than either Hispanic Americans or European Americans (Siegel et al., 2012). Although the incidence of colorectal cancer increased slightly until about 1985, the mortality rate has been declining since about 1945 (see Figures 10.2 and 10.3).

Death rates from *stomach cancer* have dropped from being the leading cause of cancer deaths for both

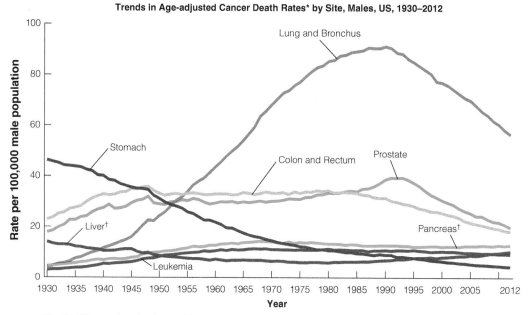

FIGURE 10.3   Cancer death rates for selected sites, men, United States, 1930–2012.

Source: The American Cancer Society. *Cancer Facts and Figures 2016.* Atlanta: American Cancer Society, Inc.

women and men to having a very low mortality rate. As we discuss later, modern refrigeration and fewer salt-cured foods probably account for most of the decrease in stomach cancer.

Cancers with Increasing Incidence and Mortality Rates

In general, incidence rates for the four leading cancers—lung, breast, prostate, and colorectal—are declining, especially for men. However, not all cancer rates are decreasing. Several cancers have increased in recent years (Siegel et al., 2012).

Liver cancer, like lung cancer, is quite lethal, with a death rate (3.6%) nearly twice as high as its incidence rate (1.7%). This cancer is the only type that is increasing among both women and men, and both incidence and death rates are higher for minorities compared with European Americans (Siegel et al., 2012). As mentioned, lung cancer continues to show a slight increase among women but a continuing decline among men.

Melanoma, a potentially fatal form of skin cancer, is increasing among both men and women. Cancer of the esophagus is increasing among men yet falling among women, possibly due to increasing rates of gastric reflux and obesity.

IN SUMMARY

Cancer is a group of diseases characterized by the presence of neoplastic cells that grow and spread without control. These new cells may form benign tumors, which tend to remain localized, or malignant tumors, which may metastasize and spread to other organs.

After more than a century of rising mortality rates, cancer deaths are declining. This decrease is most evident among the four cancers that cause most cancer deaths—lung, breast, prostate, and colorectal cancers. Since 1992, incidence and death rates among men for these four cancers have declined at a slow but steady pace, whereas women have not experienced the same magnitude of decrease. The leading cause of cancer deaths for both women and men continues to be lung cancer. The incidence of breast cancer among women and prostate cancer among men is much higher than the incidence of lung cancer, but lung cancer kills far more people in the United States than does either breast cancer or prostate cancer.

Cancer Risk Factors Beyond Personal Control

Most risk factors for cancer result from personal behavior, especially cigarette smoking. However, some factors are largely beyond personal control; these factors include both inherent and environmental risks.

Inherent Risk Factors for Cancer

Inherent risks for cancer include genetics and family history, ethnic background, and age. Many people attribute their risk of cancer to these factors, especially genetics. A survey ("Practical Nurse," 2008) indicated that 9 out of 10 people overestimated the genetic risk, and 60% of people named genetics as the primary risk for cancer. Does their perception agree with the research? How important are genetic and other inherent risk factors such as ethnicity and age?

Ethnic Background   Compared with European Americans, African Americans fare more poorly; they have a greater incidence of most cancers, and mortality is higher in almost every category (Siegel, Miller, & Jemal, 2016). However, Hispanic Americans, Asian Americans, and Native Americans have lower rates than either African Americans or European Americans for all cancer sites combined, as well as for the four most common cancers (Siegel et al., 2016). These discrepancies are most likely due to behavioral and psychosocial factors rather than to biology. For example, although Asian Americans generally have lower total cancer death rates than European Americans, they have a much higher mortality rate for stomach and liver cancer. Both cancers are caused by behavioral and environmental factors. Stomach cancer is strongly influenced by diet and chronic infection by the *Helicobacter pylori* bacteria, whereas liver cancer is strongly influenced by

infection with the hepatitis C virus (Siegel et al., 2016). Thus, behavioral factors may account for these ethnic differences.

Minority status plays a greater role in survival of cancer than it does in cancer incidence. For cancer sites with a low mortality level, the discrepancy between incidence and mortality widens with ethnic background. With breast cancer, for example, European American women have a higher incidence rate than African American women, but African American women are more likely to die from this cancer (Siegel et al., 2016).

How does minority status contribute to cancer outcomes—that is, length of survival and quality of life? Although Hispanic Americans, African Americans, Native Americans, and Asian Americans develop many cancers at a lower rate than European Americans, their diagnoses tend to come at a later stage of their cancers (Siegel et al., 2016). This difference affects survival; later diagnoses tend to lead to more advanced disease, more difficulty in treatment, and lower survival rates. An examination of survival differences between African Americans and European Americans (Du, Meyer, & Franzini, 2007) showed that controlling for socioeconomic factors erased the difference in survival rates, which suggests that social and economic factors create the disparity.

Advancing Age   The strongest risk factor for cancer— and many other diseases—is advancing age. The older people become, the greater their chances of developing and dying of cancer. Figure 10.4 shows a steep increase in cancer mortality by age for both men and women, but especially for men.

Cancer is also the second leading cause of death among children between aged 1 and 14 (exceeded only by unintentional injuries; Siegel et al., 2016). Cancers that are most common among children include leukemia, cancers of the brain and nervous system, and non-Hodgkin's lymphoma. Testicular cancer is also an exception to the general rule concerning age: The highest risk for this cancer occurs during young adulthood. These cancers are likely to have some genetic component.

Family History and Genetics   The first evidence of a genetic component for cancer came from the Nurses' Health Study (Colditz et al., 1993), which showed that women whose mothers received a breast cancer diagnosis before age 40 were more than twice as likely to develop breast cancer. A sister with breast

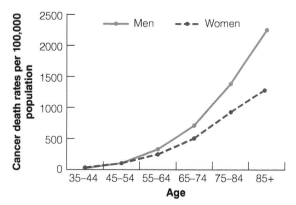

FIGURE 10.4   Cancer death rates by age and gender, United States, 2014.

Source: Data from *Health United States, 2015* (Table 24), by National Center for Health Statistics, 2016, Hyattsville, MD: U.S. Government Printing Office.

cancer also doubled the risk, and having both a sister and a mother with breast cancer increased a woman's risk about 2½ times. This research has progressed to the identification of specific genes involved in breast cancer, the *BRCA 1* and *BRCA 2* genes. These genes protect against cancer by providing the code for a protective protein (Paull, Cortez, Bowers, Elledge, & Gellert, 2001). Women who have a mutated form of *BRCA 1,* which does not allow that protective protein to develop, are as many as seven times more likely to develop breast cancer as women with the healthy form of this gene. Mutations in *BRCA 1* and *BRCA 2* have also been implicated in the development of breast cancer in men and pancreatic cancer in both women and men (Lynch et al., 2005). This gene does not create a certainty of developing cancer, but people with the mutation have a sharply increased risk.

The form of breast cancer involving *BRCA 1* and *BRCA 2* is responsible for no more than 10% of breast cancer, and the other cancers associated with *BRCA* are even less likely to arise from a gene mutation. Thus, many genes for breast cancer remain unidentified, and most of the risk for developing breast cancer comes from other sources (Oldenburg, Meijers-Heijboer, Cornelisse, & Devilee, 2007).

Across all cancers, only 5% to 10% percent are due to inherited genetic mutations (NCI, 2016), with breast, ovarian, prostate, and colorectal cancers being the types of cancer most likely to arise from inherited genetic mutations (Baker, Lichtenstein, Kaprio, & Holm, 2005).

The search for single genes that underlie the development of cancer has been largely unsuccessful (Hemminki, Försti, & Bermejo, 2006). Instead, researchers have identified configurations of genes that seem to lead to vulnerabilities for specific cancers. Furthermore, some cancers may arise from a complex interaction between genetic vulnerability and behavioral risk factors. For example, some evidence suggests that women with the *BRCA 2* mutation may be at a greater risk of alcohol-induced breast cancer compared with women without the *BRCA 2* mutation (Dennis et al., 2011). Therefore, despite the widespread publicity about genetic causes of cancer, genes play a fairly minor role in the development of cancer; environmental and behavioral factors are much more important.

Environmental Risk Factors for Cancer

Environmental risk factors for cancer include exposure to risks such as radiation and asbestos and to pollutants such as pesticides, herbicides, motor exhaust, and other chemicals (Miligi, Costantini, Veraldi, Benvenuti, & Vineis, 2006). In addition, arsenic, benzene, chromium, nickel, vinyl chloride, and various petroleum products are possible contributors to a number of cancers (Boffetta, 2004; Siemiatycki et al., 2004).

Longtime exposure to asbestos can increase risk for lung cancer, depending on the type of asbestos and the frequency and duration of exposure. A study in Sweden (Gustavsson et al., 2000) examined the possible carcinogenic effects of asbestos as well as diesel exhaust, motor exhaust, metals, welding fumes, and other environmental conditions that some workers encounter on the job. The results showed that workers with exposure to environmental carcinogens had about a 9% additional chance of developing lung cancer compared with people without exposure to these conditions. A 25-year longitudinal study of asbestos workers in China (Yano, Wang, Wang, Wang, & Lan, 2001) reported that male asbestos workers, compared with other workers, had 6.6 times the likelihood of developing lung cancer and 4.3 times the likelihood of developing any cancer.

Exposure to radiation is also a risk. Nuclear power plant workers exposed to high levels of radiation showed elevated risks for leukemia and cancers of the rectum, colon, testicles, and lung (Sont et al., 2001). Living in a community with a nuclear power plant, however, seems to present no elevated risk; the observed rate of cancer in such communities is similar to that of other communities (Boice, Bigbee, Mumma, & Blot, 2003). The radioactive gas radon also presents increased risks for lung cancer, both for miners who are exposed and for people who live in homes with high levels of this type of radiation (Krewski et al., 2006).

Some infections and chronic inflammation also present elevated risks for cancers. Infection with the bacterium *Helicobacter pylori* is widespread throughout the world and increases the risk for gastric ulcers as well as gastric cancer (McColl, Watabe, & Derakhshan, 2007). Hepatitis infection is a risk for liver cancer. Chronic inflammation is a factor in the development of bladder cancer (Michaud, 2007) and possibly in prostate cancer (De Marzo et al., 2007). However, infection and inflammation may be more attributable to behavior than to environmental exposure.

IN SUMMARY

Inherent risks for cancer include ethnic background, advancing age, and family history and genetics. African Americans have higher cancer incidence and death rates than European Americans, but people from other ethnic backgrounds have a lower incidence. These differences are due not to biology but to differences in socioeconomic status, which is related both to the incidence of cancer and to 5-year survival with the disease.

The strongest risk factor for cancer—as well as many other diseases—is advancing age. As a person gets older, the risk for cancer increases. Furthermore, men have an even greater increase than women.

Although cancer seldom develops because of a single gene, family history and genetic predisposition play a role in the development of some cancers, especially prostate and breast cancer. A woman who has a mother or sister with breast cancer has a two-to threefold higher chance of developing the disease, and mutations of the *BRCA 1* and *BRCA 2* genes place people at elevated risk for breast and pancreatic cancer. However, genetic factors play a relatively small role in the development of cancer.

Environmental risks also contribute to cancer incidence and deaths. Pollutants, pesticides, radiation exposure, and infections increase the risk for various cancers. Workers exposed to asbestos and radiation are at increased risk, as are people living in homes with high levels of radon.

Behavioral Risk Factors for Cancer

Cancer results from an interaction of genetic, environmental, and behavioral conditions, most of which are still not clearly understood. As with cardiovascular diseases, however, several behavioral cancer risk factors are clear. Recall that risk factors are not necessarily *causes* of a disease, but they do predict the likelihood that a person will develop or die from that disease. Most risk factors for cancer relate to personal behavior and lifestyle, especially smoking and diet. Other known behavioral risks include alcohol, physical inactivity, exposure to ultraviolet light, sexual behavior, and psychosocial factors.

Smoking

"If nobody smoked, 1 of every 3 cancer deaths in the United States would not happen" (U.S. Department of Health and Human Services [USDHHS], 2010d, p. 7).

The vast majority of smoking-related cancer deaths are from lung cancer, but smoking is also implicated in deaths from many other cancers, including leukemia and cancers of the stomach, bladder, upper digestive tract, esophagus, colon, and prostate (Batty et al., 2008). Smoking also increases risk for cancers of the larynx, pharynx, oral cavity, sinuses, cervix, pancreas, liver, and kidney (Gandini et al., 2008). There is not a consistent relationship between smoking and breast cancer, but women who smoke throughout adolescence may increase their risk for this type of cancer (Ha et al., 2007). The risk of cigarette smoking also applies to other countries around the world; smoking is the single largest risk for cancer mortality worldwide (Danaei, Vander Hoorn, Lopez, Murray, & Ezzati, 2005). Thus, it is a misconception that smoking causes only lung cancer. Figure 10.5 shows 15 different types of cancer associated with tobacco use.

What Is the Risk? Sufficient evidence exists for epidemiologists to conclude a causal relationship exists between cigarette smoking and lung cancer. Chapter 2 includes a review of that evidence and explains how epidemiologists can infer causation from nonexperimental studies. The strong relationship between smoking and lung cancer becomes apparent when observing the way lung cancer rates track smoking rates. About 25 to 40 years after smoking rates began to increase for men,

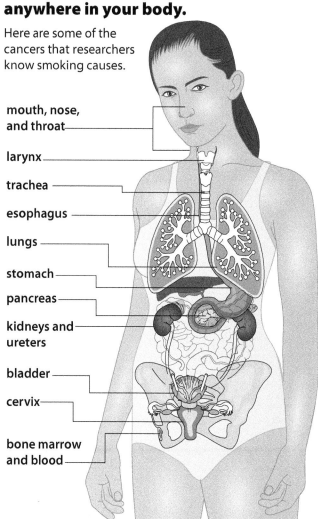

Smoking can cause cancer almost anywhere in your body.

Here are some of the cancers that researchers know smoking causes.

- mouth, nose, and throat
- larynx
- trachea
- esophagus
- lungs
- stomach
- pancreas
- kidneys and ureters
- bladder
- cervix
- bone marrow and blood

FIGURE 10.5   The many types of cancer associated with tobacco use.

Source: Adapted from U.S. Department of Health and Human Services. *A Report of the Surgeon General: How Tobacco Smoke Causes Disease: What It Means to You.* U.S. Department of Health and Human Services, Centers for Disease Control and Prevention, National Center for Chronic Disease Prevention and Health Promotion, Office of Smoking and Health, 2010.

lung cancer rates started a steep rise; about 25 to 40 years after cigarette consumption decreased for men, lung cancer death rates for men began to drop (see Figure 10.6). Women's smoking has declined more gradually, and so have their lung cancer mortality rates.

The strong relationship holds when analyzed by income. Low-income men smoke more than high-income men and they have a higher lung cancer mortality rate; low-income women smoke a little less than high-income women and they have a slightly lower rate of lung cancer mortality (Weir et al., 2003). The dose–response relationship between cigarette smoking and lung cancer and the close tracking of smoking rates and lung cancer rates provide compelling evidence for a causal relationship between smoking and the development of lung cancer.

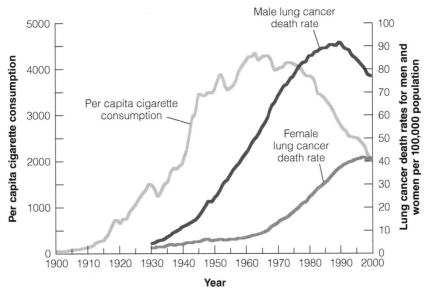

FIGURE 10.6   The parallel paths of cigarette consumption and lung cancer deaths for men and women, United States, 1900–2000.

Source: Data from *Health United States, 2011* (Table 32), by National Center for Health Statistics, 2012, Hyattsville, MD: U.S. Government Printing Office.

How high is the risk for lung cancer among cigarette smokers? The U.S. Department of Health and Human Services (USDHHS, 2014) estimated that the relative risk of lung cancer for smokers is 24.9, meaning that those who smoke are *nearly 25 times more likely to get lung cancer* than those who have never smoked. The risk that cigarette smokers have of dying of lung cancer is the strongest link between any behavior and a major cause of death.

Cigarette smoking is not the only form of tobacco use that increases risk for cancer. Smoking cigars or using smokeless tobacco—also known as "chew," "spit," or "snuff" tobacco—also increases likelihood of death from several forms of cancer, including laryngeal, oral, esophageal, and pancreatic cancer (ACS, 2012). As we discuss in greater detail in Chapter 12, there is no safe way to use tobacco products.

In addition to tobacco use, factors such as polluted air, socioeconomic level, occupation, ethnic background, and building material in one's house all link to lung cancer. Each of these has an additive or possibly a **synergistic effect** with smoking, so studies of different populations may yield quite different risk factor rates, depending on the combination of risks that cigarette smokers have in addition to their risk as a smoker. For example, Chinese men who smoke have an elevated risk for lung cancer

that increases with exposure to smoke from burning coal, which is a common practice for household heating and cooking in China (Danaei et al., 2005).

What Is the Perceived Risk?   Despite their heightened vulnerability to cancer, many smokers do not perceive that their behavior puts them at risk. They show what Neil Weinstein (1984) referred to as an *optimistic bias* concerning their chances of dying from cigarette-related causes. Both smokers and nonsmokers acknowledge that smoking is a health risk. Despite knowledge to the contrary, both high-school smokers (Tomar & Hatsukami, 2007) and adult smokers (Peretti-Watel et al., 2007) believe that, unlike other smokers, they will somehow escape the deadly effects of cigarette smoking. The adult smokers expressed their belief that smoking is dangerous at some level—but not at the level of their consumption. Sometimes, even, people who succumb to diseases associated with smoking deny the role that tobacco likely played. Rock guitarist Eddie van Halen—a smoker for over four decades—believed that his tongue and esophageal cancer were due to putting metal guitar picks in his mouth rather than smoking cigarettes.

This tendency to deny personal risk may be stronger in countries where smoking is more prevalent and attitudes toward smoking are more lenient. Denmark is such a country and Danish people are more likely to deny personal risk than Americans (Helweg-Larsen & Nielsen, 2009). This denial of risk is all the more surprising when considering that, compared with the United States, Denmark has *higher* rates of mortality due to tobacco-related diseases such as lung cancer, oral cancer, cardiovascular disease, and chronic obstructive pulmonary disease (World Health Organization [WHO], 2012). Thus, optimistic biases are common and may be tied to the cultural prevalence and acceptability of smoking.

Diet

Another risk factor for cancer is an unhealthy diet. The American Cancer Society (2012) estimates that one-third of all cancer deaths in the United States are a result of dietary choices and sedentary lifestyle. Poor dietary practices are associated with a wide variety of cancers, and good choices decrease the risks.

Foods That May Cause Cancer   Some foods are suspected of being **carcinogenic**—that is, of causing cancer, almost always because of contaminants or additives (Abnet, 2007). "Natural" foods lack preservatives, which can result in high levels of bacteria and fungi. A long list of bacteria and fungi present risks for stomach cancer. The sharp decline in this form of cancer is due in part to increased refrigeration during the last 75 years and to lower consumption of salt-cured foods, smoked foods, and foods stored at room temperature (see Figures 10.2 and 10.3). Aflatoxin is a fungus that grows on improperly stored grains and peanuts; exposure to this toxin increases the risk for liver cancer (World Cancer Research Fund/American Institute for Cancer Research [WCRF/AICR], 2007). However, food additives used as preservatives can also be carcinogenic, and toxic chemicals produced by various industries can work their way into the environment and into foods, as in the case of dioxin. Thus, foods that lack preservatives and those with preservatives may both present some risk.

In Chapter 9, we saw that dietary fat is an established risk for cardiovascular disease; a number of studies have shown that dietary fat is also a risk for cancer, especially colon cancer (Murtaugh, 2004). However, a high-fat diet is a stronger risk for cardiovascular disease than it is for cancer. Much of the research on dietary fat and cancer centers on breast cancer and suggests that dietary fat is a modest but reliable risk factor for

this form of cancer (Freedman, Kipnis, Schatzkin, & Potischman, 2008). A high-fat diet also contributes to high cholesterol levels, which appears as a risk factor for testicular cancer in men—raising the risk by 4.5 times (Dobson, 2005).

Consumption of preserved meat (such as ham, bacon, and hot dogs) raises the risk of colorectal cancer (Williams & Hord, 2005). A possible risk associated with red meat is the method of cooking; charred, smoked, or overcooked red meats may be a factor in increasing this type of risk (Alaejos, González, & Afonso, 2008), and salt-cured or heavily salted meats also raise risks for stomach cancer (WCRF/AICR, 2007).

A stronger risk for colorectal cancer comes not from any specific dietary component but from overweight and obesity (WCRF/AICR, 2007; Williams & Hord, 2005). Obesity accounts for 14% to 20% of all cancer-related deaths (ACS, 2012). Obesity is strongly related to cancer of the esophagus, breast (mostly in postmenopausal women), endometrium, and kidney. Abdominal fat is a risk not only for cardiovascular disease but also for cancer of the pancreas, endometrium, and kidney. Although eating several specific types of food increases the risk for cancers, a diet that leads to overweight or obesity is more of a risk.

Foods That May Protect Against Cancer   If specific foods and overall diet can increase the risk for cancer, might some dietary measures offer protection? One team of researchers has calculated that if people around the world were to eat an adequate amount of fruits and vegetables, as many as 2.6 million deaths per year would be eliminated (Lock, Pomerleau, Causer, Altmann, & McKee, 2005). The same researchers estimated that this fruit and vegetable-rich diet might reduce the incidence of stomach cancer by 19%, esophageal cancer by 20%, lung cancer by 12%, and colorectal cancer by 2%. Public knowledge of the benefits of a healthy diet contributed to an improvement in diet among U.S. residents from 1999 to 2012 and these improvements prevented over 1 million premature deaths (Wang, Li, Chiuve, Hu, & Willett, 2015). However, despite these improvements, the overall diet of the typical American—and many others worldwide—remains poor.

Despite these known benefits of a diet rich in fruits and vegetables, it remains unclear whether specific nutrients protect against the development or proliferation of cancer. This lack of clarity may be due to the research methods used to investigate dietary components. For example, population studies showed that people in countries with a high-fiber diet experienced lower rates of colorectal cancer than people in countries with a low-fiber diet. This result prompted research using the case–control method in which people who eat a high-fiber diet were compared with those who eat a low-fiber diet (see Chapter 2 for a description of this method). Such studies involve fewer people than population studies, so small effects of fiber in the diet may not be clear using this approach. Alternatively, other differences between the two groups may contribute to the effect of fiber in the diet, making a clear conclusion difficult. If case–control studies indicate that the nutrient has a positive effect, which they have for fiber and colorectal cancer (WCRF/AICR, 2007), researchers then perform experimental studies.

The randomized clinical trial is an experimental method that is the best method for detecting differences between groups. For dietary studies, however, this method has drawbacks (Boyd, 2007). Such studies are experimental, involving the manipulation of a factor—in this case a dietary component. Half the participants receive the component, and half do not, creating a clear comparison. However, the exposure is typically short term; few clinical trials last longer than a few years, and most have limited follow-ups. Improving a diet for 2 years may not provide sufficient exposure to have an impact on the development of cancer, which develops over years. Or participants may need to ingest nutrients during childhood or adolescence for maximum benefit, but most studies include only adult participants. In addition, randomized clinical trials usually isolate a nutrient and provide that nutrient through supplements rather than through broad changes to the diet. Taking supplements often fails to produce the benefits of eating a diet high in the same nutrients. Thus, the benefits of specific nutrients may be complex, and randomized clinical trials may miss some of those important benefits.

These limitations have restricted researchers from coming to conclusions about the cancer-preventive benefits of many nutrients. An extensive review of the evidence (WCRF/AICR, 2007) was able to place several nutrients into the category of *probable* (but not *convincing*) evidence for benefits. **Beta-carotene** is one of the carotenoids, a form of vitamin A found abundantly in foods such as carrots and sweet potatoes. Eating a diet rich in carotenoids probably lowers the risk of cancer of the mouth, larynx, pharynx, and lungs; high beta-carotene intake has a similar benefit for the risk of cancer of the esophagus, as does a diet rich in vitamin C.

People who eat foods high in folate, one of the B vitamins, probably decrease their chances of developing pancreatic cancer. Evidence for any protective power of these nutrients is weaker for other types of cancer.

Evidence concerning selenium intake is somewhat stronger (Williams & Hord, 2005). **Selenium** is a trace element found in grain products and in meat from grain-fed animals. It enters the food chain through the soil, but not all soils throughout the world contain equal amounts of selenium. In excess, selenium is toxic, but in moderate amounts, it provides some protection against colon and prostate cancers. Foods with high levels of selenium protect against colon cancer in laboratory rats (Finley, Davis, & Feng, 2000), and selenium supplements can significantly reduce cancer incidence, but only in men (Bardia et al., 2008). Calcium has received a great deal of publicity for its benefit in preventing bone mineral loss, but it may also offer some protection against colorectal cancer (WCRF/AICR, 2007).

Thus, an evaluation of the extensive research suggests that some nutrients can protect against some cancers, but the evidence of a protective effect is stronger concerning the overall diet and maintaining close to the ideal body weight. A healthy diet includes lots of fruits and vegetables, whole grains, legumes, nuts, fish and seafood, and low-fat dairy products; the amount of preserved and red meat, saturated fat, salt-cured foods, and foods made of highly processed ingredients is low. This description fits with the concept of a Mediterranean-type diet, emphasizing a plant-based diet with a variety of foods that people can adopt as part of a healthy lifestyle (Williams & Hord, 2005). Another element of the Mediterranean diet is alcohol—but in limited amounts.

Alcohol

Alcohol is not as strong a risk factor for cancer as either smoking or eating an imprudent diet. Nevertheless, alcohol does increase the risk for cancers of the mouth, esophagus, breast, and liver (WCRF/ AICR, 2007). The liver has primary responsibility for detoxifying alcohol. Therefore, persistent and excessive drinking often leads to cirrhosis of the liver, a degenerative disease that curtails the organ's effectiveness. Cancer is more likely to occur in cirrhotic livers than in healthy ones (WCRF/AICR, 2007), but alcohol abusers are likely to die of a variety of other causes before they develop liver cancer.

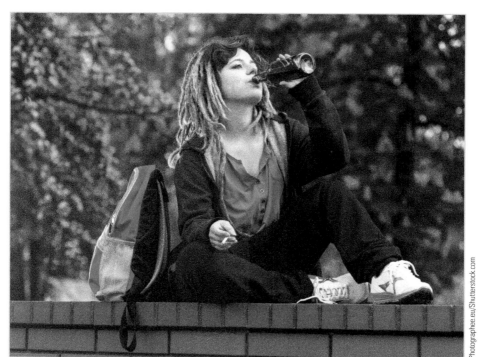

Risks from smoking, drinking, and sun exposure can have a synergistic effect, multiplying the chances of developing cancer.

Does drinking alcohol cause breast cancer? Current evaluations of the research indicate that the evidence is convincing (WCRF/AICR, 2007). The risk varies by exposure; women who consume three or more drinks per day have a moderate to strong risk for breast cancer, and women who consume as little as one to two drinks daily have some risk (Singletary & Gapstur, 2001). The risk is not equal in all countries. In the United States, about 2% of breast cancer cases can be attributed to alcohol, but in Italy, where alcohol intake is considerably higher, as many as 15% of breast cancer cases may be due to drinking. Table 10.1 summarizes the risks and benefits of specific dietary choices and alcohol consumption.

Alcohol has a synergistic effect with smoking, so people who both smoke and drink heavily have a risk for certain cancers exceeding that of the two independent risk factors added together. People who both drink and smoke and who have a family history of esophageal, stomach, or pharynx cancers have an increased risk for cancers of the digestive tract (Garavello et al., 2005). These data suggest that people who both drink heavily and smoke could substantially reduce their chances of developing cancer by giving up either smoking or drinking. Quitting both, of course, would reduce the risk still more.

Sedentary Lifestyle

A sedentary lifestyle increases the risk for some types of cancer, including cancers of the colon, endometrium, breast, lung, and pancreas (WCRF/AICR, 2007). Thus, physical activity can reduce risks for these cancers. There is strong evidence of the beneficial effect of physical activity for colon, endometrial, and breast cancer (in women after menopause); the evidence is less clear for lung and pancreatic cancer and for breast cancer in premenopausal women. Some studies (Bernstein, Henderson, Hanisch, Sullivan-Halley, & Ross, 1994; Thune, Brenn, Lund, & Gaard, 1997) suggest that women who begin a physical activity program when they are young and who continue to exercise 4 hours a week greatly reduce their risk for breast cancer. This age-sensitive effect may make the overall benefit of exercise difficult to determine for premenopausal women.

Another indirect benefit of physical activity for cancer risk is its relationship with body weight. Physical activity is important for maintaining a healthy body

TABLE 10.1   Diet and Its Effects on Cancer

Type of Food	Findings of Increased Risk	Studies
"Natural" foods with no preservatives	Grains and peanuts may be contaminated with aflatoxin, which is carcinogenic. Spoiled food increases risk for stomach cancer.	Abnet, 2007
Foods high in preservatives High-fat diet	Preservatives can be carcinogenic. Contributes to colon cancer	Abnet, 2007 Murtaugh, 2004
	Modest risk for breast cancer High cholesterol level is a strong risk for testicular cancer.	Freedman et al., 2008 Dobson, 2005
Consumption of preserved meats and red meat	Increases the risk for colorectal cancer, especially if meat is smoked or charred	WCRF/AICR*, 2007; Williams and Hord, 2005
Overweight and obesity	Strong link to colorectal, esophageal, breast, endometrial, and kidney cancer Abdominal fat is a risk for cancer of the pancreas, endometrium, and kidney.	WCRF/AICR, 2007; Williams and Hord, 2005
Alcohol	Raises the risk of cancers of the mouth, esophagus, breast, and liver, especially heavy drinking and drinking combined with smoking	WCRF/AICR, 2007
Type of Food	Findings of Decreased Risk	Studies
Diet rich in fruits and vegetables	Could reduce worldwide rates of stomach cancer by 19%, esophageal cancer by 20%, lung cancer by 12%, and colorectal cancer by 2%	Lock et al., 2005
Diet high in carotenoids, including beta-carotene	Probably lowers the risk of cancer of the mouth, larynx, pharynx, and lungs Diets high in beta-carotene (but not supplements) lower the risk for cancer of the esophagus.	WCRF/AICR, 2007
Vitamin C	Probably lowers the risk of cancer of the esophagus	WCRF/AICR, 2007
Diet high in folate	Probably lowers the risk of pancreatic cancer	WCRF/AICR, 2007
Selenium	Protects against colon cancer in laboratory rats	Finley et al., 2000
	Reduces risk of several types of cancer in men	Bardia et al., 2008
Calcium	May protect against colon cancer	WCRF/AICR, 2007
Summary	Overall diet and healthy weight are more strongly related to cancer than any one dietary component.	WCRF/AICR, 2007; Williams and Hord, 2005

*World Cancer Research Fund/American Institute for Cancer Research.

weight and a favorable level of body fat, both of which increase risk for a number of cancers. Thus, some forms of vigorous physical activity can lower cancer risk in several ways. The benefits (and potential risks) of physical activity are discussed in detail in Chapter 15. (See Would You Believe …? box to learn more about how physical activity, in addition to other cancer-prevention behaviors, reduces risk for many causes of death.)

Ultraviolet Light Exposure

Exposure to ultraviolet light, particularly from the sun, is a well-known cause of skin cancer, especially for light-skinned people (WCRF/AICR, 2007). Both cumulative exposure and occasional severe sunburn relate to subsequent risk of skin cancer. Since the mid-1970s, the incidence of skin cancer has risen in the United States.

Would You BELIEVE...? Cancer Prevention Prevents More Than Cancer

With one out of three cancer-related deaths attributable to smoking, your best way to avoid cancer is to avoid smoking. But how much do other cancer prevention behaviors matter, such as keeping a normal weight, maintaining a healthy diet, staying physically active, and drinking only in moderation (if at all)?

A recent study (McCullough et al., 2011) investigated this simple question. In the early 1990s, this research team from the American Cancer Society surveyed over 100,000 nonsmoking, older adults and asked them about their weight and height, diet, physical activity, and alcohol use. From these questions, the researchers computed a score representing the extent of adherence to the existing American Cancer Society guidelines for cancer prevention. Nearly 15 years later, the research team consulted the National Death Registry to obtain answers to two additional, important questions: Was the person dead, and if so, what was the cause of death?

One finding may not be surprising: Respondents who were the most adherent to cancer prevention guidelines had a *30% lower risk of cancer-related death* than those who were the least adherent. Thus, adhering to all the other behaviors conferred a clear benefit in preventing cancer.

However, the cancer prevention behaviors prevented much more than just cancer. The most adherent respondents had a *48% lower risk of death by cardiovascular disease* than the least adherent respondents. Taking all causes of death together, the most adherent respondents had a *42% lower risk of all-cause mortality*, compared with the least adherent respondents. Of all the behaviors this research team examined, maintaining a normal weight was the component most strongly tied to mortality.

Thus, by avoiding tobacco and following these other cancer prevention recommendations, you can reduce your odds of untimely death by nearly half.

However, because this form of cancer has a low mortality rate, it has only slightly affected total cancer mortality statistics. Not all skin cancers, however, are harmless. One form, that is, malignant melanoma, is often deadly. Malignant melanoma is especially prevalent among light-skinned people exposed to the sun.

Although we associate skin cancer with a behavioral risk (voluntary exposure to the sun over a long period), there is also a strong genetic component associated with it (Pho, Grossman, & Leachman, 2006). Light-skinned, fair-haired, blue-eyed individuals are more likely than dark-skinned people to develop skin cancer, and much of the damage occurs with sun exposure during childhood (Dennis et al., 2008). During the past 50 years, the relationship between melanoma mortality rates and geographic latitude has gradually decreased; residence in areas of the United States with high ultraviolet radiation is no longer a risk factor for melanoma but remains a risk for other types of skin cancer (Qureshi, Laden, Colditz, & Hunter, 2008). Fair-skinned people should avoid prolonged and frequent exposure to the sun by taking protective measures, including using sunscreen lotions and wearing protective clothing.

People should also avoid indoor tanning beds, which increase risk for melanoma. An international comprehensive review of research found a 75% increase in melanoma risk among people who used tanning beds in their teenage and young adult years (International Agency for Research on Cancer [IARC], 2007). Furthermore, a dose–response relationship exists: As people's frequency of tanning bed use increases, so does risk for melanoma (Lazovich et al., 2010). However, despite this clear link between tanning bed use and skin cancer, a surprising number of malignant melanoma survivors still report using tanning beds (Puthumana, Ferrucci, Mayne, Lannin, & Chagpar, 2013). Thus, the optimistic biases seen in smokers exist in many tanning bed users as well.

Not all exposure to sunlight is detrimental to health. Vitamin D derives from sun exposure and also contributes to lower rates of several types of cancer, including cancers of the breast, colon, prostate, ovary, lungs, and pancreas (Ingraham, Bragdon, & Nohe, 2008). However, the level of vitamin D necessary to protect against cancer seldom comes from diet alone. Therefore, low levels of exposure to ultraviolet light can be a healthy means of supplying vitamin D. How much sun exposure is enough but not too much? In addition to the usual dietary supply of vitamin D, as little as 5 to 10 minutes of sun exposure of the arms and legs or the arms, hands, and face two or three times a week seems sufficient (Holick, 2004). Alternatively, dietary supplementation can provide vitamin D and its protective benefits (Ingraham et al., 2008).

Sexual Behavior

Some sexual behaviors also contribute to cancer deaths, especially cancers resulting from acquired immune deficiency syndrome (AIDS). Two common forms of AIDS-related cancers are Kaposi's sarcoma and non-Hodgkin's lymphoma. Kaposi's sarcoma is a malignancy characterized by soft, dark blue or purple nodules on the skin, often with large lesions. The lesions can be so small at first as to look like a rash but can grow to be large and disfiguring. Besides covering the skin, these lesions can spread to the lung, spleen, bladder, lymph nodes, mouth, and adrenal glands. Until the 1980s, this type of cancer was quite rare and was limited mostly to older men of Mediterranean background. However, AIDS-related Kaposi's sarcoma occurs in every age group and in both men and women. Not all people with AIDS are equally susceptible to this disease; gay men with AIDS are much more likely to develop Kaposi's sarcoma than are people who developed AIDS as a result of injection drug use or heterosexual contact (Henke-Gendo & Schulz, 2004).

In non-Hodgkin's lymphoma, rapidly growing tumors spread through the circulatory or lymphatic system. Like Kaposi's sarcoma, non-Hodgkin's lymphoma can occur in AIDS patients of all ages and both genders. However, most people with non-Hodgkin's lymphoma do *not* have AIDS. The greatest risk for AIDS-related cancers continues to be unprotected sex with an HIV-positive partner.

Exposure to another sexually transmitted virus—the human papillomavirus, or HPV—increases risk for two types of cancer: cervical cancer and oral cancer. HPV is necessary for the development of cervical cancer (Baseman & Koutsky, 2005; Danaei et al., 2005). The rates of HPV infection are high, especially for sexually active young people (Datta et al., 2008). Thus, women who have had many sex partners and those whose first sexual intercourse experience occurred early in life are most vulnerable to cervical cancer because these behaviors expose them to HPV. Men's sex practices can also increase female partners' likelihood of getting cervical cancer. When men have multiple sex partners, specifically with women who have had many sex partners, their female sex partners are at increased risk of cervical cancer.

HPV is a cause of some oral cancers as well. In the last 20 years, the proportion of oral cancers associated with HPV increased dramatically, from 16% in the late 1980s to 73% in the early 2000s (Chaturvedi et al., 2011). By some estimates, new diagnoses of HPV-related oral cancer will exceed that of cervical cancers by the year 2020 (Chaturvedi et al., 2011). Furthermore, HPV-related oral cancer is twice as common in men as women (Chaturvedi, Engels, Anderson, & Gillison, 2008). Oral HPV is likely spread through oral sex, and oral HPV infections are more likely to persist among smokers (D'Souza & Dempsey, 2011). Thus, sexual behavior—in combination with tobacco use—can substantially increase the likelihood of oral cancers.

Men's sexual practices can also increase the risk of prostate cancer. Karin Rosenblatt and her associates (Rosenblatt, Wicklund, & Stanford, 2000) found a significant positive relationship between prostate cancer and lifetime number of female sex partners (but not male sex partners), early age of first intercourse, and prior infection with gonorrhea. However, they found no risk for prostate cancer associated with lifetime frequency of sexual intercourse.

Psychosocial Risk Factors in Cancer

Since the days of the Greek physician Galen (AD 131–201), people have speculated about the relationship between personality traits and certain diseases, including cancer. However, that speculation does not match the findings from scientific research. For example, a prospective study from the Swedish Twin Registry (Hansen, Floderus, Frederiksen, & Johansen, 2005) found that neither extraversion nor neuroticism—as measured by the Eysenck Personality Inventory—predicted an increased likelihood of cancer.

This study and its findings are fairly typical of attempts to relate psychosocial factors to cancer incidence and mortality. During the past 30 or 40 years, a number of researchers investigated the association between a variety of psychological factors and cancer development and prognosis. Some studies have identified various personality factors that seemed to relate to the development of cancer, but large-scale studies and reviews of the topic (Aro et al., 2005; Garssen, 2004; Levin & Kissane, 2006; Stürmer, Hasselbach, & Amelang, 2006) have found only a weak association between any psychosocial factor and cancer. Factors that show the strongest relationship come from negative emotionality and the tendency to repress (rather than express) emotion. However, these traits show a stronger relationship to response to a diagnosis of cancer than to the development of cancer.

IN SUMMARY

Cigarette smoking is the leading risk factor for lung cancer. Although not all cigarette smokers die of lung cancer and some nonsmokers develop this disease, clear evidence exists that smokers have a greatly increased chance of developing some form of cancer, particularly lung cancer. The more cigarettes people smoke per day and the more years they continue this practice, the more they are at risk.

The relationship between diet and the development of cancer is complex, with some types of food presenting dangers for the development of cancer and others offering some protection. "Natural" foods avoid the risk of preservatives but increase the likelihood of other toxins. A high-fat diet is related to colon and breast cancer, but a diet that produces overweight or obesity is a risk for a variety of cancers, including colorectal, esophageal, breast (in postmenopausal women), endometrial, and kidney cancer. Some dietary components can protect against cancer, including fruits and vegetables. The evidence for specific nutrients in foods is less persuasive, and taking supplements generally offers no protection.

Alcohol is probably only a weak risk factor for cancer. Nevertheless, it has a synergistic effect with cigarette smoking; when the two are combined, the total relative risk is much greater than the risks of the two factors added together. Lack of physical activity and high exposure to ultraviolet light are additional risk factors for cancer. Also, certain sexual behaviors, such as number of lifetime sex partners, relate to cervical, oral, and prostate cancer as well as to cancers associated with AIDS.

In general, psychosocial factors show only weak relationships to cancer incidence. Negative affect and repression of emotion may contribute to the development of cancer, but the relationship is not strong.

Living with Cancer

As Steve Jobs did in 2003, more than a million Americans receive a diagnosis of cancer each year (ACS, 2012). Most of these people receive their diagnosis with feelings of fear, anxiety, and anger, partly because they fear the disease and partly because current cancer treatments produce unpleasant effects for many cancer patients. Steve Jobs, for example, refused surgery for his pancreatic cancer for almost a year because of fears surrounding the treatment. Psychologists assist patients in coping with their emotional reactions to a cancer diagnosis, provide **social support** to patients and families, and help patients prepare for the negative side effects of some cancer treatments.

Problems with Medical Treatments for Cancer

Nearly all medical treatments for cancer have negative side effects that may add stress to the lives of cancer patients, their friends, and their families. The three most common therapies are also the three most stressful: surgery, radiation, and chemotherapy. In recent years, some **oncologists** have added hormonal treatment and immunotherapy to their arsenal of treatment regimens, but these newer treatments are generally not yet as effective as surgery, radiation, or chemotherapy.

Surgery is a common treatment recommendation when cancerous growth has not yet metastasized and when physicians have some confidence that the surgical procedure will be successful in making the tumor more manageable. Cancer patients who undergo surgery are likely to experience distress, rejection, and fears, and they often receive less emotional support than other surgery patients. These reactions are especially likely for patients with breast (Wimberly, Carver, Laurenceau, Harris, & Antoni, 2005) and prostate cancer (Couper, 2007) because of the sexual implications of their surgery. Postsurgery stress and depression lead to lower levels of immunity, which may prolong recovery time and increase vulnerability to other disorders (Antoni & Lutgendorf, 2007). Observers noted a marked decline in Steve Jobs' appearance following his liver transplant surgery in 2009, due possibly to both the cancer as well as compromised immune functioning (Lauerman, 2011).

Radiation also has severe side effects. Many patients who receive radiation therapy anticipate their treatment with fear and anxiety, dreading loss of hair, burns, nausea, vomiting, fatigue, and sterility. Most of these outcomes occur, so patients' fears are not unreasonable. However, patients are seldom adequately prepared for their radiation treatments, and thus their fears and anxieties may exaggerate the severity of these side effects.

Chemotherapy has some of the same negative side effects as radiation, and these side effects often

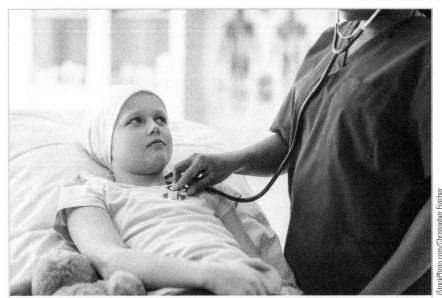

Negative side effects of chemotherapy such as hair loss add to the stress of cancer patients.

precipitate stressful reactions in cancer patients. Cancer patients treated with chemotherapy experience some combination of nausea, vomiting, fatigue, loss of coordination, decreased ability to concentrate, depression, weight change, loss of appetite, sleep problems, and hair loss. Not only do these negative effects create problems in adjusting to a diagnosis of cancer but also patients' expectations of the negative effects of chemotherapy (Olver, Taylor, & Whitford, 2005) and their beliefs about the nature of the disease (Thuné-Boyle, Myers, & Newman, 2006) contribute to distress and adjustment.

Adjusting to a Diagnosis of Cancer

Adjusting to a diagnosis of cancer is a challenge for everyone, but some people have more difficulties than others. Others, like Steve Jobs, may appear to ultimately cope well with a cancer diagnosis. Did Steve's personality—often described as confident and excessively optimistic—play a role in his adjustment to cancer?

Factors that predict a poor reaction to a diagnosis of cancer are the same factors that show some relationship to the development of cancer—negative affect and social inhibition (Verma & Khan, 2007). If negative affect is a problem for adjustment, then optimism should be an advantage, and research generally supports this hypothesis. Optimism is strongly related to adjusting well to a diagnosis of cancer (Carver et al., 2005),

but its relationship to long-term outcome is less clear (Segerstrom, 2005, 2007). This difference may arise from the difficulty of the task of adjusting to cancer treatment or from miscalculations on the part of optimists concerning the course and outcome of their treatments (Winterling, Glimelius, & Nordin, 2008). When outcomes are disappointing, optimists may find adjustment more difficult than those who have more realistic expectations. However, while being optimistic predicts better subsequent physical health among people coping with cancer (Rasmussen, Scheier, & Greenhouse, 2009), the strength of this relationship is very weak.

These findings are consistent with reviews of research on a "fighting spirit," which reflects an optimistic outlook, a belief that a cancer is controllable, and the use of active coping strategies. While a fighting spirit predicts better adjustment in early-stage cancer (O'Brien & Moorey, 2010), it appears to confer no advantage for long-term survival (Coyne & Tennen, 2010). This conclusion led one research team to advise, "People with cancer should not feel pressured into adopting particular coping styles to improve survival or reduce the risk of recurrence" (Petticrew, Bell, & Hunter, 2002, p. 1066).

After diagnosis, people with cancer show a variety of responses and different trajectories in adjusting and functioning over the course of their treatment and afterward (Helgeson, Snyder, & Seltman, 2004). Most cancer survivors report improvement in their functioning over time, but some long-term survivors attribute problems with low energy, pain, and sexual functioning to their cancers (Phipps, Braitman, Stites, & Leighton, 2008). Even 8 years after cancer diagnosis, survivors report some problems, which are much more likely to be physical complications rather than psychological problems (Schroevers, Ranchor, & Sanderman, 2006).

The same emotional factors that enhance the survival of heart disease patients may not be similarly helpful to cancer patients. That is, the calm expression of emotion that may be good advice for cardiovascular patients may not be a good choice for cancer patients; expression of emotion seems to be a better strategy. For example, for children (Aldridge & Roesch, 2007) and for men coping with prostate cancer (Roesch et al., 2005), use of emotion-focused coping did not present the disadvantages that this strategy typically does (see Chapter 5 for a discussion of coping strategies). Expression of both positive and negative emotions can be beneficial (Quartana, Laubmeier, & Zakowski, 2006). However, expressing some negative emotions may do more harm than good (Lieberman & Goldstein, 2006); expressing anger seems to lead to a better adjustment, whereas expressing fear and anxiety related to lower quality of life and higher depression. Being able to express emotions and being guided to do so in the most helpful manner require appropriate social support.

Social Support for Cancer Patients

What single factor reduces a man's chances of dying from cancer by 27%, and a woman's chances of dying from cancer by 19%?

Marriage is the factor. Both male and female cancer patients have better odds of survival if they are married than if they are not. Why?

Researchers examined this question in a longitudinal sample of over 800,000 adults diagnosed with invasive cancer (Gomez et al., 2016). One possible reason why married cancer patients fare better than their single counterparts is that marriage offers economic benefits, such as better health care options or better access to treatments. However, these researchers found that the marriage benefit had little to do with economics. Rather, it appeared that the emotional and instrumental social support that generally accompanies a marriage was responsible for the survival benefits.

Married patients are more likely to have someone available to drive them to appointments, encourage them to take medications, to offer healthy meals, or provide

emotional support. Many other studies show that social support, such as that provided by a spouse, can help cancer patients adjust to their condition, and support from other family and friends can be beneficial as well. For example, in the context of breast cancer, women with greater structural social support—that is, with larger social support networks—have slower cancer progression than women with less structural social support (Nausheen, Gidron, Peveler, & Moss-Morris, 2009). Social support is an important factor for men as well, as prostate cancer survivors who perceive more available social support from others manifest greater emotional well-being over time (Zhou et al., 2010). Unfortunately, not all social support attempts by friends and family are beneficial for people with cancer. Sometimes partners' attempts to protect spouses from the reality of their illness are not helpful (Hagedoorn et al., 2000). Thus, social support from families may or may not provide the type of support people with cancer need. Many people with cancer turn to support groups or therapists to provide emotional support.

Professionals such as psychologists, nurses, or oncologists may lead support groups, but often these groups consist of other individuals who are cancer survivors. Some studies indicate that some people profit from support groups more than others. For example, women with breast cancer who lacked adequate marital support profited more from peer group support than from support of their partners, whereas women with strong support from their partners had poorer adjustments when they participated in a peer discussion group (Helgeson, Cohen, Schulz, & Yasko, 2000). A systematic review of the value of peer support groups for cancer survivors (Hoey, Ieropoli, White, & Jefford, 2008) indicated that such groups could be but were not always helpful. In general, face-to-face support delivered by an individual and Internet groups demonstrated the best outcomes, but all types of groups can be effective for some individuals.

Psychological Interventions for Cancer Patients

Psychologists have used both individual and group techniques to help cancer patients cope with their diagnosis. To be effective, an intervention should accomplish at least one of two objectives: It should improve emotional well-being, increase survival time, or both. To what extent do psychological interventions succeed at these two objectives?

Two reviews (Edwards, Hulbert-Williams, & Neal, 2008; Manne & Andrykowski, 2006) conclude that psychological interventions generally yield short-term benefits in helping cancer patients manage the distress related to their condition. Furthermore, some psychological interventions for women with breast cancer improve physiological outcomes, such as cortisol responses and measures of immune functioning (McGregor & Antoni, 2009).

Some psychological interventions focus on cognitive behavioral stress management skills, while others focus on providing social support and an opportunity to express emotions. There is evidence that each of these types of interventions improves some outcomes (Edwards et al., 2008). For example, a program that targeted emotional regulation (Cameron, Booth, Schlatter, Ziginskas, & Harman, 2007) indicated success. However, this emphasis may not be the best approach for everyone. As one research team asked, "Does one size fit all?" (Zimmerman, Heinrichs, & Baucom, 2007, p. 225). This question highlights the need to match the characteristics and needs of people with cancer to a psychotherapy, support, educational, or multicomponent program that will be effective for each person.

Although psychological interventions can improve short-term emotional adjustment, there is less evidence that psychological interventions prolong the life span of people with cancer. The possibility that interventions could have such an effect arose when David Spiegel and colleagues (Spiegel, Bloom, Kraemer, & Gottheil, 1989) conducted a multicomponent intervention to help breast cancer patients adjust to the stressful aspects of their disease and their treatment. Not only was the intervention successful in managing pain, anxiety, and depression but also the women in the intervention group lived longer than those in the comparison group. That finding prompted researchers to examine how psychosocial and CAM (complementary and alternative medicine) interventions might prolong the life of those with cancer (see Chapter 8 for a discussion of integrative cancer treatments). Plausible mechanisms include the effect on the immune system and improvements in functioning that allow cancer patients to adhere to their medical treatment regimen (Antoni & Lutgendorf, 2007; Spiegel, 2004; Spiegel & Geise-Davis, 2003).

However, the basic finding that psychosocial interventions prolong life is now in question. Although one recent psychological intervention with women with early-stage breast cancer significantly reduced risk for recurrence and death at an 11-year follow-up (Andersen et al., 2008), large-scale reviews find little evidence that psychological interventions reliably extend survival time for breast cancer patients (Edwards, Hailey, & Maxwell, 2004; Smedslund & Ringdal, 2004). Despite a plausible mechanism for such action and despite the hope that such a benefit is possible (Coyne, Stefanek, & Palmer, 2007), little evidence exists at this point that psychological interventions prolong the life of those with cancer (Edwards et al., 2008). Thus, the value of psychological interventions lies mainly in improving the *quality* rather than the quantity of a cancer patient's life.

IN SUMMARY

After people receive a cancer diagnosis, they typically experience fear, anxiety, depression, and feelings of helplessness. The standard medical treatments for cancer—surgery, chemotherapy, and radiation—all have negative side effects that often produce added stress and discomfort. These side effects include loss of hair, nausea, fatigue, sterility, and other negative conditions. Receiving social support from family and friends, joining support groups, and receiving emotional support through psychological interventions probably help some people with cancer to increase psychological functioning, decrease depression and anxiety, manage pain, and enhance quality of life. Little evidence exists that psychotherapy can increase survival time.

Answers

This chapter has addressed five basic questions:

1. **What is cancer?**

Cancer is a group of diseases characterized by the presence of new (neoplastic) cells that grow and spread beyond control. These cells may be either benign or malignant, but both types of neoplastic cells are dangerous. Malignant cells are capable of metastasizing and spreading through the blood or lymph to other organs of the body, thus making malignancies life threatening.

2. **Are cancer death rates increasing or decreasing?**

Cancer is the second leading cause of death in the United States, accounting for about 23% of deaths. During the first nine and a half decades of the 20th century, cancer death rates in the United States rose threefold, but since the mid-1990s, death rates have begun to decline, especially for cancers of the lung, colon and rectum, breast, and prostate—the four leading sites for cancer deaths in the United States. Currently, lung cancer death rates for women are beginning to level off and may soon begin to decline.

3. **What are the inherent and environmental risk factors for cancer?**

The uncontrollable risk factors for cancer include family history, ethnic background, and advancing age. Family history is a factor in many types of cancer; inheritance of a mutated form of a specific gene increases the risk of breast cancer two- to threefold. Ethnic background is also a factor; compared with European Americans, African Americans have a significantly higher rate of mortality from cancer, but other ethnic groups have lower rates. Advancing age is the single most powerful mortality risk for cancer, but age is also the leading risk for death from cardiovascular and other diseases. Environmental exposure to airborne pollutants, radiation, and infectious organisms constitute significant risks for cancer if the exposure is heavy and prolonged.

4. **What are the behavioral risk factors for cancer?**

More than half of all cancer deaths in the United States have been attributed to either smoking or unwise lifestyle choices, such as diet and exercise. Smoking cigarettes raises the risk of lung cancer by a factor of 23, but smoking also accounts for other cancer deaths.

The relationship between diet and cancer is complex; diet can increase or decrease the risk for cancer. Toxins and contaminants in food raise the risks, but a diet high in fruits, vegetables, whole grains, low-fat dairy products, beans, and seeds and low in fat, red meat, processed meat, and salt tends to be associated with lowered risk for a variety of cancers. A diet that leads to overweight or obesity raises the risk. Alcohol is not as strong a risk for cancer as diet, but combining alcohol with smoking sharply increases the risk. A sedentary lifestyle also presents a risk, especially for breast cancer. Exposure to ultraviolet light and sexual behaviors can increase the risks for various cancers. Research has also revealed a weak link between negative affect, depression, and cancer.

5. **How can cancer patients be helped in coping with their disease?**

Cancer patients usually benefit from social support from spouse, family, and health care providers, but the type and timing of support affect its benefits. Support groups offer another type of support that is beneficial to some cancer patients, especially in allowing the expression of emotion. Therapists can use cognitive behavioral methods to assist cancer patients in coping with some of the negative aspects of cancer treatments and adjusting to their disease, thus increasing the quality of life for cancer patients, but no evidence exists that psychosocial factors can increase survival time.

Suggested Readings

American Cancer Society. (2016). *Cancer facts and figures 2016.* Atlanta, GA: American Cancer Society. This yearly publication provides extensive, updated information about cancer in the United States with some international comparisons.

Antoni, M. H., & Lutgendorf, S. (2007). Psychosocial factors in disease progression in cancer. *Current Directions in Psychological Science, 16,* 42–46. This brief article focuses on the influence of psychosocial factors and how these factors may affect the biology of cancer.

Danaei, G., Vander Hoorn, S., Lopez, A. D., Murray, C. J. L., & Ezzati, M. (2005). Causes of cancer in the world: Comparative risk assessment of nine behavioural and environmental risk factors. *Lancet, 366,* 1784–1793. For those who want an international perspective, this article examines nine behavioral and environmental factors and traces the differing rates of cancer in countries throughout the world related to these factors.

U.S. Department of Health and Human Services. (2010). *A report of the Surgeon General: How tobacco smoke causes disease: What it means to you.* Atlanta, GA: U.S. Department of Health and Human Services and Centers for Disease Control and Prevention. This short and engaging article details, in easy-to-understand language, the pathways by which tobacco increases risk for several types of cancer, as well as a multitude of other health problems.

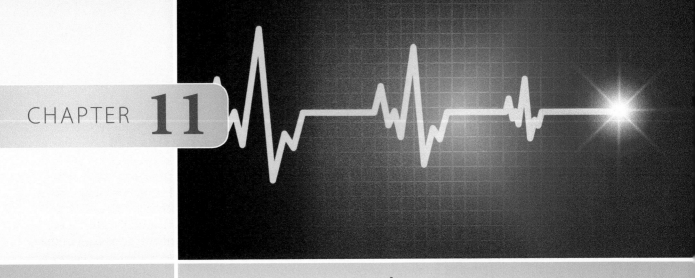

Living with Chronic Illness

CHAPTER OUTLINE

QUESTIONS

This chapter focuses on six basic questions:

1. What is the impact of chronic disease on patients and families?

2. What is the impact of Alzheimer's disease?

3. What is involved in adjusting to diabetes?

4. How does asthma affect the lives of people with this disease?

5. How can HIV infection be managed?

6. What adaptations do people make to dying and grieving?

Real-World Profile of **PRESIDENT RONALD REAGAN**

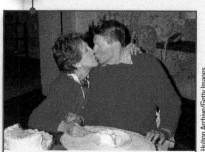

After Ronald Reagan was diagnosed with Alzheimer's disease, his wife, Nancy, learned how to cope with the consequences of living with this chronic illness.

On September 30, 1983, President Ronald Reagan declared the month of November 1983, to be National Alzheimer's Disease Month. At the time, researchers knew little about the prevalence of Alzheimer's disease. Today, we know that one in eight older Americans has Alzheimer's disease. Eleven years after Reagan declared National Alzheimer's Disease Month, he revealed to the world that he had been diagnosed with Alzheimer's disease (Alzheimer's Organization, 2004).

During the decade between the announcement of his Alzheimer's disease and his death on June 5, 2004, Reagan and his family experienced the same stresses and frustrations that millions of families endure when a family member is chronically ill. For daughter Maureen, her first realization that something was wrong with her father came in 1993, when he could not remember making one of his favorite movies (Ellis, 2004). Soon afterward, Reagan noticed that he sometimes felt disoriented. His wife, Nancy, however, said that she noticed no problems at all and was "dumbfounded" when her husband received the Alzheimer's diagnosis. Experts have commented (in Ellis, 2004) that the tendency to overlook problems is common among those closest to the patients—it's easy to deny serious problems when they present subtle symptoms.

As Reagan's symptoms became worse, Nancy was faced with the reality of his symptoms and her increasing loneliness (Ellis, 2004). Despite their resources and fame, Nancy felt isolated, a typical experience for those who are caregivers for Alzheimer's patients. She wrote, "But no one can really know what it's like unless they've traveled this path—and there are many right now traveling the same path I am. You know that it's a progressive disease and that there's no place to go but down, no light at the end of the tunnel. You get tired and frustrated, because you have no control and you feel helpless" (Reagan, 2000, p. 184).

Unlike the other millions of cases of Alzheimer's disease, Ronald Reagan's case stirred public interest, and his family's activism spurred research initiatives. The U.S. Congress passed a bill known as the Ronald Reagan Alzheimer's Breakthrough Act of 2005, which provided increased funding for Alzheimer's disease research, more help for caregivers, and greater efforts in public education and prevention. Alzheimer's disease is one of the chronic diseases that has increased in frequency and will continue to do so, unless research finds a cure or prevention.

Chronic diseases cause 7 in 10 deaths each year in the United States, and almost half of adults live with at least one chronic illness (Centers for Disease Control and Prevention [CDC], 2009). Chronic illness also affects children, with 10% to 15% having some chronic physical health problem (Bramlett & Blumberg, 2008). This chapter looks at the consequences of living with chronic illnesses such as Alzheimer's disease, diabetes, asthma, and AIDS. These and other chronic illnesses share many elements. The diseases vary in physiology, but the emotional and physical adjustments, the disruption of family dynamics, the need for continued medical care, and the necessity of self-management also apply to chronic diseases such as arthritis, heart disease, cancer, kidney disease, multiple sclerosis, head injury, and spinal cord injury.

The Impact of Chronic Disease

Chronic disease places an enormous physical and emotional burden on a patient, as well as a patient's family. Some theorists describe the diagnosis of a chronic illness as a crisis (Moos & Schaefer, 1984). Other theorists suggest that people pass through several stages in their adjustment to chronic disease, but as we will learn, there is little support for stage models of adjustment to chronic disease. Instead, adjustment seems to be a dynamic process influenced by many factors, including the characteristics of the disease, such as rapidity of progress; characteristics of the individual, such as a dispositional optimism; and characteristics of the person's social environment, such as social support. Thus, adjustment to chronic disease is a variable process, and many individual factors shape how people adjust and adapt to a chronic illness (Parker, Schaller, & Hansmann, 2003).

Impact on the Patient

Adapting to chronic disease includes dealing with the symptoms of the disease, managing the stresses of treatment, living as normal a life as possible, and facing the possibility of death. Adjustment to some chronic diseases is more difficult than others because of symptom severity and the demands of coping with symptoms. However, some chronic illnesses may influence quality of life less than healthy people imagine (Damschroder, Zikmund-Fisher, & Ubel, 2005). Research that evaluated the functioning of large groups of patients with a variety of chronic illnesses (Arnold et al., 2004; Heijmans et al., 2004) found similarities and differences among people with different chronic diseases. For some chronic diseases, such as hypertension and diabetes, people reported levels of functioning similar to those with no chronic disease. However, people with heart disease, rheumatoid arthritis, and cancer experienced more intrusive symptoms than did those with hypertension, asthma, or diabetes. Indeed, the psychological functioning appears to matter more than physical functioning in determining the quality of life of patients with chronic disease, highlighting the important role of adaptation and coping (Arnold et al., 2004). Using a variety of coping strategies allows people to deal with the stresses of chronic disease (Heijmans et al., 2004); however, active coping strategies tend to produce better results than avoidant strategies (Stanton, Revenson, & Tennen, 2007).

Receiving treatment for chronic diseases also requires adaptation. Interactions with the health care system are likely to create frustrations and problems for people with chronic illness (Parchman, Noel, & Lee, 2005). When patients must interact with the health care system, they tend to feel deprived not only of their sense of competence and mastery but also of their rights and privileges. That is, sick people begin to feel like "nonpersons" and to experience loss of personal control and threats to self-esteem (Stanton et al., 2007).

Developing and maintaining relationships with health care providers also present challenges, for both patients and practitioners. The medical system and people's experience of illness both focus on acute conditions. This experience may lead sick people to believe in the power of modern medicine and to be optimistic about cures. Physicians and other health care workers usually share this attitude (Bickel-Swenson, 2007), which may create a positive climate of trust and optimism for their treatment. Conversely, people with a chronic illness may have a hopeless and even helpless attitude toward their condition—modern medicine can offer them no cure. Health care professionals, too, tend to orient themselves toward providing cures. When they cannot do so, they may feel less positive about those whom they cannot cure (Bickel-Swenson, 2007; Turner & Kelly, 2000). These feelings can create a difficult climate for treatment, with patients questioning and resisting health care providers, and providers feeling frustrated and annoyed with patients who fail to follow treatment regimens and do not get better. Fortunately, younger physicians may be less likely to hold such negative attitudes (Lloyd-Williams, Dogra, & Petersen, 2004), which will benefit treatment and may help to counteract the growing difficulty in negotiating the U.S. health care system experienced by people with chronic conditions.

People with chronic diseases often adopt a number of coping strategies to deal with their illness. A variety of strategies can be successful, but some work better in certain situations. For example, avoidance-oriented coping, such as denial or ignoring the problem, is typically a less effective strategy than problem-focused strategies, such as planning and information seeking (Livneh & Antonak, 2005; Stanton et al., 2007). However, when events are uncontrollable, avoidance coping may be effective in easing negative emotions; when events are controllable, this strategy would be a very poor choice.

Physicians often feel inadequately prepared to help patients deal with these emotional reactions (Bickel-Swenson, 2007; Turner & Kelly, 2000). Such deficits have led to two types of supplements: psychological interventions and support groups. For many chronic illnesses, health psychologists have created interventions that emphasize the management of emotions such as anxiety and depression. Support groups also address emotional needs by providing emotional support to patients or family members who must confront an illness with little chance of a cure. These services supplement conventional health care and help chronically ill patients maintain compliance with the prescribed regimen and sustain a working relationship with health care providers. Reviews of studies dealing with the effectiveness of psychosocial interventions with cancer patients (Osborn, Demoncada, & Feuerstein, 2006) and their families (Badr & Krebs, 2013; Barlow & Ellard, 2004) indicate that cognitive behavioral interventions provide effective assistance in helping people cope with chronic diseases. Furthermore, there is also evidence that Internet-administered interventions can help alleviate distress and improve disease control across a number of chronic health conditions (Beatty & Lambert, 2013).

A major impact of chronic illness involves the changes that occur in how people think of themselves; that is, the diagnosis of a chronic disease changes self-perception. Chronic illness and treatment force many patients to reevaluate their lives, relationships, and body image (Livneh & Antonak, 2005). Being diagnosed with a chronic illness represents a loss (Murray, 2001), and people adapt to such losses through a process of grieving (Rentz, Krikorian, & Keys, 2005). Finding meaning in the experience of loss is more extensive than grieving, but developing an understanding of the meaning of the loss is a common part of coping with chronic disease. Some chronically ill people never move past the grief (Murray, 2001). Other people reconstruct the meaning of their lives in positive ways.

People with chronic diseases often find some positive aspect to their situation (Folkman & Moskowitz, 2000). Part of healthy adjustment is accepting the changes that disease brings, but some research (Fournier, de Ridder, & Bensing, 2002) found that positive expectancies and even unrealistic optimism were advantages in coping with chronic disease. As Annette Stanton and her colleagues (2007, p. 568) summarized, "A disease that disrupts life does not preclude the experience of joy." Thus, some people manage to experience personal growth through loss and grief (Hogan & Schmidt, 2002), which relates to less depression and greater well-being (Helgeson, Reynolds, & Tomich, 2006). This outcome applies not only to patients with chronic diseases but also to their families and caregivers.

Impact on the Family

Illness requires adaptation not only for patients but also for their families. Families may react with grief and feel loss during the sick person's lifetime because families see the person's loss of abilities and sometimes the sense of self.

Involving family members in psychosocial interventions benefits the well-being of both the patient (Martire, Schulz, Helgeson, Small, & Saghafi, 2010) and the family member (Martire, Lustig, Schulz, Miller, & Helgeson, 2004). However, some interventions may be more effective than others. For example, interventions that emphasize communication and interactions—especially those affecting health—provide greater benefits for patients than interventions with other components (Martire & Schulz, 2007). People with chronic illness also benefit from a type of support described as "invisible" (Bolger, Zuckerman, & Kessler, 2000). Invisible support is support that a provider reports offering, but the patient does not report receiving it; this dynamic occurs when a provider's support is given in a manner that is not perceived by the patient as an obvious attempt to help, which may help make the patient feel less helpless and more efficacious. This type of interaction may be easier to manage when a partner is not ill; a sick partner needs help, but being the obvious recipient of assistance makes that support stressful as well as helpful. Therefore, chronic illness presents difficulties even to well-intentioned, caring partners.

Although the rates of childhood diseases declined dramatically in the 20th century, a significant number of children still experience chronic diseases (Brace, Smith, McCauley, & Sherry, 2000). The majority of these illnesses are relatively minor, but many children experience severe chronic conditions such as cancer, asthma, rheumatoid arthritis, and diabetes—conditions that limit mobility and activity. These illnesses bring changes in the lives of the entire family. Parents and siblings try to "normalize" family life while coping with therapy for the sick child (Knafl & Deatrick, 2002). However, parents may experience shock, grief, and anger. Such parents face the task of providing support and care, plus the adjustments that chronically ill patients face in finding meaning in the experience of illness. Siblings also face challenges in adjusting to the illness of a family member, tending to notice the differences between their families and "normal" families and feeling some combination of sympathy for and resentment of their sick sibling (Waite-Jones & Madill, 2008a).

For adults, the changes that come with illness can alter their relationships and redefine their identity, but for children who are sick, illness can be even more distressing and disruptive. For some children, the restrictions that come with chronic illness are very difficult, leading to isolation, depression, and distress, whereas other children cope more effectively (Melamed, Kaplan, & Fogel,

2001). Younger children may have difficulty understanding the nature of their disease, and older children and adolescents may resent the restrictions that their disease imposes. Health care providers and parents can help these children make adjustments by offering alternative or modified activities.

Families of sick children face problems similar to couples: They must continue their relationships and manage the problems of caregiving (Knafl & Deatrick, 2002). A child who is ill requires a great deal of emotional support, most of which is supplied by mothers. These efforts can leave mothers so drained that they have little emotional energy left for their husbands, which can leave husbands feeling abandoned and excluded from the family. Fathers tend to cope by concealing their distress and through avoidance, which is seldom an effective coping strategy (Waite-Jones & Madill, 2008b).

Families can follow several recommendations to facilitate adjustment to a chronic disease. Families can try to be flexible and establish a routine that is as close to normal as they can manage (Knafl & Deatrick, 2002). One example of this would be to put the disease into the background and focus on the ways in which the sick child is similar to other children and other family members. Magnifying the ways that the disease makes the child different and focusing on the changes to family routine tend to lead to poorer adaptations. Families should find ways to meet sick children's needs without reinforcing their anxiety and depression (Brace et al., 2000). Like individuals with chronic illness, families tend to make a better adjustment if they focus on finding meaning and some positive aspect in their situation (Ylvén, Björck-Åkesson, & Granlund, 2006).

IN SUMMARY

Chronic diseases bring changes that require adaptation for both the person with the disease and family members. Chronically ill patients must manage their symptoms, seek appropriate health care, and adapt to the psychological changes that occur in this situation. Health care professionals may neglect the social and emotional needs of chronically ill patients, attending instead to their physical needs. Health psychologists and support groups help provide for the emotional needs associated with chronic illness. The adaptations that occur may lead to prolonged feelings of loss and grief or to changes that constitute personal growth.

Living with Alzheimer's Disease

Alzheimer's disease, a degenerative disease of the brain, is a major source of impairment among older people (Mayeaux, 2003). This disease varies in prevalence among countries but remains a major source of cognitive disability in both industrialized and developing countries. Medical researchers identified the brain abnormalities that underlie Alzheimer's disease in the late 19th century. In 1907, a German physician, Alois Alzheimer, reported on the relationship between autopsy findings of neurological abnormalities and psychiatric symptoms before death. Shortly after his report, other researchers began to call the disorder *Alzheimer's disease.*

The disease can be diagnosed definitively only through autopsy, but brain imaging technology is capable of diagnosing Alzheimer's disease with close to 90% accuracy (Vemuri et al., 2008). In addition, Alzheimer's patients show behavioral symptoms of cognitive impairment and memory loss that may lead to a provisional diagnosis (Mayeaux, 2003). During autopsy, a microscopic examination of the brain reveals "plaques" and tangles of nerve fibers in the cerebral cortex and hippocampus. These tangles of nerve fibers are the physical basis for Alzheimer's disease.

The biggest risk factor for Alzheimer's disease is age; the incidence of Alzheimer's disease rises sharply with advancing age. The prevalence of Alzheimer's disease is low for those under age 75—about 9% of people in this age group (Fitzpatrick et al., 2004; Lindsay, Sykes, McDowell, Verreault, & Laurin, 2004). However, the percentage of affected individuals doubles about every 5 years, so that by age 85, almost 50% of individuals exhibit signs of Alzheimer's disease. The increase seems not to continue at the same rate; people in their 90s who have not developed signs of the disease are not nearly as likely to do so as people between ages 65 and 85 (Hall et al., 2005). The high number of people over 85 years old who have symptoms of probable Alzheimer's disease presents a pessimistic picture for the aging population in many industrialized and some developing countries, where Alzheimer's seems destined to become a large public health problem (Wimo et al., 2013).

The underlying mechanisms in the development of the disease are not yet completely understood, but two different forms of the disease exist: an early-onset version that occurs before age 60 and a late-onset version that occurs after age 60. The early-onset type is quite rare, representing fewer than 5% of all Alzheimer's patients (Bertram & Tanzi, 2005). Early-onset Alzheimer's may arise from a genetic defect, and at least three different genes on chromosomes 1, 14, and 21 contribute.

The late-onset type has symptoms similar to the early-onset type but begins after age 60, as President Reagan's disease did. Susceptibility to this version of the disease also has a genetic component related to apolipoprotein ε, a protein involved in cholesterol metabolism (Bertram & Tanzi, 2005; Ertekin-Taner, 2007). One form of apolipoprotein, the ε4 form, affects accumulation of the amyloid ε protein, which forms the building blocks for amyloid plaque (Selkoe, 2007). This plaque seems to constitute the underlying pathology for Alzheimer's disease. The risk increases about three times for individuals who have one ε4 gene and about 15 times for individuals who have two. Older adults who do not have Alzheimer's disease but who carry the ε4 variant of this gene show lower levels of cognitive functioning than those with other variants of the gene (Small, Rosnick, Fratiglioni, & Bäckman, 2004). The ε2 form of the gene may actually offer some protection against Alzheimer's disease.

These genetic factors increase a person's susceptibility to Alzheimer's disease, rather than guarantee it. A variety of environmental and behavioral factors also play a role in the development of Alzheimer's disease, interacting with the genetics of the disease. For example, having a stroke increases the risk, and so does head injury (Pope, Shue, & Beck, 2003). These risks may apply more strongly to people who carry the ε4 form of the gene for apolipoprotein. Type 2 diabetes increases the risk for Alzheimer's disease, but the combination of ε4 apolipoprotein and diabetes raises the risk more than five times (Peila, Rodriguez, & Launer, 2002). The process of inflammation is also a risk for Alzheimer's, as it is for cardiovascular disease (Martins et al., 2006). This risk may accrue throughout life, with increased risk for people who experience prolonged bouts of inflammation, even during young or middle adulthood (Kamer et al., 2008). Fat intake during middle adulthood also increases the risk (Laitinen et al., 2006), but high cholesterol during older age has no relationship (Reitz et al., 2008). Physical activity—a protective risk factor for many other health problems—also appears to protect against the subsequent development of Alzheimer's disease (Qiu, Kivipelto, & von Strauss, 2011).

Research into risk factors for Alzheimer's disease also reveals some protective factors. Cognitive activity decreases the risk, so people whose jobs demand a high level of cognitive processing are less likely to develop Alzheimer's disease than others with less cognitively demanding jobs (see Would You Believe ...? box). Low levels of alcohol consumption cut the risk in half in one study (Ruitenberg et al., 2002). Regular doses of nonsteroidal anti-inflammatory drugs (NSAIDs) also appear to decrease the risk, especially for people who carry the ε4 form of the apolipoprotein gene (Szekely et al., 2008). Therefore, it is possible to modify the genetic risk through this behavior. Many of the risks for Alzheimer's disease overlap with those for cardiovascular disease and cancer, and so do the protective factors. That is, a healthy lifestyle may offer protection for a range of disorders. Table 11.1 presents a summary of these risks and protective factors.

TABLE 11.1   Risks and Protective Factors for the Development of Alzheimer's Disease

Risks	Protective Factors
Age—over age 65 presents increasing risk	
Inheriting apolipoprotein ε4	Inheriting apolipoprotein ε2
Stroke, head injury, or diabetes, especially for those who carry apolipoprotein ε4	
Inflammation	Taking anti-inflammatory drugs (NSAIDs)
High-fat diet during middle adulthood	
Low levels of education	Higher levels of education
Cognitively undemanding job	Cognitively demanding job
	Low-to-moderate alcohol intake
A sedentary lifestyle	Many forms of physical activity, including walking

Would You BELIEVE...?   Using Your Mind May Help Prevent Losing Your Mind

Although age and genetics contribute to the risk of developing Alzheimer's disease, not everyone of the same age or even with the same genes is at equal risk. Your intelligence, education, job, and even your television viewing habits also contribute to the risk.

People with more education have a lower risk of developing Alzheimer's disease. Because education and IQ are strongly related, separating the protective effect of education is not easy, but one study (Pavlik, Doody, Massman, & Chan, 2006) estimated that IQ score, not educational level, was a better predictor of the progression of Alzheimer's disease. This result suggests that being intelligent offers some protection against this disease. Other research, however, hints that being intelligent is by no means the whole story.

What you do with your mind may be more important than how

intelligent you are in combating Alzheimer's disease. For example, the complexity of people's jobs affects the risk. In a study of pairs of twins, in which one twin had Alzheimer's disease and the other did not (Andel et al., 2005), a distinguishing feature was the complexity of work performed by the unaffected twins. Because the study involved twins, genetic factors could not have played a role. The results indicated that those whose work involved more complexity, in terms of tasks with people or data, were likely to be unaffected by the disorder. A study of nearly 1,000 Swedish adults also confirmed this finding (Karp et al., 2009), suggesting that using your mind is protective. Would you also believe that retirement—which, for many people might mean stopping a cognitively complex job—may also increase the risk of cognitive decline? One recent study suggests

that it does (Roberts, Fuhrer, Marmot, & Richards, 2011).

Rest assured, working throughout your retirement years is not the only solution to preventing Alzheimer's disease, as work complexity is not the only type of mental activity that may offer protection. A study of leisure time activities (Lindstrom et al., 2005) found that leisure activities during middle age could be protective or risky. People who participated in intellectually stimulating leisure and social activities were at lower risk of Alzheimer's disease during their older years, whereas those who watched television were at increased risk. Indeed, each additional daily hour of television viewing raised the risk. So, using your mind during young and middle age may protect against the development of Alzheimer's disease later in life—presenting another case of "use it or lose it."

Because the symptoms of Alzheimer's include a number of behavior problems that are also symptoms of psychiatric disorders, the disease can be difficult to diagnose. These symptoms occur in a majority of people with Alzheimer's disease (Weiner, Hynan, Bret, & White, 2005). In addition to memory loss, behavioral symptoms include agitation and irritability, sleep difficulties, delusions such as suspiciousness and paranoia, inappropriate sexual behavior, and hallucinations. People with Alzheimer's disease are more likely than others to engage in dangerous behavior (Starkstein, Jorge, Mizrahi, Adrian, & Robinson, 2007). Even individuals with mild Alzheimer's disease show psychiatric symptoms similar to those with more severe cases (Shimabukuro, Awata, & Matsuoka, 2005). These behavioral symptoms can be the source of much distress to patients as well as to their caregivers, and more severe behavioral symptoms predict shorter survival times (Weiner et al., 2005).

The most common psychiatric problem among Alzheimer's patients is depression, with as many as 20% of patients exhibiting symptoms of clinical depression (van Reekum et al., 2005). Depression may even precede the development of Alzheimer's disease, serving as a risk factor. The experience of negative mood is especially common among people in the early phases of the disease and in early-onset Alzheimer's. Those who retain awareness of their problems find their deterioration distressing and respond with feelings of helplessness and depression.

The memory loss that characterizes Alzheimer's patients may first appear in the form of small, ordinary failures of memory, which represent the early stages of the disease (Morris et al., 2001). This memory loss progresses to the point that Alzheimer's patients fail to recognize family members and forget how to perform even routine self-care; former President Reagan experienced these losses. In the early phases of the disease, patients are usually aware of their memory failures, as Reagan was, making this symptom even more distressing.

The common symptoms of paranoia and suspiciousness may also relate to cognitive impairments. Alzheimer's patients may forget where they have put belongings and, because they cannot find their possessions, accuse others of taking them. However, suspicious and accusatory behaviors are not limited to misplaced belongings. Verbal aggression occurs in about 37% of Alzheimer's patients and physical aggression in about 17% (Weiner et al., 2005).

Helping the Patient

At present, Alzheimer's disease remains without a cure. However, incurability and untreatability are two different things; the physical symptoms and other accompanying disorders of Alzheimer's disease are treatable. Although researchers seek to develop drugs that prevent the disease, the primary focus of treatment is the use of drugs to slow its progress. Treatment approaches include drugs for delaying the progression of cognitive deficits and neuroleptic drugs for reducing agitation and aggression. Unfortunately, a systematic review (Seow & Gauthier, 2007) indicated that the drugs that target cognitive deficits offer only modest benefits. For some patients, these drugs slow the progress of the disease by months or even a few years, but they do not stop or cure it. One drug (donepezil) slows the loss of neurons in the hippocampus, the brain location critical for formation of new memories. This finding explains why this drug is effective for some Alzheimer's patients in delaying cognitive losses. Another drug (memantine) may improve cognitive measures and overall functioning. In addition, some researchers (Langa, Foster, & Larson, 2004) have found some benefits of statin drugs, typically prescribed for cardiovascular patients, in slowing the dementia associated with Alzheimer's disease.

Behavioral approaches can be helpful for people with Alzheimer's disease. These approaches include sensory stimulation and reality orientation to help Alzheimer's patients retain their cognitive abilities. Several reviews (Hulme, Wright, Crocker, Oluboyede, & House, 2010; O'Connor, Ames, Gardner, & King, 2009; Verkaik, Van Weert, & Francke, 2005) indicated that a few programs demonstrate effectiveness. Those that show the most promise are programs that provide pleasant stimulation, such as music, aromatherapy, exposure to sunlight, and muscle relaxation training, and programs that concentrate on cognitive skills and problem solving.

Music therapy may be more useful than other types of sensory stimulation (Svansdottir & Snaedal, 2006) and is the approach that most consistently benefits Alzheimer's patients (Hulme et al., 2010; O'Connor et al., 2009; Verkaik et al., 2005). A meta-analysis of programs that provide cognitive stimulation indicates that such programs can provide modest improvements in cognitive skills, but programs that provide cognitive training provide fewer benefits (Huntley, Gould, Smith, & Howard, 2015). However, caregivers can manage behavior problems of Alzheimer's patients through improvements in communication and modification of the environment to help decrease confusion and manage problem behaviors (O'Connor et al., 2009; Yuhas, McGowan, Fontaine, Czech, & Gambrell-Jones, 2006). For example, locking exit doors may prevent wandering. For those who get lost in their own homes, labeling the doors can be helpful.

Although none of these treatments can cure Alzheimer's disease, most will help control undesirable behaviors and alleviate some of the distressing symptoms of the disease. Any treatment that can delay symptoms of Alzheimer's disease can make a significant difference in the number of cases and in the costs of management (Haan & Wallace, 2004). In the early phases of Alzheimer's disease, both patients and their families are distressed by its symptoms, but as the patient worsens and loses awareness, the stress of Alzheimer's becomes more severe for the family. The burden of caregiving is one factor in the decision to have a family member institutionalized (Mausbach et al., 2004), which adds to the cost of this disease.

Helping the Family

As with other chronic illnesses, Alzheimer's disease affects not only patients but also family members, who bear the burden of caregiving. Some of the distressing symptoms can make caregiving difficult—caring for a spouse or parent who may be abusive and no longer recognizes you is a very difficult task. Cognitive impairments lead to changes in behavior that may make the affected one no longer seem like the same person.

Caregiving affects families in industrialized and developing countries similarly: Caring for a family member with a dementing disease such as Alzheimer's creates a burden for families (Prince, 2004). This burden is emotional and practical. The problems of taking care of an Alzheimer's patient require time, demand new skills, and greatly disrupt family routine.

In the United States (Cancian & Oliker, 2000) and around the world (Prince, 2004), the caregiver role is occupied mostly by women. By some estimates, nearly 70% of Alzheimer's caregivers are women (Yang & Levey, 2015). Unfortunately, the anger and suspiciousness that are common symptoms of Alzheimer's disease are more distressing to female than to male caregivers (Bédard et al., 2005), so that women tend to feel more burdened by providing care than men do. Their tasks may be burdensome indeed. A survey of Alzheimer's caregivers (Georges et al., 2008) indicated that these tasks may occupy more than 10 hours a day when the recipients of care are late-stage dementia patients.

The chronic stress of caregiving makes these family members of interest to psychoneuroimmunologists, who study how chronic stress affects the immune system. Janice Kiecolt-Glaser and her colleagues (Kiecolt-Glaser, McGuire, Robles, & Glaser, 2002) have studied Alzheimer's caregivers and found that they experience poorer physical and psychological health and poorer immunological function than people of similar age who are not caregivers. Also, the level of impairment of the Alzheimer's patient is directly related to the level of distress in the caregiver (Robinson-Whelen, Tada, MacCallum, McGuire, & Kiecolt-Glaser, 2001); that is, the more impaired the patient, the more distressed the caregiver. Furthermore, their distress does not decrease when their caregiving ends (Aneshensel, Botticello, & Yamamoto-Mitani, 2004). Thus, caregiving imposes severe burdens, extending even after the death of the Alzheimer's patient.

Caregivers now have more assistance available to them. For example, programs now exist to help people develop the skills they will need to be effective caregivers for someone with Alzheimer's disease (Paun, Farran, Perraud, & Loukissa, 2004). Caregivers do not feel so overwhelmed when they have the knowledge and skills to perform the necessary tasks. Reviews of such educational interventions (Beinart, Weinman, Wade, & Brady, 2012; Coon & Evans, 2009) indicate that this approach is successful in reducing stress and depression and improving self-efficacy and well-being. Support groups can also be sources of information about caring for patients and about community resources that provide respite care. Many support groups exist to provide information and emotional support for caregivers. In addition, the Internet can be a source of support. Online and telephone-based services provide support to caregivers who have difficulty obtaining assistance from other sources (Boots, de Vugt, van Knippenberg,

Kempen, & Verhey, 2014; Wilz, Schinkothe, & Soellner, 2011).

Alzheimer's caregivers frequently experience feelings of loss for the relationship that they once shared with the patient; these feelings of loss may begin with a partner's diagnosis (Robinson, Clare, & Evans, 2005). Making sense of dementia and adjusting to the loss is a strain for partner and family. However, only 19% of those caring for someone with Alzheimer's disease reported only strains (Sanders, 2005); most found positive aspects to their caregiving, such as feelings of mastery and personal and spiritual growth. In most ways, Nancy Reagan was more fortunate than the typical caregiver. She was able to hire others to help her provide care for her husband, but she and the Reagan family felt helpless and frustrated as they saw the former president progressively losing abilities (Ellis, 2004). Nancy said that she needed and appreciated the support of the many people who sent letters. Nancy's feelings of isolation and frustration were typical of caregivers for Alzheimer's patients, but Nancy and the Reagan family struggled to find meaning in their experience. One way that they did so was by becoming activists in the effort to find a cure or prevention for Alzheimer's disease.

IN SUMMARY

Alzheimer's disease is a progressive, degenerative disease of the brain that affects cognitive functioning, especially memory. Other symptoms include agitation and irritability, paranoia and other delusions, wandering, depression, and incontinence. These symptoms are also indicative of some psychiatric disorders, making Alzheimer's disease difficult to diagnose and distressing to both patients and caregivers.

Increasing age is a risk factor for Alzheimer's disease, with as many as half the people over 85 exhibiting symptoms. Both genetics and environment seem to play a role in development of the disease; both early- and late-onset varieties exist.

At this point, treatment is largely oriented toward slowing the progress of the disease, managing the negative symptoms, and helping family caregivers cope with the stress. Drug treatments intended to slow the progress of the disease have limited effectiveness but help some people. Management of symptoms can include providing sensory and cognitive stimulation to slow cognitive loss and changing the environment to make care less difficult. Training and support are also desirable for those who provide care to Alzheimer's patients because caregivers are burdened by the demands of caring for someone with this disease.

Adjusting to Diabetes

In 1989, actress Halle Berry had a role in a television sitcom and was working longer, harder hours than she ever had (Siegler, 2003). She had no opportunity to rest when she was tired or to eat a candy bar when she felt that her blood glucose level was low. Berry has **diabetes mellitus,** and her failure to take care of herself caused her to go into a coma that lasted 7 days. Despite that terrifying experience, Berry says that she left the hospital feeling better than she had in years. She sees the experience as a "wake-up call" that forced her to attend to her health. Now she is very careful about her diet, exercise, and stress. She regulated her blood glucose level by taking insulin, but in October 2007, Berry announced that she had cured herself of diabetes through a healthy diet and no longer took insulin (Goldman, 2007). Her remarks caused a furor because Berry had been diagnosed with Type 1 diabetes, for which there is no cure; if she no longer requires insulin injections, then her diabetes was really Type 2 all along. Her diagnosis, behavior, and even her misunderstanding of her disease illustrate some of the challenges presented by diabetes.

The Physiology of Diabetes

Before examining the psychological issues in the management of diabetes, let's look more closely at the physiology of the disorder. The **pancreas**, located below the stomach, produces different types of secretions. The **islet cells** of the pancreas produce several hormones, two of which, glucagon and insulin, are critically important in metabolism. **Glucagon** stimulates the release of glucose and therefore acts to elevate blood sugar levels. The action of **insulin** is the opposite. Insulin decreases the level of glucose in the blood by causing tissue cell membranes to open so glucose can enter the cells more freely. Disorders of the islet cells result in difficulties in sugar metabolism. Diabetes mellitus is a disorder caused by insulin deficiency. If the islet cells do not produce adequate insulin, sugar cannot move from the blood to the cells for use. Lack of insulin prevents the body from regulating blood sugar level. Excessive

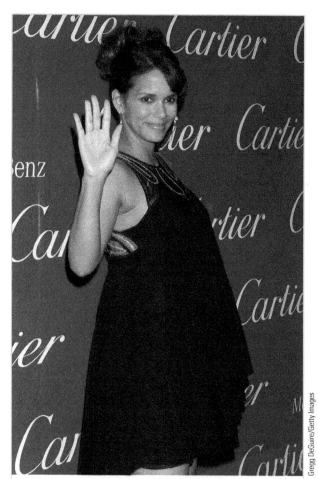

Gregg DeGuire/Getty Images

Actress Halle Berry has followed a diet and exercise regimen to control her diabetes and managed to have a healthy pregnancy.

sugar accumulates in the blood and also appears in abnormally high levels in the urine. When Halle Berry went into a coma in 1989, she thought she was going to die, and she might have. Both coma and death are possibilities for uncontrolled diabetes.

The two types of diabetes mellitus are (1) insulin-dependent diabetes mellitus (IDDM), also known as Type 1 diabetes, and (2) non-insulin-dependent diabetes mellitus (NIDDM), also known as Type 2 diabetes. Type 1 diabetes is an autoimmune disease that occurs when the person's immune system attacks the insulin-making cells in the pancreas, destroying them (Permutt, Wasson, & Cox, 2005). This process usually occurs before age 30 and leaves the person without the capability to produce insulin and thus dependent on insulin injections. Type 1 diabetes was Halle Berry's

TABLE 11.2   Characteristics of Type 1 and Type 2 Diabetes Mellitus

Type 1	Type 2
Onset occurs before age 30	Onset may occur during childhood or adulthood
Patients are often normal weight or underweight	Patients are often overweight
Patients experience frequent thirst and urination	Patients may or may not experience frequent thirst and urination
Caused primarily by genetic factors	Caused by both lifestyle factors (poor diet, low physical activity, obesity) and genetic factors
Has no socioeconomic correlates	Affects more poor than middle-class people
Management involves insulin injections and dietary change	Management involves physical activity and dietary change, medication, and sometimes insulin injections
Carries risk of kidney damage	Carries risk of cardiovascular damage
Accounts for 5% of diabetics	Accounts for 90%–95% of diabetics

diagnosis when she fell into a coma; her age and symptoms were consistent with Type 1 diabetes, but that diagnosis may have been incorrect. People with Type 1 diabetes do not recover from this disease.

Halle Berry received a diagnosis of Type 1 diabetes and followed the demands and restrictions of that regimen for years, including insulin injections, daily exercise with a personal trainer, and a low-fat/low-carbohydrate diet with lots of vegetables, fish, and chicken but few fruits and sweets. When Berry announced that she had "weaned" herself off insulin and considered herself to have Type 2 diabetes (Goldman, 2007), medical experts said that she was mistaken; no one can make a transition from Type 1 to Type 2 diabetes. It is likely that her initial diagnosis was mistaken and that she always had Type 2 diabetes.

Type 2 diabetes is the most common type of diabetes, representing 90% to 95% of all diagnosed cases of diabetes (CDC, 2011a). Until a few years ago, Type 2 diabetes was called *adult-onset diabetes* because it typically developed in people past the age of 30. However, Type 2 diabetes increasingly appears among children and adolescents, accounting for over 20% of new diabetes cases among this age group (CDC, 2014b). This trend appears not only in the United States but also in developed countries throughout the world (Malecka-Tendera & Mazur, 2006). For both children and adults, Type 2 diabetes affects ethnic minorities disproportionately, and those who develop this disease are often overweight, sedentary, and poor (Agardh, Allebeck, Hallqvist, Moradi, & Sidorchuk, 2011; CDC, 2011a).

The characteristics of both types of diabetes are shown in Table 11.2. A third type of diabetes is *gestational diabetes,* which develops in some women during pregnancy. Gestational diabetes ends when the pregnancy is completed, but the disorder complicates pregnancy and presents a risk for the development of Type 2 diabetes in the future (Reader, 2007).

The management of all types of diabetes requires lifestyle changes in order for the person to adjust to the disease and to minimize health complications. Diabetes requires daily monitoring of blood sugar levels and relatively strict compliance with both medical and lifestyle regimens to regulate blood sugar. Like other chronic diseases, diabetes can be controlled but not cured.

In addition to the danger of coma, the inability to regulate blood sugar often causes people with diabetes to have a host of other health problems. Oral or injected insulin can control the most severe symptoms of insulin deficiency but does not mimic the normal production of insulin. People with diabetes still experience elevated levels of blood sugar, which may lead to the development of (1) damage to the blood vessels, leaving diabetics prone to cardiovascular disease (diabetics are twice as likely as other people to have hypertension and to develop heart disease); (2) damage to the retina, leaving diabetics at risk for blindness (diabetics are 17 times as likely to go blind as nondiabetics); and (3) kidney diseases, leaving diabetics prone to renal failure. In addition, diabetics, compared with nondiabetics, have double the risk of cancer of the pancreas (Huxley, Ansary-Moghaddam, de González, Barzi, & Woodward, 2005).

The Impact of Diabetes

The diagnosis of any chronic disease produces an impact on patients for two reasons: First, the emotional reaction to having a lifelong incurable disease, and second, the lifestyle adjustments required by the disease. For diabetes that begins during childhood, both children and their parents must come to terms with the child's loss of health (Lowes, Gregory, & Lyne, 2005) and the management of the disorder, which includes careful restrictions in diet, insulin injections, and recommendations for regular exercise. Dietary restrictions include careful scheduling of meals and snacks as well as adherence to a set of allowed and disallowed foods.

Diabetics must test their blood sugar levels at least once (and possibly several times) a day, drawing a blood sample and using the testing equipment correctly. The results guide diabetics to appropriate levels of insulin. Injections are the standard mode of administration for Type 1 diabetics, and the daily (or more frequent) injections can be a source of fear and stress. Alternative modes of testing and insulin administration are desirable because drawing blood samples and taking injections are painful, and diabetics tend to perform less testing and fewer injections than would be optimal in managing their blood sugar. For this reason, a host of new methods for blood sugar testing are in development, including contact lenses that measure glucose in tears and transmit the data wirelessly, devices that test glucose through saliva, and devices that measure glucose through infrared laser light transmitted through the skin. These methods will not be widespread anytime soon, so diabetics still must cope with uncomfortable methods for testing and insulin administration.

Alternatives to finger-prick testing are available, but their accuracy is not as good as that of standard testing. Other modes of insulin administration exist, including external or implanted insulin pumps. Pumps are appropriate for some individuals, including children and adolescents, providing more stable blood glucose levels (Pickup & Renard, 2008). Although blood glucose testing and insulin administration are critically important, these aspects of diabetes care present difficulties for most diabetics.

Non-insulin-dependent (Type 2) diabetes often does not require insulin injections, but this type of diabetes does require lifestyle changes and oral medication. African Americans, Hispanic Americans, and Native Americans are at higher risk for Type 2 diabetes than are European Americans (CDC, 2011a), and

being overweight is a risk for all groups. Indeed, gaining weight increases and losing weight decreases the risk for Type 2 diabetes (Black et al., 2005). Even bariatric surgery, a medical treatment for extreme obesity, resolves Type 2 diabetes in a majority of diabetics who undergo the procedure (Buchwald et al., 2009). More frequently, the components of treatment for Type 2 diabetes are behavioral methods for weight loss and a healthy diet.

Type 2 diabetics must deal with dietary restrictions and attend to their schedule of oral medication. Diabetes often affects sexual functioning in both men and women, and diabetic women who become pregnant often have problem pregnancies. Halle Berry announced that she was pregnant in 2007 (Bonilla, 2007). Although Halle Berry said that she felt some fear in connection with her pregnancy, she expressed a great deal of optimism and joy. Her fame and wealth allowed her to obtain excellent medical care, and her faithful adherence to her diabetes care helped minimize the potential complications; she gave birth to a healthy baby girl in 2008.

Type 2 diabetes is more likely to cause circulatory problems, leaving these individuals prone to cardiovascular problems, which is their leading cause of death. Both women (Hu et al., 2000) and men (Lotufo et al., 2001) with Type 2 diabetes are at dramatically increased risk for death from all causes, but especially from cardiovascular disease.

Some diabetics deny the seriousness of their condition and ignore the need to restrict diet and take medication. Others acknowledge the seriousness of their problems but believe that the recommended regimen will be ineffective (Skinner, Hampson, & Fife-Schaw, 2002). Others become aggressive; they either direct their aggression outward and refuse to comply with their treatment regimen or turn their aggression inward and become depressed. Finally, many diabetics become dependent and rely on others to take care of them, thus taking no active part in their own care. All these reactions can interfere with the management of blood sugar levels and lead to serious health complications, including death.

Health Psychology's Involvement with Diabetes

Health psychologists seek to both research and treat diabetes (Gonder-Frederick, Cox, & Ritterband, 2002). Psychologist Richard Rubin became head of the American Diabetes Association in 2006, and he emphasized the role of psychology: "I want more and more people to understand that behavior and emotion play a part in diabetes and how that affects human and economic outcomes" (quoted in Dittmann, 2005, p. 35).

Researchers have concentrated on the effect of stress on glucose metabolism, the ways that diabetics understand and conceptualize their illness, the dynamics of families with diabetic children, and the factors that influence patient compliance with medical regimens. Health psychologists orient their efforts toward improving adherence to medical regimens so diabetics can control their blood glucose levels and minimize health complications.

Stress may play two roles in diabetes: as a possible cause of diabetes and as a factor in the regulation of blood sugar in diabetics. To examine the role of family stress in the development of diabetes, a team of researchers (Sepa, Wahlberg, Vaarala, Frodi, & Ludvigsson, 2005) followed a large group of infants for the first year of their lives, measuring family stress and taking blood samples to test for signs of the autoimmune response that underlies Type 1 diabetes. Indeed, stress predicted the development of this response. However, a prospective study with Native Americans (Daniels, Goldberg, Jacobsen, & Welty, 2006) found no relationship between stress during adulthood and subsequent development of Type 2 diabetes.

Clearer evidence exists showing that stress affects glucose metabolism and control among diabetics. A meta-analytic review shows that having a stress-prone personality and experiencing stressful events both predict poorer metabolic control (Chida & Hamer, 2008). A study of people with Type 2 diabetes (Surwit et al., 2002) showed that adding a stress management component to diabetes education has a small but significant effect on blood sugar levels. Depression is another factor that affects diabetics and worsens blood glucose control (Lustman & Clouse, 2005). Thus, negative emotions can adversely affect diabetes, and interventions to manage stress and depression can be a worthwhile (and cost-effective) component for diabetes management programs.

Social support appears to be particularly important for metabolic control, as poor social support is the psychosocial factor most strongly tied to poor diabetes management (Chida & Hamer, 2008). Support from family and friends may promote greater glucose monitoring and physical activity, whereas support from health professionals may increase meal plan adherence (Khan, Stephens, Franks, Rook, & Salem, 2012;

Rosland et al., 2008). Among Latinos with Type 2 diabetes, the availability of support from sources such as family, friends, health care providers, and the community together predicted better illness management and lower depression (Fortmann, Gallo, & Philis-Tsimkias, 2011). However, support need not come from face-to-face contact with another person to be helpful. For example, several recent interventions use text messaging to provide supportive information to help patients' metabolic control. These interventions are generally effective, for both adolescents and adults (Krishna & Boren, 2008; Liang et al., 2011). For example, supportive text-messaging interventions have improved metabolic control among children and adolescents with Type 1 diabetes in Scotland (Franklin, Waller, Pagliari, & Greene, 2006) and Austria (Rami, Popow, Horn, Waldhoer, & Schober, 2006).

Health psychologists also research diabetic patients' understanding of their illness and how that understanding affects their behavior. Both patients and health care workers assume that patients understand the disease and recognize the symptoms of high and low blood glucose levels. These assumptions are not always true. For example, people's perception of the risk of developing diabetes is neither accurate nor based on their existing risk factors, even for physicians (Walker, Mertz, Kalten, & Flynn, 2003). Rather, having a close friend or family member with diabetes was a circumstance that raised the perception of vulnerability (Montgomery, Erblich, DiLorenzo, & Bovbjerg, 2003). Perceptions also affect how people with diabetes care for themselves. Their conceptualizations of diabetes affect their coping behavior (Searle, Norman, Thompson, & Vedhara, 2007). For example, belief in the consequences of diabetes predicted the use of problem-focused coping strategies, and those who believed they were able to control their diabetes were more likely to use their medication.

Inaccurate beliefs can have a significant impact on self-care. In a study of the interrelationships among beliefs, personality characteristics, and self-care behavior among diabetics (Skinner et al., 2002), beliefs emerged as the most important component. The perceived effectiveness of the treatment regimen predicted all aspects of diabetes self-care. This finding emphasizes the importance of diabetes education in building adherence to the diet, exercise, and medication regimen that is necessary to control blood glucose levels.

Complete adherence to the medication and lifestyle regimen is rare (Cramer, 2004). As Chapter 4 explored, a number of factors relate to poor adherence, and diabetes combines several of these factors. First, complexity makes adherence more difficult, and second, making lifestyle changes is more difficult than taking medication. Diabetics must do both. Third, they must also perform blood sugar testing several times a day, even when they feel well. Fourth, their adherence will not cure the disease, and serious complications may be years away. Thus, poor adherence is common, and improving adherence is of primary concern to psychologists involved in providing care for diabetics.

The role of health psychology in diabetes management is likely to expand because behavioral components are important in controlling blood glucose levels. Indeed, lifestyle changes can prevent the development of diabetes in individuals who exhibit blood glucose tolerance problems (Gillies et al., 2007). For example, a lifestyle intervention conducted in China (Li et al., 2008) showed a remarkable reduction in long-term incidence of Type 2 diabetes. Diabetic adults who participated in a 6-year, group-based diet and exercise intervention reported significantly lower incidence of diabetes during the course of the intervention, as well as at a 20-year follow-up. A behavioral component can add to the effectiveness of educational programs for diabetic patients. Education alone is not adequate in helping diabetics follow their regimen (Rutten, 2005; Savage, Farrell, McManus, & Grey, 2010). Because situational factors such as stress and social pressure to eat the wrong foods affect adherence, programs with a behavioral skills training component might be a valuable addition to diabetes management training. A program that fostered feelings of control (Macrodimitris & Endler, 2001) improved diabetics' adherence to diet, exercise, and blood glucose testing, and another program (Rosal et al., 2005) used a cognitive behavioral framework to increase self-management skills in low-income, Spanish-speaking diabetics. In sum, psychosocial interventions show promise in helping diabetics stick to their management regimen (Savage et al., 2010).

IN SUMMARY

Diabetes mellitus is a chronic disease that results from failure of the islet cells of the pancreas to manufacture sufficient insulin, affecting blood glucose levels and producing effects in many organ systems. Type 1 diabetes is an autoimmune disease that typically appears during childhood; Type 2 diabetes also affects children but is more typical of people over age 30. People with diabetes must maintain a strict regimen of diet, exercise, and insulin supplements to avoid the serious cardiovascular, neurological, and renal complications of the disorder.

As with other chronic diseases, a diagnosis of diabetes mellitus produces distress for both patients and their families. Health psychologists study adjustment to the disorder and compliance with the necessary lifestyle changes. Few people with diabetes adhere to all aspects of blood glucose testing, medication, diet, and exercise that minimize the risks of health complications. Skills-training programs show some success in helping diabetics manage their disorder, but health care professionals need to find ways to encourage the development of responsibility and self-management in order to put diabetics in charge of their own health.

The Impact of Asthma

Seeing David Beckham out of breath is not unusual. The international star of soccer, a sport that requires remarkable aerobic fitness, is renowned for his two-decade long career that includes the most World Cup appearances for any player on the English national team.

In 2009, a photographer caught David Beckham out of breath on the sidelines of a soccer field, but this time it *was* unusual. David Beckham was using an asthma inhaler. Until that day, the sports world did not realize that David Beckham suffered from asthma, as he had since he was a small boy. After this photograph surfaced to the public, Beckham revealed that he takes medicine regularly to control his condition. Despite the challenges that any person with asthma faces, David Beckham remains optimistic about his health, saying "I've played 65 games a season for the last 20 years, so it doesn't affect the future" (*Daily Mail*, 2009).

Worldwide, the prevalence of asthma varies considerably across countries, with Australia, Sweden, the United Kingdom, and Netherlands having the greatest prevalence of this condition, at greater than 15% of the populations reporting asthma (To et al., 2012). In the United States, the number of people with asthma increased over the last 15 years (Moorman et al., 2012). About 26 million people in the United States have asthma (7.7%), and nearly 30% of these cases occur in children and adolescents. For all age groups, the rates

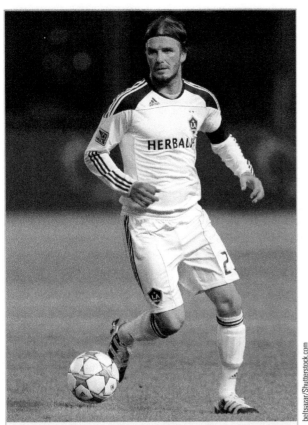

David Beckham coped with asthma throughout his life and soccer career.

are higher for African Americans than for other ethnic groups. The death rate from asthma is not high, and that mortality rate has decreased in recent years, but asthma is the largest cause of disability among children and the leading cause of missed school days, making it a serious health problem in the United States.

The Disease of Asthma

Asthma is a chronic inflammatory disease that causes constriction of the bronchial tubes, preventing air from passing freely. People experiencing an asthma attack will wheeze, cough, and have trouble breathing; such an attack can be fatal. At other times they appear to be fine, but the underlying inflammation remains (Cohn, Elias, & Chupp, 2004).

Asthma shares some features with chronic obstructive lung diseases (COLD) such as chronic bronchitis and emphysema, but asthma also differs in some ways (Barnes, 2008). All of these conditions involve inflammation, though not to the same extent or through the same immune system mechanisms. But the most important difference is that people with COLD experience constant problems, whereas people with asthma may go for long periods of time without any problems in breathing.

The cause of asthma is not understood. Indeed, asthma may not be one disease but rather a number of diseases that share symptoms yet have differences in underlying pathologies (Wenzel, 2006). Until recently, experts believed that asthma was an allergic reaction to substances in the environment, but several newer explanations involve more complex reactions of the immune system (Cohn et al., 2004; Renz, Blümer, Virna, Sel, & Garn, 2006). One view holds that a genetic vulnerability makes some infants' immune systems respond with an allergic reaction to substances in the environment that other infants' immune systems encounter without problems. This *diathesis-stress model* is a variation on the traditional view that asthma is an allergic reaction triggered by environmental allergens. These allergens include an assortment of common substances such as tobacco smoke, household dust (along with dust mites), cockroaches, animal dander, and environmental pollutants. People with the vulnerability who are exposed to the substance to which they are sensitive develop asthma; those who are not exposed fail to develop asthma or show such mild symptoms that they are not diagnosed.

Another view, called the *hygiene hypothesis,* holds that asthma is a result of the cleanliness that has become common in modern societies (von Hertzen & Haahtela, 2004). Infants have undeveloped immune systems, and in hygienic environments they encounter too little dirt and too few bacteria, leaving their immune systems underprepared to deal with these substances. Exposure then leads to overresponsiveness, which produces inflammation; this inflammation forms the basis for asthma. Support for this hypothesis comes from studies of children in rural Central Europe (Ege et al., 2011). Children who grew up on farms had greater exposure to bacteria and fungi than children who did not grow up on farms. Consistent with the hygiene hypothesis, greater exposure to microbes related to decreased risk of asthma. A refinement of the hygiene hypothesis (Martinez, 2001) combines elements of genetic vulnerability and early exposure to substances in the environment that influence immune system development to either sensitize or protect children from asthma and allergic conditions.

As the hygiene hypothesis suggests, asthma is more common in developed countries that emphasize cleanliness and a hygienic environment for infants. For example, asthma is less common in rural China than in the United States, Sweden, Australia, and New Zealand (von Hertzen & Haahtela, 2004). However, within the United States, asthma is more common in the urban inner city, where air pollution is more common, and high levels of air pollution increase the risk of developing asthma (Islam et al., 2007). In addition, asthma varies with ethnicity, and African Americans are more vulnerable than people from other ethnic groups (American Lung Association, 2007).

Other risk factors for asthma include sedentary lifestyle and obesity (Gold & Wright, 2005). People take few deep breaths when they are sedentary, which may be the link between lack of exercise and asthma. In addition, staying indoors exposes people to some of the allergens that provoke asthma attacks. The link between asthma and obesity is significant: Obese people are two to three times more likely to have asthma than non-obese people. Psychological factors also show a relationship with the development of asthma (Chida, Hamer, & Steptoe, 2008), serving as predictors of its development and appearing as a result of living with the disease. Depression is a specific psychological factor that relates to asthma (Strine, Mokdad, Balluz, Berry, & Gonzalez, 2008). Although the factors related to the development of asthma are complex and not completely understood, the triggers for attacks are better known.

Triggers are substances or circumstances that cause the development of symptoms, provoking the narrowing of the airways that causes difficulty in breathing. The substances include allergens such as mold, pollen, dust and dust mites, cockroaches, and animal dander; infections of the respiratory tract; tobacco or wood smoke; and irritants such as air pollutants, chemical sprays, or other environmental pollution (Harder, 2004). The circumstances include exercise and emotional reactions such as stress or fear. Any of these substances and experiences may provoke an attack, but most people with asthma are sensitive to only a few. Identifying an individual's triggers is part of managing asthma.

Managing Asthma

Managing asthma shows some similarities (and similar problems) to managing diabetes. Both disorders require frequent contact with the health care system, can be life threatening, affect children and adolescents, impose

restrictions on lifestyle, and pose substantial adherence problems (Elliott, 2006). People with diabetes may manage their blood sugar levels so that they have no symptoms, but even with careful management, people with asthma have attacks. The underlying inflammation of the bronchial tract is always present, but a person with asthma may go for weeks or months without an attack. Minimizing attacks is the primary goal of managing asthma. Daily attention to symptoms and status improves the chances of avoiding attacks, and behaviors are critical.

Managing asthma requires a variety of medications as well as learning personal triggers and avoiding them (Courtney, McCarter, & Pollart, 2005). To decrease the chances of an attack, people with asthma must take medication, which is usually an anti-inflammatory corticosteroid or some other medication that decreases the respiratory inflammation that underlies asthma. These drugs require daily attention and have unpleasant side effects, such as weight gain and lack of energy. The schedule may be very complicated, and as Chapter 4 detailed, complexity decreases compliance with medical regimens. The side effects also contribute to problems in adherence. Thus, adherence to their preventive medication is a major problem for people with asthma, especially for children and adolescents (Asthma Action America, 2004; Elliott, 2006).

When people with asthma have an attack, they have trouble breathing or cannot breathe. Gasping for breath, they either use a bronchodilator to inhale medication that relieves the symptoms or go to a hospital emergency room for treatment (Asthma Action America, 2004). If used improperly, bronchodilators produce a type of "high," and asthma experts believe that most people with asthma rely on bronchodilators too much and on preventive medication too little. More than 20% of people with asthma use their inhalers improperly, decreasing the effectiveness of this important device (Molimard & Le Gros, 2008). Relying on emergency rooms for managing asthma is an expensive choice and contributes to rising medical costs.

A large-scale survey (Asthma Action America, 2004) revealed widespread misunderstandings and misperceptions concerning asthma among parents and other caregivers. Misunderstandings included what underlies the condition and what constitutes adequate management; misperceptions included the frequency of children's symptoms. People with asthma also hold incorrect beliefs about the disease (Elliott, 2006). For example, they may believe that asthma is not a serious disease or that it is an intermittent disease that does not require daily care. All of these misperceptions may affect appropriate care.

Boosting self-care and increasing adherence to medication regimens are major goals for improving asthma care. A number of interventions have targeted these goals, with some success. Many of these interventions have been oriented toward education for people with asthma, assuming that when people understand the severity of the disease and the steps that are necessary to manage it, they will adhere. Research does not support those assumptions; interventions that are basically educational may increase knowledge but are not very successful in changing behavior (Bussey-Smith & Rossen, 2007; Coffman, Cabana, Halpin, & Yelin, 2008). However, a text-messaging intervention that delivered asthma information that was tailored to young adults' beliefs was effective in improving adherence (Petrie, Perry, Broadbent, & Weinman, 2012). Interventions with a behavioral component, such as developing self-care (Guevara, Wolf, Grum, & Clark, 2003) or providing a written action plan (Bhogal, Zemek, & Ducharme, 2006), tend to be more successful. Adhering to the medication and behavioral regimen to control this disorder is a challenge for people with asthma, but behavioral interventions represent a promising strategy for helping them take their medication and avoid situations that precipitate attacks.

IN SUMMARY

Asthma is a chronic disease that involves inflammation of the bronchial tubes, which leads to difficulties in breathing. Substances such as smoke or allergens and situations such as fear can trigger attacks that have symptoms of coughing, wheezing, and choking. The cause for the inflammation that underlies asthma remains unknown, but theories include a genetic component and an overreaction of the immune system that occurs in hygienic environments.

Asthma usually develops during childhood, and children and adolescents experience problems in coping with their disease. People with asthma need to take medication to decrease the chances of attacks and identify their triggers so as to avoid them. The complex schedule of medications and their unpleasant side effects contribute to adherence problems. A major goal of treatment is to help people with

asthma take medication to prevent attacks rather than rely on inhaled medications to stop symptoms or use hospital emergency room assistance. Behavioral strategies to increase compliance and self-management skills have shown some success.

Dealing with HIV and AIDS

Earvin "Magic" Johnson was the best basketball player in the world when he retired in 1991 (Beacham, 2011). That retirement came as a surprise, but his announcement that he was HIV positive was more so. Johnson learned of his HIV infection through a routine physical examination. Until that announcement, most people considered HIV infection to be a disease of gay European Americans, and Johnson was neither. Johnson's openness about his HIV status helped to change public opinion about this disease, and his celebrity status enabled him to raise money for HIV research and education. More than 25 years after his diagnosis, Johnson remains healthy and is an advocate for increasing minority participation in clinical trials. He attributes his continued health to someone who participated in a clinical trial for the many drugs developed to treat HIV infection (Gambrill, 2008).

AIDS is a disorder in which the immune system loses its effectiveness, leaving the body defenseless against bacterial, viral, fungal, parasitic, cancerous, and other opportunistic diseases. Without the immune system, the body cannot protect itself against the many organisms that can invade it and cause damage. (For a more complete discussion of the immune system and its function, see Chapter 6.) The danger from AIDS comes from the opportunistic infections that start when the immune system no longer functions effectively. In this way, AIDS is similar to the immune deficiency in children who have been born without immune system organs and are susceptible to a variety of infections.

AIDS is the result of exposure to a contagious virus, the **human immunodeficiency virus (HIV)**. So far, researchers have discovered two variants of the human immunodeficiency virus: HIV-1, which causes most AIDS cases in the United States; and HIV-2, which is responsible for most AIDS cases in Africa, although some HIV-2 cases have appeared in the United States. The progression from HIV infection to AIDS varies, and people such as Magic Johnson who are HIV positive may remain free of AIDS symptoms for many years.

Incidence and Mortality Rates for HIV/AIDS

AIDS appears to be a relatively new disease, first recognized in 1981 and identified in 1983. The disease originated in Africa in a virus that affects monkeys (Moore, 2004). Nobody knows how and when the virus came to infect humans. The first confirmed case of AIDS appeared in the Congo in 1959, but the disease was very limited. During the 1960s, the disease spread to Haiti and from there to other places in North America and the world (Gilbert et al., 2007). Both the number of new cases and the number of deaths from AIDS spread during the 1980s.

Since 2005, death rates from AIDS declined sharply worldwide (UNAIDS, 2016). Despite these improvements, AIDS remains among the leading causes of death in the world, and the leading cause of death in Africa. According to one estimate (Lamptey, 2002), AIDS is the deadliest plague in history. In 2015, over 36 million people were living with HIV; when those people die, HIV will surpass the number of people killed by the bubonic plague in the 14th century. About 2.1 million people acquire HIV infection each year, which represents a decline in the rate of infection but also poses a number that extends this plague (UNAIDS, 2016). No effective vaccine yet exists (Callaway, 2011), but drugs now extend the lives of people who are infected (UNAIDS, 2010).

In 1992, the Centers for Disease Control and Prevention (CDC, 1992) revised its definition of HIV infection so that incidence figures from 1992 and subsequent years are not directly comparable to earlier figures. The number of cases in 1992 appears to rise sharply (see Figure 11.1), but this count includes a large backlog of people who in previous years would not have been classified as having AIDS. As Figure 11.1 shows, AIDS cases reported each year (incidence) began a steady decline after 1992.

Despite these declines, HIV and AIDS disproportionately affect minority ethnic groups in the United States, especially by the epidemics affecting heterosexuals and injection drug users. African Americans are the largest segment of the U.S. population with HIV. Although African Americans represent only 14% of the U.S. population, they account for 44% of all new HIV infections (CDC, 2016b). This ethnic disparity is particularly strong among women, with 62% of new diagnoses among women in 2014 occurring in African American women (CDC, 2016b). Hispanic Americans are also disproportionately affected by HIV, with a 2013 new infection rate nearly three times as high as that of European Americans; this disparity is present mainly among men. Figure 11.2 shows the percentages of men and women of different ethnic backgrounds infected with HIV.

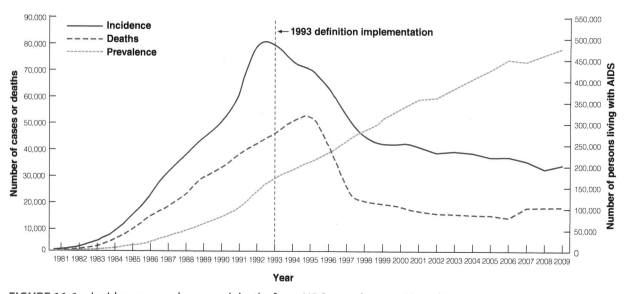

FIGURE 11.1   Incidence, prevalence, and deaths from AIDS cases by year, United States, 1981–2009.

Source: "Update, AIDS—United States, 2000," by R. M. Klevens & J. J. Neal, 2002, *Morbidity and Mortality Weekly Report,* vol. 51, no., 27, p. 593; *HIV/AIDS Surveillance Report, 2002,* by Centers for Disease Control and Prevention, 2004, vol. 14; *HIV/AIDS Surveillance Report, 2006,* by Centers for Disease Control and Prevention, 2008, vol. 18; *HIV/AIDS Surveillance Report, 2010,* by Centers for Disease Control and Prevention, 2012, vol. 22.

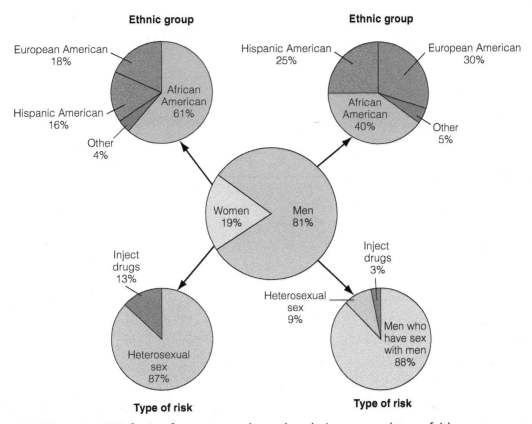

FIGURE 11.2   HIV infection for women and men, by ethnic group and type of risk.

Source: HIV/AIDS Surveillance Report, 2014, by Centers for Disease Control and Prevention, 2015, vol. 26 (Tables 1b and 3a).

Age is also a factor in HIV infection. Young adults are more likely to acquire an HIV infection than other age groups, largely due to their risky behaviors, lack of information about HIV, and lack of power to protect themselves from unsafe sex (Mantell, Stein, & Susser, 2008). For example, in the United States, more than one in five of all new HIV infections are among adolescents and young adults aged 13 to 24 (CDC, 2016b). Recent analyses indicate that this situation is improving, at least in Africa. People over age 50 are less likely to acquire an infection than younger adults, but when infected, they tend to develop AIDS more rapidly and to get more opportunistic infections (CDC, 2008).

Incidence of HIV infection increased rapidly in the United States from 1981 to 1995 and then began to decrease (Torian, Chen, Rhodes, & Hall, 2011). Mortality from AIDS dropped even more. Between 1993 and 1998, AIDS diagnoses decreased by 45%, but AIDS deaths decreased by 63%. One reason for the decline of the number of deaths from AIDS is that HIV-infected individuals now live longer. People diagnosed with AIDS in 1984 had an average survival time of 11 months (Lee, Karon, Selik, Neal, & Fleming, 2001), but more effective treatment lengthened the life expectancy of individuals who are HIV positive. Magic Johnson is an example of this increased life expectancy; Johnson has lived more than 20 years since his diagnosis.

The number of people living with AIDS (prevalence) continues to increase, as Figure 11.1 shows, but combinations of antiretroviral drugs have changed the course of HIV infection, drastically slowing the progression of infection and prolonging lives (UNAIDS, 2010). This increased survival time is a result of more effective drug therapies, early detection, and lifestyle changes. Giving up unhealthy habits such as smoking, drinking alcohol, and taking illicit drugs; becoming more vigilant about their health; and exercising more control over their treatment can help infected persons live longer and healthier lives (Chou, Holzemer, Portillo, & Slaughter, 2004). An optimistic attitude also contributes to longevity (Moskowitz, 2003).

Symptoms of HIV and AIDS

Typically, HIV progresses over a decade or more from infection to AIDS, but the progression varies. During the first phase of HIV infection, symptoms are not easily distinguishable from those of other diseases. Within a week or so of infection, people may (or may not) experience symptoms consisting of fever, sore throat, skin rash, headache, and other symptoms that resemble the flu (Cibulka, 2006). This phase lasts from a few days to 4 weeks, followed typically by a period that may last as long as 10 years, during which infected people are asymptomatic or experience only minimal symptoms. During this time, the immune systems of infected people gradually become destroyed, even though the infected individuals may remain unaware of their HIV status.

People who go untreated usually progress to symptoms, which is the beginning of HIV disease (Cibulka, 2006). Early symptomatic HIV disease occurs when a person's CD4+ T-lymphocyte cell count drops and the person's immune system becomes less able to fight infections. When the CD4+ count falls to 200 or less per cubic millimeter of blood (healthy people have a CD4+ count of 1,000), the person has AIDS. As their immune system loses its defensive capacities, people with early symptomatic HIV disease become susceptible to various opportunistic infections that a healthy immune system would resist. They may experience weight loss, persistent diarrhea, white spots in the mouth, painful skin rash, fever, and persistent fatigue.

As the supply of CD4+ T-lymphocytes depletes, the immune system loses an important mechanism for fighting infections within cells. The diseases associated with HIV are caused by a variety of agents, including viruses, bacteria, fungi, and parasites. The HIV virus damages or kills the part of the immune system that fights *viral* infections, leaving no way for the body to fight HIV. But HIV does not destroy the antibodies that the immune system has already manufactured, so the immune system response that occurs through antibodies circulating in the blood remains intact. Therefore, HIV disease does not often cause a person to develop, for example, infections with the bacterium that causes strep throat or the virus that causes influenza. Most HIV-infected people have antibodies to fight against these common agents.

As their CD4+ count falls to the level defining AIDS, people are subject to lung, gastrointestinal, nervous system, liver, bone, and brain damage from infections from otherwise rare organisms, which leads to diseases such as *Pneumocystis carinii* pneumonia, Kaposi's sarcoma, tuberculosis, and toxoplasmic encephalitis. Symptoms include greater weight loss, general fatigue, fever, shortness of breath, dry cough, purplish bumps on the skin, and AIDS-related dementia.

The Transmission of HIV

Although HIV is an infectious organism with a high fatality rate, the virus is not easily transmitted from person to person. The main routes of infection are from person to person during sex, from direct contact with blood or blood products, and from mother to child during pregnancy, birth, or breastfeeding (UNAIDS, 2007). Concentrations of HIV are especially high in the semen and blood of infected people. Therefore, contact with infected semen or blood is a risk. Other body fluids do not contain such a high concentration of HIV, making contact with saliva, urine, or tears much less of a risk. No evidence exists that any sort of casual contact spreads the infection. Eating with the same utensils or plates or drinking from the same cup as someone who is infected does not transmit HIV, nor does touching or even kissing someone who is infected. Insect bites do not spread the virus, and even being bitten by someone who is infected is not likely to infect the person who is bitten.

People most at risk for HIV infection are those affected by causes of the four epidemics: male–male sexual contact, injection drug use, heterosexual contact, and transmission from mother to baby. Each of the groups reflected by these four epidemics experiences somewhat different risks.

Male–Male Sexual Contact   In the early years of AIDS, men who had sex with men made up the majority of AIDS cases in North America and Western Europe. Male–male sexual contact is still the leading source of HIV infection in the United States. This mode of transmission declined during the 1990s but has increased slightly during the past few years; it now accounts for more than half of HIV transmissions in the United States (Prejean et al., 2011).

Among gay and bisexual men, unprotected anal intercourse is an especially risky behavior, particularly for the receptive partner. Anal intercourse can easily damage the delicate lining of the rectum, so the receptive person is at high risk if his partner is infected with HIV. The damaged rectum makes an excellent route for the virus to enter the body, and infected semen has a high concentration of HIV. Unprotected oral sex with an infected partner is also a risky practice because HIV can enter the body through any tiny cut or other lesion in the mouth.

Condom use became common among gay men, but as treatment became more effective, gay men became less concerned with contracting HIV (Kalichman et al., 2007), and a subculture of gay men are attracted to unprotected anal intercourse, despite their knowledge of its dangers (Shernoff, 2006). Using alcohol or other drugs contributes to the decision to have unprotected sex (Celentano et al., 2006). In addition, the Internet has become a meeting place for men who want to have casual sex with other men, and these encounters are less likely to include condoms than other types of meetings (Garofalo, Herrick, Mustanski, & Donenberg, 2007). Thus, risky sexual behaviors continue to put men who have sex with men in danger of HIV exposure.

Injection Drug Use   Another high-risk behavior is the sharing of unsterilized needles by injection drug users, a practice that allows the direct transmission of blood from one person to another. Injection drug use is the second most frequent source of HIV infection in the United States (CDC, 2008) and accounts for about 32% of HIV cases among women in the United States. However, in other parts of the world—such as Asia, Thailand, Pakistan, and India—injection drug use fuels the HIV epidemic (UNAIDS, 2010). Some injection drug users engage in this behavior in certain situations— for example, when intoxicated or when there is no immediate access to sterile drug equipment. Some evidence (Heimer, 2008) indicates that relatively small-scale needle exchange programs can be effective in controlling HIV infection in a variety of communities.

Transmission through injection drug use accounts for a greater percentage of infected African Americans and Hispanic Americans than European Americans (CDC, 2008). Also, a higher percentage of infected women than men are exposed to the virus through this route. Several behavioral factors relate to HIV infection for women who inject drugs, including the number of sex partners and whether they have traded sex for money or drugs. These behaviors increase the chances for transmission through heterosexual sex.

Heterosexual Contact   Heterosexual contact is the leading source of HIV infection in Africa (UNAIDS, 2007), but in the United States, heterosexual sex accounts for about 30% of cases (CDC, 2008). African Americans and Hispanic Americans are disproportionately represented among those infected through heterosexual contact, and women from these two ethnic backgrounds are in greater danger than men from heterosexual contact.

This gender asymmetry comes from ease of transmission during sexual intercourse. Although men are susceptible to HIV through sexual contact with women, male-to-female transmission is eight times more likely than female-to-male transmission. Despite women's greater likelihood of infection through heterosexual sex, they tend to see their sexual partners as safer than men do (Crowell & Emmers-Sommers, 2001).

Trust and confidence in one's partner in a heterosexual relationship may be unfounded and result in HIV infection. One study (Crowell & Emmers-Sommers, 2001) questioned HIV-positive individuals, and found many that reported a high level of trust in their past sexual partners. Another study (Klein, Elifson, & Sterk, 2003) found that women who perceived themselves to be at some risk behaved in ways that raised their risks, but half of women who felt no risk still engaged in at least some risky behaviors. Thus, people's overly trusting view of partners and failure to accept the possibility of risks lead to unprotected sex. Regular use of condoms may provide a high level of safety for heterosexual men and women, but many young heterosexual couples use condoms more as a means of preventing pregnancy than of preventing HIV (Bird, Harvey, Beckman, & Johnson, 2000).

Transmission During the Birth Process   Another group at risk for HIV infection is children born to HIV-positive women. This transmission tends to occur during the birth process. Breastfeeding can also transmit the virus (Steinbrook, 2004). Children infected with HIV during the birth process suffer from a variety of developmental disabilities, including intellectual and academic impairment, psychomotor dysfunction, and emotional and behavioral difficulties (Mitchell, 2001). In addition, many of these children are born to mothers who ingested drugs during pregnancy and thus are put at further risk for developmental difficulties.

Most individuals who are HIV positive are within their reproductive years, and knowledge of HIV-positive status does not necessarily deter people from reproduction (Delvaux & Nostlinger, 2007). Both HIV-positive women and men may wish to have children, and the family traditions of some Asian cultures push couples toward decisions to reproduce (Ko & Muecke, 2005). With people who are HIV positive, reproduction is a risk for the child. Semen carries HIV that can transmit to the fetus, and transmission during the birth process is likely unless the HIV-positive mother undergoes antiretroviral therapy. Therefore, seeking prenatal counseling and care are critically important for HIV-positive women and men who wish to start a pregnancy. Early prenatal care can reduce the risk of transmission from mother to child to about 1%.

Psychologists' Role in the HIV Epidemic

From the beginning of the AIDS epidemic, psychologists have played an important role in combating the spread of infection (Kelly & Kalichman, 2002). During the early years of the epidemic, psychologists contributed to both primary and secondary prevention efforts. Primary prevention includes changing behavior to decrease HIV transmission. Secondary prevention includes helping people who are HIV positive to live with the infection, counseling people about HIV testing, helping patients deal with social and interpersonal aspects of the disease, and helping patients adhere to their complex treatment program. Much of the improvement in length of survival of HIV-infected patients rests with the effectiveness of drug treatments, highly active antiviral therapy (HAART). This treatment consists of a combination of pills that must be taken on a strict schedule, making adherence a challenge. Psychologists' knowledge concerning adherence to medical regimens is now relevant to managing HIV infection.

Encouraging Protective Measures   Except for infants born to HIV-infected mothers, most people have some control in protecting themselves from the human immunodeficiency virus. Fortunately, HIV is not easily transmitted from person to person, making casual contact with infected persons a low risk. Health care workers who participate in surgery, emergency care, or other procedures that bring them into contact with blood should be careful to prevent infected blood from entering their body through an open wound. For example, dentists and dental hygienists wear protective gloves, and health care workers should adhere to a set of standard protective measures.

Although some risks are specific to certain professions, most people infected with HIV acquired the virus through sexual behavior or by sharing contaminated needles. People can protect themselves against HIV infection by changing those behaviors that are high risks for acquiring the infection—namely, having unprotected sexual contact or sharing needles with an infected person. Limiting the number of sex partners, using condoms, and avoiding shared needles are three behaviors that will protect the largest number of people from HIV infection. However, for people who engage in

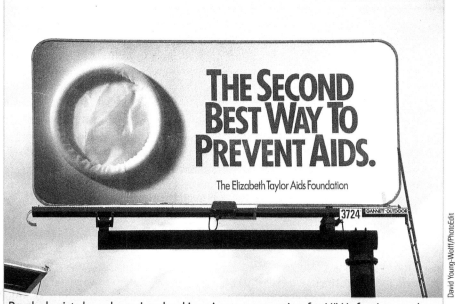

Psychologists have been involved in primary prevention for HIV infection, such as promoting condom use.

these risky behaviors, they are very difficult to change. A variety of factors contribute to this difficulty.

One factor that makes behavior change difficult is perception of risk. Most people in the United States do not perceive that they are at risk for HIV infection, and they are correct (Holtzman, Bland, Lansky, & Mack, 2001). That is, most adults do not engage in the behaviors that are primary HIV risks. However, some people are at risk and fail to perceive that risk accurately. For example, young men who have sex with men reported overly optimistic beliefs about their risk (MacKellar et al., 2007), as did college students in Nigeria (Ijadunola, Abiona, Odu, & Ijadunola, 2007). Their misperceptions play a role in their continued risky behavior, and culture is an important influence in sexual risk behaviors.

Cultures in which male dominance is supported by social custom or religion and in which women have little access to economic resources also have high rates of heterosexually transmitted HIV, such as countries in sub-Saharan Africa, the Caribbean, and Latin America (UNAIDS, 2007). When women are financially dependent on men and have limited access to economic resources, they may have little control over sexual encounters or even be vulnerable to forced or coerced sex. Thus, they may be unable to negotiate condom use, which increases their risk for infection. These dangers also apply to women in the United States. A study of HIV-positive African American women (Lichtenstein, 2005) confirmed the presence of abuse and dominance as factors in these women's HIV infection, and a large study of young adults found that alcohol use and violence contribute to HIV transmission (Collins, Orlando, & Klein, 2005).

Helping People with HIV Infection   People who believe they may be infected with HIV, as well as those who know that they are, can benefit from various psychological interventions. People who engage in high-risk behaviors may have difficulty deciding whether to be tested for HIV, and psychologists can provide both information and support for these people. Individuals from several high-risk groups have not been tested for HIV, including (1) a significant minority of gay and bisexual men, (2) a significant minority of injection drug users, and (3) a larger proportion of heterosexual men and women with multiple partners and inconsistent use of condoms (Awad, Sagrestano, Kittleson, & Sarvela, 2004). Indeed, many people who are HIV positive have not been tested and thus do not know their HIV status.

The decision to get an HIV test has both benefits and costs to the individual, but testing is considered essential to the control of HIV infection (Janssen et al., 2003). Far too many people undergo testing after their disease progresses and treatment options are less effective; a prominent part of Magic Johnson's campaign targets early testing and services for people whose tests indicate infection. Early testing for those who are HIV positive allows early treatment, which will prolong their lives and will permit them to find ways to reduce or eliminate behaviors that place others at risk.

The costs of being tested include all the problems of arranging a health care visit, plus the distress that comes with the potential for bad news. Currently, HIV testing is not part of routine health examinations, and individuals must seek testing (Clark, 2006). At least 25% of those with HIV infection are unaware of their status because they have not sought testing. In addition, many people who agree to testing never take steps to learn the results. Alternatives to the standard testing procedure, such as rapid results testing and at-home testing, increase the likelihood of learning one's HIV status (Hutchinson, Branson, Kim, & Farnham, 2006).

Learning of HIV-positive status is a traumatic event that can lead to anxiety, depression, anger, and distress. The ongoing experience of coping with HIV likewise can lead to these emotional responses, which have clear implications for disease progression. A review of over 30 prospective studies of people living with HIV concluded that emotional distress predicts a variety of indicators of HIV disease progression, including lower levels of CD4+ cells, AIDS symptoms and diagnosis, and even mortality due to AIDS (Chida & Vedhara, 2009). People's coping styles also relate to adjustment and disease progression. For example, people who take direct action to cope, maintain a positive outlook, and express emotions tend to have better physical health (Moskowitz, Hult, Bussolari, & Acree, 2009). In contrast, people who deny their illness and use disengagement coping methods such as alcohol or drug use have faster disease progression and worse physical health (Chida & Vedhara, 2009; Moskowitz et al., 2009). Some of these coping strategies may matter more in certain contexts. For example, taking direct action to cope appears to benefit physical health when it occurs soon after HIV diagnosis (Moskowitz et al., 2009). Receiving support from both health care professionals and family and friends also leads to better psychological adjustment (Moskowitz et al., 2009; Reilly & Woo, 2004).

Interventions tailored to the person's specific situation and needs have advantages over less personalized programs (Moskowitz & Wrubel, 2005). Cognitive behavioral and stress management interventions are generally effective in reducing the anxiety, depression, and distress of those who are HIV positive and improve their quality of life (Crepaz et al., 2008; Scott-Sheldon, Kalichman, Carey, & Fielder, 2008). Some cognitive behavioral stress management interventions also report beneficial effects on physiological health outcomes (Antoni et al., 1991, 2000); however, most interventions do not (Scott-Sheldon et al., 2008).

Psychologists can also help HIV patients adhere to the complex medical regimens designed to control HIV infection (Simoni, Pearson, Pantalone, Marks, & Crepaz, 2006), particularly those patients who have the greatest difficulty with adherence (Amico, Harman, & Johnson, 2006). HAART consists of a combination of antiretroviral medications; patients often take other drugs to combat side effects of the antiretroviral drugs as well as drugs to fight opportunistic infections. These regimens may include as many as a dozen drugs, all of which require precise timing. When patients do not follow the schedule, the effectiveness diminishes. Psychologists can help patients adhere to this schedule as well as facilitate their self-management skills. For example, the technique of motivational interviewing appeared to be successful in helping with the scheduling aspect of HAART adherence (DiIorio et al., 2008).

Another aspect of adjustment to HIV infection is finding meaning in the experience and developing the potential for growth and positive experiences. People with AIDS and their caregivers often succeed in finding positive experiences in their lives. In two studies (Milam, 2004; Updegraff, Taylor, Kemeny, & Wyatt, 2000), over half of individuals with HIV or AIDS had experienced positive changes, and in another study (Folkman & Moskowitz, 2000), more than 99% of AIDS patients and caregivers were able to recall a positive experience. The search for positive meaning may even influence the course of HIV infection by affecting CD4+ count (Ickovics et al., 2006). This quest for positive meaning is common to the experience of many people with chronic illness (Updegraff & Taylor, 2000), and this attitude may also appear in those who are dying.

 # Becoming Healthier

1. If you have a chronic illness, understand your condition and form a cooperative relationship with health care professionals. However, take charge of its management yourself; you are the person most affected by your condition.

2. If you are the primary caregiver for someone who is chronically ill, don't ignore your own health—both physical and psychological. Regularly schedule some time for yourself.

3. If you have Type 1 diabetes, don't try to hide your illness from your friends. Although you have a chronic disease, you can live a long and productive life, but you must adhere faithfully to a lifelong regimen that includes diet, insulin injection, and regular exercise. If you live with someone with diabetes, offer social and emotional support and encourage that person to stick with required health practices.

4. Know your blood sugar level. Type 2 diabetes can develop at any age, and this disorder may have few symptoms.

5. If you have asthma, try to minimize attacks and use of dilators. Concentrate on taking preventive medication and knowing your triggers to avoid attacks.

6. Protect yourself against HIV infection. The most common mode of transmission is sexual, and condoms make sex safer.

7. If you are the primary caregiver for someone with a terminal chronic disease such as AIDS or Alzheimer's disease, seek social and emotional support through groups specifically convened to offer such support. Take breaks from caregiving, allowing others to assume those responsibilities for a while.

8. If you have a chronic disease or if you are the caregiver for someone with such a disease, use the Internet to gain information and support. A wide variety of websites offer information, and online support groups are available for all disorders. Do not use these websites as a substitute for health care but allow these resources to supplement your knowledge and support.

IN SUMMARY

Acquired immune deficiency syndrome is the result of depletion of the immune system after infection with the human immunodeficiency virus. When the immune system fails to defend the body, a number of diseases may develop, including bacterial, viral, fungal, and parasitic infections that are uncommon in people who have functioning immune systems.

The modes of transmission of HIV are behavioral, with receptive anal intercourse and the sharing of needles for intravenous drug injection the two behaviors that have spread the infection to the most people in the United States. Unprotected heterosexual contact with an infected partner accounts for a larger proportion of people with HIV worldwide. The number of babies infected with HIV has decreased because antiretroviral drug therapies sharply decrease transmission from an infected mother during the birth process.

Psychologists use a variety of interventions to help patients reduce high-risk behaviors, cope with their illness, manage their symptoms, and adhere to the complex drug regimens that improve survival. In addition, psychologists have provided counseling services for those seeking to be tested and for those whose tests reveal infection. These programs not only encourage protective behaviors but also emphasize the role of positive health in combating AIDS.

Facing Death

Over the last century, life expectancy has increased. People do not necessarily expect a long life, but they prefer it, saying that a life of about 85 years is about right (Lang, Baltes, & Wagner, 2007). However, people also want to have control over the end of their lives, including when and how they die. This desire is consistent with the concept of "the good death," which consists of physical comfort, social support, appropriate medical care, and attempts to minimize psychological distress for the dying person and the family (Carr, 2003). What do we know about the issues that people deal with when they are dying and how people adjust to losing a loved one?

Adjusting to Terminal Illness

The experience of a "good death" is possible for many. Most of the leading causes of death in the United States and other industrialized countries are chronic diseases such as cardiovascular disease, cancer, chronic lower respiratory disease, Alzheimer's disease, kidney disease, chronic liver disease, and HIV infection. These diseases are often fatal, but death is not sudden, giving people and their families an opportunity to adjust. Even if the chronic disease does not signal terminal illness, the diagnosis entails loss and thus the need to adapt (Murray, 2001).

A common perception is that people go through several predictable stages of adaptation to a terminal illness. This perception was popularized by Elizabeth Kübler-Ross (1969). Kübler-Ross' stages included denial, anger, bargaining, depression, and acceptance. Denial is a failure to accept the validity or the severity of the diagnosis; people use this defense mechanism to deal with the anxiety they experience when they learn of their condition (Livneh & Antonak, 2005). Anger is another emotional reaction, and bargaining often takes the form of trying to negotiate a better outcome, either with God or with health care personnel. Depression is a common response of those who come to understand the progression of their disease, followed by acceptance of the situation.

Was Kübler-Ross correct? While it is true that people react to a terminal diagnosis with reactions such as denial, anger, bargaining, depression, and acceptance, there is no evidence that people respond in a set pattern (Schulz & Aderman, 1974). Nor is there any evidence that people *should* experience these reactions in a set pattern. Instead, people diagnosed with chronic diseases and people with terminal illness usually exhibit a range of negative reactions, but they may also experience positive responses oriented around growth and finding meaning in their situation.

A more useful conceptualization of adaptation to terminal illness is the notion of the dying role (Emanuel, Bennett, & Richardson, 2007). This role is an extension of the sick role, which we described in Chapter 3. Like the sick role, the dying role includes certain privileges and responsibilities and can take many forms, both healthy and unhealthy. Three key elements are involved: practical, relational, and personal. The practical element includes the tasks that people need to arrange at the end of their lives, such as arranging financial matters and making plans for medical care as the disease progresses. The relational element involves reconciling the dying role with other roles, such as caregiver, spouse, and parent. This reconciliation may be difficult: The dying role is not automatically compatible with these other roles, so the dying person must work to find ways to integrate these roles. The personal element involves "finishing one's life story" (Emanuel et al., 2007, p. 159). This element may prompt people to reexamine their life while thinking about its end and to derive new meaning from it. This new meaning may constitute a reintegration (Knight & Emanuel, 2007), or some less healthy outcome may occur.

Barriers to a good adjustment include institutional impediments and lack of access to palliative care. Institutional barriers occur when people cannot assume the dying role because health care professionals keep them in the sick role, even though it is inappropriate (Emanuel et al., 2007). Medical care is so oriented toward cures that accepting death may be difficult for medical practitioners. Appropriate care, such as hospice care or support for home care, may be unavailable, forcing people to stay in a hospital that may not serve their needs. Concentrating on the physical aspects of dying does not allow people to work toward the social and personal tasks from which they may derive a feeling of completion and reintegration.

Entry into the dying role typically meets with loss and grief (Emanuel et al., 2007). The person faces the loss of physical abilities, social relationships, and the experiences of continued life. People imagine that those in this situation are frightened of dying, but research involving people with terminal illnesses indicates otherwise (McKechnie, Macleod, & Keeling, 2007). Instead, the concerns of the dying revolve around anxiety— over their condition, whether they would be able to complete planned activities, and provisions for managing their comfort during the last stages of their disease. Because their disease imposes physical limitations on their activities, they feel unable to "live until they died" (McKechnie et al., 2007, p. 367).

In recent years, a brief psychotherapy called *dignity therapy* has been evaluated as a way to help terminal patients deal with the psychological issues of facing death. Dignity therapy provides patients with a chance to reflect on aspects of their lives that matter most, as well as to record what they would most like to be remembered for. As such, dignity therapy seeks to address the personal elements of the dying role. Randomized trials of dignity therapy in Western populations show that while it may not substantially reduce clinical indices of depression among terminal patients, it does improve self-reported end-of-life experiences, such as quality of life, dignity, spiritual well-being, and perceived appreciation from family (Chochinov et al., 2011). However, an attempt to provide dignity therapy to a sample of

Japanese terminal cancer patients encountered a number of difficulties, including a reluctance among Japanese patients to want to discuss issues of dying and death (Akechi et al., 2012). These findings highlight that fact that issues surrounding death are culturally influenced, and some of the personal elements of the dying role may be tied to Western cultural values rather than universal. For example, Western individuals tend to respond to thoughts of death by turning attention toward the self and acting in ways that preserve self-esteem, whereas Eastern individuals tend to respond to thoughts of death by turning attention toward others (Ma-Kellams & Blascovich, 2011). Thus, sensitivity to cultural differences surrounding issues of death is a challenge for those interacting with terminal patients. Regardless of culture, death influences not only the patient but also the family as well, as family members face the process of grieving the loss of a loved one.

Grieving

Loss and grief are also common to bereavement, making the reactions and processes of adaptation applicable to family and friends after the death of a loved one (Murray, 2001). Thus, a diagnosis of chronic illness, awareness of a terminal condition, and loss of a loved one provoke similar reactions, with similar possibilities for outcomes. That is, bereavement may result in care-givers' experiencing worsened symptoms or improvements (Aneshensel et al., 2004) and, eventually, growth (Hogan & Schmidt, 2002).

The similarities between those who are dying and those who are bereaved have led to similar theories of adaptation, including a stage theory of bereavement with stages of disbelief, yearning, anger, depression, and then acceptance. As with Kübler-Ross' stage theory of adaptation to dying, there is little evidence to support a stage theory of bereavement (Maciejewski, Zhang, Block, & Prigerson, 2007). People exhibit some, none, or all of these reactions. A potentially better way to describe people's reactions to bereavement is to acknowledge that some people react differently to bereavement than others. One study of over 400 German adults' reactions to bereavement (Mancini, Bonanno, & Clark, 2011) identified four different profiles of responses. Most adults exhibited a response called *resiliency,* characterized by stable levels of well-being from before a loss to 4 years after a loss of a loved one. Only 21% of the adults showed a response called *acute-recovery,* characterized by a drop in well-being at the time of loss, followed by a gradual return to normal. About 15% of adults showed *chronic low levels* of well-being that were relatively unaffected by bereavement. Surprisingly, about 5% of adults showed *improvement,* with levels of well-being that increased in the years following the death of a loved one. (Incidentally, those who showed improvement were more likely to have gained income as a result of their loss.) Clearly, people's responses to bereavement are varied and do not fit neatly into a stage model.

Bereavement typically includes negative emotions, and people have difficulty accepting such emotions as normal. Even among health care professionals, the grieving process may seem abnormal when people exhibit strong negative reactions or their feelings persist for a time considered too lengthy. Thoughts of lost loved ones and longings for their company can persist for many years (Camelley, Wortman, Bolger, & Burke, 2006). Experts suggest that it is these people who may benefit the most from psychological intervention (Mancini, Griffin, & Bonanno, 2012). In contrast, psychological intervention may have little to no benefit among people who do not show persistent and elevated levels of distress.

Even the terminology used by mental health professionals carries negative connotations. People who are adapting to the loss of a loved one are referred to as *recovering,* which implies that these individuals will go back to "normal" and that their grief reactions signal psychological problems. This tendency to "pathologize" the bereavement process should be avoided (Tedeschi & Calhoun, 2008). Some grief responses may present problems for adaptation, but like the process of adapting to chronic and terminal illness, grieving offers the promise of transformative and spiritual growth (Tedeschi & Calhoun, 2006). Thus, all three processes share essential elements.

IN SUMMARY

Facing death requires adjustment for the person who is dying and for the family. Although the process of stages of acceptance has gained popular appeal, no research supports this view. Instead, people who are dying experience a variety of negative reactions that may be better conceptualized as a role with practical, relationship, and personal elements. Some people are able to work through challenges and have access to the facilities to experience a "good death," allowing them to die without pain but with social support, appropriate medical care, and minimal psychological distress. Their adaptation may leave them with a sense of completion and even transcendence. Growth is also a possibility for those who grieve for loved ones, but the bereaved also face a process of adjustment that includes negative emotions. A wide variety of emotional responses follow bereavement, but no research suggests that people pass through predictable stages of grief. The negative emotions that are involved in grieving should not be seen as abnormal; resolving grief may take years, but this process also offers the promise of positive change.

Answers

This chapter has addressed six basic questions:

1. **What is the impact of chronic disease on patients and families?**
   Long-term chronic illnesses bring about a transition in people's lives, requiring adaptations to live with symptoms and receive medical care, changing relationships, and pushing people toward a reevaluation of themselves. Support groups and programs designed by health psychologists help people cope with the emotional problems associated with chronic illness, problems that traditional medical care often overlooks. Chronic diseases may be terminal, which forces people to consider their impending death.

2. **What is the impact of Alzheimer's disease?**
   Alzheimer's disease damages the brain and produces memory loss, language problems, agitation and irritability, sleep disorders, suspiciousness, wandering, incontinence, and loss of ability to perform routine care. The most common form of Alzheimer's disease occurs through a genetic vulnerability combined with environmental risks. Age is the main risk, with the prevalence doubling for every decade after age 65. Lifestyle factors relate to

the development of Alzheimer's disease, making prevention a possibility. Medical treatments are being developed, but the main management strategies consist of interventions to allow patients longer periods of functioning, and counseling and support groups for family members, who frequently experience more stress than the patient.

3. What is involved in adjusting to diabetes?

Diabetes, both insulin-dependent (Type 1) and non-insulin-dependent (Type 2), requires changes in lifestyle that include monitoring and adherence to a treatment regimen. Treatments include insulin injections for Type 1 diabetics and adherence to careful dietary restrictions, scheduling of meals, avoidance of certain foods, regular medical visits, and routine exercise for all diabetics. Health psychologists are involved in helping diabetics learn self-care to control the dangerous effects of their condition.

4. How does asthma affect the lives of people with this disease?

Inflammation of the bronchial tubes is the underlying basis for asthma. Combined with this inflammation, triggering stimuli or events cause bronchial constriction that produces difficulty in breathing. Asthma may be fatal, and it is the leading cause of disability among children. The origin of this process is not understood, but medication can control the inflammation and decrease the risk of attacks. People with asthma are faced with a complex medication regimen that they must follow to decrease the risk of attacks.

5. How can HIV infection be managed?

Infection with the human immunodeficiency virus depletes the immune system, leaving the body vulnerable to acquired immune deficiency syndrome and a variety of opportunistic infections. HIV epidemics affect four different populations in the United States: (1) men who have sex with men, (2) injection drug users, (3) heterosexuals, and (4) children born to HIV-positive mothers. Psychologists are involved in the HIV epidemic by encouraging protective behaviors, counseling infected people to help them cope with living with a chronic disease, and helping patients adhere to complex medical regimens that have changed HIV infection to a manageable chronic disease.

6. What adaptations do people make to dying and grieving?

People tend to react to the knowledge that they have a terminal illness with a variety of negative emotions, and the process of grieving also includes negative emotions. Contrary to popular conceptualizations, however, these reactions do not progress through a pattern of stages. Instead, dying may be conceptualized as a role that includes practical, relational, and personal elements that people encounter in their process of adaptation. Grieving can also be conceptualized as a process with negative emotions but also with the possibility of growth.

Suggested Readings

Asthma Action America. (2004). *Children and asthma in America.* Retrieved August 29, 2008, from http://www.asthmainamerica.com/frequency.html. This comprehensive survey details the impact of asthma on the lives of children and their caregivers, examining the misperceptions about the disease, the available treatments, and recommendations for more effective strategies to deal with this disease.

DeBaggio, T. (2002). *Losing my mind: An intimate look at life with Alzheimer's.* New York, NY: Free Press. When former newspaper writer Thomas DeBaggio began to recognize symptoms of Alzheimer's disease at age 57, he decided to write about his experience of "losing his mind." The result is a moving account of Alzheimer's disease from an insider's point of view.

Stanton, A. L., & Revenson, T. A. (2011). Adjustment to chronic disease: Progress and promise in research. In H. Friedman (Ed.), *The Oxford handbook of health psychology* (pp. 241–268). This chapter examines the growing body of longitudinal research on adjustment to chronic illness, exploring the important risk and protective factors that affect the process.

UNAIDS. (2010). *UNAIDS report on the global AIDS epidemic, 2010.* Geneva, Switzerland: Joint United Nations Programme on HIV/AIDS. This comprehensive report details the status of HIV infection worldwide and in each geographic area, analyzing the nature of the epidemic in each region and the progress that has been made in controlling the disease.

CHAPTER 12

Smoking Tobacco

CHAPTER OUTLINE

- Real-World Profile of President Barack Obama
- *Smoking and the Respiratory System*
- *A Brief History of Tobacco Use*
- *Choosing to Smoke*
- *Health Consequences of Tobacco Use*
- *Interventions for Reducing Smoking Rates*
- *Effects of Quitting*

QUESTIONS

This chapter focuses on five basic questions:

1. How does smoking affect the respiratory system?

2. Who chooses to smoke and why?

3. What are the health consequences of tobacco use?

4. How can smoking rates be reduced?

5. What are the effects of quitting?

☑ Check Your **HEALTH RISKS**   *Regarding Tobacco Use*

Check the items that apply to you.

☐ 1. I have not smoked more than 100 cigarettes in my life.

☐ 2. I have probably smoked between 100 and 200 cigarettes in my life, but I have not smoked at all in more than 5 years and have no desire to do so.

☐ 3. I currently smoke more than 10 cigarettes a day.

☐ 4. I currently smoke more than two packs of cigarettes a day.

☐ 5. I am a smoker who believes that the health risks of smoking have been exaggerated.

☐ 6. I am a smoker who believes that smoking is probably harmful, but I plan to stop smoking before those effects can harm me.

☐ 7. I don't smoke cigarettes, but I do smoke at least one cigar or one pipe of tobacco a day.

☐ 8. I don't smoke cigarettes, but I do use e-cigarettes.

☐ 9. I smoke cigars or a pipe because I believe that they carry a very low risk for any health problems.

☐ 10. I live with someone who smokes inside the dwelling.

☐ 11. I use smokeless tobacco (chewing tobacco) on a daily basis.

Except for the first two statements, each of these items represents a health risk from tobacco products, which account for about 480,000 deaths a year in the United States, mostly from cancer, heart disease, and chronic lower respiratory disease. Count your checkmarks for the last nine items to evaluate your risks. As you read this chapter, you will see that some of these items are riskier than others.

Real-World Profile of **PRESIDENT BARACK OBAMA**

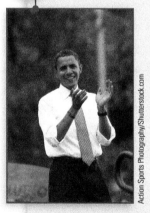

Action Sports Photography/Shutterstock.com

U.S. President Barack Obama quit smoking after years of struggling to break the habit ("Michelle Obama," 2011). Obama began smoking when he was a teenager and escalated into a heavy smoker. When he decided to run for the office of U.S. President, he promised his wife Michelle that he would quit, but he relapsed into smoking during his campaign. During a press conference President Obama held after he had signed an antismoking law, Obama admitted that he had lapsed and had begun occasional smoking ("Obama Admits," 2008). He said that he struggled to refrain from smoking but occasionally "messed up."

Obama's occasional smoking continued during the first 2 years of his presidency, but in February, 2011, First Lady Michelle Obama announced that the President had not smoked a cigarette for almost a year ("Michelle Obama," 2011). President Obama felt the pressure to quit from a number of sources, including the continued urging from his health-conscious wife, the knowledge that his smoking provided a poor role model to his children (and to other young people), and the urgings of his physician to quit for the sake of his health.

Obama's struggle to become a nonsmoker was typical of the more than a million former smokers in the United States. He began smoking as a teenager, escalated his smoking as a young adult, wanted to quit, made repeated attempts to do so, and finally succeeded.

Smoking is the most preventable cause of death in the world. In the United States, 480,000 people die every year from tobacco use (USDHHS, 2014). It's quite easy to read through the number 480,000, but let's see if we can personalize it. *Each year in the United States*, smoking kills enough people to wipe out more than half the population of Delaware. More people die every year from smoking than live within the city limits of Long Beach, California. Stated differently, an average of 1,315 people die *every day* in the United States from tobacco-related causes. Throughout the world, the deaths total is almost 6 million people per year (World Health Organization, 2011), which is equivalent to the population of Denmark. Later, we summarize the various risks from cigarette, e-cigarette, cigar, and pipe smoking, as well as from other tobacco products, including the dangers of passive smoking and smokeless tobacco. This chapter also includes information on the prevalence of smoking, the reasons why people smoke, and some methods of preventing and reducing smoking. First, however, we briefly review the effects of smoking on the respiratory system, the body system most immediately affected by smoking.

Smoking and the Respiratory System

Respiration takes oxygen into the body and expels carbon dioxide. This process draws air deep into the lungs, which routinely introduces a variety of particles into the lungs. Thus, smoking provides a pathway for lung damage and disease.

Functioning of the Respiratory System

The exchange of oxygen and carbon dioxide occurs deep in the lungs. To get air into the lungs, the diaphragm and the muscles between the ribs (intercostal muscles) contract, increasing the volume within the chest. As the space inside the chest increases, the pressure within the chest falls below atmospheric pressure, forcing air into the lungs.

Figure 12.1 illustrates where air goes on its way to the lungs. The nasal passages, pharynx, larynx, trachea, bronchi, and bronchioles conduct air into the lungs. These passages have little ability to absorb oxygen, but in the process of inhalation, the air is warmed, humidified, and cleansed. Millions of alveoli, located at the ends of the bronchioles, are the site of oxygen and carbon dioxide exchange. Air rich in oxygen is drawn into the lungs and reaches the alveoli, where an exchange of carbon dioxide and oxygen occurs in the capillaries that surround each alveolus. The blood, now oxygen rich, travels back to the heart and is pumped out to all areas of the body.

Air is an excellent medium for the introduction of foreign matter into the body. Airborne particles potentially move into the lungs with every breath. Protective mechanisms in the respiratory system, such as sneezing and coughing, expel some dangerous particles. Noxious stimulation in the nasal passages may activate the sneeze reflex, whereas stimulation in the lower respiratory system promotes the cough reflex.

Several respiratory disorders are of interest to health psychologists. All kinds of smoke as well as other types of air pollution increase mucus secretion in the respiratory system but decrease the activity of the respiratory system's protective mechanisms, thus making the system vulnerable to problems. As mucus builds up, people cough to get rid of it, but coughing may also irritate the bronchial walls. Irritation and infection of the bronchial walls may damage the respiratory system and destroy tissue in the bronchi. The formation of scar tissue in the bronchi, irritation or infection of bronchial tissue, and coughing are characteristics of **bronchitis**, one of several *chronic lower respiratory diseases* (also called chronic obstructive pulmonary disease or COPD) that are the third leading cause of death in the United States (Heron, 2016).

Acute bronchitis is caused by infection and usually responds quickly to antibiotics. When the irritation persists and the mechanism underlying the illness continues, it can become a chronic problem. Cigarette smoke is the major cause of chronic bronchitis, but environmental air pollution and occupational hazards may also underlie chronic bronchitis.

The most common of the chronic lower respiratory diseases is **emphysema**, which occurs when scar tissue and mucus obstruct the respiratory passages, bronchi lose their elasticity and collapse, and air is trapped in the alveoli. The trapped air breaks down the alveolar walls, and the remaining alveoli become enlarged. Both damaged and enlarged alveoli have reduced surface area for the exchange of oxygen and carbon dioxide. Damage also obstructs blood flow to the undamaged alveoli, and so the respiratory system

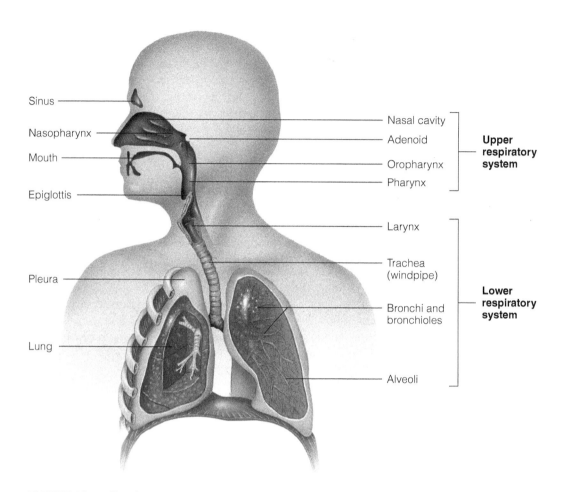

FIGURE 12.1   Respiratory system.

Source: Introduction to microbiology (p. 525), by J. L. Ingraham & C. A. Ingraham. From INGRAHAM/INGRAHAM, *Introduction to Microbiology*, 1E.

becomes restricted. The loss of efficiency in the respiratory system means that respiration delivers a limited amount of oxygen. People with emphysema experience problems with breathing and usually cannot exercise strenuously.

Chronic bronchitis, emphysema, and lung cancer are all diseases of the respiratory system associated with the inhalation of irritating, damaging particles such as smoke. Figure 12.2 shows how smoke can damage the lungs, producing bronchitis and emphysema. Cigarette smoking is of particular interest to health psychologists because it is a voluntary behavior that can be avoided, whereas air pollution and occupational hazards are social problems not under direct personal control. Thus, smoking is the target for much negative publicity

and for interventions for change. But what specifically makes inhaled smoke dangerous?

What Components in Smoke Are Dangerous?

The processed tobacco in cigarettes contains at least 4,000 compounds; at least 60 of these are known carcinogens—substances that are capable of causing cancer. All of these compounds are potentially involved in the development of disease, but cigarette smoke is a complex mixture. Analyzing the process through which cigarette smokes causes lung damage is difficult and not yet fully understood. However, nicotine is the pharmacological agent that underlies addiction to cigarette

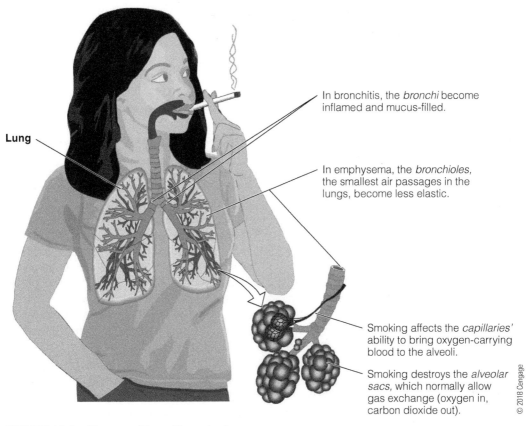

Lung

In bronchitis, the *bronchi* become inflamed and mucus-filled.

In emphysema, the *bronchioles,* the smallest air passages in the lungs, become less elastic.

Smoking affects the *capillaries'* ability to bring oxygen-carrying blood to the alveoli.

Smoking destroys the *alveolar sacs,* which normally allow gas exchange (oxygen in, carbon dioxide out).

© 2018 Cengage

FIGURE 12.2   How smoking affects the lungs.

Source: *An invitation to health* (7th ed., p. 493) by D. Hales, 1997, Pacific Grove, CA: Brooks/Cole. From HALES, *Invitation to Health*, 7E.

smoking (USDHHS, 2014). What are the effects of nicotine in the body?

Nicotine is a stimulant drug, an "upper," which affects both the central and peripheral nervous systems (USDHHS, 2014). Certain central nervous system receptor sites are specific for nicotine; that is, the brain responds to nicotine, as it does to many drugs. But smoking is a particularly effective means of delivering drugs to the brain. Nicotine, for example, can be found in the brain 7 seconds after having been ingested by smoking—faster than via intravenous injection. The half-life of nicotine, the time it takes to lose half its strength, is 30 to 40 minutes. Addicted smokers rarely go more than this length of time between "fixes."

When nicotine is delivered to the brain, it occupies receptor sites and affects the release and metabolism of several neurotransmitters, including acetylcholine, epinephrine, norepinephrine, glutamate, and dopamine (USDHHS, 2014). The overall action is to increase cortical arousal. In addition, smoking releases beta-endorphins, the brain's natural opiates. The pleasurable effects of smoking may be due to the release of these neurotransmitters. Nicotine also increases the metabolic level and decreases appetite, which explains the tendency for smokers to be thinner than nonsmokers. However, nicotine may not be the main culprit responsible for the dangerous health effects of smoking; other dangerous compounds exist in tobacco.

The term *tars* describes the water-soluble residue of tobacco smoke condensate, which is known to contain a number of compounds identified or suspected as carcinogens. Although tobacco companies have reduced the level of tars in cigarettes, no level is safe. Nevertheless, as tar levels go down, death rates from smoking-related diseases also go down. However, experienced smokers who smoke low-nicotine cigarettes tend to increase their rate of smoking and to inhale low-nicotine smoke more deeply, thus exposing themselves to more of the dangerous tars.

Additional by-products of tobacco smoke are suspected of being health risks. **Acrolein and formaldehyde** belong to a class of irritating compounds called **aldehydes.** Formaldehyde, a demonstrated carcinogen, disrupts tissue proteins and causes cell damage. **Nitric oxide and hydrocyanic acid** are gases generated in smoking tobacco that affect oxygen metabolism and therefore could be dangerous. Because tobacco companies do not provide the public with specific information about the content of cigarettes, consumers encounter this barrier when trying to know their level of health risk (USDHHS, 2014).

IN SUMMARY

The respiratory system allows oxygen to be taken into the lungs where an exchange with carbon dioxide occurs at the level of the alveoli. Along with air, other particles can enter the lungs; some of these particles can be harmful. Cigarette smoke can cause damage to the lungs, and smokers are prone to bronchitis, an inflammation of the bronchi. Cigarette smoke contributes heavily to the development of chronic lower respiratory diseases, such as chronic bronchitis and emphysema.

Several chemicals, either within the tobacco itself or produced as a by-product of smoking, can cause organic damage. Although nicotine in large doses is extremely toxic, its precise harmful effects on the average smoker are difficult to assess. This difficulty exists because the level of nicotine in commercial cigarettes varies with the level of tars, another class of potentially hazardous substances. Thus, determining what specific components of smoke connect to which sources of illness and death is difficult.

A Brief History of Tobacco Use

When Christopher Columbus and other early European explorers arrived in the Western hemisphere, they found that the Native Americans had a custom considered odd by European standards: The natives carried rolls of dried leaves, which they set afire and then "drank" the smoke. The leaves were, of course, tobacco. Those early European sailors tried smoking, liked it, and soon became quite dependent on it. Although Columbus disapproved of his sailors' using tobacco, he quickly recognized that "it was not within their power

to refrain from indulging in the habit" (Kluger, 1996, p. 9). Within a century, smoking and the cultivation of tobacco spread around the world. Despite national and international efforts (WHO, 2015a) no country where people have learned to use tobacco has ever successfully barred the habit.

The popularity of the smoking habit grew rapidly among Europeans, but it was not without its detractors. Elizabethan England adopted the use of tobacco, although Elizabeth I disapproved, as did her successor, James I. Another prominent Elizabethan, Sir Francis Bacon, spoke against tobacco and the hold it exerted over its users. Many objections to tobacco were similar—people who became addicted to it often spent money on tobacco even though they could not afford it. Because of its scarcity, tobacco was expensive; in London in 1610, it was sold for an equal weight of silver.

In 1633, the Turkish Sultan Murad IV decreed the death penalty for subjects who were caught smoking. He then conducted "sting" operations on the streets of his empire and beheaded those people who were caught using tobacco (Kluger, 1996). From the early Romanoff Empire in Russia to the 17th-century Japan, the penalties for tobacco use were also severe. Nevertheless, the habit spread. In the Spanish colonies, smoking by priests during Mass became so prevalent that the Catholic Church forbade it. In 1642 and again in 1650, tobacco was the subject of two formal papal bulls, but in 1725, Pope Benedict XIII annulled all edicts against tobacco—he liked to use snuff, which is ground tobacco.

Over the centuries, tobacco has been used in a variety of forms, including cigarettes, cigars, pipes, and snuff. Although some soldiers smoked cigarettes during the U.S. Civil War, cigarette use was not popular until the 20th century. During that time, many men considered cigarette smoking rather effeminate. Ironically, cigarette smoking was not socially acceptable for women; thus, few women smoked during the 19th century. Cigarette smoking became more popular when readymade cigarettes came on the market during the 1880s.

The development of the "blended" cigarette, a mixture of air-cured Burley and Turkish varieties of tobacco with flue-cured Virginia tobacco, came about in 1913. This blending process created a cigarette with a pleasing flavor and aroma that was also easy to inhale, prompting widespread adoption of cigarette smoking. Cigarette smoking increased in popularity during World War I, and during the 1920s, the age of the "flapper," cigarette smoking started to gain popularity among women.

From the time of Columbus until the mid-19th century, tobacco had many detractors, but the objections came from those who damned it on moral, social, xenophobic, or economic grounds rather than for scientific or medical reasons (Kluger, 1996). The tobacco industry continued to grow despite the condemnation by authorities. Not until the mid-1960s did scientific evidence on the dangerous consequences of smoking became widely recognized. Indeed, during the 1940s and 1950s, physicians often recommended the practice to their patients as a method of relaxation and stress reduction. Tobacco companies, of course, encouraged this thinking and used a variety of techniques to increase smoking rates (Proctor, 2012). Besides multiple advertising approaches, they provided free cigarettes to soldiers during World War II. At that time, only a few people suspected that smoking might have negative health consequences, and tobacco companies promoted the view that smoking was simply a personal choice.

Choosing to Smoke

Unlike many health hazards, smoking is a voluntary behavior, with each person choosing to smoke or not to smoke. What factors influence this behavior?

Several historical and social events in the United States have accompanied the increasingly popular choice not to smoke. First was the 1964 report of the Surgeon General of the United States that spelled out the adverse effects of smoking on health (U.S. Public Health Service [USPHS], 1964). Other events included placing a warning of the potential danger of cigarettes on each cigarette package, banning cigarette advertising on television, designating public buildings and spaces as smoke free, increasing the price of cigarettes, removing cigarette machines from public places, requiring identification for the purchase of cigarettes, and designing and implementing programs aimed at deterring smoking and encouraging quitting. Coincidental with these and other programs, smoking rates in the United States declined. The highest rate of per capita cigarette consumption occurred in 1966, 2 years after the first Surgeon General's report on the dangers of smoking. Figure 12.3

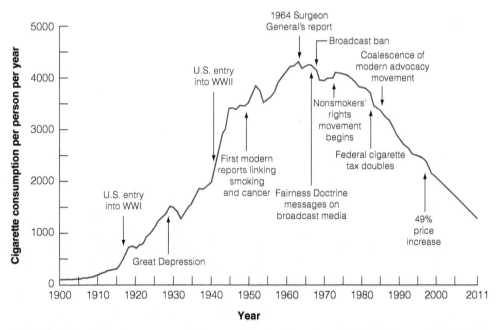

FIGURE 12.3   Cigarette consumption per person 18 and over, United States, 1900–2011.

Sources: "Surveillance for Selected Tobacco Use Behaviors—United States, 1900-1994," by G. A. Givovino et al., 1994, *Morbidity and Mortality Weekly Report, 43*, No. SS-3, pp. 6–7; National Center for Health Statistics, 2001, *Health, United States 2001*, Hyattsville, MD: U.S. Government Printing Office; "Consumption of Cigarettes and Combustible Tobacco—United States, 2000–2011," *Morbidity and Mortality Weekly Report, 61*(30), 565–569.

shows a significant decrease in the per capita consumption of cigarettes in the United States since the Surgeon General's report; it also shows historical events that may have increased or decreased the per capita consumption of cigarettes.

Who Smokes and Who Does Not?

Currently, 16.8% of adults in the United States are classified as smokers (Jamal et al., 2015), a percentage that is less than half of the 42% who smoked in 1965 (USDHHS, 2014). The number of former smokers has declined recently as the number of never-smokers has increased (see Figure 12.4); Barack Obama is now among that group of former smokers.

How Do Smokers Differ from Nonsmokers? Smokers differ from nonsmokers in gender, ethnicity, age, occupation, educational level, and a variety of other factors. By gender, about 18.8% of adult men and 14.8% of adult women in the United States are current smokers (Jamal et al., 2015). From 1965 to about 1985, the quit rate was higher for men than it was for women, thus producing a sharper decline in the number of men who smoked. During the past 25 years, the quit rates have been higher for women at time and for men at other times. Smoking rates for both have declined since 2005.

As for ethnic groups, American Indians (including Alaska Natives) have the highest rate of cigarette consumption (about 29%), and Asian Americans have the lowest percentage of smokers (fewer than 10%) (Jamal et al., 2015). Perhaps because many longtime smokers die of cigarette-related causes, smoking prevalence is lowest for people age 65 and older, with 8.5% of older people classified as smokers. Despite the high cost of cigarettes, people living below the poverty level have higher smoking rates (26.3%) than those who are wealthier (about 15%). Even for those who are not poor, smoking is inversely related to personal net wealth—smokers are poorer than nonsmokers, and poorer smokers are less likely to quit and more likely to relapse than higher-income smokers (Kendzor et al., 2010).

Finally, level of education is a good predictor of smoking rates: the higher the level of education, the lower the rate of smoking (Jamal et al., 2015). In the United States, for example, only 5.4% of people with a graduate (master's or doctoral) degree are current smokers, whereas more than 43% of people with a General

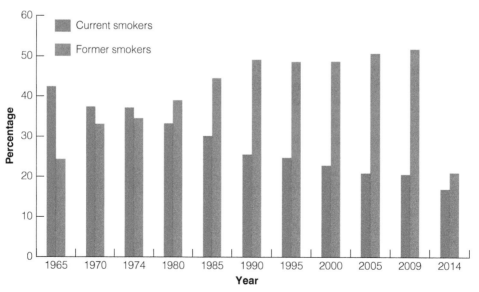

FIGURE 12.4 Percentage of current smokers and former smokers among adults, United States, 1965–2014.

Sources: "Trends in tobacco use," by American Lung Association Research and Program Services, Epidemiology and Statistics Unit, 2011, Tables 4 and 15; "Summary Health Statistics: National Health Interview Survey, 2014," National Center for Health Statistics, Table A-12. Retrieved from http://ftp.cdc.gov/pub/Health_Statistics/NCHS/NHIS/SHS/2014_SHS_Table_A-12.pdf.

Education Diploma (GED) are current smokers. This difference appears even before students enter college—college-bound high school students smoke at lower rates than those who do not plan to attend college (Miech, Johnston, O'Malley, Bachman, & Schulenberg, 2016). Figure 12.5 shows the inverse relationship between level of smoking and level of education in the United States.

The inverse relationship between level of education and level of smoking holds true for most, but not all, segments of European society. This pattern appeared in a large sample of people in Germany (Schulze & Mons, 2006), but a more complex pattern appeared in a study involving nine European countries (Schaap, van Agt, & Kunst, 2008). The relationship of smoking and education was stronger among younger people, whereas occupational status was more influential among older people in Northern Europe. The pattern was more varied for residents of Southern Europe, but education remained a predictor of smoking.

Smoking Rates Among Young People   Barack Obama started smoking when he was a teenager ("Barack Obama Quits," 2011), which makes him similar to most smokers. About 8% of ninth-grade boys and 7% of ninth-grade girls smoked at least once during the month before a survey of risky behaviors (Kann et al., 2016). Figure 12.6 shows slightly different patterns of smoking for female and male students, with male students increasing their levels of smoking throughout high school. By the time students reach 12th grade, about 8% of the boys and 6% of the girls are frequent smokers.

Many adolescents begin to experiment with tobacco during middle school and high school, but adolescence is probably not the time that young people adopt a consistent pattern of smoking. This pattern is usually established after age 18 and may consist of being a nonsmoker, a light smoker, an occasional smoker, or a heavy smoker. Recall that Obama began smoking as a teenager and escalated his smoking, becoming a heavy smoker during young adulthood.

Compared with students, young adults aged 18 to 24 have received less attention. A study from Canada (Hammond, 2005) found that the highest rate of smoking in that country was among young adults. That

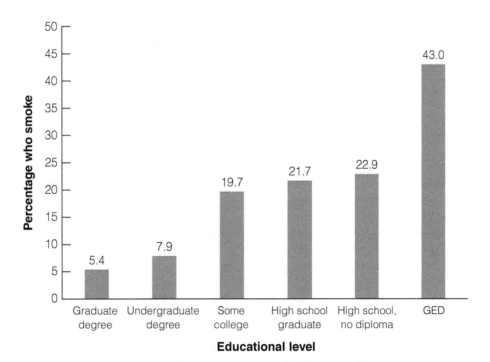

FIGURE 12.5 Percentage of persons 18 and older who are smokers, by educational level, United States, 2014.

Source: "Current cigarette smoking among adults—United States, 2005–2014," by A. Jamal, D. M. Homa, E. O'Connor, S. D. Babb, R. S. Caraballo, T. Singh, et al., 2015, *Morbidity and Mortality Weekly Report, 64*(44), p. 1236.

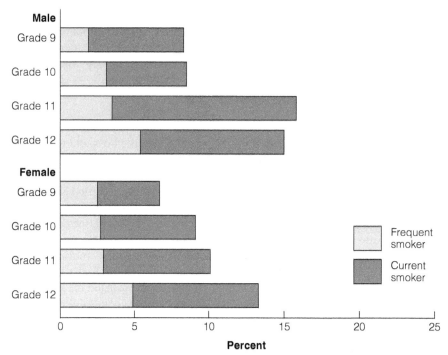

FIGURE 12.6   Current cigarette smoking among high school students by gender, frequency, and grade level, United States, 2015.

Source: L. Kann, T. McManus, W. A. Harris, S. L. Shanklin, K. H. Flint, J. Hawkins et al., "Youth risk behavior surveillance—2015," *Morbidity and Mortality Weekly Report, 65*(6), Table 31.

finding is consistent with data from the United States at that time: 28% of young men and 20.7% of young women smoked (Jamal et al., 2015). However, by 2014 the smoking rates for that age group decreased to 18.5% for young men and 14.8% for young women. This decline is consistent with the overall decrease in smoking in the United States. However, other regions of the world have higher rates (WHO, 2015a); the smoking rates in most Asian countries and many countries in Europe are higher. In addition, the gender differences in smoking rate are large in some countries in Africa, Asia, and the Middle East. These variations create complex patterns throughout the world.

Why Do People Smoke?

Despite widespread publicity linking cigarette smoking to a variety of health problems, millions of people continue to smoke. That situation is puzzling because many smokers themselves acknowledge the potential dangers of their habit. The question of why people smoke can be divided into two separate ones: Why do people begin to smoke and why do they continue?

Answers to the first question are difficult because most young people are aware of the hazards of smoking, and many of them become ill from their first attempt at smoking. The best answer to the second question seems to be that different people smoke for different reasons, and the same person may smoke for different reasons in different situations.

Why Do People Start Smoking?   Most young people are aware of the hazards of smoking (Waltenbaugh & Zagummy, 2004); since 1995 high school students in the United States have reported high disapproval ratings of smoking (Johnston, O'Malley, Miech, Bachman, & Schulenberg, 2016), but 24% said that they do not believe that there is a great deal of risk involved in smoking a pack of cigarettes a day (Miech et al., 2016). The answer in this apparent contradiction may lie in holding an optimistic bias, believing that the dangers do not apply to them. In addition, researchers have examined at least four explanations for why people begin smoking despite awareness of the dangers: genetic predisposition, peer pressure, advertising, and weight control.

Genetics   The first evidence that smoking has some genetic component appeared in the 1950s from studies on twins (Pomerleau & Kardia, 1999). These studies indicated that identical twins tended to be more similar than fraternal twins in their smoking status. More recent research has confirmed genetic factors for smoking initiation and nicotine dependence (Loukola et al., 2014; Sartor et al., 2015) as well as cessation success (Furberg et al., 2010). This research has led to the identification of a large number of genes that affect smoking, mostly through the effect of genes on neurotransmitters in the brain (Wang & Li, 2010).

Researchers have explored the involvement of several neurotransmitters in smoking initiation and in the development of dependence on nicotine. Much of that attention has focused on the monoamine class of neurotransmitters, which contains epinephrine, norepinephrine, dopamine, and serotonin. Dopamine has been of most interest, but a meta-analysis of this research (Ohmoto et al., 2013) indicated that dopamine's involvement in smoking does not extend to initiation. Another review (Hogg, 2016) examined the possibility that more than one monoamine neurotransmitter might play a role in smoking through the mechanisms that break down these neurotransmitters. Nicotine slows the breakdown of these neurotransmitters, which increases their availability. Both serotonin and dopamine relate to mood regulation, which may be more strongly related to the question of why people continue to smoke than why they begin.

The research on the genetics of smoking has confirmed a genetic component, but that research has also determined that the component provides a vulnerability to tobacco use rather than a destiny to smoke. That is, smoking is also influenced by environmental factors. In a longitudinal study of smoking initiation that controlled for genetic relatedness (Slomkowski, Rende, Novak, Lloyd-Richardson, & Niaura, 2005), both genetics and social environment contributed to smoking initiation: Adolescents who reported a closer connection to smoking siblings were more likely to become smokers.

These results highlight the interaction between social and genetic factors in the initiation of smoking.

Social Pressure   Teenagers tend to be sensitive to social pressure, and having friends, parents, or siblings who smoke increases the chances that a teen will smoke (Vitória, Salgueiro, Silva, & De Vries, 2009). Teenagers may be encouraged to smoke and to continue smoking by peers who offer them cigarettes, but overt pressure is not necessary—modeling smoking peers is more powerful than being pressured by peers; young people may begin to smoke to fit in with a social group (Harakeh & Vollebergh, 2012), a close childhood friend (Bricker et al., 2006), or a romantic partner (Kennedy, Tucker, Pollard, Go, & Green, 2011) who smokes. Young people tend to choose their friends on the basis of similar attitudes, and smoking is one such factor (Ragan, 2016). As Obama understood, parents and siblings who smoke may not encourage a teenager to start, but they furnish a model that is influential. Thus, teens in families in which parents or siblings smoke are more likely to do so than teens in nonsmoking families (O'Loughlin, Karp, Koulis, Paradis, & DiFranza, 2009), and siblings tend to be more influential than parents in starting to smoke (Mercken, Candel, Willems, & de Vries, 2007). But living with a smoker—even a stepparent—increases the risk that an adolescent will begin to smoke (Fidler, West, van Jaarsvelt, Jarvis, & Wardle, 2008).

People are not the only source of modeling for smoking; movies and other media can provide a source of social pressure. A body of evidence implicates the influence of movies in beginning smoking. John Pierce and his colleagues (Distefan, Pierce, & Gilpin, 2004; Pierce, 2005) examined the influence that movies have on young adolescents and found that viewing their favorite movie stars smoking on film has an impact on these teens. In a longitudinal study with a representative sample of adolescents in the United States (Wills, Sargent, Stoolmiller, Gibbons, & Gerrard, 2008) and in a study that used a representative sample of middle and high school students (Fulmer et al., 2015), viewing smoking in movies appeared to influence positive attitudes about smoking and prompted affiliating with friends who smoked and believing that smoking is common among peers. Social media represent another media outlet that increases exposure to tobacco messages and pushes young people toward tobacco use (Depue, Southwell, Betzner, & Walsh, 2015).

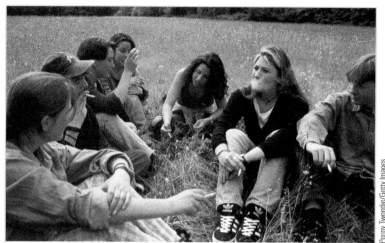

Social pressure and acceptance into a social group are factors that influence adolescents to begin smoking.

A systematic review of media influence on smoking (Nunez-Smith et al., 2010) found a strong association between media exposure and smoking.

The influence of smoking in movies extends to young people in countries other than the United States (although the movies that portray smoking are mostly from the United States). In a study of German children between ages 10 and 17 (Hanewinkel & Sargent, 2007), viewing movies with portrayals of smoking influenced the initiation and continuation of smoking. Thus, the social environment provides many sources that may influence young people to smoke or to decline; advertising is also a part of that environment.

Advertising   In addition to social pressure, tobacco companies have used advertising as a means of getting teenagers interested in smoking. John Pierce and associates (Pierce, Distefan, Kaplan, & Gilpin, 2005) studied how adolescents may become susceptible to advertising by dividing 12- to 15-year-old adolescents who had never smoked into two groups: committed never-smokers who showed no interest in smoking and susceptible never-smokers who reported some interest in smoking. An important difference between the two groups was curiosity. Committed never-smokers who lacked curiosity tended to pay little attention to tobacco ads and were unlikely to begin smoking. Thus, curiosity may be a critical ingredient in adolescents' decision to smoke or not to smoke. Advertising that arouses curiosity can be an effective means of marketing any product, including cigarettes.

Several longitudinal studies and a systematic review indicate that advertising boosts smoking, especially among young people. One longitudinal study (Henriksen, Schleicher, Feighery, & Fortmann, 2010) focused on the influence of cigarette advertising in stores and found that adolescents who often visited stores with prominent cigarette advertising were significantly more likely to begin smoking than adolescents who visited such stores less often. Another longitudinal study (Gilpin, White, Messer, & Pierce, 2007) showed that adolescents who had a favorite cigarette advertisement or were willing to use cigarette promotional items were more likely to be smokers 3 and 6 years later. The systematic review (Paynter & Edwards, 2009) evaluated the influence of advertising located where cigarettes are sold and concluded that such advertising not only makes it more likely that young people will begin to smoke but also contributes to more purchases among smokers and to relapses among those who have quit.

If prosmoking advertising is effective, can antismoking advertising be effective as well? Antismoking media campaigns can be effective, but probably not as effective as advertising to promote smoking. A mass media antismoking campaign (Flynn et al., 2010) showed little effect. Another study found that both antismoking and prosmoking advertising can be effective, but the antismoking messages were not strong enough to counteract the prosmoking appeals (Weiss et al., 2006). A study from Australia (White, Durkin, Coomber, & Wakefield, 2015) indicated that antismoking advertising can be successful, but both intensity and duration of exposure to the messages are important components. Thus, there are hints that antismoking advertising could be an antidote to tobacco company advertising.

Weight Control   Many girls and some boys begin smoking because they believe it will help them control their weight. A longitudinal study with Dutch adolescents (Harakeh, Engels, Monshouwer, & Hanssen, 2010) and another with several ethnic groups in the United States (Fulkerson & French, 2003) showed that weight concerns were positively related to smoking initiation. Young women who were dieting reported that they used smoking as a strategy to lose weight (Jenks & Higgs, 2007), including electronic cigarettes (Piñeiro et al., 2016).

However, a recent study suggests that the weight control benefit of smoking is a myth. A longitudinal study on young women with weight concerns (Stice, Marti, Rhode, & Shaw, 2015) indicated that smokers gained more weight over a 2-year follow-up than nonsmokers.

Why Do People Continue to Smoke?   Different people smoke for different reasons, including being addicted to nicotine, receiving positive and negative reinforcement, having an optimistic bias, and fearing weight gain.

Addiction   Once people begin to smoke, they quickly become dependent. The Centers for Disease Control and Prevention (CDC, 1994) surveyed smokers 10 to 22 years old and found that nearly two-thirds of those who had smoked at least 100 cigarettes during their lifetime reported that "It's really hard to quit," but only a small number of those who had smoked fewer than 100 lifetime cigarettes gave this response. In addition, nearly 90% of participants who smoked more than 15 cigarettes a day found quitting to be very hard. These results are consistent with Obama's smoking—his smoking escalated, and he became an addicted smoker who had a great deal of difficulty quitting.

When addicted smokers are restricted to low-nicotine cigarettes, they smoke more cigarettes to compensate for the scarcity of nicotine they receive from smoking. An early study by Stanley Schachter (1980) manipulated the amount of nicotine in cigarettes supplied to heavy, long-duration smokers. The participants smoked 25% more low-nicotine than high-nicotine cigarettes and took more puffs from low-nicotine cigarettes. A more recent study (Strasser, Lerman, Sandborn,

Pickworth, & Feldman, 2007) performed a similar manipulation and obtained similar results—smokers compensate when they smoke lower-nicotine cigarettes. These smokers will be willing to smoke bad-tasting cigarettes, whereas smokers who focus on pleasure or relaxation will not (Leventhal & Avis, 1976).

Nicotine addiction, however, does not explain why some people are light smokers and others smoke heavily. In addition, if nicotine were the only reason for smoking, then other modes of nicotine delivery should substitute fully for smoking. A variety of nicotine delivery systems exist, including patches, gum, nasal spray, lozenges, and electronic cigarettes (e-cigarettes), which means that smokers may receive nicotine in other (less dangerous) ways. However, smokers tend to prefer cigarettes over other delivery systems (Hughes, 2003; Sweeney, Fant, Fagerstrom, McGovern, & Henningfield, 2001). Indeed, smokers rated cigarettes with tobacco from which the nicotine has been removed as more satisfying and relaxing than nicotine inhalers (Barrett, 2010). Although nicotine may play a role in the reason people continue to smoke, this research indicates that nicotine addiction is not the entire story of continuing to smoke.

Positive and Negative Reinforcement   A second reason why people continue to smoke is that they receive either positive or negative reinforcement, or both. Behaviors are positively reinforced when they are followed immediately by a pleasant or pleasurable event. The smoking habit is strengthened by positive reinforcers such as pleasure from the smell of tobacco smoke, feelings of relaxation, and satisfaction of manual needs.

Negative reinforcement may also account for why some people continue to smoke. Behaviors are negatively reinforced when they are followed immediately by the removal of or lessening of an unpleasant condition. After smokers become addicted, they must continue to smoke to avoid the aversive effects of withdrawal; that is, when addicted smokers begin to feel tense, anxious, or depressed after not smoking for some period of time, they can remove these unpleasant symptoms by smoking another cigarette.

An experimental study using nicotine and examinations of smokers' motivations are consistent with both types of reinforcement. The experimental study demonstrated that some people who had never smoked found the effects of nicotine reinforcing (when taken in pill form), but others did not (Duke, Johnson,

Reissig, & Griffiths, 2015). This finding suggests individual differences in vulnerability to nicotine addiction. Studies with smokers provide additional confirmation. For example, smokers attending a cessation clinic (McEwen, West, & McRobbie, 2008) rated relief from stress and boredom as their top two reasons for smoking, which meets the definition of negative reinforcement. Smokers also reported pleasure and enjoyment as reasons for smoking (McEwen et al., 2008), which fit into the category of positive reinforcement.

Optimistic Bias   In addition to addiction and reinforcement, many people continue to smoke because they have an **optimistic bias** that leads them to believe that they personally have a lower risk of disease and death than do other smokers (Weinstein, 1980). For example, when asked about their chances of living to be 75 years old, people who had never smoked and those who were former and light smokers estimated fairly accurately (Schoenbaum, 1997). Heavy smokers, on the other hand, greatly overestimated their chances of living to age 75.

Neil Weinstein (2001) reviewed research on smokers' recognition of their vulnerability to harm and found that smokers showed an optimistic bias. That is, smokers do not perceive that they are at the same level of risk as other smokers. Indeed, smokers acknowledged the risk of cardiovascular disease, lung cancer, and emphysema that accompanies smoking (Waltenbaugh & Zagummy, 2004), but applied that risk to other smokers more than to themselves. Also, smokers in four countries showed an optimistic bias by rating the brand of cigarettes that they smoked as less likely to cause disease than other brands (Mutti et al., 2011). Thus, smokers tend to maintain an optimistic bias concerning their vulnerability to smoking-related dangers, which contributes to their continued smoking.

Fear of Weight Gain   Although adolescents use smoking as a means to control their weight, they are not the only age group using this strategy. Adults, too, often continue to smoke for fear of weight gain. Recall that this belief is incorrect—smokers tend to gain more weight than nonsmokers (Stice et al., 2015), but people believe that it is true and behave accordingly.

Concern about weight gain extends to a wide range of smokers, but concern varies with age, gender, and ethnicity. Weight control is a factor that influences some young people to begin smoking (Harakeh et al., 2010), and this concern continues during young adulthood

(Koval, Pedersen, Zhang, Mowery, & McKenna, 2008). In addition, weight concern plays a role in adults' choice to continue smoking (Sánchez-Johnsen, Carpentier, & King, 2011).

Gender is a strong predictor of who uses smoking for weight control. For example, college-age women with body image problems were more likely to be smokers than women without such body image problems (Stickney & Black, 2008). A study of African American and White American women and men (Sánchez-Johnsen et al., 2011) revealed weight concern as a factor in continuing to smoke for all groups, but women (and especially White women) were more concerned than men of either ethnicity. A study of women with strong weight concerns (King, Saules, & Irish, 2007) indicated that such women were much more likely to smoke (37.5%) compared with women without strong weight concerns (22%). Should women with high weight concerns quit smoking, their concerns may increase; normal-weight women who were ex-smokers expressed higher concerns over their weight than normal-weight women who had never smoked (Pisinger & Jorgensen, 2007). These results point to a factor of weight concern, which some people attempt to manage through smoking and to whom quitting presents a threat.

IN SUMMARY

The rate of smoking in the United States has declined dramatically since the mid-1960s. Presently, 14.8% of adult women and 18.8% of adult men in the United States meet the definition of smoker. Ethnic background is a factor in smoking for both adolescents and adults; Native Americans having the highest smoking rate, followed by African Americans, European Americans, Hispanic Americans, and Asian Americans. Currently, educational level is a better predictor of smoking status than gender, with highly educated people smoking at a much lower rate than those with less education.

Reasons for smoking can be divided into questions concerning why people begin to smoke and why they continue to smoke. Most smokers begin as teenagers, at a time when they are very vulnerable to peer pressure. Genetics may play a role in beginning to smoke, but social factors such as friends, siblings, and parents who smoke; advertising; and weight concerns also influence smoking initiation. The question about why people continue is a difficult one because people smoke for a variety of reasons. Nearly every smoker in the United States is familiar with the potential dangers of smoking, but many do not relate those hazards to themselves; that is, their knowledge of the dangers of smoking is influenced by an optimistic bias. For many people, smoking reduces stress, anxiety, and depression and therefore provides negative reinforcement. Some people smoke because they are addicted to the nicotine in tobacco products; others continue to smoke because they are concerned about weight gain.

Health Consequences of Tobacco Use

Tobacco use is responsible for more than 480,000 deaths yearly in the United States, or more than 1,315 deaths a day (USDHHS, 2014), and almost 6 million per year worldwide (WHO, 2015a). All forms of tobacco use have health consequences, but smoking cigarettes is the most common and thus the most hazardous. Those hazards include cardiovascular disease, cancer, chronic lower respiratory disease, and a variety of other disorders.

Cigarette Smoking

Cigarette smoking is the single deadliest behavior in the history of the United States (and possibly the world), and it is the largest preventable cause of death and disability. In Chapter 2, we discussed how scientists have found evidence to support the criteria for establishing a cause-and-effect relationship between smoking and several diseases, even though experimental research is not possible with human participants. Evidence for the harmful effects of tobacco use began to emerge as early as the 1930s, and by the 1950s, the relationship between cigarette smoking and cancer, cardiovascular disease, and chronic lower respiratory disease was well established (USDHHS, 2014). These diseases remain the three leading causes of death in the United States (Heron, 2016), and cigarette smoking contributes to all three.

Smoking and Cancer   Cancer is the second leading cause of death in the United States but the leading cause of smoking-related deaths. Smoking plays a role in the development of a long list of cancers, especially lung cancer. Sufficient evidence exists to conclude that smoking is a causal factor in cancers of the lip, pharynx, esophagus, pancreas, larynx, trachea, urinary bladder, kidney, cervix, and stomach (USDHHS, 2014). Both female and male smokers have an extremely elevated risk of dying from cancer, with men's relative risk being about 23.3 times that of nonsmokers. This risk is the strongest link established to date between any behavior and a major cause of death.

From 1950 to 1989, lung cancer deaths rose sharply, a trend that lagged about 20 to 25 years behind the rapid rise in cigarette consumption. During the mid-1960s, cigarette consumption began to drop sharply, and then about 25 to 30 years later, lung cancer deaths among men began to decline. Figure 10.5 (see Chapter 10) shows the close tracking of men's and women's deaths from lung cancer and the rise and fall of cigarette consumption in the United States. This is strong circumstantial evidence for a causal link between smoking and lung cancer.

Could other factors, including environmental pollutants, be responsible for the rapid rise in lung cancer deaths before 1990? Evidence from a prospective study (Thun, Day-Lally, Calle, Flanders, & Heath, 1995) strongly suggested that neither pollution nor any other nonsmoking factor was responsible for the increase in lung cancer deaths from 1959 to 1988. Other evidence against smoking shows that lung cancer deaths for smokers rose significantly during this period, whereas lung cancer deaths among nonsmokers remained about the same (USDHHS, 1990), thus indoor/outdoor pollution, radon, and other suspected carcinogens had little effect on increases in lung cancer mortality. These results, along with those from earlier epidemiological studies, strongly suggest that cigarette smoking is the primary contributor to lung cancer deaths.

Smoking and Cardiovascular Disease   Cardiovascular disease (including both heart disease and stroke) is the leading cause of death in the United States. Until the mid-1990s, the largest number of smoking-related deaths resulted from cardiovascular disease, but these deaths declined, whereas those from cancer have not declined so rapidly. Now, CVD is the second largest cause of tobacco-related deaths.

What is the level of risk for cardiovascular disease among people who smoke? In general, research suggests that the risk is about doubled (USDHHS, 2014). The risk is slightly higher for men than for women, but both have a significantly increased chance of both fatal and nonfatal heart attack and stroke.

What biological mechanism might explain the association between smoking and cardiovascular disease? Smoking damages the inner wall of arteries and speeds the formation of plaque within the arteries (USDHHS, 2014). Smoking is also related to formation of blood clots along the walls of arteries, which is a dangerous complication to artery damage. In addition, smoking is related to inflammation not only in the lungs but also within the entire body; growing evidence implicates the role of inflammation in the development of artery disease. Smoking has also been implicated in harmful changes in lipid metabolism, which links smoking to unfavorable cholesterol levels. Smoking also decreases the availability of oxygen to the heart muscle while at the same time increasing demand for oxygen by the heart. Nicotine itself has been implicated, and carbon monoxide is also a suspect. Thus, smoking produces a variety of physiological reactions that increase the risks for CVD.

Smoking and Chronic Lower Respiratory Disease

Chronic lower respiratory disease includes several respiratory and lung diseases; the two most deadly are emphysema and chronic bronchitis. These diseases are relatively rare among nonsmokers; most of those afflicted have been exposed to passive smoking from a spouse who smokes.

In summary, the three leading causes of death in the United States are also the three principal smoking-related causes of death. The U.S. Public Health Service has estimated that about half of all cigarette smokers eventually die from their habit (USDHHS, 1995).

Other Effects of Smoking   In addition to cancer, cardiovascular disease, and chronic lower respiratory disease, smoking is linked to a number of other problems. For example, over 600 people die each year in the United States from fires begun by cigarettes (USDHHS, 2014). In England, cigarettes and materials related to smoking (such as lighters) were the most common cause of fire fatalities for both adults and children (Mulvaney et al., 2009). Drinking alcohol interacts with smoking cigarettes to magnify the risk of fires and burns, but of course, smoking by itself contributes more to those fires than drinking by itself.

Smoking also relates to diseases of the mouth, pharynx, larynx, esophagus, pancreas, kidney, bladder, and cervix (USDHHS, 2014). Smokers also have more

than their share of periodontal disease (Bánóczy & Squier, 2004) and multiple sclerosis (Hernán et al., 2005), which may be related to the effects of smoking on inflammation and the immune system (Gonçalves et al., 2011). Smoking is also related to diminished physical strength, poorer balance, impaired neuromuscular performance (Nelson, Nevitt, Scott, Stone, & Cummings, 1994), and a variety of injuries, including motor vehicle crashes (Wen et al., 2005). Smokers are also more likely than nonsmokers to commit suicide (Miller, Hemenway, & Rimm, 2000), to develop acute respiratory disease such as pneumonia (USDHHS, 2014), to experience problems with cognitive functioning (Sabia, Marmont, Dufouil, & Singh-Manoux, 2008), and to suffer from macular degeneration (Jager, Mieler, & Miller, 2008). Smoking also has a relationship to a variety of mental illnesses (see Would You Believe …? box).

Women who smoke experience risks specific to their gender. Some research (Kiyohara & Ohno, 2010) has indicated that female smokers may be more vulnerable to lung cancer than male smokers are. Smoking at least one pack of cigarettes a day places women at double the risk for cardiovascular disease and a tenfold risk of dying from chronic lower respiratory disease. Female smokers have an increased risk of fertility problems, miscarriages, preterm delivery, birth defects, and low-birth-weight infants (USDHHS, 2014). Pregnant women who smoke double their chances of delivering a stillborn infant, and they almost triple their risk of having an infant who dies during the first year of life (Dietz et al., 2010). Children and adolescents who smoke have slower growth of lung function and begin to lose lung function at earlier ages than those who do not smoke (USDHHS, 2014).

Male smokers also experience some specific risks from their habit. Smoking not only may make men look older and less attractive (Ernster et al., 1995) but it also increases their chances of experiencing erectile dysfunction (USDHHS, 2014).

In any given year, at least 14% of smokers and former smokers will experience a chronic disease (Kahende, Woollery, & Lee, 2007), and half of smokers will die of smoking-related causes (American Cancer Society, 2016). The negative effects are not limited to individual smokers. Society, too, pays a price. Smoking-related illnesses and economic losses cost the people of the United States $176 billion annually (American Cancer Society, 2016). These costs, of course, are not limited to smokers—they affect everyone who pays health insurance premiums and everyone who pays for

Would You BELIEVE...? Smoking Is Related to Mental Illness

Most people know that smoking is a risk for a variety of physical illnesses, but smoking is also related to mental illness. In the United States between 2009 and 2011, 36% of people diagnosed with a mental illness were smokers, but only about 21% of those without any psychiatric disorder (CDC, 2013); the percentages are similar in Great Britain (Action on Smoking and Health, 2016).

The increased risk applies to a number of diagnoses, and the more serious disorders are more strongly associated with smoking. About 34% of people with phobic fears (a relatively minor type of mental disorder) smoke, but almost 60% of those who have been diagnosed with schizophrenia (a very serious mental disorder) are smokers. People who are depressed also have elevated smoking rates (Strong et al., 2010)

as do individuals with personality disorders (Zvolensky, Jenkins, Johnson, & Goodwin, 2011). Nor does the relationship between smoking and mental illness begin during adulthood: It appears during adolescence (Lawrence, Mitrou, Sawyer, & Zubrick, 2010). As the severity of the mental illness increases, so does the smoking rate (Dixon et al., 2007). In addition, people with a diagnosis of multiple mental disorders have increased chances of being heavy smokers (McClave, McKnight-Eily, Davis, & Dube, 2010).

Being a heavy smoker creates severe nicotine dependence, which means that people with serious mental disorders experience an increased risk of health problems, but they also encounter even more than the typical difficulties in quitting (Tsoi, Porwal, & Webster, 2010). One possibility for

the problems in quitting comes from medications prescribed for people with schizophrenia and bipolar disorder, which affect brain chemistry, perhaps in ways that influence nicotine receptors in the brain (Action on Smoking and Health, 2016). Another possibility is that people with mental illnesses use smoking as a form of self-medication to help them cope with their disorder. Or, the social environment of those with mental disorders may encourage and support continued smoking rather than quitting.

Despite the barriers, some people with serious mental disorders manage to quit (Dickerson et al., 2011). However, smokers with mental disorders experience increased chances for the dangers of smoking and present a difficult challenge for smoking cessation treatment.

lost worker productivity. Smokers obviously cannot legitimately argue that their smoking habit affects only themselves; their habit costs society as well as individual smokers.

Cigar and Pipe Smoking

Are cigar and pipe smoking as hazardous as cigarette smoking? People from Australia, Canada, the United Kingdom, and the United States expressed the opinion that smoking cigars or pipes is less hazardous than smoking cigarettes (O'Connor et al., 2007). The tobacco used in pipes and cigars differs somewhat from the tobacco used to make cigarettes, but pipe and cigar tobacco is similarly carcinogenic.

Whereas male, cigarette-only smokers have a risk for lung cancer of about 23 times that of nonsmokers, cigar and pipe smokers' risk is elevated only about five times that of nonsmokers (Henley, Thun, Chao, & Calle, 2004). Thus, the beliefs of lower risk for cigar and pipe smokers are correct. However, cigar and pipe smokers

experience reduced lung function and increased airflow obstruction (Rodriguez et al., 2010) but not as drastic a reduction in life expectancy—4.7 years lost for cigar or pipe smokers versus 8.8 for heavy cigarette smokers (Streppel, Boshuizen,Ocké, Kok, & Kromhout, 2007). However, cigar and pipe smokers die from heart disease, chronic lower respiratory disease, and a variety of cancers, just as cigarette smokers do. These findings suggest that cigar and pipe smoking may be less hazardous than cigarettes, but they are not safe.

The dangers of pipe smoking are of increasing concern with the increasing popularity of water pipes (hookahs) (Maziak, 2011). This practice is common in the Middle East among adults, but within the past decade, its popularity has spread around the world. The practice has become especially popular among young people. In the United States, between 6% and 34% of adolescents with Middle Eastern background and between 5% and 17% of adolescents with other ethnic backgrounds smoke tobacco in water pipes. Authorities are concerned that this trend and the spreading popularity of electronic cigarettes (e-cigarettes) may forecast a new worldwide tobacco epidemic.

E-cigarettes

Electronic cigarettes, or e-cigarettes, are electronic devices that use a heating element to vaporize a liquid mixture, which users inhale (Chang & Barry, 2015). These devices may resemble cigarettes in shape and color, complete with a glowing tip when users inhale, or they may have the shape of pipes or cigars. Some of the available liquids contain nicotine; this version of e-cigarette use is similar to smoking cigarettes, minus the other components of tobacco. Proponents of e-cigarette use argue that they provide a way to stop smoking cigarettes. Detractors argue that e-cigarettes offer increased opportunities to become addicted to nicotine.

A major controversy concerning e-cigarettes is safety. Proponents point out that these devices not only avoid tobacco but also that little evidence indicates that they are dangerous. Detractors fear that this nicotine delivery method will make nicotine use more acceptable, spurring a boom in worldwide use (Sinniah & Khoo, 2015). Although inhaling nicotine vapor should be safer than inhaling tobacco smoke, a growing body of evidence suggests that formaldehyde and other carcinogenic chemicals appear in some of the liquids used in e-cigarettes. Another line of research suggests that inhaling these vapors provides dangers to the airway and lungs, just as tobacco smoking does (Fromme & Schober, 2015). As advocates state, there is no clear evidence concerning the dangers of e-cigarettes, but the evidence is accumulating that it is not a safe habit.

Most people have heard about and accept the dangers of smoking, but the situation differs for e-cigarettes. In a study that drew a national sample of U.S. residents (Pepper, Emery, Ribisl, Rini, & Brewer, 2015), participants rated e-cigarettes as less likely to cause health problems than other forms of tobacco use. The growing evidence of dangers (Fromme & Schober, 2015) makes this acceptance disturbing. Another disturbing finding comes from their status as most common type of nicotine use among high school students (Kann et al., 2016). Indeed, e-cigarette use is replacing paper cigarette use among young people. In addition, those who use e-cigarettes are less likely to quit the habit than those who smoke cigarettes (Al-Delaimy, Myers, Lea, Strong, & Hofstetter, 2015). The combination of these findings suggests that some of the gains in lowering tobacco use may be lost due to the combination of acceptance, use, and resistance to quitting among e-cigarette users.

Passive Smoking

Many nonsmokers find the smoke of others to be a nuisance and even irritating to their eyes and nose. This annoying exposure still occurs, but laws that mandate smoke-free buildings, open spaces, and workplaces have decreased the number of people exposed to others' smoke. A survey of workplace exposure (King, Homa, Dube, & Babb, 2014) found that about 20% of participants reported that they had been exposed to secondhand smoke within the week before the survey. However, over 80% believe that they should never have that experience.

But is passive smoking, also known as environmental tobacco smoke (ETS) or secondhand smoke more than annoying—is it harmful to the health of nonsmokers? In the 1980s, some evidence began to accrue that passive smoking might be a health hazard. Specifically, secondhand smoke has been linked to several cancers, heart disease, and a variety of respiratory problems in children. In addition, the residue left behind from secondhand smoke, which is called *thirdhand smoke*, also poses health hazards by staying in the environment and interacting with other toxins (Northrup et al., 2016).

Passive Smoking and Cancer   The effect of passive smoking on lung and other cancers is difficult to determine because of problems in assessing the intensity and duration of exposure. Research has focused on workplace exposure and nonsmokers who live in households with a smoker. In general, the more environmental tobacco smoke people are exposed to and the longer the exposure, the higher the risk for cancer.

People, whose jobs expose them to high levels of smoke, have an increased risk of lung cancer mortality. One review (Siegel & Skeer, 2003) described such jobs cleverly as the "5 B's"—bars, bowling alleys, billiard halls, betting establishments, and bingo parlors. Longtime employees of these establishments had up to 18 times higher nicotine concentrations than people who worked in restaurants, residences, and offices. A meta-analysis that drew from studies worldwide (Stayner et al., 2007) found that exposed workers showed a 24% increase in lung cancer. For workers whose exposure was heavy, the risk of lung cancer was doubled.

Nonsmokers who live in a household with a smoker are also exposed to cigarette smoke unless the household has a smoking ban, which applies to an increasing number of households. Indeed, the restriction on places where smoking is allowed constitutes a major factor in the decrease in exposure to environmental tobacco smoke (Kaufmann et al., 2010). A meta-analysis of cancer risk in nonsmoking wives on three continents (Taylor, Najafi, & Dobson, 2007) revealed that risk increased between 15% and 31%, varying with geographic location. A later systematic analysis (Cao, Yang, Gan, & Lu, 2015) confirmed the elevated risk for lung and cervical cancer. Therefore, evidence from both types of individuals exposed to cigarette smoke show that this exposure increases their risk of cancer.

Passive Smoking and Cardiovascular Disease   The effect of environmental exposure to tobacco smoke increases the risk for cancer modestly, but its effects on cardiovascular disease are substantial. Exposure to smoke prompts some of the same physiological reactions as smoking—inflammation, formation of blood clots, and changes to the lining of arteries—which increases the risks for heart disease (Venn & Britton, 2007). A meta-analysis showed that the excess risk of heart disease for passive smokers is about 25% (Enstrom & Kabat, 2006), a risk similar to the risk for stroke (Lee & Forey, 2006). However, even this small elevation of risk for heart disease translates into thousands of deaths each year from passive smoking, but this large number is only about one-tenth of the number of those who die from active smoking.

Passive Smoking and the Health of Children   Infants and young children are more likely to be exposed to tobacco smoke and are more vulnerable to the hazards of tobacco smoke than adults (Kaufmann et al., 2010). The hazards can begin even before babies are born and extend into childhood. For example, smoke exposure increases the risks of sudden infant death syndrome (SIDS). Other health problems for children include decreased lung function, increased risk for chronic lower respiratory disease, and triggering of asthma attacks (Cao et al., 2015). In general, the negative effects of environmental tobacco smoke diminish as children age, but school-age children exposed to passive smoking have more than their share of wheezing, missed school days, and weaker lung function volume.

In summary, passive smoking is a health risk for lung cancer, cardiovascular disease, and many health problems of children. In general, the greater the exposure, the greater is the risk.

Smokeless Tobacco

Smokeless tobacco includes snuff and chewing tobacco, forms of tobacco that were more popular during the 19th century than at present. Currently, European American and Hispanic American male adolescents use smokeless tobacco more than any other segment of the U.S. population (USDHHS, 2014), but smokeless forms of tobacco use are common among adolescents and young men in other areas of the world, especially in the eastern Mediterranean region (Warren et al., 2008). Although many of the young people who use smokeless forms of tobacco acknowledge that it carries risks, they tend to believe that it is safer than smoking.

The belief that smokeless tobacco is safer than smoking has been a factor in its increased use throughout North America and parts of Europe. In some sense, this belief is correct; smokeless tobacco does not carry as high a risk for disease as smoking does (Colilla, 2010; USDHHS, 2014), but tobacco is still a toxin and a carcinogen with health risks. The evidence is not sufficiently strong to support a causal link, but the use of smokeless tobacco is associated with increased mortality from oral, pancreatic, and lung cancer as well as cardiovascular disease. The use of smokeless tobacco as a substitute for smoking is questionable; adolescents who begin to use smokeless tobacco are more likely to begin smoking than those who do not try this form of tobacco (Severson, Forrester, & Biglan, 2007). The risks of using smokeless tobacco are not as great as those associated with smoking cigarettes; nevertheless, chewing tobacco carries some health hazards.

IN SUMMARY

The health consequences of tobacco use are multiple and serious. Smoking is the number one cause of preventable mortality in the world. Smoking causes about 480,000 deaths a year in the United States, mostly from cancer, cardiovascular disease, and chronic lower respiratory disease. But smoking also carries a risk for nonfatal diseases and disorders such as periodontal disease, loss of physical strength, infertility among women, respiratory disorders, cognitive dysfunction, erectile dysfunction, and macular degeneration.

Many nonsmokers are bothered by the smoking of others, and rightfully so—many of these nonsmokers also have an increased risk for respiratory disease from passive smoking. Research suggests that environmental tobacco smoke raises the risk for lung cancer only slightly but boosts deaths from cardiovascular disease much more. However, children are the most serious victims of passive smoking; their risk for respiratory disorders is increased substantially.

Like cigars and pipes, smokeless tobacco is not as dangerous as cigarette smoking. Teenagers who use smokeless tobacco tend to believe that this form of tobacco is much safer than cigarette smoking. That belief also extends to e-cigarettes but growing evidence indicates that this form of nicotine use also carries dangers. Bottom line: No level of smoking or exposure to tobacco is safe.

Interventions for Reducing Smoking Rates

Although smoking rates are declining in many high-income nations, smoking rates have increased in middle- and lower-income nations, which will create increases in smoking-related diseases throughout the world. To protect against tobacco-related diseases, the WHO (2015b) has formulated a strategy to cut smoking rates through deterring young people from beginning, encouraging smokers to quit, and making smoking less accessible through restriction of availability and increased costs.

Deterring Smoking

Information alone is not an effective way to change behavior, and this generalization applies to deterring smoking. Nearly every teenager in the United States (and many other parts of the world) knows that smoking is dangerous to health, yet more than 30% of high school students in the United States have tried smoking, and more than 10% smoke at least once a month (Kann et al., 2016).

Choosing to smoke does not occur because children or adolescents lack information about the dangers of tobacco; they receive many messages about the dangers of smoking through antismoking media messages (Weiss et al., 2006), health officials, and concerned parents. By the time adolescents are 14 years old, they pay little attention to health warnings, making such warnings worthless (Siegel & Biener, 2000). Thus, information about the health dangers of smoking does not create successful prevention programs (Flay, 2009). Deterring smoking is a challenge that requires more and different types of interventions (CDC, 2014c).

The most common approach to preventing children from beginning to smoke is through school-based programs, which vary in terms of who delivers the anti-smoking message, length of intervention, and age of the target students. The most common such program is Project D.A.R.E., which is oriented to drug use but also includes tobacco. This intervention includes anti-drug messages delivered by police officers, typically once a week for a school semester. Evaluations of this program (West & O'Neal, 2004) have revealed that it is not effective in deterring smoking or other drug use. However, prevention programs can be more successful. The elements of more successful, school-based programs use interactive delivery rather than only informational lectures, build students' refusal skills, and elicit a commitment not to smoke, include at least 15 sessions that stretch into high school, integrate smoking prevention into a comprehensive health education program, and provide prevention messages in the community as well as by parents and through media messages (Flay, 2009). A systematic review of mass media campaigns aimed at young people (Brinn, Carson, Esterman, Chang, & Smith, 2010) indicated that these programs can be effective, and the more media are involved and the longer the messages persist, the more effective the campaign. Unfortunately, the evidence is more impressive for short-term than for long-term effectiveness (Dobbins, DeCorby, Manske, & Goldblatt, 2008). The elements of successful prevention must be more comprehensive than school-based programs (CDC, 2014), extending to the community in the form of mass media campaigns, legal efforts to restrict the availability of tobacco, and changes in attitudes toward tobacco use. Deterring children and adolescents from smoking is not an easy task—nor is giving up smoking.

Quitting Smoking

A second method of reducing smoking rates is for current smokers to quit. Although quitting smoking is not easy, millions of Americans have done so during the past 50 years. As a result, there are now more former smokers in the United States than there are current smokers—about 22% are former smokers and about

18% are current smokers. Figure 12.4 indicates that the decline in smoking rates is due not only to fewer people starting to smoke but also to increased cessation rates.

Nevertheless, many barriers to quitting exist. One barrier is nicotine addiction. In a study that asked people who both smoked and drank alcohol which would be the more difficult to quit, the majority reported that cigarettes would be more difficult to quit (Kozlowski et al., 1989). Despite the difficulties of quitting, smokers have been successful by quitting on their own, whereas others have done so with the assistance of pharmacological approaches, behavioral interventions, and community-wide antismoking campaigns.

Quitting Without Therapy   Most people who quit smoking have done so on their own, without the aid of formal cessation programs. In the United States, about 44% of smokers try to quit each year, and about 64% of those people used no cessation treatment (Shiffman, Brockwell, Pillitteri, & Gitchell, 2008). Who are the smokers most likely to quit on their own?

In an early study on unaided quitting, Stanley Schachter (1982) surveyed two populations: the psychology department at Columbia University and the resident population of Amaganset, New York. Schachter found a success rate of more than 60% for both groups, with an average abstinence length of more than 7 years. This rate is much higher than the quit rate from clinic studies. Schachter interpreted the high success rate, even for heavy smokers, as evidence that quitting may be easier than the clinic evaluations indicate. He suggested that people who attend clinic programs are, for the most part, those who have failed in attempts to quit on their own. Later research on the use of smoking cessation treatment confirmed this reasoning (Shiffman et al., 2008). Thus, people who attend clinics are often self-selected on the basis of previous failure. These people, therefore, do not represent the general population of smokers. Quitting on one's own is possible, but many smokers need assistance.

Using Pharmacological Approaches   Obama used nicotine gum, one type of pharmacological approach, when he was trying to quit during his first presidential campaign ("Michelle Obama," 2011). Indeed, campaign aides kept a supply of nicotine gum with them to help Obama refrain from smoking, and his physician advised him to continue to use this strategy in his efforts to quit. Several types of nicotine replacement (patch, gum, lozenge, inhaler, and nasal spray) as well as

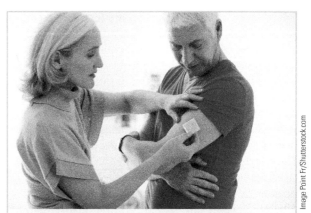

Nicotine replacement can help smokers with symptoms of withdrawal, but the effectiveness is higher when combined with behavioral techniques.

the drugs varenicline (Chantix) and bupropion (Zyban) have U.S. Food and Drug Administration approval for smoking cessation.

Nicotine replacement works by releasing small doses of nicotine into the body. Smokers work toward weaning themselves from larger doses to smaller ones until they are no longer dependent on nicotine. A systematic review of meta-analyses of drugs for smoking cessation (Cahill, Stevens, Perera, & Lancaster, 2013) indicated that nicotine replacement was effective in promoting cessation, so are varenicline and bupropion. Like all drug treatments, these pharmacological treatments have side effects, most of which are not serious; most of the side effects are substantially less dangerous than continuing to smoke. Unfortunately, the same positive results may not occur for adolescent smokers using one of these pharmacological approaches. A meta-analysis (Kim et al., 2011) found no significant effect for these approaches for adolescents. Adding other components may boost the effectiveness of all pharmacological interventions for adults, and adolescents may require some other approach to quit smoking.

Receiving a Behavioral Intervention   Behavioral approaches aimed at smoking cessation typically include a combination of strategies, such as behavior modification, cognitive behavioral approaches, contracts made by smoker and therapist in which the smoker agrees to stop smoking, group therapy, social support, relaxation training, stress management, "booster" sessions to prevent relapse, and other components.

Both individual and group counseling can be successful in helping some people quit smoking.

Psychologists, physicians, and nurses can be effective providers, but effectiveness is positively related to the amount of contact between client and therapist. For example, receiving advice from a physician to quit produces an increase in cessation (Stead, Bergson, & Lancaster, 2008), but information about the dangers of smoking is not as effective as advice that prepares smokers to quit (Gemmell & DiClemente, 2009). Face-to-face contact is not necessary; people may receive effective assistance through computer-based or web-based formats (Myung, McDonnell, Kazinets, Seo, & Moskowitz, 2009), and text messaging can be effective in helping people quit and preventing relapse (Sampson, Bhochhibhoya, Digeralamo, & Branscum, 2015).

Programs that include more sessions tend to be more effective than programs with fewer sessions. For example, counseling and behavioral programs of smoking cessation are successful for individuals who have experienced heart attacks when these programs are of sufficient duration (Barth, Critchley, & Bengel, 2008). Also, smokers who seek treatment from programs that specialize in smoking tend to be more successful than those who receive programs from providers who offer other types of services in addition to smoking cessation (Song et al., 2016). The most effective programs include both a counseling component and a pharmacological component. Each of these elements is effective, and the combination of the two improves outcomes (Hughes, 2009; Stead, Perera, Bullen, Mant, & Lancaster, 2008).

Decreasing Smoking Through Community Campaigns   Rather than targeting individuals, an alternative strategy involves campaigns that cover entire communities. Such health campaigns are not new. More than two centuries before anyone campaigned against the dangers of cigarette smoking, Cotton Mather used pamphlets and oratory to persuade the people of Boston to accept smallpox inoculations (Faden, 1987). Today, community programs exist throughout the world, a growing number of which have the goal of creating smoke-free environments (WHO, 2015b).

Such campaigns are typically sponsored by government agencies or by large corporations as an intervention designed to improve the health of large numbers of people. Interventions at the workplace level formulate and enforce a smoke-free workplace as well as encourage workers to stop smoking, often by offering cessation programs and monetary or benefits incentives. A systematic review of studies on smoke-free workplaces (Fichtenberg & Glantz, 2002) indicated that this strategy not only reduces the number of cigarettes that workers smoke but also decreases the prevalence of smoking. Another type of community intervention involves media campaigns that not only attempt to make smoking less desirable but also offer contact information to helplines, telephone- or website-based centers that offer smokers information and assistance in beginning a cessation program (CDC, 2014). Yet another community or national strategy to decrease smoking is raising the price of cigarettes, which affects smokers' willingness to purchase cigarettes.

The percentage of people who change behavior as a result of a community or media health campaign may be quite small, but if the message reaches thousands of people, then the approach results in a large number of people who quit. In addition, such campaigns have the ability to alter the acceptability of smoking, which is an important factor in decreasing smoking rates (CDC, 2014). A systematic review of media campaigns (Bala, Strzeszynski, & Cahill, 2008) indicated that such campaigns have been successful in decreasing smoking rates as well as increasing quitting. Thus, attempting to reach large numbers of people through media campaigns can be a successful strategy.

Who Quits and Who Does Not?

Who is successful at quitting, and who is not? Investigators have examined several factors that may answer this question, including age, gender, educational level, quitting other drugs, and weight concern (which we discuss in a later section). Age shows a relation to quitting. In general, younger smokers, especially those who smoke at a high level, are more likely to continue smoking than older smokers (Ferguson, Bauld, Chesterman, & Judge, 2005; Hagimoto, Nakamura, Morita, Masui, & Oshima, 2010).

Are men more likely than women to quit smoking? More men have quit smoking than women, but historically, smoking rates for men have been higher, resulting in a larger group of male smokers (USDHHS, 2014). However, some evidence is consistent with the hypothesis that women find quitting more difficult (Torchalla, Okoli, Hemsing, & Greaves, 2011), possibly because female smokers who try to quit have more obstacles to overcome. Women are not as likely as men to use pharmacological treatments in their quit attempts; for those who do, the quit rates are similar to those of men (Smith et al., 2015). The use of pharmacological treatments tends to decrease the severity of symptoms of withdrawal, and people who experience severe symptoms tend to be less successful at quitting. In addition, women tend to use smoking to manage stress, anxiety, and depression, to which they are more vulnerable. Losing a coping strategy presents difficulties, and people who use smoking as a coping strategy are less likely to quit than those who smoke for pleasure (Ferguson et al., 2005). In addition, those who live with a smoker are less likely to quit, which may affect women more than men.

Women are also less likely to receive social support for quitting, and a supportive social network is helpful in quitting. Unfortunately, only about 24% of smokers in the United States who tried to quit reported that they experienced social support (Shiffman et al., 2008). Cessation programs are more effective in maintaining abstinence when spouses of participants are trained to offer support to the partner who is trying to quit.

Does the lower rate of smokers among those with higher levels of education apply to quitting as well? Research that drew participants from 18 European countries (Schaap et al., 2008) suggested an affirmative answer. In this comparison across countries, more highly educated smokers were more likely to quit, including both women and men in all age groups.

Finally, do smokers who abuse alcohol and other drugs find it harder to give up cigarettes? Those who work in addictions treatment have long recognized the strong relationship between smoking and drinking, and the dominant view for many years was that addressing drinking problems was more urgent than smoking cessation for people who used both substances. That belief has been reevaluated; the dangers of smoking are recognized as important to address in treatment. In addition, research (Nieva, Ortega, Mondon, Ballbé, & Gual, 2011) indicates that people are capable of quitting both smoking and drinking simultaneously.

Relapse Prevention

The problem of relapse is not unique to smoking. Relapse rates are quite similar among people who have quit smoking, given up alcohol, and stopped using heroin (Hunt, Barnett, & Branch, 1971). For those who endeavor to quit, some do succeed in quitting or cutting down, but 22% go back to smoking at a higher rate than before their quit attempt (Yong, Borland, Hyland, & Siahpush, 2008).

The high rate of relapse after smoking cessation treatment prompted G. Alan Marlatt and Judith Gordon

(1980) to examine the relapse process itself. For some people who have been successful in quitting, one cigarette precipitates a full relapse, complete with feelings of total failure. Marlatt and Gordon termed this phenomenon the *abstinence violation effect*. They incorporated strategies into their treatment to cope with former smokers' despair when they violate their intention to remain abstinent. By training clients that one "slip" does not constitute a relapse, Marlatt and Gordon's technique attempts to buffer them against a full-blown relapse. Slips are common even among people who will eventually quit (Yong et al., 2008). Thus, a single slip should not discourage people from continuing their efforts to stop smoking.

Self-quitters have very high relapse rates, as many as two-thirds of smokers who quit on their own relapse after only 2 days (Hughes et al., 1992); 75% resume smoking within 6 months (Ferguson et al., 2005). A systematic review of relapse prevention (Agboola, McNeill, Coleman, & Leonardi Bee, 2010) indicated that self-help materials were effective in fighting relapse after a year for these former smokers. However, the relapse rate slows drastically after 1 year of abstinence (Herd, Borland, & Hyland, 2009), so former smokers may not be in great need of assistance past that time.

Behavioral relapse prevention techniques are most effective in the short term, between 1 and 3 months after quitting (Agboola et al., 2010), but this time is when former smokers are more vulnerable to the stress and cravings that are important in prompting relapse (McKee et al., 2011). Pharmacological treatment can be effective to prevent relapse within the important first year after quitting (Agboola et al., 2010). Thus, different approaches may be effective at different times, and researchers must work toward understanding both smoker and treatment characteristics to develop more effective ways to prevent the common problem of relapse.

IN SUMMARY

Smoking rates can be reduced either by prevention or by quitting. Providing young people with information on the dangers of smoking is not an effective strategy, and many of the school-based prevention programs have limited effects. Some of the programs are more effective when they are interactive, teach social skills to refuse smoking, and are well-integrated into the school health curriculum and the wider community. Such programs are more effective than simpler, more limited programs.

How can people quit smoking? Most people who attempt to quit do so without seeking any type of program for help, but some try pharmacological treatments or psychological interventions, whereas others are exposed to media and community campaigns to decrease smoking. Because giving up nicotine may result in withdrawal symptoms, many successful cessation programs include some form of nicotine replacement, such as a patch or gum, or a drug that affects the brain chemistry involved in smoking. Both types are more effective than a placebo or no treatment, and so are several drugs and behavioral programs; the combination is even more successful. Another approach to reducing smoking rates involves large-scale community programs, which usually include anti-tobacco mass media or workplace campaigns and also policies to limit access to cigarettes. If even a small percentage of people exposed to such campaigns stop smoking, this change can translate into thousands of people giving up tobacco.

Some studies have found that women face more barriers to quitting than men. Well-educated people are also more likely to quit than less educated ones. Many people are able to quit for months or even a year, but the problem of relapse remains a challenge. Programs aimed at relapse prevention have not demonstrated the degree of success that is needed; relapse remains a serious problem for those who quit smoking.

 # Becoming Healthier

1. If you do not smoke, don't start. College students are still susceptible to the pressure to smoke if their friends are smokers. The easiest way to be a nonsmoker is to stay a nonsmoker.

2. If you smoke, don't fool yourself into believing that the risks of smoking do not apply to you. Examine your own optimistic biases regarding smoking. Do not imagine that smoking low-tar and low-nicotine cigarettes makes smoking safe. Research indicates that these cigarettes are about as risky as any others.

3. Understand that cutting down is better than continuing to smoke at a high rate, but you will not receive the health benefits of quitting unless you quit.

4. If you smoke, try to quit. Even if you feel that quitting will be difficult, make an attempt to quit. If your first attempt is not successful, try again. Keep trying until you quit. Research indicates that people who keep trying are very likely to succeed.

5. If you have tried to quit on your own and have failed, look for a program to help you. Remember that not all programs are equally successful. Research indicates that the most effective programs combine some behavioral training with some form of pharmacological treatment.

6. The best cessation programs allow for some individual tailoring to meet personal needs. Try different techniques until you find one that works for you.

7. If you are trying to quit smoking, find a supportive network of friends and acquaintances to help you stop and to boost your motivation to quit. Avoid people who try to sabotage your attempts to quit, and be cautious in going to places or engaging in activities that have a high association with smoking.

8. Cigar smoking has undergone a resurgence in popularity. Cigar and pipe smoking are not as dangerous as cigarette smoking, but remember that no level of smoking is safe.

9. E-cigarettes are advertised as safe alternatives to cigarettes, but growing evidence does not support these advertising claims. Avoid nicotine.

10. Even if you do not smoke, remember that no level of tobacco exposure is safe. Exposure to environmental tobacco smoke is not nearly as dangerous as smoking, but it is not safe either. Smokeless tobacco use carries a number of health risks.

11. If you smoke, do not expose others to your smoke. Young children are especially vulnerable, and smoking parents can minimize the risks of respiratory disease in their children by keeping smoke away from them.

Effects of Quitting

When smokers quit, they experience a number of effects, almost all of which are positive. However, one possible negative effect is weight gain.

Quitting and Weight Gain

Many smokers fear weight gain if they give up smoking; this fear applies to men (Clark et al., 2004) as well as women (King, Matacin, White, & Marcus, 2005). Are such concerns justified? Several factors relate to the health benefits of quitting smoking and adding weight. In addition, smokers who continue to smoke gain more weight than nonsmokers (Stice et al., 2015). Thus, both continuing to smoke and quitting lead to weight gain.

The weight gain associated with quitting may be quite modest, or it may be large. Some people experience increased appetite as a symptom of nicotine withdrawal (John, Meyer, Rumpf, Hapke, & Schumann, 2006), which leads to eating more. Unfortunately, overweight ex-smokers are more likely to gain a great deal more weight than normal-weight ex-smokers (Lycett, Munafò, Johnstone, Murphy, & Aveyard, 2011). However, weight gain following smoking cessation is often fairly modest—about 6 pounds for women and about 11 for men (Reas, Nygård, & Sørensen, 2009). In addition, the weight gain may be temporary; former smokers may be heavier within a few years of quitting, but 5 years after quitting, former smokers' weight is similar to those who never smoked. Therefore, even former smokers who gain weight tend to lose the weight they have gained.

Physical activity for ex-smokers can curtail weight gain. For example, research on female smokers (Prapavessis et al., 2007) revealed that women who increased their level of exercise and used nicotine replacement after quitting smoking gained less weight than women who quit but did not become more physically active. Similarly, a study with men (Froom et al., 1999) found that those who stopped smoking had a slight increase in body mass index, but men who were active in sports gained less than sedentary ex-smokers. Although maintaining close to ideal weight and quitting smoking are both desirable, the extra weight gained by former smokers does not negate the health benefits of quitting smoking. Quitting smoking is much more beneficial to health than maintaining a lower weight (Taylor, Hasselblad, Henley, Thun, & Sloan, 2002).

Health Benefits of Quitting

Can smokers reduce their all-cause mortality by quitting smoking? An extensive review (Critchley & Capewell, 2003) compared a large group of smokers who continued to smoke with another large group who were able to stop smoking. The result: smokers who quit reduced their all-cause mortality by 36%. This reduction in mortality seems to provide solid evidence that quitting smoking can decrease mortality. To receive these health benefits, however, smokers must quit—not just cut down—the number of cigarettes smoked (Pisinger & Godtfredsen, 2007).

Two important questions for smokers considering quitting are: (1) Can smokers regain some of their life expectancy by quitting, and (2) how long must ex-smokers remain abstinent before they reverse the detrimental effects of smoking? The 1990 report of the Surgeon General (USDHHS, 1990) summarized studies on the health benefits of quitting for different levels and durations of smoking, and researchers in other countries (Bjartveit, 2009; Dresler, Leon, Straif, Baan, & Secretan, 2006; Gielkens-Sijstermans et al., 2010; Hurley & Matthews, 2007) have conducted similar analyses. The results of all reviews have been consistent: quitting improves a range of risks for health problems produced by smoking. The earlier analysis indicated that former light smokers (fewer than 20 cigarettes a day) who were able to abstain for 16 years had about the same rate of mortality as people who had never smoked. Figure 12.7 shows that after more than 15 years of abstinence, women's mortality risk decreased substantially. Figure 12.8 shows that men's mortality risk reduces steadily for up to 16 years.

Longtime smokers who quit reduce their chances of dying from heart disease much more rapidly than they lower their risk of death from lung cancer. The risk of lung cancer remains elevated for 10 years or longer, especially among men. Women also reduce their risks by quitting, and the younger they are when they quit, the less likely they will be to die of lung cancer (Zhang et al., 2005). Quitting at younger ages also lowers the risk of cardiovascular disease events (Mannan, Stevenson, Peeters, Walls, & McNeil, 2011).

These studies suggest that by quitting smoking, both male and female smokers can reduce their

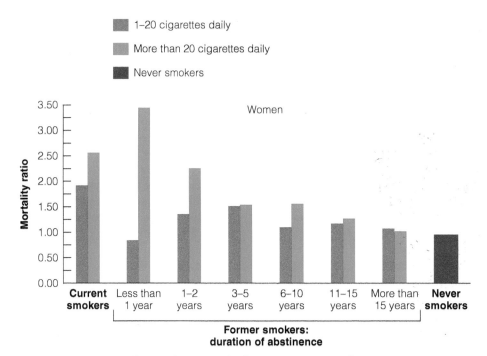

FIGURE 12.7   Overall mortality ratios for female current and former smokers compared with never smokers, by duration of abstinence.

Source: The health benefits of smoking cessation: A report of the Surgeon General (p. 78), by U.S. Department of Health and Human Services, 1990, DHHS Publication No. CDC 90–8416, Washington, DC: U.S. Government Printing Office.

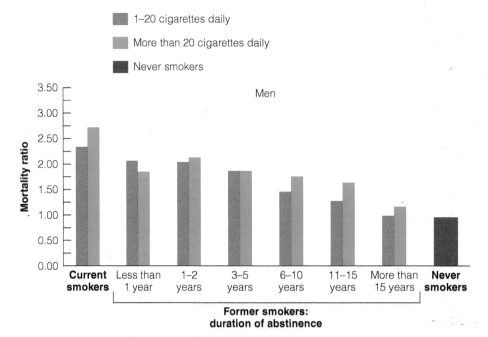

FIGURE 12.8   Overall mortality ratios for male current and former smokers compared with never smokers, by duration of abstinence.

Source: The health benefits of smoking cessation: A report of the Surgeon General (p. 78), by U.S. Department of Health and Human Services, 1990, DHHS Publication No. CDC 90–8416, Washington, DC: U.S. Government Printing Office.

risk of cardiovascular disease to that of nonsmokers, although their elevated risk of lung and other cancers declines much more slowly. Thus, never starting to smoke is healthier than quitting, but quitting has health benefits.

How much does quitting matter? For the average male and female smokers who are free of heart disease, eating a diet with no more than 10% of calories from saturated fat would extend their lives somewhere between 3 days and 3 months (Grover, Gray-Donald, Joseph, Abrahamowicz, & Coupal, 1994). By contrast, quitting smoking at age 35 would add 7 to 8 years to life expectancy. Smokers who quit earlier realize even greater extension of life expectancy, and in addition, smokers who quit also add years of healthy life, not just years of life (Hurley & Matthews, 2007).

IN SUMMARY

Many smokers fear that if they stop smoking, they will gain weight, and they may, but most people do not gain a lot of weight, and smokers who continue to smoke also gain weight. For most smokers, excessive weight is less risky than continuing to smoke. On a more positive note, stopping smoking improves health and extends life expectancy. Some evidence suggests that 16 years after quitting, former smokers' all-cause mortality rate returns to that of nonsmokers, although they may continue to have an excess risk for cancer mortality.

Answers

This chapter has addressed five basic questions:

1. How does smoking affect the respiratory system?

The respiratory system allows for the intake of oxygen and the elimination of carbon dioxide. Cigarette smoke drawn into the lungs eventually damages the lungs. Chronic bronchitis and emphysema are two chronic pulmonary diseases related to smoking. Tobacco contains several thousand compounds, including nicotine, and smoke exposes smokers to tars and other compounds that contribute to heart disease and cancer.

2. Who chooses to smoke and why?

About 17% of all U.S. adults smoke, more are former smokers, and more than half have never smoked. Slightly more men than women smoke, but gender is not as important as educational level as a predictor of smoking—higher education is associated with lower smoking rates. Most smokers start as adolescents, and genes contribute to both initiation and nicotine dependence. Additional motivation comes from peers, parents, siblings, positive media images, and advertising. Smoking is part of a risk-taking, rebellious style that is consistent with the way some adolescents want to

see themselves. No conclusive answer exists for why people continue to smoke, but the addictive properties of nicotine play a role. Smokers may derive positive reinforcement such as relaxation from smoking, or they may receive negative reinforcement from relief of withdrawal symptoms. Other smokers, especially young women, may use smoking because they believe that it will help with weight control.

3. What are the health consequences of tobacco use?

Smoking is the number one cause of preventable death in the United States, causing about 480,000 deaths a year, mostly from cancer, cardiovascular disease, and chronic lower respiratory disease. Smoking also carries a risk of nonfatal diseases and disorders such as periodontal disease, loss of physical strength and bone density, respiratory disorders, cognitive dysfunction, erectile dysfunction, and macular degeneration. Passive smoking is a slight risk for death from cancer but a greater risk for cardiovascular deaths. Environmental tobacco smoke raises young children's risk of respiratory diseases and even death. Cigar or pipe smoking is less risky than cigarette smoking, but these forms of smoking are not safe, nor are e-cigarettes. Smokeless tobacco is probably somewhat safer than cigarette smoking, but the use of smokeless tobacco is associated with increased rates of oral cancer and periodontal disease and may be related to coronary heart disease.

4. How can smoking rates be reduced?

One way to reduce smoking rates is to prevent people from starting. Such programs are often part of school programs, but to be effective, programs must be extensive, build students' refusal skills, and lead them toward a commitment to avoid smoking. Most people who quit smoking do so on their own without any formal cessation program, but relapse is a big problem for these smokers. Pharmacological treatment may take the form of nicotine replacement or drugs that influence nicotine's effects in the brain. These pharmacological treatments can be a useful component in smoking cessation but even more successful when combined with behavioral interventions. Behavioral treatment can also be effective in helping people quit, especially in the early phase of quitting. Mass media, workplace, or community-based campaigns that reach thousands of smokers are also successful in helping some smokers quit and in building a social attitude that rejects tobacco.

5. What are the effects of quitting?

Many smokers fear weight gain upon quitting, and weight gain is common but typically modest (6 to 11 pounds). Nevertheless, gaining weight is not as hazardous to a person's health as continuing to smoke. Quitting improves health and extends life, but returning to the risk level of nonsmokers takes years, and most ex-smokers will retain some elevated risk for lung cancer unless they quit smoking when they were young. Indeed, quitting while young is a health advantage.

Suggested Readings

Hughes, J. R. (2009). How confident should we be that smoking cessation treatments work? *Addiction, 104*(10), 1637–1640. In an attempt to counter the pessimism concerning the difficulty of quitting, smoking cessation authority John Hughes offers evidence that several types of cessation programs are effective. Although Hughes focuses on pharmacological treatments, he evaluates the range of treatment options and finds reason for optimism.

Proctor, R. N. (2012). *Golden holocaust: Origins of the cigarette catastrophe and the case for abolition.* Berkeley, CA: University of California Press. Robert Proctor writes about the tobacco industry and how it has created the deadliest habit in the world. His book levels harsh accusations of deception against this industry backed by an examination of the history, business, and politics of tobacco.

U.S. Department of Health and Human Services (USDHHS). (2014). *The health consequences of smoking—50 years of progress: A report of the Surgeon General.* Atlanta, GA: Author. To mark the 50th anniversary of the first Surgeon General's report on smoking and health, the Department of Health and Human Services prepared this extensive review report that traces the history and provides a current status of topics related to tobacco.

World Health Organization (WHO). (2008, 2009, 2011, 2013, 2015). *The WHO report on the global tobacco epidemic.* Geneva, Switzerland: World Health Organization. In 2008 the World Health Organization published a series of reports on their extensive program to reduce exposure to tobacco worldwide. Reports appeared in 2008, 2009, 2011, 2014, and 2015, each detailing a different facet of the program and progress in countries around the world.

CHAPTER 13

Using Alcohol and Other Drugs

CHAPTER OUTLINE

- **Real-World Profile of Charlie Sheen**
- *Alcohol Consumption—Yesterday and Today*
- *The Effects of Alcohol*
- *Why Do People Drink?*
- *Changing Problem Drinking*
- *Other Drugs*

QUESTIONS

This chapter focuses on six basic questions:

1. What are the major trends in alcohol consumption?

2. What are the health effects of drinking alcohol?

3. Why do people drink?

4. How can people change problem drinking?

5. What problems are associated with relapse?

6. What are the health effects of other drugs?

☑ Check Your **HEALTH RISKS**   *Regarding Alcohol and Drug Use*

Check the items that apply to you.

☐ 1. I have had five or more alcoholic drinks in 1 day at least once during the past month.

☐ 2. I have had five or more alcoholic drinks on the same occasion on at least five different days during the past month.

☐ 3. When I drink too much, I sometimes don't remember a lot of the things that happened.

☐ 4. I sometimes ride with a driver who has been drinking.

☐ 5. On at least one occasion during the past year, I drove a motor vehicle after having an alcoholic drink.

☐ 6. I rarely have more than two drinks in 1 day.

☐ 7. I do not drive when I am intoxicated, but I have driven an automobile after drinking.

☐ 8. I sometimes play sports or go swimming after drinking.

☐ 9. Some of my friends or family have told me that I drink too much.

☐ 10. I have tried to cut down on my drinking, but I never seem to succeed.

☐ 11. At least once in my life, I tried to completely quit drinking, but I was not successful.

☐ 12. I believe that the best way to enjoy many activities (such as a dance or a football game) is to drink alcohol.

☐ 13. After waking up with a hangover, I sometimes have a drink to feel better.

☐ 14. There are some activities that I perform better after drinking.

☐ 15. I have consumed fewer than 10 alcoholic drinks in my lifetime.

Most of these items represent a health risk related to using alcohol by increasing risk for diseases and unintentional injuries. However, agreeing with Item #6 probably reflects a healthy pattern of consumption for many people, but agreeing with #15 is not necessarily a healthy choice for everyone. As you read this chapter, you will learn that some of these items are riskier than others.

⦿ Real-World Profile of **CHARLIE SHEEN**

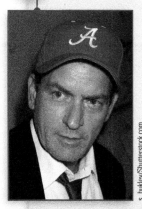

s_bukley/Shutterstock.com

A long list of celebrities has experienced alcohol and drug problems, but few have such an extensive history or made such a flamboyant impression as Charlie Sheen. Reports of his problems with alcohol and drugs surfaced in the 1990s, when his legal trouble and stints in rehabilitation clinics began ("Charlie Sheen," 2011). In December 2010, his erratic behavior escalated, his work on a popular television comedy deteriorated, and he left that show. He was the center of well-publicized incidents involving hotel rooms, cocaine, alcohol, porn stars, violence, and the neglect of his children (Brown, 2011). Unlike other celebrities who have behaved badly under the influence of drugs, Sheen was not apologetic and did not enter rehab voluntarily. His drug use was extreme but not entirely unusual. Many people who abuse drugs combine illicit drugs with alcohol (Substance Abuse and Mental Health Services Administration [SAMHSA], 2015). The results may include health problems, relationship issues (and even domestic violence), legal difficulties, and financial problems, none of which seemed to lead him to give up drugs or alcohol.

In November 2015, Sheen announced that he has another problem: He is HIV positive (Brow, 2015). In addition, he claimed that he was sober for 11 years but went back to drugs and alcohol when he learned of his diagnosis. He admitted that the strategy did not work; instead, his stress and anxiety got worse. In 2016, Sheen reported that the only drugs he takes are the antiretroviral medications to control HIV, which are working well for him. However, he did not give up drinking alcohol until after revealing his HIV status on the *Today* show (*People*, 2016). He entered rehab once again; this time, he described it as a relief.

Will Charlie Sheen finally stay away from all drugs, including alcohol? Similar to many people who abuse drugs and alcohol, he has a long history of abuse, which makes complete abstinence difficult. However, he also had a powerful motivation to lead a healthier life.

Alcohol Consumption—Yesterday and Today

Alcohol is more widely consumed than other drugs, not only in the United States but also in many other countries (Edwards, 2000), and its use both presents problems and raises questions. Charlie Sheen's drinking caused serious problems, but is all alcohol consumption dangerous? What does alcohol do in the body, and what are its risks? What drinking patterns present problems? This chapter includes answers to these questions, but first we examine the history of drinking, which reveals different attitudes about alcohol use in the past.

A Brief History of Alcohol Consumption

The history of alcohol is not easily traceable; it was discovered worldwide and repeatedly, dating back before recorded history. Producing beverage alcohol requires no sophisticated technology: The yeast that is responsible for producing alcohol is airborne, and fermentation occurs naturally in fruits, fruit juices, and grain mixtures. Even ancient cultures used beverage alcohol (Anderson, 2006). Ancient Babylonians discovered both wine (fermented grape juice) and beer (fermented grain), as did the ancient Egyptians, Greeks, Romans, Chinese, and Indians. Pre-Columbian tribes in the Americas also used fermented products.

Ancient civilizations also discovered drunkenness, of course. In several of those countries, such as Greece, drunkenness was not only allowed but also practically required on certain occasions, but these occasions were limited to festivals. This pattern resembles present-day practices in the United States, where drunkenness is condoned at some parties and celebrations. Most societies condone drinking alcohol but prohibit drunkenness or restrict it to certain occasions.

Ancient China discovered the technique of distillation, which was refined in 8th-century Arabia. The process is somewhat complex, resulting in limited availability of distilled spirits until commercial manufacture arose. In England, fermented beverages were by far the most common form of alcohol consumption until the 18th century, when England encouraged the proliferation of distilleries to stimulate commerce. Along with cheap gin came widespread consumption and widespread drunkenness. However, intoxication from distilled spirits was confined mostly to the lower and working classes; the rich drank wine, a less intoxicating beverage that was imported and thus expensive.

In colonial America, drinking was much more prevalent than it is today. Men, women, and children all drank alcohol, and that choice was acceptable for all. This image is not consistent with our present-day image of the Puritans, but nevertheless, the Puritans did not object to drinking. Rather, they considered alcohol one of God's gifts. Indeed, in those years, alcohol was often safer than unpurified water or milk, so the Puritans had a legitimate reason to condone the consumption of alcoholic beverages. Drunkenness, however, was not acceptable. The Puritans believed that alcohol, like all things, should be used in moderation. Therefore, the Puritans established severe prohibitions against drunkenness but not against drinking.

The 50 years following U.S. independence marked a transition in the way early Americans thought about alcohol (Edwards, 2000). A dedicated, vocal minority came to consider liquor a "demon" and to argue for total abstention from its use. A similar movement arose in Britain. Initially, this attitude was limited to the upper and upper-middle classes, but later, abstention came to be an accepted doctrine of the middle class and people who aspired to join the middle class. Intemperance in drinking alcohol thus became associated with the lower classes, and "respectable" people, especially women, were expected not to be heavy drinkers.

Temperance societies proliferated throughout the United States during the mid-1800s. However, the name is not quite accurate. The societies did not promote temperance—that is, the moderate use of alcohol. Rather, they advocated prohibition, the total abstinence from alcohol. Temperance societies held that liquor weakens inhibitions; loosens desires and passions; causes a large percentage of crime, poverty, and broken homes; and is powerfully addicting, so much so that even an occasional drink would put one in danger. Figure 13.1 shows a dramatic decrease in per capita alcohol consumption in the United States after 1830, a decrease due directly to the spread of this movement.

In response to the growing temperance movement, both the demographics and the location of drinking changed. Rather than being consumed in a family setting or a respectable tavern, alcohol became increasingly confined to saloons, which were patronized largely by urban industrial workers (Popham, 1978); drinking became associated with the lower and working classes. Portrayed by the temperance movement as the

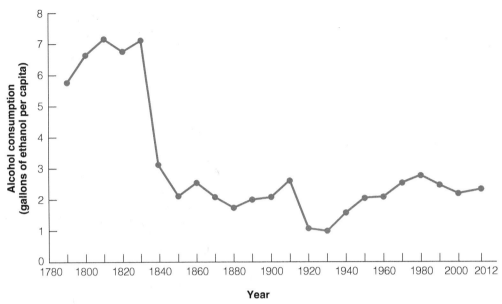

FIGURE 13.1 U.S. consumption of alcoholic beverages, 1790–2012, aged 15 and older.

Source: "The alcoholic republic: An American tradition," (p. 9), by W. J. Rorabaugh, 1979, New York: Oxford University Press. Copyright 1979 by Oxford University Press. Also "Apparent per capita alcohol consumption: National, state, and regional trends, 1977–2012" by R. A. LaVallee, T. Kim, & H.-y. Yi, Surveillance Report #98. Retrieved July 23, 2016 from http://pubs.niaaa.nih.gov/publications/surveillance98/tab1_12.htm.

personification of evil and moral degeneracy, saloons served as a focus for growing prohibitionist sentiment.

Prohibitionists were finally victorious in 1919 with the ratification of the 18th Amendment to the Constitution of the United States. This amendment outlawed the manufacture, sale, or transportation of alcoholic beverages, and per capita consumption fell drastically (as shown in Figure 13.1). The amendment was not popular and created a large illegal market for alcohol; in 1934, the 21st Amendment repealed the 18th Amendment, and Prohibition ended. Figure 13.1 shows that after the repeal of Prohibition, alcohol consumption rose sharply. Although the current per capita consumption of alcohol is considerably higher than during Prohibition, it is less than half the rate reached during the first three decades of the 19th century.

The Prevalence of Alcohol Consumption Today

About two-thirds of adults in the United States are classified as current drinkers (defined as having had at least 12 drinks during one's lifetime and one drink during the past year), about half are regular drinkers,

23% engage in binge drinking (five or more drinks on the same occasion at least once per month), and 6% are heavy drinkers (more than 14 drinks per week for men or seven per week for women) (SAMHSA, 2014). The drinking rates shown in Figure 13.2 reflect a leveling of a 20-year decline in alcohol consumption in the United States. About 2 billion people worldwide are current drinkers, which represent about half of the adult population (Anderson, 2006).

The frequency of drinking and the prevalence of heavy drinking are not equal for all demographic groups in the United States. As shown in Figure 13.3, drinking varies by ethnicity. European Americans tend to have higher rates of drinking than other ethnic groups (NCHS, 2016a, 2016b). Rates of binge and heavy drinking also vary with ethnicity. Native Americans have the highest rates of these drinking patterns, and Asian Americans have the lowest.

Age is another factor in drinking. Adults aged 25 to 44 have the highest rates of drinking, but young adults aged 18 to 24 have the highest rates of binge drinking and heavy drinking. More than a third of drinkers aged 18 to 24 are binge drinkers (NCHS, 2016a, 2016b), but they may age into more moderate drinkers, which represents a pattern that appeared in a study on adolescent binge drinkers (Tucker, Orlando, & Ellickson, 2003). However, many other patterns occur for binge drinking. A study of binge drinking adolescents in Great Britain (Viner & Taylor, 2007) indicated that their pattern of drinking predicted problem drinking in adulthood.

Binge drinking can lead to a variety of hazards (especially for inexperienced drinkers), including intoxication, poor judgment, and impaired coordination. Certain situations promote binge drinking, and college students are at particular risk, not only in the United States (Johnston et al., 2016) but also in Australia, Europe, and South America (Karam, Kypri, & Salamoun, 2007). College men face risks concerning alcohol use when they try to "man up" and match some representation of masculine norms such as risk-taking, being the "playboy," and drinking to the point of intoxication (Iwamoto, Cheng, Lee, Takamatsu, & Gordon, 2011). Men in fraternities are especially at risk; these organizations hold social norms that promote these attitudes and behaviors. However, drinking patterns tend to change when individuals are no longer affiliated. Thus, college drinking habits are not predictors of drinking problems after graduation (Jackson, Sher, Gotham, & Wood, 2001). For young people, however, binge drinking is a persistent problem that creates many hazards for unintentional injury, homicide, and suicide—the leading causes of death in this age group (Panagiotidis, Papadopoulou, Diakogiannis, Iacovides, & Kaprinis, 2008).

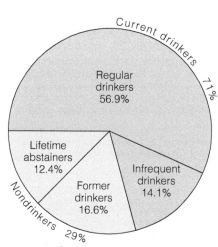

FIGURE 13.2 Types of drinkers, adults, United States, 2014.

Source: "Results from the 2014 National Survey on Drug Use and Health: Detailed Tables," SAMSHA, 2015, Table 2-41b. Retrieved August 2, 2016 from http://www.samhsa.gov/data/sites/default/files/NSDUH-DetTabs2014/NSDUH-DetTabs2014.htm#tab2-41b.

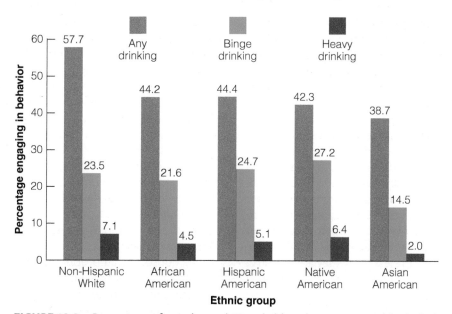

FIGURE 13.3 Percentage of people aged 12 and older who report monthly alcohol use, binge drinking, and heavy drinking, by ethnic group, United States, 2014.

Source: "Results from the 2014 National Survey on Drug Use and Health: Detailed Tables," SAMSHA, 2015, Table 2-42B. Retrieved August 2, 2016 from http://www.samhsa.gov/data/sites/default/files/NSDUH-DetTabs2014/NSDUH-DetTabs2014.htm#tab2-42b.

Among adolescents aged 12 to 17, current use of alcohol dropped dramatically after the legal age for buying alcohol was raised to 21. In 1985, more than 40% of the adolescents in this age group were current users, but by 1992, only 20% were current drinkers. The rate has drifted downward slightly during the 21st century (Miech et al., 2016). Binge drinking, however, is common among high school and college students. Among high school seniors, for example, 17.2% reported that they had five more drinks in a row within 2 weeks before the survey. Although this rate may not seem large, all of these students were drinking illegally. However, reaching the legal age for drinking—one's 21st birthday celebration—is a major occasion for a drinking binge that often prompts the highest level of drinking in which the celebrant has ever engaged (Rutledge, Park, & Sher, 2008).

When the rate for drinking among young people began to decline, authorities speculated that illicit drugs may be replacing alcohol as preferred substances. However, the evidence for this hypothesis is not clear. The Monitoring the Future Project (Johnston et al., 2016; Miech et al., 2016) found that the decreases in illicit drug use parallel the decrease in alcohol use rather than rise in compensation as drinking decreases.

Alcohol consumption rates are lowest among older adults (SAMHSA, 2015). Some people decrease their alcohol consumption as soon as they leave college with its social situations and pressures to drink. However, alcohol intake is inversely related to age—older ages are associated with lower levels of drinking. The general trend toward decreased alcohol consumption with increasing age may be a result of either people quitting or drinkers reducing the amount they drink.

Gender and educational level are also related to alcohol consumption. Men are more likely than women to be current drinkers (57% to 48%), binge drinkers (30% to 16%), and heavy drinkers (9% to 3%) (NCHS, 2016a, 2016b). These percentages suggest that men have more problems with binge and heavy drinking than do women. Educational level is another predictor of drinking behavior. In Chapter 12, we saw that the more education people have, the less likely they are to smoke cigarettes. With alcohol, however, the reverse is true: the more years of schooling, the greater the likelihood that people will drink alcohol. In 2014, about 35% of people with a college degree had a drink in the month before the survey, compared with only 9.5% of people who failed to graduate from high school (SAMHSA,

2015). After college graduation, however, individuals become less likely to be binge or drink heavily than any other educational group. High school dropouts are more likely to be heavy drinkers and to develop drinking problems when they reach their 30s (Muthen & Muthen, 2000).

These patterns of alcohol consumption are not unique to the United States, but amount and patterns of alcohol consumption vary internationally. Culture and religion have an impact on alcohol consumption. For example, in countries in the eastern Mediterranean region in which Islam is the dominant religion, alcohol consumption is low. In Europe, Canada, Australia, most countries in South America, China, and Russia, consumption is high (WHO, 2014). Across the world, men are more likely to drink than women, and people with higher educational and income levels are more likely to drink than those with lower levels of either.

Some countries, such as the United States, Canada, and the Scandinavian countries, associate alcohol with a restricted number of occasions, whereas other countries, such as France, Italy, and Greece, integrate alcohol into daily life (Bloomfield, Stockwell, Gmel, & Rehn, 2003). Drinking is more common in the latter countries, but intoxication is more common in the former. However, more numerous drinking occasions tend to be related to more numerous problems related to drinking, regardless of the pattern (Kuntsche, Plant, Plant, Miller, & Gabriel, 2008).

IN SUMMARY

People have been consuming alcohol since before recorded history, and people have probably abused alcohol for almost as long. In most ancient societies—as well as modern societies—alcohol in moderation was condoned, but drunkenness and alcohol abuse were condemned.

Alcohol consumption per capita reached a peak in the United States during the first three decades of the 19th century. From about 1830 to 1850, consumption dropped dramatically due to the efforts of early prohibitionists. Presently, alcohol consumption in the United States is stable: About half of adults are current regular drinkers, 23% are binge drinkers, and 6% are heavy drinkers. European Americans have higher rates of alcohol consumption than Hispanic Americans and African

Americans; adults aged 25 to 44 consume more than other age groups; and college graduates are much more likely to be drinkers than high school dropouts, who nevertheless are more likely to be heavy drinkers later in their lives. Drinking attitudes and patterns also vary among countries.

The Effects of Alcohol

Essentially the same thing happens to alcohol when you drink it as when you do not—it turns to vinegar (Goodwin, 1976). In the body, two enzymes turn alcohol into vinegar or acetic acid. The first enzyme, **alcohol dehydrogenase**, is located in the liver and has no other known function except to metabolize alcohol. This enzyme breaks down alcohol into aldehyde, which is a very toxic chemical. The second enzyme, **aldehyde dehydrogenase**, converts aldehyde to acetic acid.

The process of metabolizing alcohol produces at least three health-related outcomes: (1) an increase in lactic acid, which correlates with anxiety attacks; (2) an increase in uric acid, which causes gout; and (3) an increase of fat in the liver and in the blood.

The specific alcohol used in beverages is called **ethanol**. Like other alcohols, ethanol is a poison. But cases of alcohol poisoning are not common and almost always involve inexperienced drinkers who have drunk very large amounts of distilled liquor in a very short time. Otherwise, ingesting beverage alcohol is self-limiting: Intoxication usually leads to unconsciousness, preventing lethal poisoning.

Men and women are not equally affected by drinking alcohol. One factor is the difference in body weight; a 120-pound person will be more strongly affected by 3 ounces of alcohol than a 220-pound person. But body weight is not the only factor in this gender difference. Given the same blood alcohol level, men's brains are more strongly affected than women's brains (Ceylan-Isik, McBride, & Ren, 2010). However, women's stomachs tend to absorb alcohol more efficiently, producing higher blood alcohol levels with less drinking (Bode & Bode, 1997). Thus, women and men have different physiological responses to alcohol, some of which may make women more vulnerable to the effects of alcohol.

Among the problems associated with drinking are alcohol's ability to produce tolerance, dependence,

withdrawal, and addiction. Although these concepts apply to many drugs, their application to alcohol is necessary in evaluating alcohol's potential hazards.

Tolerance is a term applied to the effects of a drug when, with continued use, more and more of the drug is required to produce the same effect. Drugs with high tolerance potential may be dangerous because people who build up tolerance need to take more of the drug to produce the effect they want and expect. If this amount is progressively larger, any dangerous effects or side effects of the drug will become more of a hazard. Alcohol is a drug with generally moderate tolerance potential, but it seems to affect people differentially. For some, heavy use of alcohol for an extended period is required before noticeable tolerance begins to develop. For others, tolerance can develop within a week of moderate daily consumption. With increased tolerance comes an increased risk of the physical damage that alcohol can cause.

Dependence is separate from tolerance, and it, too, is a term that can be applied to many drugs. Dependence occurs when a drug becomes so incorporated into the functioning of the body's cells that it becomes necessary for "normal" functioning. If the drug is discontinued, the body's dependence on that drug becomes apparent and **withdrawal** symptoms develop. These symptoms are the body's signs that it is adjusting to functioning without the drug. Dependence and withdrawal are physical symptoms connected to drug use. Generally, withdrawal symptoms are the opposite of the drug's effects. Because alcohol produces mostly depressant effects, withdrawal from it produces symptoms of restlessness, irritability, and agitation (WHO, 2004).

Many drugs produce notoriously unpleasant withdrawal, and alcohol is one of the worst. How difficult the process will be depends on many factors, including the length of use and the degree of dependence. In some cases, withdrawal from alcohol can be life threatening through effects on the cardiovascular system (Bär et al., 2008) and requires careful management (Mayo-Smith et al., 2004). Usually the first symptom to appear is tremor—the "shakes." In those severely addicted, **delirium tremens** occurs, with hallucinations, disorientation, and possibly convulsions. The withdrawal process usually lasts between 2 days and a week. The physical dangers are so severe that the process is often completed in a special facility devoted to alcohol treatment.

Tolerance and dependence are independent properties. A drug may produce tolerance but not dependence; also, a person can develop dependence on a drug that has little or no tolerance potential. However, some drugs have both a tolerance and dependence potential. Tolerance and dependence are not inevitable consequences of taking drugs (Zinberg, 1984), and alcohol is a good example. Not everyone who drinks alcohol does so with sufficient frequency and in sufficient quantity to develop a tolerance and most drinkers do not become dependent.

The combination of dependence and withdrawal is sometimes described as **addiction**. Laypeople (Chassin, Presson, Rose, & Sherman, 2007) and experts (Pouletty, 2002) tend to use different definitions, but element of craving for the substance and compulsive use are part of everyone's definition (Chassin et al., 2007). Experts distinguish addiction from dependence by considering the compulsive behavior and damage done to people's life through this behavior—"loss of control of drug use or the compulsive seeking and taking of drugs despite adverse consequences" (Pouletty, 2002, p. 731). Some experts even differentiate drug abuse from addiction, defining abuse as excessive and harmful use, even if the person is not dependent or addicted. Thus, considering the properties of a drug such as alcohol includes tolerance, dependence, addiction, and abuse, each of which is separable from the others.

Some people speak of "psychological" dependence or addiction, but this term is not equivalent to dependence on a drug such as alcohol. Many behaviors become part of one's habitual manner of responding. Giving up the activity is accomplished only through much difficulty because the person has become habituated to it. This situation is common; people have great difficulty in changing behaviors such as gambling, overeating, jogging, or even watching television or shopping. Indeed, many people readily accept these behaviors as addictions. Whether this conceptualization is valid remains controversial; without a substance underlying the behavior, the analogy is not clear.

Hazards of Alcohol

Alcohol produces a variety of hazards, both direct and indirect. *Direct hazards* are the harmful physical effects of alcohol itself, exclusive of any psychological, social, or economic consequences. Individuals with severe alcohol problems have more than twice the mortality risk as those with no alcohol problems (Fichter, Quadflieg, & Fischer, 2011). *Indirect hazards* are the harmful consequences that result from psychological and physiological impairments produced by alcohol. Both direct and indirect hazards contribute to an increased mortality rate for heavy drinkers (Standridge, Zylstra, & Adams, 2004).

Direct Hazards   Alcohol affects many organ systems in the body, but liver damage is the main health consideration for long-term, heavy drinkers because the liver is mainly in charge of detoxifying alcohol. The oxidation that occurs during alcohol metabolism may be toxic, destroying cell membranes and causing liver damage (Reuben, 2008). With prolonged heavy drinking, scarring occurs, and this scarring is typically followed by **cirrhosis**, or the accumulation of nonfunctional scar tissue in the liver. Cirrhosis is an irreversible condition and a major cause of death among alcoholics. Not all alcoholics develop liver cirrhosis, and people with no history of alcohol abuse may also develop the condition, but cirrhosis has a significant association with heavy alcohol use in countries around the world (Mandayam, 2004) and is one of the 10 leading causes of death in the United States for men but not for women (Heron, 2016).

Prolonged heavy drinking is also implicated in the development of a neurological dysfunction called Korsakoff syndrome (also known as Wernicke-Korsakoff syndrome). Korsakoff syndrome is characterized by chronic cognitive impairment, severe memory problems for recent events, disorientation, and an inability to learn new information. Alcohol is related to the development of this syndrome through its interference with the absorption of thiamin, one of the B vitamins. Heavy drinkers can experience thiamin deficiency, which is worsened by their typically poor nutrition (Stacey & Sullivan, 2004). Alcohol accelerates the progression of thiamin-related brain damage, and when this process has started, vitamin supplements do not reverse the progression. Moreover, most alcoholics do not receive treatment until the process is at an irreversible stage. Although heavy, prolonged drinking is a risk factor for neurological damage, light to moderate consumption does not seem to lead to cognitive impairment (Harper & Matsumoto, 2005). Indeed, research suggests that light to moderate drinkers are less likely to develop dementia, including Alzheimer's disease (Collins, 2008).

Alcohol affects the cardiovascular system, but the effects may not all be negative. (The next section looks at the possible positive effects of moderate alcohol consumption on cardiovascular functioning.) Chronic heavy drinking or periodic heavy (binge) drinking, however, does have a direct and harmful effect on the cardiovascular system (Rehm et al., 2010; Standridge et al., 2004). In large doses, alcohol reduces oxidation of fatty acids (the heart's primary fuel source) in the myocardium. The heart directly metabolizes ethanol, producing fatty-acid ethyl esters that impair functioning of the energy-producing structures of the heart. Alcohol can also depress the myocardium's ability to contract, which can lead to abnormal cardiac functioning. Thus, heavy drinking is related to hypertensive and ischemic heart disease as well as hemorrhagic stroke (Rehm et al., 2010).

Heavy drinking also increases the risk for a wide variety of other diseases. The list includes cancers of the mouth, pharynx, esophagus, colon and rectum, liver, and breast (Nelson et al., 2013). In addition, heavy drinking is associated with increased risk for tuberculosis, seizure disorder, diabetes mellitus, and pneumonia (Rehm et al., 2010).

Alcohol has a direct and hazardous effect on pregnancy and the developing fetus in two basic ways. First, alcohol consumption reduces fertility; women who are heavy drinkers are at increased risk for infertility (Eggert, Theobald, & Engfeldt, 2004). Women who are chronic heavy users of alcohol experience amenorrhea, cessation of the menstrual cycle, which may be caused either by cirrhosis or by a direct effect of alcohol on the pituitary or the hypothalamus. Other possibilities include alcohol's effects on hormone production and regulation and interference with ovulation.

The second direct, hazardous effect of excessive drinking during pregnancy is the increased risk of developmental problems for the fetus, such as congenital malformations of the respiratory and musculoskeletal systems, which produces *fetal alcohol spectrum disorders* (Baumann, Schild, Hume, & Sokol, 2006; Rehm et al., 2010). The most severe form is **fetal alcohol syndrome (FAS)**, which affects many infants of mothers who drank heavily during pregnancy, especially those who binge drink. Some tissues in the embryo, such as neurons, are especially sensitive to alcohol, and exposure causes problems in the developing embryo. These developmental problems produce specific facial abnormalities, growth deficiencies, central nervous system disorders, and cognitive deficits. Indeed, fetal alcohol spectrum disorders are the leading cause of mental

retardation in the world (Murthy, Kudlur, George, & Mathew, 2009), but rates are not equal throughout the world; incidence is especially high in South Africa and Croatia (Roozen et al., 2016). Although heavy drinking is the main contributor to fetal alcohol syndrome, heavy smoking, stress, and poor nutrition are also involved, and combinations of these factors are not unusual in heavy drinkers.

What about moderate and even light drinking during pregnancy? Light to moderate drinking is not likely to cause fetal alcohol syndrome unless binge drinking is involved, but any level of alcohol exposure affects developing embryos. Even light drinking increases the risk for miscarriages and stillbirths (Kesmodel, Wisborg, Olsen, Henriksen, & Secher, 2002), and binge drinking during pregnancy produces deficits in cognitive functioning (Bailey et al., 2004) and increases the frequency of psychological problems (O'Leary et al., 2010). Even small amounts of alcohol, especially during the early months of pregnancy, may have direct and hazardous effects on the developing fetus (Baumann et al., 2006; Goldsmith, 2004). Unfortunately, 18% of pregnant women in the United States drink alcohol, most often during the early months of their pregnancy (SAMHSA, 2013).

Indirect Hazards   Despite the many direct hazards of drinking alcohol, the indirect hazards are even more common. Most of the indirect dangers arise from alcohol's effects on judgment, attention, and aggression. Alcohol also affects coordination and alters cognitive functioning in ways that contribute to increased chances of unintentional injury not only to the drinker but also to others (Rehm et al., 2010).

The most frequent and serious indirect hazard of alcohol consumption is the increased likelihood of unintentional injuries, the fourth leading cause of death in the United States, the leading cause of death for people under age 45 (Heron, 2016), and a leading cause of death and injury worldwide (Rehm et al., 2010). A dose–response relationship exists between alcohol consumption and unintentional fatal injuries; that is, the greater the number of drinks consumed per occasion, the greater the incidence of fatalities from unintentional injuries. About 17% of fatal unintentional injuries throughout the world involve alcohol (WHO, 2014).

Motor vehicle crashes account for the largest number of alcohol-related fatalities. In the United States, more than 130,000 people die each year from injuries resulting from motor vehicle crashes (Heron, 2016), and about 40% of such deaths are related to alcohol-impaired driving (Yi, Chen, & Williams, 2006). The National Survey on Drug Use and Health (SAMHSA, 2013) found that alcohol-impaired driving was most frequent among people 26 to 29 years old, with almost 21% reporting this behavior. However, 10.8% of 18- to 20-year-olds—who are not yet old enough to purchase alcohol legally—also said that they had driven after drinking. European Americans are more likely to drive after drinking than other ethnic groups, and men are about twice as likely as women to do so (SAMHSA, 2014). These impaired drivers are not necessarily heavy or binge drinkers; half of the drivers involved in crashes who had used alcohol were nonproblem drinkers—who became problems when they drove after drinking (Voas, Roman, Tippetts, & Durr-Holden, 2006).

For some drinkers, alcohol consumption can also lead to more aggressive behavior. Both laboratory experiments and crime statistics have shown a relationship between alcohol and aggression, but the effect does not apply to everyone. Trait anger (the disposition to experience and respond with anger) is an important factor. Not surprisingly, men with moderate or high trait anger behaved more aggressively than men with lower levels of anger (Parrott & Zeichner, 2002). However, trait anger combined with alcohol prompted these men to administer longer and higher levels of shock than their sober counterparts and provoked both women and men to engage in more aggressive verbal exchanges (Eckhardt & Crane, 2008). Alcohol may not be the underlying cause of partner violence, but it intensifies the violence (Graham, Bernards, Wilsnack, & Gmel, 2011). Jealousy combined with alcohol predicted intimate partner violence (Foran & O'Leary, 2008). Thus, some people are more likely than others to become aggressive under the influence of alcohol. Charlie Sheen's history of violence toward his wives and girlfriends is consistent with these research results.

Alcohol is also related to suicidal ideation, suicide attempts, and completed suicides (Darvishi, Farhadi, Haghtalab, & Poorolajab, 2015). In addition, alcohol use has a higher relationship to suicide attempts than other drug use (Rossow, Grøholt, & Wichstrøm, 2005).

Similarly, alcohol is related to crime. Two early studies (Mayfield, 1976; Wolfgang, 1957) indicated that either the victim or the perpetrator, or both, had been drinking in two-thirds of the homicides studied. Recent research (Felson & Staff, 2010) has confirmed this relationship and extended the findings to assaults, including sexual assaults, as well as robbery and burglary. Not only are people who commit homicides likely to be drinking but also consuming alcohol relates to increased chances of being a crime victim. These relationships, however, do not demonstrate that alcohol causes crime. Most crimes are committed by people who are not problem drinkers, and the majority of alcohol abusers do not commit violent crimes. Thus, the relationship between alcohol and crime is complex (Dingwall, 2005).

Finally, drinking alcohol can influence people's decision-making. A study of group decision-making (Sayette, Kirchner, Moreland, Levine, & Travis, 2004) showed that when group members had been drinking, the decision was riskier than when the group members were completely sober. Alterations also appear on the individual level and in nonproblem drinkers, who experienced problems in factoring several variables into a decision-making situation after drinking (George, Rogers, & Duka, 2005). Unfortunately, drinking also impairs drinkers' recognition that their decision-making capacity is impaired (Brumback, Cao, & King, 2007).

Impairment and risky decisions can be dangerous in sexual situations. For example, young men who were intoxicated expressed more interest in having unprotected sex with an attractive woman than comparable men who were not intoxicated, even when reminded of the risk (Lyvers, Cholakians, Puorro, & Sundram, 2011). Other research indicates that people who have been drinking are more likely than others to be involved in forced sexual experiences, either as victim or as perpetrator (Testa, Vazile-Tamsen, & Livingston, 2004). Thus, drinking conveys a variety of risks.

Benefits of Alcohol

Is it possible that drinking might be good for you? This question was raised as a result of several early studies that reported a U-shaped or J-shaped relationship between alcohol consumption and mortality (Room & Day, 1974; Stason, Neff, Miettinen, & Jick, 1976). That is, research indicated that people who did not drink and those who drank heavily died earlier than those who drank at low-to-moderate levels (Holahan et al., 2010; Klatsky & Udaltsova, 2007). This advantage appeared first among men, but additional research showed that this advantage applies to women (Baer et al., 2011).

The possibility of benefits for drinking has been difficult to accept, especially among those who provide treatment for those with drinking problems. Familiarity with the dangers of drinking makes these individuals reluctant to recommend drinking to anyone. This skepticism has resulted in questions concerning the methodology and validity of the studies that have shown benefits for drinking. Arguments focusing on possible flaws in these researches (Plunk, Syed-Mohammed, Cavazos-Rehg, Bierut, & Grucza, 2014) point to difficulties in defining the categories of *abstainer, moderate drinker*, and *heavy drinker*. People who misrepresent their alcohol intake could bias the results by placing themselves in the wrong category of drinking. However, this misinformation creates a bias that works both ways (Klatsky & Udalstova, 2013). For example, if individuals underreport their drinking, the *abstainer* category would include individuals who drink, which would bias the findings of disadvantage for nondrinkers. Heavier drinkers in the *light-to-moderate* category, however, would bias the findings of benefits for that category. Thus, such biases would not lead to a systematic disqualification of the results.

Another troublesome possibility is the inclusion of former drinkers in the *abstainer* category (Chikritzhs et al., 2015). This combination would mix lifelong abstainers and former drinkers who have been heavy drinkers, which would not represent individuals not exposed to alcohol. However, studies that have made this distinction still indicate benefits of drinking (Klatsky & Udaltsova, 2013). Yet another critique is the possibility that light drinkers do not gain benefits from alcohol but from their overall healthier lifestyle (Chikritzhs et al., 2015; McCulloch, 2014). That possibility is much more difficult to address; the method of study for this topic has been observational, not experimental. Thus, participants are not assigned to drinking categories, they self-select, and that selection might include many healthy lifestyle choices. However, much evidence supports the benefits of alcohol consumption.

Cardiovascular Benefits of Alcohol   Most of the health benefit from drinking comes from changes to the cardiovascular system (Klatsky, 2010; Mukamal, Chen, Rao, & Breslow, 2010) and applies to people in cultures around the world. A developing line of research indicates that alcohol affects the course of atherosclerosis, the disease condition that underlies

most CVD (Mochly-Rosen & Zakhari, 2010). Alcohol intake has a causal relationship to changes in cholesterol that are beneficial and lower the risk of cardiovascular disease (Vu et al., 2016). In addition, those changes suggest that the improvements disappear as alcohol consumption increases, which is consistent with the beneficial pattern.

The findings about alcohol and beneficial cholesterol changes are also consistent with the evidence about drinking and risk of stroke. Alcohol offers protection against ischemic stroke, which typically results from vascular disease, but raises the risk for hemorrhagic stroke, which occurs when a blood vessel in the brain ruptures and bleeds into the brain (Patra et al., 2010; Rehm et al., 2010). Also consistent with this pattern is a lowering of risk for peripheral vascular disease. That is, low-to-moderate levels of alcohol seem to be beneficial in decreasing the risk for diseases that result from restriction of blood flow through arteries. These diseases are major causes of death and disability throughout the world, so even modest benefits can have a significant effect on mortality rates.

Other Benefits of Alcohol   The effects of alcohol on cholesterol are likely to be the underlying reason for some of the other health benefits of drinking. For example, lowered risk of gallstones (Walcher et al., 2010) is likely to result from improved lipid profiles. Another example is Alzheimer's disease (Collins, 2008; Lobo et al., 2010), the most common type of dementia (see Chapter 11). Protection against dementia is a surprising effect for alcohol, considering that Korsakoff syndrome, a dementia that produces memory problems and other cognitive deficits, develops in long-term, heavy drinkers. However, this link between Alzheimer's disease and light-to-moderate drinking appears in some—but not all—studies; one meta-analysis (Cao et al., 2015) found too little evidence to conclude that drinking lowers the risk. This failure may be due to the complex risks for Alzheimer's disease, which has both genetic and nongenetic components. Among the nongenetic risk factors is high cholesterol, thus a decrease in risk for low-to-moderate drinkers is consistent with alcohol's positive effect on cholesterol (Li et al., 2015).

One health advantage that seems unrelated to cholesterol is beneficial effects on insulin sensitivity and inflammation (Mukamal et al., 2005; Rimm & Moats, 2007). The effect on insulin sensitivity explains why

TABLE 13.1   Factors That Produce Benefits for Low-to-Moderate Alcohol Consumption

Lowered Risk for	Who Benefit	Effect Occurs Through
Cardiovascular disease	Middle-aged and older people	Improved cholesterol metabolism
Ischemic stroke	Middle-aged and older people	Improved cholesterol metabolism
Gallstones		Improved cholesterol metabolism
Type 2 diabetes	Women	Influence on insulin sensitivity
Alzheimer's disease	Older people	Improved cholesterol metabolism
Inflammation	Everyone	Immune system effects

light-to-moderate drinkers experience lower chances of developing Type 2 diabetes than those who abstain (Hendriks, 2007), but alcohol also affects glucose tolerance and insulin resistance. However, a meta-analysis (Knott, Bell, & Britton, 2015) indicated that these benefits may apply only to women. The effect of alcohol on inflammation is not linear, which fits into the familiar pattern of benefits at lower levels combined with risks at higher levels of alcohol consumption (Barr, Helms, Grant, & Messaoudi, 2016). Inflammation is an underlying factor in many diseases, so a connection with alcohol may relate to lower overall mortality risk for light-to-moderate drinkers.

Who Benefits?   Despite evidence for health benefits, drinking also carries substantial risks, making an analysis of risks and benefits a necessary step. One such analysis (Rehm, Patra, & Taylor, 2007) indicated that the benefits outweigh the risks for some people, whereas others are more at risk from drinking.

Pattern of drinking and age are important factors in the dangers of drinking (Klatsky, 2010). Binge drinking brings intoxication and dangerous impairments of judgment and coordination, which overrides any possible health benefit that alcohol might confer. Age is also important; the benefits of drinking do not appear among young people but begin during middle age (Klatsky & Udaltsova, 2007; Rehm et al., 2007) and continue into older age (Downer, Jiang, Zanjani, & Fardo, 2015).

Gender is also a relevant factor: Women gain the protective effects of alcohol at lower levels of drinking than men; indeed, women may be the only beneficiaries of reduced chances of Type 2 diabetes (Knott et al., 2015). However, women experience the hazards of drinking at lower levels of alcohol intake. Table 13.1 summarizes these benefits and who benefits.

Drinking offers more health benefits than hazards for some people. However, those people who do not drink probably should not start, and those who do drink regularly (about half the people in the United States) should concentrate on keeping their drinking at low levels of consumption and avoid binge drinking to experience the health benefits. Overall, drinking presents more risks than benefits to the general population (Danaei et al., 2009).

IN SUMMARY

Alcohol consumption has both harmful and beneficial effects on health. In addition, it has some negative indirect effects on society that reach beyond an individual's physical health. The direct hazards of prolonged and heavy drinking include cirrhosis of the liver, an increased risk for some cancers, and a brain dysfunction called Korsakoff syndrome. In addition, heavy drinking during pregnancy increases the risk of fetal alcohol spectrum disorders, the most serious of which is fetal alcohol syndrome, a serious disorder that often includes growth deficiencies and severe mental retardation. Alcohol is also a risk factor for many types of violence, both intentional and unintentional. The level of alcohol consumption necessary to increase the risk is not as high as the level necessary to produce legal intoxication, but the more heavily people drink, the more likely it is that they will be involved in accidents and violence. Finally, alcohol consumption may also lead to poor decisions.

The principal positive aspect of alcohol consumption is its buffering effect against coronary heart disease, ischemic stroke, and peripheral vascular disease, but these benefits accrue only in middle-aged and older individuals. Other health benefits may include lowered risks for diabetes, gallstones, and Alzheimer's disease, but heavy or binge drinking increases these risks.

Why Do People Drink?

Investigators trying to understand drinking and alcohol abuse have proposed several models to explain behavior related to alcohol consumption. These models go beyond the pharmacological effects of alcohol and even beyond the research findings to integrate and explain drinking. To be complete, a model for drinking behavior must address at least three questions. First, why do people start drinking? Second, why do most people maintain moderate rather than excessive drinking levels? Third, why do some people drink so much that they develop serious problems? Our current conceptualizations have been shaped by the history of alcohol use.

Until the 19th century, drinking was well accepted in the United States and Europe; this attitude makes drinking the norm, thus requiring no explanation. However, drunkenness was unacceptable under most circumstances, leaving drunkenness in need of explanation. Two models arose during that time to explain drunkenness: the moral model and the medical model (Rotskoff, 2002).

The moral model appeared first, holding that people have free will to choose their behaviors, including excessive drinking. Thus, those who do so are either sinful or morally lacking in the self-discipline necessary to moderate their drinking. The moral model of alcoholism began to fade in the late 19th century with the growing prominence of medical approaches to problems. Unacceptable behaviors that were formerly cast as moral problems became medical problems and, thus, subject to scientific explanation and medical treatment. However, many people and even some alcoholism treatment staff still take a moralistic view of excessive drinking (Palm, 2004).

The medical model of alcoholism conceptualizes problem drinking as symptomatic of underlying physical problems, and the notion that alcoholism is hereditary grew from this view. The first form of this hypothesis took the view that a "constitutional weakness" ran in families, and this weakness produces alcoholics.

Problem drinking does run in families, and several types of research have explored this genetic link. One strategy involves assessing the degree of agreement in drinking behavior between twins or between adopted children and parents (Foroud, Edenberg, & Crabbe, 2010). Research generally shows a closer concordance of problem drinking for identical twins than for fraternal twins, which supports some genetic component in alcohol abuse. A second approach to establishing a hereditary factor in alcohol abuse focuses on adopted children and investigates the frequency of alcohol abuse in adoptees with an alcoholic biological parent (Ball, 2008). Results from several large-scale studies using this approach also indicate a genetic component in problem drinking. Both types of studies indicate a stronger role for genetics in the problem drinking of men than of women.

Children of problem drinkers are more likely than children of nonproblem drinkers to abuse alcohol as well as other drugs. Perhaps genetics played a role in Charlie Sheen's alcohol and drug use; his father, Martin Sheen, went through his own battle with drinking problems ("Martin Sheen," 2008), but his brother, Emilio Estevez, seems to have no such problems.

Knowing that there is a genetic component to drinking and alcohol abuse is a first step to building a comprehensive model, but it is also necessary to find underlying mechanisms that form the basis for genes to translate into behavior. Alcohol metabolism offers various possibilities for creating a vulnerability to problem drinking. For example, genes influence the functioning of neurotransmitters, such as dopamine, GABA, and serotonin, which have been linked to alcohol's effects (Foroud et al., 2010; Köhnke, 2008). A specific genetic susceptibility to problem drinking may lie in a variant of the genes that are involved with alcohol dehydrogenase, which is one enzyme involved in alcohol metabolism (Tolstrup, Nordestgaard, Rasmussen, Tybjærg-Hansen, & Grønbæk, 2008). According to this view, the speed of alcohol metabolism is related to drinking more and drinking more heavily; variants of this gene affect that speed. Other research has attempted to understand the genes involved in vulnerability to alcohol abuse (Palmer et al., 2012). One study (Thombs et al., 2011) showed that a genetic variation affected availability of the neurotransmitter serotonin in ways that related to impulsive behaviors, including drinking. Yet another approach has focused on finding the location of some of the genes involved in susceptibility to problem drinking (Ma, Fan, & Li, 2016).

However, problem drinking will not be traced to one gene pair; dozens of genes are likely involved

(Foroud et al., 2010). In addition, researchers accept the importance of a person's environment in drinking; they expect that the search for the genetic contributions to problem drinking will reveal multiple gene locations that underlie a vulnerability to problem drinking rather than a genetic determination of alcoholism. That is, researchers are looking for genetic, biological, and environmental factors that contribute to problem drinking.

The Disease Model

The disease concept of alcoholism is a variation of the medical model, holding that people with problem drinking have the disease of alcoholism. Throughout history, isolated attempts have been made to describe alcohol intoxication as a disease brought about by the physical properties of alcohol. This view became increasingly popular beginning in the late 1930s and early 1940s. The American Medical Association accepted this model in 1956, and it remains the dominant view in psychiatric and other medically oriented treatment programs in the United States (Lee, Lee, Lee, & Arch, 2010). The disease model is less influential in psychologically based treatment programs and in treatment programs in Canada, Europe, and Australia.

The disease model of alcoholism was elevated to scientific respectability by the pioneering work of E. M. Jellinek (1960), who described several different types of alcoholism and their characteristics. However, this model cast alcoholism as an incurable disease, which is too simplistic, even with the different varieties that Jellinek described.

The Alcohol Dependency Syndrome   Dissatisfaction with Jellinek's disease model led Griffith Edwards and his colleagues (Edwards, 1977; Edwards & Gross, 1976; Edwards, Gross, Keller, Moser, & Room, 1977) to advocate the alcohol dependency syndrome, which rejects the term *alcoholism*, substituting the term *alcohol dependency syndrome*. Rather than assert that alcoholics experience loss of control, Edwards and his colleagues proposed that those who are alcohol dependent have *impaired control*, suggesting that people drink heavily because, at certain times and for a variety of reasons, they do not exercise control over their drinking. The seven elements of the alcohol dependency syndrome appear in Table 13.2. This concept has influenced the "official" one that forms the basis for a diagnosis of *alcohol use disorder*, the diagnosis that appears in the *Diagnostic and Statistical Manual of Mental Disorders 5* (American Psychiatric Association, 2013).

Evaluation of the Disease Model   Despite the widespread acceptance of the disease model of alcoholism, the concept of alcoholism as a disease is difficult to validate. Even the alcohol dependency model remains controversial (Babor, 2007; Li, Hewitt, & Grant, 2007). In addition, the disease model fails to address our first question: Why do people begin to drink? Its answer to the second question about why some people continue to drink at moderate levels is hardly adequate: People

TABLE 13.2   Elements of the Alcohol Dependency Syndrome

Element	Behaviors Associated with This Element
Narrowing of drinking repertoire	Drinking the same beverage at the same time of day.
Salience of drink-seeking behavior	*Drinking begins to take precedence over other behaviors.
Increased tolerance for alcohol	*Drinkers become accustomed to performing daily tasks with high blood alcohol levels.
Withdrawal symptoms	*Restlessness, irritability, and agitation.
Avoiding withdrawal symptoms	*Additional drinking.
Personal awareness of the need to drink	*Drinkers acknowledge their need to drink.
Reinstatement of dependence after abstinence	Drinkers who have quit become dependent more rapidly when they begin to drink again; the development of dependence is inversely related to severity of prior dependence.

·ion is similar to diagnostic criterion in DSM 5.

\lcohol Dependence: Provisional Description of a Clinical Syndrome" by G. Edwards & M. M. Gross, 1976, *British Medical Journal, 1*(6017), 1058–1061.

who are not alcoholic do not develop a dependence on alcohol.

One key concept in the disease model is loss of control or impaired control—the inability to stop or moderate alcohol intake once drinking begins. This concept has been difficult to define specifically, and research has not been consistent concerning its influence (Martin, Fillmore, Chung, Easdon, & Miczek, 2006). G. Alan Marlatt and his colleagues (Marlatt, Demming, & Reid, 1973; Marlatt & Rohsenow, 1980) have conducted experiments suggesting that many effects of alcohol, including impaired control, are due more to expectancy than to any pharmacological effect of alcohol. Their experimental design, called the balanced placebo design, included four groups, two of which expect to be given alcohol and two of which do not. Two groups actually receive alcohol, and two do not. Figure 13.4 shows all four combinations.

Using the balanced placebo design, several studies (Marlatt et al., 1973; Marlatt & Rohsenow, 1980) showed that people who think they have received alcohol behave as though they have (whether they have or not). Even for those who had been in treatment for problem drinking, expectancy appeared to be the controlling factor in the craving for alcohol and in the amount consumed. These findings suggest that expectancy plays an important role in loss of control and craving for alcohol. A meta-analysis of studies on alcohol expectancy (McKay & Schare, 1999) confirmed that expectancy plays an important role in alcohol's effects.

Some investigators (Peele, 2007; Quinn, Bodenhamer-Davis, & Koch, 2004) have criticized the disease model of alcohol, arguing that it does not adequately consider environmental, cognitive, and affective determinants of abusive drinking; that is, in its emphasis on the physical properties of alcohol, the disease model neglects the cognitive and social learning aspects of drinking.

Cognitive-Physiological Theories

Of the various alternatives to the disease model, several emphasize the combination of physiological and cognitive changes that occur with alcohol use. Rather than hypothesize that alcohol use and misuse are based only on the chemical properties of alcohol, these models contend that the cognitive changes experienced by drinkers also contribute to drinking behavior.

The Tension Reduction Hypothesis   As the name suggests, the tension reduction hypothesis (Conger, 1956) holds that people drink alcohol because of its tension-reducing effects. This hypothesis has much intuitive appeal because alcohol is a sedative drug that leads to relaxation and slowed reactions.

Despite its consistency with popular belief, experimental studies have furnished limited support for the tension reduction hypothesis. Studies that have manipulated tension or anxiety to observe their effects on participants' readiness to consume alcohol have yielded contradictory results; some participants experience tension reduction,

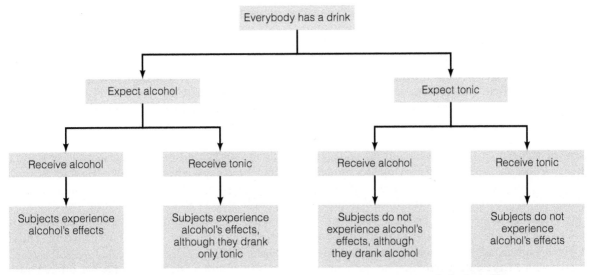

FIGURE 13.4   Balanced placebo design used in experiments on expectancy and alcohol effects.

whereas others do not (Kambouropoulos, 2003). In more naturalistic settings (Frone, 2008; Moore, Sikora, Grunberg, & Greenberg, 2007), factors other than stress and tension have been found to show a stronger relationship to drinking. One factor that complicates assessment of the tension reduction hypothesis is expectancy. When people expect to experience tension reduction, they tend to get what they expect. A large-scale study in Germany (Pabst, Baumeister, & Kraus, 2010) found that tension reduction is one of the effects that drinkers expect. Thus, tension reduction is one of many effects that may occur as a result of drinking, but expectancy may be more important than alcohol in these effects.

The realization that alcohol's effects on physiological processes are not simple led to a reformulation of the tension reduction hypothesis. A group of researchers at Indiana University (Levenson, Sher, Grossman, Newman, & Newlin, 1980; Sher, 1987; Sher & Levenson, 1982) discovered that high levels of alcohol consumption decrease the strength of responses to stress. They labeled this decrease the *stress response dampening (SRD) effect*. People who had been drinking did not respond as strongly as nondrinking participants to either physiological or psychological stressors. People whose personality profile suggested a high risk of developing problem drinking showed the strongest SRD effect, and those whose profile indicated a low risk showed a weaker effect (Sher & Levenson, 1982). This stress response–dampening effect appears in some drinkers but not in others (Zack, Poulos, Aramakis, Khamba, & MacLeod, 2007) and more strongly at higher levels of intoxication (Donohue, Curtin, Patrick, & Lang, 2007). In addition, stress response dampening tends to occur in social drinking situations (Armeli et al., 2003) and in situations with uncertain threats to a greater degree than more certain threat situations (Bradford, Shapiro, & Curtin, 2013). However, neither the original tension reduction hypothesis nor stress response dampening provides a general explanation for drinking, especially for initiating drinking.

Alcohol Myopia   Claude Steele and his colleagues (Steele & Josephs, 1990) have developed a model of alcohol use and abuse based on alcohol's psychological and physical properties. This model hypothesizes that alcohol use creates effects on social behaviors that they term *alcohol myopia*, "a state of shortsightedness in which superficially understood, immediate aspects of experience have a disproportionate influence on behavior and emotion, a state in which we can see the

tree, albeit more dimly, but miss the forest altogether" (Steele & Josephs, 1990, p. 923). According to this view, alcohol blocks out insightful cognitive processing and alters thoughts related to the self, stress, and social anxiety.

Part of alcohol myopia is *drunken excess*, the tendency for those who drink to behave more excessively. This tendency appears as increased aggression, friendliness, sexiness, and many other exaggerated behaviors. Tendencies to behave in such extreme ways are usually inhibited, but when people drink, they experience less inhibition, and their behavior becomes more extreme. Under the influence of alcohol, people tend to focus on desirable aspects of a situation rather than reasonable or feasible ones (Sevincer & Oettingen, 2013).

Another aspect of alcohol myopia is *self-inflation*, a tendency to inflate self-evaluations. When asked to rate the importance of 35 trait dimensions for their real and ideal selves, drunken participants rated themselves higher on traits that were important to them and on which they had rated themselves low when sober (Banaji & Steele, 1989). Thus, drinking allowed participants to see themselves as better than they did when they were not drinking, confirming the ability of alcohol to inflate a person's self-evaluation.

A third aspect of alcohol myopia is *drunken relief* (Steele & Josephs, 1990); that is, people who drink tend to worry less and pay less attention to their worries. When consumed in large quantities, alcohol alone may produce drunken relief, but it can also affect behavior in smaller quantities. For example, women with low self-esteem who drank alcohol interacted more with a flirtatious man after drinking than did similar women who had not been drinking and more than women with high self-esteem (Monahan & Lannutti, 2000). This finding suggests that drunken relief is not an effect entirely of alcohol but of alcohol in combination with other factors.

The alcohol myopia model has quite a bit of research support. Intoxicated people tend to analyze information at a more superficial level, are more susceptible to distraction (Ortner, MacDonald, & Olmstead, 2003), and recall fewer details of a situation they have experienced (Villalba, Ham, & Rose, 2011) than people who have not been drinking. For example, people playing an online gambling game became less focused on suggestions concerning how to maximize their winnings after they started drinking (Phillips & Ogeil, 2007).

In addition, alcohol myopia has offered a framework for interpreting a number of changes in sexual behavior that occur after drinking and also fits with behavior under the influence of other drugs (Noel, Heaton, & Brown, 2013). A review of the research on high-risk sexual behavior and alcohol (Griffin, Umstattd, & Usdan, 2010) indicated that college students' sexual decision-making is affected by intoxication. Drinking leads people to focus on specific cues in the environment, which can lead to either more or less risky decisions. For example, when intoxicated men or women focus on their sexual feelings, they tend to be more willing to engage in risky sex than those who are not intoxicated. When similarly intoxicated people's attention is focused on the perils of risky sex, they tend to be less likely to engage in risky sex than those who are sober. That is, drinkers' tendency to process information in a limited way is influenced by what cues are present rather than by a general tendency for disinhibition. Thus, many studies offer strong research support for this model.

The Social Learning Model

The social learning model provides an explanation for why people begin to drink, why they continue to drink in moderation, and why some people drink in a harmful manner. This model conceptualizes drinking as learned behavior, acquired in the same manner as other behaviors.

According to social learning theory, people begin to drink for at least three reasons. First, the taste of alcohol and its immediate effects may bring pleasure (positive reinforcement); second, drinking may allow a person to escape from an unpleasant situation (negative reinforcement); and third, the person may learn to drink through observing others (modeling). Research offers support for each of these possibilities.

First, research from countries around the world (Bergmark & Kuendig, 2008) found positive expectations for alcohol consumption. The reasons for drinking among college students in the United States (Holt et al., 2013; Read, Wood, & Capone, 2005) and in the United Kingdom (Orford, Krishnan, Balaam, Everitt, & van der Graaf, 2004) also support the role of positive reinforcement, revealing that interpersonal factors, such as social interaction and mood enhancement, are key reasons for drinking. For individuals who do not drink, social influences are also important; lifetime abstainers tended to report that they had no interest in drinking or that their religion or upbringing influenced them to abstain (Bernards, Graham, Kuendig, Hettige, & Obot, 2009).

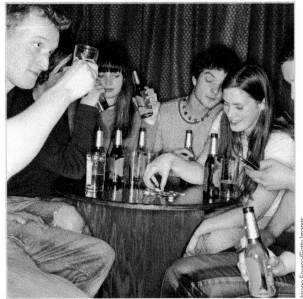

College social gatherings may encourage binge drinking.

Image Source/Getty Images

Second, modeling and social pressure are related to increases in drinking among young people. Students who were heavier drinkers put themselves in situations to receive different pressures than did students who drank less (Orford et al., 2004), and adolescents in New Zealand showed a pattern of reciprocal social influence among those whose drinking escalated (McDonough, Jose, & Stuart, 2016). A combination of modeling and expectancies of the effects of alcohol are the mechanisms hypothesized to underlie the transmission of drinking from parents to children (Campbell & Oei, 2010). People who are heavy drinkers also tend to associate with other people who have similar drinking patterns. Thus, modeling offers explanations for both the initiation of drinking and the tendency of some people to drink to excess.

A third explanation for excessive drinking offered by the social learning model is based on the principles of negative reinforcement. Dropping alcohol levels creates discomfort, and ingesting more alcohol relieves this discomfort. This process fits with the definition of negative reinforcement and provides another explanation for continuing to drink (Lowman, Hunt, Litten, & Drummond, 2000).

Social learning theory provides an explanation for why people start drinking, why some continue to drink in moderation, and why others become problem drinkers. In addition, social learning theory suggests a variety of treatment techniques to help people overcome excessive drinking habits. The treatment rationale holds that if drinking behavior is learned, then it can be unlearned or relearned, with either abstinence or moderation as a goal of therapy.

IN SUMMARY

The question of why people drink has three components: (1) Why do people begin drinking? (2) Why do some people drink in moderation? (3) Why do others drink to excess? Theories of drinking behavior should be able to offer explanations in response to each of these questions. This section discussed three theories or models, each of which has some potential explanatory ability. The disease model assumes that people drink excessively because they have the disease of alcoholism. One variation of the disease model—the alcohol dependency syndrome—assumes that alcohol-dependent people have impaired control and drink heavily for a variety of reasons. Cognitive-physiological models, including the tension reduction hypothesis and alcohol myopia, propose that people drink because alcohol produces alterations in cognitive function that allow them to escape tension or process information differently. Social learning theory hypothesizes that people acquire drinking behavior the same way that they learn other behaviors—that is, through positive or negative reinforcement and modeling. All three models offer some explanation of why some people continue to drink, but only social learning theory addresses all three components of drinking.

Changing Problem Drinking

The percentage of drinkers in the United States (about 52%) and the number of people who sought help for problem drinking (2.5 million) has remained stable over the past decade (SAMHSA, 2014). Men outnumber women by a ratio of 2:1. Women are more reluctant than men to seek treatment, and they may also seek treatment from sources that specialize in mental health treatment rather than alcohol treatment. Outpatient treatment is more common than inpatient treatment, but the most common form of treatment is attendance

at a self-help group (SAMHSA, 2014). Private, for-profit facilities emphasize inpatient treatment, but these programs may have benefits that are limited to people with the most serious problems, and the costs are much higher. Cost is a factor in treatment; almost half of those who needed but failed to receive treatment cited cost not covered by insurance as the most important factor (SAMHSA, 2014). Although adequate treatment is important for changing drinking behavior, some individuals with drinking problems are able to quit without formal treatment (Hodgins, 2005; Scarscelli, 2006).

Change Without Therapy

Some problems (and some diseases) disappear without formal treatment, and problem drinking is no exception. When a disease disappears without treatment, the term **spontaneous remission**, *natural recovery, or unassisted change* is used to describe this process. Even these terms may be somewhat misleading because people who change their drinking patterns may have the help and support of many people, including family members, employers, and friends, but have not used a formal therapy program. Changes of this type do occur (Scarscelli, 2006; Toneatto, 2013). In a study of individuals diagnosed as alcohol dependent (Dawson et al., 2005), only 25% were still in that category 1 year later, 18% were abstinent, and another 18% had moderated their drinking to nonproblem levels. Heavy drinkers who change their drinking behavior may be those who are less dependent (Cunningham, Blomqvist, Koski-Jännes, & Cordingley, 2005); others may need professional help or the assistance of traditional groups such as Alcoholics Anonymous (AA).

Presently, nearly all treatment programs in the United States are oriented toward abstinence, but programs in other countries may be oriented toward harm reduction rather than abstinence and allow for the possibility that some problem drinkers can become moderate drinkers.

Treatments Oriented Toward Abstinence

All formal treatments—even those that permit the possibility of resuming drinking—seek immediate abstinence as their goal. This section examines several treatment programs aimed at total and permanent abstinence.

Alcoholics Anonymous AA is one of the most widely used alcohol treatment programs, and it is often a component in other treatment programs. Founded in 1935 by two former alcoholics, AA has become the best known of all approaches to problem drinking. The organization follows a very strict version of the disease model and combines it with an emphasis on spirituality that is designed to bring the problem drinker into the group to receive support and mentoring from others who have experienced similar problems.

To adhere to the AA doctrine, a person must maintain total abstinence from alcohol. Part of the AA philosophy is that those who are in need of joining AA can never drink again; problem drinkers are addicted to alcohol and have no power to resist it. According to AA, alcoholics never recover but are always in the process of recovering. They will be alcoholics for life, even if they never take another drink.

AA and other 12-Step programs have attained a high level of acceptance. Each year, over 2 million people in the United States attend a self-help program such as AA for drinking or other substance use problems (SAMHSA, 2014). A majority of those individuals—perhaps as many as 75%—attend AA meetings (Magura, 2007).

The anonymity offered to those who attend AA meetings presents barriers to researchers wishing to conduct studies on the effectiveness of this program, and experimental evidence for the effectiveness of AA is lacking (Ferri, Amato, & Davoli, 2006). This lack of evidence for effectiveness was a major criticism of this approach from a review of treatment programs (CASA Columbia, 2012). The AA format does not allow for experimentation, which would involve randomly assigning participants to attend AA or some other option. However, research has indicated that AA or other support groups (Kelly, Greene, & Bergman, 2016) have the potential for offering supportive alliances between a person in need of support and a sponsor. For attendees for whom this relationship develops, support groups offer a way to replace harmful social connections that may encourage drinking (Kelly, Stout, Magill, & Tonigan, 2011). For others who do not develop such mentoring relationships, the AA 12-Step program approach is not likely to be adequate.

Alternative self-help organizations predate the development of AA and continue to proliferate around the world (White, 2004). Organizations such as Secular Organizations for Sobriety, Women for Sobriety, Self-Management and Recovery Training (SMART Recovery), Rational Recovery, and Moderation Management offer the value of support and group discussions with different philosophies than AA. For example, some do not insist on the goal of lifetime abstinence. Online groups available through the Internet offer easier access, making group support more accessible.

Psychotherapy   Nearly as many psychotherapeutic techniques have been used to treat alcohol abuse as there are psychotherapies, but some are not very effective in helping problem drinkers, whereas other techniques are much more so (CASA Columbia, 2012; Kaner et al., 2007). Many varieties of behavioral therapy exist, and cognitive behavioral therapies tend to be more effective than less directive approaches such as education about alcohol or counseling (CASA Columbia, 2012; Marlatt & Witkiewitz, 2010). Brief interventions are becoming more popular and can also be effective (Kaner et al., 2007). These techniques are designed to change motivation and may last for only a few hours, and this brevity offers advantages.

An example of both a brief intervention and one oriented toward changing motivation is motivational interviewing (Miller & Rollnick, 2002). Therapists using motivational interviewing convey their empathy with the client's situation and help clients resolve their ambivalence about their problem behavior. This process is designed to move clients toward change, making this approach a directive type of psychological intervention. Linking motivational interviewing to the transtheoretical model (see Chapter 4) provides a framework for understanding and promoting behavioral change. Reviews of motivational interviewing (Lundahl, Kunz, Brownell, Tollefson, & Burke, 2010; Rubak, Sanboek, Lauritzen, & Christensen, 2005) have revealed their effectiveness. In addition to the behavioral approaches that can be effective, some chemical treatments can also be useful in controlling problem drinking.

Chemical Treatments   Many treatment programs for problem drinking include administering drugs that reduce the urge to drink. As of 2016, only three drugs have U.S. Food and Drug Administration (FDA) approval for reducing alcohol intake, but other drugs are in the testing phase (Litten, Wilford, Falk, Ryan, & Fertig, 2016). Two of the approved drugs reduce the reward experience of drinking, and the third produces unpleasant symptoms when combined with alcohol.

Naltrexone is a drug that attaches to opiate receptors in the brain and prevents their activation. The drug acamprosate affects the neurotransmitter GABA. Both drugs may be successful in decreasing craving (Mann, 2004) and increase the chances of achieving abstinence (Carmen, Angeles, Ana, & Maria, 2004). A systematic review of studies on naltrexone as a treatment for alcoholism (Rösner et al., 2010) revealed that the effects were modest but positive. Acamprosate's effect is also modest. Both drugs are more useful in preventing relapse than helping people quit, and both are more effective when combined with some behavioral intervention (CASA Columbia, 2012).

Disulfiram (Antabuse) produces a few unpleasant effects when taken alone, but in combination with alcohol, the unpleasant effects are severe—flushing of the face, chest pains, a pounding heart, nausea and vomiting, sweating, headache, dizziness, weakness, difficulty in breathing, and a rapid decrease in blood pressure. The rationale behind the use of these drugs is to produce an aversion to drinking by building up an association between drinking and the unpleasant consequences. This process, called **aversion therapy**, applies to the use of disulfiram as well as other methods that involve aversive conditioning. Getting people to take a drug that will make them sick if they drink is a challenge, and disulfiram is only modestly successful in treating problem drinkers (Krishnan-Sarin, O'Malley, & Krysta, 2008).

Controlled Drinking

Until the late 1960s, all treatments for problem drinking were aimed at total abstinence. Then something quite unexpected happened. In 1962 in London, D. L. Davies found that 7 of the 93 recovered alcoholics whom he studied were able to drink "normally" (defined as consumption of up to 3 pints of beer or its equivalent per day) for at least a 7-year period following treatment. These moderate drinkers represented fewer than 8% of those Davies studied, but this finding was still remarkable because it opened up the possibility that problem drinkers could successfully return to nonproblem drinking. This finding provoked a controversy that continues today.

Prompted by Davies's results, several studies conducted in the United States (Armor, Polich, & Stambul, 1976; Polich, Armor, & Braiker, 1980) showed that controlled drinking occurred in a small percentage of patients who received treatment oriented toward abstinence. Publicity about this study produced a wave of criticism from those holding the position that alcoholics can never drink again, and this controversy became more heated when researchers began to design treatment programs with controlled drinking as the goal.

Problem drinkers can become moderate drinkers. Some problem drinkers in abstinence-oriented treatment programs become moderate drinkers (Miller, Walters, & Bennett, 2001; Sobell, Cunningham, & Sobell, 1996), and some who quit on their own moderate their drinking (Dawson et al., 2005). Despite the evidence concerning controlled drinking, most treatment centers in the United States have resisted the possibility that former problem drinkers can learn to moderate their use of alcohol and stick to the goal of abstinence. This attitude does not extend to other countries; in England, Wales, and Scotland, nearly all treatment centers accept continued drinking among those who have experienced drinking problems. The goal is to reduce the harm that often accompanies drinking rather than eliminate drinking itself (Heather, 2006; Rosenberg & Melville, 2005). In the United States, younger substance abuse professionals have attitudes that are more compatible with a harm reduction approach (Davis & Lauritsen, 2016), so the acceptance of moderated drinking may gain acceptance in this country as it has in others.

The thought of being able to continue drinking is appealing to most drinkers, including those whose drinking is problematic (Kosok, 2006). This appeal is one reason for the creation of a self-help group oriented toward moderating drinking, called Moderation Management. This group includes face-to-face and online meetings, and research on this approach (Hester, Delaney, & Campbell, 2011) showed that both formats can reduce problem drinking.

The Problem of Relapse

Problem drinkers who successfully complete either an abstinence-oriented or a moderation-oriented treatment program do not necessarily maintain their goals. As we saw with smoking, people who complete a treatment program usually improve quite a bit, but the problem of relapse is substantial. Interestingly, the time course and rate of relapse are similar for those who complete treatment programs for smoking, alcohol abuse, or opiate abuse (Hunt, Barnett, & Branch, 1971). Most relapses occur within 90 days after the end of the program. At 12 months after the end of treatment, only about 35% of those completing the programs remain abstinent. These similarities may be attributable to the underlying brain mechanisms involved in habitual drug use, which share some similarities regardless of differences in the pharmacological properties of the drug (Camí & Farré, 2003).

A growing view in treatment holds that alcohol abuse is a chronic illness that requires continuing care (CASA Columbia, 2012; McKay & Hiller-Sturmhöfel, 2010). Thus, treatment programs should include provisions for follow-up care to address relapse. Many inpatient treatment programs make such provisions through the requirement that participants attend AA meetings, which provide a supportive environment that discourages drinking and thus aims to deter relapse (Huebner & Kantor, 2011).

Most behavior-based treatment regimens include training for relapse prevention, taking the view that a relapse occurs in a complex environment with many sources of influence. Understanding those sources and knowing how to cope with their influence is critical; behavior change is not quick or easy (Witkiewitz & Marlatt, 2010). As discussed in Chapter 12, relapse prevention training is aimed at changing cognitions so that the addict comes to believe that one slip does *not* equal total relapse. Programs that focus on long-term goals and incorporate relapse prevention into their regimen tend to have the highest rates of success (McLellan, Lewis, O'Brien, & Kleber, 2000), but if lifetime abstinence is the goal, many relapse prevention programs do not have a high rate of success (Miller, Wilbourne, & Hettema, 2003). However, if the standard is improvement and a lower level of problems caused by drinking, then relapse is not as common; as many as 60% of people who complete a treatment program achieve this level of success.

IN SUMMARY

Despite a decline in the percentage of drinkers in the United States, the number of people seeking help for their drinking problems remains high. Some problem drinkers are able to quit without therapy; others seek treatment programs. Traditional alcohol treatment programs—such as AA, the most widely sought treatment—are oriented toward abstinence. Many problem drinkers are not able to achieve this goal; only about 25% of problem drinkers are abstinent 1 year after treatment. Drinking levels typically drop substantially, however, and so do alcohol-related problems.

Some behavioral programs are successful, including brief interventions such as motivational interviewing and cognitive behavioral therapy; these brief interventions are becoming more common. Chemical treatments such as the drugs naltrexone, acamprosate, and disulfiram have been used to curb alcohol consumption; all show modest levels of success.

Controlled drinking may be a reasonable goal for some problem drinkers. However, this goal is very controversial, and many abstinence-oriented therapists do not consider controlled drinking a viable alternative, but harm reduction has become a more common goal for treatment programs.

With all alcohol treatment approaches, relapse has been a persistent problem. Most relapses occur within 3 months after the end of treatment, and after 12 months, only 25% of those who complete programs are still abstinent. Relapse training has become a common component of both medically oriented and behaviorally oriented programs, but the goal of sustained abstinence is a difficult one.

Other Drugs

Illicit drugs have created many serious problems in the United States, but these problems are mainly social and legal. Other drugs are not the major threat to physical health that alcohol and tobacco use are. Indeed, the effects of smoking cigarettes, drinking alcohol, eating unwisely, and remaining sedentary are responsible for over 60% of deaths in the United States; deaths attributable to illicit drug use account for less than 2% (Kochanek, Xu, Murphy, Miniño, & Kung, 2011). Any death from illicit drugs is unfortunate, but all drug use—even legal drug use—poses risks. Part of that risk comes from alterations of brain function.

Researchers are beginning to understand how drugs function in the brain to alter mood and behavior. Alcohol and other drugs produce effects on neurotransmitters, the chemical basis of neural transmission. Several neurotransmitters are involved in drug actions, including GABA, glutamate, serotonin, and norepinephrine (López-Moreno, González-Cuevas, Moreno, & Navarro, 2008), but the neurotransmitter **dopamine** is especially important (Young, Gobrogge, & Wang, 2011). Dopamine may be the most important neurotransmitter in a brain subsystem that relays messages from the ventral tegmental area in the midbrain to the nucleus accumbens in the forebrain. Researchers have known for years that this area is involved in the brain's experience of reward and pleasure. However, the actions of many drugs seem to be common to the same system, not only in these two brain structures but also in the hippocampus, amygdala, and forebrain (López-Moreno et al., 2008). That is, drugs seem to activate the brain circuits that underlie reward. Indeed, experiences such as gambling may activate the same brain mechanisms (Martin & Petry, 2005).

All psychoactive drugs do not act in the same way in this subsystem, but all affect the availability of neurotransmitters, especially dopamine. Alterations of these neurotransmitters produce temporary changes in brain chemistry but rarely damage neurons. Changing the brain's chemistry carries risks, but brain damage is not a health effect associated with most drugs (see Would You Believe …? box).

Would You BELIEVE...?   Brain Damage Is Not a Common Risk of Drug Use

Despite the vivid media images of a brain "fried" by drug use, most psychoactive drugs do not cause damage to neurons. Indeed, some of the drugs that can most wreck a person's life are among the *least* likely to damage the brain. For example, opiate drugs such as heroin, morphine, oxycodone, and hydrocodone produce both tolerance and dependence. Repeated use of these drugs results in compulsive drug taking and a pattern of use in which social relationships and responsibilities become unimportant. People who are dependent on opiate drugs usually experience major problems, but brain damage is not among them.

Like other psychoactive drugs, opiates cross the blood–brain barrier, where they occupy receptors for endorphins, the body's own analgesics (Advokat, Comaty, & Julien, 2014). Thus, these drugs are compatible with the brain's existing neurochemistry; they occupy these receptors without causing damage. Their repeated use produces a host of physiological effects, some of which can be very dangerous, but damage to the nervous system is unlikely.

Marijuana also acts by occupying brain receptors for neurochemicals called endocannabinoids (Pope, Mechoulam, & Parsons, 2010). The discovery of these neurochemicals suggested that the brain makes its own marijuana-like chemicals and also explained some of the actions that marijuana takes in the brain. Marijuana also produces a wide variety of physiological and behavioral effects, some of which may be dangerous. However, those effects do not include damage to neurons in the brain. Indeed, recent research (Pope et al., 2010) has suggested that endocannabinoids may exert protective effects in the nervous system.

Both publicity and public service announcements have decried the dangers of the drug Ecstasy, but the research that formed the basis for these claims was withdrawn by the researcher because of inaccuracies (Holden, 2003). Use of Ecstasy may not pose the risk to life that some feared (Cole, 2014), but the drug is not without dangers (Halpern et al., 2011). However, the only evidence that implicates this drug in neural damage comes from combinations with alcohol or stimulants, and then only as a possibility (Gouzoulis-Mayfrank & Daumann, 2006).

However, some drugs do carry risks of damage to the nervous system. Those risks typically occur with heavy, long-term use to those who fit into the category of abusers. For example, the potential for brain damage as a result of extended alcohol abuse is well known (Harper & Matsumoto, 2005). Some evidence has also suggested that the abuse of stimulants such as cocaine (Rosenberg, Grigsby, Dreisbach, Busenbark, & Grigsby, 2002) and amphetamines (Chang et al., 2002) produces toxic neurological effects. The evidence for brain damage from the use of household solvents is strong (Rosenberg et al., 2002). These chemicals act to alter consciousness not through changes to neurotransmitters but through oxygen restriction to the brain, so, of course, these substances cause brain damage.

The greatest risks from drug use are not neurological damage but rather the ability of these drugs to alter perception, decision-making, and coordination. These effects increase the risk for unintentional injuries, which are a far more likely result than brain damage.

Health Effects

Even though most drugs do not damage neurons, both legal and illegal drugs pose potential health hazards. However, illegal drugs present certain risks not found with legal drugs, regardless of pharmacological effects. Illegal drugs may be sold as one drug when they are actually another, buyers have no assurance as to dosage, and illegally manufactured drugs may have impurities that can be dangerous chemicals themselves. In addition, the sources of illegal drugs can be dangerous people. Legal drugs are free from these risks, but they are not harmless and not always safe.

All drugs have potential hazards, but drugs termed *safe* are tested by the U.S. FDA and defined as safe when potential benefits outweigh potential hazards. Many drugs, such as antibiotics, have been approved although they produce severe side effects in some people. The more potentially beneficial a drug is, the more likely it is to be labeled *safe* despite unpleasant or even dangerous side effects.

The FDA classifies drugs into five categories, based on their potential for abuse and their potential medical benefits. Table 13.3 summarizes this schedule, presents the restrictions on availability, and gives examples of drugs in each category. This classification has evolved somewhat haphazardly over more than 100 years and represents legislative and social convention rather than scientific findings.

A classification of drugs based on the action of the drugs is more useful than a classification based on legal availability. A classification according to the effects of

the drugs would have major sections for sedatives, stimulants, hallucinogens, marijuana, and anabolic steroids. **Sedatives** are drugs that induce relaxation and sometimes intoxication by lowering the activity of the brain, neurons, muscles, and heart, and even by slowing the metabolic rate (Advokat et al., 2014). The types of drugs classified as sedatives include barbiturates, tranquilizers, opiates, and alcohol. In low doses, these drugs tend to make people feel relaxed and even euphoric. In high doses, they cause loss of consciousness and can produce coma and death as a result of their inhibitory effect on the brain center that controls respiration. These risks represent the most common hazards of sedative use. Table 13.4 shows the types of drugs that fit into this category, their effects, and their risks.

Stimulants are another main category of psychoactive drugs. All drugs in the stimulant category tend to produce alertness, reduce feelings of fatigue, elevate mood, and decrease appetite. Stimulant drugs include caffeine, nicotine, amphetamines, and cocaine. Caffeine, found in coffee, tea, and many types of sodas, is so widely consumed that many people do not think of it as a drug, but it produces the effects typical of stimulant drugs. **Amphetamines** are a class of powerful stimulant drug that includes methamphetamines and crystal methamphetamine that are often abused because of their mood-altering effects. Another stimulant drug, **cocaine**, is extracted from the coca plant. Cocaine is sold in powder form and as crack cocaine, which can be smoked. Using cocaine in combination with alcohol enhances the dangers of each drug by producing a third chemical, *cocaethylene* (Hearn et al., 1991;

TABLE 13.3   FDA Drug Schedules, Restrictions, and Examples of Drugs in Each Category

Schedule	Description	Restriction on Availability	Examples
I	High abuse potential; no medical uses	Not legally available under U.S. federal law	LSD, marijuana, heroin
II	High abuse potential but with medical uses	Prescription only	Morphine, oxycontin, barbiturates, amphetamines, cocaine
III	Moderate or low dependence; medical uses	Prescription only	Codeine, some tranquilizers
IV	Low dependence, low abuse potential; medical uses	Prescription only	Phenobarbital, most tranquilizers
V	Less abuse potential than drugs in Schedule IV	Over the counter	Aspirin, antacids, antihistamines, and others

TABLE 13.4 Summary of Characteristics of Psychoactive Drugs

Name	Tolerance	Dependence	Effects	Risks
Sedatives/Depressants				
Barbiturates	Yes	Yes	Relaxes, intoxicates	Unconsciousness, coma, death
Tranquilizers	Yes	Yes	Relaxes, intoxicates	Altered judgment, impaired coordination, coma
Opiates Opium derivatives, oxycodone, hydrocodone	Yes	Yes	Produces analgesia, euphoria, sedation	Coma, respiratory arrest, death
Alcohol	Yes	Yes	Relaxes, intoxicates	Impaired judgment and coordination, unconsciousness
Stimulants				
Caffeine	Yes	Yes	Increased alertness, reduced fatigue	Increased nervousness
Cocaine	Yes	Yes	Euphoria, suppressed appetite	Heart arrhythmia, heart attack
Amphetamines (Methamphetamine, crystal meth)	Yes	Yes	Produces alertness, reduces fatigue	Heart attack, feelings of paranoia, increased violence
Nicotine (Tobacco products)	Yes	Yes	Increases alertness, decreases appetite, elevates blood pressure	Increased heart disease and cancer
Hallucinogens				
Ecstasy (MDMA)	No	No	Produces feelings of well-being	Temperature regulation problems
LSD	No	No	Produces perceptual distortions, intoxicates	Altered perception and judgment
Marijuana				
Marijuana	No	Yes	Relaxes, intoxicates	Impaired judgment, coordination, respiratory problems (if smoked)
Steroids				
Anabolic steroids	Yes	No	Builds muscles, increases blood pressure, reduces immune system functioning	Testicular atrophy, increased aggression, lowered immune function

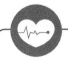

Becoming Healthier

1. Avoid binge drinking—that is, drinking five or more drinks on any one occasion. There are no health benefits associated with binge drinking, and there are many risks.

2. Avoiding alcohol may not be the healthiest choice for middle-aged and older individuals, but if you do not drink and are comfortable with that choice, do not start drinking. If you are younger than 40, drinking is not likely to confer health benefits.

3. Occasional drinking—either light or heavy—presents some risks but does not convey many benefits. The pattern that confers the most benefits is daily (or almost daily) light drinking.

4. One or two drinks per day can impair judgment and coordination. These dangers are the biggest risk of alcohol consumption, and people who drink should find ways to manage this risk.

5. Do not drive, operate machinery, or swim after drinking.

6. Do not escalate your drinking; keep to one or two drinks per day (not an average of one or two).

7. The safest level of alcohol for pregnant women is none.

8. If one or both of your parents experienced drinking problems, you may be at elevated risk. Manage this risk by moderating your drinking or by not drinking.

9. If you have an extremely pleasant experience with any drug (including alcohol) the first time you try it, be aware that future use of this drug may present problems for you.

10. Don't combine drugs; drugs in combination are more dangerous than taking one drug.

11. Drugs that produce dependence are more dangerous than those that do not. Even if you have a prescription, be aware and cautious about using alcohol and nicotine as well as opiates, barbiturates, and amphetamines.

12. Illegal drugs, even those without tolerance or dependence potential, can be dangerous because they are illegal.

Herbst et al., 2011). This chemical is hazardous (Huq, 2007) and may boost the user's risk for cardiac problems (Tacker & Okorodudu, 2004). Table 13.4 also summarizes these drugs and their characteristics.

Methylenedioxymethamphetamine (MDMA)—Ecstasy—is a derivative of methamphetamine, but people use it for its mild hallucinogenic effects, including feelings of peace and empathy with others. These feelings come from a massive release of the neurotransmitter *serotonin*, which depletes the supply of serotonin, but this depletion tends to be temporary (Buchert et al., 2004). Other hallucinogenic drugs such as lysergic acid diethylamide (LSD), mescaline, and psilocybin exert more complex effects on neurotransmitters, but serotonin is also involved in the effects of these drugs (Halberstadt & Geyer, 2011).

Marijuana has some hallucinogenic properties but lacks most other characteristics of hallucinogens. The intoxicating ingredient in marijuana, delta-9-tetrahydrocannabinol (THC), comes from the resin of the *Cannabis sativa* plant. The brain contains receptors for cannabinoids in many locations, which results in a variety of effects from ingesting marijuana, including altered thought processes, memory impairment, feelings of relaxation and euphoria, increased appetite, and impaired coordination (Nicoll & Alger, 2004). Its potential for serious health consequences is still debated, but so are its medical benefits. A growing body of evidence supports a variety of medical benefits of marijuana (Koppel et al., 2014), and growing public acceptance has resulted in an increasing number of states passing "medical marijuana" laws that allow access to marijuana for those who have a prescription. However, like all drug use, marijuana use poses risks. Its effects on cognition, judgment, and coordination boost the risk of unintentional injuries. In addition, users who smoke marijuana face increased risks for respiratory problems and possibly even lung cancer (Joshi, Joshi, & Bartter, 2014).

Anabolic steroids (ASs) are synthetic hormones used to enhance athletic performance (King & Pace, 2005). The effects of anabolic steroids include thickening of the vocal cords, enlargement of the larynx, increase of muscle bulk, and decrease of body fat. These last two properties make ASs attractive to athletes, bodybuilders, and people who wish to alter their

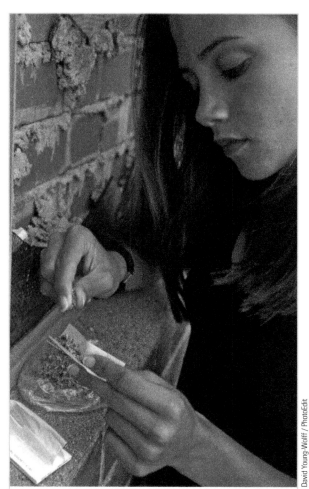

Marijuana is the most commonly used illicit drug, with higher use among adolescents and young adults.

David Young-Wolff / PhotoEdit

appearance. Unfortunately, use of anabolic steroids can upset the chemical balance in the body, produce toxicity, and shut off the body's production of its own steroids, leaving the person more susceptible to stress and infection and altering reproductive functioning. In addition, behavioral problems include aggression, euphoria, mood swings, distractibility, and confusion. Table 13.4 presents a summary of anabolic steroids and other psychoactive drug characteristics.

How common is the use of these illicit drugs? Is drug use increasing or decreasing? Illicit drug use in the United States has varied over the past 40 years, reaching a peak in the late 1970s, followed by a decline in the 1980s (Johnston et al., 2015). Another increase occurred in the early 1990s and another decrease in the late 1990s. This overall pattern is similar across age groups, but levels of use are not: Young people use illicit drugs more often than older people. Indeed, trends in drug use among high school students often predict societal drug use several years later.

Illicit drug use has varied little overall within the past decade, with fluctuations from year to year and from drug to drug (SAMHSA, 2015). (The use of alcohol and nicotine has also varied, but the percentage of people who use these legal drugs is higher than those who use illicit drugs.) Marijuana remains the most commonly used illicit drug, with levels of use far above any other type of illicit drug. The next most commonly used classification is the nonmedical use of therapeutic drugs such as painkillers (oxycontin, hydrocodone), stimulants (methamphetamines), tranquilizers, and sedatives. Cocaine use has not increased over the past 10 years, but cocaine remains one of the most commonly used illicit drugs. Ecstasy use has not increased. As Table 13.5 shows, the level of use of these drugs is much lower than marijuana use. Although these percentages represent occasional use by some people, some people misuse and others abuse these drugs.

Drug Misuse and Abuse

Most people believe that some drugs are acceptable and even desirable because of the medical benefits they confer. But all *psychoactive* drugs—drugs that cross the blood–brain barrier and alter mental functioning—pose potential health risks. Most have the capacity for tolerance or dependence (see Table 13.4). Even drugs that are not psychoactive have the potential for unpleasant side effects. For example, penicillin can cause nausea, vomiting, diarrhea, swelling, and skin eruptions. In addition, people who have allergies to penicillin can die from ingesting it. Caffeine, a drug commonly found in coffee and cola drinks, also creates dependence. A review of studies on caffeine withdrawal (Juliano & Griffiths, 2004) confirmed that people who habitually consume caffeine experience withdrawal symptoms that include headache, difficulty concentrating, and depressed mood. These risks are less serious than the substance use disorders listed in *DSM-5* (American Psychiatric Association, 2013), but all drug use carries some risks.

Almost all drugs that have potential medical or health benefits also have the potential for misuse and abuse. The moderate use of alcohol, for instance, is related to decreased cardiovascular mortality. The *misuse* of alcohol—defined as inappropriate but not

TABLE 13.5   Lifetime, Past Year, and Past Month Use of Various Drugs, Including Nonmedical Use of Legal Drugs, Persons Aged 12 Years and Older, United States, 2014

Drug	Lifetime Use (%)	Use During Past Year (%)	Use During Past Month (%)
Alcohol	82.1	66.6	52.7
Cigarettes	61.0	24.8	20.8
Smokeless tobacco	17.1	4.4	3.3
Sedatives	3.0	0.3	0.1
Tranquilizers	9.4	2.0	0.7
Heroin	1.8	0.3	0.2
Pain relievers	13.6	3.9	1.6
Stimulants	8.5	1.4	0.6
Cocaine	14.8	1.7	0.6
Crack cocaine	3.6	0.3	0.1
Marijuana	44.2	13.2	8.4
LSD	9.4	0.5	0.1
Ecstasy	6.6	0.9	0.2

Source: *Results from the 2014 National Survey on Drug Use and Health: Detailed Tables*, by Substance Abuse and Mental Health Services Administration, 2015, Tables 1.1B and 2.1B. Retrieved July 24, 2016, from http://www.samhsa.gov/data/sites/default/files/NSDUH-DetTabs2014/NSDUH-DetTabs2014.pdf.

health-threatening levels of consumption—can result in social embarrassment, violent acts, and injury. And abuse of alcohol—defined as frequent, heavy consumption to the point of addiction—can lead to cirrhosis, brain damage, heart attack, and fetal alcohol syndrome.

Not all individuals who use drugs or alcohol are equally likely to become abusers. Genetic and situational factors contribute to the risks of substance abuse, but another major risk is the presence of psychopathology. Individuals with schizophrenia and bipolar disorder who use illicit drugs tend to have more severe symptoms and to respond more poorly to treatment than individuals with the same disorders who do not use illicit drugs (Ringen et al., 2008).

Treatment for Drug Abuse

Treatment for the use and abuse of illegal drugs is similar to the treatment of alcohol abuse, both in the philosophy and in the administration of treatment (Schuckit, 2000). In the United States and many other countries, the goal of treatment for all types of illegal drug use is total abstinence. In many cases, the programs that treat drug abusers coexist physically (as well as philosophically) with treatment programs for alcohol abuse, and patients who are receiving treatment for their drug problems participate in the same therapy as those who

are receiving therapy for their alcohol problems. The philosophy that guides AA led to the development of Narcotics Anonymous, an organization devoted to helping drug users abstain from using drugs. Self-help groups are common components in treating drug abuse, as they are in dealing with alcohol abuse (Margolis & Zweben, 2011).

The reasons for entering drug abuse treatment programs are often similar to those for entering treatment for alcohol abuse, and those reasons are primarily social. The abuse of illegal drugs leads to legal, financial, and interpersonal problems, just as alcohol abuse does. Like alcohol, most illegal drugs produce impairments of judgment that lead to unintentional injury and death, making such injury the leading health risk from drug abuse. The abuse of most illegal drugs does not produce as many direct health hazards as alcohol abuse. However, when health problems occur, they are likely to be major and life threatening. Such crises may precipitate a person's decision to seek treatment or lead family members to enforce treatment. Charlie Sheen has been in treatment for his drug abuse several times, but his father was instrumental in that treatment ("Martin Sheen," 2008). His several stays in inpatient treatment facilities were typical of such facilities in the United States—their goal is complete abstinence, and its philosophy is the same as AA's.

Inpatient treatment programs for drug abuse differ from programs for alcohol abuse in several minor ways. The detoxification phase of inpatient hospitalization is typically shorter and less severe for most types of drug use than it is for alcohol, for which withdrawal can be life threatening. Alcohol is a depressant drug, as are barbiturates, tranquilizers, and opiates. Therefore, all these drugs have similar symptoms during withdrawal, including agitation, tremor, gastric distress, and possibly perceptual distortions (Advokat et al., 2014). Stimulants such as amphetamines and cocaine produce different withdrawal symptoms—namely, lethargy and depression. These differences necessitate different medical care during detoxification.

After detoxification, additional care is important for success. Frequently, this continued care comes from joining a support group such as Narcotics Anonymous. Getting substance abusers to attend such groups is a challenge, and the low rate of success for such interventions is a problem. Other interventions show better results. A meta-analysis of psychosocial interventions (Dutra et al., 2008) identified several types as effective, including contingency management and cognitive behavioral therapy. Such interventions were most effective for people who used marijuana and least effective for those who abused several substances. Unfortunately, relapse prevention interventions were not among the more effective programs.

One similarity between drug and alcohol abuse treatment is the high rate of relapse. As noted earlier, alcohol, smoking, and opiate treatment all share a high rate of relapse (Hunt et al., 1971), and the first 6 months after treatment are critical. Recognizing substance abuse as a chronic problem is important to changes that will improve effectiveness (CASA Columbia, 2012). A one-size-fits-all approach may not be successful for relapse prevention because people relapse for different reasons (Zywiak et al., 2006). Some people are provoked to relapse by negative feelings, and others cannot withstand cravings, whereas others succumb to social pressure from their drug-using friends. Addressing individual concerns and weaknesses through interventions that are specific to individuals may improve the situation.

Charlie Sheen provides an excellent example of the problem of relapse. He experienced trouble staying in treatment, and after completing the program, he relapsed several times. His behavior in early 2011 was a dramatic example of relapse and resisting treatment for an obvious problem ("Charlie Sheen," 2011). Sheen's 2016 rehab may have been successful (*People*, 2016).

Preventing and Controlling Drug Use

Chapter 12 presented information on attempts to decrease smoking in children and adolescents by various interventions aimed at discouraging their experimentation with cigarettes and smokeless tobacco. Similar efforts have been applied to the use of alcohol and other drugs (Botvin & Griffin, 2015; Lemstra et al., 2010; Roe & Becker, 2005; Soole, Mazerolle, & Rombouts, 2008). The prevention attempts aimed at keeping children and adolescents from experimenting with drugs are intended to delay or inhibit the initiation of drug use. As with efforts to prevent smoking (see Chapter 12), those aimed at preventing drug use do not have an impressive success rate. Programs that rely on scare tactics, moral training, factual information about drug risks, and boosting self-esteem are generally ineffective. For example, the popular Drug Abuse Resistance Education (DARE) program has minimal effects (West & O'Neal, 2004).

However, some types of prevention programs are more effective than others. The Life Skills Training program (Botvin & Griffin, 2015) has demonstrated both short-term and long-term effectiveness. This program teaches social skills, both to resist social pressure to use drugs and to enhance decision-making skills as well as social and personal competence. In addition, some evidence (Springer et al., 2004) indicates that prevention programs that are tailored to be culturally compatible with the targeted groups are more effective than more general programs. Systematic reviews of prevention programs (Lemstra et al., 2010; Roe & Becker, 2005; Soole et al., 2008) have indicated that school programs that are interactive, intensive, and focus on life skills are more effective than programs that lack these components. Aiming prevention efforts at children aged between 11 and 13 is most effective, but programs aimed at children and adolescents are not the only approach to controlling drug use.

A more common control technique is to limit availability. This strategy is common in all Western countries through laws that limit legal access to drugs. However, legal restriction of drugs has a number of side effects, some of which create other social problems (Robins, 1995). For example, when the United States legally prohibited the manufacture and sale of alcohol, illegal manufacture and distribution flourished, creating a large criminal enterprise, huge profits, loss of tax revenue, and corruption among law enforcement agencies. Thus, limiting availability has negative as well as positive consequences, and the extent to which this approach should be continued is a controversy currently applicable to the availability of marijuana.

Another strategy is control of the harm of drug use. This strategy assumes that people will use psychoactive drugs, sometimes unwisely, but that reducing the health consequences of drug use should be the first priority (Heather, 2006; O'Hare, 2007; Peele, 2002). Rather than taking a moralistic stand on drug use, this strategy takes a practical approach to minimizing the dangers of drug use. An example of the *harm reduction strategy* is helping injection drug users exchange used needles for sterile ones, thus slowing the spread of HIV infection. Another example is encouraging the designated driver approach to avoiding vehicle injuries. The controversy surrounding such programs is representative of the debate over the harm reduction strategy. However, a systematic review of harm reduction (Ritter & Cameron, 2006) concluded that the evidence indicates that this approach should be adopted as a policy for illicit drugs. Furthermore, some experts in the field (Lee, Engstrom, & Petersen, 2011) have contended that the approaches

oriented toward abstinence are not as incompatible with harm reduction as the controversy suggests. Both approaches may have a place in controlling drug use.

IN SUMMARY

Abuse of alcohol is a serious health problem in most developed nations, but other drugs—including depressants, stimulants, hallucinogens, marijuana, and anabolic steroids—are also potentially harmful to health. Although abuse of these drugs often leads to a number of personal and social problems, their consumption levels are lower and thus health risks are much less than those associated with cigarettes or alcohol. Treatments for drug abuse are similar to those for alcohol abuse, and programs aimed at prevention are similar to those aimed at preventing smoking. A strategy of *harm reduction* aims at decreasing the social and health risks of taking drugs by changing treatment goals and drug policies.

Answers

This chapter has addressed six basic questions:

1. What are the major trends in alcohol consumption?

People have consumed alcohol worldwide since before recorded history. Alcohol consumption in the United States reached a peak during the early 1800s, dropped sharply during the mid-1800s as a result of the "temperance" movement, and continued at a steady rate until a sharp decline during Prohibition. Currently, rates of alcohol consumption in the United States are holding steady after a period of slow decline. About two-thirds of adults drink; half are classified as current, regular drinkers, including 23% as binge drinkers and 7% as heavy drinkers. Adult European Americans have higher rates of drinking than members of other ethnic groups, but the patterns of alcohol consumption vary in countries around the world.

2. What are the health effects of drinking alcohol?

Drinking has both positive and negative health effects. Prolonged heavy drinking of alcohol often

leads to cirrhosis of the liver and other serious health problems, such as heart disease and brain dysfunction. Moderate drinking may have certain long-range health benefits, including reduced heart disease and lowered probability of developing gallstones, Type 2 diabetes, and Alzheimer's disease, but these advantages apply to middle-aged and older individuals who maintain a light level of drinking. Younger people experience no health benefits from alcohol intake. Overall, the risks of alcohol outweigh the benefits.

3. Why do people drink?

Models for drinking behavior should explain why people begin drinking, why some can drink in moderation, and why others drink to excess. The disease model assumes that people drink excessively because they have the disease of alcoholism. Cognitive-physiological models, including the tension reduction hypothesis and alcohol myopia, propose that people drink because alcohol allows them to escape tension and negative self-evaluations. Social learning theory proposes that people acquire drinking behavior through positive or negative reinforcement, modeling, and cognitive mediation. Research evidence supports a genetic component to problem drinking, which interacts with social and individual factors to push individuals toward abstinence, moderate, or problem drinking.

4. **How can people change problem drinking?**

Some problem drinkers seem to be able to quit without therapy, and treatment programs are moderately effective in helping people who do not succeed in quitting on their own. In the United States and many other countries, most treatment programs are oriented toward abstinence, which is a difficult criterion to attain. Alcoholics Anonymous is the most popular but not the most effective treatment program. Brief interventions oriented toward enhancing motivation, such as motivational interviewing, and cognitive behavioral interventions are more effective. Pharmacological treatments such as naltrexone, acamprosate, and disulfiram can also be useful components in a treatment program and are more effective when combined with behavioral techniques. The goal of harm reduction rather than abstinence is becoming a more accepted goal of treatment.

5. **What problems are associated with relapse?**

Relapse is common among heavy drinkers who have quit, although many are able to maintain abstinence or to decrease their alcohol intake. Most relapses occur during the first 3 months after quitting. After a year, about 65% of all successful quitters have resumed drinking, some in a harmful manner. The knowledge of frequent relapse has led to the creation of follow-up relapse prevention treatment and the growing opinion that problem drinking should be considered a chronic condition.

6. **What are the health effects of other drugs?**

Other drugs—including depressants, stimulants, hallucinogens, marijuana, and anabolic steroids—have had some medical use, but they are also potentially harmful to health. The principal problems from most of these drugs are social, but the use of any drug brings physical risks, which may include coma, heart attack, or respiratory failure. Treatments for drug abuse are similar to those for alcohol abuse, and programs aimed at prevention are similar to those aimed at preventing smoking.

Suggested Readings

Botvin, G. J., & Griffin, K. W. (2015). Life Skills Training: A competence enhancement approach to tobacco, alcohol, and drug abuse prevention. In L. M. Scheier (Ed.), *Handbook of adolescent drug use prevention: Research, intervention strategies, and practice* (pp. 177–196). Washington, DC: American Psychological Association. This chapter summarizes the components of one successful prevention program and the evidence for its effectiveness.

Heather, N. (2006). Controlled drinking, harm reduction and their roles in the response to alcohol-related problems. *Addiction Research and Theory, 14*, 7–18. Heather discusses the controlled drinking controversy, presenting the difference between the harm reduction approach that is common in Europe and the strategy of decreasing drug/alcohol use to a controlled level.

Lee, P. R., Lee, D. R., Lee, P., & Arch, M. (2010). 2010: U.S. drug and alcohol policy, looking back and moving forward. *Journal of Psychoactive Drugs, 42*(2), 99–114. This article provides an examination of the history of drug and alcohol policy that can lead to an understanding of U.S. laws and policies that govern alcohol and drugs. The efforts to control these substances and the treatment options and their availability are also included.

Nestler, E. J., & Malenka, R. C. (2004, March). The addicted brain. *Scientific American, 290*, 78–85. This article details the brain mechanisms that underlie reward and addiction, pointing out the commonalities among all compulsive drug use.

Rehm, J., Baliunas, D., Borges, G. L. G., Graham, K., Irving, H., Kehoe, T., ... Taylor, B. (2010). The relation between different dimensions of alcohol consumption and burden of disease: An overview. *Addiction, 105*(5), 817–843. This review presents a comprehensive view of the harm that alcohol does in creating disease, including an examination of the pathways through which alcohol creates disease and the patterns of drinking that are most dangerous.

Eating and Weight

CHAPTER OUTLINE

QUESTIONS

This chapter focuses on six basic questions:

1. How does the digestive system function?
2. What factors are involved in weight maintenance?
3. What is obesity, and how does it affect health?
4. Is dieting a good way to lose weight?
5. What is anorexia nervosa, and how can it be treated?
6. What is bulimia, and how does it differ from binge eating?

☑ Check Your **HEALTH RISKS** *Regarding Eating and Controlling Your Weight*

☐ 1. I feel comfortable with my present weight.

☐ 2. Although I don't eat much, I stay heavier than I would like.

☐ 3. I have lost 15 pounds or more over the past 2 years.

☐ 4. I have gained 15 pounds or more over the past 2 years.

☐ 5. I am more than 30 pounds overweight.

☐ 6. My weight has fluctuated about 5 or 10 pounds during the past 2 years, but I'm not concerned about it.

☐ 7. If I were thinner, I would be happier.

☐ 8. My waist is as big as or bigger than my hips.

☐ 9. I have been on at least 10 different diet programs in my life.

☐ 10. I have fasted, used laxatives, or used diet drugs to lose weight.

☐ 11. My family has been concerned that I am too thin, but I disagree.

☐ 12. A coach, instructor, or trainer has suggested that weighing less could improve my athletic performance.

☐ 13. I sometimes lose control over eating and eat far more than I planned.

☐ 14. I would like to have liposuction or gastric bypass surgery to lose weight.

☐ 15. I have vomited after eating as a way to control my weight.

☐ 16. Food is a danger that can be managed by careful thought and mental preparation in order not to eat too much.

Items 1 and 6 reflect a healthy attitude toward weight, but each of the other items represents a health risk from unhealthy eating or attitudes concerning eating. Unhealthy eating not only relates to the development of several diseases but also preoccupation with weight and frequent dieting can be unhealthy.

Real-World Profile of **DANNY CAHILL**

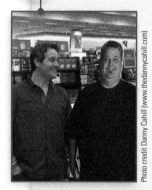

Photo credit Danny Cahill (www.thedannycahill.com)

Danny Cahill was the biggest loser of the eighth season of the television show *The Biggest Loser*. Danny weighed 430 pounds when he began the competition and ended at 191; he had lost more weight than any other contestant in the program's history (Kolata, 2016). But over the next several years, he gained back 100 pounds, and other contestants also admitted that they had not maintained the lower weight that they attained during their time on the show.

This situation prompted obesity researcher Kevin Hall and his colleagues to study as many of the contestants as they could (Fothergill et al., 2016). Hall enlisted these contestants in a 6-year study to track their weight as well as their metabolic rate. Years ago, researchers had established that weight loss is accompanied by a slowing of the metabolic rate, but Hall and his colleagues want to determine how much time was necessary for dieters' metabolism to return to normal. The results surprised them: Dieters' metabolic rate remained slow, even after years. That slow metabolic rate is certainly a factor in the weight gain that happened to so many contestants—and to millions of other dieters.

This chapter examines in detail the four major problems of eating—overeating and dieting, anorexia nervosa, bulimia, and binge eating—each related to difficulties in weight maintenance. To put these in context, we first consider the organs and functions of the digestive system.

The Digestive System

The human body can digest a wide variety of plant and animal tissues, converting these foods into usable proteins, fats, carbohydrates, vitamins, and minerals. The digestive system takes in food, processes it into particles that can be absorbed, and excretes the undigested wastes. The particles that are absorbed through the digestive system are transported through the bloodstream so as to be available to all body cells. These molecules nourish the body by providing the energy for activity as well as the materials for body growth, maintenance, and repair.

The digestive tract is a modified tube, consisting of a number of specialized structures. Also included in the digestive system are several accessory structures connected to the digestive tract by ducts. These ducted glands produce substances that are essential for digestion, and the ducts provide a way for these substances to enter the digestive system. Figure 14.1 shows the digestive system.

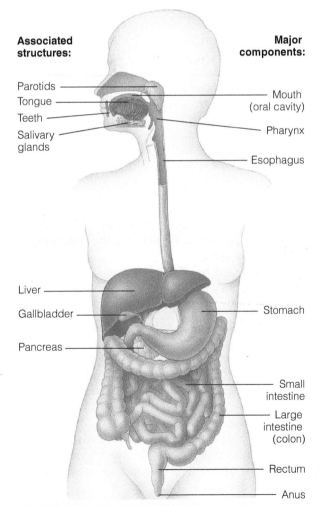

Associated structures:
- Parotids
- Tongue
- Teeth
- Salivary glands
- Liver
- Gallbladder
- Pancreas

Major components:
- Mouth (oral cavity)
- Pharynx
- Esophagus
- Stomach
- Small intestine
- Large intestine (colon)
- Rectum
- Anus

FIGURE 14.1   The digestive system.

Source: Introduction to microbiology (p. 556), by J. L. Ingraham & C. A. Ingraham. From INGRAHAM/INGRAHAM, *Introduction to Microbiology*, 1E. © 1995 Cengage Learning.

In humans and other mammals, some digestion begins in the mouth. The teeth tear and grind food, mixing it with saliva. Several **salivary glands** furnish the moisture that allows the food to be tasted. Without such moisture, the taste buds on the tongue do not function. Saliva also contains an enzyme that digests starch, so some digestion actively begins before food particles leave the mouth.

Swallowing is a voluntary action, but once food is swallowed, its progress through the **pharynx** and **esophagus** is largely involuntary. **Peristalsis,** the rhythmic contraction and relaxation of the circular muscles of structures in the digestive system, propels food through the digestive system, beginning with the esophagus. In the stomach, rhythmic contractions mix the food with **gastric juices** secreted by the stomach and the glands that empty into the stomach. Little absorption of nutrients occurs in the stomach; only alcohol, aspirin, and some fat-soluble drugs are absorbed through the stomach lining. The major function of the stomach is to mix food particles with gastric juices, preparing the mixture for absorption in the small intestine.

The mixture of food particles and gastric juices moves into the small intestine a little at a time. The high acidity of the gastric juices results in a very acidic mixture, and the small intestine cannot function in high acidity. To reduce the level of acidity, the pancreas secretes several acid-reducing enzymes into the small intestine. These **pancreatic juices** are also essential for digesting carbohydrates and fats.

The digestion of starch that begins in the mouth is completed in the small intestine. The upper third of the small intestine absorbs starch and other carbohydrates. Protein digestion, initiated in the stomach, is also completed when proteins are absorbed in the upper portion of the small intestine. Fats, however, enter the small intestine almost entirely undigested. **Bile salts** produced in the **liver** and stored in the **gall bladder** break down fat molecules into a form that is acted on by a pancreatic enzyme. Absorption of fats occurs in the middle third of the small intestine. The bile salts that aid the process are reabsorbed later in the lower third of the small intestine.

Large quantities of water pass through the small intestine. In addition to the water that people drink, digestive juices increase the fluid volume. Of all the water that passes into the small intestine, 90% is absorbed. This absorption process also causes vitamins and electrolytes to pass into the body at this point in digestion.

From the small intestine, digestion proceeds to the large intestine. As with other portions of the digestive system, movement through the large intestine occurs through peristalsis. However, the peristaltic movement in the large intestine is more sluggish and irregular than in the small intestine. Bacteria inhabit the large intestine and manufacture several vitamins. Although the large intestine has absorptive capabilities, it typically absorbs only water, a few minerals, and the vitamins manufactured by its bacteria.

Feces consist of the materials left after digestion has taken place. Feces are composed of undigested fiber, inorganic material, undigested nutrients, water, and bacteria. Peristalsis carries the feces through the large intestine, through the **rectum**, and finally through the **anus**, where they are eliminated.

In summary, the digestive system turns food into nutrients by a process that begins in the mouth with the breakdown of food into smaller particles. Digestive juices continue to act on food particles in the stomach, but digestion of most types of nutrients occurs in the small intestine. Digestion is completed with the elimination of the undigested residue. The digestive system is plagued by more diseases and disorders than any other body system. Many digestive disorders are not of active concern to health psychology, but several, such as obesity, anorexia nervosa, bulimia, and binge eating, have important behavioral components. In addition, maintaining a stable weight depends on behaviors—eating and activity.

Factors in Weight Maintenance

Stable weight occurs when the calories absorbed from food equal those expended for body metabolism plus physical activity. This balance is not a simple calculation but, rather, the result of a complex set of actions and interactions. Caloric content varies with foods; fat has more calories per volume than carbohydrates or proteins. The degree of absorption depends on how rapidly food passes through the digestive system and even the nutrient composition of the foods. Furthermore, metabolic rates can differ from person to person and from time to time, as Danny Cahill's has done. Activity level is another source of variability, with greater activity requiring greater caloric expenditures.

To obtain calories, people (and other animals) eat. Eating and weight balance have regulating components in the nervous system. A variety of hormones and neurotransmitters form a short-term and a long-term regulation system (Blundell, Gibbons, Caudwell, Finlayson, & Hopkins, 2015). **Leptin**, a protein hormone discovered in 1994, is produced by white adipose tissue (fat) and acts on receptors in the central nervous system as part of a signaling system involved in the long-term regulation of weight. Low leptin levels signal low fat stores, prompting eating. High levels signal adequate fat stores and satiation. *Insulin* is a second hormone involved in weight maintenance. Produced by the pancreas, this hormone allows body cells to take in glucose for their use. (Deficiency in insulin production or use results in diabetes, which is covered in Chapter 11.) High insulin production leads to the intake of more glucose than cells can use, and the excess is converted into fat in the body. In the brain, insulin acts on the **hypothalamus**, sending signals of satiation and decreasing appetite.

The hormone **ghrelin**, a peptide hormone discovered in 1999, also plays a role in eating (Blundell et al., 2015). This hormone is produced by cells in the stomach wall, and its level rises before and falls after meals. Thus ghrelin seems to be involved in the short-term regulation of food intake by prompting eating. Ghrelin also acts in the hypothalamus to activate *neuropeptide Y*, which secretes *Agouti-related peptide*. This peptide stimulates appetite and decreases metabolism, thus affecting the weight balance equation in two ways.

In addition to the hormones that prompt eating, a variety of hormones is related to feelings of satiation and thus tends to decrease or terminate eating. The hormone **cholecystokinin (CCK)**, a peptide hormone produced by the intestines, acts on the brain to produce feelings of satiation. CCK, *glucagon-like peptide 1*, and *peptide YY* are all produced in the intestines but act on the hypothalamus to signal satiation (Blundell et al., 2015). Thus, the picture of hormone and neurotransmitter action in relation to hunger and eating is very complex and not yet fully understood. One system appears to initiate eating, and one seems to produce satiation and thus decrease eating. Table 14.1 lists each set of hormones and shows where they are produced. Notice that many are produced in the hypothalamus and all may act on different nuclei in the hypothalamus to form a complex mechanism for the short-term and long-term regulation of weight.

To understand the complexities of weight metabolism and weight maintenance, consider an extreme example: an experiment in which participants were systematically starved.

TABLE 14.1   Hormones Involved in Appetite and Satiation

Hormones That Increase Appetite		Hormones That Increase Satiation	
Hormone	Produced in	Hormone	Produced in
Ghrelin	Stomach	Leptin	Adipose tissue
Neuropeptide Y	Hypothalamus	Insulin	Pancreas
Orexins	Hypothalamus	Cholecystokinin	Intestines
Agouti-related peptide	Hypothalamus	Glucagon-like peptide 1	Intestines
Melanin-concentrating hormone (MCH)	Hypothalamus	Peptide YY	Intestines

Experimental Starvation

More than 60 years ago, Ancel Keys and his colleagues (Keys, Brozek, Henschel, Mickelsen, & Taylor, 1950) began a study on the physical effects of human starvation. The research took place during World War II; the participants were conscientious objectors who volunteered to be part of the study as an alternative to military service. In most ways these volunteers were quite normal young men; their weights were normal, their IQs were in the normal to bright range, and they were emotionally stable.

For the first 3 months of the project, the 36 volunteers ate regularly to establish their normal caloric requirements. Next, the men received half their previous rations, with the goal of reducing their body weight to 75% of previous levels. Although the researchers cut the participants' caloric intake in half, they were careful to give them adequate nutrients so that the men were never in any danger of actually starving. However, the men were hungry almost constantly.

At first the men lost weight rapidly, but the initial pace of weight loss did not last. To continue losing weight, the men had to consume even fewer calories, which led to considerable suffering. Nevertheless, most stayed with the project through the entire 6 months, and most met their goal of losing 25% of their body weight.

The behaviors that accompanied the semistarvation were quite surprising to Keys and his colleagues. The men were optimistic and cheerful initially, but these feelings soon vanished. The men became irritable, aggressive, and began to fight among themselves—behavior that was completely out of character. Although the men continued this bellicose behavior throughout the 6 months of the starvation phase, they also became apathetic and avoided physical activity as much as they could. They became neglectful of their dormitory, their own physical appearance, and their girlfriends.

The men became increasingly obsessed with thoughts of food. Mealtimes became the center of their lives; they tended to eat very slowly and to be very sensitive to the taste of their food. At the beginning of the period of caloric reduction, the researchers saw no need to place physical restrictions on the men to prevent them from cheating on their diets. But about 3 months into the starvation, the men said that they should not

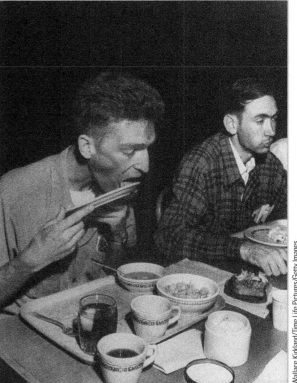

Experimental starvation produced an obsession with food and a variety of negative changes in the behavior of these volunteers.

Wallace Kirkland/Time Life Pictures/Getty Images

leave the dormitory alone because they feared they would cheat. As a result, they were allowed to go out only in pairs or in larger groups. These dedicated, polite, normal, stable young men had become abnormal and unpleasant under conditions of semistarvation.

Obsession with food and a continuing negative outlook also characterized the refeeding phase of the project. The plan for refeeding was for the men to regain the weight they had lost over a 3-month period. This phase was to have lasted 3 months, with food introduced at gradually increasing levels. The men objected so strongly that the pace of refeeding was accelerated. As a result, the men ate as much and as often as they could, some as many as five large meals a day. By the end of the refeeding period, most men had regained their pre-experimental weight; indeed, many were slightly heavier. About half were still preoccupied with food, and for many, their prestarvation optimism and cheerfulness had not completely returned.

Experimental Overeating

The counterpart to experimental starvation is experimental overeating, which seems like a much more attractive option. Ethan Allen Sims and his associates (Sims, 1974, 1976; Sims et al., 1973; Sims & Horton, 1968) found a group of people who should have been especially interested and appreciative—prisoners. Inmates at the Vermont State Prison volunteered to gain 20 to 30 pounds as part of an experiment on overeating. Sims interest was analogous to Keys'—an understanding of the physical and psychological components of overeating. These prisoners had special living arrangements, including plentiful and delicious food. In addition, the experiment included a restriction of physical activity to make weight gain easier.

Increased calories and decreased physical activity would seem to assure weight gain. Did these men gain weight? At first they gained fairly easily. But soon the rate of weight gain slowed, and the participants had to eat more and more to continue gaining. As with the men in the starvation study, these men needed about 3,500 calories to maintain their weight at normal levels, but many had to double that amount to continue gaining. Not all the men were able to attain their weight goals, regardless of how much they ate. One man did not reach his goal even though he ate more than 10,000 calories per day.

Were the overeating prisoners as miserable as the starving conscientious objectors? No, but they did find overeating unpleasant. Food became repulsive to them,

despite the excellent quality and preparation. They had to force themselves to eat, and many considered dropping out of the study.

When the weight gain phase of the study was over, the prisoners cut down their food intake dramatically and lost weight. Not all lost as quickly as others, and two had some trouble returning to their original weight. An examination of these two men's medical backgrounds revealed some family history of obesity, although the men themselves had never been overweight. These results indicate that normal weight people have trouble increasing their weight substantially and that, even if they do, the increased weight is difficult to maintain.

IN SUMMARY

Weight maintenance depends largely on two factors: the number of calories absorbed through food intake and the number expended through body metabolism and physical activity. Underlying this balance is a complex set of hormones and neurotransmitters that have selective effects on various brain sites, including the hypothalamus. Weight gain occurs when more nutrients are present than are required for maintenance of body metabolism and physical activity. Weight loss occurs when insufficient nutrients are present to furnish the necessary energy for body metabolism and activity. An experiment in starvation showed that loss of too much weight leads to irritability, aggression, apathy, lack of interest in sex, and preoccupation with food. Another experiment in overeating showed that some people find gaining weight almost as difficult as losing it.

Overeating and Obesity

Overeating is not the sole cause of obesity, but it is an important part of the weight maintenance equation. As the studies on experimental starvation and overeating show, metabolic-level changes with food intake as well as with energy output alter the efficiency of nutrient use by the body. Thus, individual variations in body metabolism allow some people to burn calories faster than others. Two people who eat the same amount may have different weights.

Although many overweight people report that they eat less than others, these self-reports tend to be inaccurate; objective measurements usually indicate that

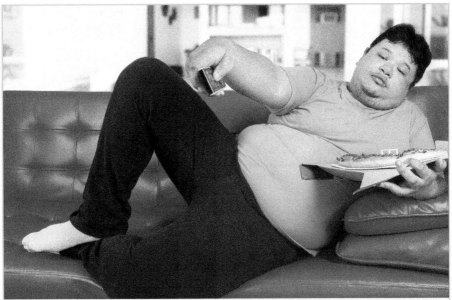

The weight maintenance equation is complex, but overeating is a cause of obesity.

overweight people eat more (Jeffery & Harnack, 2007; Pietiläinen et al., 2010). They are especially likely to eat food rich in fat, which has a higher caloric density than carbohydrates or protein. That is, they may eat less food but more calories. Overweight individuals also have a tendency to be less physically active than leaner people, which contributes to overweight. These behaviors contribute to obesity and its related health consequences, but the underlying reasons for obesity and even its definition remain controversial.

What Is Obesity?

Answers to the question of what obesity is vary by personal and social standards. Should obesity be defined in terms of health? Appearance? Body mass? Percentage of body fat? Weight charts? Total weight? No good definition of obesity would consider only body weight, because some individuals have a small skeletal frame, whereas others are larger, and some people's weight is in muscle, whereas others carry weight in fat. Muscle tissue and bone weigh more than fat, so some people can be heavier yet leaner, as athletes often are.

Determining percentage and distribution of body fat is not easy, and several different assessment methods exist (Mazić et al., 2014). Many new technologies for imaging the body—ultrasound, magnetic resonance imaging, and potassium-40 analysis—can be applied to

assessing fat content, but these methods have the drawbacks of being very expensive and relatively inaccessible. Simpler methods include the skinfold technique, which involves measuring the thickness of a pinch of skin, and bioelectrical impedance measurement, which involves sending a harmless level of electrical current through the body to measure levels of fat in various parts of the body. Neither of these approaches is as accurate as the more expensive measurements.

The most common assessment is even easier: consulting a chart. Height–weight charts were popular, but the **body mass index (BMI)** is now the most important approach. BMI is defined as body weight in kilograms (kg) divided by height in meters squared (m^2)—that is, BMI = kg/m^2. Although BMI does not consider a person's age, gender, or body build, this measurement began to gain popularity in the early 1990s. Neither weight charts nor BMI measures body fat, but this index can provide a standard for measuring overweight and obesity (National Task Force on the Prevention and Treatment of Obesity, 2000). Overweight is usually defined as a BMI of 25 through 29.9 and obesity as a BMI of 30 or more. (A 5' 10" man with a BMI of 30 would weigh 207 pounds, and a 5' 4" woman with a BMI of 30 would weigh 174.) Table 14.2 shows a sample of BMI levels and their corresponding heights and weights.

Another measure that can be useful in assessing overweight is fat distribution, measured as the

TABLE 14.2 Body Mass Index Scores and Their Corresponding Heights and Weights

	Body Mass Index (kg/m²)							
	17[a]	21	23	25	27	30	35	40[b]
Height in Inches	Weight in Pounds							
60	88	107	118	128	138	153	179	204
61	90	111	122	132	143	158	185	211
62	93	115	126	136	147	164	191	218
63	96	118	130	141	152	169	197	225
64	99	122	134	145	157	174	202	232
65	102	126	138	150	162	180	210	240
66	106	130	142	155	167	186	216	247
67	109	134	146	159	172	191	223	255
68	112	138	151	164	177	197	230	262
69	115	142	155	169	182	203	236	270
70	119	146	160	174	188	207	243	278
71	122	150	165	179	193	215	250	286
72	125	154	169	184	199	221	258	294
73	129	159	174	189	204	227	265	302
74	132	163	179	194	210	233	272	311
75	136	168	184	200	216	240	279	319
76	140	172	189	205	221	246	287	328

[a]BMI of 17 after intentional starvation meets one World Health Organization definition of anorexia nervosa.

[b]BMI of 40 is considered morbid obesity by Bender, Trautner, Spraul, & Berger (1998).

ratio of waist to hip size. People who have waists that approach the size of their hips tend to have fat distributed around their middles, whereas people who have large hips compared with their waists have lower hip-to-waist ratios.

Regardless of the definitions that researchers have used to study obesity, overweight is often defined in terms of social standards and fashion. These definitions usually have little to do with health and are subject to variations by culture and time. Numerous examples come from human history. During times when food supply was uncertain (the most frequent situation throughout history), carrying some supply of fat on the body was a type of insurance and thus often considered attractive (Nelson & Morrison, 2005). Fat could also be considered a mark of prosperity; fat advertised to the world that a person could afford an ample supply of food. Only in very recent history has this standard changed. Before 1920, thinness was considered unattractive, possibly due to its association with diseases or poverty.

Thinness is no longer considered unattractive. Indeed, today it is as highly desirable as plumpness was in previous centuries, especially for women. Early studies that examined changes in the body weight of *Playboy* centerfolds and Miss America candidates from 1959 to 1978 (Garner, Garfinkel, Schwartz, & Thompson, 1980), from 1979 to 1988 (Wiseman, Gray, Mosimann, & Ahrens, 1992), and another from 1922 to 1999 (Rubenstein & Caballero, 2000) found that weights for both groups had decreased relative to average weight of the general population. More recent analysis of centerfolds (Seifert, 2005; Sypeck et al., 2006) confirmed this trend toward thinness over the past 50 years. These ideal bodies are so thin that 99% of centerfolds and 100% of Miss America winners fall into the underweight range (Spitzer, Henderson, & Zivian, 1999).

This thin ideal for women's bodies has become so widely accepted that even normal weight women often consider themselves too heavy (Maynard, Serdula, Galuska, Gillespie, & Mokdad, 2006). The acceptance of thinness as attractive for women begins as early as age 3 (Harriger, Calogero, Witherington, & Smith, 2010), is established by age 5 (Damiano et al., 2015), and persists into adulthood (Brown & Slaughter, 2011).

Clearly, obesity, like beauty, is in the eye of the beholder, and the ideal body has become thinner over the past 50 years.

Despite the emphasis on thinness, obesity has become epidemic. In the United States, adult obesity increased by 50% from the early 1980s to the late 1990s (NCHS, 2011) and has remained high (NCHS, 2016). A similar increase occurred worldwide during the same time frame (WHO, 2016b). In the United States, extreme obesity more than doubled during the 1990s and continued to grow among women through 2014 (NCHS, 2016). Nor is the increase in obesity confined to adults or even to humans; other animals such as dogs, cats, and rats that live in close proximity to humans have also become fatter over the past several decades (Klimentidis, 2011). There are now more people in the world who are obese than underweight (WHO, 2016b). As Barry Popkin (2009) concluded, "The world is fat."

If obesity is defined as having a BMI of 30 or higher, then 37.8% of U.S. adults are obese, and an additional 32.6% are overweight, defined as a BMI of 25.0 to 29.9 (NCHS, 2016). The rates of obesity are lower in children (13.4%) and adolescents (20.6%), but these rates are higher than 25 years ago. Obesity and overweight occurs in both genders, all ethnic groups, all geographic regions, and all educational levels. As Figure 14.2 shows, however, the rates of obesity and overweight vary by gender and ethnic background.

Overweight and obesity rates in the United States rank among the highest in the world (WHO, 2016a), but in many other countries, the rate of overweight is also over 50%. For example, all of the countries in the Americas have a rate this high, and so do all of the countries in Europe. Indeed, many countries have a rate of over 60%. However, in no country in Southeast Asia is the rate of overweight 50% or higher, and many countries in Africa also have low rates. Of course, obesity rates are lower than rates of overweight, but countries with high rates of overweight also have high obesity rates.

Why Are Some People Obese?

Researchers have proposed several reasons for the dramatic increase in obesity over the past two decades, including an increase in consumption of fast food and sweetened sodas, growing portion sizes, and a decrease in physical activity. These factors apply not only to people in the United States (Pereira et al., 2005) but also those in many other countries, including low-income countries (Popkin, 2009). A lifestyle of fast food and television viewing is related to a larger body mass index and to weight gain. Indeed, adolescents whose schools are located within half a mile of a fast-food restaurant are more likely to be overweight compared with those without a fast-food restaurant so close to their school (Davis & Carpenter, 2009).

The consumption of sugar-sweetened sodas is another behavior that studies have related to increased incidence of overweight (Bermudez & Gao, 2011; Bray, 2004; Must, Barrish, & Bandini, 2009). Large portion size also contributes to increasing obesity, and despite pleas by health authorities, fast-food restaurants continue to "supersize" meals (Young & Nestle, 2007), which tends to supersize diners. This trend affects high-income countries more than middle- or low-income countries, but obesity is a growing epidemic around the world (WHO, 2016a, 2016b).

However, in all countries, some people are obese, whereas others stay thin.

To account for this variation, researchers have examined a complex set of biological and environmental factors and have developed several models. These models, which should be able to explain both the development and the maintenance of obesity, include the set-point model, genetic explanations, and the positive incentive model.

The Set-Point Model   The set-point model holds that weight is regulated around a **set-point**, a type of internal thermostat. When fat levels rise above or fall

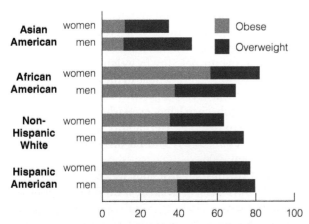

FIGURE 14.2   Percentage of U. S. women and men who are overweight and obese, by ethnic group.

Source: Data from Statistical Abstract of the United States adults and national health interview survey, 1009, 2010, by J.R. Plei, B. W. word and J. Wlucas, National center for health statistics. Vital health statistics, 10(249) Table 31, p. 106.

below a certain level, physiological and psychological mechanisms are activated that encourage a return to set-point. The discovery of leptin and the other hormones related to weight regulation is consistent with this view. Body fat produces leptin, which acts as a signaling system to the hypothalamus in the brain. The findings from the study on experimental starvation, the studies on experimental overeating, and the contestants on *The Biggest Loser* who regained weight are also consistent with the concept of a set-point, which predicts that deviations from normal weight in either direction are achieved only with difficulty, and dieters encounter additional difficulty in maintaining a different body weight. When fat levels fall below set-point, the body takes action to preserve its fat stores. Part of that action includes slowing the metabolic process to require fewer calories, which Fothergill et al. (2016) found in tracking the metabolic changes in *The Biggest Loser* contestants. People on diets have difficulty in continuing to lose weight because their bodies fight against the depletion of fat stores. With conditions of prolonged and serious starvation, this slowed metabolism is expressed behaviorally as listlessness and apathy—both of which were exhibited by Keys' starving volunteers.

Increased hunger is the body's other corrective action when fat supplies fall below set-point. Again, this mechanism seems to be consistent with the action of leptin, the results of the Keys et al. study on starvation, and Danny Cahill and other contestants. When fat stores fall, leptin levels decrease, which activates the hypothalamus in ways that result in hunger (Blundell et al., 2015). In Keys' study, the men became miserable as they dieted, and they stayed that way until they were back to their original weight. During the time they were below their normal weight (which would be below set-point), they were obsessed with food. When they were allowed to eat, they preferred the high-calorie foods that tended to increase their fat stores most rapidly, a situation that is consistent with set-point theory. They acted as though they were receiving messages from their bodies to eat. *The Biggest Loser* contestants tried to ignore these messages; some failed, but some succeeded in keeping the weight off, which is not consistent with set-point theory.

The experiment on overeating also fits with set-point theory. The prisoners who tried to gain more than their normal weight were fighting their natural set-point, possibly through the leptin signaling system, which should have translated into something like "Stop eating." The prisoners' bodies heard the signal—they would have preferred to eat less.

Questions remain concerning the set-point model, including why the set-point should vary so much from person to person and why some people have a set-point that is set at obese. One answer may be that the set-point is at least partly established through a hereditary component.

Genetic Explanations of Obesity   One genetic explanation of obesity looks to human prehistory to explain why people have a tendency to put on weight, hypothesizing that humans (and other animals) have evolved a "thrifty" metabolism that tends to store fat (Cummings & Schwartz, 2003). This tendency would be adaptive if food supplies were scarce, as they have been throughout most of history and prehistory. With the plentiful supply of food available to most people in high- and middle-income countries, this thrifty metabolism pushes people toward overweight and obesity. Indeed, some speculation holds that this availability makes obesity almost inevitable (Walker, Walker, & Adam, 2003). However, not all people are obese, and within any environment, some individuals are fatter than others. Some of that variation must be attributable to factors other than a general tendency to store fat.

Obesity tends to run in families, which suggests the possibility of a specific genetic basis. However, eating patterns are also shared in families, so researchers have studied twins and adopted children to disentangle genetic and environmental influences in weight. Results from early studies on adopted children (Stunkard et al., 1986) and identical twins reared together or apart (Stunkard, Harris, Pedersen, & McClean, 1990) suggested a role for heredity in weight. Adopted children's weights were more similar to their biological parents' than to their adoptive parents', and the weights of twins were highly correlated, even when the twins had not been raised together. Heritability also affects BMI (Schousboe et al., 2004) and fat distribution on the body (Fox et al., 2004).

These studies suggest that weight and fat distribution have strong genetic components, but no authorities claim that any single gene determines most human obesity (Cummings & Schwartz, 2003). Indeed, even researchers who claim a strong genetic influence for weight are focusing on the interaction among many genes and various environmental circumstances to understand weight regulation and

Would You BELIEVE...? — You May Need a Nap Rather Than a Diet

Would you believe that sleep deprivation is related to obesity? It's not that being awake longer creates more opportunities for eating (which may be true) or that nighttime snacking may lead to obesity (which it may; Coles, Dixon, & O'Brien, 2007). Rather, sleep may be related to weight regulation, and missing sleep may produce problems in this system.

A suggestion of the importance of sleep for weight regulation came from the observation that sleep deprivation has become increasingly common for large numbers of people, which has coincided with increasing obesity. Researchers began to wonder: Is this relationship a coincidence or is there some underlying connection?

First, researchers attended to the basic question: Does inadequate sleep correlate with overweight? An examination of the sleep habits of a representative sample of the U.S. population (Wheaton et al., 2011) led to the conclusion that individuals who get less than 7 hours of sleep per night are more likely to be overweight or obese than people who sleep more. This relationship also occurs in obese children (Seegers et al., 2011). Research has also established that short sleep duration precedes weight gain (Lyytikäinen, Rahkonen, Lahelma, & Lallukka, 2011), which is a necessary link in establishing any causal relationship.

Next, researchers attempted to connect lack of sleep with hormonal mechanisms that might underlie the relationship between sleep deprivation and obesity. Reviews of that research (Knutson & van Cauter, 2008; Leger, Bayon, & de Sanctis, 2015) support the conclusion that the type of partial sleep deprivation that has become so common is also capable of altering the regulation of the hormones involved in appetite and eating in ways that may cause weight gain and insulin resistance. Specifically, sleep deprivation increases ghrelin, which stimulates eating, and decreases leptin, which acts as a satiation signal (Knutson & van Cauter, 2008). Individuals who sleep less than 6 hours a night are at elevated risk of overweight and obesity (Leger et al., 2015). Thus, getting adequate sleep may be more beneficial than keeping you well rested—sleeping may protect against obesity.

obesity (Levin, 2010; Morrison, 2008; Rooney & Ozanne, 2011; Wells, 2011). Some combinations of genes may function in faulty ways that disregulate the set-point system and produce obesity. Another possibility emphasizes maternal overnutrition during late pregnancy and nursing, which may activate genes that produce permanent changes in metabolism. Other possibilities include combinations of many genes that respond to the food environment (such as availability of high-fat or sweetened food) and create obesity.

This emphasis on the food environment is well founded—obesity occurs in a specific context; a person cannot be obese without an adequate food supply, regardless of genetics. Although the genetic components of obesity may explain some of the variation in weight among people in a given environment, the increase in obesity that is occurring around the world has developed too rapidly to be the result of genes. Researchers must look beyond inheritance to attain a complete explanation of obesity. (See Would You Believe ...? box for another suggestion of an environmental influence on the development of obesity.)

The Positive Incentive Model The shortcomings of set-point theory and genetics in explaining all factors related to eating and obesity led to the formulation of the *positive incentive model*. This model holds that the positive reinforcement of eating has important consequences for weight maintenance. This view suggests that people have several types of motivation to eat, including personal pleasure and social context as well as food deprivation and hormone production (Pinel, Assanand, & Lehman, 2000). The personal pleasure factors revolve around the pleasures from the type and taste of food. The social context of eating includes the cultural background of the person eating as well as the surroundings, the presence of others, and whether or not they are eating. Biological factors include the length of time since eating and blood glucose and ghrelin levels. In addition, some proponents of the positive incentive theory (Pinel et al., 2000) take an evolutionary view, contending that humans have an evolved tendency to eat in the presence of food. Scarcity of food has built animals that survived when they laid on fat, making eating and the selection of food an important evolved ability. Therefore, this model includes biological factors but holds that eating is a process involving self-regulation, with important individual, learned, and cultural components (Epstein, Leddy, Temple, & Faith, 2007; Finlayson, King, & Blundell, 2007).

The set-point model ignores the factors of taste, learning, and social context in eating, and these factors are unquestionably important (Bessesen, 2011; Rozin, 2005; Stroebe, Papies, & Aarts, 2008). For each person in each instance, the act of choosing something to eat has a long history of personal experience and cultural learning. But a preferred food will not be equally appealing under all circumstances. For example, some foods—such as pickles and ice cream—do not seem to go together (at least for most people), even if both foods are individually tasty.

Social setting is important to eating, which is often a social activity. People tend to eat more in the presence of others, unless they believe that the others are judging them, and then they eat less (Vartanian, Herman, & Polivy, 2007), suggesting that social norms govern eating situations (Herman & Polivy, 2005). Culture provides an even wider context for eating, and various cultures have restrictions (and requirements) on what, when, and how much to eat. People tend to get hungry on a schedule that corresponds to mealtimes, but people in the United States are much more likely to eat cereal for breakfast than for dinner. In contrast, people in Spain lack a cultural tradition for this type of food, which made marketing cereal difficult in that country (Visser, 1999). These cultural and learned factors also affect the caloric value of chosen foods and how much a person eats, and these choices influence body weight. For example, when people choose "comfort foods," they often choose either food that carries personal nostalgic emotions or food that represents a personal indulgence (Locher, Yoels, Maurer, & Van Ells, 2005).

The positive incentive view predicts a variety of body weights, depending on food availability, individual experience with food, cultural encouragement to eat various foods, and the cultural ideal for body weight. Thus, the availability of an abundant food supply is necessary but not sufficient to produce obesity. People must overeat to become obese, and the quantity of food a person eats is related to how palatable the food is. Some tastes, such as sweet, are innately determined through the action of taste buds, and an overabundance of sweet food may be a factor in the disregulation of body weight (Swithers, Martin, Clark, Laboy, & Davidson, 2010).

In high-income countries, a huge food industry promotes food products as desirable through massive advertising campaigns, and many of these foods

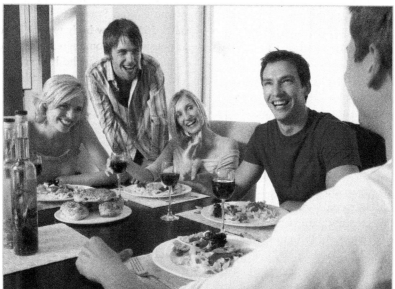

Eating is often a social activity, and social factors may contribute to overeating.

are high in sugar and fat. This situation influences individual food choices that promote population-wide obesity (Brownell & Horgen, 2004). Indeed, even rats eat more when food cues are abundant in the environment (Polivy, Coelho, Hargreaves, Fleming, & Herman, 2007).

Another factor that promotes overeating is the availability of a variety of foods. Eating a very desirable food leads to a decreased evaluation of how pleasant that food is (Brondel et al., 2009); that is, people become satiated for any particular food. When food supplies are limited in variety (but not in quantity), this factor can lead to lower levels of food consumption, but a new taste can tempt someone who is full to eat more. Indeed, if eating a sufficient amount terminated a meal, dessert would not be so popular (Pinel, 2014).

Variety is important in boosting eating, even in rats. A large body of research (Ackroff et al., 2007; Raynor & Epstein, 2001; Sclafani, 2001) indicates that variety is important in the amount eaten, for rats and for humans. An early study (Sclafani & Springer, 1976) showed that a "supermarket" diet produced weight gains of 269% in laboratory rats. The diet consisted of a changing variety of foods chosen from the supermarket, including chocolate chip cookies, salami, cheese, bananas, marshmallows, chocolate, peanut butter, and sweetened condensed milk. The combination of high fat and high sugar plus the changing variety led to enormous weight gain.

Are humans very different? The availability of a wide variety of tasty food should produce widespread obesity, which is exactly the situation that exists in a number of countries today. This wide variety of foods allows people to always have some foods that furnish a new taste, and people in such situations never become satiated for all available foods.

However, fat may be more important than other ingredients in producing obesity. Not only is fat denser in calories, but some evidence indicates that fat intake is also capable of affecting the biology of weight regulation. One hypothesis (Niswender, Daws, Avison, & Galli, 2011) holds that ingestion of foods high in fat and sugar disrupts satiation signals and boosts appetite signals in the brain. Thus, eating a diet high in fat and sugar increases appetite rather than leading to satiation. Results from a twin study (Rissanen et al., 2002) support this contention. To control for genetics, this study examined twin pairs in which one twin was obese and the other was normal weight. This procedure assured that the weight difference was due to environmental

rather than genetic factors. The analysis indicated that the obese twins not only ate a diet higher in fat than their leaner twins but also reported memories of preferences for such foods from adolescence and young adulthood.

Thus, the positive incentive theory of eating and weight maintenance takes into account factors that the set-point model ignores, including individual food preferences, cultural influences on eating, cultural influences on body composition, and the relationship between food availability and obesity. Both models draw on biological factors and inheritance, and many advocates of the set-point theory acknowledge that the factors highlighted by the positive incentive theory are important to weight regulation and contribute to obesity.

How Unhealthy Is Obesity?

Overweight and obesity are undesirable from a fashion point of view, but how much does overweight endanger health? These effects depend partly on the degree of overweight and the distribution of fat on the body. Being slightly overweight is not much of a health risk (McGee, 2005), but increasing overweight increases risks, and being obese places a person at an elevated risk for health problems and premature death.

A U-shaped relationship has appeared between weight and poor health; that is, the very thinnest and the very heaviest people seem to be at greatest risk for all-cause mortality in Europe (Pischon et al., 2008) and in the United States (Flegal, Kit, Orphana, & Graubard, 2013). Low body weight is not as much of a risk as obesity, and some researchers (Fontana & Hu, 2014) have argued that low body weight can be healthier than normal weight; observational studies that show a risk for low body weight are confounded by the inclusion of thin people who were thin because they were sick. The risk for people who are overweight but not obese is also controversial (Fontana & Hu, 2014), but without any question, obesity is a mortality risk. A summary of these levels of risk appears in Table 14.3.

Other studies show similar results: Obesity is associated not only with increased mortality but also with increased use of medical care (Bertakis & Azari, 2005) and increased chances for developing Type 2 diabetes (Lotta et al., 2015), osteoarthritis (Reyes et al., 2016), stroke and hypertension (Fontana & Hu, 2014), heart attack (Zhu et al., 2014), and a variety of cancers (Brenner, 2014). Obesity also raises the risks for gallbladder disease (Smelt, 2010); migraine headache (Peterlin,

TABLE 14.3   Categories of Obesity and Risks for All-Cause Mortality Based on Body Mass Index (BMI)

Degree of Obesity	BMI Range	Risk for Men	Relative Risk	Risk for Women	Relative Risk
Moderate	25 to 32	None	1.0	Slightly elevated	1.1
Obese	32 to 36	Low	1.3	Low	1.2
Gross	36 to 40	High	1.9	Low	1.3
Morbid	40>	Very high	3.1	Very high	2.3

Source: Based on Bender et al. (1998).

Rosso, Rapoport, & Scher, 2010); kidney stones (Taylor, Stampfer, & Curhan, 2005); and sleep apnea, respiratory problems, liver disease, osteoarthritis, reproductive problems in women, and colon cancer (National Task Force on the Prevention and Treatment of Obesity, 2000). A large-scale study in Europe found that mortality risk was lowest for women with a BMI of 24.3 and for men with a BMI of 25.3 (Pischon et al., 2008).

Both age and ethnicity complicate the interpretation of risk from obesity. For young and middle-aged adults, being obese is a risk for all-cause mortality and especially for death due to cardiovascular disease (McGee, 2005). Indeed, being overweight during childhood and adolescence predicts increased morbidity (Llewellyn, Simmonds, Owen, & Woolacott, 2016) and mortality (Bjørge, Engeland, Tverdal, & Smith, 2008) during adulthood. For older adults, being slightly overweight poses less risk than being thin (Winter, MacInnis, Wattanapenpaiboon, & Nowson, 2014).

Another weight-related factor associated with morbidity and mortality is weight distribution. People who accumulate excess weight around their abdomen are at greater risk than people who carry their excess weight on their hips and thighs, and the tendency for this distribution has a genetic component (Fox et al., 2004). A variety of studies have shown that patterns of body weight and the waist-to-hip ratio may be better predictors of all-cause mortality than the body mass index (Fontana & Hu, 2014; Pischon et al., 2008). Excess abdominal fat also raises the risk for Type 2 diabetes.

The dangers of "beer bellies" were noted more than 30 years ago (Hartz, Rupley, & Rimm, 1984), but more recently this pattern of fat distribution has been integrated into a pattern of risk factors called the *metabolic syndrome*, a collection of factors proposed to elevate the risk for cardiovascular disease and diabetes. In addition to excess abdominal fat, components of the metabolic syndrome include elevated blood pressure, insulin resistance, and problems with the levels of two components of cholesterol. A large waistline is the most visible symptom of this syndrome, and research has indicated that abdominal fat is positively related to the metabolic syndrome, but fat on the thighs has a negative relationship (Goodpaster et al., 2005).

In conclusion, obese people have heightened risks of developing certain health problems, especially diabetes, gallstones, and cardiovascular disease. Table 14.4 summarizes studies showing that obesity and fat distributed around the waist both relate to increased mortality rates, especially from heart disease.

IN SUMMARY

Obesity can be defined in terms of health or social standards, and the two are not always the same. Assessment of body fat requires complex technology for accurate measurement, so the body mass index is often used as the assessment for overweight and obesity. Social standards, however, have dictated a standard of thinness with a lower body weight than is ideal for health.

Obesity has been explained by the set-point model, genetic factors, and the positive incentive model. Set-point theory explains weight regulation in terms of biological control systems that are sensitive to body fat. This model hypothesizes that obesity is a defect in this control mechanism. Such a defect is the primary component of genetic models of obesity, which hypothesize that obesity occurs when a person inherits some configuration of defective genes that affect the neurochemicals that signal hunger or satiation. However, neither of these models takes learned and environmental factors of eating into account, but the positive incentive model does. This view holds that people (and other animals) gain weight when they have ready access to an abundant and varied supply of tasty food.

TABLE 14.4   The Relationship Between Weight and Disease or Death

Results	Sample	Authors
Effects of Obesity		
Obesity is a risk for all-cause mortality.	U.S. population	Flegal et al., 2013
Obesity and underweight are risks for all-cause mortality.	Adults from nine countries in Europe	Pischon et al., 2008
Obese adults sought health care more often than normal-weight adults.	Obese and normal-weight adults	Bertakis & Azari, 2005
Obesity is a risk for Type 2 diabetes	Systematic review	Lotta et al., 2016
Headaches are more common among obese, especially those with abdominal obesity.	Large sample of U.S. adults	Peterlin et al., 2010
Obesity is a risk for kidney stones.	Men, older women, younger women	Taylor et al., 2005
Obesity increases risk for all-cause mortality.	Young and middle-aged adults	Flegal et al., 2013; McGee, 2005
Overweight and obesity increase risk for heart attack.	Meta-analysis of five studies	Zhu et al., 2014
Overweight was slightly protective of mortality for older adults.	U.S. adults	Winter et al., 2014
Overweight during childhood and adolescence raises the risk for later mortality.	Overweight children and adolescents; systematic review	Bjørge et al., 2008; Llewellyn et al., 2016
Effects of Abdominal Fat		
Abdominal fat is strongly associated with all-cause mortality.	Adults from nine countries in Europe	Pischon et al., 2008
Abdominal fat is related to the metabolic syndrome.	Older women and men	Goodpaster et al., 2005

Dieting

Many people in the United States have some knowledge of the risks of obesity and even know about the risks of an unfavorable waist-to-hip ratio, but media portrayals of idealized thin bodies are even more influential in the motivation to diet (Wiseman, Sunday, & Becker, 2005). Despite the idealization of thinness, obesity in the United States rose sharply during the 1990s and has not decreased significantly since (NCHS, 2016). Acceptance of the ideal body as thin, combined with the growing prevalence of overweight, produces a situation in which dieting and weight loss are the subjects of a great many people's concern. What are people doing to try to lose weight, and how well do these strategies work?

People are inundated with messages about diets—television, magazine, newspapers, and Internet pop-ups are filled with advertisements for miracle diets that take off pounds almost effortlessly. Those diets may seem too good to be true, and they are. In September 2002, the U.S. Federal Trade Commission issued a report that described how widespread false and misleading diets have become ("Federal Trade Commission," 2002). Despite the customer testimonials and the before-and-after photos, these "miracle" diets do not work. As U.S. Surgeon General Richard Carmona said, "There is no such thing as a miracle pill for weight loss. The surest and safest way to weight loss and healthier living is by combining healthful eating and exercising" ("Federal Trade Commission," 2002, p. 8). This seemingly simple plan is far from simple to follow.

Unwise decisions abound in choice of diet. The trend toward dieting has become more severe in the past few decades. During the mid-1960s, only 10% of overweight adults were dieting (Wyden, 1965), but during subsequent years those percentages steadily increased; in 2015, 60% of high-school girls and 31% of high-school boys were trying to lose weight (Kann et al., 2016). Adults, on the other hand, are less likely to diet than 20 years ago (NPD Group, 2013). The decline has been more apparent among women; in 2012 only 23% of women reported that they were on a diet, whereas 38% were dieting 10 years earlier (Kruger, Galuska, Serdula, & Jones, 2004).

Approaches to Losing Weight

To lose weight or keep from gaining weight, people have several choices. They can (1) reduce portion size, (2) restrict the types of food they eat, (3) increase their level of exercise, (4) rely on drastic medical procedures such as fasting, diet pills, or surgery, or (5) use a combination of these approaches. Regardless of the approach, *all diets that prompt weight loss do so through restriction of calories.*

Restricting Types of Food   Maintaining a diet consisting of a variety of foods with smaller portions is a reasonable and healthy strategy. A number of commercial diet programs take this approach, and a meta-analysis of these programs (Johnston et al., 2014) indicated that all are similarly effective in producing weight loss. However, a healthy, balanced diet is not the most common diet approach; many programs rely on restricting types of foods.

Common approaches to restricting types of food include restricting carbohydrates (such at the Atkins diet) or restricting fat (LEARN diet). A meta-analysis comparison of low-carbohydrate and low-fat diets (Sackner-Bernstein, Kanter, & Kaul, 2015) also indicated comparable effectiveness. Both approaches showed success, and despite warnings from nutritionists about the dangers of low-carbohydrate diet plans, people who follow these diets have not experienced unfavorable changes in cholesterol levels or risks for cardiovascular disease. In addition, these diets tend to produce lower dropout rates than low-fat diets (Hession, Rolland, Kulkarni, Wise, & Broom, 2009). All of the diets produced significant weight loss compared to individuals who did not diet, but long-term weight loss is modest—in the 10- to 12-pound range.

Some diets are more extreme, restricting the dieter to a limited group of foods or even a single food. All-fruit diets, egg diets, cabbage soup diet, and even the ice cream diet fall into this category. Of course, such diets are nutritional disasters. They produce weight loss by restricting calories; dieters get tired of the monotony of one food and eat less than they would if they were eating a variety. "All the hard-boiled eggs you want" turns out to be not many!

Taking monotony a step further are the liquid diets, which exist in a variety of forms and under various brand names. Liquid diets have the advantage of being nutritionally more balanced than most restricted food diets. Still, liquid diets and their equivalent meals in the form of shakes or bars have the disadvantage of being monotonous and repetitive, and tend to be low in fiber. Like all other diets, these work by restricting calorie intake. Although current researchers may disagree on the advantages of low-fat or low-carbohydrate diets, they are likely to agree that diets high in fiber from fruits and vegetables are good choices (Schenker, 2001). However, even this approach can be successful. An intensive behavioral program using meal replacements (Anderson, Conley, & Nicholas, 2007) was successful for very overweight people, producing weight losses of 50 to 100 pounds, with better maintenance rates than most diet programs.

In conclusion, all food restriction strategies can be successful in producing weight loss, but many are bad approaches. Most of these diets fail to teach new eating habits that people can maintain over the long term. This problem was a factor for Danny Cahill; he lost over 200 pounds but gained 100 of them back. The metabolic slowdown that Cahill and other *Biggest Loser* contestants experienced made it difficult to maintain their weight loss, but so did their previous eating habits.

Behavior Modification Programs   Although dieting should be seen as a permanent modification in one's eating habits, such change is difficult. The behavior modification approach toward treating weight loss begins with the assumption that eating is a behavior that is subject to change. This application of behavioral theory was originated by Richard Stuart (1967), who reported a much higher success rate than that achieved through previous diet approaches. Most behavior modification programs focus on eating and exercise, helping overweight people to monitor and change their behavior. Clients in these programs often keep eating diaries to focus their awareness on the types of foods they eat and under what circumstances, as well as to provide data the therapist can use to devise a personal plan for changing unhealthy eating habits. The outcome of one weight loss trial (Hollis et al., 2008) indicated that dieters who kept a diary lost twice as much weight as those on the same program who did not. In addition, exercise goals are a typical component of behavior modification programs. The most common format for these programs is a group setting with weekly meetings that include instruction in nutrition and in self-monitoring to attain individual goals (Wing & Polley, 2001). Almost all weight control programs include some modification of eating, physical activity, or both, and these programs may be referred to as behavioral or behavior modification programs (Wadden, Crerand, & Brock, 2005).

Because weight loss is not a behavior, these behavioral programs tend to reinforce good eating habits rather than the number of pounds lost—behaviors, not the consequences, are the targets for reward and change. People who are overweight to moderately obese may be fairly successful in these types of programs (Moldovan & David, 2011). The goal is typically gradual weight loss and maintenance of that loss. The average amount of weight lost is about 20 pounds over 6 months, but dieters maintain only about 60% of that loss over a year (Wing & Polley, 2001). Thus, even moderate, gradual weight loss may be difficult to maintain.

Exercise   The importance of exercise in weight loss has become increasingly apparent (Wu, Gao, Chen, & van Dam, 2009). Exercise alone is not as effective for weight loss as dieting (Verheggen et al., 2016), but adding physical activity to a program to change eating is important. Because metabolic rate slows down when food intake decreases, physical activity can counteract this metabolic slowdown and thus may be an indispensable part of weight reduction programs. A large-scale survey of dieters ("Federal Trade Commission weighs in on losing weight," 2002) found that 73% of successful dieters exercised at least three times a week, and a meta-analysis of successful components in a diet program (Wu et al., 2009) indicated that physical activity was such a component. Exercise can also change body composition, adding muscle while dieting decreases fat levels (Verheggen et al., 2016). (The role of exercise is discussed more fully in Chapter 15.)

Drastic Methods of Losing Weight   People sometimes take drastic measures to lose weight, and physicians sometimes recommend drastic measures for severely obese patients. Even with medical supervision, some weight reduction programs present risks, sometimes to the point of being life threatening.

One approach that has turned out to carry substantial risks is taking drugs to reduce appetite. In the 1950s and 1960s, amphetamines were widely prescribed as diet pills to increase the activity of the nervous system, speed up metabolism, and suppress appetite. Unfortunately, the effects are short term, and dependence may become a more serious problem than obesity. Increasing evidence of the dangers of amphetamines led to the development of other diet drugs, but the quest for a safe, effective drug that helps people lose weight has proven difficult. Currently available drugs in the United States include sibutramine (Meridia), orlistat (Xenical), naltrexone-bupropion (Contrave), phentermine-topiramate (Qsymia), and liraglutide (Saxenda), which offer the possibility of statistically significant yet modest weight loss (Khera et al., 2016). The developing knowledge of hormones and neurochemicals related to weight regulation suggests that more effective drugs are possible, but that promise has not developed into a safe drug that is effective for major weight loss. Thus, a growing number of obese people are turning to surgery as a way to manage their weight.

Several types of surgery can affect weight, but most current surgeries either restrict the size of the stomach by gastric banding (placing a band around the stomach), sleeve gastrectomy (decreasing the size of the stomach), or gastric bypass (routing food around most of the stomach and part of the intestines). People are candidates for these surgeries if their BMI is 40 or higher or if their BMI is 35 or higher and they have health problems that make weight loss imperative. These procedures are successful in promoting drastic weight loss and changing eating behaviors (Chang et al., 2014). Like any surgery, these procedures carry some risks, and patients typically must be prepared to monitor their food intake and to take nutritional supplements for the rest of their lives (Tucker, Szomstein, & Rosenthal, 2007). However, the benefits outweigh the risks for many obese individuals. These changes in weight and metabolism improve diabetes, hypertension, and other risk factors for cardiovascular disease. In 2015, 196,000 people in the United States underwent some type of bariatric surgery (American Society for Metabolic and Bariatric Surgery, 2016).

Another surgical approach to weight loss is to remove adipose tissue through a fat-suctioning technique called liposuction. The technique produces a recontouring of the body rather than an overall weight loss (Sattler, 2005). This procedure is not useful in controlling the health complications of obesity; rather, it is a cosmetic procedure to change body shape, not a way to lose weight or affect health. Despite the discomfort and expense of the surgery, liposuction is the most common type of plastic surgery (American Society for Aesthetic Plastic Surgery, 2014). Like all surgery, it presents risks such as infection and reactions to anesthesia.

Drastic means of losing weight are poor solutions to obesity for most people. However, they are fairly common. High-school girls reported using drastic strategies for weight loss such as fasting (18.7%), taking appetite suppressant drugs (6.6%), and using laxatives or purging (6.6%); a large majority (62.6%) reported that they were dieting (Kann et al., 2014). Having a friend who uses these methods increases adolescent girls' risks for doing so (Eisenberg, Neumark-Sztainer, Story, & Perry, 2005), and being overweight raises the percentages of those who have used such methods to 40% for girls and 20% for boys (Neumark-Sztainer et al., 2007). All these drastic means of losing weight can be dangerous. In addition, all are difficult to maintain long enough to produce significant weight loss. Even when dieters succeed with these strategies, they usually regain the weight they have lost because these approaches do not enable them to learn how to make good diet choices for permanent weight loss. As Danny Cahill and other *Biggest Loser* contestants have experienced, keeping weight off is a major challenge, regardless of weight loss method.

Maintaining Weight Loss   In Chapters 12 and 13, we saw that about two-thirds of the people who initially quit smoking or stop drinking will relapse. For people who succeed in losing weight, maintaining that loss is comparably difficult. One systematic review of commercial weight loss programs (Tsai & Wadden, 2005) indicated that people who managed to lose weight on these programs (not all do) had a high probability of regaining 50% of the weight they lost within 1 to 2 years. Results from another meta-analysis (Johnston et al., 2014) found that dieters regained less than 20% of the weight they lost after 12 months.

Effective formal weight reduction interventions typically include posttreatment programs to help dieters maintain weight loss, which makes these programs more successful than those that lack a posttreatment phase. For example, a comparison of two follow-up interventions in dieters who had completed a 6-month weight loss program (Svetkey et al., 2008) included three groups of dieters. One group received no follow-up, one received an intervention that involved brief personal contact on a monthly basis, and another consisted of an interactive, technology-based intervention. The personal follow-up was more effective, but both interventions produced dieters who weighed less than before they started the program. Thus, the follow-up need not be intensive or complex; simple procedures can be effective. For example, people who lost weight and weighed themselves daily were less likely to regain the lost weight than those who did not step on the scales so often (Wing et al., 2007).

A survey by *Consumer Reports* ("The Truth About Dieting," 2002) supplied information about more than 32,000 dieters, both successful and unsuccessful. This number confirmed that people have problems both with losing weight and with maintaining weight loss, but it also showed that some people are successful.

Most of the dieters in the *Consumer Reports* survey lost weight on their own rather than through a formal weight loss program. Those who were successful tended to use a variety of approaches, including exercising and increasing physical activity, eating fewer fatty and sweet foods, increasing consumption of fruits and vegetables, and cutting down on portion size. Not surprisingly, those dieters who were successful in maintaining their weight loss rarely used any of the drastic means of losing weight reviewed in the prior section, except for surgery; individuals who undergo surgery to lose weight tend to lose large amounts of weight and maintain some of that weight loss (Douketis, Macie, Thabane, & Williamson, 2005). People who lose weight without surgery and keep it off tend to alter their eating and physical activity, forming new habits that they are able to maintain.

Childhood obesity has increased, even among children as young as preschool age, and has become a worldwide epidemic and thus of great concern (Spruijt-Metz, 2011). Interventions may include strategies for preventing the development of overweight, dietary programs, family interventions, physical activity programs, school-based programs, or some combination of these elements. Although dietary modification can result in reducing weight among overweight children, a physical activity component boosts effectiveness (Vissers, Hens, Hansen, & Taeymans, 2016). A meta-analysis of programs for children and adolescents (Altman & Wilfley,

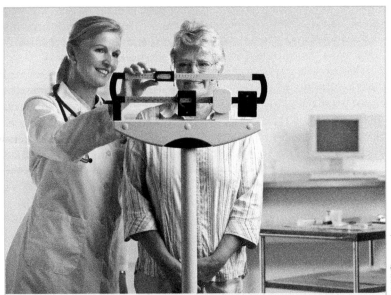

Dieting is common, even among those who do not need to lose weight for health reasons.

2015) indicated that family-based behavioral interventions and parent-guided behavioral interventions for children have well-established efficacy. Other types of interventions may also be effective, even interventions for overweight toddlers. However, all effective programs include multiple components that target behavioral and lifestyle changes and involve the family.

Is Dieting a Good Choice?

Although dieting can produce weight loss, it may not be a good choice for everyone. Dieting has psychological costs, may not be effective in improving health, and may be a signal of body dissatisfaction that is a risk for eating disorders. A group of dieters rated their overall experience as positive early in their diet (Jeffery, Kelly, Rothman, Sherwood, & Boutelle, 2004), but as the dieting continued, positive feelings decreased. Some dieters exhibit strong reactions, behaving very much like starving people: They are irritable, obsessed with food, finicky about taste, easily distractible, and hungry. These behavioral reactions make dieting foolish for those who are close to the best weight for their health.

For those who are sufficiently overweight to endanger their health, dieting may still be an unwise choice. As the analysis of *The Biggest Loser* contestants (Fothergill et al., 2016) showed, dieting may produce changes in metabolism that make it very difficult to maintain the weight loss. Developing reasonable and healthy eating patterns is a far better choice than dieting. That is, dieting is not the same as eliminating overeating (Herman, van Strien, & Polivy, 2008). The former is not a good choice for many people, whereas the latter is a good choice for everyone.

Ironically, weight loss may be a health risk for some people yet a health benefit for others. Involuntary weight loss is often associated with disease, so the association between unintentional weight loss and mortality is no surprise. Older people are more likely to lose weight due to illness, and studies that considered participants' age indicated that younger people are at risk from overweight but that after age 65, overweight is no longer a predictor of mortality (Kuk & Ardern, 2009); indeed, slight overweight may be an advantage (Winter et al., 2014). However, when overweight and obese adults were assigned randomly to a weight loss program (Shea et al., 2010), those who lost weight did not experience any increase in mortality; indeed, their risk was lowered.

Thus, the benefits of weight loss may not apply equally to all people. Even modest weight loss can be important for individuals who are obese and who can maintain the loss. However, the risks of dieting may be greater than the risks of moderate, stable overweight (Gaesser, 2003). Obesity, however, is not healthy.

IN SUMMARY

The near obsession with thinness in our culture has led to a plethora of diets, many of which are neither safe nor permanently effective. Most diets produce some initial weight loss in response to the restriction of caloric intake, but maintaining the reduced weight levels is a matter of permanent changes in basic eating habits and activity levels. Despite attempts to be thin, people in the United States are now heavier than ever because they have increased the number of calories they consume and lowered their amount of physical activity.

Losing weight is easier than maintaining weight loss, but programs that include posttreatment and frequent follow-up can be successful in helping people maintain a healthy weight. Whether part of a formal program or a personal attempt, eating a variety of healthy foods and maintaining physical activity are more likely than drastic programs to result in long-term weight loss. Like programs for adults, programs for obese children and adolescents face similar challenges and include the same effective components—healthy food choices and physical activity.

Dieting is a good choice for some people but not for others. Obese people and those with a high waist-to-hip ratio should try to lose weight and keep it off. However, most people who diet for cosmetic reasons would be healthier (and happier) if they did not diet, and even people who are slightly overweight may not benefit from dieting.

Eating Disorders

The eating disorders that have received the most attention, both in the popular media and in the scientific literature, are anorexia nervosa and bulimia, but binge eating is also an eating disorder diagnosis (American Psychiatric Association [APA], 2013). An **eating disorder** is a serious and habitual disturbance in eating behavior that produces unhealthy consequences. This definition of eating disorders excludes starvation resulting from the inability to find suitable food supplies and also unhealthy eating resulting from inadequate information about nutrition. Included are disturbances in eating behavior such as pica, or the eating of non-nutritive substances such as plastic and wood, and rumination disorder—that is, regurgitation

of food without nausea or gastrointestinal illness. Neither of these disorders presents serious health problems, and they are of relatively minor importance in health psychology.

The term *anorexia nervosa* literally means lack of appetite due to a nervous or psychological condition; *bulimia* means continuous, morbid hunger. Neither meaning, however, is quite accurate. Anorexia nervosa is an eating disorder that includes intentional starvation and a distorted body image. People with anorexia nervosa have not lost their appetite. Ordinarily, they are perpetually hungry, but they insist that they do not wish to eat.

Bulimia has come to mean more than continuous, morbid hunger. The chief identifying mark of this eating disorder is repeated bingeing and purging, the purge usually coming after eating huge quantities of food, typically high in calories and loaded with carbohydrates, fat, or both. Eating large quantities of food is critical to the definition of binge eating; people with this disorder binge but do not purge, resulting in overweight and obesity.

These three eating disorders obviously have much in common. Indeed, some authorities regard anorexia and bulimia as two dimensions of the same illness. Others see the three as separate but related disorders (Polivy & Herman, 2002). For example, binge eating is common to all three. In addition, the core components of all three include body dissatisfaction combined with preoccupation with food, weight, and body shape. The basis for body dissatisfaction is easy to understand: Overweight and obesity have become more common, yet the ideal body is thin. This combination has created a discontent that touches everyone in the culture. Children as young as early elementary school age express body dissatisfaction (Brown & Slaughter, 2011; Damiano et al., 2015), and discontent with body shape is so common among women that it is the norm (Grogan, 2007; Rodin, Silberstein, & Striegel-Moore, 1985). However, only a small percentage of people with body dissatisfaction develop eating disorders, indicating that other factors operate to produce these disorders (Tylka, 2004).

Janet Polivy and Peter Herman (2002, 2004) suggested that body dissatisfaction constitutes an essential precursor to the development of eating disorders, but those who develop eating problems must also come to see being thin as a solution to other problems in their lives. People who channel their distress into body concerns and focus on their bodies as a way to change their dissatisfaction have the cognitions that lead to eating disorders (Evans, 2003). Such cognitions include the feeling that being thin will lead to happiness.

Other risks for eating disorders include family and personality correlates such as a great deal of negative family interaction; a history of sexual abuse during childhood; low self-esteem; and high levels of negative mood, anxiety, and depression (Polivy & Herman, 2002). In addition, some genetic or neuroendocrine predisposition may contribute to the development of eating disorders; the neurotransmitter serotonin has been implicated (Kaye, 2008), and leptin exerts a variety of actions in the brain (Zupancic & Mahajan, 2011). Test of factors related to unhealthy weight control strategies (Liechty, 2010; Neumark-Sztainer, Wall, Story, & Perry, 2003) show that concern about body weight appears to be a primary factor in eating disorders.

Anorexia Nervosa

Despite the current focus on anorexia, neither the disorder nor the term is new. The first two documented cases of intentional self-starvation were reported by Richard Morton in 1689 (Sours, 1980). Morton wrote about an 18-year-old English girl who had died of the effects of anorexia some 25 years earlier and about an 18-year-old boy who had survived. Both had shown a remarkable indifference to starvation, and both had been described as sad and anxious. In London, Sir William Gull (1874) studied several cases of intentional self-starvation during the 1860s. He regarded the condition as a psychological disorder and coined the term *anorexia nervosa* to indicate loss of appetite due to "nervous" causes—that is, psychological factors.

During the 1940s and 1950s, psychiatrists who took a psychoanalytic view hypothesized that the ailment was a denial of femininity and a fear of motherhood. Other theorists suggested that it represented an attempt on the part of the young woman to re-establish unity with her mother. Unfortunately, none of these hypotheses expanded the scientific understanding of anorexia nervosa. The past six decades have seen a shift away from this sort of speculation and a turn toward the view that anorexia involves a complex of sociocultural, family, and biological factors (Polivy & Herman, 2002). Recent emphasis has been on describing the disorder in terms of behaviors and their physiological effects, demographic correlates, and effective treatment procedures.

What Is Anorexia?   Anorexia nervosa is an eating disorder characterized by intentional self-starvation or semistarvation, sometimes to the point of death. People with anorexia are extremely afraid of gaining weight and have a distorted body image, seeing themselves as being too heavy even though they are exceedingly thin. Research using brain imaging (Sachdev, Mondraty, Wen, & Gulliford, 2008) has revealed that women who are anorexic process images of their own bodies differently than they do images of other women's bodies— even when the two bodies are the same weight.

The *Diagnostic and Statistical Manual of Mental Disorders* (5th edition [*DSM-5*], APA, 2013) defines *anorexia nervosa* as intentional weight loss to a point that the person weighs less than a normal weight for a person with similar age, sex, and developmental status, along with a fear of being fat, and a distorted body image.

The *DSM-5* (APA, 2013) identifies two subtypes of anorexia: the restricting type and the binge–purge type. Individuals with the restricting type eat almost nothing, losing weight by dieting, fasting, exercising, or a combination of these strategies. Those with the binge–purge type may eat large quantities of food and use vomiting or laxatives to purge the food they have eaten. Alternatively, these anorexics may eat small amounts of food and purge. Research has confirmed that these two subtypes are distinct (Kaye, 2008). Purging is typical of bulimia, and binge eating occurs in binge eating disorder, but bulimics use purging to maintain a normal body weight. Anorexics purge to lose weight.

Anorexia is not confined to any demographic group, but young women are at higher risk than older women or men of any age. Typically, they are preoccupied with food, may like to cook for others and insist that others eat their food, but eat almost nothing themselves. They lose from 15% to 50% of their body weight, yet continue to see themselves as overweight. These young women tend to be ambitious, perfectionist, from high-achieving families, and unhappy with their bodies. People with anorexia are preoccupied with body fat, which usually leads to a strenuous program of exercise—dancing, jogging, doing calisthenics, or playing tennis. Excessively active and energetic behavior continues until their weight loss reaches a level that produces fatigue and weakness, making further activity difficult.

After substantial weight loss has occurred, individual differences tend to disappear, and accounts of individuals with the disorder are remarkably similar. Interestingly, many of the characteristics match the sketch of starving conscientious objectors drawn by Keys et al. (1950). Thus, these characteristics are probably an effect of starvation and not its cause. As weight loss reaches more than 25% of one's previous normal weight, the person constantly feels chilled, grows a soft, downy covering of body hair, loses scalp hair, loses interest in sex, and develops an unusual preoccupation with food. As starvation nears a perilous level, the anorexic individual becomes more hostile toward family and friends who try to reverse the weight loss.

Many authorities, including Hilde Bruch (1973, 1978, 1982), have regarded anorexia nervosa as a means of gaining control. Bruch, who spent more than 40 years studying eating disorders and the effects of starvation, reported that prior to dieting, anorexics typically are troubled girls who feel incapable of changing their lives. These young women often see their parents as overdemanding and in absolute control of their life, yet they remain too compliant to rebel openly. They try to seize control of their life in the most personal manner possible: by changing the shape of their body. Short of force-feeding, no one can stop these young women from controlling their own body size and shape. Anorexics take great pleasure and pride in doing something that is difficult and often compare their superior willpower with that of others who are overweight or who shun exercise. Bruch (1978) reported that anorexics enjoy being hungry and eventually regard any food in the stomach as dirty or damaging.

Who Has Anorexia?   Although anorexia is associated with Western culture, it appears in non-Western cultures around the world (Keel & Klump, 2003) and cuts across ethnic groups (Marques et al., 2011). This diagnosis was once more common among upper-middle-class and upper-class women of European ancestry in North America and Europe, but an assessment of many ethnic groups (Marques et al., 2011) showed that the prevalence of anorexia is similar in Hispanic American, Asian American, and African American women. Anorexia has become more common than it was 50 years ago (Keel & Klump, 2003), but anorexia nervosa is still a very rare disorder. An estimate of its prevalence among adolescent girls—the group with the most common occurrence—was less than 1% (Stice, Marti, & Rohde, 2013), with similar low figures for young women in Australia (Hay, Girosi, & Mond, 2015). However, among some groups the incidence rates are much higher. For example, 26% of young women who had competed in beauty pageants reported that they believed they had or had received a diagnosis of an eating disorder (Thompson & Hammond, 2003). The competitive, weight-conscious

atmosphere of professional schools for dance and modeling prompt the development of anorexia, and 6.5% of dance students and 7% of modeling students met the diagnostic criteria for anorexia nervosa (Garner & Garfinkel, 1980). A survey of college students involved in theater, dance, cheerleading, and athletics (Robles, 2011) indicated that 12% had been treated for eating disorders. Female athletes who participate in sports that emphasize appearance, thin body type, or low body fat are especially at risk (Torstveit, Rosenvinge, & Sundgot-Borgen, 2008). Level of involvement in these activities may be more at risk; for example, more elite dancers experience more frequent and severe symptoms of eating disorders (Thomas, Keel, & Heatherton, 2005).

Individuals with anorexia often report family difficulties, but it is difficult to determine if the difficulties precede the onset of eating problems or are a result of them (Polivy & Herman, 2002). Family environment is important in several ways. Families with children who have eating disorders tend to include a lot of negative emotion and little emotional support. Family violence—either as an observer or a target—is a risk for eating disorders for both men and women (Bardy, 2008). In addition, a family member with an eating disorder raises the risk for others in the family (Tylka, 2004), but so does having friends with unhealthy weight control practices (Eisenberg et al., 2005) or joining a sorority (Basow, Foran, & Bookwala, 2007). Thus, disordered eating is affected by social context as well as family dynamics. In addition, physical or sexual abuse is a more common experience in the history of those who are anorexic than for individuals who eat normally (Rayworth, 2004).

Over the years, a large majority of those diagnosed as anorexic have been women, who have been the focus of research and treatment. The estimates that women have 90% of eating disorders come from diagnoses and clinical impressions rather than complete population data. Reviews of eating disorders in men (Jones & Morgan, 2010; Wooldridge & Lemberg, 2016) claim that more representative assessments of eating disorders reveal much higher numbers, with men constituting at least 20% of cases (Hudson, Hiripi, Pope, & Kessler, 2007). Thus, this eating disorder may be more common among men than the clinical impressions suggest.

Male anorexics are quite similar to female anorexics in terms of social class and family configuration, symptoms, treatment, and prognosis, but they differ in terms of the factors that pushed them toward disordered

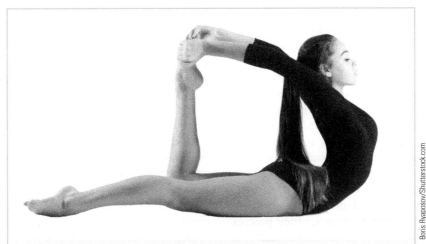

Eating disorders are more common among models, dancers, and athletes whose sports demand thinness.

eating (Ricciardelli, McCabe, Williams, & Thompson, 2007). For example, some studies have found that sexual orientation is a factor—more male anorexics are gay (Boisvert & Harrell, 2009), but a comparison of symptoms and characteristics (Crisp et al., 2006) revealed many more similarities than differences.

Boys and young men may take drastic measures to achieve their ideal body, just as girls and young women do (Olivardia, Pope, & Phillips, 2000; Wooldridge & Lemberg, 2016). The ideal body for boys is muscular, and escaping this indoctrination is as difficult as avoiding the thin body ideal is for girls (Mosley, 2009). However, both ideals share the abhorrence of fat. Thus, both women and men have concerns about body shape and size that may appear as disordered eating.

Treatment for Anorexia   Two unfortunate situations exist concerning treatment for anorexia: This disorder has the highest mortality rate of any psychiatric diagnosis, but no treatment has demonstrated a high degree of effectiveness (Cardi & Treasure, 2010). About 3% of all anorexics die from causes related to their disorder (Keel & Brown, 2010). Most die of cardiac arrhythmia, but suicide is also a frequent cause of death for those with the bingeing–purging type of anorexia (Foulon et al., 2007). Unfortunately, anorexia nervosa remains one of the most difficult behavior disorders to treat. About 75% of anorexics recover (Keel & Brown, 2010). Of those who do not recover, some improve but struggle with eating-related body image problems, obsessive-compulsive disorder, or depression. Between 9% and 18% continue

to exhibit symptoms of anorexia; those who are treated on an inpatient basis fare more poorly than those who receive community-based treatment.

An initial complication for treatment is that most people with anorexia are focused on losing weight, resent suggestions that they are too thin, and resist any attempt to change their eating. That attitude appears on a number of websites hosted by individuals who are anorexic and promote it as a lifestyle alternative rather than a disorder (Davis, 2008). Readiness for change predicts more successful treatment (McHugh, 2007). Motivating anorexics to seek treatment is thus a major challenge that may be addressed by the application of motivational interviewing (Hogan & McReynolds, 2004). This technique is a directive intervention to change attitudes about problems and make people more willing to work toward change.

As starvation continues, anorexia leads to fatigue, exhaustion, and possible physical collapse, and forced treatment. This situation seems undesirable, but even those who have been subjected to involuntary treatment later agreed that the intervention was justified (Tan, Stewart, Fitzpatrick, & Hope, 2010). The immediate aim of almost any treatment program for those who require hospitalization is medical stabilization of any physical dangers from starvation. Then, individuals with anorexia need to work toward restoration of normal weight, healthy eating, and improved body image. Recommendations concerning the methods of achieving these goals are not universally accepted, and systematic reviews have yet to reach firm conclusions concerning what treatments are most effective for people with anorexia. However, one meta-analysis indicated that both family-based behavioral treatment and individual behavioral therapy showed comparable effectiveness (Couturier, Kimber, & Szatmari, 2013).

Since the mid-1970s, cognitive behavioral therapy has become increasingly popular as a treatment for anorexia nervosa, and it has shown some success in changing both cognitive distortions that accompany body image problems and eating behavior (Fairburn & Harrison, 2003). Cognitive behavioral therapists attack these irrational beliefs while maintaining a warm and accepting attitude toward patients. Anorexics are taught to discard the absolutist, all-or-nothing thinking pattern expressed in such self-statements as "If I gain one pound, I'll go on to gain a hundred." Addressing cognitive distortions may be an important component of therapy—a developing body of research indicates that anorexics experience significant cognitive distortions that apply to the processing of food-related words (Nikendei et al., 2008). In addition, people with anorexia are more likely than others to believe that they cannot control their thoughts, and half reported that they used cognitive strategies to make themselves feel worse (Woolrich, Cooper, & Turner, 2008). The cognitive component of cognitive behavioral therapy has the potential to address these problems.

Cognitive behavioral therapy is not greatly more effective than other types of psychological and multimodal interventions such as the standard programs for anorexia, which consist of individual and group therapy plus supervised meals, meal planning, and nutrition education (Williamson, Thaw, & Varnado-Sullivan, 2001). Such programs are effective for some individuals with anorexia. Unfortunately, none of the treatments for anorexia show impressive success rates (Hay & de M. Claudino, 2010), and researchers are searching for improvements, especially in treating adults with anorexia.

For adolescents, the picture is somewhat more optimistic. An approach developed at the Maudsley Hospital in London emphasizes the role of family and family involvement in treatment for anorexia (Locke, le Grange, Agras, & Dare, 2001). Rather than treat parents as part of the problem, this approach accepts them as an essential part of the solution. Acknowledging that it is relatively easy to get anorexics to gain weight in the hospital, this approach focuses on helping them eat at home by equipping parents with strategies to get their children to eat. The value of including families in treatment of anorexia in adolescents has become well accepted (Cardi & Treasure, 2010; Couturier, Kimber, & Szatmari, 2013).

Treatment of anorexia may also include drugs. However, evidence is lacking for the effectiveness of any drug, including antidepressants, antipsychotics, and mood stabilizers (Tortorella, Fabrazzo, Monteleone, Steardo, & Monteleone, 2014). Thus, the arsenal for treating this difficult disease remains understocked.

Relapse always remains a possibility. Even with intensive therapy that targets irrational eating patterns and distorted body image, some people treated for anorexia retain elements of these maladaptive thought processes. Some slip back to self-starvation, some attempt suicide, some become depressed, and some develop other eating disorders (Carter, Blackmore, Sutandar-Pinnock, & Woodside, 2004; Castellini et al., 2011). Follow-up care is often included in comprehensive programs, and cognitive behavioral therapy seems especially important in preventing relapses (Pike, Timothy, Vitousek, Wilson, & Bauer, 2003).

Bulimia

Bulimia is often regarded as a companion disorder to anorexia nervosa, and some cases have been identified of individuals who have moved from one diagnosis to the other (Eddy et al., 2007). Unlike those with anorexia, who rely mostly on strict fasts to lose more and more weight, individuals with bulimia consume huge quantities of food in an uncontrolled manner (binge) and then purge, either by vomiting or by taking laxatives. The seemingly bizarre practice of binge eating followed by purging is not new. The ancient Romans sometimes indulged in very similar eating rituals. After they had feasted on great quantities of rich food, these Romans would retire to the vomitorium, empty their stomachs, and then return to eat some more (Friedländer, 1968). Unlike bulimia, this practice may not have been oriented toward weight control. Today, bulimia is defined as an eating disorder and affects millions of people.

What Is Bulimia?   As defined by the *Diagnostic and Statistical Manual of Mental Disorders* of the American Psychiatric Association (APA, 2013), *bulimia nervosa* involves recurrent episodes of binge eating, a sense of lack of control over eating, and inappropriate, drastic measures to compensate for the binge. Some bulimics fast or exercise excessively, but most use self-induced vomiting or laxatives to maintain a relatively normal weight.

One factor that distinguishes bulimia from anorexia is lack of impulse control (Farstad, McGeown, & von Ranson, 2016), although this characteristic may apply to some people who are bulimic more strongly than to others (Myers et al., 2006). Bulimics often experience problems related to impulsivity, such as a history of alcohol or drug abuse, sexual promiscuity, suicide attempts, and stealing or shoplifting. This factor may be critical; a person may become bulimic rather than anorexic if she or he cannot resist the impulse to eat, yet feels the body dissatisfaction that is common to both of these disorders.

Childhood experiences with sexual abuse, physical abuse, and posttraumatic stress are additional correlates of bulimia (Rayworth, 2004; Treur, Koperdák, Rózsa, & Füredi, 2005). In addition, recent involvement with sexual assault raises the risk (Fischer, Stojek, & Hartzell, 2010). A survey of a representative sample of bulimic women in the United States (Wonderlich, Wilsnack, Wilsnack, & Harris, 1996) revealed that nearly one-fourth of all female victims of childhood sexual abuse displayed bulimic behaviors later on. These women tend to have more severe symptoms than others (Treur et al., 2005). A relationship also exists between bulimia and depression, but childhood sexual abuse is also related to depression, as are suicide attempts. Body image and eating disorders tend to precede the development of depression in adolescent girls (Kaye, 2008; Salafia & Gondoli, 2011), which suggests a developmental sequence and may allow the establishment of a chain of causality for the development of bulimia.

Who Is Bulimic?   In at least one way, the population of bulimics is quite similar to that of anorexics: Both eating disorders occur far more often in women than in men. Bulimia occurs with equal prevalence in various social classes and ethnic groups in the United States (Franko et al., 2007).

How prevalent is bulimia? Is its incidence increasing or decreasing? Approximately 1.5% of American women and 0.5% of men meet the current diagnostic criteria for bulimia (Hudson et al., 2007), making this disorder much more common than anorexia. In a survey of high-school students (Kann et al., 2014), 6.6% of girls and 2.2% of boys said that they had vomited or used laxatives to lose or avoid gaining weight. These percentages reflect a high rate of these behaviors, which suggests a

growing prevalence of bulimia. An analysis of the history of this disorder (Keel & Klump, 2003) indicated a substantial increase during the second half of the 20th century. Furthermore, bulimia differs from anorexia in its occurrence: Bulimia is restricted to Western cultures and those cultures influenced by Western values.

Is Bulimia Harmful?   To many people, bingeing and purging may seem an acceptable means of controlling weight. For others, guilt is a nearly inevitable part of bulimia, and some mental health problems accompany this disorder. However, the question remains: Is bulimia harmful to physical health? Unlike anorexia nervosa, which has a mortality rate of 3% (Keel & Brown, 2010), bulimia is very seldom fatal (Steinhausen & Weber, 2010). Nevertheless, bulimia has serious health consequences.

The combination of binge eating and purging is harmful in several ways. First, the intake of large quantities of sweets can result in **hypoglycemia**, or a deficiency of sugar in the blood. This may seem paradoxical because the typical binge eater consumes huge amounts of sugar, but the metabolism of sugar prompts insulin release, which drives down blood sugar levels. Low blood sugar results in dizziness, fatigue, depression, and cravings for more sugar, which may prompt another binge. Second, binge eaters seldom eat a balanced diet, and poor nutrition may lead to lethargy and depression. Third, binge eating is expensive. Bulimics can spend more than $100 a day on food and this expense can lead to other problems, such as financial difficulties or stealing. Also, binge eaters are preoccupied with food in an obsessive way, thinking and planning the next binge. This obsession may leave bulimics with limited time to attend to other activities (Polivy & Herman, 2002).

Purging also leads to several physical problems (Mehler, 2011). One of the most common consequences of frequent vomiting is damaged teeth; hydrochloric acid from the stomach erodes the enamel that protects the teeth. Many longtime bulimics need extensive dental work. Indeed, dentists are sometimes the first health care professionals to see evidence of bulimia. Hydrochloric acid may also lead to damage in the mouth and esophagus. Bleeding and tearing of the esophagus are not common among bulimics but are very dangerous. Some longtime sufferers report reverse peristalsis, an involuntary regurgitation of food, often after eating quite moderately. Other potential dangers of frequent purging include **anemia**, a reduction in the number of red blood cells; **electrolyte imbalance** caused by the loss of minerals such as sodium, potassium, magnesium, and calcium; and **alkalosis**, an abnormally high level of alkaline in the body tissues resulting from the loss of hydrochloric acid. These conditions may lead to weakness and fatigue. Purging through excessive use of laxatives and diuretics may lead to kidney damage, dehydration, and a spastic colon or the loss of voluntary control over excretory functions. In addition, ingredients in the substances used as laxatives may have toxic properties, adding to the dangers (Steffen, Mitchell, Roerig, & Lancaster, 2007). In summary, bulimia is not a harmless weight control strategy but a serious disorder with a multitude of potential dangers.

Treatment for Bulimia   Treatment of bulimia has a critical advantage over therapy programs for anorexia nervosa—those with bulimia are more likely to be motivated to change their eating behaviors. Unfortunately, this motivation does not guarantee that those with bulimia will seek therapy.

Cognitive behavioral therapy is the preferred treatment for bulimia (Cardi & Treasure, 2010). Cognitive behavioral therapists work toward changing both distorted cognitions, such as obsessive body concerns, and behaviors, such as bingeing, vomiting, and laxative use. Specific techniques may include keeping a diary on the factors related to bingeing and on feelings after purging, monitoring caloric intake, eating slowly, eating regular meals, and clarifying distorted views of eating and weight control. A systematic review of treatments for bulimia (Shapiro et al., 2007) revealed that cognitive behavioral treatment is effective, including assessments at long-term follow-up.

Interpersonal psychotherapy has also been used successfully in treating bulimia (Tanofsky-Kraff & Wilfley, 2010). Interpersonal psychotherapy is a nonintrospective, short-term therapy that originated as a treatment for depression. It focuses on present interpersonal problems and not on eating, taking the approach that eating problems tend to appear in late adolescence when interpersonal issues present major developmental challenges. In this view, eating problems represent maladaptive attempts to cope. The success rate of interpersonal therapy is comparable to that of cognitive behavioral therapy, but it does not work as quickly. Factors that relate to success include positive changes early in therapy, lower depression, fewer binge episodes, and motivation to change (Vall & Wade, 2015).

Although the antidepressant drugs are not very effective in treating anorexia, the results for bulimia are more positive (Tortorella et al., 2014). Psychotherapy is a better choice for most patients than drugs alone, but the combination of drugs and psychotherapy may be a good choice for some people with bulimia.

Therapy for bulimia is usually successful (Keel & Brown, 2010); about 70% of bulimics recover as a result of therapy, and others improve. However, between 11% and 14% do not respond positively to therapy, and these individuals experience continuing problems with bingeing and purging, which may continue for years.

Preventing bulimia would be more desirable than treatment, and some programs attempt to change the attitudes that put people at risk. These programs are aimed at young women with the risk factors of low self-esteem, poor body image, high acceptance of the thin body ideal, a strong need for perfection, a history of repeated dieting, and other dysfunctional eating behaviors or attitudes. Some programs are school based, whereas others target young women at high risk. One typical strategy is psychoeducational, which attempts to change the acceptance of the thin body ideal and boost self-esteem. Adding a weight control component oriented toward building healthy eating while controlling weight has resulted in better success (Stice, Presnell, Groesz, & Shaw, 2005; Stice, Trost, & Chase, 2003). The Body Project is another successful strategy, which involves attempting to create dissonance by encouraging participants to critique the thin ideal (Stice, Rohde, & Shaw, 2013). Thus, programs that address the cognitive component of bulimia and offer a healthy way to manage body concerns may be more successful in averting this disorder.

Binge Eating Disorder

Many people eat too much at times, such as parties or holidays, but binge eating disorder is more than an occasional overindulgence. Binge eating consists of the same type of out-of-control eating that is symptomatic of bulimia, but without any form of compensation. Binge eating appeared as an official diagnosis in *DSM-5* (APA, 2013). To be diagnosed with this disorder, people must exhibit frequent binge eating episodes (an average of at least once a week for at least 3 months) with feelings of a lack of control, and they must experience distress over this behavior.

Becoming Healthier

1. Develop your eating competence (Stotts et al., 2007) by getting good information about nutrition and using that information in deciding on a healthy diet that you will enjoy.
2. Give up dieting, but also give up overeating.
3. Consult a chart that contains body mass index rather than a fashion magazine to determine what is the correct weight for you.
4. Be more concerned with eating a healthy diet than with your weight.
5. Concentrate less on food restriction and more on exercise as a way to change your body shape.
6. Do not skip meals as a way to lose weight, especially breakfast;

people who eat breakfast are less likely to be overweight than those who skip it (Purslow et al., 2008).
7. Do not compare your body to those of models and actors or actresses. These images furnish unrealistic and unattainable body images that tend to make people unhappy with their own bodies.
8. Understand that losing weight will not solve all your problems.
9. If you lose weight, know when to stop. Listen to people who tell you that you have lost enough.
10. Do not hide how little you weigh from friends or family by wearing baggy clothing.

11. When you make dietary changes, find ways to keep eating a pleasurable activity. Feelings of deprivation and going without favorite foods can make you too miserable to care about eating correctly.
12. Do not use diet drugs, fast, or go on a very low-calorie diet to lose weight, even if you are very obese.
13. Do not vomit as a way to keep from gaining weight.
14. Learn how to see someone who is normal weight or slightly overweight as attractive. Look for such people in the news and in the media.

Who Are Binge Eaters? Eating large quantities of food would seem to be a risk for obesity, and it is (Stice, Presnell, & Spangler, 2002). Many individuals who are obese experience binge eating. An examination of women with eating disorders (Striegel-Moore et al., 2004) revealed that binge eaters had higher BMIs than women with other eating disorders and experienced an even greater degree of body dissatisfaction. Binge eating is common to bulimia and, to a lesser degree, to anorexia; thus, it is not surprising that individuals with any of these eating disorders exhibit similar self-esteem, body dissatisfaction, and weight concerns (Decaluwé & Braet, 2005; Grilo et al., 2008). Alcohol problems are also common to both bulimics and binge eaters (Krahn, Kurth, Gomberg, & Drewnowski, 2005).

As with individuals who have anorexia, binge eaters are more likely to be female (3.5%) than male (2.0%), but binge eating is more common among men than anorexia or bulimia is (Hudson et al., 2007). Some researchers (Striegel, Bedrosian, Wang, & Schwartz, 2012) contend that men have been excluded from research on this disorder, creating an inaccurate impression; the prevalence is actually equal in men and

women. Children younger than 12 (Tanofsky-Kraff, Marcus, Yanovski, & Yanovski, 2008) and adolescents (Goldschmidt et al., 2008) are also affected by the loss of control that characterizes binge eating, which poses a major factor in obesity for these age groups. In addition, all ethnic groups are represented, and binge eating occurs in non-Western societies at rates that are similar to those in the United States and Europe (Becker, Burwell, Navara, & Gilman, 2003). Binge eating is also more common than either anorexia or bulimia—the estimated prevalence is at least 2% of the population. As with other eating disorders, most people with symptoms are not diagnosed and thus do not receive treatment.

Like others with eating disorders, people who experience eating binges also tend to have other behavioral or psychiatric problems, which complicates the diagnosis of this disorder (Hilbert et al., 2011; Stunkard & Allison, 2003). Indeed, the presence of personality disorders is one criterion that distinguishes binge eaters from those who are obese but do not binge (Farstad et al., 2016; van Hanswijck de Jonge, van Furth, Lacey, & Waller, 2003). Table 14.5 presents a comparison of anorexia, bulimia, and binge eating.

TABLE 14.5 Comparison of Anorexia, Bulimia, and Binge Eating

	Anorexia	Bulimia	Binge Eating
Body weight	<17 BMI	Normal	Overweight
Distorted body image	Yes	Yes	Yes
Percent affected			
Women	0.9%	1.5%	3.5%
Men	0.3%	0.5%	2.0%
Vulnerability			
Gender	Women	Women	Women
Age	Adolescent and young adult	Adolescent and young adult	Adults
Ethnicity	European and European American	All	All
Prominent characteristics	Ambitious, perfectionist, anxiety disorders	Impulsive, sensation-seeking	Personality disorders
Alcohol or drug abuse problems	Not common	Common	Common
Obsessive thoughts	Body fat and control	Food and next binge	Food and next binge
Health risks	3% mortality	Hypoglycemia, anemia, electrolyte imbalance	Obesity
Treatment success	75%; relapse is a risk	80%; relapse is a risk	Good success for binges but weight loss is difficult

Treatment for Binge Eating Treatments for binge eating face the challenge of changing an established eating pattern plus helping binge eaters lose weight. Cognitive behavioral therapy has demonstrated effectiveness in helping people control binge eating, but it is not as effective in promoting weight loss (Striegel-Moore et al., 2010; Yager, 2008). Nor are obese binge eaters good candidates for weight loss surgery; this intervention does not help in managing binges (Yager, 2008).

Thus, researchers have searched for a component to add to therapy programs. One consideration was SSRI (selective serotonin reuptake inhibitor) antidepressant drugs, which has some use in managing bulimia. These drugs produce a significant decrease in binge eating (Leombruni et al., 2008) but do not prompt weight loss. Adding the weight loss drug orlistat produced a modest weight loss (Reas & Grilo, 2008); the weight loss drug sibutramine may be more effective (Yager, 2008). However, these results highlight the difficulties of addressing the two problem components that binge eaters encounter.

Perception of the problem also plays a role in treatment for binge eaters. Some people who experience binges seek treatment for the bingeing behavior, whereas others see their main problem as overweight. Those who focus on their binge eating tend to choose cognitive behavioral therapy; those who see their problem as weight are more likely to choose a therapy with that goal (Brody, Masheb, & Grilo, 2005). This type of tailoring is an advantage not only for binge eating but also for many therapies and problems.

An application of the concept of mindfulness meditation (see Chapter 8) to binge eating appears to be a more effective treatment than others. Mindfulness-Based Eating Awareness (Kristeller & Wolever, 2011) aims to address the emotional component that is prominent in binge eating by helping binge-eaters to develop an awareness of the emotional underpinnings of their eating, become aware of physiologically based (rather than emotionally based) hunger, and exert conscious control over their eating behavior. A systematic review of the effectiveness of this intervention (Godfrey, Gallo, &

Afari, 2015) indicated moderate-to-large effects for this approach.

IN SUMMARY

Some people begin a weight loss program that seemingly gets out of control and turns into an almost total fasting regimen. This eating disorder, called anorexia nervosa, is uncommon but most prevalent among young, high-achieving women who have high body dissatisfaction and believe that being thin will solve their problems. Anorexia is very difficult to treat successfully because people with this disorder continue to see themselves as too fat and thus resist attempts to change their eating habits. A type of family therapy and cognitive behavioral therapy are more effective than other approaches.

Bulimia is an eating disorder characterized by uncontrolled binge eating, usually accompanied by guilt and followed by vomiting or other purgative methods. In general terms, people with bulimia are more likely than others to be depressed and impulsive, which may lead to alcohol and other drug abuse as well as stealing. In addition, they are more likely to have been victims of childhood sexual or family abuse, to be dissatisfied with their bodies, and to use food as a coping strategy.

Treatment for bulimia has generally been more successful than treatment for anorexia, partly because of bulimics' greater motivation to change. The more successful programs for eating disorders are those that include cognitive behavioral techniques, which seek to change not only eating patterns but also the pathological concerns about weight and eating, and interpersonal therapy, which focuses on relationship issues. Antidepressant drugs may also be useful in treating bulimia.

Binge eating appeared in *DSM-5* as an eating disorder. Those who experience binges are often overweight or obese and share impulse control and other psychological problems common to those with bulimia. Women are more likely to be binge eaters, but more men have this than any other eating disorder. Treatment faces the problems of altering maladaptive eating patterns and body image problems as well as promoting weight loss. Cognitive behavioral therapy is effective with the former, but losing weight is a difficult problem for binge eaters. Mindfulness-Based Eating Awareness is a new approach that appears to be more successful than others for Binge Eating Disorder.

Answers

This chapter has addressed six basic questions:

1. How does the digestive system function?

The digestive system turns food into nutrients by breaking down food into particles that can be absorbed. The process of breaking down food begins in the mouth and continues in the stomach, but absorption of most nutrients occurs in the small intestine. A complex signaling system involves hormones produced in the body and brain and received by the hypothalamus and other brain structures to control eating and weight. Hormones such as ghrelin, neuropeptide Y, agouti-related peptide, and melanin-concentrating hormone increase appetite and feelings of hunger, whereas leptin, insulin, cholecystokinin, glucagon-like peptide 1, and peptide YY are involved in satiation.

2. What factors are involved in weight maintenance?

Weight maintenance depends largely on two factors: the number of calories absorbed through food intake and the number expended through body metabolism and physical activity. Experimental starvation has demonstrated that losing weight leads to irritability, aggression, apathy, lack of interest in sex, and preoccupation with food. Initial weight loss may be easy, but the slowing of metabolic rate makes drastic weight loss difficult. Experimental overeating has demonstrated that gaining weight can be almost as difficult and unpleasant as losing it.

3. What is obesity, and how does it affect health?

Obesity can be defined in terms of percent body fat, body mass index, or social standards, all of which yield different estimates for the prevalence of obesity. Over the past 25 years, obesity has become more common in countries around the world, but in many Western countries, the ideal body has become thinner. The difficulty of either losing or gaining weight and the discovery of leptin, ghrelin, and other hormones involved in weight regulation are consistent with the notion of a natural setpoint for weight maintenance. Obesity seems to be a deviation from this regulation that has genetic components, but the recent rapid growth of obesity is not compatible with a genetic model. An alternative view holds that positive aspects of eating lead people to overeat when a variety of tasty foods are available, which is the situation in the United States and other high-income countries.

Obesity is associated with increased mortality, heart disease, Type 2 diabetes, and digestive tract diseases. The very heaviest—but also the very thinnest—people are at the greatest risk for death. Severe obesity and carrying excess weight around the waist rather than hips are both risks of death from several causes, especially heart disease.

4. Is dieting a good way to lose weight?

A cultural obsession with thinness has led to a plethora of diets, many of which are neither safe nor permanently effective. Changing from overeating to healthier eating patterns and incorporating physical activity are wise choices for weight change, whereas liposuction, diet drugs, fasting, and very low-calorie diets are not.

5. What is anorexia nervosa, and how can it be treated?

Anorexia nervosa is an eating disorder characterized by self-starvation. This disorder is most prevalent among young, high-achieving women with body image problems, but anorexia is uncommon, affecting less than 1% of the population. Individuals with anorexia are very difficult to treat successfully because they continue to see themselves as too fat and thus lack the motivation to change their eating habits. Cognitive behavioral therapy and a specific type of family therapy are more effective than other approaches.

6. What is bulimia, and how does it differ from binge eating?

Bulimia is an eating disorder characterized by uncontrolled binge eating, usually accompanied by guilt and followed by vomiting or other purgative methods. Bulimia is more common than anorexia, affecting between 1% and 2% of the population. Their motivation to change eating patterns has made people with bulimia better therapy candidates than those with anorexia. Treatment for bulimia, especially cognitive behavioral therapy and interpersonal therapy, has generally been successful.

Binge eating is similar to bulimia in terms of binges, but binge eaters do not purge. Thus, they are often overweight or obese, whereas bulimics tend to be normal weight. Binge eating is also more common than bulimia, especially among men. The two disorders are similar in terms of impulsivity, history of family violence, and coexisting personality disorders. Binge eating is a challenge for treatment because therapy must address both binge eating and weight problems.

Suggested Readings

Brownell, K. D., & Horgen, K. B. (2004). *Food fight: The inside story of the food industry, America's obesity crisis, and what we can do about it*. New York, NY: McGraw-Hill. In this controversial book, Kelly Brownell and Katherine Horgen contend that obesity is the result not of a lack of willpower but of a "toxic food environment" created by the food industry.

Hurley, D. (2011, June). The hungry brain. *Discover, 32*(5), 53–59. Hurley's readable story reviews research on the complexities of the physiology and neurochemistry of eating and obesity.

Polivy, J., & Herman, C. P. (2004). Sociocultural idealization of thin female body shapes: An introduction to the special issues on body image and eating disorders. *Journal of Social and Clinical Psychology, 23*, 1–6. These prominent researchers provide an interesting perspective on eating and eating disorders, which summarizes the findings of articles from a special issue devoted to this topic.

Popkin, B. (2009). *The world is fat: The fads, trends, policies, and products that are fattening the human race*. New York, NY: Avery/Penguin. Barry Popkin takes a worldwide view of eating and obesity, examining how obesity has become a more urgent problem than hunger.

CHAPTER **15**

Exercising

CHAPTER OUTLINE

QUESTIONS

This chapter focuses on six basic questions:

1. What are the different types of physical activity?

2. Does physical activity benefit the cardiovascular system?

3. What are some other health benefits of physical activity?

4. Can physical activity be hazardous?

5. How much is enough but not too much?

6. What are effective interventions for improving physical activity?

☑ Check Your **HEALTH RISKS** *Regarding Exercise and Physical Activity*

1. Whenever the urge to exercise comes over me, I sit down until the urge goes away.

2. My family history of heart disease means that I am going to have a heart attack whether I exercise or not.

3. When it comes to exercise, I subscribe to the motto "No pain, no gain."

4. I have changed jobs in order to have more time to train for competitive athletic events.

5. I use exercise along with diet as a means of controlling my weight.

6. People have advised me to start an exercise program, but I just never seem to have the time or energy.

7. One of the reasons I exercise is that I believe that a person can't be too thin and that exercise will help me continue to lose weight.

8. I may begin an exercise program when I'm older, but now I'm young and in good shape.

9. I'm too old and out of shape to begin exercising.

10. I'd probably have a heart attack if I started to jog or run.

11. I'd like to exercise, but I can't run, and walking isn't strenuous enough to be good exercise.

12. I try not to let injuries interfere with my regular exercise routine.

Except for item 5, each of these items represents a health risk from either too little or too much exercise. Count your checkmarks to evaluate your risks. As you read this chapter, you will learn that some of these items are riskier than others.

Real-World Profile of **RICKY GERVAIS**

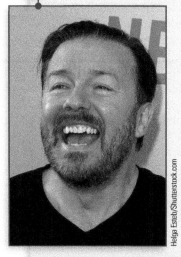

Helga Esteb/Shutterstock.com

Soon after Christmas, at the age of 48, comedian and actor Ricky Gervais realized he needed to change his habits. It wasn't a health scare, a new acting role, or the desire to look fit that led him to this conclusion. Rather, he looked down on an empty plate, a plate that not long before had 11 sausages on it. Ricky had eaten all of them in short time. He felt horribly ill, "like a snake just trying to digest it." Ricky thought to himself, "That's ridiculous… I hit 14 stone" (the equivalent of 200 pounds). "Things were getting out of control" ("Ricky Gervais had sausage binge," 2010).

Ricky changed his behavior, but he didn't focus his attention on losing weight or going on a diet. Rather, he focused on exercising. He began a regimen that involved 55 minutes a day of exercising. His choice of 55 minutes was deliberate: "It's a psychological thing. If it's under an hour, you don't feel it's taking up a huge amount of your day and you can do other stuff" ("MH Interview: Ricky Gervais," 2012).

Although his aim was not necessarily to lose weight, the public saw a different image of Ricky when he hosted the 2010 Golden Globe Awards. Ricky looked thinner, he looked fitter. He had dropped 20 pounds.

Gervais did not change his diet by much, saying that his aim in increasing exercise was to "stay alive and eat more cheese and drink more wine" (Men's Health, 2012).

Now, Gervais can often be seen jogging daily around the neighborhoods of New York or London, a habit he has kept up for years. "I would love to lose more weight actually but not by cutting calories. I will do it, if I can, by upping my workout even more. If this doesn't work, then fine. I will be fit and heavy" (Gervais, 2010).

Weight loss is one possible consequence of physical activity, as Ricky Gervais discovered. Weight loss is one of the most commonly reported reasons for why people initiate a physical activity routine. However, as you will learn in this chapter, physical activity has a multitude of benefits, aside from slimming one's waistline. Physical activity can reduce common health risks, improve mood, reduce stress, and improve cognitive functioning. Despite these benefits, many people do not adhere to recommendations for physical activity, and we will describe some strategies that help people stick to physical activity goals. Also, in this chapter, you will learn that the benefits of physical activity persist across the lifetime. So, as Ricky Gervais noted, "It's never too late, never ever too late" to begin a lifestyle of physical activity.

Types of Physical Activity

Although exercise can include hundreds of different kinds of physical activities, physiologically there are only five types of exercise: isometric, isotonic, isokinetic, anaerobic, and aerobic. Each has different goals, different activities, and different advocates. Each can contribute to some aspect of fitness or health, but only aerobic exercise produces benefits for cardiorespiratory health.

Isometric exercise involves contracting muscles against an immovable object. Although the body does not move in isometric exercise, muscles push hard against each other or against an immovable object and thus produce increases in strength. Pushing hard against a solid wall is an example of isometric exercise. This type of physical activity can improve muscle strength, which can be especially important for older people in preserving independent living.

Isotonic exercise requires the contraction of muscles and the movement of joints. Weight lifting and many forms of calisthenics fit into this category. Programs based on isotonic exercise can improve muscle strength and muscle endurance if the program is sufficiently lengthy. Again, older people can benefit from isotonic exercise, but many people in a weight-lifting program are bodybuilders interested in improving the appearance of their body rather than improving health.

Isokinetic exercise is similar to isotonic exercise, except that isokinetic exercise involves exerting effort to move muscles and joints against a variable amount of resistance. This type of exercise requires specialized equipment that adjusts the amount of resistance according to the amount of force applied. People who suffer muscle injuries often receive prescriptions to perform isokinetic exercise as a way to restore muscle strength and endurance. Isokinetic exercise is an important adjunct in physical rehabilitation, helping injured people to regain strength and flexibility with more safety than other types of exercise.

Anaerobic exercises require short, intensive bursts of energy but no increased amount of oxygen use. This form of exercise includes short-distance running, some calisthenics, softball, and other exercises that require intense, short-term energy. Such exercises improve speed and endurance, but they may carry risks for people with coronary heart disease.

Aerobic exercise is any exercise that requires dramatically increased oxygen consumption over an extended period of time. Aerobic exercise includes jogging, walking at a brisk pace, cross-country skiing, dancing, rope skipping, swimming, cycling, and other activities that increase oxygen consumption.

The important characteristics of aerobic exercise are intensity and duration. Exercise must be intense enough to elevate the heart rate into a certain range, based on a person's age and maximum possible heart rate. This type of program requires elevated oxygen use and provides a workout for both the respiratory system, which furnishes the oxygen, and the coronary system, which pumps the blood. Of the various approaches to fitness, aerobic activity is superior to other types of exercise in developing cardiorespiratory health.

Current recommendations call for a person to engage in some aerobic exercise at least three times a week. However, any aerobic exercise is better than none.

Reasons for Exercising

People exercise for a variety of reasons, some that are consistent with good health and some that are not. Reasons for adhering to a physical activity program include physical fitness, weight control, cardiovascular health, increased longevity, protection against cancer, prevention of osteoporosis, control of diabetes, better cognitive functioning, and as a buffer against depression, anxiety, and stress. This chapter looks at evidence relating to each of these reasons as well as to the potential hazards of physical activity.

Physical Fitness

Does physical activity help people become physically fit? The effects of exercise on fitness depend both on the duration and intensity of the exercise and on the definition of fitness. To most exercise physiologists, fitness is a complex condition consisting of muscle strength, muscle endurance, flexibility, and cardiorespiratory (aerobic) fitness. Each of the five types of exercise can contribute to these four different aspects of fitness, but no one type fulfills all the requirements.

In addition, fitness has both organic and dynamic aspects. *Organic fitness* is the capacity for action and movement that is determined by inherent characteristics of the body. These organic factors include genetic endowment, age, and health limitations. *Dynamic fitness* arises through physical activity, whereas organic fitness does not. A person can have a good level of organic fitness and yet be "out of shape" and perform poorly. Another person may train and improve dynamic fitness but still be unable to win races because of relatively poor organic fitness. Athletes who want to be champions need to have been very selective about choosing their biological parents in order to have inherited a high level of organic fitness. Aspiring champions must train in order to gain the dynamic fitness necessary for optimal athletic performance. Michael Phelps, the champion swimmer and holder of the most Olympic medals of all time, had an excellent balance of organic and dynamic fitness—he inherited a body suited to swimming, but he needed to work hard to break records. The rest of this chapter deals almost exclusively with dynamic fitness and its components, because this type of fitness arises from exercise, whereas organic fitness does not.

Muscle Strength and Endurance   Two components of physical fitness are muscle strength and muscle endurance. Muscle strength is a measure of how strongly a muscle can contract. This type of fitness can come from isometric, isotonic, isokinetic, and to a lesser extent, anaerobic exercise. All these types of exercise have the capability to increase muscle strength because they involve contracting muscles.

Muscle endurance differs from muscle strength in that it requires continued performance. Some strength is necessary for muscle endurance, but the opposite is not true: A muscle may be strong but not have the endurance to continue its performance. Exercises that improve strength require greater exertion for limited repetitions; exercises that improve endurance require less exertion but more frequent repetition (Knuttgen, 2007). Both muscle strength and muscle endurance improve through similar types of exercises, including isometric, isotonic, and isokinetic.

Flexibility   Flexibility is the range-of-motion capacity of a joint. The types of exercises that develop muscle strength and muscle endurance generally do not improve flexibility. Moreover, flexibility is specific to each joint, so that exercises designed to develop flexibility are varied. In addition to being a component of fitness, flexibility also decreases the likelihood of injury in other types of physical activity, especially aerobic and anaerobic exercise.

Slow and sustained stretching exercises promote muscle flexibility. In contrast, fast, jerky, bouncing movements cause muscle soreness and injury. Flexibility training is typically not as intense as strength and endurance training. Yoga and tai chi provide the types of movements that increase flexibility.

Aerobic Fitness   Of all the types of physical activity, aerobic exercise contributes most to cardiorespiratory fitness. When people acquire aerobic fitness, they improve cardiorespiratory health in several ways. First, they increase the amount of oxygen available during strenuous exercise, and second, they increase the amount of blood pumped with each heartbeat. These changes result in a lowering of both resting heart rate and resting blood pressure and increase the efficiency of the cardiovascular system (Cooper, 2001). This type of exercise helps protect both men and women from heart disease and a variety of other diseases (Murphy, Nevill, Murtagh, & Holder, 2007).

Weight Control

Obesity continues to be a worldwide problem. Many people adopt a sedentary lifestyle, spending much of their time watching television, viewing videos, playing computer games, surfing the Internet, and talking on cell phones. There is a link between these two phenomena, as research shows that physical activity contributes to weight control.

Most experts see obesity as a long-term accumulation of excess body fat (Forbes, 2000; Hansen, Shriver, & Schoeller, 2005). Obesity can arise over time, when a person's dietary caloric intake exceeds his or her expenditure of energy through physical activity. However, the level of exercise needed for cardiovascular health is not necessarily the same as that needed for weight control. For example, 15 minutes of walking or cycling to and from work can be enough to reduce both cardiovascular mortality and all-cause mortality (Barengo et al., 2004). However, the amount of exercise necessary to prompt weight loss is far greater. Some authorities (Hill & Wyatt, 2005; Jakicic & Otto, 2005) recommend that obese people need to spend at least 60 minutes a day engaged in moderate-to-heavy physical activity to bring about initial weight loss and to maintain that loss. Thus, longer and more intense physical activity is required for long-lasting weight control, which exceeds the amount of physical activity needed for cardiovascular health.

Exercise can also serve as a means for sculpting an ideal body shape. Unfortunately, exercise is limited as a method of spot reduction. Muscle and fat have little to do with one another, and a person can have both in the same part of the body. If people exercise during weight reduction, they build muscle tissue while losing fat, which may build a more attractive body shape. Spot reduction appears to be the result because fat tends to be lost from the places where it was most abundant. However, fat distribution is under strong genetic control, and people with large hips or thighs in relation to other body parts will have large hips or thighs after they lose weight. Despite some exercise promoters' claims, a particular calisthenic exercise will not reduce fat in a specific part of the body.

Inactive people who are concerned about weight and who have recently stopped smoking should strongly consider beginning a physical activity program. Steven Blair and Tim Church (2004) claimed that such an exercise program would be at least as effective as dieting in controlling weight and much better than dieting in changing the ratio of fat to muscle tissue. An early study supported this view. Investigators randomly assigned sedentary, obese men to one of three groups: dieters, runners, or controls (Wood et al., 1988). The dieters did not exercise, the runners did not diet, and the controls did neither. After a year, people in both the exercise group and the dieting group had lost about the same amount of weight, and both of these groups had lost more than people in the control group. However, some important differences emerged in comparing the dieters and the runners. Although both groups had lost an equal amount of weight, the dieters lost both fat and lean tissue, whereas the runners lost only fat tissue and retained more lean muscle tissue.

Exercise does not produce much weight loss through burning calories; for example, more than 30 minutes of tennis is required to work off the

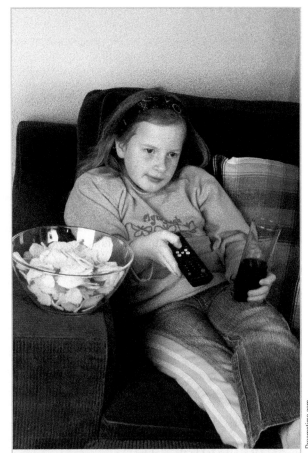

Sedentary leisure activities add to the problem of childhood obesity.

calories in two doughnuts! However, sitting and eating doughnuts is a risk for obesity in two ways—the sitting and the eating. Sitting is a health risk independent of one's level of moderate and vigorous physical activity (Biswas et al., 2015; Koster et al., 2012; Patel et al., 2010); that is, one may engage in regular bouts of physical activity, but there may be risks to spending the rest of the time sitting in a car, in front of a computer, or in front of a television. However, the risks of sedentary behavior are greater when it is accompanied by few to no episodes of physical activity (Biswas et al., 2015). Thus, sitting presents its own health risks. Most of the weight loss associated with exercise comes from elevation of the metabolic rate, the rate at which the body metabolizes calories. Thus, physical activity can promote weight loss because the resulting increase in the number of calories burned can produce changes in weight that exceed the number of calories spent in any activity.

IN SUMMARY

Five basic categories subsume all forms of physical activity: isometric, isotonic, isokinetic, anaerobic, and aerobic. Each of these five exercise types has advantages and disadvantages for improving physical fitness, but only aerobic exercise benefits cardiorespiratory health.

People have a variety of reasons for maintaining an exercise regimen, including physical fitness, aerobic health, and weight control. The various types of exercise can increase dynamic fitness, strengthen muscles, improve endurance, and increase flexibility. Aerobic fitness reduces death not only from cardiovascular disease (CVD) but also from all causes.

One popular reason for remaining physically active is to control weight and achieve a sculpted body. Physical activity can help people lose weight, but its capacity for spot reduction is very limited. Overweight people can lose weight through moderate physical activity, highly active thin people can maintain lean body mass through proper diet, and people of moderate weight can increase lean body weight without an overall weight gain.

Physical Activity and Cardiovascular Health

Nowadays, most people recognize the health benefits of physical activity. This knowledge, however, did not exist until relatively recently. During the early years of the 20th century, physicians often advised patients with heart disease to avoid strenuous physical activity, based on the belief that too much physical activity could damage the heart and threaten a person's life. (Figure 9.7 in Chapter 9 paints a dramatic picture of the rise and fall of death rates from CVD throughout the 20th century.) During the middle of the 20th century, some cardiologists rethought this advice and recommended aerobic exercise both as an adjunct to standard treatment and as a protection against heart disease. Later in this section, we describe the cardiovascular benefits of exercise, but first we look briefly at the history of studies that examined exercise and cardiovascular health.

Early Studies

Jeremy Morris and his colleagues (Morris, Heady, Raffle, Roberts, & Parks, 1953) made history with their observation of a link between physical activity and CVD. This observation took place in England and involved London's famous double-decker buses. Morris and his colleagues discovered that physically active male conductors differed from the sedentary drivers in their incidence of heart disease. Ten years later, Harold Kahn (1963) investigated the relationship between physical activity and heart disease among postal workers in Washington, D.C. Kahn found lower coronary heart disease (CHD) death rates among the physically active men. These studies, of course, did not prove that physical activity decreased the risk of CHD, because the high- and low-activity workers may also have differed on the basis of body type, personality, or some other factor associated with a high or low risk of CHD.

Ralph Paffenbarger, a professor of epidemiology at Stanford University School of Medicine and the Harvard School of Public Health, built upon this earlier work with the publication of several landmark studies on the relationship between physical activity and CHD. The first studies followed a group of San Francisco longshoremen in 1951 and tracked CHD deaths over time (Paffenbarger, Gima, Laughlin, & Black, 1971; Paffenbarger, Laughlin, Gima, & Black, 1970). In general, they found that CHD death rates were much higher for workers with low versus high activity. In these studies, all workers in both the high- and low- activity groups had begun their employment with at least 5 years of strenuous cargo handling; thus, all workers were likely in good shape at the start of the study. Yet, physical activity level emerged as a significant predictor of subsequent risk for CHD death.

In the late 1970s, Paffenbarger and his associates (Paffenbarger, Wing, & Hyde, 1978) published a landmark epidemiological study based on extensive medical records of former Harvard University students, their weekly total energy expenditure, and a composite physical activity index that took into account all activity, both on and off the job. With these data, Paffenbarger and his colleagues divided the Harvard alumni into high- and low-activity groups. Of those men whose energy levels could be determined, about 60% expended fewer than 2,000 kcal per week and placed in the low-activity group; the 40% who expended more than 2,000 kcal made up the high-activity group. (Note that 2,000 kcal of energy is approximately that expended in 20 miles of jogging or its equivalent.) The results showed that the least active Harvard alumni had an increased risk of heart attack over their more

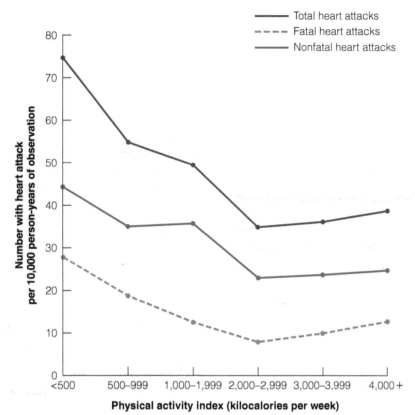

FIGURE 15.1 Age-adjusted first heart attack rates by physical activity index in a 6- to 10-year follow-up of male Harvard alumni.

Source: Adapted from "Physical activity as an index of heart attack risk in college alumni," by R. S. Paffenbarger, Jr., A. L. Wing, and R. T. Hyde, 1978, *American Journal of Epidemiology*, 108, p. 166. Copyright © 1978 by The Johns Hopkins University School of Hygiene and Public Health.

physically active classmates, with 2,000 kcal per week as the breaking point. In addition, exercise benefited men who smoked, had a history of hypertension, or both. Beyond the 2,000 kcal per week expenditure, increased exercise paid no dividends in terms of reduced risk of fatal or nonfatal heart attacks. Figure 15.1 shows this relationship.

Later Studies

Dozens of more recent studies have examined the relationship between physical activity and cardiovascular mortality. A systematic review of these studies shows that physical activity confers a 35% reduction in risk of death due to cardiovascular causes (Nocon et al., 2008). The same review concludes that physical activity confers a 33% reduction in risk of death due to all causes. Furthermore, both men and women benefit from physical activity, but risk reductions may be larger for women than for men (Nocon et al., 2008). More recent reviews confirm this link, with a dose–response relationship observed between levels of vigorous physical activity and reduced risk of all-cause mortality (Samitz, Egger, & Zwahlen, 2011), and a large reduction in risk when comparing people who report no activity to those who report low levels of light-to-moderate physical activity (Woodcock, Franco, Orsini, & Roberts, 2011). Thus, some activity is far better than none, but there are still benefits adding more activity to some activity.

Evidence also shows cardiovascular benefits among people from a variety of nations and different ethnic groups. For example, many Mexican Americans are at risk for obesity, high cholesterol, and other cardiovascular risk factors, which suggests that they can probably profit from a routine exercise program. A study of Mexican Americans in the San Antonio Heart Study (Rainwater et al., 2000) found that changes in physical activity over a 5-year period tended to mirror changes in CVD risk factors.

Thus, it is unmistakably clear that physical activity protects against CVD (Myers, 2000; Nocon et al., 2008; Schlicht, Kanning, & Bos, 2007). First, people who are already active receive some gains by increasing their level of activity, but the largest gains occur when people go from a sedentary lifestyle to an active one. Second, walking, especially for older people, confers protection against CVD (Murphy et al., 2007). Third, an inactive lifestyle is equal to diabetes, high cholesterol level, smoking, and high blood pressure as a CVD risk factor. Fourth, physically fit men and women in all age groups can reduce their CVD risk through leisure-time activities. Fifth, exercise accumulated several years ago does not provide much current protection against all-cause mortality. Similarly, people who survive a heart attack and who include physical activity as part of their cardiac rehabilitation program decrease their all-cause mortality as well as their risk for a subsequent heart attack. However, those benefits disappear after 5 years if participants stop exercising. Thus, because previous physical activity loses its benefit after a few years, heart attack survivors should maintain their exercise program.

Exercise also offers protection against stroke. Researchers from the Nurses' Health Study (Hu et al., 2000) found that the most active women, compared with sedentary women, reduced their risk of death from ischemic stroke by about 34%, compared with sedentary women. Furthermore, there was a dose–response relationship between levels of physical activity and protection from ischemic stroke. Individuals who had a stroke were less physically active than others, including less physical activity in the week preceding their stroke (Krarup et al., 2007). Similarly, a meta-analysis (Wendel-Vos et al., 2004) found that high levels of occupational and leisure-time physical activity reduce the risk of both ischemic stroke and hemorrhagic stroke.

These and other reports on CVD suggest that a lifestyle that includes at least some physical activity can help protect people against premature CVD, including stroke. Even small amounts of activity can help, but more is better, at least to a point. (In a later section, we discuss how much is enough without being too much.)

Do Women and Men Benefit Equally?

All the early studies on the cardiovascular effects of exercise had one important limitation: They focused exclusively on men. To complete the picture of the health benefits of exercise, later researchers extended their investigations to women. Gender differences in degree of physical activity, leisure-time activity, and job-related activity might suggest differences between men and women in their level of protection against CVD and all-cause mortality.

Do the benefits of physical activity extend to women as well as men? Paffenbarger and his associates (Oguma, Sesso, Paffenbarger, & Lee, 2002) looked at 37 prospective cohort studies and one retrospective study that dealt with the association between all-cause mortality and both physical activity and physical fitness in women. The results indicated that women can gain about as much as men from physical activity, a finding confirmed in a more recent review (Nocon et al., 2008). Inactive women were much more likely than active women to have died during the study period. More recent reviews suggest that women may have even a greater reduction in all-cause mortality risk through physical activity than men (Samitz et al., 2011). (See Figure 15.1 for a relationship between level of kilocalories and first heart attack in men.)

In summary, both women and men can improve their cardiovascular health and live longer with light-to-moderate exercise. Physically active people can expect an average increase in longevity of about 2 years (Blair, Cheng, & Holder, 2001). A cynic might note that a person would need to jog a total of about 2 years between the ages of 20 and 80 to increase longevity by 2 years. Why live another 2 years if one must spend that time exercising? However, physical activity does more than simply add quantity to a person's life span; it adds *quality* to those years as well, by improving well-being, mental health, and cognitive functioning (as we will discuss later in this chapter).

Physical Activity and Cholesterol Levels

How does exercise protect against CVD? Exercise increases high-density lipoprotein (HDL, or "good" cholesterol) while decreasing LDL ("bad" cholesterol; Hausenloy & Yellen, 2008). The combination of raising HDL and lowering LDL may leave total cholesterol the same, but the ratio of total cholesterol to HDL becomes more favorable, and the risk for heart disease decreases. Thus, physical activity can benefit cardiac patients in two ways: by lowering LDL and by raising HDL (Szapary, Bloedon, & Foster, 2003).

Moderate levels of exercise, with or without dietary changes, bring about a favorable ratio of total cholesterol to HDL. Reviews of studies from the Toronto symposium (Leon & Sanchez, 2001; Williams, 2001) generally found that moderate exercise, such as walking and gardening, increases HDL and less frequently decreases both LDL and triglycerides. The combination of a low-fat diet and exercise is even more effective (Varady & Jones, 2005). Thus, moderate activity may lead to a more favorable ratio of total cholesterol to HDL, but prolonged strenuous physical activity does not seem to confer additional protection against heart disease; that is, there is inconsistent evidence for a dose–response relationship between levels of physical activity and death from heart disease (Leon & Sanchez, 2001).

If adults can improve their lipid numbers through moderate exercise, could children and adolescents also benefit from regular physical activity? Identifying the link between fitness and cardiovascular risk factors in children is difficult, as many children and adolescents who are sedentary are also overweight or obese. Despite this challenge, low fitness is related to high cholesterol levels and other cardiovascular risk factors for children in Europe (Andersen et al., 2008) and the United States (Eisenmann, Welk, Wickel, & Blair, 2007). Programs to improve these risk factors typically include both weight loss and exercise, yielding little research that evaluates only the influence of physical activity on cardiovascular risk factors (Kelley & Kelley, 2007).

In general, physically active children can benefit from exercise, but probably not as much as adults (Tolfrey, 2004). However, children as young as 4 can profit from an enhanced exercise program (Sääkslahti et al., 2004). This research looked at 4- to 7-year-old children and found that both girls and boys with highly active play time had low levels of total cholesterol, high levels of HDL cholesterol, and a favorable ratio between total cholesterol and HDL cholesterol. A study of preadolescent and early adolescent children showed results similar to studies with adults; that is, exercise

seems to lower LDL while raising HDL and leaving total cholesterol basically unchanged (Tolfrey, Jones, & Campbell, 2000). Regular aerobic exercise may protect against heart disease in both adults and children by increasing HDL and by improving the ratio of total cholesterol to HDL.

IN SUMMARY

Accumulating evidence suggests that physical activity reduces the incidence of coronary heart disease. Early research had many flaws and tended to include only men. However, more recent research confirms a strong association between a regimen of moderate physical activity and cardiovascular health, including heart disease and stroke. In addition, physical activity can raise HDL, thereby improving the ratio of total cholesterol to HDL. As a result, regular activity may add as much as 2 years to one's life while decreasing disability, especially in later years.

Other Health Benefits of Physical Activity

Although most people who exercise do so for physical fitness, weight control, or cardiovascular health, other benefits accrue to those who adopt a physical activity regimen, including protection against some kinds of cancer, prevention of bone density loss, control of diabetes, and improved psychological health.

Protection Against Cancer

Several reviews (Miles, 2007; Thune & Furberg, 2001) examine the connection between physical activity and various cancers. Of the hundreds of studies evaluated, most focused on cancers of the colon and rectum, breast, endometrium, prostate, and lung. Physical activity offers protection against each of these types of cancer, with the strongest evidence for colorectal and breast cancer. The protective effects for colorectal cancer seem as strong for women as for men (Wolin, Yan, Colditz, & Lee, 2009), and exercise appears to protect postmenopausal more than premenopausal women from breast cancer (Friedenreich & Cust, 2008). Furthermore, exercise may be more likely to protect non-Caucasian women against breast cancer better than Caucasian women (Friedenreich & Cust, 2008). Results from a meta-analysis (Tardon et al., 2005) are consistent with the systematic reviews, suggesting that moderate to high levels of physical activity reduce incidence of lung cancer in both women and men, but the relationship is stronger for women.

How does physical activity lower risk for cancer? Although the answer is unclear, physical activity may do so by influencing tumor initiation and growth (Rogers, Colbert, Greiner, Perkins, & Hursting, 2008). Furthermore, physical activity affects proinflammatory cytokines, which are involved in the development of both CVD (Stewart et al., 2007) and cancer. Thus, research has not only established the protective benefits of physical activity for cancer but also has begun to show how those benefits may occur.

Exercise may also be helpful for people with cancer. Cancer patients undergoing chemotherapy benefit from physical activity training by increasing strength, aerobic fitness, and weight (Quist et al., 2006). A systematic review (Speck, Courneya, Masse, Duval, & Schmitz, 2010) also indicates that exercise helps manage the fatigue that often accompanies cancer treatment. Thus, physical activity is effective in preventing several types of cancer and is helpful in managing some of the distressing side effects of cancer treatment.

Prevention of Bone Density Loss

Exercise also protects against osteoporosis, a disorder characterized by a reduction in bone density due to calcium loss that results in brittle bones. Physical activity can protect both men and women against loss of bone mineral density (BMD), especially those who were active during their youth. Bone minerals accrue during childhood and early adolescence, and activity during those years may be especially important for bone health (Hind & Burrows, 2007). For example, one comparison of retired athletes and a comparison group found that the former athletes retained more BMD and had fewer fractures at age 60 than those who had not been athletes.

Both men and women can benefit from high-impact exercise such as running and jumping. However, this type of exercise may leave people (especially older individuals) vulnerable to injuries. We discuss these and other injuries later in this chapter, but as the Would

You Believe...? box explains, both older and young people benefit from exercise. An experimental study (Vainionpää, Korpelainen, Leppäluoto, & Jämsä, 2005) indicated that young, premenopausal women in the experimental (high-impact) group had significantly higher BMD than young women in the control group. However, an intervention featuring walking (Palombaro, 2005) and another using tai chi (Wayne et al., 2007) did not demonstrate effectiveness as clearly as the program with high-impact exercise (Zehnacker & Bemis-Dougherty, 2007).

Control of Diabetes

Because obesity is a factor in Type 2 diabetes and because exercise is an established means of controlling weight, it follows that physical activity may be a useful weapon in the control of diabetes. Systematic reviews of research on this topic confirm the benefits of exercise for improvement of insulin resistance (Plasqui & Westerterp, 2007), for prevention of Type 2 diabetes (Jeon, Lokken, Hu, & van Dam, 2007), for the management of this condition (Kavookjian, Elswick, & Whetsel, 2007), and for reduction in mortality risk among diabetics (Sluik et al., 2012). Thus, the benefits of exercise for Type 2 diabetes are well established.

Does physical activity protect Type 1 diabetics? A meta-analysis of behavior change interventions (Conn et al., 2008) shows that exercise is an important component in managing Type 1 diabetes. Physically active adolescents with Type 1 diabetes exhibit lower cardiovascular risk factors than those who are less active (Herbst, Kordonouri, Schwab, Schmidt, & Holl, 2007). Although these studies reported a modest protective benefit for physical activity, they do not suggest that exercise is a panacea for the control of diabetes. Nevertheless, they do indicate that physical activity can be a useful component in the treatment of insulin-dependent diabetes and can offer some protection against the development of non-insulin-dependent diabetes.

Psychological Benefits of Physical Activity

As stated earlier, physical activity increases not only the quantity of life but also its quality. The gains from regular physical activity extend to psychological benefits, including a defense against depression, a reduction of anxiety, a buffer against stress, and

Would You BELIEVE...?

It's Never Too Late—or Too Early

Physical activity is a healthy habit, but would you believe that it's never too late in the life span to start exercising? Or too early?

Older adults benefit from being physically active in many ways. Cardiovascular benefits include lower blood pressure, improved symptoms of congestive heart failure, and decreased risk for cardiovascular disease (Karani, McLaughlin, & Cassel, 2001). In addition, physically active older adults have lower risk for diabetes, osteoporosis, osteoarthritis, and depression. All of these benefits result in lowered sickness and death among physically active older adults (Everett, Kinser, & Ramsey, 2007).

Despite these many benefits, 56% of Americans over age 75 are sedentary (USCB, 2011). People tend to become less active as they age, and they also reduce their exercising when they experience pain (Nied & Franklin, 2002). For example, arthritis causes knee and hip joint pain that makes older people less willing to exercise. Also, people who have had a stroke may experience balance or weakness problems that make them feel uneasy about even normal levels of activity. Older people are more likely than younger ones to fall, and resulting broken bones may make a permanent change in their mobility and independence. Although

all of these concerns have some foundation, the risks are manageable. Physical activity offers more benefits than risks for older people, even for those over age 85 and for those who are frail. They may need supervision for their exercise, but older adults benefit from physical activity. Exercise such as tai chi even helps quell fears and risks of falling (Sattin, Easley, Wolf, Chen, & Kutner, 2005; Zijlstra et al., 2007). Almost all older people can decrease health risks and gain mobility from exercising.

It's also never too early to begin an active lifestyle. Physical activity furnishes lifetime benefits, and even young children benefit. Very young children may not seem to be at any risk from inactivity, but they are. To maintain their goals of safety and convenience, parents and caregivers often confine infants in strollers, infant seats, or playpens that limit their movement (National Association for Sport and Physical Education [NASPE], 2002). These experiences not only limit mobility during infancy but also may delay developmental goals such as crawling and walking. Lack of physical activity during toddlerhood can lead to a sedentary childhood. Inactive children may also lag in developing motor skills and join the growing number of overweight and

obese children in the United States (Floriani & Kennedy, 2008).

The National Association for Sport and Physical Education (NASPE, 2002) proposed guidelines for physical activity, beginning during infancy. For all children, NASPE emphasized supervision and safety. The recommendations for infants included allowing them to experience settings in which they can move while maintaining safety and playing a variety of games such as peekaboo and hide-and-seek. NASPE recommended at least 30 minutes a day of structured physical activity for toddlers and 60 minutes for preschool children. Scott Roberts (2002) went a step further, recommending workouts for children. He argued that the prohibitions against weight lifting and other types of strength training for children have no research basis. On the contrary, Roberts maintained that children experience the same benefits from this type of exercise as do adults, including protection against cardiovascular disease, hypertension, and obesity as well as improved strength, flexibility, and posture.

Remember, physical activity brings lifetime benefits, so it's never too early—or too late—to begin a lifetime exercise program.

a contributor to better cognitive functioning. People who exercise regularly often say it improves their mood, reduces stress, and helps them focus. Does the evidence support these claims?

In general, the link between physical activity and psychological functioning is less clearly established than the link between physical activity and physiological

health. In addition, any evaluation of the therapeutic effects of exercise on psychological disorders must consider the problems raised by the placebo effect. For this reason, quality research is difficult, and some areas lack adequate research to evaluate the effects (Larun, Nordheim, Ekeland, Hagen, & Heian, 2006). Nevertheless, evidence suggests that a regular exercise regimen can decrease depression, reduce anxiety, buffer stress, and improve cognitive functioning.

Decreased Depression   The *Diagnostic and Statistical Manual of Mental Disorders*, 5th edition, of the American Psychiatric Association (APA, 2013) defines a major depressive episode as a period of at least 2 weeks during which there is either depressed mood or the loss of interest or pleasure in nearly all activities. During a lifetime, as many as 25% of women and 12% of men may suffer from major depression (APA, 2000). If physical activity can relieve major depression, then millions of people can benefit from a therapy that is easily available to nearly everyone.

People who exercise regularly are generally less depressed than sedentary people (Martinsen, 2005). When researchers compare groups of exercisers with groups of sedentary people on different measures of depression, they find that highly active people are usually less depressed. One possible explanation is that, rather than improved mood, exercising may be restricted to healthy people. Depressed people may simply be less motivated to exercise.

Experimental studies aim to determine the direction of causation. For example, one randomized controlled trial (Annesi, 2005) divided moderately depressed individuals into an experimental group that performed 10 weeks of moderate physical activity three times a week for 20 to 30 minutes and a control group that did not exercise. Clear differences emerged between the two groups, with those who exercised experiencing much lower levels of depression than participants in the control group. Furthermore, a similar research design (Dunn, Trivedi, Kampert, Clark, & Chambliss, 2005) found evidence for a dose–response relationship between physical activity and relief from depressive symptomatology. Recent reviews of research confirm that physical activity does reduce symptoms of depression (Silveira et al., 2013), although well-controlled studies tend to show less of a benefit than more poorly designed studies (Cooney et al., 2013).

Exercise is certainly more effective than no treatment and may be comparable to cognitive therapy (Donaghy, 2007) or antidepressant medication (Daley, 2008). The long-term effects of physical activity on depression, however, have not been substantiated. Nevertheless, an evaluation of the significance of exercise programs (Rethorst, Wipfli, & Landers, 2007) determined that such programs produced not only statistically significant differences but also clinically significant effects. Thus, the body of research supports an early statement by Rod Dishman (2003), who explained: "I am not proposing that exercise is a replacement for psychotherapy or drug therapy, but these findings about exercise are not trivial and suggest that physical activity may be an important addition or complement to standard treatment for mild depression" (p. 45).

Reduced Anxiety   Many people report that they exercise to feel more relaxed and less anxious. Does exercise play a role in anxiety reduction? The answer may depend on the type of anxiety under study. **Trait anxiety** is a general personality characteristic or trait that manifests itself as a more or less constant feeling of dread or uneasiness. **State anxiety** is a temporary, affective condition that stems from a specific situation. Feelings of worry or concern over a final examination or a job interview are examples of state anxiety. Physiological changes such as increased perspiration and heart rate typically accompany this type of anxiety.

Research on the effects of physical activity on state anxiety suffers from many of the same methodological limitations as research on physical activity and depression; that is, only a few of the studies have had an adequate number of participants and have used random assignment to experimental and control groups (Dunn, Trivedi, & O'Neal, 2001). A meta-analysis of randomized controlled trials (Wipfli, Rethorst, & Landers, 2008) indicated that exercise is more effective than no treatment and has comparable or superior effects to other forms of therapy. Furthermore, physical activity is also effective in reducing anxiety symptoms among chronic illness patients (Herring, O'Connor, & Dishman, 2010).

How does physical activity reduce anxiety? One hypothesis is that exercise simply provides a change of pace—a chance to relax and forget one's troubles. In support of this change-of-pace hypothesis, exercise demonstrated no stronger therapeutic effect than meditation (Bahrke & Morgan, 1978). Studies show that other techniques to reduce anxiety, including biofeedback, transcendental meditation, "time-out" therapy, and even beer drinking in a pub atmosphere, can also be effective (Morgan, 1981). Each of these interventions provides a change of pace, and all are associated with reduced levels of state anxiety.

Another hypothesis involves changes in brain chemistry. Studies with rats (Greenwood et al., 2005) show that exercise changes the transport of the neurotransmitter serotonin, which is related to positive mood. Studies with humans (Broocks et al., 2003) also suggest that changes occur in the metabolism of this neurotransmitter after exercise. Thus, physical activity may reduce anxiety by providing a change of pace, by altering neurotransmitter activity, or through some combination of the two.

Buffer Against Stress   Two questions arise in relation to exercise and stress: (1) Can exercise enhance psychological well-being? (2) Can it protect people against the harmful effects of stress? Research on the first question has generally produced an affirmative answer. For example, older adults who exercise more regularly report greater well-being as well as greater quality of life than older adults who do not (Paxton, Motl, Aylward, & Nigg, 2010). Furthermore, a meta-analysis (Netz, Wu, Becker, & Tenenbaum, 2005) finds that physical activity relates to psychological well-being, but longer exercise duration does not always lead to continuing increases in feelings of well-being. Thus, moderate exercise may be enough to boost well-being.

Answers to the second question are more difficult because a direct causal link between stress and subsequent physical illness has not yet been established (see Chapter 6 on stress and disease). However, several studies suggest that physical activity helps people deal with stress. Fitness appears to act as a buffer for both physical and psychological stress (Ensel & Lin, 2004); individuals who are more fit experience less distress.

Why might fitness reduce feelings of stress? One pathway may involve cardiovascular responses to stress, as exercise moderates the increase in blood pressure that accompanies psychological stress (Hamer, Taylor, & Steptoe, 2006). A second pathway may involve immune responses, as the effect of stress on the release of proinflammatory cytokines is moderated in fit individuals (Hamer & Steptoe, 2007). Thus, exercise acts to decrease stress, on both a psychological and a physiological level.

The duration of exercise required to produce positive effects is not extreme; as little as 10 minutes of moderately strenuous exercise is capable of elevating mood (Hansen, Stevens, & Coast, 2001). The results of the studies on stress buffering do not indicate a strong effect for exercise, but physical activity is a strategy that many people use to help them manage stress. Figure 15.2 shows some of the positive effects of exercise.

Better Cognitive Functioning   Physical activity may make you feel better, but can it also make you think better? Earlier we said (mischievously, perhaps) that you could extend your life by 2 years by spending 2 years exercising. However, time spent in physical activity could be more worthwhile when considering the rewards it brings to cognitive functioning. One recent study of nearly 1,000 older adults showed that those who engaged in high amounts of physical activity had, at a 5-year follow-up, cognitive skills characteristic of individuals *10 years younger* compared to those who engaged in little to no physical activity (Willey et al., 2016). Thus, while more research is needed to confirm these findings, they do suggest that physical activity could make one's living years *smarter*, not just more numerous.

Cognitive functioning includes diverse abilities such as the ability to focus attention, the speed of processing new information, and memory. Cognitive functioning also includes executive functioning, which refers to the ability to plan for and successfully pursue goals.

Aging often brings about a decline in cognitive functioning. Consequently, most research that focuses on the link between physical activity and cognitive functioning involves adults, particularly older adults. Indeed, a recent review of 29 exercise intervention studies (Smith, Blumenthal, et al., 2010) concludes that adults who participate in regular physical activity programs show greater attention, processing speed, memory, and executive functioning than adults who do not participate in physical activity programs. Moreover, physical activity appears to reduce some of the cognitive declines that occur with aging. For example, physical activity interventions show a stronger protective effect on memory among older adults than among younger adults, as well as among adults who are at greatest risk for Alzheimer's disease. Aerobic fitness training also contributes to increases in brain volume among older adults, but not younger adults (Colcombe et al., 2006).

One Australian study focused on older adults who reported memory problems that were indicative of risk for Alzheimer's disease (Lautenschlager et al., 2008). Through random assignment, some of these adults participated in a 6-month, home-based physical activity intervention; others adults did not. At an 18-month follow-up, the adults assigned to the intervention *improved* in their cognitive functioning. In contrast, those who did not receive the physical activity intervention showed no change in cognitive functioning.

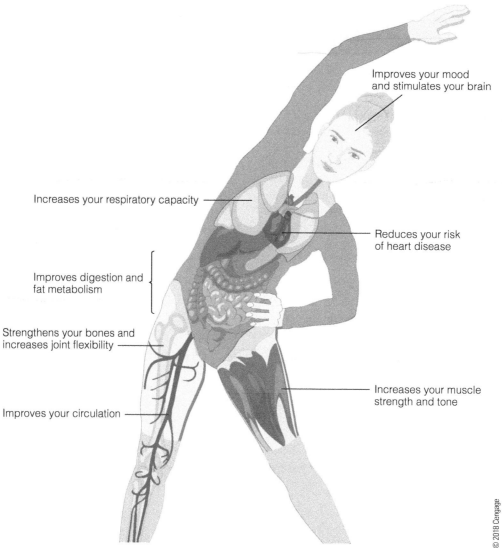

Improves your mood
and stimulates your brain

Increases your respiratory capacity

Reduces your risk
of heart disease

Improves digestion and
fat metabolism

Strengthens your bones and
increases joint flexibility

Increases your muscle
strength and tone

Improves your circulation

© 2018 Cengage

FIGURE 15.2   Some of the physical and psychological benefits of exercise.

Source: An invitation to health (7th ed., p. 493), by D. Hales, 1997, Pacific Grove, CA: Brooks/Cole. Copyright © 1997 by Brooks/Cole Publishing Company.

Can physical activity also improve cognitive function in children? Recent research suggests it can. Children who are physically fit show better memory performance than those who are less fit, as well as greater volume of the hippocampus, a brain structure that plays an important role in memory (Chaddock et al., 2010). Intervention research also shows this link between physical activity and cognitive functioning. For example, a 3-month physical activity intervention program for overweight and sedentary children led to greater planning abilities as well as greater performance on a standardized math test (Davis et al., 2011).

Why does physical activity improve cognitive functioning? While the exact reason remains unknown, researchers speculate that these benefits may derive from increased cerebral blood flow or increased expression of brain-derived neurotrophic factor (BDNF), a protein that contributes the growth and differentiation of neurons in the brain (Brown et al., 2010; Smith et al., 2010).

Would You BELIEVE...?   Exercise Can Help You Learn

What plays in the earplugs of people you see working out? Perhaps it's an inspiring "power song," perhaps a podcast, or maybe even a recording of a TV show. Would it seem strange if you learned that a person was listening to a class lecture while running, or a foreign language lesson while riding a bike?

Physical activity can improve cognitive functioning, and new research is examining whether physical activity can help people learn new information.

Researchers from Germany (Schmidt-Kassow et al., 2013) asked young adult women to learn new vocabulary terms under one of three conditions. One condition had the women learn the words while resting in a comfortable chair. Another condition had the women learn the words immediately after riding a stationary bicycle for 30 minutes. The third condition had the women learn the words *while* riding the stationary

bicycle. For those who rode the bike, the researchers ensured that the women's exertion was of a light-to-moderate intensity. All women then completed a test to assess how many of the new vocabulary terms they could correctly remember.

The major difference that the researchers found was that the women who were exposed to the new words *while* riding the bike had significantly better memory of the words than those who were exposed to the words while relaxing. Interestingly, this difference was largest for those women who were initially identified as poor vocabulary learners. These findings suggest that for some kinds of learning tasks, exposure to the information *while* engaging in low-to-moderate intensity activity could improve learning.

Another study examined whether physical activity *following* a learning task could improve memory (van Dongen, Kersten,

Wagner, Morris, & Fernandez, 2016). In this study, all participants were exposed to a set of pictures and locations. Then, the participants were assigned to one of three conditions: no aerobic exercise, aerobic exercise immediately following the learning task, and aerobic exercise 4 hours following the learning task. The researchers found superior memory for the picture-location associations among those who exercised 4 hours after the learning task.

While the exact biological mechanisms for these findings remain unclear, they do suggest that light-to-moderate physical activity can promote learning of new information. So, if you have new information to learn and you also want to do some light-to-moderate exercise, you could use physical activity to your advantage: listen to the class lecture or lesson while exercising, or make sure you follow up your studying with an exercise session.

IN SUMMARY

During the past 50 years, research supports the hypothesis that physical activity improves health and psychological functioning. Regular moderate physical activity can reduce the incidence of CVD, including heart disease and stroke. Exercise improves both blood pressure and cholesterol profile, showing some ability to raise HDL. Physical activity also shows benefits for decreasing the risk for the development of diabetes and several types of cancer, including colon and breast cancer. Exercise can also promote bone growth in young people and slow the loss of bone minerals in older individuals. Moreover, physical activity shows psychological benefits. Indeed, exercise may be a useful intervention for depression. Benefits also

appear for reducing anxiety, buffering stress, and improving cognitive functioning.

An earlier section of this chapter examined several reasons why people exercise. Table 15.1 lists some of these reasons, summarizes research evidence, and cites at least one study pertaining to each reason.

Hazards of Physical Activity

Although physical activity can enhance physical functioning, reduce anxiety, stress, and depression, and improve cognitive functioning, it also poses hazards to one's physical and psychological health. Some athletes overtrain to the point of staleness and, as a consequence,

TABLE 15.1   Reasons for Exercising and Research Supporting These Reasons

Reasons for Exercising	Findings	Principal Source(s)
Weight control	Obesity can be reduced through exercise; 60 to 90 minutes a day may be necessary.	Hill & Wyatt, 2005; Jakicic & Otto, 2005
	Exercise is as effective as dieting; sculpting the perfect body won't work.	Blair & Church, 2004; Wood et al., 1988
Heart disease and aerobic fitness	Light-to-moderate exercise provides sufficient protection.	Barengo et al., 2004; Paffenbarger et al., 1978
	Both physical fitness and physical activity have a dose–response relationship with aerobic health.	Blair et al., 2001
	Walking confers benefits for older people.	Murphy et al., 2007
Stroke	Active women reduce risk of stroke.	Hu et al., 2000
	Inactive people are more likely to have strokes.	Krarup et al., 2007
	Physical activity can reduce two types of stroke.	Wendel-Vos et al., 2004
All-cause mortality	Nurses' Health Study reviewed 37 prospective cohort studies.	Oguma et al., 2002
	Dose–response relationship between vigorous physical activity and mortality risk	Samitz et al., 2011
	Largest reduction in mortality risk when comparing no physical activity to some physical activity	Woodcock et al., 2011
Cholesterol level	Exercise increases HDL and decreases LDL.	Hausenloy & Yellen, 2008; Szapary et al., 2003
	Exercise reduces LDL and triglycerides.	Leon & Sanchez, 2001
	Low fitness is related to high cholesterol in children and adolescents.	Andersen et al., 2008; Eisenmann et al., 2007
	Exercise relates to low cholesterol in children.	Sääkslahti et al., 2004; Tolfrey, 2004; Tolfrey et al., 2000
Cancer	Meta-analyses show inverse relationship between exercise and cancer of various sites.	Miles, 2007; Thune & Furberg, 2001
	Exercise reduces risk for lung cancer, with a stronger relationship for women.	Tardon et al., 2005
	Exercise may protect against both tumor initiation and growth.	Rogers et al., 2008
	Physical activity helps people with cancer manage the effects of cancer treatment.	Quist et al., 2006; Speck et al., 2010
Bone density loss (osteoporosis)	Exercise helps build bone mass in children and adolescents.	Hind & Burrows, 2007
	Retired male athletes retain much of bone mineral density.	Nordström et al., 2005
	High-impact activity can delay loss of bone minerals in women.	Vainionpää et al., 2005
	Low-impact activities are not as effective as high-impact exercise.	Palombaro, 2005; Wayne et al., 2007; Zehnacker et al., 2007

TABLE 15.1 *(Continued)*

Reasons for Exercising	Findings	Principal Source(s)
Diabetes	Exercise improves insulin resistance.	Plasqui & Westerterp, 2007
	Exercise lowers risk for Type 2 diabetes.	Jeon et al., 2007
	Exercise can help in managing Type 2 diabetes.	Kavookjian et al., 2007
	Exercise is an important component in managing Type 1 diabetes.	Conn et al., 2008
	Exercise lowers risk for CVD in individuals with Type 1 diabetes.	Herbst et al., 2007
	Exercise lowers mortality risk in diabetics.	Sluik et al., 2012
Decreased depression	Moderate exercise three times a week for 20 to 30 minutes reduces depression.	Annesi, 2005; Silveira et al., 2013
	A dose–response relationship occurs with exercise and depression.	Dunn et al., 2005
	Exercise compares with cognitive therapy and antidepressant medication in effectiveness.	Daley, 2008; Donaghy, 2007
	Benefits of exercise are clinically significant.	Rethorst et al., 2007
Reduced anxiety	Moderate exercise can reduce state anxiety.	Dunn et al., 2001; Wipfli et al., 2008
	Physical activity is effective in reducing anxiety among chronic illness patients.	Herring et al., 2010
Buffer against stress	Exercise enhances mood, feelings of well-being, and quality of life.	Ensel & Lin, 2004; Hansen et al., 2001; Paxton et al., 2010
	Exercise increases well-being, but more is not always better.	Netz et al., 2005
	Exercise affects blood pressure and immune system response to stress.	Hamer et al., 2006; Hamer & Steptoe, 2007
Better cognitive functioning	Exercise is linked to greater attention, processing speed, memory, and executive functioning in adults.	Smith et al., 2010
	Aerobic fitness training is linked to increases in brain volume among older adults.	Colcombe et al., 2006
	Very physically active older adults have cognitive skills far superior to inactive older adults.	Wiley et al., 2016
	Six month exercise program led to improved cognitive functioning.	Lautenschlager et al., 2008
	Children who exercise more show better memory, planning, and math performance.	Chaddock et al., 2010; Davis et al., 2011

suffer from negative mood, fatigue, and depression (Tobar, 2005). In addition, some highly active people suffer from exercise-related injuries. Other people allow exercise to assume an almost addictive importance in their lives. In this section, we look at some of these potential hazards related to physical activity.

Exercise Addiction

Some people become so involved with exercise that they ignore injuries to continue exercising or allow their exercise regimen to interfere with other parts of their lives such as work or family responsibilities. Others may think these people have an *exercise addiction,* but their behavior may not match the description of an addiction. In Chapter 13, we saw that addictions produce tolerance, dependence, and withdrawal symptoms.

William Morgan (1979) compared the process of excessive exercising to the development of other addictions. Initially, the tolerance for running is low, and it has many unpleasant side effects. But persistence eases the unpleasant aspects, and the pleasure of meeting goals becomes a powerful reinforcer. Like most social drinkers who have a casual, nonobsessive relationship with alcohol, most exercisers are able to incorporate physical activity into their lives without drastic changes in lifestyle. Other exercisers, however, cannot. Those who continue to increase their exercise must make changes in their lives to accommodate the time required, with consequences for other responsibilities and activities.

A high level of commitment to exercise is not the same as addiction (Terry, Szabo, & Griffiths, 2004). Some people's exercise habits reflect a high degree of commitment, whereas others fit the description of dependence, showing a strong emotional attachment to exercise (Ackard, Brehm, & Steffen, 2002) and exhibiting withdrawal symptoms such as depression and anxiety when prevented from exercising (Hausenblas & Symons Downs, 2002a, 2002b). Committed exercisers tend to have rational reasons for their exercise behavior such as extrinsic rewards, whereas addicted exercisers tend to use exercise as a way to manage negative emotions and problems in their lives (Warner & Griffiths, 2006). Some research opens up the possibility that exercise may be analogous to other types of addiction (Hamer & Karageorghis, 2007). This contention remains controversial, however, and some authorities prefer the term *obligatory exercise* or *exercise dependence* rather than exercise addiction.

Obligatory exercisers share several characteristics with people with eating disorders, especially anorexia. For example, they continue their chosen activity even when they are injured, continuing behavior that is harmful and even self-destructive. They also show a progressive self-absorption, with a great deal of concentration on internal experiences. In addition, many people who are anorexic experience a compulsion to exercise excessively (Klein et al., 2004). This observation prompted the proposal that teenage female anorexics and addicted male runners are analogous (Davis & Scott-Robertson, 2000); both show the need for mastery of the body, unusually high expectations of self, tolerance, or denial of physical discomfort and pain, and a single-minded commitment to endurance. Other researchers (Ackard et al., 2002) found that obligatory exercisers exhibited body obsession, were more likely to have eating disorders, and showed symptoms of other psychological problems. The motivation for excessive exercise is a critical mediating factor that connects exercise to eating disorders (Cook & Hausenblas, 2008). For these individuals, the connection between exercising and eating disorders is a strong emotional attachment to exercise. These individuals experience injuries yet continue to exercise, neglect their personal relationships, and shortchange their jobs to devote time to exercise. Perhaps this fanaticism can be best expressed in the words of one obligatory runner:

> One day last spring I was having an exceptionally good run. I was running about 10 miles a day at that time and on this particular day I had decided to extend my workout. I was around the 14-mile point and I was preparing to cross a one-lane bridge when all of a sudden a large cement mixer turned the corner and began to cross the bridge. I never thought for a second about stopping and letting the truck pass. I simply continued and said to myself, "Come on you son-of-a-bitch and I'll split you right down the middle—there will be concrete all over the road!" The driver slammed on the brakes and swerved to the side as I sailed by. That was really scary afterward, but at the time I really felt good. I have felt equally strong and indestructible many times since, but never have taken on a cement truck again. (Morgan, 1979, pp. 63, 67)

Injuries from Physical Activity

Excluding head-to-head challenges with cement trucks, what are the chances of experiencing injuries from

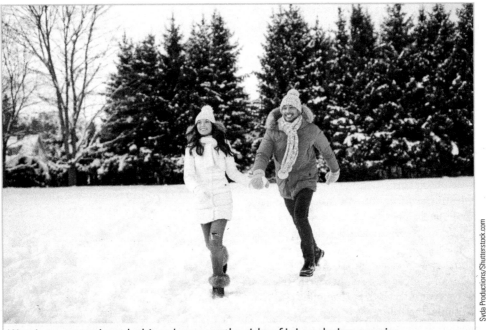

Wearing appropriate clothing decreases the risks of injury during exercise.

exercise? Many people with a regular exercise program accept minor injuries and soreness as an almost inevitable component of their program. However, irregular exercise produces even more injuries and more discomfort, with "weekend athletes" accounting for a disproportional number of injuries.

Musculoskeletal injuries are common, and the greater the frequency and intensity of exercise, the more likely it is that people will injure themselves (Powell, Paluch, & Blair, 2011). The Surgeon General's report (USDHHS, 1996) found that about half of runners had experienced an injury during the past year. This review also found, as expected, that the injury rate was lower for walkers than for joggers and that previous injury is a risk factor for subsequent injury. Physical activity is the source of 83% of all musculoskeletal injuries, and at least one-fourth of exercisers must interrupt their regimen because of such injuries (Hootman et al., 2002). The decision to decrease exercise in response to injury is a wise one; "working through the pain" is an exercise myth that is associated with further injury.

Besides muscular and skeletal injuries, avid exercisers encounter a number of other health hazards. Heat, cold, dogs, and drivers can all be sources of danger. During exercise, body temperature rises. Both heat and cold present problems, some of which can be dangerous (Roberts, 2007). Fluid intake before, after, and even during exercise can protect against overheating by allowing cooling through sweating. However, conditions of extremely high air temperature, high humidity, and sunlight can combine to raise body temperature and prevent sweat from evaporating from the skin surface. If the body cannot cool itself, dangerous overheating may occur. Managing the risks for heat stress is a challenge for those who manage sports teams (Cleary, 2007).

Cold temperatures can also be dangerous for outdoor exercising (Roberts, 2007), but proper clothing can provide protection. Layered clothing for the body and gloves, hat, and even a face mask can protect against temperatures of 20 °F and below (Pollock, Wilmore, & Fox, 1978). Temperatures below zero, especially when combined with wind, can be dangerous even to people who are not exercising.

Death During Exercise

Many patients who have had a heart attack go into cardiac rehabilitation programs that include an exercise program, which generally includes close supervision. Although these coronary patients are at elevated risk during exercise, the cardiovascular benefit they gain from exercising ordinarily outweighs the risk (USDHHS, 1996). Nevertheless, individuals diagnosed with coronary heart disease should undertake exercise only with a physician's permission and under the supervision of specialists in cardiac rehabilitation.

What about people who have no known disease? Is it possible for a person who looks and feels well to die unexpectedly during exercise? Yes—but it is also possible to die unexpectedly while watching TV or sleeping. However, exercise increases the risk of such sudden death (Thompson et al., 2007). A 12-year follow-up analysis of male physicians (Albert et al., 2000) showed that sudden death was more than 16 times more likely during or immediately after vigorous physical exertion than during other times. However, the risk was very low for any specific episode of exercise—one death per 1.5 million episodes of exercise. This study also showed that the benefits of exercise outweighed the risks: Men who exercised regularly were less likely to die during exercise than those who were unaccustomed to exertion. Although the men in this follow-up study (Albert et al., 2000) did not identify themselves as having CVD when the study began, either they were affected without their knowledge or developed this disease during the 12 years of the study. Indeed, most sudden deaths during exercise are the result of some type of heart disease, but people may be unaware of their risks.

Under most circumstances, exercise shows benefits for the cardiovascular system, but for those with CVD or other heart problems and for those who have exercised heavily for years of their lives (Raum, Rothenbacher, Ziegler, & Brenner, 2007), this pattern of physical activity is a risk. Even seemingly healthy, young people may be vulnerable to sudden cardiac death during exercise (Virmani, Burke, & Farb, 2001). Professional basketball player Reggie Lewis, who died during a practice game at the age of 28 due to a previously undiagnosed heart condition, is one of many seasoned athletes who have died during or shortly after periods of exercise. In children, adolescents, and young adults, the cause of sudden cardiac death is most often congenital heart abnormalities or arrhythmias (abnormal heartbeat patterns). Among adults, about 60% of sudden cardiac deaths are due to blood clots that precipitate heart attacks, the typical case of the most frequent cause of death in the United States. Thus, most sudden deaths during exercise are those of individuals who had underlying cardiovascular problems, whether they knew it or not.

Reducing Exercise Injuries

Adequate caution can decrease the probability of injury. For people who have or are at risk for CVD, supervised training is a wise precaution, especially when initiating an exercise program. Others, such as people who have been sedentary for a long time, may also benefit from supervision or training. With the guidance of a trainer, people will be less likely to attempt exercise that is inappropriate for their fitness level or to continue to exercise for too long as they start a program. In addition, an exercise professional will teach proper warm-up and stretching routines that are important in preventing injuries (Cooper, 2001).

Regardless of the level of fitness, the use of appropriate equipment decreases injuries. For example, proper running shoes are a necessity for running, jogging, or even exercise walking (Cooper, 2001). The correct type and amount of clothing are also important, either to allow for cooling or to retain heat. In addition to dressing properly for heat or cold, exercisers need to recognize the symptoms of heat stress. These include dizziness, weakness, nausea, muscle cramps, and headache. Each of these symptoms is a signal to stop exercising.

IN SUMMARY

Exercise has hazards as well as benefits. Potential hazards include exercise addiction—that is, a compulsive need to devote long periods of time to strenuous physical activity. Also, exercise may lead to injuries, the majority of which are musculoskeletal and relatively minor. Exercisers should avoid working out in extreme temperatures, and they should know how to avoid dogs, drivers, and darkness.

Death during exercise is a possibility. Those most vulnerable are individuals with CVD, who are often older, but young people with heart abnormalities are also at risk. Nevertheless, people who exercise regularly are much less likely than sporadic exercisers to die of a heart attack during intense physical exertion. Exercise-related injuries can be reduced by appropriate preparation such as choosing the appropriate level of exercise, using appropriate equipment, and recognizing signs of trouble and reacting appropriately.

How Much Is Enough But Not Too Much?

How much physical activity is enough but not too much? Table 15.2 lists the current physical activity recommendations, by age group. In recent years, estimates have decreased for the amount of exercise that produces health benefits. In 2011, the American College of Sports Medicine revised its recommendations for the amount and type of activity for health benefits (Garber et al., 2011). These recommendations clarified earlier recommendations, taking new research into account. According to this official view, a healthy adult under age 65 should participate in 30 minutes of moderately vigorous activity five times a week or vigorous activity 20 minutes three times a week. In addition, people should engage in 8 to 10 strength training exercises for 12 repetitions at least twice a week. These experts described this level of exercise as adequate to protect against chronic disease, including CVD.

The moderately vigorous activity recommendations reflect the evidence that less intense exercise produces health benefits and that vigorous exercise is not necessary. For example, a program of walking decreased cardiovascular risk factors in previously sedentary individuals (Murphy et al., 2007). Indeed, moderate exercise may be superior to more intense activity for some cardiovascular risk factors (Johnson et al., 2007). However, moderately vigorous activity three times

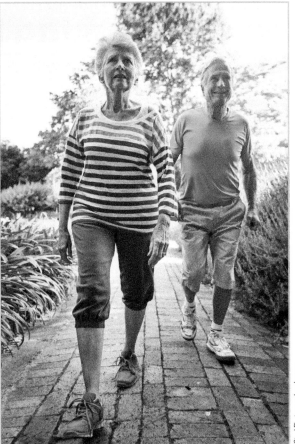

Walking is one form of physical activity that offers more advantages than hazards for most people.

TABLE 15.2 Current Physical Activity Recommendations

Age Group	Recommendation
Children and adolescents (aged 6–17)	1 hour of aerobic physical activity every day; most of this activity should be of moderate-to-vigorous intensity. Muscle-strengthening and bone-strengthening activity on at least 3 days per week.
Adults (aged 18–64)	2.5 hours of moderate-intensity aerobic activity per week, or 1.25 hours of vigorous-intensity aerobic activity per week. Muscle-strengthening activities on at least 2 days per week.
Older adults (aged 65 and older)	Same recommendations as for adults, or as much as abilities allow. Exercise that maintains or improves balance is recommended as well.

Source: Garber, C. E., Blissmer, B., Deschenes, M. R., Franklin, B. A., Lamonte, M. J., Lee, I.-M., Nieman, D. C., & Swain, D. P. (2011). Quantity and quality of exercise for developing and maintaining cardiorespiratory, musculoskeletal, and neuromotor fitness in apparently healthy adults: Guidance for prescribing exercise. *Medicine & Science in Sports & Exercise, 43,* 1334–1359; U.S. Department of Health and Human Services (USDHHS). (2008). *Physical activity guidelines for Americans.* Retrieved February 20, 2012, from http://www.health.gov/PAGuidelines/factsheetprof.aspx

Becoming Healthier

1. If you don't exercise, make specific plans to start a program of regular physical activity, concentrating on choosing an activity that is convenient and that you feel capable of performing (and even enjoying).
2. If you are overweight and over 40, consult a physician before beginning.
3. Don't start too fast. Once you have determined that you are ready to begin an exercise program, start slowly. The first day you may feel as though you can run a mile. Don't give in to that temptation.

4. Exercising too vigorously on the first day will result in injuries or at least sore muscles. If you are stiff and sore the next day, you overdid it, and you won't feel like exercising.
5. If you are exercising for weight control, don't weigh yourself every day, and try not to become preoccupied with your weight or body shape.
6. If you are in the process of quitting smoking, use exercise as a way to prevent weight gain.
7. Social support helps. Enlist a friend to exercise with you, or join a team or group exercise program.

8. If you jog or cycle in a location unfamiliar to you, check out your surroundings before you begin. Dogs, ditches, and dangerous detours may be in your path.
9. Remember that in order to receive maximum health benefits from your exercise program, you must stick to it. Don't expect quick or dramatic results.
10. To acquire muscle tone as well as aerobic fitness, include a combination of types of exercise such as working out with weights or other isotonic exercise as well as aerobics.

a week will not prompt weight loss or maintain weight loss; those goals require more lengthy and more intense exercise (Garber et al., 2011). Therefore, how much is enough depends on the health goals.

Improving Adherence to Physical Activity

Adherence to nearly all medical and health regimens is a serious problem (see Chapter 4), and exercise is no exception. Only 33% of adults in the United States get regular physical activity at either a moderate or vigorous intensity (USCB, 2011); the percentage is similar in the European Union (Sjöström, Oja, Hagströmer, Smith, & Bauman, 2006). For individuals who participate in prescribed exercise regimens, the dropout rates closely parallel the relapse rates reported in smoking and alcohol cessation programs.

Everybody could use some extra motivation to get up off the couch and exercise. For some people, a membership at a health club, a personal trainer, or an opportunity to be a contestant on *The Biggest Loser* provides the motivation. Unfortunately, with so much of the population being sedentary, interventions are

needed that do not require such costly face-to-face contact with a fitness professional. Thus, interventions that aim to improve physical activity often rely on other methods and channels, such as the computers and the Internet, telephone, mass media, and changes to the environment. In this section, we review some of these interventions and describe their effectiveness. As you will learn, one of the challenges in improving adherence to physical activity is maintaining the activity over time. Furthermore, you will learn that even some of the simplest interventions can have surprising effects.

Informational Interventions   Informational interventions seek to raise public awareness of the importance of physical activity and its benefits, as well as highlight opportunities to engage in exercise. These informational interventions take a variety of forms, ranging from mass media campaigns to "point-of-decision" prompts.

Mass media campaigns use widespread media channels such as television and radio commercials, newspaper and magazine advertisements, billboards, and bus wraps to inform people about the importance of physical activity. A recent review of 18 mass media interventions—implemented in a variety of countries, including the United States, New Zealand, Australian, Canada, Columbia, and Brazil—finds that these mass media campaigns are generally successful at raising awareness, as measured by people's ability to recall information from the campaign (Leavy, Bull, Rosenberg, & Bauman, 2011).

Does this awareness translate into increases in physical activity? The evidence regarding this question is mixed. While some of these mass media campaigns led to greater levels of self-reported physical activity, other interventions did not. Furthermore, there is little evidence that any mass media campaign has effects on physical activity that persist long after a campaign ends (Leavy et al., 2011). Thus, the effectiveness of mass media campaigns on adoption of physical activity remains unclear.

Informational interventions can occur in simpler and less expensive forms, such as through "point-of-decision" prompts. When you need to get to a higher floor in a building, do you take the elevator or do you take the stairs? This is a choice that many people make on an everyday basis, and taking the stairs is an opportunity to inject physical activity into an otherwise sedentary day. Yet, most people choose the elevator. Dozens of studies show that signs placed near stairs— whether they be in the workplace, shopping malls, or subway exits—motivate people to make the physically active choice. In fact, reviews of research on these point-of-decision prompts show that they increase stair use by approximately 50% (Nocon, Müller-Riemenschneider, Nitzschke, & Willich, 2010; Soler et al., 2010). Furthermore, people who are obese are more likely than normal-weight individuals to respond to these signs by taking the stairs (Webb & Cheng, 2010).

These point-of-decision prompts may also be cost effective. One team of British researchers (Olander & Eves, 2011) compared the effects of two interventions aimed at increasing stair use on a university campus. One intervention, called "Workplace Well-being Day," placed research staff at an information booth in the center of campus at midday, where informational leaflets were handed out to over 1,000 people. The other intervention simply had point-of-decision signs strategically placed between the elevators and the stairs of several buildings. How much did these interventions cost? The "Workplace Wellbeing Day" cost almost $800 to implement and had no effect on stair use. In contrast, the point-of-decision signs cost merely $30 to implement and significantly increased stair use. Thus, informational interventions can work, particularly when people are exposed to the information at the point of decision (Wakefield, Loken, & Hornik, 2010).

However, informational interventions seek to raise awareness or generate positive attitudes toward physical activity. These are only the first steps toward maintaining an activity regimen; changing behavior patterns is much more difficult.

Behavioral and Social Interventions   Behavioral interventions attempt to teach people the skills necessary for adoption and maintenance of physical activity. Social interventions aim to create a social environment that makes adoption and maintenance of physical activity more successful. These types of interventions range from school-based physical education programs, to interventions designed to increase social support, to individually tailored health behavior change programs.

School-based physical education programs are often a mix of structured physical activity and education about the benefits of regular exercise. There is strong evidence that school-based physical activity programs increase the amount of time that students spend in moderate-to-vigorous physical activity, and this increased activity often leads to improvements in aerobic fitness (Kahn et al., 2002). However, these benefits are largely due to the physical activity incorporated directly into these programs, rather than the educational aspect. For example, classroom-based educational programs that focus on reducing sedentary behaviors—such as watching television and playing video games—do not reliably increase physical activity (Kahn et al., 2002). Furthermore, school-based physical education programs are less effective at increasing physical activity outside of school hours than they are at increasing physical activity during school hours (Cale & Harris, 2006). Thus, school-based physical education programs are moderately successful at increasing students' physical activity but do not appear to teach skills that enable students to increase physical activity on their own time.

Social support interventions focus on changing physical activity by building and maintaining social relationships that can facilitate behavior change. Examples of these interventions include developing a "buddy system," making a contract with another person to exercise for a specific period of time, or participating in a group exercise program. A systematic review of social support interventions (Kahn et al., 2002) concludes that they are effective. Social support interventions generally increase the amount of time spent in physical activity, increase the frequency of exercise, and lead to improvements in aerobic fitness

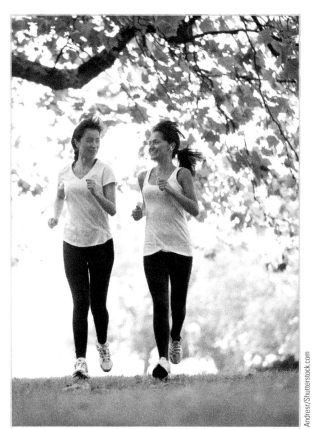

Andresr/Shutterstock.com

The "buddy system" can make physical activity easier and more enjoyable.

and decreases in body fat. Thus, the power of social support is clear in the context of physical activity; enlisting the support of a friend, family member, or coworker can increase a person's likelihood of staying physically active.

Individually tailored health behavior change programs constitute a third form of behavioral intervention for physical activity. These typically involve information and activities that address goal setting, self-monitoring, reinforcement, development of self-efficacy, problem solving, and relapse prevention; in other words, many of the successful behavior change strategies described in Chapter 4. Individually tailored health behavior change programs are also generally successful, as they are associated with increases in time spent in physical activity and increases in aerobic fitness (Kahn et al., 2002).

However, individually tailored health behavior change programs can be expensive if delivered in person by a trained counselor. Therefore, many individually tailored programs are delivered via telephone, Internet, or computer. Interventions delivered through these channels generally yield significant increases in physical activity during the intervention period (Goode, Reeves, & Eakin, 2012; Hamel, Robbins, & Wilbur, 2011; Neville, O'Hara, & Milat, 2009) and can be as successful as face-to-face programs (Mehta & Sharma, 2012).

People are increasingly turning to smartphone "apps" and other technologies such as wearable fitness trackers to monitor and encourage physical activity. At present, there are few studies that rigorously assess whether these technologies improve physical activity over long periods of time, but the few studies that exist suggest that people who use them do increase their physical activity, at least temporarily (Bort-Roig, Gilson, Puig-Ribera, Contreras, & Trost, 2014; Fanning, Mullen, & McAuley, 2012; Stephens & Allen, 2013). Many of these technologies incorporate features that provide effective behavior change strategies (see Chapter 4), such as self-monitoring of behavior, goal setting, and feedback (Direito et al., 2014). Some smartphone apps—such as the "Pokemon Go" game— take a different approach, by "gamifying" physical activity and providing virtual rewards for exploring one's community on foot. Obviously, such technologies are only available to people who can afford them, so may not reach large segments of a population.

Unfortunately, individually tailored health behavior change programs suffer the problem that many interventions have: They are generally not successful at maintaining physical activity post-intervention (Goode et al., 2012; Hamel et al., 2011; Neville et al., 2009). One phenomenon that contributes to the problem of relapse is the **abstinence violation effect** (Marlatt & Gordon, 1980). When people go 5 or 6 days without exercising, they tend to adopt the attitude "I'm out of shape now. It would take too much energy and pain to start over again." As with the smoker or the abuser of alcohol, this exerciser is allowing one lapse to turn into a full-blown relapse. Research with dropouts from an exercise program (Sears & Stanton, 2001) attempted to warn participants that they may be tempted to permanently quit exercising after a period of inactivity but that resuming exercise is a better choice than continued inactivity. The abstinence violation effect is an example of one of many psychological factors that influences adherence to physical activity recommendations. However, it would be shortsighted to believe that only psychological factors matter; the physical environment influences adherence as well.

Environmental Interventions   Physical activity can be far easier and far more enjoyable if it takes place in a pleasing environment, such as a hike on a trail, a jog on a neighborhood sidewalk, or a stroll through a park. Thus, characteristics of a person's neighborhood can predict the likelihood of physical activity.

A large study of over 11,000 adults living in 11 different countries confirms the link between characteristics of neighborhood environments and physical activity (Sallis et al., 2009). People are more likely to meet physical activity guidelines if their neighborhoods have sidewalks on most streets, plenty of shops, bicycle facilities, and free or low-cost recreational facilities. The importance of the neighborhood environment for physical activity among children is critical as well. Children who live in neighborhoods with access to playgrounds, parks, and recreational facilities tend to be more active and less obese (Veugelers, Sithole, Zhang, & Muhajarine, 2008). These associations may emerge for two reasons. First, easier access to recreational locations makes it easier to exercise. Second, people are more likely to be physically active when they see other people doing the same. For example, simply viewing people engaging in physical activity in and around one's neighborhood can motivate exercise (Kowal & Fortier, 2007).

Thus, one way to increase levels of physical activity is through enhancing access to places that encourage physical activity. These kinds of interventions may include providing access to fitness equipment in the workplace or in community centers, creating trails, or improving park amenities and facilities. Environmental interventions do work, in terms of increasing the physical activity and fitness of those working or living nearby (Kahn et al., 2002). However, these types of interventions can be quite expensive, and there is limited evidence available regarding their cost effectiveness. Regardless, it is important to recognize the key role that the physical environment plays in physical activity.

IN SUMMARY

In the United States and other industrialized countries, a sedentary lifestyle is more common than a physically active one; about 67% of adults fail to comply with recommendations for regular, vigorous exercise. Interventions for improving physical activity include: informational interventions, behavioral and social interventions, and environmental interventions. Informational interventions, such as mass media campaigns, have little effectiveness in changing behavior, unless "point-of-decision" prompts are used. Behavioral and social interventions are more successful in improving physical activity but do not have a good record of maintaining physical activity after the intervention concludes. Environmental interventions may be effective in changing behavior long-term, but the cost effectiveness of environmental interventions is not clear.

Answers

This chapter has addressed six basic questions:

1. **What are the different types of physical activity?**

All physical activity can be subsumed under one or more of five basic categories: isometric, isotonic, isokinetic, anaerobic, and aerobic. Each of these five exercise types has advantages and disadvantages for improving physical fitness. Most people who exercise do so for the benefits from one or another of these five types of physical activity, but no one type of exercise promotes all types of fitness.

2. **Does physical activity benefit the cardiovascular system?**

Most results on the health benefits of exercise have confirmed a positive relationship between regular physical activity and enhanced cardiovascular health, including weight control and a favorable cholesterol ratio. This research suggests that a regimen of moderate, brisk physical activity should be prescribed as one of several components in a program of coronary health.

3. **What are some other health benefits of physical activity?**

In addition to improving cardiovascular health, regular physical activity may protect against some kinds of cancer, especially colon and breast cancer; help prevent bone density loss, thus lowering one's risk of osteoporosis; prevent and control Type 2 diabetes and help manage Type 1 diabetes; and help people live longer.

Besides improving physical fitness and health, regular exercise can confer certain psychological benefits. Specifically, research has demonstrated that exercises can decrease depression, reduce anxiety, buffer against the harmful effects of stress, and improve cognitive functioning.

4.   Can physical activity be hazardous?

Several hazards accompany both regular and occasional exercise. Some runners appear to be addicted to exercise, becoming obsessed with body image and fearful of being prevented from following their exercise regimen. Injuries are frequent among those who exercise regularly, especially if they train intensively. However, the most serious hazard is sudden death while exercising, which almost always occurs in people with cardiovascular disease. People who exercise regularly are much less likely than occasional exercisers to die of a heart attack during heavy physical exertion.

5.   How much is enough but not too much?

The current pronouncement from the American College of Sports Medicine allowed for two routes to achieve acceptable levels of physical activity. One possibility is moderately vigorous exercise for 30 minutes five times per week, and the other involves intense exercise for 20 minutes three times a week. In addition, individuals should participate in strength training. Although the less intense program of physical activity is not sufficient to promote a high level of fitness, health benefits occur at lower levels of exercise. For cardiovascular health, almost any amount of exercise is better than no exercise.

6.   What are effective interventions for improving physical activity?

More than 50% of adults in the United States are too sedentary for good health. One simple and effective intervention for improving physical

activity is using "point-of-decision" prompts, which highlight opportunities for people to engage in exercise—such as using stairs instead of an elevator. Social and behavioral interventions are also effective in promoting adoption of physical activity; these interventions can be delivered in person, as well as through the computer, telephone, and Internet. However, the effects of social and behavioral interventions may not be maintained for long after the intervention concludes. One challenge in maintaining physical activity over time is the abstinence violation effect, when people give up on a regimen after a short setback.

Suggested Readings

Burfoot, A. (2005, August). Does running lower your risk of cancer? *Runner's World, 40*, 60–61. In this article, Amby Burfoot looks at some of the research on exercise and cancer and takes issue with Ken Cooper's statement that anyone who exercises more than the equivalent of 15 miles a week is running for something other than health. Burfoot considers the growing evidence that physical activity may protect against cancer as well as help people recover from cancer.

Powell, K. E., Paluch, A. E., & Blair, S. N. (2011). Physical activity for health: What kind? How much? How intense? On top of what? *Annual Review of Public Health, 32*, 349–365. This excellent and up-to-date review chapter summarizes a number of key concepts important in understanding the relationship between physical activity and health, such as the intensity of activity, the dose–response relationship, and the importance of initiating even light-intensity activity to improve health.

Silver, J. K., & Morin, C. (Eds.). (2008). *Understanding fitness: How exercise fuels health and fights disease.* Westport, CT: Praeger Publishers/Greenwood Publishing Group. This book provides an explanation of the biological processes that occur when people exercise, including a review of the many diseases that exercise can help prevent.

CHAPTER 16

Future Challenges

CHAPTER OUTLINE

- Real-World Profile of Dwayne and Robyn
- *Challenges for Healthier People*
- *Outlook for Health Psychology*
- *Making Health Psychology Personal*

QUESTIONS

This chapter focuses on three basic questions:

1. What role does health psychology play in contributing to the goals of *Healthy People 2020*?

2. What is the outlook for the future of health psychology?

3. How can you use health psychology to cultivate a healthier lifestyle?

Real-World Profile of **DWAYNE AND ROBYN**

Dwayne Brown* is a 21-year-old college junior who seldom thinks about his health—either his present or future health. Dwayne feels good, believes that his present lack of obvious illness is a sign that he is in good health, and assumes that he will always be free of disease and disability.

Dwayne has a number of habits that have consequences for his health. One of these is his diet, which consists mostly of fast-food burgers, with an occasional fried fish sandwich for variety. However, variety is not a high priority for Dwayne, who eats three meals a day, 6 days a week at the same fast-food restaurant. Breakfast usually consists of a biscuit, scrambled eggs, sausage, and a soft drink (because he doesn't like coffee). For lunch, he has a burger, fries, and another soft drink. Dinner is a repeat of lunch. He also snacks and often chooses ice cream and candy bars. Despite his "junk food" diet, Dwayne is not overweight.

Dwayne holds other attitudes, beliefs, and behaviors that present risks. He seldom exercises or wears seat belts and has few close friends. He believes that his future health is beyond his personal control—that genetics and fate are the underlying determinants of heart disease, cancer, and accidents. Thus, he has thought little about ways of maintaining his health or decreasing his chances of chronic illness or premature death. He does not see a physician regularly. When he feels ill, he takes over-the-counter medication, hoping that he will feel better.

However, Dwayne does some things right. He does not smoke cigarettes or drink alcohol and considers his life as low stress. His abstinence from drinking stems from his religious rather than health beliefs, and his avoidance of smoking comes from an incident during his adolescence when he smoked a cigarette and became sick. His score on the Social Readjustment Rating Scale (Holmes & Rahe, 1967; see Chapter 5) was as low as anyone's could be, including only one stressful life event—Christmas. Dwayne sees himself as a healthy person.

Robyn Green* is also a 21-year-old college junior, but her attitudes and behaviors concerning health differ a great deal from Dwayne's. Her differences include a basic attitude—that she has the primary responsibility for her health. Consistent with this attitude, Robyn has adopted a lifestyle that she believes will keep her healthy. Like Dwayne, she does not smoke; she took a puff from a cigarette when she was in fourth grade and coughed for a long time, which discouraged her from smoking. Her father was a smoker during her childhood and adolescence, but she and her mother convinced him to stop smoking in their home. To further avoid exposure to secondhand smoke, Robyn avoids enclosed places where people are smoking. Unlike Dwayne, Robyn drinks alcohol. Her drinking is moderate, and she does not binge drink. Her parents are also moderate drinkers, and Robyn's home was one in which alcohol was consumed but not abused.

Robyn's diet differs dramatically from Dwayne's diet. She seldom eats eggs, whole milk products, beef, or pork; she concentrates on eating lots of fruits and vegetables (yet is not vegetarian). She occasionally allows herself a dessert. Robyn is careful about choosing a low-fat diet because she is concerned about cholesterol. Her grandfather died of heart disease at age 63, and she believes that his smoking and high-fat, high-cholesterol diet hastened his death. Robyn also follows an exercise program, which she finds somewhat difficult to maintain with her school schedule. She takes an aerobic dance class 3 days a week; she walks 30 minutes a day on those days with no dance class. So far, she has been faithful in maintaining this workout schedule. Robyn sees herself as a healthy person.

*The names have been changed to protect these persons' privacy.

How do Dwayne's and Robyn's health habits and attitudes compare with yours? Dwayne is less knowledgeable and concerned with his health than most college students, whereas Robyn is more so. Both Dwayne and Robyn see themselves as healthy people; yet, you should know by now that Robyn is more likely to maintain her health, whereas Dwayne is likely to see his deteriorate if his habits persist. In this chapter, we will examine some health issues specific to college students and hope to convince you of health psychology's relevance to your life. But first, let's look at health care and the challenges facing not only health psychologists but also all health care providers in the United States and around the world.

Challenges for Healthier People

People in the United States, Canada, and other high-income countries are inundated with health information telling about the dangers of smoking, abusing alcohol, eating improperly, and not exercising regularly. As you learned in Chapters 3 and 4, knowledge does not always translate into action, and people have difficulty in adopting these healthy habits. Still, over the past 35 years U.S. residents have managed to make some healthy changes in their lifestyles, and these changes contribute to the declining mortality for heart disease, stroke, cancer, homicide, and unintentional injuries (USCB, 2011). However, unhealthy and risky behaviors still contribute to an increasing rate of obesity, diabetes, and lower respiratory disease.

What are the most current public health goals of the United States? *Healthy People 2020* (USDHHS, 2010a) is a report that establishes the U.S. health objectives for the years 2010 through 2020. These objectives include 40 focus areas and nearly 600 specific goals, along with 12 leading indicators, which appear in Table 16.1. Notice that most of these indicators are major areas of concern to health psychologists. In addition, two overarching goals summarize the focus of the *Health People 2020* report: to increase quality and

TABLE 16.1   Leading Health Indicators for Healthy People 2020

Nutrition, physical activity, and obesity
- Increase number of adults who meet physical activity guidelines
- Reduce number of children, adolescents, and adults who are obese
- Increase total vegetable intake in children, adolescents, and adults

Oral health
- Increase number of children and adults who use oral health services regularly

Tobacco use
- Reduce number of adults who are current cigarette smokers
- Reduce number of adolescents who smoked in past 30 days

Substance abuse
- Reduce number of adolescents who use alcohol or illicit drugs
- Reduce number of adults engaging in binge drinking

Reproductive and sexual health
- Increase number of sexually active females who receive reproductive health services
- Increase number of persons living with HIV who know their HIV status

Mental health
- Reduce suicides
- Reduce number of adolescents who experience major depressive episodes

(Continued)

TABLE 16.1   *(Continued)*

Injury and violence
- Reduce fatal injuries
- Reduce homicides

Environmental quality
- Increase air quality
- Reduce number of children exposed to secondhand smoke

Access to health services
- Increase number of people with medical insurance
- Increase number of people with a usual primary care provider

Clinical preventive services
- Increase number of adults who receive colorectal cancer screenings
- Increase number of adults with hypertension whose blood pressure is under control
- Increase number of adult diabetics with good glycemic control
- Increase number of children who receive recommended vaccinations

Maternal, infant, and child health
- Reduce infant mortality
- Reduce number of preterm births

Social determinants of health
- Increase number of students who graduate with a high-school equivalency diploma

years of healthy life and to eliminate health disparities. Although these goals are ambitious and have presented challenges in the past (USDHHS, 2007), the United States has progressed toward or met many prior *Healthy People* goals (USDHHS, 2010a).

Increasing the Span of Healthy Life

The first goal—to increase the span of healthy life—is a bit different from increasing life expectancy. Rather than striving for longer lives, many people are now trying to increase their number of well-years. A well-year is "the equivalent of a year of completely well life, or a year of life free of dysfunction, symptoms, and health-related problems" (Kaplan & Bush, 1982, p. 64). A concept closely related to well-years is health expectancy, defined as the number of years a person can anticipate spending free from disability (Robine & Ritchie, 1991). For example, life expectancy in the United States is about 76 for men and 81 for women,

but health expectancy is about 68 for men and 70 for women, leaving both men and women with a discrepancy of about 8 to 11 years of disability (WHO, 2016c). Japan boasts both the highest life expectancy (84) and the highest health expectancy (75) of any country; even in Japan, people can expect approximately 9 years of disability (WHO, 2016a, 2016b).

In the United States, years of life are increasing, but years of life without chronic illness are declining (USDHHS, 2007). U.S. residents are not benefiting from increases in healthy life expectancy as much as residents of many other countries (Mathers et al., 2004). Although people in the United States may expect 70 years of healthy life, this figure ranks 36th in the world in terms of disability-free life expectancy. The United States trails most other industrialized countries because of high rates of smoking-related disease, violence, and AIDS-related health problems. Although the decline in tobacco use in recent decades improves Americans' healthy life expectancy, these gains will

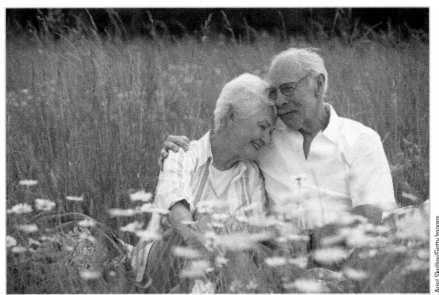

Increasing the span of healthy life is a goal for health psychologists.

likely be offset by the increasing rate of obesity in the United States (Stewart, Cutler, & Rosen, 2009). Table 16.2 shows the healthy life expectancy for a selection of countries with both high and low values. As other industrialized countries have health expectancy much greater than the United States, improvements should be possible in the United States.

What explains the difference between life expectancy and health expectancy? Economic factors play an important role. The differences between life expectancy and health expectancy are even larger when comparing the richest and poorest countries or even the richest and poorest segments of the population within a country (Jagger et al., 2009; Mathers et al., 2004; McIntosh, Fines, Wilkins, & Wolfson, 2009). Wealthy people not only live longer but also have more years of healthy life.

The changing nature of disease also accounts for the difference between life expectancy and health expectancy. Diseases that kill people will influence life expectancy; diseases that compromise health will influence health expectancy. For example, circulatory disorders head both lists, but disorders producing restricted movement and respiratory disorders are responsible for producing lost health expectancy, whereas cancer and accidents are major sources of lost life expectancy. Depression also compromises health expectancy more so than it compromises life expectancy (Reynolds, Haley, & Kozlenko, 2008). Thus, interventions aimed at increasing life expectancy will not necessarily improve health expectancy and quality of life. For this reason, experts recommend using a population's health expectancy as an indicator of overall population health (Steifel, Perla, & Zell, 2010).

Reducing Health Disparities

Healthy People 2020 defines a health disparity as "a particular type of health difference that is closely linked with social, economic, and/or environmental disadvantage" (USDHHS, 2008b). Disparities exist based on race and ethnicity, education, income, gender, sexual orientation, disability status, special health care needs, and geographic location. All of these disparities are important to understand and reduce; however, racial and ethnic disparities are the most documented health disparities in the United States. In the United States, ethnicity is not separable from social, economic, and educational factors that contribute to disease as well as to seeking and receiving medical care (Kawachi, Daniels, & Robinson, 2005). Being poor with a low educational level elevates risks for many diseases and provides a poorer prognosis for those who are ill. These disadvantages also apply to children in these socioeconomic groups (Wen, 2007). African Americans, Hispanic Americans, and Native Americans have lower average educational levels and incomes than

TABLE 16.2   Healthy Life Expectancy for Selected Nations, 2015

Country	Healthy Life Expectancy
Japan	75
Singapore	74
Italy	73
Iceland	73
Switzerland	73
Australia	72
Sweden	72
Canada	72
Germany	71
United Kingdom	71
Costa Rica	70
USA	69
Cuba	69
China	69
Mexico	67
Vietnam	67
Brazil	66
Colombia	65
Russian Federation	63
Iraq	60
India	60
Rwanda	57
Haiti	55
Afghanistan	52
Sierra Leone	44

Source: Data from *World Health Statistics 2015*, by World Health Organization. Retrieved August 22, 2016, from www.who.int/gho.

European Americans and Asian Americans (USCB, 2011), and education relates to income. Thus, the racial and ethnic disparities are intertwined with income and education disparities, complicating our understanding of the underlying reasons for health disparities among people of different ethnic backgrounds.

Racial and Ethnic Disparities. African Americans, compared with European Americans, have a shorter life expectancy as well as a higher infant mortality rate, more homicide deaths, higher rates of cardiovascular disease, higher cancer mortality, and more tuberculosis and diabetes (USCB, 2011). They also experience lower health expectancy (USDHHS, 2007). Inadequate medical treatment may be a factor: African Americans receive poorer care than European Americans on nearly half of the quality measures of medical care (AHRQ, 2011). But even when equating for income (De Lew & Weinick, 2000) and access to medical care (Schneider, Zaslavsky, & Epstein, 2002), African Americans have poorer outcomes than European Americans. Part of the discrepancy may be due to limited **health literacy**, the ability to read and understand health information to make health-related decisions (Paasche-Orlow, Parker, Gazmararian, Nielsen-Bohlman, & Rudd, 2005; Rudd, 2007). Disparities in health literacy account for some ethnic health disparities, such as ethnic differences in vaccination (Bennett, Chen, Soroui, & White, 2009), HIV and diabetes management (Osborn, White, Cavanaugh, Rothman, & Wallston, 2009; Waldrop-Valverde et al., 2010), and medication use (Bailey et al., 2009). The Would You Believe ...? box discusses the importance of health literacy and some ways that health psychologists can increase people's understanding of health information.

Discrimination may also be a factor contributing to inadequate medical treatment for African Americans (Brown et al., 2008; Smiles, 2002). For example, African Americans receive less aggressive treatment for symptoms of coronary heart disease, are less likely to be referred to a cardiologist than European Americans, are less likely to receive kidney dialysis, and are less likely to receive the most effective treatments for HIV infection (Institute of Medicine [IOM], 2002). Many physicians believe that race or ethnicity plays no role in the care they provide (Lillie-Blanton, Maddox, Rushing, & Mensah, 2004), but these results and the reports of African Americans (Brown et al., 2008) indicate otherwise.

Low economic status, lack of access to medical care, and poor health literacy affect Native Americans at least as strongly as African Americans (AHRQ, 2011; USDHHS, 2007). Native Americans have a shorter life expectancy, a higher mortality rate, higher infant mortality, and higher rates of infectious illness than European Americans (Hayes-Bautista et al., 2002). Many Native Americans receive medical care from the Indian Health Service, but that organization has a history of poor funding as well as mistreatment of Native American patients that has led to mistrust (Keltner, Kelley, & Smith, 2004). In addition, many Native Americans live in rural settings in which medical care services are limited. These circumstances contribute to decreased access to medical care, which is related to poor health,

Would You BELIEVE...?
Health Literacy Can Improve by "Thinking Outside the Box"

Sometimes, even the most well-intentioned health interventions may not work for one simple reason: People do not understand the information presented. This is a problem faced not merely by people with low levels of health literacy. It is a problem likely faced by you.

In the 1990s, several countries—including the United States, Canada, Mexico, and United Kingdom—passed laws requiring food manufacturers to post a "Nutrition Facts" box on food packaging. The governments' goal with this legislation was to help consumers make healthier and more informed food choices. In the United States, the "Nutrition Facts" box typically appears on the back of the product and reports information such as serving size, calories, fat, cholesterol, sodium, vitamins, and minerals.

If you are like most people, you probably do not pay much attention to—or even understand—the information presented in these boxes. People's use of nutrition information boxes declined from 1996 to 2006 (Todd & Variyam, 2008). Why? Despite the government's best efforts to design a box that would be easy to read, many people find it difficult to interpret all the numerical information (IOM, 2012). How much fat is too much fat? How big is a serving size? Is one snack food more or less healthy than another snack food? These are the kinds of questions that consumers need answers to, but current nutrition boxes effectively hide this information by tacking it to the back of a package and presenting it as a list of nearly indecipherable numbers.

Most experts think the cause of this problem is not people's lack of health literacy, but rather, problems with how the labels are designed. For example, experts in health literacy know that images often convey information better than numbers do (Houts, Doak, Doak, & Loscalzo, 2006). Recently, a group of health psychologists, public health experts, marketers, and nutritionists convened to recommend broad changes to food nutrition labels (IOM, 2012). This group concluded that consumers should be able to make better food choices when nutrition information appears on the *front* of the package, and use symbols and images rather than numbers to convey important information. Furthermore, the symbols should represent only the most essential nutrition information, such as calories, saturated and *trans* fats, sodium, and added sugars. An example of a front-of-package nutrition symbol system designed by the United Kingdom appears in this box. It uses standard traffic light colors to inform consumers that a product is high, medium, or low in a particular element. Which system is easier for you to understand: the current U.S. fact box or the redesigned UK symbols? In a laboratory experiment, researchers found that the UK labels were effective in guiding healthy food choices, even though people tended to avoid the "reds" (unhealthy choices) more than they chose the "greens" (healthy choices) (Scarborough et al., 2015).

This is one example of how health psychologists can address literacy issues by rethinking how marketers and interventions present information. Another example of an innovative approach to addressing health literacy issues is the use of *telenovelas* to communicate health information to Latino populations. Telenovelas are short, dramatic "soap operas," immensely popular in Latino culture, that focus on romantic and middle class issues. Some health psychologists created "entertainment interventions" using the *telenovela* format to communicate to Spanish-speaking audiences about the importance of breast screening (Wilkin et al., 2007) and HIV testing (Olshefsky, Zive, Scolari, & Zuniga, 2007). Both interventions were deemed successful, largely because they presented health information in a format that the audience was familiar with and could easily understand.

Thus, addressing disparities in health literacy is a public health challenge and will require extensive efforts to ensure that people understand important information. With more "thinking outside of the box," efforts to address disparities in health literacy may be more successful.

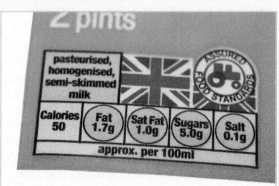

The UK Traffic Light system of nutrition labeling makes it easier for people to understand important health information.

Libby Welch/Alamy Stock Photo

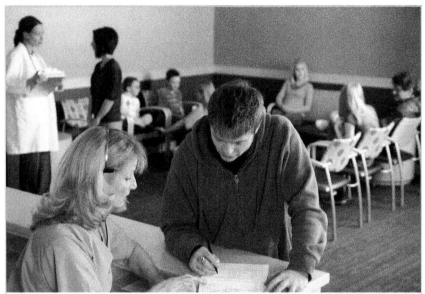

Many people in the United States face barriers in obtaining medical care.

but Native Americans who live in urban areas also experience poor health and limited access to medical care (Castor et al., 2006). Native Americans also exhibit many risky behaviors that influence their health, including high rates of smoking and alcohol abuse, poor diet, and behaviors that increase injuries and deaths from violence. Native Americans, then, are one of the groups poorly served by the current system of medical care and health education in the United States.

Many Hispanic Americans also experience low income and educational status. However, Hispanics in the United States include a variety of groups, and their health and longevity tend to vary with income and education. Cuban Americans generally have higher education and economic levels than Mexican Americans or Puerto Ricans, and Cuban Americans are more likely to have access to regular medical care and physician visits (LaVeist, Bowie, & Cooley-Quille, 2000). Cubans have better health, and Puerto Ricans tend to have poorer health, than other groups of Hispanics in the United States (Borrell, 2005).

Hispanic Americans are much more likely to develop diabetes, obesity, and hypertension than European Americans (USDHHS, 2000). Hispanic American young men are at sharply increased risk of violent death (Hayes-Bautista et al., 2002), which may be the reason for the overall lower life expectancy of Hispanic Americans. In other age groups, Hispanics fare about the same as or better than European Americans on some health and mortality measures. Hispanic Americans have a lower death rate than many other ethnic groups, including European Americans, for heart disease, stroke, and lung cancer (NCHS, 2011). These low death rates seem puzzling, given the high rates of smoking, obesity, and hypertension among Hispanic Americans. The poor health habits of Hispanic Americans, combined with their low disease prevalence, may reflect a transition in which immigrants adopt American lifestyles but have not yet had time to develop the chronic diseases typical of the United States (Borrell, 2005).

Asian Americans have lower infant mortality, longer life expectancy, fewer lung and breast cancer deaths, and lower cardiovascular death rates than other ethnic groups (NCHS, 2011). Like Hispanic Americans, Asian Americans come from a variety of ethnicities, including Chinese, Korean, Japanese, Vietnamese, and Cambodian. Many Asian cultures share values that promote good health, such as strong social and family ties, but other factors present barriers to good health. For example, Vietnamese and Cambodian cultures show a higher tolerance for family violence than European American culture (Weil & Lee, 2004). Overall, Asian Americans have the longest life expectancy and best health of any ethnic group in the United States.

Educational and Socioeconomic Disparities Low income has an obvious connection to lower standards of medical care. After adjusting for poverty, many of the health disadvantages of ethnicity disappear (Krieger, Chen,

Waterman, Rehkopf, & Subramanian, 2005). One medical care disadvantage related to poverty is lack of insurance, which makes access to medical care more difficult in the United States. However, universal access to medical care does not completely remove the disparities among socioeconomic groups (Lasser, Himmelstein, & Woolhandler, 2006; Martikainen, Valkonen, & Martelin, 2001). Even in countries that have universal access to medical care, health disparities between poor and wealthy people persist, suggesting that factors other than access to medical care are involved in maintaining health.

Education and socioeconomic level are two factors that may influence health status—independent of access to medical care. Across ethnic groups and in countries around the world, people who have higher education and income also have better health and longevity than those with lower education and income (Crimmins & Saito, 2001; Mackenbach et al., 2008). As the Chapter 1 Would You Believe …? box detailed, people who attend college have many health advantages. Compared with those with a high school education or less, those who attend college live longer and healthier, with lower rates of infectious and chronic diseases and unintentional injuries (NCHS, 2011). These advantages should not be surprising, considering the low rate of smoking among those who attend or graduate from college compared with people with fewer than 12 years of education; smoking is a leading contributor to ill health and death.

In addition, people with low education and low socioeconomic status are more likely to have risky health habits, such as eating a high-fat diet and leading a sedentary life, than people with higher incomes and more education. Although improved access to medical care and decreased discrimination in medical care delivery will probably eliminate some of the health disparities among ethnic groups, changes in health-related behaviors, affordable and accessible options for healthy behavior, and improved living conditions will also be necessary to achieve the goal of eliminating health disparities in the United States.

IN SUMMARY

People in the United States and other industrialized countries are becoming more health conscious, and both government policy and individual behavior reflect this concern. *Healthy People 2020* states two overarching goals for the U.S. population: (1) to increase the quality and years of healthy life and (2) to eliminate health disparities. The first goal includes increasing the number of well-years or health expectancy—that is, years free of dysfunction, disease symptoms, and health-related problems. The second goal—eliminating disparities in health care—is far from being met, in part because people at the upper socioeconomic level continue to make greater gains in health status than do those at the lower levels. Ethnicity remains a factor in health and medical care, not only in the United States but also in other countries. In the United States, African Americans and Native Americans experience great disadvantages compared with Asian Americans and European Americans. Some Hispanics experience health advantages, and others disadvantages. The factors of education and income are intertwined with ethnicity, complicating understanding of the source of disparities in health.

Outlook for Health Psychology

Since the founding of health psychology more than 30 years ago, the field has blossomed, prompting a plethora of research and clinical applications to a variety of health-related behaviors and outcomes. That progress has touched many areas of health care, but social and economic forces will influence the future of the field.

Progress in Health Psychology

Until the 1970s, very few psychologists focused on physical health as an area of research (APA Task Force on Health Research, 1976). However, during the past 40 years, psychology research on health issues accelerated to the point that it has changed the field of psychology, making health-related issues common topics in psychology journals. Health psychologists are now frequent contributors to journals in medicine and health care.

Despite the growth of health psychology and its ability to contribute to health care, the field faces several challenges. One major challenge is acceptance by other health care practitioners, an acceptance that continues to grow. Like physicians and patients, health psychologists also face the most serious problem within medical care—namely, escalating costs. In an environment of limited resources, psychologists will need to justify the costs that their services add to health care (Thielke, Thompson, & Stuart, 2011; Tovian, 2004). Although the diagnostic and therapeutic techniques used by health psychologists have demonstrated effectiveness, these procedures also have financial costs. Health psychology must justify its costs by offering services that meet the needs of individuals and society while fitting within a troubled health care system (IOM, 2010).

Future Challenges for Health Care

Health and medical care in the United States face enormous challenges. The two goals of *Healthy People 2020*—to add years of healthy life and to eliminate disparities in providing health care—will be difficult to achieve. Adding years of healthy life to an aging population is a daunting task. As the population ages, chronic illnesses and chronic pain become more common.

In 1900, only 4% of the population was over 65; in 2006, more than 13% of U.S. citizens had reached that age (USCB, 2011). During this same period, life expectancy increased from 47 to 78 years. Experts project that life expectancy in the United States will reach 80 years by the year 2020 (see Figure 16.1), with more than 19 million people, or 6.1% of the total population, over age 75.

As the population continues to age during the next few decades, psychology will play an important role in helping older people achieve and maintain healthy and productive lifestyles and adjust to the problems of chronic illness. As we have seen, health psychology plays an important role in preventing illness, promoting healthy aging, and helping people cope with pain. In old age, lifestyles can still be changed to help prevent illness, but health psychology's alliance with gerontology will more likely produce an emphasis on promoting and maintaining health, managing pain, and formulating health care policy.

The elimination of health disparities based on gender, ethnicity, age, income, educational level, and disability will also prove difficult, and increasing diversity will continue to challenge the health care system. As we discussed earlier in this chapter, many ethnic disparities trace back to economic, educational, and health literacy differences among ethnic groups (Lasser et al., 2006; USDHHS, 2007). The health disparity attributable to gender is not so easy to understand. Women receive poorer health care yet have longer life expectancies. This survival advantage was small in 1900, grew to more than 7 years during the 1970s, and has declined to about 5 years (USCB, 2011). Efforts to trace this gender

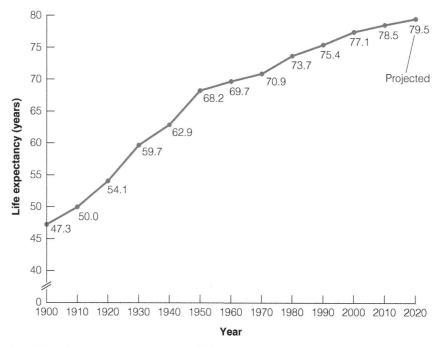

FIGURE 16.1 Actual and projected life expectancy, United States, 1900–2020.

Sources: Data from *Historical statistics of the United States: Colonial times to 1970* (p. 55), by U.S. Department of Commerce, Bureau of the Census, 1975, Washington, DC: U.S. Government Printing Office; *Statistical abstracts of the United States: 2001* (p. 73); *Statistical abstracts of the United States, 2012*, by U.S. Bureau of the Census, 2011, Washington, DC: U.S. Government Printing Office.

difference to biology have been largely unsuccessful, but health-related behaviors, social support, and coping strategies favor women (Whitfield, Weidner, Clark, & Anderson, 2002). Importantly, the escalating costs of medical care in the United States will place limits on the extent that health care policies and interventions can successfully address disparities.

Controlling Health Care Costs   The richest nation in the world is having trouble paying its medical bills. Health and medical care costs in the United States have escalated at a higher rate than inflation and other costs of living (Bodenheimer, 2005a; Mongan, Ferris, & Lee, 2008), leaving many people unable to afford medical care and others in the position of fearing that they will not be able to do so in the future.

A number of factors contribute to the high costs. These factors include the proliferation of expensive technology, a large proportion of physicians who are specialists, inefficient administration, inappropriate treatments, and a profit-oriented system that resists controls (IOM, 2010).

Figure 16.2 shows where health care dollars go. Hospitals receive 38% and physicians 25% of the dollars spent (NCHS, 2015). Although physicians receive less of the health care dollar than hospitals, their fees contribute

significantly to the high cost of health care (Boden-heimer, 2005c). Managed care curtailed physicians' fees during the late 1980s and early 1990s, but the backlash against managed care loosened these restrictions, and physicians' fees began to increase again in the late 1990s. The number of specialists adds to the cost of medical care, and the scarcity of primary care/family practitioners (and the lack of incentive for going into primary care) also plays a role (Sepulveda, Bodenheimer, & Grundy, 2008). Ironically, more physicians created competition, but rather than decreasing costs, this situation has contributed to higher costs (Weitz, 2010).

Administrative costs also contribute to the high health care costs in the United States (Bodenheimer, 2005a; Mongan et al., 2008). The complex system of insurance, private physicians, private and public hospitals, and government-supported medical programs such as Medicare produced different procedures, forms, payment plans, expenses allowed, maximum payments, and deductibles involved in payment for medical services. Thus, payment is a complex matter, which adds to people's frustration in dealing with the medical care system and creates possibilities for errors and fraud.

Health care reform is an urgent priority for the United States, but many conflicting interests have prevented widespread changes (Bodenheimer, 2005c;

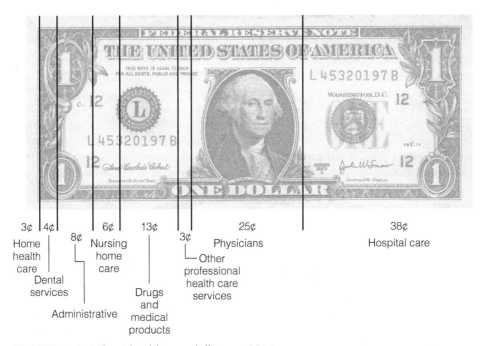

FIGURE 16.2 Where health care dollars go, 2014.

Source: Health, United States, 2015, 2016, by National Center for Health Statistics, Hyattsville, MD. Table 94.

Mongan et al., 2008). During the 1980s, health maintenance organizations (HMOs) proliferated as a way to control costs (Weitz, 2010). Originally, HMOs were nonprofit organizations oriented toward preventive care, but corporations entered the HMO market and profit became a motive. The growth of HMOs and the restriction of care received through these organizations contributed to slowing the medical care cost escalation. A backlash against the restrictions on care imposed by HMOs produced patients' rights movements, which have edged the system back toward high spending.

Can the United States provide quality medical care more efficiently? Other industrialized countries such as Canada, Japan, Australia, the countries of Western Europe, and Scandinavia share certain factors with the United States—aging populations with high rates of cardiovascular disease, cancer, and other chronic diseases—that pose similar challenges for their medical care systems (Bodenheimer, 2005b). Many of these countries do a better job of providing medical care to a larger percentage of their residents at lower cost than does the U.S. system. Their longer life expectancies and health expectancies are testimony to the effectiveness of their systems.

Germany, Canada, Japan, and Great Britain all face the problem of escalating medical care costs, and these nations also struggle to contain rising costs (Weitz, 2010). The history of medical care costs in these countries and the United States appears in Figure 16.3. These countries have managed to contain expenditures by controlling at least some of the factors that account for the rise in medical costs in the United States: Canada has a single-payer system, which minimizes administrative costs; Great Britain limits access to high-technology medicine; and Germany imposes some limits on payments to physicians and limits hospitals' purchases of high-technology equipment. Japan has an insurance system as the United States does, but insurers do not compete with one another, as the government regulates the cost of services and fees. Japan, however, has lower rates of obesity than many other countries, which contributes to a healthier population.

All of the strategies for cost containment have drawbacks. For example, people have quicker access to medical procedures such as MRIs, mammograms, and knee replacement surgery in the United States than in Canada, but these procedures are significantly more expensive in the United States (Bodenheimer, 2005b). Time delays for some services may pose risks, but in other cases, patients in the United States are overtreated, and limiting access could minimally influence health

outcomes (IOM, 2010) or may actually boost health and life expectancy (Emanuel & Fuchs, 2008; Research and Policy Committee, 2002). Canadians' longer life expectancy suggests that the delays they experience do not pose major threats (Lasser et al., 2006).

By devising systems in which all people have access to health care, Germany, Canada, Great Britain, and Japan have diminished competitive profit making, which remains a central feature of the U.S. system (Mahar, 2006). These four countries have different systems for paying for medical care, and all have experienced cost problems, but each has universal coverage, whereas a growing percentage of people in the United States have limited access to medical care. In 2010, U.S. President Barack Obama signed into law the Patient Protection and Affordable Care Act, which requires all Americans to maintain health insurance coverage, while also establishing a marketplace in which Americans choose from various health care insurance plans and coverage. Implementation of this reform plan has been challenged on a number of grounds, including its constitutionality. In 2012, the U.S. Supreme Court upheld the constitutionality of most of this law, and its provisions are gradually being enacted. Still, health care reform has been—and remains—an urgent issue in the United States (IOM, 2010).

The Importance of Prevention   About 70% of the cost of medical care is spent on 10% of the population, whereas healthy people (about 50% of the population) account for about 3% of medical care expenditures (Bodenheimer & Fernandez, 2005). These statistics highlight the importance of maintaining and promoting health as a way to contain medical care costs. Thus, health psychologists can have a role in reducing medical care costs because unhealthy behaviors contribute to the chronic diseases that generate the majority of expenses, such as cardiovascular disease, cancer, diabetes, and chronic lower respiratory disease. Those with good health habits have lifetime medical costs of about *half* those for people with poor health habits. However, people who live longer have years to accrue medical costs, so even good health can be costly in the long run (van Baal et al., 2008). Promotion of good health habits is an important way to decrease the need for medical services in the short run.

Reducing the demand for medical services is another approach to controlling medical care costs (Fries, 1998), which may be a good strategy to move people toward self-care. The availability of a wide range

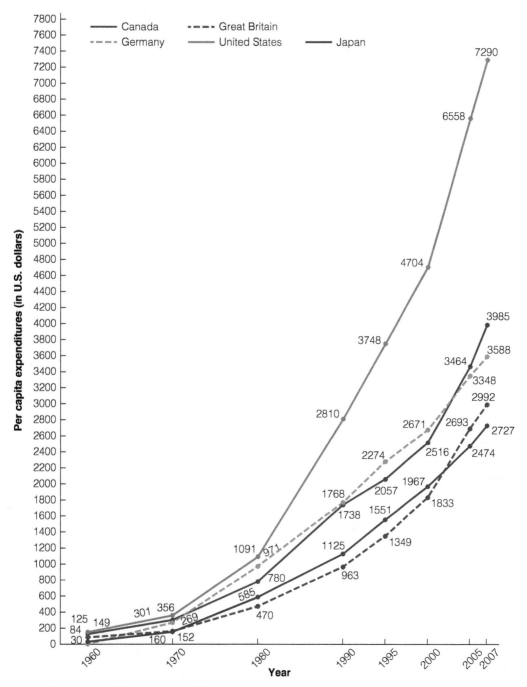

FIGURE 16.3 Health care expenditures in Canada, Germany, Great Britain, Japan, and the United States, 1960–2007.

Source: Health, United States, 2010, 2011, by National Center for Health Statistics, Hyattsville, MD: U.S. Government Printing Office, Table 121.

of medical technology has led to the widespread belief that modern medicine can cure any disease, and this belief fosters an overreliance on medicine to heal rather than a reliance on good health habits to avoid disease and on self-management for people with chronic conditions. As we discussed in Chapter 4, building feelings of personal efficacy for health—such as the beliefs that Robyn held—can help reduce the demand for medical services, and this approach has potential benefits for health in U.S. society. For example, encouraging individuals with chronic health problems to join self-help groups may reduce their need for intensive medical care (Humphreys & Moos, 2007). Additional research in this area may reveal that this approach can be a good strategy for containing medical care costs.

Controlling medical care costs will require substantial changes in the U.S. health care system. Insurance companies, hospitals, and physicians are all affected by health care reform and have all fought against changes (Mongan et al., 2008). As our examination of health care systems in other countries showed, no system can provide the best quality of medical care for low costs, but many countries do a better job than the United States.

Adapting to Changing Health Care Needs   Chronic illnesses now are the leading cause of death and disability in the United States and other industrialized countries. Yet, the medical care system remains oriented toward providing acute care for sick people rather than providing services that will prevent, ameliorate, or manage chronic conditions. That is, the medical care system has not responded to meet the needs created by changed patterns of disease that occurred during the 20th century (Bodenheimer, 2005c). Controlling chronic illness can occur through two routes: management to control these disabling conditions and prevention to avoid them.

Management of chronic illness is a current need and will become even more important in the future. Cardiovascular disease, cancer, chronic lower respiratory disease, and diabetes account for nearly 70% of deaths in the United States (USCB, 2011). However, medical care for these and other chronic illnesses is plagued by undertreatment, overtreatment, and mistreatment. For example, overtreatment occurred with 30% of individuals attending a primary care clinic, who were diagnosed with asthma and prescribed inhaled corticosteroids despite a lack of evidence for symptoms of asthma (Lucas, Smeenk, Smeele, & van Schayck, 2008). Undertreatment occurred in an analysis of management of

hypertension in patients who had experienced a stroke (Elkins, 2006), 20% to 30% of who did not receive treatment for diagnosed hypertension. Mistreatment occurs when health care providers make medical errors, which occurs with alarming frequency (HealthGrades, 2011). A system that provides more effective management of chronic illnesses will demand a shift from hospital- and physician-based care to a team approach that includes access to medical care and patient education to improve monitoring and self-care.

Self-care—rather than medical care—is a priority for prevention, which is a strategy that can reduce the need for medical services. In general, primary prevention offers more savings than secondary prevention. *Primary prevention* consists of immunizations and programs that encourage lifestyle changes; this type of prevention is usually a good bargain. Immunizations have some potential for harm but remain good choices unless the risk from side effects of the immunization is comparable to the risk of catching the disease. Programs that encourage people to quit smoking, eat properly, exercise, and moderate their drinking generally have low cost and little potential to do harm (Clark, 2008). In addition, some of these behaviors, such as smoking and inactivity, are risks for many health problems, and efforts oriented toward changing these behaviors can pay off by decreasing risks for several disorders. For example, a study of people who led a life that included the recommended exercise, body mass index, eating habits, and no history of smoking (Fraser & Shavlike, 2001) concluded that healthy lifestyle can add 10 years of life. Thus, primary prevention efforts pose few risks and offer many potential benefits.

Most prevention efforts target young and middle-aged adults who feel the need to change their behavior for health reasons. Such people are generally more responsive to prevention efforts than adolescents because adults generally recognize greater susceptibility to disease. Health habits begun later in life can add health years to life (Siegler, Bastian, Steffens, Bosworth, & Costa, 2002), but lifelong health habits should reap greater rewards. Thus, broadening prevention efforts to adolescents and young adults would be even more advantageous, but this group has been even more neglected in terms of lifestyle interventions (Williams, Holmbeck, & Greenley, 2002). Most of the health research and interventions for adolescents center on injury prevention and smoking deterrence, but adolescents build a foundation for a lifetime of health-related behaviors. Thus, primary prevention efforts tailored for people throughout the life span have the potential to improve health and life expectancy.

Secondary prevention consists of screening people at risk for developing a disease in order to find potential problems in their early and more treatable stages. However, such efforts can be costly because the number of people at risk may be much larger than the number who will develop the disease. Based on the economic considerations of cost–benefit analysis—that is, how much money is spent and how much is saved—secondary prevention may cost more than it saves.

However, neither hospitals' nor physicians' primary focus is on prevention services. Hospitals focus on acute care, and physicians' time is too expensive to focus on health education. Public health agencies, health educators, and health psychologists can provide health education in a more cost-effective manner than hospitals and physicians. Broadening the role of these entities in the health care system may provide better care as well as offer the potential for controlling medical care costs.

Will Health Psychology Continue to Grow?

The problems in the U.S. health care system influence people in clinical health psychology and behavioral medicine because these practitioners must work within that troubled system and demonstrate that the services they provide have value (IOM, 2010; Tovian, 2004). However, health psychologists are also working to reform the system. Their commitment to the biopsychosocial model has helped to promote this model as a more comprehensive view of health and to end the false dichotomy between mental and physical health (Suls & Rothman, 2004). Clinical health psychologists have firmly established their expertise as consultants, but health psychologists may become even more prominent as health care providers. Kaiser Permanente of Northern California designated psychologists as primary health care providers in its health maintenance facilities more than a decade ago (Bruns, 1998), and programs are currently in place for training health psychologists to be primary providers (McDaniel & le Roux, 2007). These psychologists typically become behavioral health or behavioral medicine specialists and serve as part of teams that implement an integrated care approach to health care services. Psychologists are increasingly involved in team-based approaches to primary care (Nash, McKay,

Vogel, & Masters, 2012), a trend that is likely to continue as long as the cost effectiveness of the psychologist's role can be demonstrated (Thielke et al., 2011).

Technological and medical advances create not only new opportunities to improve health but also new issues for health psychology to address. One of the greatest scientific achievements of the last decade was the mapping of the human genome, which allowed researchers unprecedented opportunity to identify the genes that predispose people to various health conditions. As the genetic basis of health conditions becomes clearer, genetic tests will become increasingly available to the public. Health psychologists are ideally poised to help the health care system find ways to improve people's understanding of genetic risk information, to understand their emotional responses to test results, and to encourage high-risk individuals to maintain a healthy lifestyle (Saab et al., 2004). Other technological advances such as the Internet and smartphones allow for new methods of intervention, as these channels are being used to facilitate smoking cessation (Wetter et al., 2011), pain management (Rosser & Eccleston, 2011), and diabetes self-management (Arsand, Tatara, Ostengen, & Hartvigsen, 2010). Given their expertise in understanding health behavior, health literacy, and risk communication, psychologists will play an important role in designing and evaluating technology-based interventions for health behavior.

IN SUMMARY

Health psychology has made significant contributions to health care research and practice, but must meet a number of challenges to continue to grow. Several of these challenges relate to the troubled health care system in the United States. Medical care costs have risen in the United States more rapidly than in other industrialized countries, many of which manage to provide health care to a wider segment of their population and with a better outcome in terms of life expectancy and health expectancy. The United States needs to reform its inefficient medical care system so that a larger segment of the population can receive quality health care services.

The future of health care will demand better management of chronic illnesses and a greater emphasis on prevention. The aging population will increase the need for management of chronic conditions that are more common among older people. Prevention may be the key both to better health and to controlling medical care costs. Health psychology has a role to play in both the management and prevention of chronic illness, as reflected in the growth of the field of primary care psychology. Technological and medical advances such as genetic testing and smartphone technology present new opportunities for psychologists to contribute to the changing landscape of health care.

Making Health Psychology Personal

At the beginning of this chapter, we met Dwayne Brown and Robyn Green, two college students with varying attitudes toward health and differing health-related behaviors. You may see similarities and differences between Dwayne's and Robyn's behavior and your own. By contrasting their behavior with that of typical college students and analyzing their actions and attitudes, you may be able to understand your risks and form a plan to adopt health behaviors that will lead you to a healthier and longer life.

Understanding Your Risks

Like Dwayne and Robyn, nearly 90% of college students rate their health as good, if not excellent (American College Health Association [ACHA], 2016). That perception is consistent with statistics on morbidity and mortality (USCB, 2011); young adults have a lower incidence of disease and death than older adults. The perception of good health may be beneficial, but that view may also create hazards by leading young adults (like Dwayne) to believe that their good health will continue, regardless of their behavior. This view is dangerously incorrect and may even increase the risks for the leading cause of death to this age group—unintentional injury (accidents). Indeed, both unintentional injury and intentional violence are leading causes of injury and death for people before age 45.

Injury and Violence   As the leading killers of young people, injuries and violence lead to more lost years of life than any other source. For example, each cancer-related death accounts for an average of 19 lost years of life, but each death due to unintentional injury steals an average of 33 years from a person's life expectancy (USCB, 2011). Sadly, most deaths among college students result from behaviors that contribute to either unintentional or intentional injuries.

Automobile crashes are by far the leading cause of fatal injuries among adolescents and young adults; they account for about two-thirds of fatalities from unintentional injuries for young people 15 to 24 (USCB, 2011). Nearly half of these deaths are due to drinking and driving (Hingson, Heeren, Winter, & Wechsler, 2005). In the United States, young adults aged 21 to 24 lead all other age groups in a frightening statistic: fatalities due to drunk driving (USCB, 2011). In countries around the world, driving after drinking is an unfortunately common practice for college students, and countries with higher rates of this practice also have higher rates of traffic fatalities (Steptoe et al., 2004). The university environment appears to contribute to this dangerous behavior; college students are more likely than their nonstudent peers to drive after drinking (Hingson et al., 2005). College students are also more likely than their peers to use cell phones while driving, which is another behavior that sharply increases the risk of a crash (Cramer, Mayer, & Ryan, 2007). In the United States, the percentage of traffic fatalities due to such distracted driving nearly doubled from 2005 to 2009 (USCB, 2011)!

Failure to use seat belts also contributes to the injury and death rate for automobile crashes; unrestrained drivers are five times more likely to be injured than those using restraints (Bustamante, Zhang, O'Connell, Rodriguez, & Borroto-Ponce, 2007). A substantial difference appears for male and female college students in driving-related risks. College men and women are equally as likely to report using seat belts (ACHA, 2016). However, women are more likely to use cell phones while driving (Cramer et al., 2007).

College students are also victims (and perpetrators) of intentional violence, including assaults, robberies, rapes, and murders, but at a lower rate than nonstudents of comparable age (Carr, 2007). Crime rates in general have decreased in the United States, and that trend has also appeared on college campuses; only about one-fourth of campus injuries are the result of intentional violence. However, many campus crimes go unreported, and people fail to report sexual and partner violence more often than they report these acts of violence.

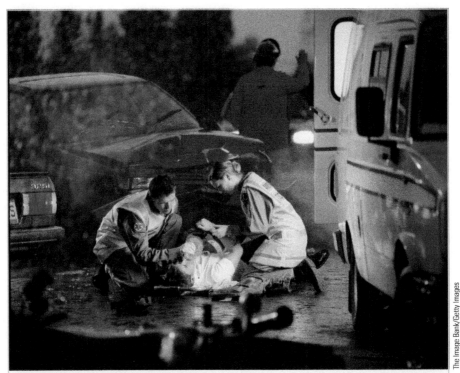

Automobile crashes are the leading cause of fatal injuries for adolescents and young adults in the United States.

Three percent of college women and 1% of college men have been raped within the past school year (ACHA, 2016); nearly twice as many women report being the target of an attempted rape. These percentages are small but represent thousands of people per year. In addition, the percentage is cumulative; by the end of college life, the chance of a college woman experiencing a rape or attempted rape is more than 20% (Carr, 2007). Unwanted sexual touching and threats are much more common. Sexual victimization relates to a variety of health risks for women, including smoking, drug use, thoughts of suicide, and eating disorders (Gidycz, Orchowski, King, & Rich, 2008). Thus, sexual violence can initiate a cascade of health problems.

Dating violence is also a common experience during college, although emotionally abusive relationships are much more common (10% within the past year) than physically abusive ones (2% within the past year) (ACHA, 2016). Women who are involved in physically abusive relationships are at increased risk for sexual violence and for victimization by a stalker, a form of victimization that is

more common among college students than other groups. However, both women and men are perpetrators as well as victims of dating violence. A large, international study of dating violence (Straus, 2008) revealed that women are almost as likely as men to initiate dating violence. Couples in which one partner is more dominant than the other are at increased risk for violent behavior.

Suicide and suicide attempts are other forms of intentional violence that occur among college students. About 11% of college women and 8% of college men have seriously considered suicide within the past school year (ACHA, 2016); 2% had attempted suicide within that time span. Feelings of hopelessness and depression; involvement in an abusive relationship; and being lesbian, gay, or bisexual increase the risk for suicidal thoughts and suicide attempts (Carr, 2007). As Joetta Carr (2007) commented, "Some campus violence is a reflection of society's sexism, racism, and homophobia" (p. 311). Drinking, drug use, and mental health problems magnify the risks for all types of campus violence. However, college campuses are safer environments than most places, and students are safer on campus than in most communities.

Lifestyle Choices   Although young adulthood presents hazards due to intentional and unintentional violence, it is also a time during which individuals adopt health-related behaviors that influence their health for decades. These health behaviors contribute to the risks for the leading causes of death during middle age and later. Dwayne and Robyn exhibit both risky and protective health behaviors, the most important of which is their status as nonsmokers. The choice to be a nonsmoker is typical of college students; a lower percentage of college students smoke than of those who have not attended college (Wetter et al., 2005). Indeed, education is currently the best predictor of smoking status. Thus, it may not be surprising that individuals with a college education live longer and experience better health than others.

Dwayne's abstention from alcohol and Robyn's social drinking are patterns that appear among college students, but many students choose less wisely and engage in binge drinking. Binge drinking represents the most dangerous pattern of drinking among young people. Such behavior can bring many health problems, and almost 4% of college students report that drinking interfered with their academic performance (ACHA, 2016). Even occasional binge drinking is risky because of its association with injury and violence. Over 40% of those between ages 18 and 25 engage in binge drinking (NCHS, 2011), and college students are more likely than others to do so.

College students often fail to eat a healthy diet. When students begin college, they often enter a new living situation in which they make dietary choices rather than eat at home. A study of college students in Greece (Papadaki, Hondros, Scott, & Kapsokefalou, 2007) found that students who moved away from home tended to change their diet to less healthy choices that included more sugar, alcohol, and fast food. Those who continued to live at home made few changes. Like Dwayne, few college students in the United States meet the guidelines for fruit and vegetable consumption (Adams & Colner, 2008). Like Robyn, those who do tend to adhere to other healthy behaviors, including using seat belts, engaging in physical activity, and sleeping well, along with decreased chances of smoking and driving after drinking.

College students are less likely than the general population to be overweight and more likely to engage in physical exercise; yet, significant percentages of students fall short of those health goals. One study of eating, weight, and physical activity among college students (Burke, Lofgren, Morrell, & Reilly, 2007) indicated that 33% of male and 22% of female college students were overweight; 11% and 7% were obese. A third of the women and 23% of the men accumulated less than 30 minutes of physical activity per day. As we would expect, these students had elevated cholesterol and blood pressure, laying the foundations for cardiovascular disease. Neither Dwayne nor Robyn is overweight, but Dwayne's diet and lack of exercise put him at greater risk for high cholesterol and high blood pressure than Robyn, who does not want to repeat her grandfather's experience with heart disease.

College students also encounter stress, with a majority reporting more than average or a tremendous amount of stress (ACHA, 2016). Robyn's rating of her stress is more typical than Dwayne's rating, which was very low. Most college students report many more sources of stress, which is the most frequently named reason for academic problems (ACHA, 2016). Thus, stress is a major challenge for college students, but developing problem-focused strategies to manage stress is important (Largo-Wight, Peterson, & Chen, 2005). Indeed, college students can lead healthy lives during their college years by cultivating a healthy lifestyle, and these habits provide the basis for a longer life as well as a healthier one.

What Can You Do to Cultivate a Healthy Lifestyle?

Health psychologists and other health researchers generate a massive amount of information about health and health-related behaviors. Electronic media, including television and the Internet, inundate people with health information; some of this information may come from valid sources, but some may not. People are often confused by what they perceive as an overwhelming amount of information, which even seems contradictory at times (Kickbusch, 2008). Evaluating all the information and translating it into personal terms is a substantial task, which requires *health literacy*—the ability to read and understand health information to make health decisions. This ability is related, of course, to literacy in general but goes further to include an understanding and evaluation of scientific information related to health (White, Chen, & Atchison, 2008; Zaarcadoolas, Pleasant, & Greer, 2005).

Increase Your Health Literacy   Despite their educational level, college students do not necessarily have a high degree of health literacy. They actively seek health information but tend to consult friends and family rather than more expert sources (Baxter, Egbert, & Ho, 2008). To increase your health literacy, begin to evaluate health claims critically, considering the source of the claim (Chapter 2 presents useful tips for evaluating the trustworthiness of information on the Internet). Expertise matters, so listen to the experts. Health research has produced a large body of evidence that allows health researchers to make recommendations. The massive research findings from health psychology represent an authoritative source, with recommendations on smoking, drinking alcohol, eating a healthy diet, exercising, decreasing the risk of unintentional injury, and managing stress.

Adopt Good Health Behaviors—Now   One way to summarize the recommendations from health research is to work toward integrating the findings from the Alameda County study into your life. Recall from Chapter 2 that this study identified five behaviors that led to better health and lower mortality (Belloc, 1973; Berkman & Breslow, 1983): (1) refraining from smoking cigarettes, (2) engaging in regular physical exercise, (3) drinking alcohol in moderation or not at all, (4) maintaining a healthy weight, and (5) sleeping 7 to 8 hours per night.

Of these habits, avoiding tobacco is probably the most important health behavior you can adopt, as it is the health behavior most strongly linked to longevity (Ford, Bergmann, Boeing, Li, & Capewell, 2012; Ford, Zhao, Tsai, & Li, 2011). The damage from tobacco takes years to become apparent, but smoking cigarettes and exposure to secondhand smoke are both hazardous. The evidence is also overwhelming concerning the benefits of adopting an active lifestyle. For individuals of any age, physical activity boosts health and prevents disease and disability. Physical activity can also improve cognitive functioning, mood, and learning—outcomes that may be more immediate than long-term health benefits. These two health habits are more important for long-term health benefits than for immediate ones, but nonsmokers who exercise regularly experience short-term health advantages as well as longer life expectancies.

Moderating alcohol intake is also an important health behavior. Light drinkers are healthier than those who drink more, and probably than those who do not

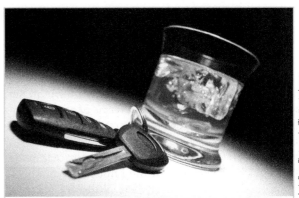

Alcohol is a significant contributor to motor vehicle crashes, and college students are more likely than others to binge drink.

Andy Dean Photography/Shutterstock.com

drink at all. However, these findings apply to older adults more strongly than to younger ones. For college students, light drinking can often turn into binge drinking, which presents many serious risks to college students. Thus, good advice for college students is to work toward moderating drinking and avoiding the hazards of mixing alcohol and motor vehicles. Also, alcohol increases the risk of all types of violence, which is the leading cause of death for young adults. Avoiding heavy or binge drinking is the wise choice for college students.

Maintaining a healthy weight is important, but so are food choices. The foundation for cardiovascular disease begins during adolescence and young adulthood, and food choices are important. A high-fat diet is a component in this process. Even if you are able to maintain close to an ideal weight while eating a high-fat diet (as Dwayne was), this choice is a bad one. Strong evidence shows that a diet with lots of fruits and vegetables provides many health benefits. Choosing such a diet while balancing work, school, and personal demands is not an easy task but will lead to short-term benefits through weight maintenance and long-term advantages through decreasing the risks for cardiovascular disease, diabetes, and cancer. How much do these health habits matter? People who do not smoke, get adequate physical activity, moderate their alcohol consumption, and keep a healthy diet can benefit from an estimated *14 more years of life* than those who do not practice these four behaviors (Khaw et al., 2008)!

The fifth recommendation from the Alameda County study may be the most difficult for college students to follow: Get 7 to 8 hours of sleep a night. Only 5% of college students say they always get enough sleep so they feel rested when they wake up, and most college students only feel rested 3 out of 7 days of the week (ACHA, 2016). People who sleep more than 8 or less than 6 hours per night experience higher death rates than those who get 7 to 8 hours of sleep (Patel et al., 2004). Setting a priority on sleep may be difficult but will also pay off immediately in terms of energy, concentration, and perhaps even improved immune function (Motivala & Irwin, 2007).

A final recommendation from the Alameda County study emphasized the importance of social support (Camacho & Wiley, 1983; Wiley & Camacho, 1980). People with a social network are healthier than those with few social contacts. College students have many opportunities to form a social network of friends, which they may add to their families as sources of social support. Remember that social support provides one type of coping strategy, but it is wise to cultivate a range of such strategies, including problem-focused as well as emotion-focused strategies, and use them appropriately.

The combination of these health behaviors will extend your life and improve your health, not only in the future but also during your college years. We (Linda, Jess, and John) sincerely wish you a healthy and happy future.

IN SUMMARY

Improving the health of college students requires understanding the risks specific to this group and finding ways to diminish those risks, including changes in their health-related behaviors. Injuries from intentional and unintentional violence are major health threats to young adults, including college students. Vehicle crashes are the most common threat, but injuries and deaths occur as a result of assault, rape, partner violence, suicide, and homicide. Alcohol is a factor in all of those types of violence.

Health habits adopted during young adulthood lay the foundation for health or disease in later years. To make healthy choices, individuals need to develop their health literacy so that they can evaluate the health information that that they receive from others and from the media. A good guideline for cultivating a healthy lifestyle comes from the Alameda County study, which found that people are healthier and live longer if they (1) refrain from smoking cigarettes, (2) engage in physical activity regularly, (3) drink alcohol in moderation or not at all, (4) maintain a healthy weight, and (5) sleep 7 to 8 hours per night. In addition, developing a social support network enhances health.

Answers

This chapter has addressed three basic questions:

1. **What role does health psychology play in contributing to the goals of *Healthy People 2020*?**

Health psychology is one of several disciplines that have a role in helping the nation achieve the goals and objectives of *Healthy People 2020*. The two broad goals of this document are (1) increasing the span of healthy life and (2) eliminating health disparities among various ethnic groups. Health psychologists emphasize adding healthy years of life, not merely more years. They cooperate with other health professionals in understanding and reducing health discrepancies among different ethnic groups, but this goal has proven difficult to accomplish.

2. **What is the outlook for the future of health psychology?**

Health psychology faces challenges in the 21st century. Finding ways to control health care costs is a major goal for all health care providers. Health psychologists can contribute to that goal through their expertise in understanding and treating the chronic diseases that have become the leading causes of death in industrialized countries. Even more important, health psychologists have advocated for prevention, which has the potential to decrease the need for health care. Prevention through behavior change can help in controlling health care costs. To be included in future health care, health psychologists must continue to add to both the research and practice components of the field: Build a research base and develop more effective strategies for behavior change.

3. **How can you use health psychology to cultivate a healthier lifestyle?**

The habits that you adopt during young adulthood form a foundation for your health-related behavior throughout middle and older adulthood, so the choices you make now are important for your future health. Health psychology offers suggestions concerning how to cultivate healthy choices in terms of smoking, drinking and drug use, diet, exercise, and stress management. Increasing your health literacy and relying on research rather than information from the media or from friends provide a strategy for making good health choices.

Suggested Readings

Kickbusch, I. (2008). Health literacy: An essential skill for the twenty-first century. *Health Education,* *108*, 101–104. This article examines the challenges to developing health literacy and emphasizes the importance of doing so in light of the ever-increasing complexity of health research.

Mongan, J. J., Ferris, T. G., & Lee, T. H. (2008). Options for slowing the growth of health care costs. *New England Journal of Medicine, 358*, 1509–1514. This recent article examines some possibilities for controlling health care costs without a drastic overhaul of the U.S. health care system.

Whitfield, K. E., Weidner, G., Clark, R., & Anderson, N. B. (2002). Sociodemographic diversity in behavioral medicine. *Journal of Consulting and Clinical Psychology, 70*, 463–481. Keith Whitfield and his colleagues provide a comprehensive review of ethnic, gender, and economic factors that affect health and life expectancy, analyzing the risks and protective factors associated with each demographic group.

GLOSSARY

A-beta fibers Large sensory fibers involved in rapidly transmitting sensation and possibly in inhibiting the transmission of pain. (Chapter 7)

absolute risk A person's chances of developing a disease or disorder independent of any risk that other people may have for that disease or disorder. (Chapter 2)

abstinence violation effect Feelings of guilt and loss of control often experienced after a person lapses into an unhealthy habit after a period of abstinence. (Chapters 12, 15)

acceptance and commitment therapy (ACT) A type of therapy that teaches people to notice and accept unwanted thoughts and feelings, while also committing to valued goals and activities. (Chapter 7)

acetylcholine One of the major neurotransmitters of the autonomic nervous system. (Chapter 5)

acquired immune deficiency syndrome (AIDS) An immune deficiency caused by viral infection and resulting in vulnerability to a wide range of bacterial, viral, and malignant diseases. (Chapter 6)

acrolein A yellowish or colorless, pungent liquid produced as a byproduct of tobacco smoke; one of the aldehydes. (Chapter 12)

acupressure The application of pressure rather than needles to the points used in acupuncture. (Chapter 8)

acupuncture An ancient Chinese form of analgesia that consists of inserting needles into specific points on the skin and continuously stimulating the needles. (Chapter 8)

acute pain Short-term pain that results from tissue damage or other trauma. (Chapter 7)

addiction Dependence on a drug such that stopping its use results in withdrawal symptoms. (Chapter 13)

A-delta fibers Small sensory fibers that are involved in the experience of "fast" pain. (Chapter 7)

adherence A patient's ability and willingness to follow recommended health practices. (Chapter 4)

adrenal cortex The outer layer of the adrenal glands; secretes glucocorticoids. (Chapter 5)

adrenal glands Endocrine glands, located on top of each kidney, that secrete hormones and affect metabolism. (Chapter 5)

adrenal medulla The inner layer of the adrenal glands; secretes epinephrine and norepinephrine. (Chapter 5)

adrenocortical response The response of the adrenal cortex, prompted by ACTH, that results in the release of glucocorticoids, including cortisol. (Chapter 5)

adrenocorticotropic hormone (ACTH) A hormone produced by the anterior portion of the pituitary gland that acts on the adrenal gland and is involved in the stress response. (Chapter 5)

adrenomedullary response The response of the adrenal medulla, prompted by sympathetic nervous system activation, that results in the release of epinephrine. (Chapter 5)

aerobic exercises Exercises that require an increased amount of oxygen consumption over an extended period of time. (Chapter 15)

afferent neurons Sensory neurons that relay information from the sense organs toward the brain. (Chapter 7)

alarm reaction The first stage of the general adaptation syndrome (GAS), in which the body's defenses are mobilized against a stressor. (Chapter 5)

alcohol dehydrogenase A liver enzyme that metabolizes alcohol into aldehyde. (Chapter 13)

aldehyde dehydrogenase An enzyme that converts aldehyde to acetic acid. (Chapter 13)

aldehydes A class of organic compounds obtained from alcohol by oxidation and also found in cigarette smoke; they cause mutations and are related to the development of cancer. (Chapter 12)

alkalosis An abnormally high level of alkaline in the body. (Chapter 14)

allergies Immune system responses characterized by an abnormal reaction to a foreign substance. (Chapter 6)

allostasis The concept that different circumstances require different levels of physiological activation. (Chapter 5)

allostatic load The term refers to the "wear and tear" of the body due to prolonged activation of physiological stress responses. (Chapter 5)

alternative medicine A group of diverse medical and health care systems, practices, and products that are not currently considered part of conventional medicine and are used as alternatives to conventional treatment. (Chapter 8)

amphetamines One type of stimulant drug. (Chapter 13)

anabolic steroids Steroid drugs that increase muscle bulk and decrease body fat but also have toxic effects. (Chapter 13)

anaerobic exercises Exercises that require short, intensive bursts of energy but do not require an increased amount of oxygen use. (Chapter 15)

analgesic drugs Drugs that decrease the perception of pain. (Chapter 7)

anemia A low level of red blood cells, leading to generalized weakness and lack of vitality. (Chapter 14)

angina pectoris A disorder involving a restricted blood supply to the myocardium, which results in chest pain and restricted breathing. (Chapter 9)

anorexia nervosa An eating disorder characterized by intentional starvation, distorted body image, excessive amounts of energy, and an intense fear of gaining weight. (Chapter 14)

antibodies Protein substances produced in response to a specific invader or antigen, marking it for destruction and thus creating immunity to that invader. (Chapter 6)

antigens Substances that provoke the immune system to produce antibodies. (Chapter 6)

anus Opening through which feces are eliminated. (Chapter 14)

arteries Vessels carrying blood away from the heart. (Chapter 9)

arterioles Small branches of an artery. (Chapter 9)

arteriosclerosis A condition marked by loss of elasticity and hardening of arteries. (Chapter 9)

asthma A chronic disease that causes constriction of the bronchial tubes, preventing air from passing freely and causing wheezing and difficulty breathing during attacks. (Chapters 6, 11)

atheromatous plaques Deposits of cholesterol and other lipids, connective tissue, and muscle tissue. (Chapter 9)

atherosclerosis The formation of plaque within the arteries. (Chapter 9)

autoimmune diseases Disorders that occur as a result of the immune system's failure to differentiate between body cells and foreign cells, resulting in the body's attack and destruction of its own cells. (Chapter 6)

autonomic nervous system (ANS) The part of the peripheral nervous system that primarily serves internal organs. (Chapter 5)

aversion therapy A type of behavioral therapy, based on classical conditioning techniques, that uses some aversive stimulus to countercondition the patient's response. (Chapter 13)

Ayurveda A system of medicine that originated in India more than 2,000 years ago; it emphasizes the attainment of health through balance and connection with all things in the universe. (Chapter 8)

B-cells The type of lymphocytes that attacks invading microorganisms. (Chapter 6)

behavior modification Shaping behavior by manipulating reinforcement in order to obtain a desired behavior. (Chapter 7)

behavioral medicine An interdisciplinary field concerned with developing and integrating behavioral and biomedical sciences. (Chapter 1)

behavioral willingness A person's motivation in a given situation to engage in a risky behavior, often as a reaction to social and situational pressures. (Chapter 4)

benign Limited in cell growth to a single tumor. (Chapter 10)

beta-carotene A form of vitamin A found in abundance in vegetables such as carrots and sweet potatoes. (Chapter 10)

bile salts Salts produced in the liver and stored in the gall bladder that aid in digestion of fats. (Chapter 14)

biofeedback The process of providing feedback information about the status of a biological system to that system. (Chapter 8)

biomedical model A perspective that considers disease to result from exposure to a specific disease-causing organism. (Chapter 1)

biopsychosocial model The approach to health that includes biological, psychological, and social influences. (Chapter 1)

body mass index (BMI) An estimate of obesity determined by body weight and height. (Chapter 14)

bronchitis Any inflammation of the bronchi. (Chapter 12)

bulimia An eating disorder characterized by periodic bingeing and purging, the latter usually taking the form of self-induced vomiting or laxative abuse. (Chapter 14)

C fibers Small-diameter nerve fibers that provide information concerning slow, diffuse, lingering pain. (Chapter 7)

cancer A group of diseases characterized by the presence of new cells that grow and spread beyond control. (Chapter 10)

capillaries Very small vessels that connect arteries and veins. (Chapter 9)

carcinogenic Cancer-inducing. (Chapter 10)

carcinomas Cancers of the epithelial tissues. (Chapter 10)

cardiac rehabilitation A complex of approaches designed to restore heart patients to cardiovascular health. (Chapter 9)

cardiologists Medical doctors who specialize in the diagnosis and treatment of heart disease. (Chapter 9)

cardiovascular disease (CVD) Disorders of the circulatory system, including coronary artery disease and stroke. (Chapter 9)

cardiovascular reactivity (CVR) An increase in blood pressure and heart rate as a reaction to frustration or harassment. (Chapter 9)

cardiovascular system The system of the body that includes the heart, arteries, and veins. (Chapter 9)

case–control studies Retrospective epidemiological studies in which people affected by a given disease (cases) are compared with others not affected (controls). (Chapter 2)

catecholamines A class of chemicals containing epinephrine and norepinephrine. (Chapter 5)

catharsis The spoken or written expression of strong negative emotion, which may result in improvement in physiological or psychological health. (Chapter 5)

central control trigger A nerve impulse that descends from the brain and influences the perception of pain. (Chapter 7)

central nervous system (CNS) All the neurons within the brain and spinal cord. (Chapter 5)

cholecystokinin (CCK) A peptide hormone released by the intestines that may be involved in feelings of satiation after eating. (Chapter 14)

chronic diseases Long-lasting diseases that can be controlled but not cured. (Chapters 1, 11)

chronic pain Pain that endures beyond the time of normal healing; frequently experienced in the absence of detectable tissue damage. (Chapter 7)

chronic recurrent pain Alternating episodes of intense pain and no pain. (Chapter 7)

cirrhosis A liver disease resulting in the production of nonfunctional scar tissue. (Chapter 13)

clinical trial A research design that tests the effects of medical treatment. Many clinical trials are randomized controlled trials that allow researchers to determine whether a new treatment is or is not effective. (Chapter 2)

cluster headache A type of severe headache that occurs in daily clusters for 4 to 16 weeks. Symptoms are similar to migraine, but duration is much briefer. (Chapter 7)

cocaine A stimulant drug extracted from the coca plant. (Chapter 13)

cognitive behavioral therapy (CBT) A type of therapy that aims to develop beliefs, attitudes, thoughts, and skills to make positive changes in behavior. (Chapter 5)

cognitive therapy A type of therapy that aims to change attitudes and beliefs, assuming that behavior change will follow. (Chapter 7)

complementary medicine A group of diverse medical and health care systems, practices, and products that are not currently considered part of conventional medicine and are used in addition to conventional techniques. (Chapter 8)

conscientiousness A personality trait marked by a tendency to be planful and goal-oriented, to delay gratification, and to follow norms and rules. (Chapter 4)

continuum theories Theories that explain adherence with a single set of factors that should apply equally to all people. (Chapter 4)

control group In an experiment or clinical trial, the group of participants who do not receive an active treatment. The control group serves as a comparison to the experimental group. (Chapter 2)

coping Strategies that individuals use to manage the distressing problems and emotions in their lives. (Chapter 5)

coronary artery disease (CAD) A disorder of the myocardium arising from atherosclerosis and/or arteriosclerosis. (Chapter 9)

coronary heart disease (CHD) Any damage to the myocardium resulting from insufficient blood supply. (Chapter 9)

correlation coefficient Any positive or negative relationship between two variables. Correlational evidence cannot prove causation, but only that two variables vary together. (Chapter 2)

correlational studies Studies designed to yield information concerning the degree of relationship between two variables. (Chapter 2)

cortisol A type of glucocorticoid that provides a natural defense against inflammation and regulates carbohydrate metabolism. (Chapter 5)

cross-sectional studies Research designs in which subjects of different ages are studied at one point in time. (Chapter 2)

cytokines Chemical messengers secreted by cells in the immune system, forming a communication link between the nervous and immune systems. (Chapter 6)

daily hassles Everyday events that people experience as harmful, threatening, or annoying. (Chapter 5)

delirium tremens A condition induced by alcohol withdrawal and characterized by excessive trembling, sweating, anxiety, and hallucinations. (Chapter 13)

dependence A condition in which a drug becomes incorporated into the functioning of the body's cells so that it is needed for "normal" functioning. (Chapters 7, 13)

dependent variable In an experiment or clinical trial, the variable that represents the effect or outcome of interest. (Chapter 2)

diabetes mellitus A disorder caused by insulin deficiency. (Chapters 6, 11)

diastolic pressure A measure of blood pressure between contractions of the heart. (Chapter 9)

diathesis–stress model A theory of stress that suggests that some individuals are vulnerable to stress-related illnesses because they are genetically predisposed to those illnesses. (Chapter 6)

disulfiram A drug that causes an aversive reaction when taken with alcohol; used to treat alcoholism; Antabuse. (Chapter 13)

dopamine A neurotransmitter that is especially important in mediating the reward associated with taking psychoactive drugs. (Chapter 13)

dorsal horns The part of the spinal cord away from the stomach that receives sensory input and that may play an important role in the perception of pain. (Chapter 7)

dose–response relationship A direct, consistent relationship between an independent variable, such as a behavior, and a dependent variable, such as an illness. For example, the greater the number of cigarettes one smokes, the greater the likelihood of lung cancer. (Chapter 2)

double-blind design An experimental design in which neither the subjects nor those who dispense the treatment condition have knowledge of who receives the treatment and who receives the placebo. (Chapter 2)

eating disorder Any serious and habitual disturbance in eating behavior that produces unhealthy consequences. (Chapter 14)

e-cigarettes Handheld electronic devices wherein a heating element vaporizes a liquid mixture that users inhale; also known as electronic cigarettes. (Chapter 12)

efferent neurons Motor neurons that convey impulses away from the brain. (Chapter 7)

electrolyte imbalance A condition caused by loss of body minerals. (Chapter 14)

electromyograph (EMG) biofeedback Feedback that reflects activity of the skeletal muscles. (Chapter 8)

electronic cigarettes Handheld electronic devices wherein a heating element vaporizes a liquid mixture that users inhale. Electronic cigarettes are also known as e-cigarettes. (Chapter 12)

emotional disclosure A therapeutic technique whereby people express their strong emotions by talking or writing about the events that precipitated them. (Chapter 5)

emotion-focused coping Coping strategies oriented toward managing the emotions that accompany the perception of stress. (Chapter 5)

emphysema A chronic lung disease in which scar tissue and mucus obstruct the respiratory passages. (Chapter 12)

endocrine system The system of the body consisting of ductless glands. (Chapter 5)

endorphins Naturally occurring neurochemicals whose effects resemble those of the opiates. (Chapter 7)

environmental tobacco smoke (ETS) The smoke of spouses, parents, or coworkers to which nonsmokers are exposed; passive smoking. (Chapter 12)

epidemiology A branch of medicine that investigates the various factors that contribute either to positive health or to the frequency and distribution of a disease or disorder. (Chapter 2)

epinephrine A chemical manufactured by the adrenal medulla that accounts for much of the hormone production of the adrenal glands; sometimes called adrenaline. (Chapter 5)

esophagus The tube leading from the pharynx to the stomach. (Chapter 14)

essential hypertension Elevations of blood pressure that have no known cause. (Chapter 9)

ethanol The variety of alcohol used in beverages. (Chapter 13)

ex post facto design A scientific study in which the values of the independent variable are not manipulated, but selected by the experimenter after the groups have naturally divided themselves. (Chapter 2)

exhaustion stage The final stage of the general adaptation syndrome (GAS), in which the body's ability to resist a stressor has been depleted. (Chapter 5)

experimental group In an experiment or clinical trial, the group of participants who receive an active treatment. (Chapter 2)

feces Any materials left over after digestion. (Chapter 14)

fetal alcohol syndrome (FAS) A pattern of physical and psychological symptoms found in infants whose mothers drank heavily during pregnancy. (Chapter 13)

fibromyalgia A chronic pain condition characterized by tender points throughout the body; this condition produces symptoms of fatigue, headache, cognitive difficulties, anxiety, and sleep disturbances. (Chapter 7)

formaldehyde A colorless, pungent gas found in cigarette smoke; it causes irritation of the respiratory system and has been found to be carcinogenic; one of the aldehydes. (Chapter 12)

gall bladder A sac on the liver in which bile is stored. (Chapter 14)

gastric juices Stomach secretions that aid in digestion. (Chapter 14)

gate control theory A theory of pain holding that structures in the spinal cord act as a gate for sensory input that is interpreted as pain. (Chapter 7)

ghrelin A peptide hormone produced primarily in the stomach, the level of which rises before and falls after meals. (Chapter 14)

glucagon A hormone secreted by the pancreas that stimulates the release of glucose, thus elevating blood sugar level. (Chapter 11)

granulocytes A type of lymphocytes that acts rapidly to kill invading organisms. (Chapter 6)

health disparity A difference in a health condition that exists between specific population groups. (Chapter 16)

health expectancy The period of life that a person spends free from disability. (Chapter 16)

health literacy The ability to read and understand health information to make health decisions. (Chapter 16)

health psychology A field of psychology that contributes to both behavioral medicine and behavioral health; the scientific study of behaviors that relate to health enhancement, disease prevention, and rehabilitation. (Chapter 1)

high-density lipoprotein (HDL) A form of lipoprotein that confers some protection against coronary artery disease. (Chapter 9)

hormones Chemical substances released into the blood and having effects on other parts of the body. (Chapter 5)

human immunodeficiency virus (HIV) A virus that attacks the human immune system, depleting the body's ability to fight infection; the infection that causes AIDS. (Chapter 11)

hydrocyanic acid A poisonous acid produced by treating a cyanide with an acid; one of the products of cigarette smoke. (Chapter 12)

hypertension Abnormally high blood pressure, with either a systolic reading in excess of 160 or a diastolic reading in excess of 105. (Chapter 9)

hypoglycemia Deficiency of sugar in the blood. (Chapter 14)

hypothalamic-pituitary-adrenal (HPA) A set of signals and relationships that exist among the hypothalamus, the pituitary gland, and the adrenal glands. (Chapter 5)

hypothalamus A small structure beneath the thalamus, involved in the control of eating, drinking, and emotional behavior. (Chapter 14)

illness behavior Those activities undertaken by people who feel ill and who wish to discover their state of health, as well as suitable remedies. Illness behavior precedes formal diagnosis. (Chapter 3)

immunity A response to foreign microorganisms that occurs with repeated exposure and results in resistance to a disease. (Chapter 6)

implementational intentions Detailed plans that link a specific situation with a goal that a person wants to achieve. (Chapter 4)

incidence A measure of the frequency of new cases of a disease or disorder during a specified period of time. (Chapter 2)

independent variable In an experiment or clinical trial, the variable that represents the presumed cause of an effect or outcome. (Chapter 2)

induction The process of being placed into a hypnotic state. (Chapter 8)

inflammation A general immune system response that works to restore damaged tissue. (Chapter 6)

insulin A hormone that enhances glucose intake to the cells. (Chapter 11)

integrative medicine The approach to treatment that attempts to integrate techniques from both conventional and alternative medicine. (Chapter 8)

interneurons Neurons that connect sensory neurons to motor neurons; association neurons. (Chapter 7)

ischemia Restriction of blood flow to tissue or organs; often used with reference to the heart. (Chapter 9)

islet cells The part of the pancreas that produces glucagon and insulin. (Chapter 11)

isokinetic exercise Exercise requiring exertion for lifting and additional effort for returning weight to the starting position. (Chapter 15)

isometric exercise Exercise performed by contracting muscles against an immovable object. (Chapter 15)

isotonic exercise Exercise that requires the contraction of muscles and the movement of joints, as in weight lifting. (Chapter 15)

Kaposi's sarcoma A malignancy characterized by multiple soft, dark blue or purple nodules on the skin, with hemorrhages. (Chapter 10)

laminae Layers of cell bodies. (Chapter 7)

lay referral network The network of family and friends from whom a person may first seek medical information and advice. (Chapter 3)

leptin A protein hormone produced by fat cells in the body that is related to eating and weight control. (Chapter 14)

leukemias Cancers originating in blood or blood-producing cells. (Chapter 10)

life events Major events in a person's life that require change or adaptation. (Chapter 5)

life expectancy The expected number of years of life that remain for a person of a given age. (Chapters 1, 16)

lipoproteins Substances in the blood consisting of lipid and protein. (Chapter 9)

liver The largest gland in the body; it aids digestion by producing bile, regulates organic components of the blood, and acts as a detoxifier of blood. (Chapter 14)

longitudinal studies Research designs in which one group of participants is studied over a period of time. (Chapter 2)

low-density lipoprotein (LDL) A form of lipoprotein found to be positively related to coronary artery disease. (Chapter 9)

lymph node Small nodules of lymphatic tissue spaced throughout the lymphatic system that help clean lymph of debris. (Chapter 6)

lymph Tissue fluid that has entered a lymphatic vessel. (Chapter 6)

lymphatic system System that transports lymph through the body. (Chapter 6)

lymphocytes A response to foreign microorganisms that occurs with repeated exposure and results in resistance to a disease. (Chapter 6)

lymphoma Cancer of the lymphoid tissues, including lymph nodes. (Chapter 10)

macrophages A type of lymphocytes that attacks invading organisms. (Chapter 6)

malignant Having the ability not only to grow but also to spread to other parts of the body. (Chapter 10)

marijuana A drug derived from the resin of the cannabis sativa plant. The effects of marijuana abuse include memory impairment, altered thought process, feelings of relaxation and euphoria, impaired coordination, and increased appetite. (Chapter 13)

medulla The structure of the hindbrain just above the spinal cord. (Chapter 7)

meta-analysis A statistical technique for combining results of several studies when these studies have similar definitions of variables. (Chapter 2)

metastasize To undergo metastasis, the spread of malignancy from one part of the body to another by way of the blood or lymph systems. (Chapter 10)

migraine headaches Recurrent headaches originally believed to be caused by constriction and dilation of the vascular arteries but now accepted as involving neurons in the brain stem. (Chapter 7)

mindfulness Quality of awareness that is brought about by focusing on the present moment and accepting the thoughts in a nonjudgmental manner. (Chapter 7)

motivational interviewing A therapeutic approach that originated within substance abuse treatment that attempts to change a client's motivation and prepares the client to enact changes in behavior. (Chapter 4)

motivational phase In the health action process approach, the stage in which a person develops an intention to pursue a health-related goal. (Chapter 4)

myelin A fatty substance that acts as insulation for neurons. (Chapter 7)

myocardial infarction Heart attack. (Chapter 9)

myocardium The heart muscle. (Chapter 9)

natural killer (NK) cells The type of lymphocytes that attacks invading organisms. (Chapter 6)

negative reinforcement Removing an unpleasant or negatively valued stimulus from a situation, thereby strengthening the behavior that precedes this removal. (Chapter 4)

neoplastic Characterized by new, abnormal growth of cells. (Chapter 10)

neuroendocrine system Those endocrine glands that are controlled by and interact with the nervous system. (Chapter 5)

neurons Nerve cells. (Chapter 5)

neuroticism A personality trait marked by a tendency to experience negative emotional states. (Chapter 3)

neurotransmitters Chemicals that are released by neurons and that affect the activity of other neurons. (Chapter 5)

nitric oxide A colorless gas prepared by the action of nitric acid on copper and also produced in cigarette smoke; it affects oxygen metabolism and may be dangerous. (Chapter 12)

nocebo effect Adverse effect of a placebo. (Chapter 2)

nociception The process wherein sensory nerve cells are stimulated in response to harmful stimuli resulting in the perception of pain. (Chapter 7)

nociceptors Sensory receptors in the skin and organs that are capable of responding to various types of stimulation that may cause tissue damage. (Chapter 7)

non-Hodgkin's lymphoma A malignancy characterized by rapidly growing tumors that are spread through the circulatory or lymphatic systems. (Chapter 10)

nonnarcotic analgesics Drugs that help in relieving pain without causing loss of consciousness and comprises of nonsteroidal anti-inflammatory drugs and acetaminophen. (Chapter 7)

norepinephrine One of two major neurotransmitters of the autonomic nervous system. (Chapter 5)

oncologists Physicians who specialize in the treatment of cancer. (Chapter 10)

opiate painkillers Substances such as morphine, codeine, oxycodone, and hydrocodone that help relieve pain. (Chapter 7)

optimistic bias The belief that other people, but not oneself, will develop a disease, have an accident, or experience other negative events. (Chapters 4, 9, 12)

optimists People who have a positive outlook on life and expect good things to happen to them. (Chapter 5)

osteoarthritis Progressive inflammation of the joints. (Chapter 7)

osteoporosis A disease characterized by a reduction in bone density, brittleness of bones, and a loss of calcium from the bones. (Chapter 15)

outcome expectations The beliefs that carrying out a specific behavior will lead to valued outcomes. (Chapter 4)

pancreas An endocrine gland, located below the stomach, that produces digestive juices and hormones. (Chapter 11)

pancreatic juices Acid-reducing enzymes secreted by the pancreas into the small intestine. (Chapter 14)

parasympathetic nervous system A division of the autonomic nervous system that promotes relaxation and functions under normal, nonstressful conditions. (Chapter 5)

passive smoking The exposure of nonsmokers to the smoke of spouses, parents, or coworkers; environmental tobacco smoke. (Chapter 12)

pathogen Any disease-causing organism. (Chapter 1)

periaqueductal gray An area of the midbrain that, when stimulated, decreases pain. (Chapter 7)

peripheral nervous system (PNS) The nerves that lie outside the brain and spinal cord. (Chapter 5)

peristalsis Contractions that propel food through the digestive tract. (Chapter 14)

personal control Confidence that people have in their ability to control the events that shape their lives. (Chapter 5)

phagocytosis The process of engulfing and killing foreign particles. (Chapter 6)

phantom limb pain The experience of chronic pain in an absent body part. (Chapter 7)

pharynx Part of the digestive tract between the mouth and the esophagus. (Chapter 14)

pituitary gland An endocrine gland that lies within the brain and whose secretions regulate many other glands. (Chapter 5)

placebo An inactive substance or condition that has the appearance of an active treatment and that may cause improvement or change because of people's belief in the placebo's efficacy. (Chapter 2)

plasma cells Cells, derived from B-cells, that secrete antibodies. (Chapter 6)

population density A physical condition in which a large population occupies a limited space. (Chapter 5)

positive reinforcement Adding a positively valued stimulus to a situation, thereby strengthening the behavior it follows. (Chapter 4)

positive reinforcers Positively valued stimuli that, when added to a situation, strengthens the behavior it follows. (Chapter 7)

posttraumatic stress disorder (PTSD) An anxiety disorder caused by experience with an extremely traumatic event and characterized by recurrent and intrusive reexperiencing of the event. (Chapters 5, 6)

prechronic pain Pain that endures beyond the acute phase but has not yet become chronic. (Chapter 7)

prevalence The proportion of a population that has a disease or disorder at a specific point in time. (Chapter 2)

primary afferents Sensory neurons that convey impulses from the skin to the spinal cord. (Chapter 7)

primary appraisal One's initial appraisal of a potentially stressful event (Lazarus and Folkman). (Chapter 5)

problem-focused coping Coping strategies aimed at changing the source of the stress. (Chapter 5)

proinflammatory cytokine A chemical secreted by the immune system that promotes inflammation, and is associated with feelings of sickness, depression, and social withdrawal. (Chapter 6)

prospective studies Longitudinal studies that begin with a disease-free group of subjects and follow the occurrence of disease in that population or sample. (Chapter 2)

psychoneuroimmunology (PNI) A multidisciplinary field that focuses on the interactions among behavior, the nervous system, the endocrine system, and the immune system. (Chapter 6)

punishment The presentation of an aversive stimulus or the removal of a positive one. Punishment sometimes, but not always, weakens a response. (Chapter 4)

Raynaud's disease A vasoconstrictive disorder characterized by inadequate circulation in the extremities, especially the fingers or toes, resulting in pain. (Chapter 8)

reappraisal One's nearly constant reevaluation of stressful events (Lazarus and Folkman). (Chapter 5)

reciprocal determinism Bandura's model that includes environment, behavior, and person as mutually interacting factors. (Chapter 4)

rectum The end of the digestive tract leading to the anus. (Chapter 14)

referred pain Pain perceived at a place that is different from the place of the stimulus. Visceral pain is often *referred* to sites on the skin. (Chapter 7)

relative risk The risk a person has for a particular disease compared with the risk of other people who do not have that person's condition or lifestyle. (Chapter 2)

reliability The extent to which a test or other measuring instrument yields consistent results. (Chapter 2)

resistance stage The second stage of the general adaptation syndrome (GAS), in which the body adapts to a stressor. (Chapter 5)

retrospective studies Longitudinal studies that look back at the history of a population or sample. (Chapter 2)

rheumatoid arthritis An autoimmune disorder characterized by a dull ache within or around a joint. (Chapters 6, 7)

risk factor Any characteristic or condition that occurs with greater frequency in people with a disease than it does in people free from that disease. (Chapter 2)

salivary glands Glands that furnish moisture that helps in tasting and digesting food. (Chapter 14)

sarcomas Cancers of the connective tissues. (Chapter 10)

secondary appraisal One's perceived ability to control or cope with harm, threat, or challenge (Lazarus and Folkman). (Chapter 5)

sedatives Drugs that induce relaxation and sometimes intoxication by lowering the activity of the brain, the neurons, the muscles, the heart, and even by slowing the metabolic rate. (Chapter 13)

selenium A trace element found in grain products and in meat from grain-fed animals. (Chapter 10)

self-efficacy The belief that one is capable of performing the behaviors that will produce desired outcomes in any particular situation. (Chapter 4)

self-selection A condition of an experimental investigation in which subjects are allowed, in some manner, to determine their own placement in either the experimental or the control group. (Chapter 2)

set-point A hypothetical ratio of fat to lean tissue at which a person's weight will tend to stabilize. (Chapter 14)

sick role behavior Those activities undertaken by people who have been diagnosed as sick that are directed at getting well. (Chapter 3)

single-blind design A design in which the participants do not know if they are receiving the active or inactive treatment, but the providers are not blind to treatment conditions. (Chapter 2)

social contacts Number and kinds of people with whom one associates; members of one's social network. (Chapter 5)

social isolation The absence of specific role relationships. (Chapter 5)

social network The number and kinds of people with whom one associates; social contacts. (Chapter 5)

social support Both tangible and intangible support a person receives from other people. (Chapters 4, 5)

somatic nervous system The part of the PNS that serves the skin and voluntary muscles. (Chapter 5)

somatosensory cortex The part of the brain that receives and processes sensory input from the body. (Chapter 7)

spleen A large organ near the stomach that serves as a repository for lymphocytes and red blood cells. (Chapter 6)

spontaneous remission Disappearance of problem behavior or illness without treatment. (Chapter 13)

stage theories Theories that propose that people pass through discrete stages as they attempt to change a health behavior. Stage theories propose that different factors become important at different times, depending on a person's stage. (Chapter 4)

state anxiety A temporary condition of dread or uneasiness stemming from a specific situation. (Chapter 15)

stimulants Psychoactive drugs such as cocaine, amphetamines, nicotine, and caffeine that tend to elevate mood, arouse action, reduce feelings of fatigue, and decrease appetite. (Chapter 13)

subject variable A variable chosen (rather than manipulated) by a researcher to provide levels of comparison for groups of subjects. (Chapter 2)

substantia gelatinosa Two layers of the dorsal horns of the spinal cord. (Chapter 7)

sympathetic nervous system A division of the autonomic nervous system that mobilizes the body's resources in emergency, stressful, and emotional situations. (Chapter 5)

synaptic cleft The space between neurons. (Chapter 5)

syndrome A cluster of symptoms that characterize a particular condition. (Chapter 7)

synergistic effect The combined effect of two or more variables that exceeds the sum of their individual effects. (Chapter 10)

systolic pressure A measure of blood pressure generated by the heart's contraction. (Chapter 9)

T-cells The cells of the immune system that produce immunity. (Chapter 6)

telomere A region at the end of a chromosome where repetitive nucleotide sequences appear acting as a protective cap and preventing chromosomes from deterioration. (Chapter 6)

tension headaches Pain produced by sustained muscle contractions in the neck, shoulders, scalp, and face, as well as by activity in the central nervous system. (Chapter 7)

thalamus Structure in the forebrain that acts as a relay center for incoming sensory information and outgoing motor information. (Chapter 7)

theory A set of related assumptions from which testable hypotheses can be drawn. (Chapter 2)

thermal biofeedback Feedback concerning changes in skin temperature. (Chapter 8)

thermistor A temperature-sensitive resistor used in thermal biofeedback. (Chapter 8)

thymosin A hormone produced by the thymus. (Chapter 6)

thymus An organ located near the heart that secretes thymosin and thus processes and activates T-cells. (Chapter 6)

tolerance The need for increasing levels of a drug in order to produce a constant level of effect. (Chapters 7, 13)

tonsils Masses of lymphatic tissue located in the pharynx. (Chapter 6)

trait anxiety A personality characteristic that manifests itself as a more or less constant feeling of dread or uneasiness. (Chapter 15)

transcutaneous electrical nerve stimulation (TENS) Treatment for pain involving electrical stimulation of neurons from the surface of the skin. (Chapter 7)

triglycerides A group of molecules consisting of glycerol and three fatty acids; one of the components of serum lipids that has been implicated in the formation of atherosclerotic plaque. (Chapter 9)

urban press The many environmental stressors that affect city living, including noise, crowding, crime, and pollution. (Chapter 5)

validity Accuracy; the extent to which a test or other measuring instrument measures what it is supposed to measure. (Chapter 2)

veins Vessels that carry blood to the heart. (Chapter 9)

venules The smallest veins. (Chapter 9)

volitional phase In the health action process approach, the stage in which a person pursues a health-related goal. (Chapter 4)

well-year The equivalent of a year of complete wellness. (Chapter 16)

withdrawal Adverse physiological reactions exhibited when a drug-dependent person stops using that drug; the withdrawal symptoms are typically unpleasant and opposite to the drug's effects. (Chapter 13)

Abbott, R. B., Hui, K.-K., Hays, R. D., Li, M.-D., & Pan, T. (2007). A randomized controlled trial of tai chi for tension headaches. *Evidence Based Complementary and Alternative Medicine, 4*, 107–113.

Abi-Saleh, B., Iskandar, S. B., Elgharib, N., & Cohen, M. V. (2008). C-reactive protein: The harbinger of cardiovascular diseases. *Southern Medical Journal, 101*, 525–533.

Abnet, C. C. (2007). Carcinogenic food contaminants. *Cancer Investigation, 25*, 189–196.

Ackard, D. M., Brehm, B. J., & Steffen, J. J. (2002). Exercise and eating disorders in college-aged women: Profiling excessive exercisers. *Eating Disorders, 10*, 31–47.

Ackroff, L., Bonacchi, K., Magee, M., Yijn, Y.-M., Graves, J. V., & Sclafani, A. (2007). Obesity by choice revisited: Effects of food availability, flavor variety and nutrient composition on energy intake. *Physiology and Behavior, 92*, 468–478.

Action on Smoking and Health. (2016). *Fact sheet: Smoking and mental health*. Retrieved June 24, 2016, from http://ash.org.uk/files/documents/ASH_120.pdf

Adams, B., Aranda, M. P., Kemp, B., & Takagi, K. (2002). Ethnic and gender differences in distress among Anglo American, African American, Japanese American, and Mexican American spousal caregivers of persons with dementia. *Journal of Clinical Geropsychology, 8*, 279–301.

Adams, T. B., & Colner, W. (2008). The association of multiple risk factors with fruit and vegetable intake among a nationwide sample of college students. *Journal of American College Health, 56*, 455–461.

Adamson, J., Ben-Shlomo, Y., Chaturvedi, N., & Donovan, J. (2003). Ethnicity, socio-economic position and gender: Do they affect reported health-care seeking behavior? *Social Science and Medicine, 47*, 895–904.

Ader, R., & Cohen, N. (1975). Behaviorally conditioned immunosuppression. *Psychosomatic Medicine, 37*, 333–340.

Advokat, C. D., Comaty, J. E., & Julien, R. M. (2014). *Julien's primer of drug action: A comprehensive guide to the actions, uses, and side effects of psychoactive drugs* (13th ed.). New York, NY: Worth.

Agardh, E., Allebeck, P., Hallqvist, J., Moradi, T., & Sidorchuk, A. (2011). Type 2 diabetes incidence and socio-economic position: A systematic review and meta-analysis. *International Journal of Epidemiology, 40*, 804–818.

Agboola, S., McNeill, A., Coleman, T., & Leonardi Bee, J. (2010). A systematic review of the effectiveness of smoking relapse prevention interventions for abstinent smokers. *Addiction, 105*(8), 1362–1380.

Agency for Healthcare Research and Quality (AHRQ). (2011). *2010 National healthcare disparities report* (AHRQ Publication No. 11-0005). Rockville, MD: U.S. Department of Health and Human Services.

Agid, O., Siu, C. O., Potkin, S. G., Kapur, S., Watsky, E., Vanderburg, D., Zipursky, R. B., & Remington, G. (2013). Meta-regression analysis of placebo response in antipsychotic trials, 1970–2010. *American Journal of Psychiatry, 170*, 1335–1344.

Aiken, L. S. (2006). Angela Bryan: Award for distinguished scientific early career contributions to psychology. *American Psychologist, 61*, 802–804.

Aiken, L. S., West, S. G., Woodward, C. K., Reno, R. R., & Reynolds, K. D. (1994). Increasing screening mammography in asymptomatic women: Evaluation of a second-generation, theory-based program. *Health Psychology, 13*, 526–538.

Ajzen, I. (1985). From intentions to actions: A theory of planned behavior. In J. Kuhland & J. Beckman (Eds.), *Action-control: From cognitions to behavior* (pp. 11–39). Heidelberg, Germany: Springer.

Ajzen, I. (1991). The theory of planned behavior. *Organizational Behavior and Human Decision Processes, 50*, 179–211.

Akechi, T., Akazawa, T., Komori, Y., Morita, T., Otani, H., Shinjo, T., Okuyama, T., & Kobayashi, M. (2012). Dignity therapy: Preliminary cross-cultural findings regarding implementation among Japanese advanced cancer patients. *Palliative Medicine, 26*(5), 768–769.

Alaejos, M. S., González, V., & Afonso, A. M. (2008). Exposure to heterocyclic aromatic amines from the consumption of cooked red meat and its effect on human cancer risk: A review. *Food Additives and Contaminants, 25*, 2–24.

Albert, C. M., Mittleman, M. A., Chae, C. U., Lee, I.-M., Hennekens, C. H., & Manson, J. E. (2000). Triggering of sudden death from cardiac causes by vigorous exertion. *New England Journal of Medicine, 343*, 1355–1361.

Al-Delaimy, W. K., Myers, M. G., Leas, E. C., Strong, D. R., & Hofstetter, C. R. (2015). E-cigarette use in the past and quitting behavior in the future: A population-based study. *American Journal of Public Health, 105*(6), 1213–1219.

Aldana, S. G., Greenlaw, R., Salberg, A., Merrill, R. M., Hager, R., & Jorgensen, R. B. (2007). The effects of an intensive lifestyle modification program on carotid artery intima-media thickness: A randomized trial. *American Journal of Health Promotion, 21*, 510–516.

Aldridge, A. A., & Roesch, S. C. (2007). Coping and adjustment in children and cancer: A meta-analytic study. *Journal of Behavioral Medicine, 30*, 115–129.

Alexander, F. (1950). *Psychosomatic medicine*. New York, NY: Norton.

Alfaro, A. (2014). Correlaton of acupuncture point sensitivity and lesion location in 259 horses. *American Journal of Traditional Chinese Veterinary Medicine, 9*(1), 83–87.

Allen, K. (2003). Are pets a healthy pleasure? The influence of pets on blood pressure. *Current Directions in Psychological Science, 12*, 236–239.

Allen, K., Blascovich, J., & Mendes, W. B. (2002). Cardiovascular reactivity and the presence of pets, friends, and spouses: The truth about cats and dogs. *Psychosomatic Medicine, 64*, 727–739.

Alper, J. (1993). Ulcers as infectious diseases. *Science, 260*, 159–160.

Altman, M., & Wilfley, D. E. (2015). Evidence update on the treatment of overweight and obesity in children and adolescents. *Journal of Clinical Child and Adolescent Psychology, 44*(4), 521–537.

Alzheimer's Organization. (2004). *Text of President Reagan's letter announcing his own Alzheimer's diagnosis, November 5, 1994*. Retrieved July 1, 2005, from http://www.alz.org/Media/news releases/ronaldreagan/reaganletter.asp

Amante, D. J., Hogan, T. P., Pagoto, S. L., English, T. M., & Lapane, K. L. (2015). Access to care and use of the internet to search for health information: Results from the US National Health Interview Survey. *Journal of Medical Internet Research, 17*(4), e106.

Amanzio, M., Corazzini, L. L., Vase, L., & Benedetti, F. (2009). A systematic review of adverse events in placebo groups of anti-migraine clinical trials. *Pain, 146*, 261–269.

Amato, P. R., & Hohmann-Marriott, B. (2007). A comparison of high-and low-distress marriages that end in divorce. *Journal of Marriage and Family, 69*, 621–638.

American Cancer Society. (2012). *Cancer facts and figures 2012*. Atlanta, GA: Author.

American Cancer Society. (2016). *Cancer facts & figures*. Atlanta, GA: Author.

American College Health Association. (2016). *American College Health Association-National College Health Assessment II: Undergraduate Students Reference Group Data Report Fall 2015*. Hanover, MD: Author.

American Lung Association. (2007). *Trends in asthma morbidity and mortality*. Retrieved August 3, 2008, from http://www.lungusa.org/site/c.dvLUK9O0E/b.33347/

American Psychiatric Association (APA). (2000). *Diagnostic and Statistical Manual of Mental Disorders* (4th ed., text revision). Washington, DC: Author.

American Psychiatric Association. (2013). *Diagnostic and statistical manual of mental disorders: DSM-5*. Washington, DC: Author.

American Psychological Association (APA). (2002). Ethical principles of psychologists and code of conduct. *American Psychologist, 57*, 1060–1073.

American Psychological Association (APA) Task Force on Health Research. (1976). Contributions of psychology to health research: Patterns, problems, and potentials. *American Psychologist, 31*, 263–274.

American Society for Aesthetic Plastic Surgery. (2014). *Statistics, surveys & trends*. Retrieved August 12, 2016, from http://www.surgery.org/media/news-releases/the-american-society-for-aesthetic-plastic-surgery-reports-americans-spent-largest-amount-on-cosmetic-surger

American Society for Metabolic and Bariatric Surgery. (2016). *Estimate of bariatric surgery numbers, 2011-2015*. Retrieved August 12, 2016, from https://asmbs.org/resources/estimate-of-bariatric-surgery-numbers

Amico, R., Harman, J. J., & Johnson, B. T. (2006). Efficacy of antiretroviral therapy adherence interventions: A research synthesis of trials, 1996 to 2004. *Journal of Acquired Immune Deficiency Syndromes, 41*, 285–297.

Anand, S. S., Islam, S., Rosengren, A., Franzosi, M. G., Steyn, K., Yusufali, A. H., … Interheart Investigators. (2008). Risk factors for myocardial infarction in women and men: Insights from the INTER-HEART study. *European Heart Journal, 29*, 932–940.

Andel, R., Crowe, M., Pedersen, N. L., Mortimer, J., Crimmins, E., Johansson, B., … Gatz, M. (2005). Complexity of work and risk of Alzheimer's disease: A population-based study of Swedish twins. *Journal of Gerontology Series B: Psychological Sciences and Social Sciences, 60B*(5), 251–258.

Andersen, B. L., Yang, H.-C. Y., Farrar, W. B., Golden-Kreutz, D. M., Emery, C. F., Thornton, L. M., … Carson, W. E. (2008). Psychologic intervention improves survival for breast cancer patients: A randomized clinical trial. *Cancer, 113*, 3450–3458.

Andersen, L. B., Sardinha, L. B., Froberg, K., Riddoch, C. J., Page, A. S., & Andersen, S. A. (2008). Fitness, fatness and clustering of cardiovascular risk factors in children from Denmark, Estonia and Portugal: The European Youth Heart Study. *International Journal of Pediatric Obesity, 3*(Suppl. 1), 58–66.

Anderson, J. L., Horne, B. D., Jones, H. U., Reyna, S. P., Carlquist, J. F., Bair, T. L., … Muhlestein J. B. (2004). Which features of the metabolic syndrome predict the prevalence and clinical outcomes of angiographic coronary artery disease? *Cardiology, 101*, 185–193.

Anderson, J. W., Conley, S. B., & Nicholas, A. S. (2007). One hundred pound weight losses with an intensive behavioral program: Changes in risk factors in 118 patients with long-term follow-up. *American Journal of Clinical Nutrition, 86*, 301–307.

Anderson, K. O., Green, C. R., & Payne, R. (2009). Racial and ethnic disparities in pain: Causes and consequences of unequal care. *The Journal of Pain, 10*, 1187–1204.

Anderson, K. O., Syrjala, K. L., & Cleeland, C. S. (2001). How to assess cancer pain. In D. C. Turk & R. Melzack (Eds.), *Handbook of pain assessment* (2nd ed., pp. 579–600). New York, NY: Guilford Press.

Anderson, P. (2006). Global use of alcohol, drugs and tobacco. *Drug and Alcohol Review, 25*, 489–502.

Andersson, K., Melander, A., Svensson, C., Lind, O., & Nilsson, J. L. G. (2005). Repeat prescriptions: Refill adherence in relation to patient and prescriber characteristics, reimbursement level and type of medication. *European Journal of Public Health, 15*, 621–626.

Andrasik, F. (2001). Assessment of patients with headache. In D. C. Turk & R. Melzack (Eds.), *Handbook of pain assessment* (2nd ed., pp. 454–474). New York, NY: Guilford Press.

Andrasik, F. (2003). Behavioral treatment approaches to chronic headache. *Neurological Science, 24*, S80–S85.

Andrews, J. A., Hampson, S. E., Barckley, M., Gerrard, M., & Gibbons, F. X. (2008). The effect of early cognitions on cigarette and alcohol use during adolescence. *Psychology of Addictive Behaviors, 22*, 96–106.

Aneshensel, C. S., Botticello, A. L., & Yamamoto-Mitani, N. (2004). When caregiving ends: The course of depressive symptoms after bereavement. *Journal of Health and Social Behavior, 45*, 422–440.

Anisman, H., Merali, Z., Poulter, M. O., & Hayley, S. (2005). Cytokines as a precipitant of depressive illness: Animal and human studies. *Current Pharmaceutical Design, 11*, 963–972.

Annesi, J. J. (2005). Changes in depressed mood associated with 10 weeks of moderate cardiovascular exercise in formerly sedentary adults. *Psychological Reports, 96*, 855–862.

Antall, G. F., & Kresevic, D. (2004). The use of guided imagery to manage pain in an elderly orthopaedic population. *Orthopaedic Nursing, 23*, 335–340.

Antoni, M. H., Baggett, L., Ironson, G., LaPerriere, A., August, S., Klimas, N., … Fletcher, M. A. (1991). Cognitive-behavioral stress management intervention buffers distress responses and immunologic changes following notification of HIV-1 seropositivity. *Journal of Consulting and Clinical Psychology, 59*, 906–915.

Antoni, M. H., Cruess, D. G., Cruess, S., Lutgendorf, S., Kumar, M., Ironson, G., … Schneiderman, N. (2000). Cognitive-behavioral stress management intervention effects on anxiety, 24-hr urinary norepinephrine output, and T-cytotoxic/suppressor cells over time among symptomatic HIV-infected gay men. *Journal of Consulting and Clinical Psychology, 68*, 31–45.

Antoni, M. H., Ironson, G., & Scheiderman, N. (2007). *Cognitive-behavioral stress management workbook*. New York, NY: Oxford University Press.

Antoni, M. H., Lechner, S., Diaz, A., Vargas, S., Holley, H., Phillips, K., … Blomberg, B. (2009). Cognitive behavioral stress management effects on psychosocial and physiological adaptation in women undergoing treatment for breast cancer. *Brain, Behavior, and Immunity, 23*, 580–591.

Antoni, M. H., & Lutgendorf, S. (2007). Psychosocial factors in disease progression in cancer. *Current Directions in Psychological Science, 16*, 42–46.

Apkarian, A. V., Bushnell, M. C., Treede, R.-D., & Zubieta, J.-K. (2005). Human brain mechanisms of pain perception and regulation in health and disease. *European Journal of Pain, 9*, 463–484.

Applebaum, A. J., Richardson, M. A., Brady, S. M., Brief, D. J., & Keane, T. M. (2009). Gender and other psychosocial factors as predictors of adherence to highly active antiretroviral therapy (HAART) in adults with comorbid HIV/AIDS, psychatric and substance-related disorder. *AIDS and Behavior, 13*, 60–65.

Arbisi, P. A., & Seime, R. J. (2006). Use of the MMPI-2 in medical settings. In J. N. Butcher (Ed.), *MMPI-2: A practitioner's guide* (pp. 273–299). Washington, DC: American Psychological Association.

Armeli, S., Tennen, H., Todd, M., Carney, A., Mohr, C., Affleck, G., … Hromi, A. (2003). A daily process examination of the stress-response dampening effects of alcohol consumption. *Psychology of Addictive Behaviors, 17*, 266–276.

Armitage, C. J. (2004). Evidence that implementation intentions reduce dietary fat intake: A randomized trial. *Health Psychology, 23*, 319–323.

Armitage, C. J. (2009). Is there utility in the transtheoretical model? *British Journal of Health Psychology, 14*, 195–210.

Armitage, C. J., & Conner, M. (2000). Social cognition models and health behaviour: A structured review. *Psychology and Health, 15*, 173–189.

Armitage, C. J., Sheeran, P., Conner, M., & Arden, M. A. (2004). Stages of change or changes of stage? Predicting transitions in transtheoretical model stages in relation to healthy food choice. *Journal of Consulting and Clinical Psychology, 72,* 491–499.

Armor, D. J., Polich, J. M., & Stambul, H. B. (1976). *Alcoholism and treatment.* Santa Monica, CA: Rand.

Armour, B. S., Woollery, T., Malarcher, A., Pechacek, T. F., & Husten, C. (2005). Annual smoking-attributable mortality, years of potential life lost, and productivity losses—United States, 1997–2001. *Mortality and Morbidity Weekly Reports, 54*(25), 625–628.

Armstrong, B., & Doll, R. (1975). Environmental factors and cancer incidence and mortality in different countries, with special reference to dietary practices. *International Journal of Cancer, 15*(4), 617–631.

Arnold, R., Ranchor, A. V., Sanderman, R., Kempen, G. I. J. M., Ormel, J., & Suurmeijer, T. P. B. M. (2004). The relative contribution of domains of quality of life to overall quality of life for different chronic diseases. *Quality of Life Research, 13,* 883–896.

Arntz, A., & Claassens, L. (2004). The meaning of pain influences its experienced intensity. *Pain, 109,* 20–25.

Aro, A. R., De Koning, H. J., Schreck, M., Henriksson, M., Anttila, A., & Pukkala, E. (2005). Psychological risk factors of incidence of breast cancer: A prospective cohort study in Finland. *Psychological Medicine, 35,* 1515–1521.

Arora, N. K., Rutten, L. J. F., Gustafson, D. H., Moser, R., & Hawkins, R. P. (2007). Perceived helpfulness and impact of social support provided by family, friends, and health care providers to women newly diagnosed with breast cancer. *Psycho-Oncology, 16,* 474–486.

Arsand, E., Tatara, N., Ostengen, G., & Hartvigsen, G. (2010). Mobile phone-based self-management tools for type 2 diabetes: The Few Touch application. *Journal of Diabetes Science and Technology, 4,* 328–336.

Arthur, C. M., Katkin, E. S., & Mezzacappa, E. S. (2004). Cardiovascular reactivity to mental arithmetic and cold pressor in African Americans, Caribbean Americans, and White Americans. *Annals of Behavioral Medicine, 27,* 31–37.

Ashton, W., Nanchahal, K., & Wood, D. (2001). Body mass index and metabolic risk factors for coronary heart disease in women. *European Health Journal, 22,* 46–55.

Aspden, P., Wolcott, J., Bootman, J. L., & Cronenwett, L. R. (Eds.). (2007). *Preventing medication errors: Quality chasm series.* Washington, DC: National Academies Press.

Aspinwall, L. G., & Taylor, S. E. (1992). Modeling cognitive adaptation: A longitudinal investigation of the impact of individual differences and coping on college adjustment and performance. *Journal of Personality and Social Psychology, 63*(6), 989–1003.

Associated Press. (2004). Clinton leaves hospital after surgery. *Associated Press Heart Health.* Retrieved June 16, 2005, from http://www.msnbc.msn.com/id/5906976/

Asthma Action America. (2004). *Children and asthma in America.* Retrieved July 7, 2005, from http://www.asthmainamerica.com/frequency.html

Astin, J. A. (1998). Why patients use alternative medicine. *Journal of the American Medical Association, 279,* 1548–1553.

Astin, J. A. (2004). Mind-body therapies for the management of pain. *Clinical Journal of Pain, 20,* 27–32.

Atkinson, N. L., Saperstein, S. L., & Pleis, J. (2009). Using the Internet for health-related activities: Findings from a national probability sample. *Journal of Medical Internet Research, 11,* e4.

Aune, D., Chan, D. S., Vieira, A. R., Rosenblatt, D. A. N., Vieira, R., Greenwood, D. C., … Norat, T. (2013). Red and processed meat intake and risk of colorectal adenomas: A systematic review and meta-analysis of epidemiological studies. *Cancer Causes and Control, 24*(4), 611–627.

Averbuch, M., & Katzper, M. (2000). A search for sex differences in response to analgesia. *Archives of Internal Medicine, 160,* 3424–3428.

Awad, G. H., Sagrestano, L. M., Kittleson, M. J., & Sarvela, P. D. (2004). Development of a measure of barriers to HIV testing among individuals at high risk. *AIDS Education and Prevention, 16,* 115–125.

Ayers, S. L., & Kronenfeld, J. J. (2011). Using zero-inflated models to explain chronic illness, pain, and complementary and alternative medicine use. *American Journal of Health Behavior, 35*(4), 447–457.

Babor, T. F. (2007). We shape our tools, and thereafter our tools shape us: Psychiatric epidemiology and the Alcohol Dependence Syndrome concept. *Addiction, 102*(10), 1534–1535.

Back, S. E., Gentilin, S., & Brady, K. T. (2007). Cognitive-behavioral stress management for individuals with substance use disorders: A pilot study. *Journal of Nervous and Mental Disease, 195,* 662–668.

Badr, H., & Krebs, P. (2013). A systematic review and meta-analysis of psychosocial interventions for couples coping with cancer. *Psycho-Oncology, 22*(8), 1688–1704.

Baer, H. A. (2008). The growing legitimation of complementary medicine in Australia: Successes and dilemmas. *Australian Journal of Medical Herbalism, 20,* 5–11.

Baer, H. J., Glynn, R. J., Hu, F. B., Hankinson, S. E., Willett, W. C., Colditz, G. A., … Rosner, B. (2011). Risk factors for mortality in the Nurses' Health Study: A competing risk analysis. *American Journal of Epidemiology, 173*(3), 319–329.

Bahrke, M. S., & Morgan, W. P. (1978). Anxiety reduction following exercise and meditation. *Cognitive Therapy and Research, 2,* 323–334.

Bailey, B. N., Delaney-Black, V., Covington, C. Y., Ager, J., Janisse, J., Hannigan, J. H., … Sokol, R. J. (2004). Prenatal exposure to binge drinking and cognitive and behavioral outcomes at age 7 years. *American Journal of Obstetrics and Gynecology, 191,* 1037–1042.

Bailey, S. C., Pandit, A. U., Yin, S., Federman, A., Davis, T. C., Parker, R. M., … Wolf, M. S. (2009). Predictors of misunderstanding pediatric liquid medication instructions. *Family Medicine, 41,* 715–721.

Bailis, D. S., Segall, A., Mahon, M. J., Chipperfield, J. G., & Dunn, E. M. (2001). Perceived control in relation to socioeconomic and behavioral resources for health. *Social Science and Medicine, 52,* 1661–1676.

Baker, S. G., Lichtenstein, P., Kaprio, J., & Holm, N. (2005). Genetic susceptibility to prostate, breast, and colorectal cancer among Nordic twins. *Biometrics, 61,* 55–63.

Bala, M., Strzeszynski, L., & Cahill, K. (2008). Mass media interventions for smoking cessation in adults. *Cochrane Database of Systematic Reviews,* Cochrane Art. No.: CD004704, DOI: 10.1002/14651858.CD004704.pub2.

Baliki, M. N., Geha, P. Y., Apkarian, A. V., & Chialvo, D. R. (2008). Beyond feeling: Chronic pain hurts the brain, disrupting the default-mode network dynamics. *Journal of Neuroscience, 28,* 1398–1403.

Balkrishnan, R., & Jayawant, S. S. (2007). Medication adherence research in populations: Measurement issues and other challenges. *Clinical Therapeutics, 29,* 1180–1183.

Ball, D. (2008). Addiction science and its genetics. *Addiction, 103,* 360–367.

Banaji, M. R., & Steele, C. M. (1989). The social cognition of alcohol use. *Social Cognition, 7,* 137–151.

Bandura, A. (1986). *Social foundations of thought and action: A social cognitive theory.* Englewood Cliffs, NJ: Prentice-Hall.

Bandura, A. (1997). *Self-efficacy: The exercise of control.* New York, NY: Freeman.

Bandura, A. (2001). Social cognitive theory: An agentic perspective. *Annual Review of Psychology, 52,* 1–26.

Bánóczy, J., & Squier, C. (2004). Smoking and disease. *European Journal of Dental Education, 8,* 7–10.

Bär, K.-J., Boettger, M. K., Schulz, S., Neubauer, R., Jochum, T., Voss, A., … Yeragani, V. K. (2008). Reduced cardio-respiratory coupling in acute alcohol withdrawal. *Drug & Alcohol Dependence, 98*(3), 210–217.

"Barack Obama Quits." (2011, Feb. 9). Barack Obama quits smoking after 30 years. *The Telegraph.* Retrieved June 2, 2011, from http://www.telegraph.co.uk/news/worldnews/barackobama/8314049/Barack-Obama-quits-smoking-after-30-years.html

Barber, J. (1996). A brief introduction to hypnotic analgesia. In J. Barber (Ed.), *Hypnosis and suggestion in the treatment of pain: A clinical guide* (pp. 3–32). New York, NY: Norton.

Barber, T. X. (1984). Hypnosis, deep relaxation, and active relaxation: Data, theory, and clinical applications. In R. L. Woolfolk & P. M. Lehrer (Eds.), *Principles and practice of stress management.* New York, NY: Guilford Press.

Barber, T. X. (2000). A deeper understanding of hypnosis: Its secrets, its nature, its essence. *American Journal of Clinical Hypnosis, 42,* 208–272.

Bardia, A., Tleyjeh, I. M., Cerhan, J. R., Sood, A. K., Limburg, P. J. Erwin, P. J., … Montori, V. M. (2008). Efficacy of antioxidant supplementation in reducing primary cancer incidence and mortality: Systematic review and meta-analysis. *Mayo Clinic Proceedings, 83,* 23–34.

Bardy, S. S. (2008). Lifetime family violence exposure is associated with current symptoms of eating disorders among both young men and women. *Journal of Traumatic Stress, 21,* 347–351.

Barengo, N. C., Hu, G., Lakka, T. A., Pekkarinen, H., Nissinen, A., & Tuomilehto, J. (2004). Low physical activity as predictor for total and cardiovascular disease mortality in middle-aged men and women in Finland. *European Heart Journal, 25,* 2204–2211.

Barlow, J. H., & Ellard, D. R. (2004). Psycho-educational interventions for children with chronic disease, parents and siblings: An overview of the research evidence base. *Child: Care, Health and Development, 30,* 637–645.

Barnes, P. J. (2008). Immunology of asthma and chronic obstructive pulmonary disease. *Nature Reviews Immunology, 8,* 183–192.

Barnett, R. C., & Hyde, J. S. (2001). Women, men, work, and family: An expansionist theory. *American Psychologist, 56,* 781–796.

Barr, T., Helms, C., Grant, K., & Messaoudi, I. (2016). Opposing effects of alcohol on the immune system. *Progress in Neuro-Psychopharmacology & Biological Psychiatry, 65,* 242–251.

Barrett, S. P. (2010). The effects of nicotine, denicotinized tobacco, and nicotine-containing tobacco on cigarette craving, withdrawal, and self-administration in male and female smokers. *Behavioural Pharmacology, 21*(2), 144–152.

Barron, F., Hunter, A., Mayo, R., & Willoughby, D. (2004). Acculturation and adherence: Issues for health care providers working with clients of Mexican origin. *Journal of Transcultural Nursing, 15,* 331–337.

Barth, J., Critchley, J., & Bengel, J. (2008). Psychosocial interventions for smoking cessation in patients with coronary heart disease. *Cochrane Database of Systematic Reviews,* Cochrane Art. No.: CD006886, DOI: 10.1002/14651858.CD006886.

Barth, K. R., Cook, R. L., Downs, J. S., Switzer, G. E., & Fischhoff, B. (2002). Social stigma and negative consequences: Factors that influence college students' decisions to seek testing for sexually transmitted infections. *Journal of American College Health, 50*(4), 153–159.

Barton-Donovan, K., & Blanchard, E. B. (2005). Psychosocial aspects of chronic daily headache. *Journal of Headache and Pain, 6,* 30–39.

Baseman, J. G., & Koutsky, L. A. (2005). The epidemiology of human papillomavirus infections. *Journal of Clinical Virology, 32,* 16–24.

Basow, S. A., Foran, K. A., & Bookwala, J. (2007). Body objectification, social pressure, and disordered eating behavior in college women: The role of sorority membership. *Psychology of Women Quarterly, 31*(4), 394–400.

Bassman, L. E., & Uellendahl, G. (2003). Complementary/alternative medicine: Ethical, professional, and practical challenges for psychologists. *Professional Psychology: Research and Practice, 34,* 264–270.

Batty, G. D., Kivimaki, M., Gray, L., Smith, G. D., Marmot, M. G., & Shipley, M. J. (2008). Cigarette smoking and site-specific cancer mortality: Testing uncertain associations using extended follow-up of the original Whitehall study. *Annals of Oncology, 19,* 996–1002.

Batty, G. D., Shipley, M. J., Mortensen, L. H., Boyle, S. H., Barefoot, J., Grønbæk, M., … Deary, I. J (2008). IQ in late adolescence/early adulthood, risk factors in middle age and later all-cause mortality in men: The Vietnam Experience Study. *Journal of Epidemiology and Community Health, 62,* 522–531.

Baum, A., Perry, N. W., Jr., & Tarbell, S. (2004). The development of psychology as a health science. In R. G. Frank, A. Baum, & J. L. Wallander (Eds.), *Handbook of clinical health psychology* (Vol. 3, pp. 9–28). Washington, DC: American Psychological Association.

Baumann, L. J., Cameron, L. D., Zimmerman, R. S., & Leventhal, H. (1989). Illness representations and matching labels with symptoms. *Health Psychology, 8,* 449–469.

Baumann, P., Schild, C., Hume, R. F., & Sokol, R. J. (2006). Alcohol abuse—A persistent preventable risk for congenital anomalies. *International Journal of Gynecology and Obstetrics, 95,* 66–72.

Baxter, L., Egbert, N., & Ho, E. (2008). Everyday health communication experiences of college students. *Journal of American College Health, 56,* 427–436.

Beacham, G. (2011). Magic Johnson still beating HIV 20 years later. *USA Today,* September 7, 2011.

Beaglehole, R., Bonita, R., & Kjellström, T. (1993). *Basic epidemiology.* Geneva, Switzerland: World Health Organization.

Beatty, L., & Lambert, S. (2013). A systematic review of internet-based self-help therapeutic interventions to improve distress and disease-control among adults with chronic health conditions. *Clinical Psychology Review, 33*(4), 609–622.

Beck, A. T. (1976). *Cognitive therapy and the emotional disorders.* New York, NY: International Universities Press.

Beck, A. T., Ward, C. H., Mendelson, M., Mock, J., & Erbaugh, J. (1961). An inventory for measuring depression. *Archives of General Psychiatry, 4,* 561–571.

Becker, A. E., Burwell, R. A., Navara, K., & Gilman, S. E. (2003). Binge eating and binge eating disorder in a small-scale, indigenous society: The view from Fiji. *International Journal of Eating Disorders, 34,* 423–431.

Becker, M. H., & Rosenstock, I. M. (1984). Compliance with medical advice. In A. Steptoe & A. Mathews (Eds.), *Health care and human behavior* (pp. 135–152). London: Academic Press.

Bédard, M., Kuzik, R., Chambers, L., Molloy, D. W., Dubois, S., & Lever, J. A. (2005). Understanding burden differences between men and women caregivers: The contribution of care-recipient problem behaviors. *International Psychogeriatrics, 17,* 99–118.

Beecher, H. K. (1946). Pain of men wounded in battle. *Annals of Surgery, 123,* 96–105.

Beecher, H. K. (1955). The powerful placebo. *Journal of the American Medical Association, 149,* 1602–1607.

Beecher, H. K. (1956). Relationship of significance of wound to pain experience. *Journal of the American Medical Association, 161,* 1609–1613.

Beecher, H. K. (1957). The measurement of pain. *Pharmacological Review, 9,* 59–209.

Beetz, A., Kotrschal, K., Turner, D. C., Hediger, K., Uvnäs-Moberg, K., & Julius, H. (2011). The effect of a real dog, toy dog, and friendly person on insecurely attached children during a stressful task: An exploratory study. *Anthrozoos: A Multidisciplinary Journal of the Interactions of People & Animals, 24,* 349–368.

Beilin, L., & Huang, R.-C. (2008). Childhood obesity, hypertension, the metabolic syndrome and adult cardiovascular disease. *Clinical and Experimental Pharmacology and Physiology, 35,* 409–411.

Beinart, N., Weinman, J., Wade, D., & Brady, R. (2012). Caregiver burden and psychoeducational interventions in Alzheimer's disease: A review. *Dementia and Geriatric Cognitive Disorders Extra, 2*(1), 638–648.

Bekke-Hansen, S., Trockel, M., Burg, M. M., & Taylor, C. B. (2012). Depressive symptom dimensions and cardiac prognosis following myocardial infarction: Results from the ENRICHD clinical trial. *Psychological Medicine, 42,* 51–60.

Bélanger-Gravel, A., Godin, G., & Amireault, S. (2011). A meta-analytic review of the effect of implementation intentions on physical activity. *Health Psychology Review,* DOI: 10.1080/17437199.2011.560095.

Belar, C. D. (1997). Clinical health psychology: A specialty for the 21st century. *Health Psychology, 16,* 411–416.

Belar, C. D. (2008). Clinical health psychology: A health care specialty in professional psychology. *Professional Psychology: Research and Practice, 39,* 229–233.

Bell, R. A., Kravitz, R. L., Thom, D., Krupat, E., & Azari, R. (2001). Unsaid but not forgotten: Physician-patient relationship. *Archives of Internal Medicine, 161,* 1977–1983.

Bell, R. A., Kravitz, R. L., Thom, D., Krupat, E., & Azari, R. (2002). Unmet expectations for care and the patient-physician relationship. *Journal of General Internal Medicine, 17,* 817–824.

Belloc, N. (1973). Relationship of health practices and mortality. *Preventive Medicine, 2,* 67–81.

Ben-Arye, E., Frendel, M., Klein, A., & Scharf, M. (2008). Attitudes toward integration of complementary and alternative medicine in primary care: Perspectives of patients, physicians and complementary practitioners. *Patient Education and Counseling*, *70*(3), 395–402.

Benaim, C., Froger, J., Cazottes, C., Gueben, D., Porte, M., Desnuelle, C., ... Pelissier, J. Y. (2007). Use of the Faces Pain Scale by left and right hemispheric stroke patients. *Pain*, *128*, 52–58.

Bendapudi, N. M., Berry, L. L., Frey, K. A., Parish, J. T., & Rayburn, W. L. (2006). Patients' perspectives on ideal physician behaviors. *Mayo Clinic Proceedings*, *81*, 338–344.

Bender, R., Trautner, C., Spraul, M., & Berger, M. (1998). Assessment of excess mortality in obesity. *American Journal of Epidemiology*, *147*, 42–48.

Benedetti, F. (2006). Placebo analgesia. *Neurological Sciences*, *27*(Suppl. 2), S100–S102.

Benight, C. C., Ruzek, J. I., & Waldrep, E. (2008). Internet interventions for traumatic stress: A review and theoretically based example. *Journal of Traumatic Stress*, *21*, 513–520.

Bennett, G. G., Merritt, M. M., Sollers, J. J., III, Edwards, C. L., Whitfield, K. E., Brandon, D. T., ... Tucker, R. D. (2004). Stress, coping, and health outcomes among African-Americans: A review of the John Henryism hypothesis. *Psychology and Health*, *19*, 369–383.

Bennett, I. M., Chen, J., Soroui, J. S., & White, S. (2009). The contribution of health literacy to disparities in self-rated health status and preventive health behaviors in older adults. *Annals of Family Medicine*, *7*, 204–211.

Benyamini, Y., Leventhal, E. A., & Leventhal, H. (2000). Gender differences in processing information for making self-assessments of health. *Psychosomatic Medicine*, *62*, 354–364.

Beresford, S. A., Johnson, K. C., Ritenbaugh, C., Lasser, N. L., Snetselaar, L. G., Black, ... Whitlock, E. (2006). Low-fat dietary pattern and risk of colorectal cancer: The Women's Health Initiative Randomized Controlled Dietary Modification Trial. *JAMA*, *295*(6), 643–654.

Bergmark, K. H., & Kuendig, H. (2008). Pleasures of drinking: A cross-cultural perspective. *Journal of Ethnicity and Substance Abuse*, *7*(2), 131–153.

Berkman, L. F., Blumenthal, J., Burg, M., Carney, R. M., Catellier, D., Cowan, M. J., ... Enhancing Recovery in Coronary Heart Disease Patients Investigators (ENRICHD). (2003). Effects of treating depression and low perceived social support on clinical events after myocardial infarction: The Enhancing Recovery in Coronary Heart Disease Patient (ENRICHD) randomized trial. *Journal of the American Medical Association*, *289*, 3106–3116.

Berkman, L. F., & Breslow, L. (1983). *Health and ways of living: The Alameda County Study.* New York, NY: Oxford University Press.

Berkman, L. F., & Syme, S. L. (1979). Social networks, host resistance, and mortality: A nine-year follow-up study of Alameda County residents. *American Journal of Epidemiology*, *109*, 186–204.

Berman, J. D., & Straus, S. E. (2004). Implementing a research agenda for complementary and alternative medicine. *Annual Review of Medicine*, *55*, 239–254.

Bermudez, O. I., & Gao, X. (2011). Greater consumption of sweetened beverages and added sugars is associated with obesity among US young adults. *Annals of Nutrition & Metabolism*, *57*(3/4), 211–218.

Bernards, S., Graham, K., Kuendig, H., Hettige, S., & Obot, I. (2009). 'I have no interest in drinking': A cross-national comparison of reasons why men and women abstain from alcohol use. *Addiction*, *104*(10), 1658–1668.

Berne, R. M., & Levy, M. N. (2000). *Principles of physiology* (3rd ed.). St. Louis, MO: Mosby.

Bernstein, L., Henderson, B. E., Hanisch, R., Sullivan-Halley, J., & Ross, R. K. (1994). Physical exercise and reduced risk of breast cancer in young women. *Journal of the National Cancer Institute*, *86*, 1403–1408.

Bertakis, K. D., & Azari, R. (2005). Obesity and the use of health care services. *Obesity Research*, *13*, 372–379.

Bertram, L., & Tanzi, R. E. (2005). The genetic epidemiology of neurodegenerative disease. *Journal of Clinical Investigation*, *115*, 1449–1457.

Bessesen, D. H. (2011). Regulation of body weight: What is the regulated parameter? *Physiology & Behavior*, *104*(4), 599–607.

Betsch, C., Brewer, N. T., Brocard, P., Davies, P., Gaissmaier, W., Haase, N., ... Stryk, M. (2012). Opportunities and challenges of Web 2.0 for vaccination decisions. *Vaccine*, *30*(25), 3727–3733.

Bhat, V. M., Cole, J. W., Sorkin, J. D., Wozniak, M. A., Malarcher, A. M., Giles, W. H., ... Kittner, S. J. (2008). Dose-response relationship between cigarette smoking and risk of ischemic stroke in young women. *Stroke*, *39*, 2439–2443.

Bhatt, S. P., Luqman-Arafath, T. K., & Guleria, R. (2007). Non-pharmacological management of hypertension. *Indian Journal of Medical Sciences*, *61*, 616–624.

Bhogal, S., Zemek, R., & Ducharme, F. M. (2006). Written action plans for asthma in children. *Cochrane Database of Systematic Reviews*, Cochrane Art. No.: CD005306, DOI: 10.1002/14651858.CD005306. pub2.

Bianchini, K. J., Etherton, J. L., Greve, K. W., Heinly, M. T., & Meyers, J. E. (2008). Classification accuracy of MMPI-2 validity scales in the detection of pain-related malingering: A known-groups study. *Assessment*, *15*, 435–449.

Bickel-Swenson, D. (2007). End-of-life training in U.S. medical schools: A systematic literature review. *Journal of Palliative Medicine*, *10*, 229–235.

Bigal, M. E., & Lipton, R. B. (2008a). Concepts and mechanisms of migraine chronification. *Headache*, *48*, 7–15.

Bigal, M. E., & Lipton, R. B. (2008b). The epidemiology and burden of headaches. In M. Levin (Ed.), *Comprehensive review of headache medicine* (pp. 39–59). New York, NY: Oxford University Press.

Bigatti, S., & Cronan, T. A. (2002). A comparison of pain measures used with patients with fibromyalgia. *Journal of Nursing Measurement*, *10*, 5–14.

Bird, S. T., Harvey, S. M., Beckman, L. J., & Johnson, C. H. (2000). Getting your partner to use condoms: Interviews with men and women at risk of HIV/STDs. *Journal of Sex Research*, *38*, 233–240.

Biron, C., Brun, J., Ivers, H., & Cooper, C. L. (2006). At work but ill: Psychosocial work environment and well-being determinants of presenteeism propensity. *Journal of Public Mental Health*, *5*, 26–37.

Birtane, M., Uzunca, K., Tastekin, N., & Tuna, H. (2007). The evaluation of quality of life in fibromyalgia syndrome: A comparison with rheumatoid arthritis by using SF-36 Health Survey. *Clinical Rheumatology*, *26*, 679–684.

Bisson, J., & Andrew, M. (2007). Psychological treatment of post-traumatic stress disorder (PTSD). *Cochrane Database of Systematic Reviews*, Cochrane Art. No.: CD003388, DOI: 10.1002/14651858. CD003388.pub3.

Biswas, A., Oh, P. I., Faulkner, G. E., Bajaj, R. R., Silver, M. A., Mitchell, M. S., ... Alter, D. A. (2015). Sedentary time and its association with risk for disease incidence, mortality, and hospitalization in adults: A systematic review and meta-analysis. *Annals of Internal Medicine*, *162*(2), 123–132.

Bjartveit, K. (2009). Health consequences of sustained smoking cessation. *Tobacco Control*, *18*(3), 197–205.

Bjørge, T., Engeland, A., Tverdal, A., & Smith, G. D. (2008). Body mass index in adolescence in relation to cause-specific mortality: A follow-up to 230,000 Norwegian adolescents. *American Journal of Epidemiology*, *168*, 30–37.

Black, E., Holst, C., Astrup, A., Toubro, S., Echwald, S., Pedersent, O., ... Sørensen, T. I. (2005). Long-term influences of body-weight changes, independent of the attained weight, on risk of impaired glucose tolerance and Type 2 diabetes. *Diabetic Medicine*, *22*, 1100–1205.

Black, L. I., Clarke, T. C., Barnes, P. M., Stussman, B. J., & Nahin, R. L. (2015). Use of complementary health approaches among children aged 4-17 years in the United States: National Health Interview Survey, 2007-2012. *National Health Statistics Report*, *78*, 1–18.

Black, P. H. (2003). The inflammatory response is an integral part of the stress response: Implications for atherosclerosis, insulin resistance, Type II diabetes and metabolic syndrome X. *Brain, Behavior and Immunity*, *17*, 350–364.

Blackmore, E. R., Stansfeld, S. A., Weller, I., Munce, S., Zagorski, B. M., & Stewart, D. E. (2007). Major depressive episodes and work stress: Results from a national population survey. *American Journal of Public Health*, *97*, 2088–2093.

Blair, S. N., Cheng, Y., & Holder, J. S. (2001). Is physical activity or physical fitness more important in defining health benefits? *Medicine and Science in Sports & Exercise*, *33*, S379–S399.

Blair, S. N., & Church, T. (2004). The fitness, obesity, and health equation: Is physical activity the common denominator? *Journal of the American Medical Association, 292,* 1232–1234.

Blalock, J. E., & Smith, E. M. (2007). Conceptual development of the immune system as a sixth sense. *Brain, Behavior and Immunity, 21,* 23–33.

Blanchard, C. M., Kupperman, J., Sparling, P. B., Nehl, E., Rhodes, R. E., Courneya, K. S., … Baker, F. (2009). Do ethnicity and gender matter when using the theory of planned behavior to understand fruit and vegetable consumption? *Appetite, 52,* 15–20.

Blanchard, E. B., & Andrasik, F. (1985). *Management of chronic headaches: A psychological approach.* New York, NY: Pergamon Press.

Blanchard, E. B., Appelbaum, K. A., Radniz, C. L., Morrill, B., Michultka, D., Kirsch, C., … Barron, K. D. (1990). A controlled evaluation of thermal bio-feedback and thermal biofeedback combined with cognitive therapy in the treatment of vascular headache. *Journal of Consulting and Clinical Psychology, 58,* 216–224.

Blanchard, J., & Lurie, N. (2004). R-E-S-P-E-C-T: Patient reports of disrespect in health care setting and its impact on care. *Journal of Family Practice, 53,* 721–730.

Blascovich, J., Spencer, S. J., Quinn, D., & Steele, C. (2001). African Americans and high blood pressure: The role of stereotype threat. *Psychological Science, 12,* 225–229.

Bleil, M. E., Gianaros, P. J., Jennings, J. R., Flory, J. D., & Manuck, S. B. (2008). Trait negative affect: Toward an integrated model of understanding psychological risk for impairment in cardiac autonomic function. *Psychosomatic Medicine, 70,* 328–337.

Blodgett Salafia, E. H., & Gondoli, D. M. (2011). A 4-year longitudinal investigation of the processes by which parents and peers influence the development of early adolescent girls' bulimic symptoms. *Journal of Early Adolescence, 31*(3), 390–414.

Bloomfield, K., Stockwell, T., Gmel, G., & Rehn, N. (2003). *International comparison of alcohol consumption.* National Institute of Alcoholism and Alcohol Abuse. Retrieved April 12, 2005, from http://www.niaaa. nih.gov/publications/arh27–1/95-109.htm

Bloor, M. (2005). Observations of shipboard illness behavior: Work discipline and the sick role in a residential work setting. *Qualitative Health Research, 15,* 766–777.

Blundell, J. E., Gibbons, C., Caudwell, P., Finlayson, G., & Hopkins, M. (2015). Appetite control and energy balance: Impact of exercise. *Obesity Reviews,* (Suppl. 16), 67–76.

Bode, C., & Bode, J. C. (1997). Alcohol absorption, metabolism, and production in the gastrointestinal tract. *Alcohol Health & Research World, 21,* 82–83.

Bodenheimer, T. (2005a). High and rising health care costs: Part 1. Seeking an explanation. *Archives of Internal Medicine, 142,* 847–854.

Bodenheimer, T. (2005b). High and rising health care costs: Part 2. Technologic innovation. *Archives of Internal Medicine, 142,* 932–937.

Bodenheimer, T. (2005c). High and rising health care costs: Part 3. The role of health care providers. *Archives of Internal Medicine, 142,* 996–1002.

Bodenheimer, T., & Fernandez, A. (2005). High and rising health care costs: Part 4. Can costs be controlled while preserving quality? *Archives of Internal Medicine, 143,* 26–31.

Bodenmann, G., Meuwly, N., Germann, J., Nussbeck, F. W., Heinrichs, M., & Bradbury, T. N. (2015). Effects of stress on the social support provided by men and women in intimate relationships. *Psychological Science, 26*(10), 1584–1594.

Bodhi, B. (2011). What does mindfulness really mean? A canonical perspective. *Contemporary Buddhism, 12*(1), 19–39.

Boffetta, P. (2004). Epidemiology of environmental and occupational cancer. *Oncogene, 23,* 6392–6403.

Bogart, L. M., & Delahanty, D. L. (2004). Psychosocial models. In T. J. Boll, R. G. Frank, A. Baum, & J. L. Wallander (Eds.), *Handbook of clinical health psychology: Vol. 3. Models and perspectives in health psychology* (pp. 201–248). Washington, DC: American Psychological Association.

Bogg, T., & Roberts, B. W. (2004). Conscientiousness and health-related behaviors: A meta-analysis of the leading behavioral contributors to mortality. *Psychological Bulletin, 130,* 887–919.

Bogg, T., & Roberts, B. W. (2013). The case for conscientiousness: Evidence and implications for a personality trait marker of health and longevity. *Annals of Behavioral Medicine, 45*(3), 278–288.

Boice, J. D., Jr., Bigbee, W. L., Mumma, M. T., & Blot, W. J. (2003). Cancer mortality in counties near two former nuclear materials processing facilities in Pennsylvania, 1950–1995. *Health Physics, 85,* 691–700.

Boisvert, J. A., & Harrell, W. A. (2009). Homosexuality as a risk factor for eating disorder symptomatology in men. *Journal of Men's Studies, 17*(3), 210–225.

Boldt, E. (2016). Veterinary acupuncture and chiropractic: What, when, who? *Horse Health.* Retrieved May 12, 2016, from http://www.aaep. org/info/horse-health?publication=697

Bolger, N., Zuckerman, A., & Kessler, R. C. (2000). Invisible support and adjustment to stress. *Journal of Personality and Social Psychology, 79,* 953–961.

Bolognesi, M., Nigg, C. R., Massarini, M., & Lippke, S. (2006). Reducing obesity indicators through brief physical activity counseling (PACE) in Italian primary care settings. *Annals of Behavioral Medicine, 31,* 179–185.

Bonica, J. J. (1990). Definitions and taxonomy of pain. In J. J. Bonica (Ed.), *The management of pain* (2nd ed., pp. 18–27). Malvern, PA: Lea & Febiger.

Bonilla, K. (2007, June 29). Diabetes, pregnancy and Halle Berry. *MyDiabetesCentral.com.* Retrieved June 29, 2008, from http://www.health central.com/diabetes/c/5868/13828/halle-berry/

Boots, L. M. M., de Vugt, M. E., Knippenberg, R. J. M., Kempen, G. I. J. M., & Verhey, F. R. J. (2014). A systematic review of Internet-based supportive interventions for caregivers of patients with dementia. *International Journal of Geriatric Psychiatry, 29*(4), 331–344.

Borrell, L. N. (2005). Racial identity among Hispanics: Implications for health and well-being. *American Journal of Public Health, 95,* 379–381.

Bort-Roig, J., Gilson, N. D., Puig-Ribera, A., Contreras, R. S., & Trost, S. G. (2014). Measuring and influencing physical activity with smartphone technology: A systematic review. *Sports Medicine, 44*(5), 671–686.

Bos, V., Kunst, A. E., Garssen, J., & Mackenbach, J. P. (2005). Socioeconomic inequalities in mortality within ethnic groups in the Netherlands, 1995–2000. *Journal of Epidemiology and Community Health, 59,* 329–335.

Bosch-Capblanch, S., Abba, K., Prictor, M., & Garner, P. (2007). Contracts between patients and healthcare practitioners for improving patients' adherence to treatment, prevention and health promotion activities. *Cochrane Database of Systematic Reviews,* Cochrane Art. No.: CD004808, DOI: 10.1002/14651858.CD004808.pub3.

Bottonari, K. A., Roberts, J. W., Ciesla, J. A., & Hewitt, R. G. (2005). Life stress and adherence to antiretroviral therapy among HIV-positive individuals: A preliminary investigation. *AIDS Patient Care and STDs, 19,* 719–727.

Bottos, S., & Dewey, D. (2004). Perfectionists' appraisal of daily hassles and chronic headache. *Headache, 44,* 772–779.

Botvin, G. J., & Griffin, K. W. (2015). Life Skills Training: A competence enhancement approach to tobacco, alcohol, and drug abuse prevention. In L. M. Scheier (Ed.), *Handbook of adolescent drug use prevention: Research, intervention strategies, and practice* (pp. 177–196). Washington, DC: American Psychological Association.

Boudreaux, E. D., & O'Hea, E. L. (2004). Patient satisfaction in the emergency department: A review of the literature and implications for practice. *The Journal of Emergency Medicine, 26,* 13–26.

Bowe, S., Adams, J., Lui, C.-W., & Sibbritt, D. (2015). A longitudinal analysis of self-prescribed complementary and alternative medicine use by a nationally representative sample of 19,783 Australian women, 2006-2010. *Complementary Therapies in Medicine, 23*(5), 699–704.

Bowers, S. L., Bilbo, S. D., Dhabhar, F. S., & Nelson, R. J. (2008). Stress-or-specific alterations in corticosterone and immune responses in mice. *Brain, Behavior, and Immunity, 22,* 105–113.

Boyd, D. B. (2007). Integrative oncology: The last ten years—A personal retrospective. *Alternative Therapies in Health and Medicine, 13,* 56–64.

Brace, M. J., Smith, M. S., McCauley, E., & Sherry, D. D. (2000). Family reinforcement of illness behavior: A comparison of adolescents with chronic fatigue syndrome, juvenile arthritis, and healthy controls. *Journal of Developmental and Behavioral Pediatrics, 21,* 332–339.

Bradford, D. E., Shaprio, B. L., & Curtin, J. H. (2013). How bad could it be? Alcohol dampens stress responses to threat of uncertain intensity. *Psychological Science, 24*(12), 2541–2549.

Bramlett, M. D., & Blumberg, S. J. (2008). Prevalence of children with special health care needs in metropolitan and micropolitan statistical areas in the United States. *Maternal and Child Health Journal, 12,* 488–498.

Bray, G. A. (2004). The epidemic of obesity and changes in food intake: The fluoride hypothesis. *Physiology and Behavior, 82,* 115–121.

Brecher, E. M. (1972). *Licit and illicit drugs.* Boston, MA: Little, Brown.

Breibart, W., & Payne, D. (2001). Psychiatric aspects of pain management in patients with advanced cancer. In H. Chochinov & W. Breibart (Eds.), *Handbook of psychiatry in palliative medicine* (pp. 131–199). New York, NY: Oxford University Press.

Brenner, D. R. (2014). Cancer incidence due to excess body weight and leisure-time physical inactivity in Canada: Implications for prevention, *Preventive Medicine, 66,* 131–139.

Breuer, B., Fleishman, S. B., Cruciani, R. A., & Portenoy, R. K. (2011). Medical oncologists' attitudes and practice in cancer pain management: A national survey. *Journal of Clinical Oncology, 29,* 4769–4775.

Breuer, J., & Freud, S. (1955). *Studies on hysteria.* In J. Strachey (Ed. and Trans.), *The standard edition of the complete psychological works of Sigmund Freud* (Vol. 2). London: Hogarth Press. (Original work published 1895)

Bricker, J. B., Petersen, A. V., Andersen, M. R., Rajan, K. B., Leroux, B. G., & Sarason, I. G. (2006). Childhood friends who smoke: Do they influence adolescents to make smoking transitions? *Addictive Behaviors, 31,* 889–900.

Brinn, M. P., Carson, K. V., Esterman, A. J., Chang, A. B., & Smith, B. J. (2010). Mass media interventions for preventing smoking in your people. *Cochrane Database of Systematic Reviews,* Cochrane Art No.: CD001006.

Briones, T. L. (2007). Psychoneuroimmunology and related mechanisms in understanding health disparities in vulnerable populations. *Annual Review of Nursing Research, 25,* 219–256.

Brissette, I., Scheier, M. F., & Carver, C. S. (2002). The role of optimism in social network development, coping, and psychological adjustment during a life transition. *Journal of Personality and Social Psychology, 82*(1), 102–111.

Broadbent, E., Kahokeher, A., Booth, R. J., Thomas, J., Windsor, J. A., Buchanan, C. M., … Hill, A. G. (2012). A brief relaxation intervention reduces stress and improves surgical wound healing response: A randomized trial. *Brain, Behavior, and Immunity, 26,* 212–217.

Brody, M. L., Masheb, R. M., & Grilo, C. M. (2005). Treatment preferences of patients with binge eating disorder. *International Journal of Eating Disorders, 37,* 352–356.

Brondel, L., Van Wymelbeke, V., Pineau, N., Jiang, T., Hanus, C., & Rigaud, D. (2009). Variety enhances food intake in humans: Role of sensory-specific satiety. *Physiology & Behavior, 97*(1), 44–51.

Broocks, A., Meyer, T., Opitz, M., Bartmann, U., Hillmer-Vogel, U., George, A., … Bandelow, B. (2003). 5-HT-1A responsivity in patients with panic disorder before and after treatment with aerobic exercise, clomipramine or placebo. *European Neuropsychopharmacology, 13,* 153–164.

Brooks, V. L., Haywood, J. R., & Johnson, A. K. (2005). Translation of salt retention to central activation of the sympathetic nervous system in hypertension. *Clinical and Experimental Pharmacology and Physiology, 32,* 426–432.

Brow, J. (2015, Nov. 17). Charlie Sheen insists he's not doing drugs but is he still drinking? *Hollywood Life.* Retrieved July 3, 2016, from http://hollywoodlife.com/2015/11/17/charlie-sheen-drugs-use-stopped-drinking-hiv-clean/

Brown, A. D., McMorris, C. A., Longman, R. S., Leigh, R., Hill, M. D., Friedenreich, C. M., … Pouolin, M. J. (2010). Effects of cardiorespiratory fitness and cerebral blood flow on cognitive outcomes in older women. *Neurobiology of Aging, 31,* 2047–2057.

Brown, B. (1970). Recognition of aspects of consciousness through association with EEG alpha activity represented by a light signal. *Psycho-physics, 6,* 442–446.

Brown, D. (2011, March 2). In Charlie Sheen rants, mental-health and drug experts see lessons for others. *The Denver Post.* Retrieved June 19, 2011, from http://www.denverpost.com/recommended/ci_17515950

Brown, D. R., Hernández, A., Saint-Jean, G., Evans, S., Tafari, I., Brewster, L. G., … Page, J. B. (2008). A participatory action research pilot study on urban health disparities using rapid assessment response and evaluation. *American Journal of Public Health, 98,* 28–38.

Brown, F. L., & Slaughter, V. (2011). Normal body, beautiful body: Discrepant perceptions reveal a pervasive 'thin ideal' from childhood to adulthood. *Body Image, 8*(2), 119–125.

Brown, I., Sheeran, P., & Reuber, M. (2009). Enhancing antiepileptic drug adherence: A randomized controlled trial. *Epilepsy & Behavior, 16,* 634–639.

Brownell, K. D., & Horgen, K. B. (2004). *Food fight: The inside story of the food industry, America's obesity crisis, and what we can do about it.* New York, NY: McGraw-Hill.

Bruch, H. (1973). *Eating disorders. Obesity, anorexia nervosa and the person within.* New York, NY: Basic Books.

Bruch, H. (1978). *The golden cage: The enigma of anorexia nervosa.* Cambridge, MA: Harvard University Press.

Bruch, H. (1982). Anorexia nervosa: Therapy and theory. *American Journal of Psychiatry, 139,* 1531–1538.

Brugts, J. J., Yetgin, T., Hoeks, S. E., Gotto, A. M., Shepherd, J., Westendorp, R. G. J., … Deckers, J. W. (2009). The benefits of statins in people without established cardiovascular disease but with cardiovascular risk factors: Meta-analysis of randomized controlled trials. *British Medical Journal, 338,* 2376.

Brumback, T., Cao, D., & King, A. (2007). Effects of alcohol on psychomotor performance and perceived impairment in heavy binge social drinkers. *Drug and Alcohol Dependence, 91,* 10–17.

Brummett, B. H., Barefoot, J. C., Siegler, I. C., Clapp-Channing, N. E., Lytle, B. L., Bosworth, H. B., … Mark, D. B. (2001). Characteristics of socially isolated patients with coronary artery disease who are at elevated risk for mortality. *Psychosomatic Medicine, 63,* 267–272.

Bruns, D. (1998). Psychologists as primary care providers: A paradigm shift. *Health Psychologist, 20*(4), 19.

Bryan, A., Fisher, J. D., & Fisher, W. A. (2002). Tests of the mediational role of preparatory safer sexual behavior in the context of the theory of planned behavior. *Health Psychology, 21,* 71–80.

Buchert, R., Thomasius, R., Wilke, F., Petersen, K., Nebeling, B., Obrocki, J., … Clausen, M. (2004). A voxel-based PET investigation of the long-term effects of "Ecstasy" consumption on brain serotonin transporters. *American Journal of Psychiatry, 161*(7), 1181–1189.

Buchwald, H., Estok, R., Fahrbach, K., Banel, D., Jensen, M. D., Pories, W. J., … Sledge, I. (2009). Weight and Type 2 diabetes after bariatric surgery: Systematic review and meta-analysis. *The American Journal of Medicine, 122,* 248–256.

Buffington, A. L. H., Hanlon, C. A., & McKeown, M. J. (2005). Acute and persistent pain modulation of attention-related anterior cingulate fMRI activations. *Pain, 113,* 172–184.

Burckhardt, C. S., & Jones, K. D. (2003a). Adult measures of pain: Short-Form McGill Pain Questionnaire (SF-MPQ). *Arthritis & Rheumatism: Arthritis Care & Research, 49*(S5), S98–S99.

Burckhardt, C. S., & Jones, K. D. (2003b). Adult measures of pain: Short-Visual Analog Scale (VAS). *Arthritis & Rheumatism: Arthritis Care & Research, 49*(S5), S100–S101.

Burgess, D. J., Ding, Y., Hargreaves, M., van Ryn, M., & Phelan, S. (2008). The association between perceived discrimination and underutilization of needed medical and mental health care in a multi-ethnic community sample. *Journal of Health Care for the Poor and Underserved, 19,* 1049–1089.

Burke, A., Nahin, R. L., & Stussman, B. J. (2015). Limited health knowledge as a reason for non-use of four common complementary health practices. *PLoS One, 10*(6), 1–18.

Burke, A., & Upchurch, D. M. (2006). Patterns of acupuncture use: Highlights from the National Health Interview Survey. *American Acupuncturist, 37,* 30–31.

Burke, A., Upchurch, D. M., Dye, C., & Chyu, L. (2006). Acupuncture use in the United States: Findings from the National Health Interview Survey. *Journal of Alternative and Complementary Medicine, 12,* 639–648.

Burke, J. D., Lofgren, I. E., Morrell, J. S., & Reilly, R. A. (2007). Health indicators, body mass index and food selection practices in college age students. *FASEB Journal, 21,* A1063.

Burschka, J. M., Keune, P. M., Oy, U. H, Oschmann, P., & Kuhn, P. (2014). Mindfulness-based interventions in multiple sclerosis: Beneficial effects of tai chi on balance, coordination, fatigue and depression. *BMC Neurology, 14,* 165.

Bussey-Smith, K. L., & Rossen, R. D. (2007). A systematic review of randomized control trials evaluating the effectiveness of interactive computerized asthma patient education programs. *Annals of Allergy, Asthma and Immunology, 98,* 507–516.

Bustamante, M. X., Zhang, G., O'Connell, E., Rodriguez, D., & Borroto-Ponce, R. (2007). Motor vehicle crashes and injury among high school and college aged drivers. Miami–Dade County, FL 20005. *Annals of Epidemiology, 17,* 742.

Cahill, K., Stevens, S., Perera, R., & Lancaster, T. (2013). Pharmacological interventions for smoking cessation: An overview and network meta-analysis. *Cochrane Database of Systematic Reviews,* Cochrane Art. No. CD009329. DOI: 10.1002/14651858.CD009329.pub2.

Cahill, S. P., & Foa, E. B. (2007). PTSD: Treatment efficacy and future directions. *Psychiatric Times, 24,* 32–34.

Cale, L., & Harris, J. (2006). Interventions to promote young people's physical activity: Issues, implications and recommendations for practice. *Health Education Journal, 65,* 320–337.

Calhoun, J. B. (1956). A comparative study of the social behavior of two inbred strains of house mice. *Ecological Monogram, 26,* 81.

Calhoun, J. B. (1962, February). Population density and social pathology. *Scientific American, 206,* 139–148.

Calipel, S., Lucaspolomeni, M.-M., Wodey, E., & Ecoffey, C. (2005). Pre-medication in children: Hypnosis versus midazolam. *Pediatric Anesthesia, 15,* 275–281.

Callaway, E. (2011, September 16). Clues emerge to explain first successful HIV vaccine trial. *Nature.* DOI: 10.1038/news.2011.541.

Callister, L. C. (2003). Cultural influences on pain perceptions and behavior. *Home Health Care Management and Practice, 15,* 207–211.

Camacho, T. C., & Wiley, J. A. (1983). Health practices, social networks, and change in physical health. In L. F. Berkman & L. Breslow (Eds.), *Health and ways of living: The Alameda County Study* (pp. 176–209). New York, NY: Oxford University Press.

Camelley, K. B., Wortman, C. B., Bolger, N., & Burke, C. T. (2006). The time course of brief reactions to spousal loss: Evidence from a national probability sample. *Journal of Personality and Social Psychology, 91,* 476–492.

Cameron, L. D., Booth, R. J., Schlatter, M., Ziginskas, D., & Harman, J. E. (2007). Changes in emotion regulation and psychological adjustment following use of a group psychosocial support program for women recently diagnosed with breast cancer. *Psycho-Oncology, 16,* 171–180.

Cameron, L. D., Leventhal, E. A., & Leventhal, H. (1995). Seeking medical care in response to symptoms and life stress. *Psychosomatic Medicine, 57,* 37–47.

Cameron, L. D., Petrie, K. J., Ellis, C., Buick, D., & Weinman, J. A. (2005). Symptom experiences, symptom attributions, and causal attributions in patients following first-time myocardial infarction. *International Journal of Behavioral Medicine, 12,* 30–38.

Camhi, J. (2012). Health problems plague city cab drivers. *Gotham Gazette.* Retrieved July 29, 2016, from http://www.gothamgazette.com/index.php/city/1149-health-problems-plague-city-cab-drivers

Camí, J., & Farré, M. (2003). Drug addiction. *New England Journal of Medicine, 349,* 975–986.

Campbell, J. M., & Oei, T. P. (2010). A cognitive model for the intergenerational transference of alcohol use behavior. *Addictive Behaviors, 35*(2), 73–83.

Cancian, F. M., & Oliker, S. J. (2000). *Caring and gender.* Thousand Oaks, CA: Pine Forge Press.

Cannon, W. (1932). *The wisdom of the body.* New York, NY: Norton.

Cao, L., Tan, L., Wang, H.-F., Jiang, T., Zhu, X.-C., Lu, H., ... Yu, J.-T. (2015, Nov. 9). Dietary patterns and risk of dementia: A systematic review and meta-analysis of cohort studies. *Molecular Neurobiology.* DOI: 10.1007/s12035-015-9516-4.

Cao, S., Yang, C., Gan, Y., & Lu, Z. (2015). The health effects of passive smoking: An overview of systematic reviews based on observational epidemiological evidence. *PLoS One, 10*(10), 1–12.

Cardi, V., & Treasure, J. (2010). Treatments in eating disorders: Towards future directions. *Minerva Psichiatrica, 51*(3), 191–206.

Carlson, L. E., Speca, M., Faris, P., & Patel, K. D. (2007). One year prepost intervention follow-up of psychological, immune, endocrine and blood pressure outcomes of mindfulness-based stress reduction (MBSR) in breast and prostate cancer outpatients. *Brain, Behavior, and Immunity, 21*(8), 1038–1049.

Carmen, B., Angeles, M., Ana, M., & Maria, A. J. (2004). Efficacy and safety of naltrexone and acamprosate in the treatment of alcohol dependence: A systematic review. *Addiction, 99*(7), 811–829.

Carmody, J., & Baer, R. A. (2008). Relationships between mindfulness practice and level of mindfulness, medical and psychological symptoms and well-being in a mindfulness-based stress reduction program. *Journal of Behavioral Medicine, 31,* 23–33.

Carmody, J., & Baer, R. A. (2009). How long does a mindfulness-based stress reduction program need to be? A review of class contact hours and effect sizes for psychological distress. *Journal of Clinical Psychology, 65*(6), 627–638.

Carpenter, C. J. (2010). A meta-analysis of the effectiveness of health belief model variables in predicting behavior. *Health Communication, 25,* 661–669.

Carr, D. (2003). A "good death" for whom? Quality of spouse's death and psychological distress among older widowed persons. *Journal of Health and Social Behavior, 44,* 215–232.

Carr, J. L. (2007). Campus violence white paper. *Journal of American College Health, 55,* 304–319.

Carrillo, J. E., Carrillo, V. A., Perez, H. R., Salas-Lopez, D., Natale-Pereira, A., & Byron, A. T. (2011). Defining and targeting health care access barriers. *Journal of Health Care for the Poor and Underserved, 22,* 562–575.

Carter, C. J., Blackmore, E., Sutandar-Pinnock, K., & Woodside, D. B. (2004). Relapse in anorexia nervosa: A survival analysis. *Psychological Medicine, 34,* 671–679.

Carter-Harris, L., Hermann, C. P., Schreiber, J., Weaver, M. T., & Rawl, S. M. (2014, May). Lung Cancer Stigma Predicts Timing of Medical Help-Seeking Behavior. In *Oncology nursing forum* (Vol. 41, No. 3, p. E203). NIH Public Access.

Carver, C. S., Pozo, C., Harris, S. D., Noriega, V., Scheier, M. F., Robinson, D. S., ... Clark, K. (1993). How coping mediates the effect of optimism on distress: A study of women with early stage breast cancer. *Journal of Personality and Social Psychology, 65*(2), 375–390.

Carver, C. S., Smith, R. G., Antoni, M. H., Petronis, V. M., Weiss, S., & Derhagopian, R. P. (2005). Optimistic personality and psychosocial well-being during treatment predict psychosocial well-being among long-term survivors of breast cancer. *Health Psychology, 24,* 508–516.

Caspi, A., Harrington, H., Moffitt, T. E., Milne, B. J., & Poulton, R. (2006). Socially isolated children 20 years later. *Archives of Pediatric Adolescent Medicine, 160,* 805–811.

Caspi, A., Sugden, K., Moffitt, T. E., Taylor, A., Craig, I. W., Harrington, H., ... Poulton, R. (2003). Influence of life stress on depression: Moderation by a polymorphism in the 5-HTT gene. *Science, 301,* 386–389.

Cassidy, E. L., Atherton, R. J., Robertson, N., Walsh, D. A., & Gillett, R. (2012). Mindfulness, functioning and catastrophizing after multidisciplinary pain management for chronic low back pain. *Pain, 153*(3), 644–650.

Castellini, G., Lo Sauro, C., Mannucci, E., Ravaldi, C., Rotella, C. M., Faravelli, C., ... Ricca, V. (2011). Diagnostic crossover and outcome predictors in eating disorders to DSM-IV and DSM-V proposed criteria: 6-year follow-up study. *Psychosomatic Medicine, 73*(3), 270–279.

Castor, M. L., Smyser, M. S., Taualii, M. M., Park, A. N., Lawson, S. A., & Forquera, R. A. (2006). A nationwide population-based study identifying health disparities between American Indians/Alaska Natives and the general populations living in select urban counties. *American Journal of Public Health, 96*, 1478–1484.

Castro, C. M., Wilson, C., Wang, F., & Schillinger, D. (2007). Babel babble: Physicians' use of unclarified medical jargon with patients. *American Journal of Health Behavior, 31*, S85–S95.

Celebrity Central: Lindsay Lohan. (2011). *People.* Retrieved November 17, 2011, from http://www.people.com/people/lindsay_lohan

Celentano, D. D., Valleroy, L. A., Sifakis, F., MacKellar, D. A., Hylton, J., Thiede, H., … Torian, L. V. (2006). Associations between substance use and sexual risk among very young men who have sex with men. *Sexually Transmitted Diseases, 33*, 265–271.

Center on Addiction and Substance Abuse at Columbia (CASA). (2012). *Addiction medicine: Closing the gap between science and practice.* New York, NY: National Center on Addiction and Substance Abuse at Columbia University.

Centers for Disease Control and Prevention (CDC). (1992). 1993 revised classification system for HIV infection and expanded surveillance case definition for AIDS among adolescents and adults. *Morbidity and Mortality Weekly Report, 41*, No. RR-17.

Centers for Disease Control and Prevention (CDC). (1994). Reasons for tobacco use and symptoms of nicotine withdrawal among adolescent and young adult tobacco users—United States, 1993. *Morbidity and Mortality Weekly Report, 43*, 745–750.

Centers for Disease Control and Prevention (CDC). (2008). *HIV/AIDS surveillance report, 2006* (Vol. 18). Atlanta, GA: U.S. Department of Health and Human Services, Centers for Disease Control and Prevention. Retrieved August 3, 2008, from http://www.cdc.gov/hiv/topics/surveillance/resources/reports/

Centers for Disease Control and Prevention (CDC). (2009). *Chronic diseases—The power to prevent, the call to control: At a glance, 2009.* Atlanta, GA: U.S. Department of Health and Human Services, Centers for Disease Control and Prevention. Retrieved March 20, 2012, from http://www.cdc.gov/chronicdisease/resources/publications/aag/ pdf/chronic.pdf

Centers for Disease Control and Prevention (CDC). (2010a). *HIV among gay, bisexual and other men who have sex with men (MSM).* Atlanta, GA: U.S. Department of Health and Human Services, Centers for Disease Control and Prevention. Retrieved March 20, 2012, from http://www.cdc.gov/hiv/topics/msm/pdf/msm.pdf

Centers for Disease Control and Prevention (CDC). (2010b). Vital signs: Current cigarette smoking among adults ≥18 years—United States, 2009. *Morbidity and Mortality Weekly Report, 59*(35), 1135–1140.

Centers for Disease Control and Prevention (CDC) and NCHS. (2010c). *Health, United States, 2010. Chartbook, special feature on death and dying.* Hyattsville, MD: Author.

Centers for Disease Control and Prevention (CDC). (2011a). *National diabetes fact sheet, 2011.* Atlanta, GA: U.S. Department of Health and Human Services, Centers for Disease Control and Prevention. Retrieved March 20, 2012, from http://www.cdc.gov/diabetes/pubs/pdf/ndfs_2011.pdf

Centers for Disease Control and Prevention (CDC). (2011b). *Safe on the outs.* Retrieved April 18, 2012, from http://www.cdc.gov/hiv/topics/research/prs/resources/factsheets/safe-on-the-outs.htm

Centers for Disease Control and Prevention (CDC). (2013). Vital signs: Current cigarette smoking among adults aged ≥18 years with mental illness—United States, 2009-2011. *Morbidity and Mortality Weekly Reports, 62*(5), 81–87.

Centers for Disease Control and Prevention (CDC). (2014a). Opioid painkiller prescribing. Retrieved July 17, 2015, from http://www.cdc.gov/vitalsigns/opioid-prescribing/

Centers for Disease Control and Prevention (CDC). (2014b). *National Diabetes Statistics Report, 2014.* Retrieved August 16, 2016, from http://www.cdc.gov/diabetes/pubs/statsreport14/national-diabetes-report-web.pdf

Centers for Disease Control and Prevention (CDC). (2014c). *Best practices for tobacco control programs—2014.* Atlanta, GA: Author.

Centers for Disease Control and Prevention (CDC). (2016). *HIV among African Americans.* Retrieved August 16, 2016, from http://www.cdc.gov/hiv/group/racialethnic/africanamericans/index.html

Centers for Disease Control and Prevention (CDC). (2016a). *Wide-ranging online data for epidemiologic research (WONDER).* Atlanta, GA: CDC, National Center for Health Statistics. Retrieved from http://wonder.cdc.gov

Centers for Disease Control and Prevention (CDC). (2016b). *HIV among youth.* Retrieved March 20, 2012, from http://www.cdc.gov/hiv/youth/pdf/youth.pdf

Centola, D. (2011). An experimental study of homophily in the adoption of health behavior. *Science, 334*(6060), 1269–1272.

Centola, D., & van de Rijt, A. (2015). Choosing your network: Social preferences in an online health community. *Social Science and Medicine, 125*, 19–31.

Central Intelligence Agency (CIA). (2016). *World factbook, 2016-2017.* Washington, DC: Author.

Cepeda, M. S., Berlin, J. A., Gao, Y., Wiegand, F., & Wada, D. R. (2012). Placebo response changes depending on the neuropathic pain syndrome: Results of a systematic review and meta-analysis. *Pain Medicine, 13*, 575–595.

Ceylan-Isik, A. F., McBride, S. M., & Ren, J. (2010). Sex difference in alcoholism: Who is at a greater risk for development of alcoholic complication? *Life Sciences, 87*(5/6), 133–138.

Cha, E. S., Doswell, W. M., Kim, K. H., Charron-Prochownik, D., & Patrick, T. E. (2007). Evaluating the Theory of Planned Behavior to explain intention to engage in premarital sex amongst Korean college students: A questionnaire survey. *International Journal of Nursing Studies, 44*, 1147–1157.

Chaddock, L., Erickson, K. I., Prakash, R. S., Kim, J. S., Voss, M. W., VanPatter, M., … Kramer, A. F. (2010). A neuroimaging investigation of the association between aerobic fitness, hippocampal volume, and memory performance in preadolescent children. *Brain Research, 1358*, 172–183.

Chakrabarty, S., & Zoorob, R. (2007). Fibromyalgia. *American Family Physician, 76*, 247–254.

Chandrashekara, S., Jayashree, K., Veeranna, H. B., Vadiraj, H. S., Ramesh, M. N., Shobha, A., … Vikram, Y. K. (2007). Effects of anxiety on TNF-a levels during psychological stress. *Journal of Psychosomatic Research, 63*, 65–69.

Chang, A. Y., & Barry. M. (2015). The global health implications of e-cigarettes. *Journal of the American Medical Association, 314*(7), 663–664.

Chang, E. C., Sanna, L. J., Hirsch, J. K., & Jeglic, E. L. (2010). Loneliness and negative life events as predictors of hopelessness and suicidal behaviors in Hispanics: Evidence for a diathesis-stress model. *Journal of Clinical Psychology, 66*(12), 1242–1253.

Chang, L., Ernst, T., Speck, O., Patel, H., DeSilva, M., Leonido-Yee, M., … Miller, E. N. (2002). Perfusion MRI and computerized cognitive test abnormalities in abstinent methamphetamine users. *Psychiatry Research: Neuroimaging Section, 114*, 65–79.

Chang, S. H., Stoll, C. R., Song, J., Varela, J. E., Eagon, C. J., & Colditz, G. A. (2014). The effectiveness and risks of bariatric surgery: An updated systematic review and meta-analysis. *Journal of the American Medical Association Surgery, 149*(3), 275–287.

Chapman, C. R., Nakamura, Y., & Flores, L. Y. (1999). Chronic pain and consciousness: A constructivist perspective. In R. J. Gatchel & D. C. Turk (Eds.), *Psychosocial factors in pain: Critical perspectives* (pp. 35–55). New York, NY: Guilford Press.

Chapman, R. H., Petrilla, A. A., Benner, J. S., Schwartz, J. S., & Tang, S. S. K. (2008). Predictors of adherence to concomitant antihypertensive and lipid-lowering medications in older adults: A retrospective, cohort Study. *Drugs and Aging, 25*, 885–892.

Charlee, C., Goldsmith, L. J., Chambers, L., & Haynes, R. B. (1996). Provider-patient communication among elderly and nonelderly patients in Canadian hospitals: A national survey. *Health Communication, 8*, 281–302.

"Charlie Sheen." (2011, February 14). Charlie Sheen. *Famous and celebrity drug addicts.* Retrieved June 19, 2011, from http://www.famous celebritydrugaddicts.com/charlie-sheen.htm

Chassin, L., Presson, C. C., Rose, J., & Sherman, S. J. (2007). What is addiction? Age-related differences in the meaning of addiction. *Drug and Alcohol Dependence, 87,* 30–38.

Chaturvedi, A. K., Engels, E. A., Anderson, W. F., & Gillison, M. L. (2008). Incidence trends for human papillomavirus-related and -unrelated oral squamous cell carcinomas in the United States. *Journal of Clinical Oncology, 26,* 612–619.

Chaturvedi, A. K., Engels, E. A., Pfeiffer, R. M., Hernandez, B. Y., Xiao, W., Kim, E., … Gillison, M. L. (2011). Human papillomavirus and rising oropharyngeal cancer incidence in the United States. *Journal of Clinical Oncology, 29,* 4294–4301.

Chei, C. L., Iso, H., Yamagishi, K., Inoue, M., & Tsugane, S. (2008). Body mass index and weight change since 20 years of age and risk of coronary heart disease among Japanese: The Japan Public Health Center–Based Study. *International Journal of Obesity, 32,* 144–151.

Chen, E., Cohen, S., & Miller, G. E. (2010). How low socioeconomic status affects 2-year hormonal trajectories in children. *Psychological Science, 21*(1), 31–37.

Chen, E., & Miller, G. E. (2007). Stress and inflammation in exacerbations of asthma. *Brain, Behavior and Immunity, 21,* 993–999.

Chen, E., Strunk, R. C., Bacharier, L. B., Chan, M., & Miller, G. E. (2010). Socioeconomic status associated with exhaled nitric oxide responses to acute stress in children with asthma. *Brain, Behavior and Immunity, 24,* 444–450.

Chen, H. Y., Shi, Y., Ng, C. S., Chan, S. M., Yung, K. K., Lam, Z., … Zhang, Q. L. (2007). Auricular acupuncture treatment for insomnia: A systematic review. *Journal of Alternative and Complementary Medicine, 13,* 669–676.

Chen, J. Y., Fox, S. A., Cantrell, C. H., Stockdale, S. E., & Kagawa-Singer, M. (2007). Health disparities and prevention: Racial/ethnic barriers to flu vaccinations. *Journal of Community Health, 32,* 5–20.

Cheng, B. M. T., Lauder, I. J., Chu-Pak, L., & Kumana, C. R. (2004). Meta-analysis of large randomized controlled trials to evaluate the impact of statins on cardiovascular outcomes. *British Journal of Clinical Pharmacology, 57,* 640–651.

Cheng, T. Y. L., & Boey, K. W. (2002). The effectiveness of a cardiac rehabilitation program on self-efficacy and exercise. *Clinical Nursing Research, 11,* 10–19.

Cherkin, D. C., Sherman, K. J., Kahn, J., Wellman, R., Cook, A. J., Johnson, E., … Deyo, R. A. (2011). A comparison of the effects of 2 types of massage and usual care on chronic low-back pain: A randomized, controlled trial. *Annals of Internal Medicine, 155*(1), 1–9.

Cherkin, D. C., Sherman, K. J., Balderson, B. H., Cook, A. J., Anderson, M. L., Hawkes, R. J., Hansen, K. E., & Turner, J. A. (2016). Effect of mindfulness-based stress reduction vs cognitive behavioral therapy or usual care on back pain and functional limitations in adults with chronic low back pain: A randomized clinical trial. *JAMA, 315*(12), 1240–1249.

Chia, L. R., Schlenk, E. A., & Dunbar-Jacob, J. (2006). Effect of personal and cultural beliefs on medication adherence in the elderly. *Drugs and Aging, 23,* 191–202.

Chiaramonte, G. R., & Friend, R. (2006). Medical students' and residents' gender bias in the diagnosis, treatment, and interpretation of coronary heart disease symptoms. *Health Psychology, 25*(3), 255.

Chida, T., Hamer, M., & Steptoe, A. (2008). A bidirectional relationship between psychosocial factors and atopic disorders: A systematic review and meta-analysis. *Psychosomatic Medicine, 70,* 102–116.

Chida, Y., & Hamer, M. (2008). An association of adverse psychosocial factors with diabetes mellitus: A meta-analytic review of longitudinal cohort studies. *Diabetologia, 51,* 2168–2178.

Chida, Y., Hamer, M., Wardle, J., & Steptoe, A. (2008). Do stress-related psychosocial factors contribute to cancer incidence and survival? *Nature Reviews Clinical Oncology, 5*(8), 466–475.

Chida, Y., & Mao, X. (2009). Does psychosocial stress predict symptomatic herpes simplex virus recurrence? A meta-analytic investigation on prospective studies. *Brain, Behavior, and Immunity, 23,* 917–925.

Chida, Y., & Steptoe, A. (2008). Positive psychological well-being and mortality: A quantitative review of prospective observational studies. *Psychosomatic Medicine, 70,* 741–756.

Chida, Y., & Steptoe, A. (2009). The association of anger and hostility with future coronary heart disease: A meta-analytic review of prospective evidence. *Journal of the American College of Cardiology, 53,* 936–946.

Chida, Y., & Vedhara, K. (2009). Adverse psychological factors predict poorer prognosis in HIV disease: A meta-analytic review of prospective investigations. *Brain, Behavior, and Immunity, 23,* 434–445.

Chiesa, A., & Serretti, A. (2010). A systematic review of neurobiological and clinical features of mindfulness meditations. *Psychological Medicine, 40*(8), 1239–1252.

Chikritzhs, T., Stockwell, T., Naimi, T., Andreasson, S., Dangardt, F., & Liang, W. (2015). Has the leaning tower of presumed health benefits from 'moderate' alcohol use finally collapsed? *Addiction, 110*(5), 726–727.

Chithiramohan, A., & George, S. (2015). Pharmacological interventions for alcohol relapse prevention. *Internet Journal of Medical Update, 10*(2), 41–45.

Chochinov, H. M., Kristjanson, L. J., Breitbart, W., McClement, S., Hack, T. F., Hassard, T., … Harlos, M. (2011). Effect of dignity therapy on distress and end-of-life experience in terminally ill patients: A randomised controlled trial. *The Lancet Oncology, 12*(8), 753–762.

Cholesterol Treatment Trialists' (CTT) Collaboration, Baigent, C., Blackwell, L., Emberson, J., Holland, L. E., Reith, C., … Collins, R. (2010). Efficacy and safety of more intensive lowering of LDL cholesterol: A meta-analysis of data from 170,000 participants in 26 randomised trials. *The Lancet, 376,* 1670–1681.

Chong, C. S., Tsunaka, M., Tsang, H. W., Chan, E. P., & Cheung, W. M. (2011). Effects of yoga on stress management in healthy adults: A systematic review. *Alternative Therapies in Health and Medicine, 17*(1), 32–38.

Chou, F., Holzemer, W. L., Portillo, C. J., & Slaughter, R. (2004). Self-care strategies and sources of information for HIV/AIDS symptom management. *Nursing Research, 53,* 332–339.

Chou, R., Qaseem, A., Snow, V., Casey, D., Cross, J. T., Jr., Shekelle, P., … American Pain Society Low Back Pain Guidelines Panel. (2007). Diagnosis and treatment of low back pain: A joint clinical practice guideline from the American College of Physicians and the American Pain Society. *Annals of Internal Medicine, 147,* 478–491, W118–W120.

Chow, C. K., Islam, S., Bautista, L., Rumboldt, Z., Yusufali, A., Xie, C., … Yusuf, S. (2011). Parental history and myocardial infarction risk across the world. *Journal of the American College of Cardiology, 57,* 619–627.

Chow, G., Liou, K. T., & Heffron, R. C. (2016). Making whole: Applying the principles of integrative medicine to medical education. *Rhode Island Medical Journal, 99*(3), 16–19.

Christakis, N. A., & Fowler, J. H. (2007). The spread of obesity in a large social network over 32 years. *New England Journal of Medicine, 357*(4), 370–379.

Christakis, N. A., & Fowler, J. H. (2008). The collective dynamics of smoking in a large social network. *New England Journal of Medicine, 358*(21), 2249–2258.

Christenfeld, N., Glynn, L. M., Phillips, D. P., & Shrira, I. (1999). Exposure to New York City as a risk factor for heart attack mortality. *Psychosomatic Medicine, 61,* 740–743.

Chung, M. L., Moser, D. K., Lennie, T. A., Worrall-Carter, L., Bentley, B., Trupp, R., …Amentano, D. S. (2006). Gender differences in adherence to the sodium-restricted diet in patients with heart failure. *Journal of Cardiac Failure, 12,* 628–634.

Cibulka, N. J. (2006). HIV infection. *American Journal of Nursing, 106,* 59.

Ciesla, J. A., & Roberts, J. E. (2007). Rumination, negative cognition, and their interactive effects on depressed mood. *Emotion, 7,* 555–565.

Cintron, A., & Morrison, R. S. (2006). Pain and ethnicity in the United States: A systematic review. *Journal of Palliative Medicine, 9,* 1454–1473.

Clark, A. D. (2008). The new frontier of wellness. *Benefits Quarterly, 24,* 23–28.

Clark, A. M., Whelan, H. K., Barbour, R., & MacIntyre, P. D. (2005). A realist study of the mechanisms of cardiac rehabilitation. *Journal of Advanced Nursing*, 52, 362–371.

Clark, L., Jones, K., & Pennington, K. (2004). Pain assessment practices with nursing home residents. *Western Journal of Nursing Research*, 26, 733–750.

Clark, M. M., Decker, P. A., Offord, K. P., Patten, C. A., Vickers, K. S., Croghan, I. T., … Dale, L. C. (2004). Weight concerns among male smokers. *Addictive Behaviors*, 29, 1637–1641.

Clark, P. A. (2006). The need for new guidelines for AIDS testing and counseling: An ethical analysis. *Internet Journal of Infectious Diseases*, 5(2), 8.

Clark, R. (2003). Self-reported racism and social support predict blood pressure reactivity in Blacks. *Annals of Behavioral Medicine*, 25, 127–136.

Clarke, T. C., Black, L. I., Stussman, B. J., Barnes, P. M., & Nahin, R. L. (2015). Trends in the use of complementary health approaches among adults: United States, 2002-2012. *National Health Statistics Reports*, 79, 1–9.

Clark-Grill, M. (2007). Questionable gate-keeping: Scientific evidence for complementary and alternative medicines (CAM): Response to Malcolm Parker. *Journal of Bioethical Inquiry*, 4, 21–28.

Claxton, A. J., Cramer, J., & Pierce, C. (2001). A systematic review of the association between dose regimens and medication compliance. *Clinical Therapeutics*, 23, 1296–1310.

Claydon, L. S., Chesterton, L. S., Barlas, P., & Sim, J. (2011). Dose-specific effects of transcutaneous electrical nerve stimulation (TENS) on experimental pain: A systematic review. *Clinical Journal of Pain*, 27, 635–647.

Cleary, M. (2007). Predisposing risk factors on susceptibility to exertional heat illness: Clinical decision-making considerations. *Journal of Sport Rehabilitation*, 16, 204–214.

Cleland, J. A., Palmer, J. A., & Venzke, J.W. (2005). Ethnic differences in pain perception. *Physical Therapy Reviews*, 10, 113–122.

Clements, K., & Turpin, G. (1996). The life events scale for students: Validation for use with British samples. *Personality and Individual Differences*, 20(6), 747–751.

Clever, S. L., Jin, L., Levinson, W., & Meltzer, D. O. (2008). Does doctor-patient communication affect patient satisfaction with hospital care? Results of an analysis with a novel instrumental variable. *Health Services Research*, 43, 1505–1519.

Clinton, W. J. (2005, September 25). I was a heart attack waiting to happen. *Parade Magazine*, 4–5.

Coe, C. L., & Laudenslager, M. L. (2007). Psychosocial influences on immunity, including effects on immune maturation and senescence. *Brain, Behavior and Immunity*, 21, 1000–1008.

Coffman, J. M., Cabana, M. D., Halpin, H. A., & Yelin, E. H. (2008). Effects of asthma education on children's use of acute care services: A meta-analysis. *Pediatrics*, 121, 575–586.

Cohen, S. (2005). Keynote presentation at the eighth International Congress of Behavioral Medicine. *International Journal of Behavioral Medicine*, 12(3), 123–131.

Cohen, S., Alper, C. M., Doyle, W. J., Treanor, J. J., & Turner, R. B. (2006). Positive emotional style predicts resistance to illness after experimental exposure to rhinovirus or influenza A virus. *Psychosomatic Medicine*, 68, 809–815.

Cohen, S., Doyle, W. J., Alper, C. M., Janicki-Deverts, D., & Turner, R. B. (2009). Sleep habits and susceptibility to the common cold. *Archives of Internal Medicine*, 169, 62–67.

Cohen, S., Doyle, W. J., Skoner, D. P., Rabin, B. S., & Gwaltney, J. M., Jr. (1997). Social ties and susceptibility to the common cold. *Journal of the American Medical Association*, 277, 1940–1944.

Cohen, S., Doyle, W. J., Turner, R., Alper, C. M., & Skoner, D. P. (2003). Sociability and susceptibility to the common cold. *Psychological Science*, 14, 389–395.

Cohen, S., Frank, E., Doyle, W. J., Skoner, D. P., Rabin, B. S., & Gwaltney, J. M., Jr. (1998). Types of stressors that increase susceptibility to the common cold in healthy adults. *Health Psychology*, 17, 214–223.

Cohen, S., Janicki-Deverts, D., Turner, R. B., Casselbrant, M. L., Li-Korotky, H. S., Epel, E. S., … Doyle, W. J. (2013a). Association between telomere length and experimentally induced upper respiratory viral infection in healthy adults. *JAMA*, 309(7), 699–705.

Cohen, S., Janicki-Deverts, D., Turner, R. B., Marsland, A. L., Casselbrant, M. L., Li-Korotky, H. S., Epel, E. S., … Doyle, W. J. (2013b). Childhood socioeconomic status, telomere length, and susceptibility to upper respiratory infection. *Brain, Behavior, and Immunity*, 34, 31–38.

Cohen, S., Kamarck, T., & Mermelstein, R. (1983). A global measure of perceived stress. *Journal of Health and Social Behavior*, 24, 385–396.

Cohen, S., Tyrrell, D. A. J., & Smith, A. P. (1991). Psychological stress and susceptibility to the common cold. *New England Journal of Medicine*, 325, 606–612.

Cohen, S., Tyrrell, D. A. J., & Smith, A. P. (1993). Negative life events, perceived stress, negative affect, and susceptibility to the common cold. *Journal of Personality and Social Psychology*, 64, 131–140.

Cohn, L., Elias, J. A., & Chupp, G. L. (2004). Asthma: Mechanisms of disease persistence and progression. *Annual Review of Immunology*, 22, 789–818.

Colcombe, S. J., Erickson, K. I., Scalf, P. E., Kim, J. S., Prakash, R., McAuley, E., …Kramer, A. F. (2006). Aerobic exercise training increases brain volume in aging humans. *The Journals of Gerontology: Series A*, 61, 1166–1170.

Colditz, G. A., Willett, W. C., Hunter, D. J., Stampfer, M. J., Manson, J. E., Hennekens, C. H., … Rosner, B. A. (1993). Family history, age, and risk of breast cancer. *Journal of the American Medical Association*, 270, 338–343.

Cole, J. C. (2014). MSMA and the "ecstacy paradigm." *Journal of Psychoactive Drugs*, 46(1), 44–56.

Cole, S. W., Naliboff, B. D., Kemeny, M. E., Griswold, M. P., Fahey, J. L., & Zack, J. A. (2001). Impaired response to HAART in HIV-infected individuals with high autonomic nervous system activity. *Proceedings of the National Academy of Sciences of the United States of America*, 98, 12695–12700.

Coles, S. L., Dixon, J. B., & O'Brien, P. E. (2007). Night eating syndrome and nocturnal snacking: Association with obesity, binge eating and psychological distress. *International Journal of Obesity*, 31, 1722–1730.

Colilla, S. A. (2010). An epidemiologic review of smokeless tobacco health effects and harm reduction potential. *Regulatory Toxicology and Pharmacology*, 56(2), 197–211.

Collins, M. A. (2008). Protective mechanisms against neuroinflammatory proteins induced by preconditioning braincultures with moderate ethanol concentrations. *Neurotoxicity Research*, 13, 130.

Collins, R. L., Orlando, M., & Klein, D. J. (2005). Isolating the nexus of substance use, violence and sexual risk for HIV infection among young adults in the United States. *AIDS and Behavior*, 9, 73–87.

Colloca, L., Lopiano, L., Lanotte, M., & Benedetti, F. (2004). Overt versus covert treatment for pain, anxiety, and Parkinson's disease. *The Lancet: Neurology*, 3, 679–684.

Committee on the Use of Complementary and Alternative Medicine by the American Public, Institute of Medicine. (2005). *Complementary and alternative medicine in the United States*. Washington, DC: National Academic Press.

Conger, J. (1956). Reinforcement theory and the dynamics of alcoholism. *Quarterly Journal of Studies on Alcohol*, 17, 296–305.

Conn, V. S., Hafdahl, A. R., LeMaster, J. W., Ruppar, T. M., Cochran, J. E., & Nielsen, P. J. (2008). Meta-analysis of health behavior change interventions in Type 1 diabetes. *American Journal of Health Behavior*, 32, 315–392.

Cook, A. J., Roberts, D. A., Henderson, M. D., Van Winkle, L. C., Chastain, D. C., & Hamill-Ruth, R. J. (2004). Electronic pain questionnaires: A randomized, crossover comparison with paper questionnaires for chronic pain assessment. *Pain*, 110, 310–317.

Cook, B. J., & Hausenblas, H. A. (2008). The role of exercise dependence for the relationship between exercise behavior and eating pathology: Mediator or moderator? *Journal of Health Psychology*, 13, 495–502.

Coon, D. W., & Evans, B. (2009). Empirically based treatments for family caregiver distress: What works and where do we go from here? *Geriatric Nursing*, 30, 426–436.

Cooney, G. M., Dwan, K., Greig, C. A., Lawlor, D. A., Rimer, J., Waugh, F. R., McMurdo, M., & Mead, G. E. (2013). Exercise for depression. *Cochrane Database of Systematic Reviews, 9,* CD004366.

Cooper, B. (2001, March). Long may you run. *Runner's World, 36*(3), 64–67.

Cooper, K. L., Harris, P. E., Relton, C., & Thomas, K. J. (2013). Prevalence of visits to five types of complementary and alternative medicine practitioners by the general population: A systematic review. *Complementary Therapies in Clinical Practice, 19*(4), 214–220.

Corasaniti, M. T., Amantea, D., Russo, R., & Bagetta, G. (2006). The crucial role of plasticity in pain and cell death. *Cell Death and Differentiation, 13,* 534–536.

Cornford, C. S., & Cornford, H. M. (1999). 'I'm only here because of my family': A study of lay referral networks. *The British Journal of General Practice, 49,* 617–620.

Costa, L. C. M., Maher, C. G., McAuley, J. H., & Costa, L. O. P. (2009). Systematic review of cross-cultural adaptations of McGill Pain Questionnaire reveals a paucity of clinimetric testing. *Journal of Clinical Epidemiology, 62,* 934–943.

Cottington, E. M., & House, J. S. (1987). Occupational stress and health: A multivariate relationship. In A. Baum & J. E. Singer (Eds.), *Handbook of psychology and health: Vol. 5. Stress* (pp. 41–62). Hillsdale, NJ: Erlbaum.

Couper, J. W. (2007). The effects of prostate cancer on intimate relationships. *Journal of Men's Health and Gender, 4,* 226–232.

Courtney, A. U., McCarter, D. F., & Pollart, S. M. (2005). Childhood asthma: Treatment update. *American Family Physician, 71,* 1959–1968.

Cousins, N. (1979). *Anatomy of an illness as perceived by the patient: Reflections on healing and regeneration.* New York, NY: Norton.

Coussons-Read, M. E., Okun, M. L., & Nettles, C. D. (2007). Psychosocial stress increases inflammatory markers and alters cytokine production across pregnancy. *Brain, Behavior and Immunity, 21,* 343–350.

Couturier, J., Kimber, M., & Szatmari, P. (2013). Efficacy of family-based treatment for adolescents with eating disorders: A systematic review and meta-analysis. *International Journal of Eating Disorders, 46*(1), 3–9.

Covington, E. C. (2000). The biological basis of pain. *International Review of Psychiatry, 12,* 128–147.

Coyne, J. C., Stefanek, M., & Palmer, S. C. (2007). Psychotherapy and survival in cancer: The conflict between hope and evidence. *Psychological Bulletin, 133,* 367–394.

Coyne, J. C., & Tennen, H. (2010). Positive psychology in cancer care: Bad science, exaggerated claims, and unproven medicine. *Annals of Behavioral Medicine, 39,* 16–26.

Craciun, C., Schüz, N., Lippke, S., & Schwarzer, R. (2012). Facilitating sunscreen use in women by a theory-based online intervention: A randomized controlled trial. *Journal of Health Psychology, 17,* 207.

Craig, A. D. (2003). Pain mechanisms: Labeled lines versus convergence in central processing. *Annual Review of Neuroscience, 26,* 1–30.

Cramer, H., Lauche, R., Paul, A., & Dobos, G. (2012). Mindfulness-based stress reduction for breast cancer—a systematic review and meta-analysis. *Current Oncology, 19*(5), 343–352.

Cramer, J. A. (2004). A systematic review of adherence with medications for diabetes. *Diabetes Care, 27,* 1218–1224.

Cramer, S., Mayer, J., & Ryan, S. (2007). College students use cell phones while driving more frequently than found in government study. *Journal of American College Health, 56,* 181–184.

Crandall, C. S., Preisler, J. J., & Aussprung, J. (1992). Measuring life event stress in the lives of college students: The Undergraduate Stress Questionnaire (USQ). *Journal of Behavioral Medicine, 15,* 627–662.

Crepaz, N., Passin, W. F., Herbst, J. H., Rama, S. M., Malow, R. M., Purcell, D. W., … HIV/AIDS Prevention Research Synthesis Team. (2008). Meta-analysis of cognitive-behavioral interventions on HIV-positive persons' mental health and immune functioning. *Health Psychology, 27,* 4–14.

Crimmins, E. M., Ki Kim, J., Alley, D. E., Karlamangla, A., & Seeman, T. (2007). Hispanic paradox in biological risk profiles. *American Journal of Public Health, 97,* 1305–1310.

Crimmins, E. M., & Saito, Y. (2001). Trends in healthy life expectancy in the United States, 1970–1990: Gender, racial, and educational differences. *Social Science and Medicine, 52,* 1629–1642.

Crisp, A., Gowers, S., Joughin, N., McClelland, L., Rooney, B., Nielsen, S., … Clifton, A. (2006). Anorexia nervosa in males: Similarities and differences to anorexia nervosa in females. *European Eating Disorders Review, 14*(3), 163–167.

Crispo, A., Brennan, P., Jockel, K.-H., Schaffrath-Rosario, A., Wichman, H.-E., Nyberg, F., … Darby, S. (2004). The cumulative risk of lung cancer among current, ex- and never-smokers in European men. *British Journal of Cancer, 91,* 1280–1286.

Critchley, J. A., & Capewell, S. (2003). Mortality risk reduction associated with smoking cessation in patients with coronary heart disease: A systematic review. *Journal of the American Medical Association, 290,* 86–97.

Croft, P., Blyth, F. M., & van der Windt, D. (2010). The global occurrence of chronic pain: An introduction. In P. Croft, F. M. Blyth, & D. van der Windt (Eds.), *Chronic pain epidemiology: From Aetiology to public health* (pp. 9–18). New York, NY: Oxford University Press.

Crowell, T. L., & Emmers-Sommer, T. M. (2001). "If I knew then what I know now": Seropositive individuals' perceptions of partner trust, safety and risk prior to HIV infection. *Communication Studies, 52,* 302–323.

Cruess, D. G., Petitto, J. M., Leserman, J., Douglas, S. D., Gettes, D. R., Ten Have, T. R., … Evans, D. L. (2003). Depression and HIV infection: Impact on immune function and disease progression. *CNS Spectrums, 8,* 52–58.

Cummings, D. E., & Schwartz, M. W. (2003). Genetics and pathophysiology of human obesity. *Annual Review of Medicine, 54,* 453–471.

Cunningham, J. A., Blomqvist, J., Koski-Jännes, A., & Cordingley, J. (2005). Maturing out of drinking problems: Perceptions of natural history as a function of severity. *Addiction Research and Theory, 13,* 79–84.

Cutrona, C. E., Russell, D. W., Brown, P. A., Clark, L. A., Hessling, R. M., & Gardner, K. A. (2005). Neighborhood context, personality, and stressful life events as predictors of depression among African American women. *Journal of Abnormal Psychology, 114,* 3–15.

Cutting Edge Information. (2004). *Pharmaceutical patient compliance and disease management.* Retrieved July 18, 2004, from http://www.pharmadiseasemanagement.com/metrics.htm

Czerniecki, J. M., & Ehde, D. M. (2003). Chronic pain after lower extremity amputation. *Critical Reviews in Physical and Rehabilitation Medicine, 15,* 309–332.

Dagenais, S., Caro, J., & Haldeman, S. (2008). A systematic review of low back pain cost of illness studies in the United States and internationally. *Spine Journal, 8,* 8–20.

Dalal, H. M., Zawada, A., Jolly, K., Moxham, T., & Taylor, R. S. (2010). Home based versus centre based cardiac rehabilitation: Cochrane systematic review and meta-analysis. *British Medical Journal, 340,* b5631.

Daley, A. (2008). Exercise and depression: A review of reviews. *Journal of Clinical Psychology in Medical Settings, 15,* 140–147.

Damiano, S. R., Paxton, S. J., Wertheim, E. H., McLean, S. A., & Gregg, K. J. (2015). Dietary restraint of 5-year-old girls: Associations with internalization of the thin ideal and maternal, media, and peer influences. *International Journal of Eating Disorders, 48*(8), 1166–1169.

D'Amico, D., Grazzi, L., Usai, S., Raggi, A., Leonardi, M., & Bussone, G. (2011). Disability in chronic daily headache: State of the art and future directions. *Neurological Sciences, 32,* 71–76.

Damjanovic, A. K., Yang, Y., Glaser, R., Kiecolt-Glaser, J. K., Huy, N., Laskowski, B., … Weng, N. P. (2007). Accelerated telomere erosion is associated with a declining immune function of caregivers of Alzheimer's disease patients. *Journal of Immunology, 179,* 4249–4254.

Damschroder, L. J., Zikmund-Fisher, B. J., & Ubel, P. A. (2005). The impact of considering adaptation in health state valuation. *Social Science and Medicine, 61,* 267–277.

Danaei, G., Ding, E. L., Mozffarian, D., Taylor, B., Rehm, J., Murray, C. J. L., … Ezzati, M. (2009). The preventable causes of death in the United States: Comparative risk assessment of dietary, lifestyle, and metabolic risk factors. *PLoS Medicine, 6*(4), 1–23.

Danaei, G., Vander Hoorn, S., Lopez, A. D., Murray, C. J. L., & Ezzati, M. (2005). Causes of cancer in the world: Comparative risk assessment of nine behavioural and environmental risk factors. *Lancet, 366,* 1784–1793.

Daniels, M. C., Goldberg, J., Jacobsen, C., & Welty, T. K. (2006). Is psychological distress a risk factor for the incidence of diabetes among American Indians? The Strong Heart Study. *Journal of Applied Gerontology, 25*(S1), 60S–72S.

Dansinger, M. L., Gleason, J. A., Griffith, J. L., Selker, H. P., & Schaefer, E. J. (2005). Comparison of the Atkins, Ornish, Weight Watchers, and Zone diets for weight loss and heart disease risk reduction: A randomized trial. *JAMA, 293*(1), 43–53.

Dantzer, R., O'Connor, J. C., Freund, G. G., Johnson, R. W., & Kelley, K. W. (2008). From inflammation to sickness and depression: When the immune system subjugates the brain. *Nature Reviews Neuroscience, 9*, 46–57.

D'Arcy, Y. (2005). Conquering pain: Have you tried these new techniques? *Nursing, 35*(3), 36–42.

Darvishi, N., Farhadi, M., Haghtalab, T., & Poorolajal, J. (2015). Alcohol-related risk of suicidal ideation, suicide attempt, and completed suicide: A meta-analysis. *PLoS One, 10*(5), e0126870.

Datta, S. D., Koutsky, L. A., Ratelle, S., Unger, E. R., Shlay, J., McClain, T., … Weinstock, H. (2008). Human papillomavirus infection and cervical cytology in women screened for cervical cancer in the United States, 2003–2005. *Annals of Internal Medicine, 148*, 493–501.

"David Beckham's biggest secret revealed as star admits he has asthma." (2009, November 25). David Beckham's biggest secret revealed as star admits he has asthma. *Daily Mail.* Retrieved April 19, 2012, from http://www.dailymail.co.uk/tvshowbiz/article-1230404/

Davidson, K., MacGregor, M. W., Stuhr, J., Dixon, K., & MacLean, D. (2000). Constructive anger verbal behavior predicts blood pressure in a population-based sample. *Health Psychology, 19*, 55–64.

Davidson, K. W., & Mostofsky, E. (2010). Anger expression and risk of coronary heart disease: Evidence from the Nova Scotia Health Survey. *American Heart Journal, 159*, 199–206.

Davies, D. L. (1962). Normal drinking in recovered alcohol addicts. *Quarterly Journal of Studies on Alcohol, 24*, 321–332.

Davis, A. K., & Lauritsen, K. J. (2016). Acceptability of non-abstinence goals among students enrolled in addiction studies programs across the United States. *Substance Abuse, 37*(1), 2014–2208.

Davis, B., & Carpenter, C. (2009). Proximity of fast-food restaurants to schools and adolescent obesity. *American Journal of Public Health, 99*(3), 505–510.

Davis, C., & Scott-Robertson, L. (2000). A psychological comparison of females with anorexia nervosa and competitive male body-builders: Body shape ideals in the extreme. *Eating Behaviors, 1*, 33–46.

Davis, C. L., Tomporowski, P. D., McDowell, J. E., Austin, B. P., Miller, P. H., Yanasak, N. E., … Naglieri, J. A. (2011). Exercise improves executive function and achievement and alters brain activation in overweight children: A randomized, controlled trial. *Health Psychology, 30*, 91–98.

Davis, J. (2008). Pro-anorexia sites—A patient's perspective. *Child and Adolescent Mental Health, 13*, 97.

Davis, K. D. (2000). Studies of pain using functional magnetic resonance imaging. In K. L. Casey & M. C. Bushnell (Eds.), *Pain imaging: Progress in pain research and management* (pp. 195–210). Seattle, WA: IASP Press.

Davis, M. C., Zautra, A. J., Younger, J., Motivala, S. J., Attrep, J., & Irwin, M. R. (2008). Chronic stress and regulation of cellular markers of inflammation in rheumatoid arthritis: Implications for fatigue. *Brain, Behavior and Immunity, 22*, 24–32.

Dawson, D. A., Grant, B. F., Stinson, F. S., Chou, P. S., Huang, B., & Ruan, W. J. (2005). Recovery from DSM-IV alcohol dependence: United States, 2001–2002. *Addiction, 100*, 281–292.

Deandrea, S., Montanari, M., Moja, L., & Apolone, G. (2008). Prevalence of undertreatment in cancer pain: A review of published literature. *Annals of Oncology, 19*, 1985–1991.

De Andrés, J., & Van Buyten, J.-P. (2006). Neural modulation by stimulation. *Pain Practice, 6*, 39–45.

DeBar, L. L., Stevens, V. J., Perrin, N., Wu, P., Pearson, J., Yarborough, B. J., … Lynch, F. (2012). A primary care-based, multicomponent lifestyle intervention for overweight adolescent females. *Pediatrics, 129*, e611–e620.

De Benedittis, G. (2003). Understanding the multidimensional mechanisms of hypnotic analgesia. *Contemporary Hypnosis, 20*, 59–80.

de Bloom, J., Geurts, S. A. E., Taris, T. W., Sonnentag, S., de Weerth, C., & Kompier, M. A. J. (2010). Effects of vacation from work on health and well-being: Lots of fun, quickly gone. *Work and Stress, 2*, 196–216.

de Bloom, J., Kompier, M., Geurts, S., de Weerth, C., Taris, T., & Sonnentag, S. (2009). Do we recover from vacation? Meta-analysis of vacation effects on health and well-being. *Journal of Occupational Health, 51*, 13–25.

de Brouwer, S. J. M., Kraaimaat, F. W., Sweep, F. C. G. J., Creemers, M. C. W., Radstake, T. R. D. J., Laarhoven, A. I. M., … Evers, A. W. M. (2010). Experimental stress in inflammatory rheumatic diseases: A review of psychophysiological stress responses. *Arthritis Research and Therapy, 12*, R89.

Decaluwé, V., & Braet, C. (2005). The cognitive behavioural model for eating disorders: A direct evaluation in children and adolescents with obesity. *Eating Behaviors, 6*, 211–220.

De Civita, M., & Dobkin, P. L. (2005). Pediatric adherence: Conceptual and methodological considerations. *Children's Health Care, 34*, 19–34.

DeFulio, A., & Silverman, K. (2012). The use of incentives to reinforce medication adherence. *Preventive Medicine, 55*, S86–S94.

Dehle, C., Larsen, D., & Landers, J. E. (2001). Social support in marriage. *American Journal of Family Therapy, 29*, 307–324.

de Leeuw, R., Schmidt, J. E., & Carlson, C. R. (2005). Traumatic stressors and post-traumatic stress disorder symptoms in headache patients. *Headache, 45*, 1365–1374.

DeLeo, J. A. (2006). Basic science of pain. *Journal of Bone and Joint Surgery, 88*(Suppl. 2), 58–62.

De Lew, N., & Weinick, R. M. (2000). An overview: Eliminating racial, ethnic, and SES disparities in health care. *Health Care Financing Review, 21*(4), 1–7.

DeLongis, A., Folkman, S., & Lazarus, R. S. (1988). The impact of daily stress on health and mood: Psychological and social resources as mediators. *Journal of Personality and Social Psychology, 54*, 486–495.

Delvaux, T., & Nostlinger, C. (2007). Reproductive choice for women and men living with HIV: Contraception, abortion and fertility. *Reproductive Health Matters, 15*(S29), 46–66.

De Marzo, A. M., Platz, E. A., Sutcliffe, S., Xu, J., Grönberg, H., Drake, C. G., … Nelson, W. G. (2007). Inflammation in prostate carcinogenesis. *Nature Reviews Cancer, 7*, 256–269.

Dembroski, T. M., MacDougall, J. M., Williams, R. B., Haney, T. L., & Blumenthal, J. A. (1985). Components of Type A, hostility, and anger-in: Relationship to angiographic findings. *Psychosomatic Medicine, 47*, 219–233.

Deniz, O., Aygül, R., Koçak, N., Orhan, A., & Kaya, M. D. (2004). Precipitating factors of migraine attacks in patients with migraine with and without aura. *Pain Clinic, 16*, 451–456.

Dennis, J., Krewski, D., Côté, F.-S., Fafard, E., Little, J., & Ghadirian, P. (2011). Breast cancer risk in relation to alcohol consumption and BRCA gene mutations: A case-only study of gene-environment interaction. *The Breast Journal, 17*, 477–484.

Dennis, L. K., Vanbeek, M. J., Freeman, L. E. B., Smith, B. J., Dawson, D. V., & Coughlin, J. A. (2008). Sunburns and risk of cutaneous melanoma: Does age matter? A comprehensive meta-analysis. *Annals of Epidemiology, 18*, 614–627.

de Oliveira, C., Watt, W., & Hamer, M. (2010). Toothbrushing, inflammation, and risk of cardiovascular disease: Results from Scottish Health Survey. *British Medical Journal, 340*, c2451.

Depue, J. B., Southwell, B. G., Betzner, A. E., & Walsh, B. M. (2015). Encoded exposure to tobacco use in social media predicts subsequent smoking behavior. *American Journal of Health Promotion, 29*(4), 259–261.

Derogatis, L. R. (1977). *Manual for the Symptom Checklist-90, Revised.* Baltimore, MD: Johns Hopkins University School of Medicine.

deRuiter, W. K., Cairney, J., Leatherdale, S. T., & Faulkner, G. E. (2014). A longitudinal examination of the interrelationship of multiple health behaviors. *American Journal of Preventive Medicine, 47*(3), 283–289.

Dettmer, A. M., Novak, M. A., Meyer, J. S., & Suomi, S. J. (2014). Population density-dependent hair cortisol concentrations in rhesus monkeys (Macaca mulatta). *Psychoneuroendocrinology, 42*, 59–67.

DeVoe, J. E., Baez, A., Angier, H., Krois, L., Edlund, C., & Carney, P. A. (2007). Insurance + access ≠ health care: Typology of barriers to health care access for low-income families. *Annals of Family Medicine, 5*, 511–518.

DeVries, A. C., Glasper, E. R., & Detillion, C. E. (2003). Social modulation of stress responses. *Physiology and Behavior, 79*, 399–407.

DeWall, C. N., MacDonald, G., Webster, G. D., Masten, C. L., Baumeister, R. F., Powell, C., … Eisenberger, N. I. (2010). Acetaminophen reduces social pain: Behavioral and neural evidence. *Psychological Science, 21*, 931–937.

Dewaraja, R., & Kawamura, N. (2006). Trauma intensity and posttraumatic stress: Implications of the tsunami experience in Sri Lanka for the management of future disasters. *International Congress Series, 1287*, 69–73.

Dhanani, N. M., Caruso, T. J., & Carinci, A. J. (2011). Complementary and alternative medicine for pain: An evidence-based review. *Current Pain and Headache Reports, 15*(1), 39–46.

Dickerson, F., Bennett, M., Dixon, L., Burke, E., Vaughan, C., Delahanty, J., … DiClemente, C. (2011). Smoking cessation in persons with serious mental illnesses: The experience of successful quitters. *Psychiatric Rehabilitation Journal, 34*(4), 311–316.

Dickerson, S. S., & Kemeny, M. E. (2004). Acute stressors and cortisol responses: A theoretical integration and synthesis of laboratory research. *Psychological Bulletin, 130*, 355–391.

Dietz, P. M., England, L. J., Shapiro-Mendoza, C. K., Tong, V. T., Farr, S. L., & Callaghan, W. M. (2010). Infant morbidity and mortality attributable to prenatal smoking in the U.S. *American Journal of Preventive Medicine, 39*(1), 45–52.

DiIorio, C., McCarty, F., Resnicow, K., Holstad, M. M., Soet, J., Yeager, K., … Lundberg, B. (2008). Using motivational interviewing to promote adherence to antiretroviral medications: A randomized controlled study. *AIDS Care, 20*, 273–283.

Dillard, J., with Hirchman, L. A. (2002). *The chronic pain solution.* New York, NY: Bantam.

DiMatteo, M. R. (2004a). Social support and patient adherence to medical treatment: A meta-analysis. *Health Psychology, 23*, 207–218.

DiMatteo, M. R. (2004b). Variations in patients' adherence to medical recommendations: A quantitative review of 50 years of research. *Medical Care, 42*, 200–209.

DiMatteo, M. R., & DiNicola, D. D. (1982). *Achieving patient compliance: The psychology of the medical practitioner's role.* New York, NY: Pergamon Press.

DiMatteo, M. R., Giordani, P. J., Lepper, H. S., & Croghan, T. W. (2002). Patient adherence and medical treatment outcomes: A meta-analysis. *Medical Care, 40*, 794–811.

DiMatteo, M. R., Haskard, K. B., & Williams, S. L. (2007). Health beliefs, disease severity, and patients adherence: A meta-analysis. *Medical Care, 45*, 521–528.

DiMatteo, M. R., Lepper, H. S., & Croghan, T. W. (2000). Meta-analysis of the effects of anxiety and depression on patient adherence. *Archives of Internal Medicine, 160*, 2101–2107.

Dimsdale, J. E., Eckenrode, J., Haggerty, R. J., Kaplan, B. H., Cohen, F., & Dornbusch, S. (1979). The role of social supports in medical care. *Social Psychiatry, 14*, 175–180.

Dingwall, G. (2005). *Alcohol and crime.* Cullompton, UK: Willan Publishing.

DiNicola, D. D., & DiMatteo, M. R. (1984). Practitioners, patients, and compliance with medical regimens: A social psychological perspective. In A. Baum, S. E. Taylor, & J. E. Singer (Eds.), *Handbook of psychology and health: Vol. 4. Social psychological aspects of health* (pp. 55–84). Hillsdale, NJ: Erlbaum.

Direito, A., Dale, L. P., Shields, E., Dobson, R., Whittaker, R., & Maddison, R. (2014). Do physical activity and dietary smartphone applications incorporate evidence-based behaviour change techniques? *BMC Public Health, 14*(1), 1.

di Sarsina, R. (2007). The social demand for a medicine focused on the person: The contribution of CAM to healthcare and health genesis. *Evidence-Based Complementary and Alternative Medicine, 4*(Suppl. 1), 45–51.

Dishman, R. K. (2003). The impact of behavior on quality of life. *Quality of Life Research, 12*(Suppl. 1), 43–49.

Distefan, J. M., Pierce, J. P., & Gilpin, E. A. (2004). Do favorite movie stars influence adolescent smoking initiation? *American Journal of Public Health, 94*, 239–244.

Dittmann, M. (2005). Publicizing diabetes' behavioral impact. *Monitor on Psychology, 36*(7), 35–36.

Dixon, L., Medoff, D. R., Wohlheiter, K., DiCelmente, C., Goldberg, R., Kreyenbuhl, J., … Davin, C. (2007). Correlates of severity of smoking among persons with severe mental illness. *American Journal of Addictions, 16*(2), 101–110.

Dobbins, M., DeCorby, K., Manske, S., & Goldblatt, E. (2008). Effective practices for school-based tobacco use prevention. *Preventive Medicine, 46*, 289–297.

Dobson, R. (2005). High cholesterol may increase risk of testicular cancer. *British Medical Journal, 330*, 1042.

Doevendans, P. A., Van der Smagt, J., Loh, P., De Jonge, N., & Touw, D. J. (2003). Prognostic implications of genetics in cardiovascular disease. *Current Pharmacogenomics, 1*, 217–228.

Donaghy, M. E. (2007). Exercise can seriously improve your mental health: Fact or fiction? *Advanced in Physiology, 9*(2), 76–88.

Donohue, K. F., Curtin, J. J., Patrick, C. J., & Lang, A. R. (2007). Intoxication level and emotional response. *Emotion, 7*, 103–112.

Dorenlot, P., Harboun, M., Bige, V., Henrard, J.-C., & Ankri, J. (2005). Major depression as a risk factor for early institutionalization of dementia patients living in the community. *International Journal of Geriatric Psychiatry, 20*, 471–478.

Dorn, J. M., Genco, R. J., Grossi, S. G., Falkner, K. L., Hovey, K. M., Iacoviello, L., … Trevisan, M. (2010). Periodontal disease and recurrent cardiovascular events in survivors of myocardial infarction (MI): The Western New York Acute MI Study. *Journal of Periodontology, 81*, 502–511.

Dorr, N., Brosschot, J. F., Sollers, J. J., & Thayer, J. F. (2007). Damned if you do, damned if you don't: The differential effect of expression and inhibition of anger on cardiovascular recovery in Black and White males. *International Journal of Psychophysiology, 66*, 125–134.

Doty, H. E., & Weech-Maldonado, R. (2003). Racial/ethnic disparities in adult preventive dental care use. *Journal of Health Care for the Poor and Underserved, 14*, 516–534.

Dougall, A. L., & Baum, A. (2001). Stress, health, and illness. In A. Baum, T. A. Revenson, & J. E. Singer (Eds.), *Handbook of health psychology* (pp. 321–337). Mahwah, NJ: Erlbaum.

Douketis, J. D., Macie, C., Thabane, L., & Williamson, D. F. (2005). Systematic review of long-term weight loss studies in obese adults: Clinical significance and applicability to clinical practice. *International Journal of Obesity, 29*, 1153–1167.

Dovidio, J. F., Penner, L. A., Albrecht, T. L., Norton, W. E., Gaertner, S. L., & Shelton, J. N. (2008). Disparities and distrust: The implications of psychological processes for understanding racial disparities in health and health care. *Social Science and Medicine, 67*, 478–486.

Dowell, D, Haegerich, T. M., & Chou, R. (2016). CDC guideline for prescribing opioids for chronic pain—United States, 2016. *JAMA, 315*(15), 1624–1645.

Downer, B., Jiang, Y., Zanjani, F., & Fardo, D. (2015). Effects of alcohol consumption on cognition and regional brain volumes among older adults. *American Journal of Alzheimer's Disease and Other Dementias, 30*(4), 364–374.

Dresler, C. M., Leon, M. E., Straif, K., Baan, R., & Secretan, B. (2006). Reversal of risk upon quitting smoking. *Lancet, 368*, 348–349.

D'Souza, G., & Dempsey, A. (2011). The role of HPV in head and neck cancer and review of the HPV vaccine. *Preventive Medicine, 53*, S5–S11.

Du, X. L., Meyer, T. E., & Franzini, L. (2007). Meta-analysis of racial disparities in survival in association with socioeconomic status among men and women with color cancer. *Cancer, 109*, 2161–2170.

Duangdao, K. M., & Roesch, S. C. (2008). Coping with diabetes in adulthood: A meta-analysis. *Journal of Behavioral Medicine, 31*, 291–300.

Duke, A., Johnson, M., Reissig, C., & Griffiths, R. (2015). Nicotine reinforcement in never-smokers. *Psychopharmacology, 232*(23), 4243–4252.

Dunbar, H. F. (1943). *Psychosomatic diagnosis.* New York, NY: Hoeber.

Dunkel-Schetter, C. (2011). Psychological science on pregnancy: Stress processes, biopsychosocial models, and emerging research issues. *Annual Review of Psychology, 62,* 531–58.

Dunn, A. L., Trivedi, M. H., Kampert, J. B., Clark, C. G., & Chambliss, H. O. (2005). Exercise treatment for depression: Efficacy and dose response. *American Journal of Preventive Medicine, 28,* 1–8.

Dunn, A. L., Trivedi, M. H., & O'Neal, H. A. (2001). Physical activity dose-response effects on outcomes of depression and anxiety. *Medicine and Science in Sports and Exercise, 33,* S587–S597.

Dunton, G. F., Liao, Y., Intille, S. S., Spruijt-Metz, D., & Pentz, M. (2011). Investigating children's physical activity and sedentary behavior using ecological momentary assessment with mobile phones. *Pediatric Obesity, 19,* 1205–1212.

Dusseldrop, E., van Elderen, T., Maes, S., Meulman, J., & Kraaj, V. (1999). A meta-analysis of psychoeducational programs for coronary heart disease patients. *Health Psychology, 18,* 506–519.

Dutra, L., Stathopoulou, G., Basden, S. L., Leyro, T. M., Powers, M. B., & Otto, M. W. (2008). A meta-analytic review of psychosocial interventions for substance use disorders. *American Journal of Psychiatry, 165,* 179–187.

Dwan, K., Altman, D. G., Arnaiz, J. A., Bloom, J., Chan, A.-W., Cronin, E., … Williamson, P. R. (2008). Systematic review of the empirical evidence of study publication bias and outcome reporting bias. *PLoS One, 3,* e3081.

Eaker, E. D., Sullivan, L. M., Kelly-Hayes, M., D'Agostino, R. B., Sr., & Benjamin, E. J. (2007). Marital status, marital strain, and risk of coronary heart disease or total mortality: The Framingham Offspring Study. *Psychosomatic Medicine, 69,* 509–513.

Ebrecht, M., Hextall, J., Kirtley, L.-G., Taylor, A., Dyson, M., & Weinman, J. (2004). Perceived stress and cortisol levels predict speed of wound healing in healthy male adults. *Psychoneuroendocrinology, 29,* 798–809.

Eckhardt, C. I., & Crane, C. (2008). Effects of alcohol intoxication and aggressivity on aggressive verbalizations during anger arousal. *Aggressive Behavior, 34,* 428–436.

Eddy, K. T., Dorer, D. J., Franko, D. L., Tahilani, K., Thompson-Brenner, H., & Herzog, D. B. (2007). Should bulimia nervosa be subtyped by history of anorexia nervosa? A longitudinal validation. *International Journal of Eating Disorders, 40*(S3), S67–S71.

Edwards, A. G. K., Hailey, S., & Maxwell, M. (2004). Psychological interventions for women with metastatic breast cancer. *Cochrane Database of Systematic Reviews,* Cochrane AN: CD004253.

Edwards, A. G. K., Hulbert-Williams, N., & Neal, R. D. (2008). Psychological interventions for women with metastatic breast cancer. *Cochrane Database of Systematic Reviews,* Cochrane Art. No.: CD004253. DOI: 10.1002/14651858.CD004253.pub3.

Edwards, C. L., Fillingim, R. B., & Keefe, F. (2001). Race, ethnicity and pain. *Pain, 94,* 133–137.

Edwards, G. (1977). The alcohol dependence syndrome: Usefulness of an idea. In G. Edwards & M. Grant (Eds.), *Alcoholism: New knowledge and new responses.* London: Croom Helm.

Edwards, G. (2000). *Alcohol: The world's favorite drug.* New York, NY: Thomas Dunne Books.

Edwards, G., & Gross, M. M. (1976). Alcohol dependence: Provisional description of a clinical syndrome. *British Medical Journal, 1,* 1058–1061.

Edwards, G., Gross, M. M., Keller, M., Moser, J., & Room, R. (1977). *Alcohol-related disabilities* (WHO Offset Pub. No. 32). Geneva, Switzerland: World Health Organization.

Edwards, L. M., & Romero, A. J. (2008). Coping with discrimination among Mexican descent adolescents. *Hispanic Journal of Behavioral Sciences, 30,* 24–39.

Ege, M. J., Mayer, M., Normand, A.-C., Genuneit, J., Cookson, W. O. C. M., Braun-Fahrlander, C., … von Mutius, E. (2011). Exposure to environmental microorganisms and childhood asthma. *The New England Journal of Medicine, 364,* 701–709.

Eggert, J., Theobald, H., & Engfeldt, P. (2004). Effects of alcohol consumption on female fertility during an 18-year period. *Fertility and Sterility, 81,* 379–383.

Ehrlich, G. E. (2003). Low back pain. *Bulletin of the World Health Organization, 81,* 671–676.

Eisenberg, M. E., Neumark-Sztainer, D., Story, M., & Perry, C. (2005). The role of social norms and friends' influences on unhealthy weight-control behaviors among adolescent girls. *Social Science and Medicine, 60,* 1165–1173.

Eisenberger, N. I., Gable, S. L., & Lieberman, M. D. (2007). Functional magnetic resonance imaging responses relate to differences in real-world social experience. *Emotion, 7,* 745–754.

Eisenberger, N. I., Inagaki, T. K., Mashal, N. M., & Irwin, M. R. (2010). Inflammation and social experience: An inflammatory challenge induces feelings of social disconnection in addition to depressed mood. *Brain, Behavior, and Immunity, 24,* 558–563.

Eisenberger, N. I., & Lieberman, M. D. (2004). Why rejection hurts: A common neural alarm system for physical and social pain. *Trends in Cognitive Sciences, 8,* 294–300.

Eisenberger, N. I., Lieberman, M. D., & Williams, K. D. (2003). Does rejection hurt? An fMRI study of social exclusion. *Science, 302,* 290–292.

Eisenmann, J. C., Welk, G. J., Wickel, E. E., & Blair, S. N. (2007). Combined influence of cardiorespiratory fitness and body mass index on cardiovascular disease risk factors among 8–18 year old youth: The Aerobics Center Longitudinal Study. *International Journal of Pediatric Obesity, 2*(2), 66–72.

Ekelund, U., Brage, S., Franks, P. W., Hennings, S., Emms, S., & Wareham, N. J. (2005). Physical activity energy expenditure predicts progression toward the metabolic syndrome independently of aerobic fitness in middle-aged healthy Caucasians. *Diabetes Care, 28,* 1195–1200.

Elbel, B., Gyamfi, J., & Kersh, R. (2011). Child and adolescent fast-food choice and the influence of calorie labeling: A natural experiment. *International Journal of Obesity, 35,* 493–500.

Elkins, J. S. (2006). Management of blood pressure in patients with cere-brovascular disease. *Johns Hopkins Advanced Studies in Medicine, 6*(8), 363–369, 349–350.

Eller, N. H., Netterstrøm, B., & Hansen, Å. M. (2006). Psychosocial factors at home and at work and levels of salivary cortisol. *Biological Psychology, 73,* 280–287.

Elliott, R. A. (2006). Poor adherence to anti-inflammatory medication in asthma: Reasons, challenges, and strategies for improved disease management. *Disease Management and Health Outcomes, 14,* 223–233.

Ellis, A. (1962). *Reason and emotion in psychotherapy.* New York, NY: Stuart.

Ellis, D. A., Podolski, C.-L., Frey, M., Naar-King, S., Wang, B., & Moltz, K. (2007). The role of parental monitoring in adolescent health outcomes: Impact on regimen adherence in youth with Type 1 diabetes. *Journal of Pediatric Psychology, 32,* 907–917.

Ellis, L. (2004). Thief of time. *InteliHealth.* Retrieved July 1, 2005, from http://www.intelihealth.com/IH/ihtIH/WSIHW000/8303/24299.html

Emanuel, A. S., McCully, S. N., Gallagher, K. M., & Updegraff, J. A. (2012). Theory of planned behavior explains gender difference in fruit and vegetable consumption. *Appetite. 59*(3), 693–697.

Emanuel, E. J., & Fuchs, V. R. (2008). The perfect storm of over-utilization. *Journal of the American Medical Association, 299,* 2789–2791.

Emanuel, L., Bennett, K., & Richardson, V. E. (2007). The dying role. *Journal of Palliative Medicine, 10,* 159–168.

Empana, J.-P., Jouven, X., Lemaitre, R., Sotoodehnia, N., Rea, T., Raghunathan, T., … Siscovick, D. (2008). Marital status and risk of out-of-hospital sudden cardiac arrest in the population. *European Journal of Preventive Cardiology, 15,* 577–582.

Endresen, G. K. M. (2007). Fibromyalgia: A rheumatologic diagnosis? *Rheumatology International, 27,* 999–1004.

Engler, M. B., & Engler, M. M. (2006). The emerging role of flavonoid-rich cocoa and chocolate in cardiovascular health and disease. *Nutrition Reviews, 64,* 109–118.

Ensel, W. M., & Lin, N. (2004). Physical fitness and the stress process. *Journal of Community Psychology, 32*, 81–101.

Enstrom, J. E., & Kabat, G. C. (2006). Environmental tobacco smoke and coronary heart disease mortality in the United States—A meta-analysis and critique. *Inhalation Toxicology, 18*(3), 199–210.

Epel, E. S., Blackburn, E. H., Lin, J., Dhabhar, F. S., Adler, N. E., Morrow, J. D., & Cawthon, R. M. (2004). Accelerated telomere shortening in response to life stress. *Proceedings of the National Academy of Sciences of the United States of America, 101*(49), 17312–17315.

Ephraim, P. L., Wegener, S. T., MacKenzie, E. J., Dillingham, T. R., & Pezzin, L. E. (2005). Phantom pain, residual limb pain, and back pain in amputees: Results of a national survey. *Archives of Physical Medicine and Rehabilitation, 86*, 1910–1919.

Epstein, L. H., Leddy, J. J., Temple, J. L., & Faith, M. S. (2007). Food reinforcement and eating: A multilevel analysis. *Psychological Bulletin, 133*, 884–906.

Ernster, V. L., Grady, D., Müke, R., Black, D., Selby, J., & Kerlikowske, K. (1995). Facial wrinkling in men and women by smoking status. *American Journal of Public Health, 85*, 78–82.

Ertekin-Taner, N. (2007). Genetics of Alzheimer's disease: A centennial review. *Neurologic Clinics, 25*, 611–667.

European Vertebral Osteoporosis Study Group. (2004). Variation in back pain between countries: The example of Britain and Germany. *Spine, 29*, 1017–1021.

Evans, D., & Norman, P. (2009). Illness representations, coping and psychological adjustment to Parkinson's disease. *Psychology and Health, 24*, 1181–1197.

Evans, G. W., & Stecker, R. (2004). Motivational consequences of environmental stress. *Journal of Environmental Psychology, 24*, 143–165.

Evans, G. W., & Wener, R. E. (2007). Crowding and personal space invasion on the train: Please don't make me sit in the middle. *Journal of Environmental Psychology, 27*(1), 90–94.

Evans, P. C. (2003). "If only I were thin like her, maybe I could be happy like her": The self-implications of associating a thin female ideal with life success. *Psychology of Women Quarterly, 27*, 209–214.

Everett, M. D., Kinser, A. M., & Ramsey, M. W. (2007). Training for old age: Production functions for the aerobic exercise inputs. *Medicine and Science in Sports and Exercise, 39*, 2226–2233.

Evers, A., Klusmann, V., Ziegelmann, J. P., Schwarzer, R., & Heuser, I. (2011). Long-term adherence to a physical activity intervention: The role of telephone-assisted vs. self-administered coping plans and strategy use. *Psychology and Health. 27*(7), 784–797.

Everson, S. A., Lynch, J. W., Kaplan, G. A., Lakka, T. A., Sivenius, J., & Salonen, J. T. (2001). Stress-induced blood pressure reactivity and incident stroke in middle-aged men. *Stroke, 32*, 1263–1270.

Ezekiel, J. E., & Miller, F. G. (2001). The ethics of placebo-controlled trials: A middle ground. *New England Journal of Medicine, 345*, 915–920.

Ezzo, J., Streitberger, K., & Schneider, A. (2006). Cochrane systematic reviews examine p6 acupuncture-point stimulation for nausea and vomiting. *Journal of Complementary and Alternative Medicine, 12*, 489–495.

Faden, R. R. (1987). Ethical issues in government sponsored public health campaigns. *Health Education Quarterly, 14*, 27–37.

Fairburn, C. G., & Harrison, P. J. (2003). Eating disorders. *Lancet, 361*, 407–416.

Fairhurst, M., Wiech, K., Dunckley, P., & Tracey, I. (2007). Anticipatory brainstem activity predicts neural processing of pain in humans. *Pain, 128*, 101–110.

Falagas, M. E., Zarkadoulia, E. A., Pliatsika, P. A., & Panos, G. (2008). Socioeconomic status (SES) as a determinant of adherence to treatment in HIV infected patients: A systematic review of the literature. *Retrovirology, 5*, 13.

Fang, C. V., & Myers, H. F. (2001). The effects of racial stressors and hostility on cardiovascular reactivity in African American and Caucasian men. *Health Psychology, 20*, 64–70.

Fanning, J., Mullen, S. P., & McAuley, E. (2012). Increasing physical activity with mobile devices: A meta-analysis. *Journal of Medical Internet Research, 14*(6), e161.

Farley, J. J., Rodrigue, J. R., Sandrik, L. L., Tepper, V. J., Marhefka, S. L., & Sleasman, J. W. (2004). Clinical assessment of medication adherence among HIV-infected children: Examination of the Treatment Interview Protocol (TIP). *AIDS Care, 16*, 323–337.

Farrell, S. P., Hains, A. A., Davies, W. H., Smith, P., & Parton, E. (2004). The impact of cognitive distortions, stress, and adherence on metabolic control in youths with Type 1 diabetes. *Journal of Adolescent Health, 34*, 461–467.

Farstad, S. M., McGeown, L. M., & von Ranson, K. M. (2016). Eating disorders and personality, 2004-2016: A systematic review and meta-analysis. *Clinical Psychology Review, 46*, 91–105.

Favier, I., Haan, J., & Ferrari, M. D. (2005). Chronic cluster headache: A review. *Journal of Headache and Pain, 6*, 3–9.

Federal Trade Commission weighs in on losing weight. (2002). *FDA Consumer, 36*, 8.

Feist, J., & Feist, G. J. (2006). *Theories of personality* (6th ed.). Boston, MA: McGraw-Hill.

Feldman, P. J., Cohen, S., Gwaltney, J. M., Jr., Doyle, W. J., & Skoner, D. P. (1999). The impact of personality on the reporting of unfounded symptoms and illness. *Journal of Personality and Social Psychology, 77*, 370–378.

Feldt, K. (2007). Pain measurement: Present concern and future directions. *Pain Medicine, 8*, 541–543.

Felson, R. B., & Staff, J. (2010). The effects of alcohol intoxication on violent versus other offending. *Criminal Justice and Behavior, 37*(12), 1343–1360.

Ferguson, J., Bauld, L., Chesterman, J., & Judge, K. (2005). The English smoking treatment services: One-year outcomes. *Addiction, 100*(Suppl. 2), 59–69.

Ferlay, J., Parkin, D. M., & Steliarova-Foucher, E. (2010). Estimates of cancer incidence and mortality in Europe in 2008. *European Journal of Cancer, 46*, 765–781.

Fernandez, E., & Sheffield, J. (1996). Relative contributions of life events versus daily hassles to the frequency and intensity of headaches. *Headache, 36*, 595–602.

Fernandez, R., Griffiths, R., Everett, B., Davidson, P., Salamonson, Y., & Andrew, S. (2007). Effectiveness of brief structured interventions on risk factor modification for patients with coronary heart disease: A systematic review. *International Journal of Evidence-Based Healthcare, 5*, 370–405.

Ferri, M., Amato, L., & Davoli, M. (2006). Alcoholics Anonymous and other 12-step programmes for alcohol dependence. *Cochrane Database of Systematic Reviews*, Cochrane Art. No.: CD005032, DOI: 10.1002/14651858.CD005032.pub2.

Fichtenberg, C. M., & Glantz, S. A. (2002). Effect of smoke-free workplaces on smoking behaviour. Systematic review, *British Journal of Medicine, 325*, 188–195.

Fichter, M., Quadflieg, N., & Fischer, U. (2011). Severity of alcohol-related problems and mortality: Results from a 20-year prospective epidemiological community study. *European Archives of Psychiatry and Clinical Neuroscience, 261*(4), 293–302.

Fidler, J. A., West, R., van Jaarsveld, C. H. M., Jarvis, M. J., & Wardle, J. (2008). Smoking status of step-parents as a risk factor for smoking in adolescence. *Addiction, 103*(3), 496–501.

Fifield, J., Mcquillan, J., Armeli, S., Tennen, H., Reisine, S., & Affleck, G. (2004). Chronic strain, daily work stress and pain among workers with rheumatoid arthritis: Does job stress make a bad day worse? *Work and Stress, 18*, 275–291.

Fillingim, R. B., King, C. D., Ribeiro-Dasilva, M. C., Rahim-Williams, B., & Riley, J. L. (2009). Sex, gender, and pain: A review of recent clinical and experimental findings. *The Journal of Pain, 10*, 447–485.

Finkelstein, A., Taubman, S., Wright, B., Bernstein, M., Gruber, J., Newhouse, J. P., …The Oregon Health Study Group. (2011). *The Oregon Health Insurance Experiment: Evidence from the first year* (NBER Working Paper No. 17190). Washington, DC: National Bureau of Economic Research.

Finlayson, G., King, N., & Blundell, J. E. (2007). Liking vs. wanting food: Importance for human appetite control and weight regulation. *Neuroscience and Biobehavioral Reviews, 31*, 987–1002.

Finley, J. W., Davis, C. D., & Feng, Y. (2000). Selenium from high selenium broccoli protects rats from colon cancer. *Journal of Nutrition, 130*, 2384–2389.

Firenzuoli, F., & Gori, L. (2007). Herbal medicine today: Clinical and research issues. *Evidence Based Complementary and Alternative Medicine, 4*(Suppl. 1), 37–40.

Fischer, S., Stojek, M., & Hartzell, E. (2010). Effects of multiple forms of childhood abuse and adult sexual assault on current eating disorder symptoms. *Eating Behaviors, 11*(3), 190–192.

Fishbain, D. A., Cole, B., Lewis, J., Rosomoff, H. L., & Rosomoff, R. S. (2008). What percentage of chronic nonmalignant pain patients exposed to chronic opioid analgesic therapy develop abuse/addiction and/or aberrant drug-related behaviors? A structured evidence-based review. *Pain Medicine, 9,* 444–459.

Fitzgerald, T. E., Tennen, H., Affleck, G., & Pransky, G. S. (1993). The relative importance of dispositional optimism and control appraisals in quality of life after coronary artery bypass surgery. *Journal of Behavioral Medicine, 16*(1), 25–43.

Fitzpatrick, A. L., Kuller, L. H., Ives, D. G., Lopez, O. L., Jagust, W., Breitner, J. C. S., ... Dulberg, C. (2004). Incidence and prevalence of dementia in the Cardiovascular Health Study. *Journal of the American Geriatrics Society, 52,* 195–204.

Fjorback, L. O., Arendt, M., Ørnbøl, E., Fink, P., & Walach, H. (2011). Mindfulness-based stress reduction and mindfulness-based cognitive therapy—A systematic review of randomized controlled trials. *Acta Psychiatrica Scandinavica, 124*(2), 102–119.

Flay, B. R. (2009). The promise of long-term effectiveness of school-based smoking prevention programs: A critical review of reviews. *Tobacco Induced Diseases, 5*(7), 1–12.

Flegal, K. M., Carroll, M. D., Kit, B. K., & Ogden, C. L. (2012). Prevalence of obesity and trends in the distribution of body mass index among US adults, 1999–2010. *Journal of the American Medical Association, 307,* 491–497.

Flegal, K. M., Kit, B. K., Orpana, H., & Graubard, B. I. (2013). Association of all-cause mortality with overweight and obesity using standard body mass index categories: A systematic review and meta-analysis. *Journal of the American Medical Association, 309*(1), 71–82.

Fleshner, M., & Laudenslager, M. L. (2004). Psychoneuroimmunology: Then and now. *Behavioral and Cognitive Neuroscience Reviews, 3,* 114–130.

Flor, H. (2001). Psychophysiological assessment of the patient with chronic pain. In D. C. Turk & R. Melzack (Eds.), *Handbook of pain assessment* (2nd ed., pp. 70–96). New York, NY: Guilford Press.

Flor, H., Nikolajsen, L., & Staehelin Jensen, T. (2006). Phantom limb pain: A case of maladaptive CNS plasticity? *Nature Reviews Neuroscience, 7,* 873–881.

Flores, G. (2006). Language barriers to health care in the United States. *New England Journal of Medicine, 355,* 229–231.

Floriani, V., & Kennedy, C. (2008). Promotion of physical activity in children. *Current Opinion in Pediatrics, 20,* 90–95.

Flynn, B. S., Worden, J. K., Bunn, J. Y., Solomon, L. J., Ashikaga, T., Connolly, S. W., ... Ramirez, A. G. (2010). Mass media interventions to reduce youth smoking prevalence. *American Journal of Preventive Medicine, 39*(1), 53–62.

Folkman, S., & Lazarus, R. S. (1980). An analysis of coping in a middle-aged community sample. *Journal of Health and Social Behavior, 21,* 219–239.

Folkman, S., & Moskowitz, J. T. (2000). Positive affect and the other side of coping. *American Psychologist, 55,* 647–654.

Folkman, S., & Moskowitz, J. T. (2004). Coping: Pitfalls and promise. *Annual Review of Psychology, 55,* 745–774.

Foltz, V., St. Pierre, Y., Rozenberg, S., Rossignol, M., Bourgeois, P., Joseph, L., ... Fautrel, B. (2005). Use of complementary and alternative therapies by patients with self-reported chronic back pain: A nationwide survey in Canada. *Joint Bone Spine, 72,* 571–577.

Fontana, L., & Hu, F. B. (2014). Optimal body weight for health and longevity: Bridging basic, clinical, and population research. *Aging Cell, 13*(3), 391–400.

Foran, H., & O'Leary, K. (2008). Problem drinking, jealousy, and anger control: Variables predicting physical aggression against a partner. *Journal of Family Violence, 23,* 141–148.

Forbes, G. B. (2000). Body fat content influences the body composition response to nutrition and exercise. *Annals of the New York Academy of Sciences, 904,* 359–368.

Ford, E. S., Ajani, U. A., Croft, J. B., Critchley, J. A., Labarthe, D. R., Kottke, T. E., ... Capewell, S. (2007). Explaining the decrease in U. S. deaths from coronary disease, 1980–2000. *New England Journal of Medicine, 356,* 2388–2398.

Ford, E. S., Bergmann, M. M., Boeing, H., Li, C., & Capewell, S. (2012). Healthy lifestyle behaviors and all-cause mortality among adults in the United States. *Preventive Medicine, 55,* 23–27.

Ford, E. S., Zhao, G., Tsai, J., & Li, C. (2011). Low-risk lifestyle behaviors and all-cause mortality: Findings from the National Health and Nutrition Examination Survey III Mortality Study. *American Journal of Public Health, 101,* 1922–1929.

Fordyce, W. E. (1974). Pain viewed as learned behavior. In J. J. Bonica (Ed.), *Advances in neurology* (Vol. 4, pp. 415–422). New York, NY: Raven Press.

Fordyce, W. E. (1976). *Behavioral methods for chronic pain and illness.* St. Louis, MO: Mosby.

Forlenza, J. J., & Baum, A. (2004). Psychoneuroimmunology. In R. G. Frank, A. Baum, & J. L. Wallander (Eds.), *Handbook of clinical health psychology* (Vol. 3, pp. 81–114). Washington, DC: American Psychological Association.

Foroud, T., Edenberg, H. J., & Crabbe, J. C. (2010). Genetic research: Who is at risk for alcoholism? *Alcohol Research and Health, 33*(1/2), 64–75.

Fortmann, A., Gallo, L. C., & Philis-Tsimkas, A. (2011). Glycemic control among Latinos with Type 2 diabetes: The role of social-environmental support resources. *Health Psychology, 30,* 251–258.

Fothergill, E., Guo, J., Howard, L., Kerns, J. C., Knuth, N. D., Brychta, R., ... Hall, K. D. (2016). Persistent metabolic adaptation 6 years after "The Biggest Loser" competition. *Obesity, 24*(8), 1612–1619.

Foulon, C., Guelfi, J. D., Kipman, A., Adès, J., Romo, L., Houdeyer, K., ... Gorwood, P. (2007). Switching to the bingeing/purging subtype of anorexia nervosa is frequently associated with suicidal attempts. *European Psychiatry, 22,* 513–519.

Fournier, J. C., DeRubeis, R. J., Hollon, S. D., Dimidjian, S., Amsterdam, J. D., Shelton, R. C., ... Fawcett, J. (2010). Antidepressant drug effects and depression severity: A patient-level meta-analysis. *Journal of the American Medical Association, 303,* 47–53.

Fournier, M., de Ridder, D., & Bensing, J. (2002). Optimism and adaptation to chronic disease: The role of optimism in relation to self-care options for Type 1 diabetes mellitus, rheumatoid arthritis and multiple sclerosis. *British Journal of Health Psychology, 7,* 409–432.

Fox, C. S., Heard-Costa, N. L., Wilson, P. W. F., Levy, D., D'Agostino, R. B., Sr., & Atwood, L. D. (2004). Genome-wide linkage to chromosome 6 for waist circumference in the Framingham Heart Study. *Diabetes, 53,* 1399–1402.

Frank, E., Ratanawongsa, N., & Carrera, J. (2010). American medical students' beliefs in the effectiveness of alternative medicine. *International Journal of Collaborative Research on Internal Medicine and Public Health, 2*(9), 292–305.

Franklin, V. L., Waller, A., Pagliari, C., & Greene, S. A. (2006). A randomized controlled trial of Sweet Talk, a text-messaging system to support young people with diabetes. *Diabetic Medicine, 23,* 1332–1338.

Franko, D. L., Becker, A. E., Thomas, J. J., & Herzog, D. B. (2007). Cross-ethnic differences in eating disorder symptoms and related distress. *International Journal of Eating Disorders, 40,* 156–164.

Franks, H. M., & Roesch, S. C. (2006). Appraisals and coping in people living with cancer: A meta-analysis. *Psycho-Oncology, 15,* 1027–1037.

Fraser, G. E., & Shavlik, D. J. (2001). Ten years of life: Is it a matter of choice? *Archives of Internal Medicine, 161,* 1645–1652.

Frattaroli, J. (2006). Experimental disclosure and its moderators: A meta-analysis. *Psychological Bulletin, 132,* 823–865.

Frattaroli, J., Thomas, M., & Lyubomirsky, S. (2011). Opening up in the classroom: Effects of expressive writing on graduate school entrance exam performance. *Emotion, 11,* 691–696.

Frattaroli, J., Weidner, G., Merritt-Worden, T. A., Frenda, S., & Ornish, D. (2008). Angina pectoris and atherosclerotic risk factors in the Multisite Cardiac Lifestyle Intervention Program. *American Journal of Cardiology, 101,* 911–918.

Fredrickson, B. L., & Levenson, R. W. (1998). Positive emotions speed recovery from the cardiovascular sequelae of negative emotions. *Cognition and Emotion, 12*(2), 191–220.

Freedman, D. H. (2011). The triumph of new-age medicine. *The Atlantic, 308*(1), 90–100.

Freedman, D. S., Khan, L. K., Dietz, W. H., Srinivasan, S. R., & Berenson, G. S. (2001). Relationship of childhood obesity to coronary heart disease risk factors in adulthood: The Bogalusa Heart Study. *Pediatrics, 108*, 712–718.

Freedman, L. S., Kipnis, V., Schatzkin, A., & Potischman, N. (2008). Methods of epidemiology: Evaluating the fat-breast cancer hypothesis—Comparing dietary instruments and other developments. *Cancer Journals, 14*(2), 69–74.

Friedenreich, C. M., & Cust, A. E. (2008). Physical activity and breast cancer risk: Impact of timing, type and dose of activity and population subgroup effects. *British Journal of Sports Medicine, 42*, 636–647.

Friedländer, L. (1968). *Roman life and manners under the early empire.* New York, NY: Barnes and Noble.

Friedman, B., Veazie, P. J., Chapman, B. P., Manning, W. G., & Duberstein, P. R. (2013). Is personality associated with health care use by older adults? *Milbank Quarterly, 91*(3), 491–527.

Friedman, M., & Rosenman, R. H. (1974). *Type A behavior and your heart.* New York, NY: Knopf.

Friedman, E., & Thomas, S. A. (1995). Pet ownership, social support, and one-year survival after acute myocardial infarction in the Cardiac Arrhythmia Suppression Trial (CAST). *The American Journal of Cardiology, 76*, 1213–1217.

Friedson, E. (1961). *Patients' views of medical practice.* New York, NY: Russell Sage.

Fries, J. F. (1998). Reducing the need and demand for medical services. *Psychosomatic Medicine, 60*, 140–142.

Frisina, P. G., Borod, J. C., & Lepore, S. J. (2004). A meta-analysis of the effects of written emotional disclosure on the health outcomes of clinical populations. *Journal of Nervous and Mental Disease, 192*, 629–634.

Fromme, H., & Schober, W. (2015). Waterpipes and e-cigarettes: Impact of alternative smoking techniques on indoor air quality and health. *Atmospheric Environment, 106*, 429–441.

Frone, M. R. (2008). Are work stressors related to employee substance use? The importance of temporal context assessment of alcohol and illicit drug use. *Journal of Applied Psychology, 93*, 199–206.

Froom, P., Kristal-Boneh, E., Melamed, S., Gofer, D., Benbassat, J., & Ribak, J. (1999). Smoking cessation and body mass index of occupationally active men: The Israeli CORDIS Study. *American Journal of Public Health, 89*, 718–722.

Fuertes, J. N., Mislowack, A., Bennett, J., Paul, L., Gilbert, T. C., Fontan, G., ... Boylan, L. S. (2007). The physician-patient working alliance. *Patient Education and Counseling, 66*, 29–36.

Fujino, Y., Tamakoshi, A., Iso, H., Inaba, Y., Kubo, T., Ide, R., ... JACC Study Group. (2005). A nationwide cohort study of educational background and major causes of death among the elderly population in Japan. *Preventive Medicine, 40*, 444–451.

Fulkerson, J. A., & French, S. A. (2003). Cigarette smoking for weight loss or control among adolescents: Gender and racial/ethnic differences. *Journal of Adolescent Health, 32*, 306–313.

Fulmer, E. B., Neilands, T. B., Dube, S. R., Kuiper, N. M., Arrazola, R. A., & Glantz, S. A. (2015). Protobacco media exposure and youth susceptibility to smoking cigarettes, cigarette experimentation, and current tobacco use among US youth. *PLoS One, 10*(8), e0134734.

Fumal, A., & Schoenen, J. (2008). Tension-type headache: Current research and clinical management. *Lancet Neurology, 7*, 70–83.

Fung, T. T., Chiuve, S. E., McCullough, M. L., Rexrode, K. M., Logroscino, G., & Hu, F. B. (2008). Adherence to a DASH-style diet and risk of coronary heart disease and stroke in women. *Archives of Internal Medicine, 168*, 713–720.

Furberg, H., YunJung, K., Dackor, J., Boerwinkle, E., Franceschini, N., Ardissinio, D., ... Sullivan, P. F. (2010). Genome-wide meta-analyses identify multiple loci associated with smoking behavior. *Nature Genetics, 42*(5), 441–447.

Furlan, A. D., Imamura, M., Dryden, T., & Irvin, E. (2008). Massage for low-back pain. *Cochrane Database of Systematic Reviews 2008*, Issue 4, Cochrane Art. No.: CD001929, DOI: 10.1002/14651858. CD001929. pub2.

Furlan, A. D., Yazdi, F., Tsertsvadze, A., Gross, A., Van Tulder, M., Santaguida, L., ... Tsouros, S. (2012). A systematic review and meta-analysis of efficacy, cost-effectiveness, and safety of selected complementary and alternative medicine for neck and low-back pain. *Evidence-based Complementary and Alternative Medicine, 2012*, 1–61.

Furnham, A. (2007). Are modern health worries, personality and attitudes to science associated with the use of complementary and alternative medicine? *British Journal of Health Psychology, 12*, 229–243.

Gaab, J., Sonderegger, L., Scherrer, S., & Ehlert, U. (2007). Psychoneuroendocrine effects of cognitive-behavioral stress management in a naturalistic setting—A randomized controlled trial. *Psychoneuroendocrinology, 31*, 428–438.

Gabriel, R., Ferrando, L., Cortón, E. S., Mingote, C., García-Camba, E., Liria, A. F., ...Gale, S. (2007). Psychopathological consequences after a terrorist attack: An epidemiological study among victims, the general population, and police officers. *European Psychiatry, 22*, 339–346.

Gaesser, G. A. (2003). Weight, weight loss, and health: A closer look at the evidence. *Healthy Weight Journal, 17*, 8–11.

Gagliese, L., Weizblit, N., Ellis, W., & Chan, V. W. S. (2005). The measurement of postoperative pain: A comparison of intensity scales in younger and older surgical patients. *Pain, 117*, 412–420.

Galdas, P. M., Cheater, F., & Marshall, P. (2005). Men and health help-seeking behavior: Literature review. *Journal of Advanced Nursing, 49*, 616–623.

Gallagher, B. (2003). Tai chi chuan and qigong. *Topics in Geriatric Rehabilitation, 19*, 172–182.

Galland, L. (2006). Patient-centered care: Antecedents, triggers, and mediators. *Alternative Therapies, 12*, 62–70.

Gallegos-Macias, A. R., Macias, S. R., Kaufman, E., Skipper, B., & Kalishman, N. (2003). Relationship between glycemic control, ethnicity and socioeconomic status in Hispanic and white non-Hispanic youths with Type 1 diabetes mellitus. *Pediatric Diabetes, 4*, 19–23.

Galloway, G. P., Coyle, J. R., Guillén, J. E., Flower, K., & Mendelson, J. E. (2011). A simple, novel method for assessing medication adherence: Capsule photographs taken with cellular telephones. *Journal of Addiction Medicine, 5*, 170–174.

Gambrill, S. (2008, April). Magic Johnson—Celebrity spokesperson for minority patient recruitment? *Clinical Trials Today.* Retrieved June 30, 2008, from http://www.clinicaltrialstoday.com/2008/04/magic-johnsonce.html

Gan, T. J., Gordon, D. B., Bolge, S. C., & Allen, J. G. (2007). Patient-controlled analgesia: Patient and nurse satisfaction with intravenous delivery systems and expected satisfaction with transdermal delivery systems. *Current Medical Research and Opinion, 23*, 2507–2516.

Gandini, S., Botteri, E., Iodice, S., Boniol, M., Lowenfels, A. B., Maison-neuve, P., ... Boyle, P. (2008). Tobacco smoking and cancer: A meta-analysis. *International Journal of Cancer, 122*, 155–164.

Gans, J. A., & McPhillips, T. (2003). Medication compliance-adherence-persistence. *Medication Compliance-Adherence-Persistence (CAP) Digest, 1*, 1–32.

Gao, L., Weck, M. N., Stegmaier, C., Rothenbacher, D., & Brenner, H. (2010). Alcohol consumption, serum gamma-glutamyltransferase, and Helicobacter pylori infection in a population-based study among 9733 adults. *Annals of Epidemiology, 20*(2), 122–128.

Garavello, W., Negri, E., Talamini, R., Levi, F., Zambon, P., Dal Maso, L., ... La Vecchia, C. (2005). Family history of cancer, its combination with smoking and drinking, and risk of squamous cell carcinoma of the esophagus. *Cancer Epidemiology, Biomarkers, and Prevention, 14*, 1390–1393.

Garber, C. E., Blissmer, B., Deschenes, M. R., Franklin, B. A., Lamonte, M. J., Lee, I.-M., ... Swain, D. P. (2011). Quantity and quality of exercise for developing and maintaining cardiorespiratory, musculoskeletal, and neuromotor fitness in apparently healthy adults: Guidance for prescribing exercise. *Medicine and Science in Sports and Exercise, 43,* 1334–1359.

Garber, M. C. (2004). The concordance of self-report with other measures of medication adherence: A summary of the literature. *Medical Care, 42,* 649–652.

García, J., Simón, M. A., Durán, M., Canceller, J., & Aneiros, F. J. (2006). Differential efficacy of a cognitive-behavioral intervention versus pharmacological treatment in the management of fibromyalgic syndrome. *Psychology, Health and Medicine, 11,* 498–506.

Garcia, K., & Mann, T. (2003). From "I wish" to "I will": Social-cognitive predictors of behavioral intentions. *Journal of Health Psychology, 8,* 347–360.

Garland, E. L., Gaylord, S. A., Palsson, O., Faurot, K., Mann, J. D., & Whitehead, W. E. (2012). Therapeutic mechanisms of a mindfulness-based treatment for IBS: Effects on visceral sensitivity, catastrophizing, and affective processing of pain sensations. *Journal of Behavioral Medicine, 35*(6), 591–602.

Garner, D. M., & Garfinkel, P. E. (1980). Social-cultural factors in the development of anorexia nervosa. *Psychological Medicine, 10,* 647–656.

Garner, D. M., Garfinkel, P. E., Schwartz, D., & Thompson, M. (1980). Cultural expectations of thinness in women. *Psychological Reports, 47,* 483–491.

Garofalo, R., Herrick, A., Mustanski, B. S., & Donenberg, G. R. (2007). Tip of the iceberg: Young men who have sex with men, the Internet, and HIV risk. *American Journal of Public Health, 97,* 1113–1117.

Garssen, B. (2004). Psychological factors and cancer development. Evidence after 30 years of research. *Clinical Psychology Review, 24,* 115–338.

Gatchel, R. J. (2005). The biopsychosocial approach to pain assessment and management. In R. J. Gatchel (Ed.), *Clinical essentials of pain management* (pp. 23–46). Washington, DC: American Psychological Association.

Gatchel, R. J., & Epker, J. (1999). Psychosocial predictors of chronic pain and response to treatment. In R. J. Gatchel & D. C. Turk (Eds.), *Psychosocial factors in pain: Critical perspectives* (pp. 412–434). New York, NY: Guilford Press.

Gatchel, R. J., Peng, Y. B., Peters, M. L., Fuchs, P. N., & Turk, D. C. (2007). The biopsychosocial approach to chronic pain: Scientific advances and future directions. *Psychological Bulletin, 133*(4), 581.

Gatzounis, R., Schrooten, M. G., Crombez, G., & Vlaeyen, J. W. (2012). Operant learning theory in pain and chronic pain rehabilitation. *Current Pain and Headache Reports, 16*(2), 117–126.

Geary, D. C., & Flinn, M. V. (2002). Sex differences in behavioral and hormonal response to social threat: Commentary on Taylor et al. (2000). *Psychological Review, 109,* 745–750.

Geisser, M. E., Ranavaya, M., Haig, A. J., Roth, R. S., Zucker, R., Ambroz, C., … Caruso, M. (2005). A meta-analytic review of surface electromyography among persons with low back pain and normal, healthy controls. *Journal of Pain, 6,* 711–726.

Gelhaar, T., Seiffge-Krenke, I., Borge, A., Cicognani, E., Cunha, M., Loncaric, D., … Metzke, C. W. (2007). Adolescent coping with everyday stressors: A seven-nation study of youth from central, eastern, southern, and northern Europe. *European Journal of Developmental Psychology, 4,* 129–156.

Gellad, W. F., Haas, J. S., & Safran, D. G. (2007). Race/ethnicity and non-adherence to prescription medications among seniors: Results of a national study. *Journal of General Internal Medicine, 22,* 1572–1578.

Gemmell, L., & DiClemente, C. C. (2009). Styles of physician advice about smoking cessation in college students. *Journal of American College Health, 58*(2), 113–119.

George, S., Rogers, R. D., & Duka, T. K. (2005). The acute effect of alcohol on decision making in social drinkers. *Psychopharmacology, 182,* 160–169.

Georges, J., Jansen, S., Jackson, J., Meyrieux, A., Sadowska, A., & Selmes, M. (2008). Alzheimer's disease in real life—The dementia carer's survey. *International Journal of Geriatric Psychiatry, 23,* 546–553.

Gerteis, J., Izrael, D., Deitz, D., LeRoy, L., Ricciardi, R., Miller, T., & Basu, J. (2014). *Multiple chronic conditions chartbook.* Rockville, MD: Agency for Healthcare Research and Quality (AHRQ) Publications.

Gervais, R. (2010, March/April). *Week one hundred and twelve* [Web log comment]. Retrieved from http://www.rickygervais.com/thissideofthetruthc.php

Gibbons, F. X., Gerrard, M., Blanton, H., & Russell, D. W. (1998). Reasoned action and social reaction: Willingness and intention as independent predictors of health risk. *Journal of Personality and Social Psychology, 74,* 1164–1180.

Gibney, A. (director). (2013). *The Armstrong Lie [Motion picture].* United States: Sony Pictures Classics.

Gidycz, C. A., Orchowski, L. M., King, C. R., & Rich, C. L. (2008). Sexual victimization and health-risk behaviors: A prospective analysis of college women. *Journal of Interpersonal Violence, 23,* 744–763.

Gielkens-Sijstermans, C. M., Mommers, M. A., Hoogeveen, R. T., Feenstra, T. L., de Vreede, J., Bovens, F. M., … van Schayck, O. C. (2010). Reduction of smoking in Dutch adolescents over the past decade and its health gains: A repeated cross-sectional study. *European Journal of Public Health, 20*(2), 146–150.

Giggins, O., Persson, U. M., & Caulfield, B. (2013). Biofeedback in rehabilitation. *Journal of NeuorEngineering and Rehabilitation, 10*(1), 1–11.

Gilbert, M. T. P., Rambaut, A., Wlasiuk, G., Spira, T. J., Pitchenik, A. E., & Worobey, M. (2007). The emergence of HIV/AIDS in the Americas and beyond. *Proceedings of the National Academy of Sciences of the United States of America, 104,* 18566–18570.

Gillies, C. L., Abrams, K. R., Lambert, P. C., Cooper, N. J., Sutton, A. J., & Hsu, R. T. (2007). Pharmacological and lifestyle interventions to prevent or delay Type 2 diabetes in people with impaired glucose tolerance: Systematic review and meta-analysis. *British Medical Journal, 334,* 299–302.

Gilpin, E. A., White, M. M., Messer, K., & Pierce, J. P. (2007). Receptivity to tobacco advertising and promotions among young adolescents as a predictor of established smoking in young adulthood. *American Journal of Public Health, 97,* 1489–1495.

Ginsberg, J., Mohebbi, M. H., Patel, R. S., Brammer, L., Smolinski, M. S., & Brilliant, L. (2009). Detecting influenza epidemics using search engine query data. *Nature, 457,* 1012–1014.

Glaser, R. (2005). Stress-associated immune dysregulation and its importance for human health: A personal history of psychoneuroimmunology. *Brain, Behavior and Immunity, 19,* 3–11.

Glassman, A. H., Bigger, T., & Gaffney, M. (2009). Psychiatric characteristics associated with long-term mortality among 361 patients having an acute coronary syndrome and major depression. *Archives of General Psychiatry, 66,* 1022–1029.

Glueckauf, R. L., Ketterson, T. U., Loomis, J. S., & Dages, P. (2004). Online support and education for dementia caregivers: Overview, utilization, and initial program evaluation. *Telemedicine Journal and e-Health, 10*(2), n.p.

Godfrey, J. R. (2004). Toward optimal health: The experts discuss therapeutic humor. *Journal of Women's Health, 13,* 474–479.

Godfrey, K., Gallo, L., & Afari, N. (2015). Mindfulness-based interventions for binge eating: A systematic review and meta-analysis. *Journal of Behavioral Medicine, 38*(2), 348–362.

Goffaux, P., Redmond, W. J., Rainville, P., & Marchand, S. (2007). Descending analgesia: When the spine echoes what the brain expects. *Pain, 130,* 137–143.

Gold, D. R., & Wright, R. (2005). Population disparities in asthma. *Annual Review of Public Health, 26,* 89–113.

Goldman, R. (2007, November 6). Halle Berry says she cured herself of Type 1 diabetes, but doctors say that's impossible. *ABC News on Call.* Retrieved June 28, 2008, from http://abcnews.go.com/Health/DiabetesResource/Story?id=3822870&page=1

Goldring, M. B., & Goldring, S. R. (2007). Osteoarthritis. *Journal of Cellular Physiology, 213,* 626–634.

Goldschmidt, A. B., Jones, M., Manwaring, J. L., Luce, K. H., Osborne, M. I., Cunning, D., … Taylor, C. B. (2008). The clinical significance of loss of control over eating in overweight adolescents. *International Journal of Eating Disorders, 41,* 153–158.

Goldsmith, C. (2004). Fetal alcohol syndrome: A preventable tragedy. *Access, 18*(5), 34–38.

Goldstein, A. (1976). Opioid peptides (endorphins) in pituitary and brain. *Science, 193,* 1081–1086.

Goldston, K., & Baillie, A. J. (2008). Depression and coronary heart disease: A review of the epidemiological evidence, explanatory mechanisms and management approaches. *Clinical Psychology Review, 28*, 289–307.

Gomez, S. L., Hurley, S., Canchola, A. J., Keegan, T. H., Cheng, I., Murphy, J. D., … Martínez, M. E. (2016). Effects of marital status and economic resources on survival after cancer: A population-based study. *Cancer, 122*(10), 1618–1625.

Gonçalves, R. B., Coletta, R. D., Silvério, K. G., Benevides, L., Casati, M. Z., da Silva, J. S., … Nociti, F. H., Jr. (2011). Impact of smoking on inflammation: Overview of molecular mechanisms. *Inflammation Research, 60*(5), 409–424.

Gonder-Frederick, L. A., Cox, D. J., & Ritterband, L. M. (2002). Diabetes and behavioral medicine: The second decade. *Journal of Consulting and Clinical Psychology, 70*, 611–625.

Gonzalez, J. S., Penedo, F. J., Antoni, M. H., Durán, R. E., Fernandez, M. I., McPherson-Baker, S., … Schneiderman, N. (2004). Social support, positive states of mind, and HIV treatment adherence in men and women living with HIV/AIDS. *Health Psychology, 23*, 413–418.

Gonzalez, J. S., Peyrot, M., McCarl, L. A., Collins, E. M., Serpa, L., Mimiaga, M. J., … Safren, S. A. (2008). Depression and diabetes treatment nonadherence: A meta-analysis. *Diabetes Care, 31*, 2398–2403.

Gonzalez, R., Nolen-Hoeksema, S., & Treynor, W. (2003). Rumination reconsidered: A psychometric analysis. *Cognitive Therapy and Research, 27*, 247–259.

Goode, A. D., Reeves, M. M., & Eakin, E. G. (2012). Telephone-delivered interventions for physical activity and dietary behavior change: An updated systematic review. *American Journal of Preventive Medicine, 42*, 81–88.

Goodpaster, B. H., Krishnaswami, S., Harris, T. B., Katsiaras, A., Kritchevsky, S. B., Simonsick, E. M., … Newman, A. B. (2005). Obesity, regional body fat distribution, and the metabolic syndrome in older men and women. *Archives of Internal Medicine, 165*, 777–783.

Goodwin, D. G. (1976). *Is alcoholism hereditary?* New York, NY: Oxford University Press.

Gottfredson, L. S., & Deary, I. J. (2004). Intelligence predicts health and longevity, but why? *Current Directions in Psychological Science, 13*, 1–4.

Gouzoulis-Mayfrank, E., & Daumann, J. (2006). The confounding problem of polydrug use in recreational ecstasy/MDMA users: A brief overview. *Journal of Psychopharmacology, 20*, 188–193.

Goyal, M., Singh, S., Sibinga, E. M., Gould, N. F., Rowland-Seymour, A., Sharma, R., … Haythornthwaite, J. A. (2014). Meditation programs for psychological stress and well-being: A systematic review and meta-analysis. *JAMA Internal Medicine, 174*(3), 357–368.

Grafton, K. V., Foster, N. E., & Wright, C. C. (2005). Test-retest reliability of the Short-Form McGill Pain Questionnaire: Assessment of intraclass correlation coefficients and limits of agreement in patients with osteoarthritis. *Clinical Journal of Pain, 21*, 73–82.

Graham, J. E., Christian, L. M., & Kiecolt-Glaser, J. K. (2006). Marriage, health, and immune function. In S. R. H. Beach, M. Z. Wamboldt, N. J. Kaslow, R. E. Heyman, M. B. First, L. G. Underwood … D. Reiss (Eds.), *Relational processes and DSM-V: Neuroscience, assessment, prevention, and treatment* (pp. 61–76). Washington, DC: American Psychiatric Association.

Graham, J. E., Glaser, R., Loving, T. J., Malarkey, W. B., Stowell, J. R., & Kiecolt-Glaser, J. K. (2009). Cognitive word use during marital conflict and increases in proinflammatory cytokines. *Health Psychology, 28*, 621–630.

Graham, K., Bernards, S., Wilsnack, S. C., & Gmel, G. (2011). Alcohol may not cause partner violence but it seems to make it worse: A cross national comparison of the relationship between alcohol and severity of partner violence. *Journal of Interpersonal Violence, 26*(8), 1503–1523.

Graig, E. (1993). Stress as a consequence of the urban physical environment. In L. Goldberger & S. Breznitz (Eds.), *Handbook of stress: Theoretical and clinical aspects* (2nd ed., pp. 316–332). New York, NY: Free Press.

Grant, B. F., Hasin, D. S., Chou, S. P., Stinson, F. S., & Dawson, D. A. (2004). Nicotine dependence and psychiatric disorders in the United States. *Archives of General Psychiatry, 61*, 1107–1115.

Grant, J. A., Courtemanche, J., Duerden, E. G., Duncan, G. H., & Rainville, P. (2010). Cortical thickness and pain sensitivity in Zen Meditators. *Emotion, 10*(1), 43–53.

Greenwood, B. N., Foley, T. E., Day, H. E. W., Burhans, D., Brooks, L., Campeau, S., … Fleshner, M. (2005). Wheel running alters serotonin (5-HT) transporter, 5-HT1A, 5-HT1B, and alpha1b-adrenergic receptor mRNA in the rat raphe nuclei. *Biological Psychiatry, 57*, 559–568.

Griffin, J. A., Umstattd, M. R., & Usdan, S. L. (2010). Alcohol use and high-risk sexual behavior among collegiate women: A review of research on alcohol myopia theory. *Journal of American College Health, 58*(6), 523–532.

Griffing, S., Lewis, C. S., Chu, M., Sage, R. E., Madry, L., & Primm, B. J. (2006). Exposure to interpersonal violence as a predictor of PTSD symptomatology in domestic violence survivors. *Journal of Interpersonal Violence, 21*, 936–954.

Grilo, C. M., Hrabosky, J. I., White, M. A., Allison, K. C., Stunkard, A. J., & Masheb, R. M. (2008). Overvaluation of shape and weight in binge eating disorder and overweight controls: Refinement of a diagnostic construct. *Journal of Abnormal Psychology, 117*, 414–419.

Groenewald, C., Beals-Erickson, S., Ralston-Wilson, J., Rabbitts, J., & Palermo, T. (2016). Complementary and alternative medicine use among children with pain in the United States: Patterns, predictors, and perceived benefits. *Journal of Pain, 17*(4), S113.

Grogan, S. (2007). *Body image: Understanding body dissatisfaction in men, women, and children* (rev. ed.). New York, NY: Routledge.

Grossman, P., Niemann, L., Schmidt, S., & Walach, H. (2004). Mindfulness-based stress reduction and health benefits: A meta-analysis. *Journal of Psychosomatic Research, 57*, 35–43.

Grover, S. A., Gray-Donald, K., Joseph, L., Abrahamowicz, M., & Coupal, L. (1994). Life expectancy following dietary modification or smoking cessation. *Archives of Internal Medicine, 154*, 1697–1704.

Grundy, S. M. (2007). Cardiovascular and metabolic risk factors: How can we improve outcomes in the high-risk patient? *American Journal of Medicine, 120*(Suppl. 1), S3–S8.

Grundy, S. M., Cleeman, J. I., Bairey Merz, C. N., Brewer, B., Jr., Clark, L. T., Hunninghake, D. B., … Stone, N. J. (2004). Implications of recent clinical trials for the National Cholesterol Education Program Adult Treatment Panel III guidelines. *Circulation, 110*, 227–239.

Grzywacz, J. G., Almeida, D. M., Neupert, S. D., & Ettner, S. L. (2004). Socioeconomic status and health: A micro-level analysis of exposure and vulnerability to daily stressors. *Journal of Health and Social Behavior, 45*, 1–16.

Gu, J., Strauss, C., Bond, R., & Cavanagh, K. (2015). How do mindfulness-based cognitive therapy and mindfulness-based stress reduction improve mental health and wellbeing? A systematic review and meta-analysis of mediation studies. *Clinical Psychology Review, 37*, 1–12.

Guck, T. P., Kavan, M. G., Elsasser, G. N., & Barone, E. J. (2001). Assessment and treatment of depression following myocardial infarction. *American Family Physician, 64*, 641–656.

Guevara, J. P., Wolf, F. M., Grum, C. M., & Clark, N. M. (2003). Effects of educational interventions for self-management of asthma in children and adolescents: Systematic review and meta-analysis. *British Medical Journal, 326*, 1308–1309.

Guillot, J., Kilpatrick, M., Hebert, E., & Hollander, D. (2004). Applying the transtheoretical model to exercise adherence in clinical settings. *American Journal of Health Studies, 19*, 1–10.

Gull, W. W. (1874). Anorexia nervosa (apepsia hysterica, anorexia hysterica). *Transactions of the Clinical Society of London, 7*, 22–28. [Reprinted in R. M. Kaufman & M. Heiman (Eds.), *Evolution of psychosomatic concepts: Anorexia nervosa, a paradigm*. New York: International University Press, 1964.]

Günes, C., & Rudolph, K. L. (2013). The role of telomeres in stem cells and cancer. *Cell, 152*(3), 390–393.

Guo, Q., Johnson, C. A., Unger, J. B., Lee, L., Xie, B., Chou, C.-P., … Pentz, M. (2007). Utility of the theory of reasoned action and theory of planned behavior for predicting Chinese adolescent smoking. *Addictive Behaviors, 32*, 1066–1081.

Guo, X., Zhou, B., Nishimura, T., Teramukai, S., & Fukushima, M. (2008). Clinical effect of qigong practice on essential hypertension: A meta-analysis of randomized controlled trials. *Journal of Alternative and Complementary Medicine, 14*, 27–37.

Gustafson, E. M., Meadows-Oliver, M., & Banasiak, N. C. (2008). Asthma in childhood. In T. P. Gullotta & G. M. Blau (Eds.), *Handbook of childhood behavioral issues: Evidence-based approaches to prevention and treatment* (pp. 167–186). New York, NY: Routledge/Taylor and Francis.

Gustavsson, P., Jakobsson, R., Nyberg, F., Pershagen, G., Järup, L., & Schéele, P. (2000). Occupational exposure and lung cancer risk: A population-based case-referent study in Sweden. *American Journal of Epidemiology, 152*, 32–40.

Ha, M., Mabuchi, K., Sigurdson, A. J., Freedman, D. M., Linet, M. S., & Doody, M. M. (2007). Smoking cigarettes before first childbirth and risk of breast cancer. *American Journal of Epidemiology, 166*, 55–61.

Haak, T., & Scott, B. (2008). The effect of qigong on fibromyaliga (FMS): A controlled randomized study. *Disability and Rehabilitation, 30*, 625–633.

Haan, M. N., & Wallace, R. (2004). Can dementia be prevented? Brain aging in a population-base. *Annual Review of Public Health, 25*, 1–24.

Haas, M., Spegman, A., Peterson, D., Aickin, M., & Vavrek, D. (2010). Dose response and efficacy of spinal manipulation for chronic cervi-cogenic headache: A pilot randomized controlled trial. *Spine Journal, 10*(2), 117–128.

Haberer, J. E., Kiwanuka, J., Nansera, D., Ragland, K., Mellins, C., & Bangsberg, D. R. (2012). Multiple measures reveal antiretroviral adherence successes and challenges in HIV-infected Ugandan children. *PLoS One, 7*(5), e36737.

Hagedoorn, M., Kujer, R. G., Buuk, B. P., DeJong, G. M., Wobbes, T., & Sanderman, R. (2000). Marital satisfaction in patients with cancer: Does support from intimate partners benefit those who need it the most? *Health Psychology, 19*, 274–282.

Hagger, M. S., & Orbell, S. (2003). A meta-analytic review of the commonsense model of illness representations. *Psychology and Health, 18*, 141–184.

Hagimoto, A., Nakamura, M., Morita, T., Masui, S., & Oshima, A. (2010). Smoking cessation patterns and predictors of quitting smoking among the Japanese general population: A 1-year follow-up study. *Addiction, 105*(1), 164–173.

Haimanot, R. T. (2002). Burden of headache in Africa. *Journal of Headache and Pain, 4*, 47–54.

Halberstadt, A. L., & Geyer, M. A. (2011). Multiple receptors contribute to the behavioral effects of indoleamine hallucinogens. *Neuropharmacology, 61*(3), 364–381.

Hale, C. J., Hannum, J. W., & Espelage, D. L. (2005). Social support and physical health: The importance of belonging. *Journal of American College Health, 53*, 276–284.

Hale, S., Grogan, S., & Willott, S. (2007). Patterns of self-referral in men with symptoms of prostate disease. *British Journal of Health Psychology, 12*, 403–419.

Hall, C. B., Verghese, J., Sliwinski, M., Chen, Z., Katz, M., Derby, C., … Lipton, R. B. (2005). Dementia incidence may increase more slowly after age 90: Results from the Bronx Aging Study. *Neurology, 65*, 882–886.

Hall, J. A., Blanch-Hartigan, D., & Roter, D. L. (2011). Patients' satisfaction with male versus female physicians: A meta-analysis. *Medical Care, 49*, 611–617.

Hall, M. A., & Schneider, C. E. (2008). Patients as consumers: Courts, contracts, and the new medical marketplace. *Michigan Law Review, 106*, 643–689.

Halpern, P., Moskovich, J., Avrahami, B., Bentur, Y., Soffer, D., & Peleg, K. (2011). Morbidity associated with MDMA (ecstacy) abuse: A survey of emergency department admissions. *Human and Experimental Toxicology, 30*(4), 259–266.

Hamel, L. M., Robbins, L. B., & Wilbur, J. (2011). Computer- and web-based interventions to increase preadolescent and adolescent

physical activity: A systematic review. *Journal of Advanced Nursing, 67*, 251–268.

Hamer, M., & Karageorghis, C. (2007). Psychobiological mechanisms of exercise dependence. *Sports Medicine, 37*, 477–485.

Hamer, M., & Steptoe, A. (2007). Association between physical fitness, parasympathetic control, and proinflammatory responses to mental stress. *Psychosomatic Medicine, 69*, 660–666.

Hamer, M., Taylor, A., & Steptoe, A. (2006). The effect of acute aerobic exercise on stress related blood pressure responses: A systematic review and meta-analysis. *Biological Psychology, 71*, 183–190.

Hammond, D. (2005). Smoking behaviour among young adults: Beyond youth prevention. *Tobacco Control, 14*, 181–185.

Hanewinkel, R., & Sargent, J. D. (2007). Exposure to smoking in popular contemporary movies and youth smoking in Germany. *American Journal of Preventive Medicine, 32*, 466–473.

Hanley, M. A., Jensen, M. P., Smith, D. G., Ehde, D. M., Edwards, W. T., & Robinson, L. R. (2007). Preamputation pain and acute pain predict chronic pain after lower extremity amputation. *Journal of Pain, 8*, 102–109.

Hann, K. E., & McCracken, L. M. (2014). A systematic review of randomized controlled trials of Acceptance and Commitment Therapy for adults with chronic pain: Outcome domains, design quality, and efficacy. *Journal of Contextual Behavioral Science, 3*(4), 217–227.

Hansen, C. J., Stevens, L. C., & Coast, J. R. (2001). Exercise duration and mood state: How much is enough to feel better? *Health Psychology, 20*, 267–275.

Hansen, K., Shriver, T., & Schoeller, D. (2005). The effects of exercise on the storage and oxidation of dietary fat. *Sports Medicine, 35*, 363–373.

Hansen, P. E., Floderus, B., Frederiksen, K., & Johansen, C. B. (2005). Personality traits, health behavior, and risk for cancer: A prospective study of a Swedish twin cohort. *Cancer, 103*, 1082–1091.

Hanson-Turton, T., Ryan, S., Miller, K., Counts, M., & Nash, D. B. (2007). Convenient care clinics: The future of accessible health care. *Disease Management, 10*(2), 61–73.

Hanvik, L. J. (1951). MMPI profiles in patients with low back pain. *Journal of Consulting and Clinical Psychology, 15*, 350–353.

Harakeh, Z., Engels, R. C. M. E., Monshouwer, K., & Hanssen, P. F. (2010). Adolescent's weight concerns and the onset of smoking. *Substance Use and Misuse, 45*(12), 1847–1860.

Harakeh, Z., & Vollebergh, W. A. M. (2012). The impact of active and passive peer influence on young adult smoking: An experimental study. *Drug and Alcohol Dependence, 121*(3), 220–223.

Harburg, E., Julius, M., Kaciroti, N., Gleiberman, L., & Schork, M. A. (2003). Expressive/suppressive anger-coping responses, gender, and types of mortality: A 17–year follow-up (Tecumseh, Michigan, 1971–1988). *Psychosomatic Medicine, 65*, 588–597.

Harder, B. (2004). Asthma counterattack. *Science News, 166*, 344–345.

Harper, C., & Matsumoto, I. (2005). Ethanol and brain damage. *Current Opinion in Pharmacology, 5*, 73–78.

Harriger, J., Calogero, R., Witherington, D., & Smith, J. (2010). Body size stereotyping and internalization of the thin ideal in preschool girls. *Sex Roles, 63*(9/10), 609–620.

Harrington, A. (2008). *The cure within: A history of mind-body medicine.* New York, NY: Norton.

Harrington, J., Noble, L. M., & Newman, S. P. (2004). Improving patients' communication with doctors: A systematic review of intervention studies. *Patient Education and Counseling, 52*, 7–16.

Harris, M. I. (2001). Racial and ethnic differences in health care access and health outcomes for adults with Type 2 diabetes. *Diabetes Care, 24*, 454–459.

Harrison, B. J., Olver, J. S., Norman, T. R., & Nathan, P. J. (2002). Effects of serotonin and catecholamine depletion on interleukin-6 activation and mood in human volunteers. *Human Psychopharmacology: Clinical and Experimental, 17*, 293–297.

Harter, J. K., & Stone, A. A. (2012). Engaging and disengaging work conditions, momentary experiences and cortisol response. *Motivation and Emotion, 36*(2), 104–113.

Hartz, A., Kent, S., James, P., Xu, Y., Kelly, M., & Daly, J. (2006). Factors that influence improvement for patients with poorly controlled

Type 2 diabetes. *Diabetes Research and Clinical Practice, 74,* 227–232.

Hartz, A. J., Rupley, D. C., & Rimm, A. A. (1984). The association of girth measurements with disease in 32,856 women. *American Journal of Epidemiology, 119,* 71–80.

Harvie, D. S., Broecker, M., Smith, R. T., Meulders, A., Madden, V. J., & Moseley, G. L. (2015). Bogus visual feedback alters onset of movement-evoked pain in people with neck pain. *Psychological Science, 26*(4), 385–392.

Hasin, D. S., Keyes, K. M., Hatzenbuehler, M. L., Aharonovich, E. A., & Alderson, D. (2007). Alcohol consumption and posttraumatic stress after exposure to terrorism: Effects of proximity, loss, and psychiatric history. *American Journal of Public Health, 97,* 2268–2275.

Hass, N. (2012). Hope Solo drops her guard. *Smithsonian Magazine,* July 2012. Retrieved September 22, 2016, from http://www.smithsonianmag.com/people-places/hope-solo-drops-her-guard-138385366/

Hatfield, J., & Job, R. F. S. (2001). Optimism bias about environmental degradation: The role of the range of impact of precautions. *Journal of Environmental Psychology, 21,* 17–30.

Hausenblas, H. A., & Symons Downs, D. (2002a). Exercise dependence: A systematic review. *Psychology of Sport and Exercise, 3,* 89–123.

Hausenblas, H. A., & Symons Downs, D. (2002b). Relationship among sex, imagery, and exercise dependence symptoms. *Psychology of Addictive Behaviors, 16,* 169–172.

Hausenloy, D. J., & Yellon, D. M. (2008). Targeting residual cardiovascular risk: Raising high-density lipoprotein cholesterol levels. *Heart, 94,* 706–714.

Hawkley, L. C., & Cacioppo, J. T. (2003). Loneliness and pathways to disease. *Brain, Behavior and Immunity, 17,* 98–105.

Hawkley, L. C., & Cacioppo, J. T. (2007). Aging and loneliness: Downhill quickly? *Current Directions in Psychological Science, 16,* 187–191.

Hay, P., Girosi, F., & Mond, J. (2015). Prevalence and sociodemographis correlates of DSM-5 eating disorders in the Australian population. *Journal of Eating Disorders, 3,* 19.

Hay, P. J., & de M. Claudino, A. (2010). Evidence-based treatment for eating disorders. In W. S. Agras (Ed.), *The Oxford handbook of eating disorders* (pp. 452–479). New York, NY: Oxford University Press.

Hayes, S., Bulow, C., Clarke, R., Vega, E., Vega-Perez, E., Ellison, L., … Stover, K. (2000). Incidence of low back pain in women who are pregnant. *Physical Therapy, 80,* 34.

Hayes-Bautista, D. E., Hsu, P., Hayes-Bautista, M., Iniguez, D., Chamberlin, C. L., Rico, C., … Solorio, R. (2002). An anomaly within the Latino epidemiological paradox: The Latino adolescent male mortality peak. *Archives of Pediatrics and Adolescent Medicine, 156,* 480–484.

Haynes, R. B. (1976). Strategies for improving compliance: A methodologic analysis and review. In D. L. Sackett & R. B. Haynes (Eds.), *Compliance with therapeutic regimens* (pp. 69–82). Baltimore, MD: Johns Hopkins University Press.

Haynes, R. B. (1979). Introduction. In R. B. Haynes, D. W. Taylor, & D. L. Sackett (Eds.), *Compliance in health care* (pp. 1–7). Baltimore, MD: Johns Hopkins University Press.

Haynes, R. B. (2001). Improving patient adherence: State of the art, with a special focus on medication taking for cardiovascular disorders. In L. E. Burke & I. S. Ockene (Eds.), *Compliance in healthcare and research* (pp. 3–21). Armonk, NY: Futura.

Haynes, R. B., Ackloo, E., Sahota, N., McDonald, H. P., & Yao, X. (2008). Interventions for enhancing medication adherence. *Cochrane Database of Systematic Reviews,* Cochrane Art. No.: CD000011, DOI: 10.1002/14651858.CD000011.pub3.

Haynes, R. B., McDonald, H. P., & Garg, A. X. (2002). Helping patients follow prescribed treatment: Clinical applications. *Journal of the American Medical Association, 288,* 2880–2883.

He, D. (2005). An introduction to Chinese medical qi gong. *New England Journal of Traditional Chinese Medicine, 4,* 42–44.

HealthGrades. (2011). *Eighth annual patient safety in American hospitals study.* Retrieved November 2, 2011, from http://www.healthgrades.com

Hearn, W. L., Flynn, D. D., Hime, G. W., Rose, S., Cofino, J. C., Mantero-Atienza, E., … Mash, D. C. (1991). Cocaethylene: A unique cocaine metabolite displays high affinity for the dopamine transporter. *Journal of Neurochemistry, 56,* 698–701.

Heather, N. (2006). Controlled drinking, harm reduction and their roles in the response to alcohol-related problems. *Addiction Research and Theory, 14,* 7–18.

Heijmans, M., Rijken, M., Foets, M., de Ridder, D., Schreurs, K., & Bensing, J. (2004). The stress of being chronically ill: From disease-specific to task-specific aspects. *Journal of Behavioral Medicine, 27,* 255–271.

Heikkilä, K., Nyberg, S. T., Theorell, T., Fransson, E. I., Alfredsson, L., Bjorner, J. B., … Kivimaki, M. (2013). Work stress and risk of cancer: Meta-analysis of 5700 incident cancer events in 116 000 European men and women. *BMJ, 346,* f165.

Heimer, R. (2008). Community coverage and HIV prevention: Assessing metrics for estimating HIV incidence through syringe exchange. *International Journal of Drug Policy, 19*(Suppl. 1), S65–S73.

Heinrich, K. M., Lee, R. E., Regan, G. R., Reese-Smith, J. Y., Howard, H. H., Haddock, C. K., … Ahluwalia, J. S. (2008). How does the built environment relate to body mass index and obesity prevalence among public housing residents? *American Journal of Health Promotion, 22,* 187–194.

Held, C., Iqbal, R., Lear, S. A., Rosengren, A., Islam, S., Mathew, J., … Yusuf, S. (2012). Physical activity levels, ownership of goods promoting sedentary behavior and risk of myocardial infarction: Results of the INTERHEART study. *European Heart Journal, 33,* 452–466.

Helgeson, V. S. (2003). Cognitive adaptation, psychological adjustment, and disease progression among angioplasty patients: 4 years later. *Health Psychology, 22,* 30–38.

Helgeson, V. S., Cohen, S., Schulz, R., & Yasko, J. (2000). Group support interventions for women with breast cancer: Who benefits from what? *Health Psychology, 19,* 107–114.

Helgeson, V. S., Reynolds, K. A., Tomich, P. L. (2006). A meta-analytic review of benefit finding and growth. *Journal of Consulting and Clinical Psychology, 74,* 797–816.

Helgeson, V. S., Snyder, P., & Seltman, H. (2004). Psychological and physical adjustment of breast cancer over 4 years: Identifying distinct trajectories of change. *Health Psychology, 23,* 3–15.

Helweg-Larsen, M., & Nielsen, G. (2009). Smoking cross-culturally: Risk perceptions among young adults in Denmark and the United States. *Psychology and Health, 24,* 81–93.

Hembree, E. A., & Foa, E. B. (2003). Interventions for trauma-related emotional disturbances in adult victims of crime. *Journal of Traumatic Stress, 16,* 187–199.

Hemminki, K., Försti, A., & Bermejo, J. L. (2006). Gene-environment interactions in cancer. *Annals of the New York Academy of Science, 1076,* 137–148.

Henderson, L. A., Gandevia, S. C., & Macefield, V. G. (2008). Gender differences in brain activity evoked by muscle and cutaneous pain: A retrospective study of singe-trial fMRI data. *NeuroImage, 39,* 1867–1876.

Hendriks, H. F. J. (2007). Moderate alcohol consumption and insulin sensitivity: Observations and possible mechanisms. *Annals of Epidemiology, 17*(5 Suppl.), S40–S42.

Heneghan, C. J., Glasziou, P., & Perera, R. (2007). Reminder packaging for improving adherence to self-administered long-term medications. *Cochrane Database of Systematic Reviews,* Cochrane Art. No.: CD005025, DOI: 10.1002/14651858.CD005025.pub2.

Henke-Gendo, C., & Schulz, T. F. (2004). Transmission and disease association of Kaposi's sarcoma–associated herpes virus: Recent developments. *Current Opinion in Infectious Diseases, 17,* 53–57.

Henley, S. J., Thun, M. J., Chao, A., & Calle, E. E. (2004). Association between exclusive pipe smoking and mortality from cancer and other diseases. *Journal of the National Cancer Institute, 96,* 853–861.

Henriksen, L., Schleicher, N. C., Feighery, E. C., & Fortmann, S. P. (2010). A longitudinal study of exposure to retail cigarette advertising and smoking initiation. *Pediatrics, 126*(2), 232–238.

Henschke, N., Ostelo, R. W. J. G., van Tulder, M. W., Vlaeyen, J. W. S., Morley, S., Assendelft, W. J. J., … Main, C. J. (2010). Behavioural treatment for chronic low-back pain. *Cochrane Database of Systematic Reviews*, Cochrane Art. No.: CD002014, DOI: 10.1002/14651858.CD002014. pub3.

Herbst, E. D., Harris, D. S., Everhart, E. T., Mendelson, J., Jacob, P., & Jones, R. T. (2011). Cocaethylene formation following ethanol and cocaine administration by different routes. *Experimental and Clinical Psychopharmacology*, *19*(2), 95–104.

Herbst, A., Kordonouri, O., Schwab, K. O., Schmidt, F., & Holl, R. W. (2007). Impact of physical activity on cardiovascular risk factors in children with Type 1 diabetes. *Diabetes Care*, *30*, 2098–2100.

Herd, N., Borland, R., & Hyland, A. (2009). Predictors of smoking relapse by duration of abstinence: Findings from the International Tobacco Control (ITC) Four Country Survey. *Addiction*, *104*(12), 2088–2099.

Herman, C. P., & Polivy, J. (2005). Normative influences on food intake. *Physiology and Behavior*, *86*, 762–772.

Herman, C. P., van Strien, T., & Polivy, J. (2008). Undereating or eliminating overeating? *American Psychologist*, *63*, 202–203.

Hernán, M. A., Jick, S. S., Logroscino, G., Olek, M. J., Ascherio, A., & Jick, H. (2005). Cigarette smoking and the progression of multiple sclerosis. *Brain*, *128*(Pt. 6), 1461–1465.

Heron, M. (2016). Deaths: Leading causes for 2013. *National Vital Statistics Reports*, *65*(2), 1–95.

Herring, M. P., O'Connor, P. J., & Dishman, R. K. (2010). The effect of exercise training on anxiety symptoms among patients: A systematic review. *Archives of Internal Medicine*, *170*, 321–331.

Herrmann, S., McKinnon, E., John, M., Hyland, N., Martinez, O. P., Cain, A., … Mallal, S. (2008). Evidence-based, multifactorial approach to addressing non-adherence to antiretroviral therapy and improving standards of care. *Internal Medicine Journal*, *38*, 8–15.

Herzog, T. (2008). Analyzing the transtheoretical model using the framework of Weinstein, Rothman, and Sutton (1998). The example of smoking cessation. *Health Psychology*, *27*, 548–556.

Hession, M., Rolland, C., Kulkarni, U., Wise, A., & Broom, J. (2009). Systematic review of randomized controlled trials of low-carbohydrate vs. low fat/low calorie diets in the management of obesity and its comorbidities. *Obesity Reviews*, *10*(1), 36–50.

Hester, R. K., Delaney, H. D., & Campbell, W. (2011). ModerateDrinking.com and moderation management: Outcomes of a randomized clinical trial with non-dependent problems drinkers. *Journal of Consulting and Clinical Psychology*, *79*(2), 215–224.

Hilbert, A., Pike, K. M., Wilfley, D. E., Fairburn, C. G., Dohm, F.-A., & Striegel-Moore, R. H. (2011). Clarifying boundaries of binge eating disorder and psychiatric comorbidity: A latent structure analysis. *Behaviour Research and Therapy*, *49*(3), 202–211.

Hilgard, E. R. (1978). Hypnosis and pain. In R. A. Sternbach (Ed.), *The psychology of pain* (p. 219). New York, NY: Raven Press.

Hilgard, E. R., & Hilgard, J. R. (1994). *Hypnosis in the relief of pain* (rev. ed.). Los Altos, CA: Kaufmann.

Hill, J. O., & Wyatt, H. R. (2005). Role of physical activity in preventing and treating obesity. *Journal of Applied Physiology*, *99*, 765–770.

Hill, P. L., & Roberts, B. W. (2011). The role of adherence in the relationship between conscientiousness and perceived health. *Health Psychology*, *30*, 797–804.

Himmelstein, D. U., Thorne, D., Warren, E., & Woolhandler, S. (2009). Medical bankruptcy in the United States, 2007: Results of a national study. *The American Journal of Medicine*, *122*, 741–746.

Hind, K., & Burrows, M. (2007). Weight-bearing exercise and bone mineral accrual in children and adolescents: A review of controlled trials. *Bone*, *40*, 14–27.

Hingson, R., Heeren, T., Winter, M., & Wechsler, H. (2005). Magnitude of alcohol-related mortality and morbidity among U.S. college students ages 18–24: Changes from 1998 to 2001. *Annual Review of Public Health*, *26*, 259–279.

Hochbaum, G. (1958). *Public participation in medical screening programs* (DHEW Publication No. 572, Public Health Service). Washington, DC: U.S. Government Printing Office.

Hodgins, D. (2005). Can patients with alcohol use disorders return to social drinking? Yes, so what should we do about it? *Canadian Journal of Psychiatry*, *50*(5), 264–265.

Hoey, L. M., Ieropoli, S. C., White, V. M., & Jefford, M. (2008). Systematic review of peer-support programs for people with cancer. *Patient Education and Counseling*, *70*, 315–337.

Hoeymans, N., van Lindert, H., & Westert, G. P. (2005). The health status of the Dutch population as assessed by the EQ-6D. *Quality of Life Research*, *14*, 655–643.

Hoffman, B. M., Papas, R. K., Chatkoff, D. K., & Kerns, R. D. (2007). Meta-analysis of psychological interventions for chronic low back pain. *Health Psychology*, *26*, 1–9.

Hofmann, S. G., Sawyer, A. T., Witt, A. A., & Oh, D. (2010). The effect of mindfulness-based therapy on anxiety and depression: A meta-analytic review. *Journal of Consulting and Clinical Psychology*, *78*(2), 169.

Hogan, B. E., & Linden, W. (2004). Anger responses styles and blood pressure: At least don't ruminate about it! *Annals of Behavioral Medicine*, *27*, 38–49.

Hogan, E. M., & McReynolds, C. J. (2004). An overview of anorexia nervosa, bulimia nervosa, and binge eating disorders: Implications for rehabilitation professionals. *Journal of Applied Rehabilitation Counseling*, *35*(4), 26–34.

Hogan, N. S., & Schmidt, L. A. (2002). Testing the grief to personal growth model using structural equation modeling. *Death Studies*, *26*, 615–634.

Hogg, R. C. (2016). Contribution of monoamine oxidase inhibition to tobacco dependence: A review of the evidence. *Nicotine and Tobacco Research*, *18*(5), 509–523.

Holahan, C. J., Schutte, K. K., Brennan, P. L., Holahan, C. K., Moos, B. S., & Moos, R. H. (2010). Late-life alcohol consumption and 20-year mortality. *Alcoholism: Clinical and Experimental Research*, *34*(11), 1061–1071.

Holden, C. (2003, September 8). Party drug paper pulled. *Science Now*, 1–2.

Holick, M. F. (2004). Sunlight and vitamin D for bone health and prevention of autoimmune disease, cancers, and cardiovascular disease. *American Journal of Clinical Nutrition*, *80*(Suppl. 6), S1678–S1688.

Hollis, J. F., Gullion, C. M., Stevens, V. J., Brantley, P. J., Appel, L. J., Ard, J. D., …Weight Loss Maintenance Trial Research Group. (2008). Weight loss during the intensive intervention phase of the weight-loss maintenance trial. *American Journal of Preventive Medicine*, *35*, 118–126.

Holman, E. A., Silver, R. C., Poulin, M., Andersen, J., Gil-Rivas, V., & McIntosh, D. N. (2008). Terrorism, acute stress, and cardiovascular health: A 3-year national study following the September 11th attacks. *Archives of General Psychiatry*, *65*, 73–80.

Holmes, T. H., & Rahe, R. H. (1967). The Social Readjustment Rating Scale. *Journal of Psychosomatic Research*, *11*, 213–218.

Holsti, L., & Grunau, R. E. (2007). Initial validation of the Behavioral Indicators of Infant Pain (BIIP). *Pain*, *132*, 264–272.

Holt, L. J., Armeli, S., Tennen, H., Austad, C. S., Raskin, S. A., Fallahi, … Pearlson, G. D. (2013). A person-centered approach to understanding negative reinforcement drinking among first year college students. *Addictive Behaviors*, *38*(12), 2937–2944.

Holt-Lunstad, J., Birmingham, W., & Jones, B. Q. (2008). Is there something unique about marriage? The relative impact of marital status, relationship quality, and network social support on ambulatory blood pressure and mental health. *Annals of Behavioral Medicine*, *35*, 239–244.

Holt-Lunstad, J., Smith, T. B., & Layton, J. B. (2010). Social relationships and mortality risk: A meta-analytic review. *PLoS Med*, *7*(7), e1000316.

Holtzman, D., Bland, S. D., Lansky, A., & Mack, K. A. (2001). HIV-related behaviors and perceptions among adults in 25 states: 1997 Behavioral Risk Factor Surveillance System. *American Journal of Public Health*, *91*, 1882–1888.

Hölzel, B. K., Carmody, J., Vangel, M., Congleton, C., Yerramsetti, S. M., Gard, T., … Lazar, S. W. (2011). Mindfulness practice leads to increases in regional brain gray matter density. *Psychiatry Research: Neuroimaging*, *191*(1), 36–43.

Hootman, J. M., Macera, C. A., Ainsworth, B. E., Addy, C. L., Martin, M., & Blair, S. N. (2002). Epidemiology of musculoskeletal injuries among sedentary and physically active adults. *Medicine and Science in Sports and Exercise, 34*, 838–844.

Horne, R., Buick, D., Fisher, M., Leake, H., Cooper, V., & Weinman, J. (2004). Doubts about necessity and concerns about adverse effects: Identifying the types of beliefs that are associated with non-adherence to HAART. *International Journal of STD and AIDS, 15*, 38–44.

Horowitz, S. (2010). Health benefits of meditation: What the newest research shows. *Alternative and Complementary Therapies, 16*(4), 223–228.

Houts, P. S., Doak, C. C., Doak, L. G., & Loscalzo, M. J. (2006). The role of pictures in improving health communication: A review of research on attention, comprehension, recall, and adherence. *Patient Education and Counseling, 61*, 173–190.

"How Ricky Gervais totally lost it" (2012, January 25). Retrieved from http://www.menshealth.com/weight-loss/ricky-gervais

Howe, G. W., Levy, M. L., & Caplan, R. D. (2004). Job loss and depressive symptoms in couples: Common stressors, stress transmission, or relationship disruption? *Journal of Family Psychology, 18*, 639–650.

Hróbjartsson, A., & Gøtzsche, P. C. (2010). Placebo interventions for all clinical conditions. *The Cochrane Database of Systematic Reviews*, Cochrane Art. No.: CD003974, DOI: 10.1002/14651858.CD003974. pub3.

Hsiao, A.-F., Ryan, G. W., Hays, R. D., Coulter, I. D., Andersen, R. M., & Wenger, N. S. (2006). Variations in provider conceptions of integrative medicine. *Social Science and Medicine, 62*, 2973–2987.

Hsiao, A.-F., Wong, M. D., Goldstein, M. S., Becerra, L. S., Cheng, E. M., & Wenger, N. S. (2006). Complementary and alternative medicine use among Asian-American subgroups: Prevalence, predictors, and lack of relationship to acculturation and access to conventional health care. *Journal of Alternative and Complementary Medicine, 12*, 1003–1010.

Hsu, C., BlueSpruce, J., Sherman, K., & Cherkin, D. (2010). Unanticipated benefits of CAM therapies for back pain: An exploration of patient experiences. *Journal of Alternative and Complementary Medicine, 16*(2), 157–163.

Hu, B., Li, W., Wang, X., Liu, L., Teo, K., & Yusuf, S. (2012). Marital status, education, and risk of acute myocardial infarction in mainland China: The INTERHEART study. *Journal of Epidemiology, 22*, 123–129.

Hu, F. B., Stampfer, M. J., Colditz, G. A., Ascherio, A., Rexrode, K. M., Willett, W. C., ... Manson, J. E. (2000). Physical activity and risk of stroke in women. *Journal of the American Medical Association, 283*, 7961–7967.

Huang, J.-Q., Sridhar, S., & Hunt, R. H. (2002). Role of *Helicobacter pylori* infection and non-steroidal anti-inflammatory drugs in pepticulcer disease: A meta-analysis. *Lancet, 359*, 14–21.

Hudson, J. I., Hiripi, E., Pope, H. G., Jr., & Kessler, R. C. (2007). The prevalence and correlates of eating disorders in the National Comorbidity Survey replication. *Biological Psychiatry, 61*, 348–358.

Huebner, D. M., & Davis, M. C. (2007). Perceived antigay discrimination and physical health outcomes. *Health Psychology, 26*, 627–634.

Huebner, R. B., & Kantor, L. W. (2011). Advances in alcoholism treatment. *Alcohol Research and Health, 33*(4), 295–299.

Hufford, D. J. (2003). Evaluating complementary and alternative medicine: The limits of science and of scientists. *Journal of Law, Medicine and Ethics, 31*, 198–212.

Hughes, J. (1975). Isolation of an endogenous compound from the brain with pharmacological properties similar to morphine. *Brain Research, 88*, 295–308.

Hughes, J. (2003). Motivating and helping smokers to stop smoking. *Journal of General Internal Medicine, 18*, 1053–1057.

Hughes, J., Gulliver, S. B., Fenwick, J. W., Valliere, W. A., Cruser, K., Pepper, S., ... Flynn, B. S. (1992). Smoking cessation among self-quitters. *Health Psychology, 11*, 331–334.

Hughes, J. R. (2009). How confident should we be that smoking cessation treatments work? *Addiction, 104*(10), 1637–1640.

Hughes, J. W., Fresco, D. M., Myerscough, R., van Dulmen, M., Carlson, L. E., & Josephson, R. (2013). Randomized controlled trial of mindfulness-based stress reduction for prehypertension. *Psychosomatic Medicine, 75*(8), 721–728.

Huizinga, M. M., Bleich, S. N., Beach, M. C., Clark, J. M., & Cooper, L. A. (2010). Disparity in physician perception of patients' adherence to medications by obesity status. *Obesity, 18*(10), 1932–1937.

Hulme, C., Wright, J., Crocker, T., Oluboyede, Y., & House, A. (2010). Non-pharmacological approaches for dementia that informal carers might try or access: A systematic review. *International Journal of Geriatric Psychiatry, 25*, 756–763.

Humane Society of the United States. (2011). *U.S. pet ownership statistics*. Retrieved August 31, 2012, from http://www.humanesociety.org/ issues/pet_overpopulation/facts/pet_ownership_ statistics.html

Humphrey, L. L., Fu, R., Buckley, D. I., Freeman, M., & Helfand, M. J. (2008). Periodontal disease and coronary heart disease incidence: A systematic review and meta-analysis. *Journal of General Internal Medicine, 23*, 2079–2020.

Humphreys, K., & Moos, R. H. (2007). Encouraging posttreatment self-help group involvement to reduce demand for continuing care services: Two-year clinical and utilization outcomes. *Alcoholism: Clinical and Experimental Research, 31*, 64–68.

Hunt, W. A., Barnett, L. W., & Branch, L. G. (1971). Relapse rates in addiction programs. *Journal of Clinical Psychology, 27*, 455–456.

Huntley, J. D., Gould, R. L., Liu, K., Smith, M., & Howard, R. J. (2015). Do cognitive interventions improve general cognition in dementia? A meta-analysis and meta-regression. *BMJ Open, 5*(4), e005247.

Huq, F. (2007). Molecular modeling analysis of the metabolism of cocaine. *Journal of Pharmacology and Toxicology, 2*, 114–130.

Hurley, S. F., & Matthews, J. P. (2007). The quit benefits model: A Markov model for assessing the health benefits and health care cost savings of quitting smoking. *Cost Effectiveness and Resource Allocation, 5*, 2–20.

Hurt, R. D., Weston, S. A., Ebbert, J. O., McNallan, S. M., Croghan, I. T., Schroeder, D. R., & Roger, V. L. (2012). Myocardial infarction and sudden cardiac death in Olmsted County, Minnesota, before and after smoke-free workplace laws. *Archives of Internal Medicine, 172*(21), 1635–1641.

Hutchinson, A. B., Branson, B. M., Kim, A., & Farnham, P. G. (2006). A meta-analysis of the effectiveness of alternative HIV counseling and testing methods to increase knowledge of HIV status. *AIDS, 20*, 1597–1604.

Huth, M. M., Broome, M. E., & Good, M. (2004). Imagery reduces children's post-operative pain, *Pain, 110*, 439–448.

Huxley, R., Ansary-Moghaddam, A., de González, A. B., Barzi, F., & Woodward, M. (2005). Type-II diabetes and pancreatic cancer: A meta-analysis of 36 studies. *British Journal of Cancer, 92*, 2076–2083.

Huxley, R. R., & Neil, H. A. W. (2003). The relation between dietary flavonol intake and coronary heart disease mortality: A meta-analysis of prospective cohort studies. *Journal of Clinical Nutrition, 57*, 904–908.

Iagnocco, A., Perella, C., Naredo, E., Meenagh, G., Ceccarelli, F., Tripodo, E., ... Valesini, G. (2008). Etanercept in the treatment of rheumatoid arthritis: Clinical follow-up over one year by ultrasonography. *Clinical Rheumatology, 27*, 491–496.

Iannotti, R. J., Schneider, S., Nansel, T. R., Haynie, D. L., Plotnick, L. P., Clark, L. M., ... Simons-Morton, B. (2006). Self-efficacy, outcome expectations, and diabetes self-management in adolescents with Type 1 diabetes. *Journal of Developmental and Behavioral Pediatrics, 27*, 98–105.

Ickovics, J. R., Milan, S., Boland, R., Schoenbaum, E., Schuman, P., Vlahov, D. ... HIV Epidemiology Research Study (HERS) Group. (2006). Psychological resources protect health: 5-year survival and immune function among HIV-infected women from four US cities. *AIDS, 20*, 1851–1860.

Iglesias, S. L., Azzara, S., Squillace, M., Jeifetz, M., Lores Arnais, M. R., Desimone, M. F., ... Diaz, L. E. (2005). A study on the effectiveness of a stress management programme for college students. *Pharmacy Education, 5*, 27–31.

Ijadunola, K. T., Abiona, T. C., Odu, O. O., & Ijadunola, M. Y. (2007). College students in Nigeria underestimate their risk of contacting HIV/AIDS infection. *European Journal of Contraception and Reproductive Health Care, 12*, 131–137.

Ilies, R., Schwind, K. M., Wagner, D. T., Johnson, M. D., DeRue, D. S., & Ilgen, D. R. (2007). When can employees have a family life? The effects of daily workload and affect on work-family conflict and social behaviors at home. *Journal of Applied Psychology, 92,* 1368–1379.

Imes, R. S., Bylund, C. L., Sabee, C. M., Routsong, T. R., & Sanford, A. A. (2008). Patients' reasons for refraining from discussing Internet health information with their healthcare providers. *Health Communication, 23,* 538–547.

Ingersoll, K. S., & Cohen, J. (2008). The impact of medication regimen factors on adherence to chronic treatment: A review of the literature. *Journal of Behavioral Medicine, 31,* 213–224.

Ingraham, B. A., Bragdon, B., & Nohe, A. (2008). Molecular basis for the potential of vitamin D to prevent cancer. *Current Medical Research and Opinion, 24,* 139–149.

Innes, K. E., & Vincent, H. K. (2007). The influence of yoga-based programs on risk profiles in adults with Type 2 diabetes mellitus: A systematic review. *Evidence Based Complementary and Alternative Medicine, 4,* 469–486.

Institute of Medicine (IOM). (2002). *Unequal treatment: Confronting racial and ethnic disparities in health care.* Washington, DC: Author.

Institute of Medicine (IOM). (2010). *Value in health care: Accounting for cost, quality, safety, outcomes, and innovations: Workshop summary.* Washington, DC: Author.

Institute of Medicine (IOM). (2011). *Relieving pain in America: A blueprint for transforming prevention, care, education, and research.* Washington, DC: Author.

Institute of Medicine (IOM). (2012). *Front-of-package nutrition rating systems and symbols: Promoting healthier choices.* Washington, DC: Author.

International Agency for Research on Cancer Working Group on artificial ultraviolet (UV) light and skin cancer (IARC). (2007). The association of use of sunbeds with cutaneous malignant melanoma and other skin cancers: A systematic review. *International Journal of Cancer, 120,* 1116–1122.

International Association for the Study of Pain (IASP), Subcommittee on Taxonomy. (1979). Pain terms: A list with definitions and notes on usage. *Pain, 6,* 249–252.

Iqbal, R., Anand, S., Ounpuu, S., Islam, S., Zhang, X., Rangarajan, S., … INTERHEART Study Investigators. (2008). Dietary patterns and the risk of acute myocardial infarction in 52 countries: Results of the INTERHEART study. *Circulation, 118,* 1929–1937.

Iribarren, C., Darbinian, J. A., Lo, J. C., Fireman, B. H., & Go, A. S. (2006). Value of the sagittal abdominal diameter in coronary heart disease risk assessment: Cohort study in a large, multiethnic population. *American Journal of Epidemiology, 164,* 1150–1159.

Iribarren, C., Sidney, S., Bild, D. E., Liu, K., Markovitz, J. H., Roseman, J. M., … Matthews, K. (2000). Association of hostility with coronary artery calcification in young adults. *Journal of the American Medical Association, 283,* 2546–2551.

Ironson, G., Weiss, S., Lydston, D., Ishii, M., Jones, D., Asthana, D., … Antoni, M. (2005). The impact of improved self-efficacy on HIV viral load and distress in culturally diverse women living with AIDS: The SMART/ EST women's project. *AIDS Care, 17,* 222–236.

Irwin, D. E., Milsom, I., Kopp, Z., Abrams, P., & EPIC Study Group. (2008). Symptom bother and health care-seeking behavior among individuals with overactive bladder. *European Urology, 53,* 1029–1039.

Irwin, M. R. (2008). Human psychoneuroimmunology: 20 years of discovery. *Brain, Behavior and Immunity, 22,* 129–139.

Irwin, M. R., Pike, J. L., Cole, J. C., & Oxman, M. N. (2003). Effects of a behavioral intervention, tai chi chih, on varicella-zoster virus specific immunity and health functioning in older adults. *Psychosomatic Medicine, 65,* 824–830.

Isaacson, W. (2011). *Steve Jobs.* New York, NY: Simon and Schuster.

Islam, T., Gauderman, W. J., Berhane, K., McConnell, R., Avol, E., Peters, J. M., … Gilliland, F. D. (2007). Relationship between air pollution, lung function and asthma in adolescents. *Thorax, 62,* 957–963.

Iso, H., Rexrode, K. M., Stampfer, M. J., Manson, J. E., Colditz, G. A., Speizer, F. E., … Willett, W. C. (2001). Intake of fish and omega-3 fatty acids and risk of stroke in women. *Journal of the American Medical Association, 285,* 304–312.

Ito, T., Takenaka, K., Tomita, T., & Agari, I. (2006). Comparison of ruminative responses with negative rumination as a vulnerability factor for depression. *Psychological Reports, 99,* 763–772.

Ivanovski, B., & Malhi, G. S. (2007). The psychological and neurophysiological concomitants of mindfulness forms of meditation. *Acta Neuropsychiatrica, 19*(2), 76–91.

Iwamoto, D. K., Cheng, A., Lee, C. S., Takamatsu, S., & Gordon, D. (2011). "Man-ing" up and getting drunk: The role of masculine norms, alcohol intoxication and alcohol-related problems among college men. *Addictive Behaviors, 36*(9), 906–911.

Jackson, G. (2004). Treatment of erectile dysfunction in patients with cardiovascular disease: Guide to drug selection. *Drugs, 64,* 1533–1545.

Jackson, K. M., Sher, K. J., Gotham, H. J., & Wood, P. K. (2001). Transitioning into and out of large-effect drinking in young adulthood. *Journal of Abnormal Psychology, 110,* 378–391.

Jacobs, G. D. (2001). Clinical applications of the relaxation response and mind-body interventions. *Journal of Alternative and Complementary Medicine, 7*(Suppl. 1), 93–101.

Jacobson, E. (1938). *Progressive relaxation: A physiological and clinical investigation of muscle states and their significance in psychology and medical practice* (2nd ed.). Chicago, IL: University of Chicago Press.

Jager, R. D., Mieler, W. F., & Miller, J. W. (2008). Age-related macular degeneration. *New England Journal of Medicine, 358,* 2606–2617.

Jagger, C., Gillies, C., Moscone, F., Cambois, E., Van Oyen, H., Nusselder, W., … EHLEIS Team. (2009). Inequalities in healthy life years in the 25 countries of the European Union in 2005: A cross-national meta-regression analysis. *The Lancet, 372,* 2124–2131.

Jahnke, R., Larkey, L., Rogers, C., & Etnier, J. (2010). A comprehensive review of health benefits of qigong and tai chi. *American Journal of Health Promotion, 24*(6), e1–e25.

Jakicic, J. M., & Otto, A. D. (2005). Physical activity considerations for the treatment and prevention of obesity. *American Journal of Clinical Nutrition, 82*(Suppl. 1), 226S–229S.

Jamal, A., Homa, D. M., O'Connor, E., Babb, S. D., Caraballo, R. S., Singh, T., … King, B. A. (2015). Current cigarette smoking among adults—United States, 2005-2014. *Morbidity and Mortality Weekly Report, 64*(44), 1233–1240.

Janssen, R. S., Onorato, I. M., Valdiserri, R. O., Durham, T. M., Nichols, W. P., Seiler, E. M., … Jaffe, H. W. (2003). Advancing HIV prevention: New strategies for a changing epidemic—United States, 2003. *Morbidity and Mortality Weekly Report, 52,* 329–332.

Janssen, S. A. (2002). Negative affect and sensitization to pain. *Scandinavian Journal of Psychology, 43,* 131–137.

Jay, S. M., Elliott, C. H., Woody, P. D., & Siegel, S. (1991). An investigation of cognitive-behavior therapy combined with oral valium for children undergoing painful medical procedures. *Health Psychology, 10,* 317–322.

Jeffery, R. W., & Harnack, L. J. (2007). Evidence implicating eating as a primary driver for the obesity epidemic. *Diabetes, 56,* 2673–2676.

Jeffery, R. W., Kelly, K. M., Rothman, A. J., Sherwood, N. E., & Boutelle, K. N. (2004). The weight loss experience: A descriptive analysis. *Annals of Behavioral Medicine, 27,* 100–106.

Jellinek, E. M. (1960). *The disease concept of alcoholism.* New Haven, CT: College and University Press.

Jenkins, S., & Armstrong, L. (2001). *It's not about the bike: My journey back to life.* New York, NY: Penguin Books.

Jenks, R. A., & Higgs, S. (2007). Associations between dieting and smoking-related behaviors in young women. *Drug and Alcohol Dependence, 88,* 291–299.

Jensen, M. P., & Karoly, P. (2001). Self-report scales and procedures for assessing pain in adults. In D. C. Turk & R. Melzack (Eds.), *Handbook of pain assessment* (2nd ed., pp. 15–34). New York, NY: Guilford Press.

Jeon, C. Y., Lokken, R. P., Hu, F. B., & van Dam, R. M. (2007). Physical activity of moderate intensity and risk of Type 2 diabetes: A systematic review. *Diabetes Care, 30,* 744–752.

Jha, A. P., Krompinger, J., & Baime, M. J. (2007). Mindfulness training modifies subsystems of attention. *Cognitive, Affective and Behavioral Neuroscience, 7,* 109–119.

John, U., Meyer, C., Rumpf, H.-J., Hapke, U., & Schumann, A. (2006). Predictors of increased body mass index following cessation of smoking. *American Journal of Addictions, 15,* 192–197.

Johnson, A., Sandford, J., & Tyndall, J. (2007). Written and verbal information versus verbal information only for patients being discharged from acute hospital settings to home. *Cochrane Database of Systematic Reviews,* Cochrane Art. No.: CD003716, DOI: 10.1002/14651858. CD003716.

Johnson, J. L., Slentz, C. A., Houmard, J. A., Samsa, G. P., Duscha, B. D., Aiken, L. B., … Kraus, W. E. (2007). Exercise training amount and intensity effects on metabolic syndrome (from Studies of a Targeted Risk Reduction Intervention through Defined Exercise). *American Journal of Cardiology, 100,* 1759–1766.

Johnson, L. W., & Weinstock, R. S. (2006). The metabolic syndrome: Concepts and controversy. *Mayo Clinic Proceedings, 81,* 1615–1621.

Johnson, M. I. (2006). The clinical effectiveness of acupuncture for pain relief—You can be certain of uncertainty. *Acupuncture in Medicine, 24,* 71–79.

Johnson, S. S., Driskell, M.-M., Johnson, J. L., Dyment, S. J., Prochaska, J. O., Prochaska, J. M., … Bourne, L. (2006). Transtheoretical model intervention for adherence to lipid-lowering drugs. *Disease Management, 9,* 102–114.

Johnston, B. C., Kanters, S., Bandayrel, K., Wu, P., Naji, F., Siemieniuk, R. A., … Mills, E. J. (2014). Comparison of weight loss among named diet programs in overweight and obese adults: A meta-analysis. *Journal of the American Medical Association, 312*(9), 923–933.

Johnston, L. D., O'Malley, P. M., Bachman, J. G., & Schulenberg, J. E. (2007). *Monitoring the Future: National survey results on drug use, 1975–2006: Vol. 2. College students and adults ages 19–45* (NIH Publication No. 07-6206). Bethesda, MD: National Institute on Drug Abuse.

Johnston, L. D., O'Malley, P. M., Miech, R. A., Bachman, J. D., & Schulenberg, J. E. (2016). *Monitoring the Future: National survey results on drug use, 1975-2015: Overview, key findings on adolescent drug use.* Ann Arbor, MI: Institute for Social Research, The University of Michigan.

Jolliffe, C. D., & Nicholas, M. K. (2004). Verbally reinforcing pain reports: An experimental test of the operant model of chronic pain. *Pain, 107,* 167–175.

Jones, D. W., Chambless, L. E., Folsom, A. R., Heiss, G., Hutchinson, R. G., Sharrett, A. R., … Taylor, H. A., Jr. (2002). Risk factors for coronary heart disease in African Americans: The Atherosclerosis Risk in Communities Study, 1987–1997. *Archives of Internal Medicine, 162,* 2565–2571.

Jones, W. R., & Morgan, J. F. (2010). Eating disorders in men: A review of the literature. *Journal of Public Mental Health, 9*(2), 23–31.

Jorgensen, R. S., & Kolodziej, M. E. (2007). Suppressed anger, evaluative threat, and cardiovascular reactivity: A tripartite profile approach. *International Journal of Psychophysiology, 66,* 102–108.

Joshi, M., Joshi, A., & Bartter, T. (2014). Marijuana and lung disease. *Current Opinion in Pulmonary Medicine, 20*(2), 173–179.

Juliano, L. M., & Griffiths, R. R. (2004). A critical review of caffeine withdrawal: Empirical validation of symptoms and signs, incidence, severity, and associated features. *Psychopharmacology, 176,* 1–29.

Julien, R. M., Advokat, C., & Comaty, J. E. (2010). *A primer of drug action* (12th ed.). New York, NY: Worth.

Juster, R. P., McEwen, B. S., & Lupien, S. J. (2010). Allostatic load bio-markers of chronic stress and impact on health and cognition. *Neuroscience and Biobehavioral Reviews, 35,* 2–16.

Kabat-Zinn, J. (1993). Mindfulness meditation: Health benefits of an ancient Buddhist practice. In D. Goleman & J. Gurin (Eds.), *Mind/body medicine: How to use your mind for better health* (pp. 259–275). Yonkers, NY: Consumer Reports Books.

Kahende, J. W., Woollery, T. A., & Lee, C.-W. (2007). Assessing medical expenditures on 4 smoking-related diseases, 1996–2001. *American Journal of Health Behavior, 31,* 602–611.

Kahn, E. B., Ramsey, L. T., Brownson, R. C., Heath, G. W., Howze, E. H., Powell, K. E., … Corso, P. (2002). The effectiveness of interventions to increase physical activity: A systematic review. *American Journal of Preventive Medicine, 22,* 73–107.

Kahn, H. A. (1963). The relationship of reported coronary heart disease mortality to physical activity of work. *American Journal of Public Health, 53,* 1058–1067.

Kaholokula, J. K., Saito, E., Mau, M. K., Latimer, R., & Seto, T. B. (2008). Pacific Islanders' perspectives on heart failure management. *Patient Education and Counseling, 70,* 281–291.

Kalichman, S. C., Eaton, L., Cain, D., Cherry, C., Fuhrel, A., Kaufman, M., … Kalichman, M. O. (2007). Changes in HIV treatment beliefs and sexual risk behaviors among gay and bisexual men, 1997–2005. *Health Psychology, 26,* 650–656.

Kamarck, T. W., Muldoon, M. F., Shiffman, S. S., & Sutton-Tyrrell, K. (2007). Experiences of demand and control during daily life are predictors of carotid atherosclerotic progression among healthy men. *Health Psychology, 26,* 324–332.

Kambouropoulos, N. (2003). The validity of the tension-reduction hypothesis in alcohol cue-reactivity research. *Australian Journal of Psychology, 55*(S1), 6.

Kamer, A. R., Craig, R. G., Dasanayke, A. P., Brys, M., Glodzik-Sobanska, L., & de Leon, M. J. (2008). Inflammation and Alzheimer's disease: Possible role of periodontal diseases. *Alzheimer's and Dementia, 4,* 242–250.

Kamiya, J. (1969). Operant control of the EEG alpha rhythm and some of its reported effects on consciousness. In C. Tart (Ed.), *Altered states of consciousness* (pp. 519–529). New York, NY: Wiley.

Kaner, E. F. S., Beyer, F., Dickinson, H. O., Pienaar, E., Campbell, F., Schlesinger, C., … Burnand, B. (2007). Effectiveness of brief alcohol interventions in primary care populations. *Cochrane Database of Systematic Reviews,* Cochrane Art. No.: CD004148, DOI: 10.1002/14651858. CD004148.pub3.

Kann, L., Kitchen, S., Shanklin, S. L., Flint, K. H., Hawkins, J., Harris, W. A., … Zaza, S. (2014). Youth risk behavior surveillance—2013. *Morbidity and Mortality Weekly Report, 63*(4), 1–168.

Kann, L., McManus, T., Harris, W. A., Shanklin, S. L., Flint, K. H., Hawkins, J., … Zaza, S. (2016). Youth risk behavior surveillance—2015. *Morbidity and Mortality Weekly Report, 65*(6), 1–174.

Kanner, A. D., Coyne, J. C., Schaefer, C., & Lazarus, R. S. (1981). Comparison of two modes of stress measurement: Daily hassles and uplifts versus major life events. *Journal of Behavioral Medicine, 4,* 1–39.

Kaʻopua, L. S. I., & Mueller, C. W. (2004). Treatment adherence among Native Hawaiians living with HIV. *Social Work, 49,* 55–62.

Kaplan, R. M., & Bush, J. W. (1982). Health-related quality of life measurement for evaluation research and policy analysis. *Health Psychology, 1,* 61–80.

Kaptchuk, T., Eisenberg, D., & Komaroff, A. (2002). Pondering the placebo effect. *Newsweek, 140*(23), 71, 73.

Kaptchuk, T. J., Friedlander, E., Kelley, J. M., Sanchez, M. N., Kokkotou, E., Singer, J. P., … Lembo, A. J. (2010). Placebos without deception: A randomized controlled trial in irritable bowel syndrome. *PLoS One, 5,* e15591.

Karam, E., Kypri, K., & Salamoun, M. (2007). Alcohol use among college students: An international perspective. *Current Opinion in Psychiatry, 20,* 213–221.

Karani, R., McLaughlin, M. A., & Cassel, C. K. (2001). Exercise in the healthy older adult. *American Journal of Geriatric Cardiology, 10,* 269–273.

Karavidas, M. K., Tsai, P.-S., Yucha, C., McGrady, A., & Lehrer, P. M. (2006). Thermal biofeedback for primary Raynaud's phenomenon: A review of the literature. *Applied Psychophysiology and Biofeedback, 31,* 203–216.

Karl, A., Mühlnickel, W., Kurth, R., & Flor, H. (2004). Neuroelectric source imaging of steady-state movement-related cortical potentials in human upper extremity amputees with and without phantom limb pain. *Pain, 110,* 90–102.

Karlamangla, A. S., Singer, B. H., Williams, D. R., Schwartz, J. E., Matthews, K. A., Kiefe, C. I., … Seeman, T. E. (2005). Impact of socioeconomic status on longitudinal accumulation of cardiovascular risk in young adults: The CARDIA Study (USA). *Social Science and Medicine, 60,* 999–1015.

Karoly, P., & Ruehlman, L. S. (2007). Psychosocial aspects of pain-related life task interference: An exploratory analysis in a general population sample. *Pain Medicine, 8,* 563–572.

Karp, A., Andel, R., Parker, M., Wang, H.-X., Winblad, B., & Fratiglioni, L. (2009). Mentally stimulating activities at work during midlife and dementia risk after 75: Follow-up study from the Kungsholmen project. *The American Journal of Geriatric Psychiatry*, 17, 227–236.

Karvinen, K. H., Courneya, K. S., Plotnikoff, R. C., Spence, J. C., Venner, P. M., & North, S. (2009). A prospective study of the determinants of exercise in bladder cancer survivors using the Theory of Planned Behavior. *Supportive Care in Cancer*, 17, 171–179.

Kasl, S. V., & Cobb, S. (1966a). Health behavior, illness behavior, and sick role behavior: I. Health and illness behavior. *Archives of Environmental Health*, 12, 246–266.

Kasl, S. V., & Cobb, S. (1966b). Health behavior, illness behavior, and sick role behavior: II. Sick role behavior. *Archives of Environmental Health*, 12, 531–541.

Kato, M., Noda, M., Inoue, M., Kadowaki, T., & Tsugane, S. (2009). Psychological factors, coffee and risk of diabetes mellitus among middle-aged Japanese: A population-based prospective study in the JPHC study cohort. *Endocrine Journal*, 56, 459–468.

Katon, W. J., Russo, J. E., Heckbert, S. R., Lin, E. H. B., Ciechanowski, P., Ludman, E., … Von Korff, M. (2010). The relationship between changes in depression symptoms and changes in health risk behaviors in patients with diabetes. *International Journal of Geriatric Psychiatry*, 25, 466–475.

Kaufmann, R. B., Babb, S., O'Halloran, A., Asman, K., Bishop, E., Tynan, M., … Wang, L. (2010). Vital signs: Nonsmokers' exposure to secondhand smoke—United States, 1999-2008. *Morbidity and Mortality Weekly Report*, 59(35), 1141–1146.

Kaur, S., Cohen, A., Dolor, R., Coffman, C. J., & Bastian, L. A. (2004). The impact of environmental tobacco smoke on women's risk of dying from heart disease: A meta-analysis. *Journal of Women's Health*, 13, 888–897.

Kavookjian, J., Elswick, B. M., & Whetsel, T. (2007). Interventions for being active among individuals with diabetes: A systematic review of the literature. *Diabetes Educator*, 33, 962–988.

Kawachi, I., Daniels, N., & Robinson, D. E. (2005). Health disparities by race and class: Why both matter. *Health Affairs*, 24, 343–352.

Kaye, W. (2008). Neurobiology of anorexia and bulimia nervosa. *Physiology and Behavior*, 94, 121–135.

Keefe, F. J. (1982). Behavioral assessment and treatment of chronic pain: Current status and future directions. *Journal of Consulting and Clinical Psychology*, 50, 896–911.

Keefe, F. J., & Smith, S. J. (2002). The assessment of pain behavior: Implications for applied psychophysiology and future research directions. *Applied Psychophysiology and Biofeedback*, 27, 117–127.

Keefe, F. J., Smith, S. J., Buffington, A. L. H., Gibson, J., Studts, J. L., & Caldwell, D. S. (2002). Recent advances and future directions in the biopsychosocial assessment and treatment of arthritis. *Journal of Consulting and Clinical Psychology*, 70, 640–655.

Keel, P. K., & Brown, T. A. (2010). Update on course and outcome in eating disorders. *International Journal of Eating Disorders*, 43(3), 195–204.

Keel, P. K., & Klump, K. L. (2003). Are eating disorders culture-bound syndromes? Implications for conceptualizing their etiology. *Psychological Bulletin*, 129, 747–769.

Keith, V., Kronenfeld, J., Rivers, P., & Liang, S. (2005). Assessing the effects of race and ethnicity on use of complementary and alternative therapies in the USA. *Ethnicity and Health*, 10, 19–32.

Keller, A., Hayden, J., Bombardier, C., & van Tulder, M. (2007). Effect sizes of non-surgical treatments of non-specific low-back pain. *European Spine Journal*, 16, 1776–1788.

Kelley, G. A., & Kelley, K. S. (2007). Aerobic exercise and lipids and lipoproteins in children and adolescents: A meta-analysis of randomized controlled trials. *Atherosclerosis*, 191, 447–453.

Kelley, K. W., Bluthé, R.-M., Dantzer, R., Zhou, J.-H., Shen, W.-H., Johnson, R. W., … Broussard, S. R. (2003). Cytokine-induced sickness behavior. *Brain, Behavior, and Immunity*, 17(S1), 112–118.

Kelly, J. A., & Kalichman, S. C. (2002). Behavioral research in HIV/AIDS primary and secondary prevention: Recent advances and future directions. *Journal of Consulting and Clinical Psychology*, 70, 626–639.

Kelly, J. F., Greene, M. C., & Bergman, B. G. (2016). Recovery benefits of the "therapeutic alliance" among 12-step mutual-help organization attendees and their sponsors. *Drug and Alcohol Dependence*, 162, 64–71.

Kelly, J. F., Stout, R. L., Magill, M., & Tonigan, J. S. (2011). The role of Alcoholics Anonymous in mobilizing adaptive social network changes: A prospective lagged mediational analysis. *Drug and Alcohol Dependence*, 114(2/3), 119–126.

Keltner, B., Kelley, F. J., & Smith, D. (2004). Leadership to reduce health disparities. *Nursing Administration Quarterly*, 28, 181–190.

Kemeny, M. E. (2003). The psychobiology of stress. *Current Directions in Psychological Science*, 12, 124–129.

Kemeny, M. E., & Schedlowski, M. (2007). Understanding the interaction between psychosocial stress and immune-related diseases: A stepwise progression. *Brain, Behavior and Immunity*, 21, 1009–1018.

Kendler, K. S., Gatz, M., Gardner, C. O., & Pedersen, N. L. (2007). Clinical indices of familial depression in the Swedish Twin Registry. *Acta Psychiatrica Scandinavica*, 115, 214–220.

Kendzor, D. E., Businelle, M. S., Costello, T. J., Castro, Y., Reitzel, L. R., Cofta-Woerpel, L. M., … Wetter, D. W. (2010). Financial strain and smoking cessation among racially/ethnically diverse smokers. *American Journal of Public Health*, 100(4), 702–706.

Kennedy, D. P., Tucker, J. S., Pollard, M. S., Go, M.-H., & Green, H. D. (2011). Adolescent romantic relationships and change in smoking status. *Addictive Behaviors*, 36(4), 320–326.

Keogh, E., Bond, F. W., & Flaxman, P. E. (2006). Improving academic performance and mental health through a stress management intervention: Outcomes and mediators of change. *Behaviour Research and Therapy*, 44, 339–357.

Kerns, R. D., Turk, D. C., & Rudy, T. E. (1985). The West Haven–Yale Multidimensional Pain Inventory. *Pain*, 23, 345–356.

Kerse, N., Buetow, S., Mainous, A. G., III, Young, G., Coster, G., & Arroll, A. (2004). Physician-patient relationship and medication compliance: A primary care investigation. *Annals of Family Medicine*, 2, 455–461.

Kertesz, L. (2003). The numbers behind the news. *Healthplan*, 44(5), 10–14, 16, 18.

Kesmodel, U., Wisborg, K., Olsen, S. F., Henriksen, T. B., & Secher, N. J. (2002). Moderate alcohol intake during pregnancy and the risk of stillbirth and death in the first year of life. *American Journal of Epidemiology*, 155, 305–312.

Kessler, R. C., Berglund, P., Delmer, O., Jin, R., Merikangas, K. R., & Walters, E. E. (2005). Lifetime prevalence and age-of-onset distributions of DSM-IV disorders in the National Comorbidity Survey Replication. *Archives of General Psychiatry*, 62, 593–602.

Keys, A., Brozek, J., Henschel, A., Mickelsen, O., & Taylor, H. L. (1950). *The biology of human starvation* (2 Vols.). Minneapolis, MN: University of Minnesota Press.

Khan, C. M., Stephens, M. A. P., Franks, M. M., Rook, K. S., & Salem, J. K. (2012). Influences of spousal support and control on diabetes management through physical activity. *Health Psychology*. DOI: 10.1037/a0028609.

Kharbanda, R., & MacAllister, R. J. (2005). The atherosclerosis time-line and the role of the endothelium. *Current Medicinal Chemistry—Immunology, Endocrine, and Metabolic Agents*, 5, 47–52.

Khaw, K.-T., Wareham, N., Bingham, S., Luben, R., Welch, A., & Day, N. (2004). Association of hemoglobin A1c with cardiovascular disease and mortality in adults: The European Prospective Investigation Into Cancer in Norfolk. *Annals of Internal Medicine*, 141, 413–420.

Khaw, K.-T., Wareham, N., Bingham, S., Welch, A., Luben, R., & Day, N. (2008). Combined impact of health behaviours and mortality in men and women: The EPIC-Norfolk prospective population study. *PLoS Med*, 5, e12.

Khera, R., Murad, M. H., Chandar, A. K., Dulai, P. S., Zhen W., Prokop, L. J., … Wang, Z. (2016). Association of pharmacological treatments for obesity with weight loss and adverse events: A systematic review and meta-analysis. *Journal of the American Medical Association*, 315(22), 2424–2434.

Kickbusch, I. (2008). Health literacy: An essential skill for the twenty-first century. *Health Education*, 108, 101–104.

Kiecolt-Glaser, J. K. (1999). Stress, personal relationships, and immune function: Health implications. *Brain, Behavior and Immunity, 13*, 61–72.

Kiecolt-Glaser, J. K., Dura, J. R., Speicher, C. E., Trask, O. J., & Glaser, R. (1991). Spousal caregivers of dementia victims: Longitudinal changes in immunity and health. *Psychosomatic Medicine, 53*(4), 345–362.

Kiecolt-Glaser, J. K., Malarkey, W. B., Cacioppo, J. T., & Glaser, R. (1994). Stressful personal relationships: Immune and endocrine function. In R. Glaser & J. K. Kiecolt-Glaser (Eds.), *Handbook of human stress and immunity* (pp. 321–339). San Diego, CA: Academic Press.

Kiecolt-Glaser, J. K., Marucha, P. T., Malarkey, W. B., Mercado, A. M., & Glaser, R. (1995). Slowing of wound healing by psychological stress. *Lancet, 346*, 1194–1196.

Kiecolt-Glaser, J. K., McGuire, L., Robles, T. F., & Glaser, R. (2002). Emotions, morbidity, and mortality: New perspectives from psychoneuroimmunology. *Annual Review of Psychology, 53*, 83–108.

Kiecolt-Glaser, J. K., & Newton, T. L. (2001). Marriage and health: His and hers. *Psychological Bulletin, 127*, 472–503.

Kim, D., Kawachi, I., Hoorn, S. V., Ezzati, M. (2008). Is inequality at the heart of it? Cross-country associations of income inequality with cardiovascular diseases and risk factors. *Social Science and Medicine, 66*, 1719–1732.

Kim, H., Neubert, J. K., Rowan, J. S., Brahim, J. S., Iadarola, M. J., & Dionne, R. A. (2004). Comparison of experimental and acute clinical pain responses in humans as pain phenotypes. *Journal of Pain, 5*, 377–384.

Kim, H. S., Sherman, D. K., & Taylor, S. E. (2008). Culture and social support. *American Psychologist, 63*, 518–526.

Kim, Y., Myung, S.-K., Jeon, Y.-J., Lee, E.-H., Park, C.-H., Seo, H. G., … Huh, B. Y. (2011). Effectiveness of pharmacologic therapy for smoking cessation in adolescent smokers: Meta-analysis of randomized controlled trials. *American Journal of Health-System Pharmacy, 68*(3), 219–226.

Kimball, C. P. (1981). *The biopsychosocial approach to the patient.* Baltimore, MD: Williams and Wilkins.

King, B. A, Homa, D. M., Dube, S. R., & Babb, S. D. (2014). Exposure to secondhand smoke and attitudes toward smoke-free workplaces among employed U.S. adults: Findings from the National Adult Tobacco Survey. *Nicotine and Tobacco Research, 16*(10), 1307–1318.

King, D., & Pace, L. (2005, April). Sports, steroids, and scandals. *Information Today, 22*, 25–27.

King, J., & Henry, E. (2004, September 4). Bill Clinton awaits heart surgery next week. *CNN Washington Bureau.* Retrieved June 16, 2005, from http://www.cnn.com/2004/ALLPOLITICS/09/03/clinton.tests/

King, L., Saules, K. K., & Irish, J. (2007). Weight concerns and cognitive style: Which carries more "weight" in the prediction of smoking among college women? *Nicotine and Tobacco Research, 9*, 535–543.

King, T. K., Matacin, M., White, K. S., & Marcus, B. H. (2005). A prospective examination of body image and smoking cessation in women. *Body Image, 2*, 19–28.

Kirschbaum, C., Tietze, A., Skoluda, N., & Dettenborn, L. (2009). Hair as a retrospective calendar of cortisol production: Increased cortisol incorporation into hair in the third trimester of pregnancy. *Psychoneuroendocrinology, 34*, 32–37.

Kivlinghan, K. T., Granger, D. A., & Booth, A. (2005). Gender differences in testosterone and cortisol response to competition. *Psychoneuroendocrinology, 30*, 58–71.

Kiyohara, C., & Ohno, Y. (2010). Sex differences in lung cancer susceptibility: A review. *Gender Medicine, 7*(5), 381–401.

Klatsky, A. L. (2010). Alcohol and cardiovascular health. *Physiology and Behavior, 100*(1), 76–81.

Klatsky, A. L., & Udaltsova, N. (2007). Alcohol drinking and total mortality risk. *Annals of Epidemiology, 17*(S5), S63–S67.

Klatsky, A. L., & Udaltsova, A. (2013). Abounding confounding. *Addiction, 108*(9), 1549–1552.

Klein, D. A., Bennett, A. S., Schebendach, J., Foltin, R. W., Devlin, M. J., & Walsh, B. T. (2004). Exercise "addiction" in anorexia nervosa: Model development and pilot data. *CNS Spectrums, 9*, 531–537.

Klein, H., Elifson, K. W., & Sterk, C. E. (2003). "At risk" women who think that they have no chance of getting HIV: Self-assessed perceived risks. *Women and Health, 38*, 47–63.

Klimentidis, Y. C. (2011). Canaries in the coal mine: A cross-species analysis of the plurality of obesity epidemics. *Proceedings of the Royal Society B: Biological Sciences, 278*(1712), 1626–1632.

Kloberdanz, K. (2016). Taxi drivers: Years of living dangerously. *HealthDay.* Retrieved October 1, 2016, from https://consumer.healthday.com/encyclopedia/work-and-health-41/occupational-health-news-507/taxi-drivers-years-of-living-dangerously-646377.html

Klonoff, E. A., & Landrine, H. (2000). Is skin color a marker for racial discrimination? Explaining the skin color–hypertension relationship. *Journal of Behavioral Medicine, 23*, 329–338.

Kluger, R. (1996). *Ashes to ashes: America's hundred-year cigarette war, the public health and the unabashed triumph of Philip Morris.* New York, NY: Knopf.

Knafl, K. A., & Deatrick, J. A. (2002). The challenge of normalization for families of children with chronic conditions. *Pediatric Nursing, 28*, 49–54.

Knight, S. J., & Emanuel, L. (2007). Processes of adjustment to end-of-life losses: A reintegration model. *Journal of Palliative Medicine, 10*, 1190–1198.

Knott, C., Bell, S., & Britton, A. (2015). Alcohol consumption and the risk of type 2 diabetes: A systematic review and dose-response meta-analysis of more than 1.9 million individuals from 38 observational studies. *Diabetes Care, 38*(9), 1804–1812.

Knutson, K. L., & van Cauter, E. (2008). Associations between sleep loss and increased risk of obesity and diabetes. *Annals of the New York Academy of Sciences, 1129*(Suppl. 1), 287–304.

Knuttgen, H. G. (2007). Strength training and aerobic exercise: Comparison and contrast. *Journal of Strength and Conditioning, 21*, 973–978.

Ko, N.-Y., & Muecke, M. (2005). Reproductive decision-making among HIV-positive couples in Taiwan. *Journal of Nursing Scholarship, 37*, 41–47.

Kochanek, K. D., Xu, J., Murphy, S. L., Miniño, A. M., & Kung, H.-C. (2011). Deaths: Preliminary data for 2009. *National Vital Statistics Reports, 59*(4), 1–68.

Kofman, O. (2002). The role of prenatal stress in the etiology of developmental behavioural disorders. *Neuroscience and Biobehavioral Reviews, 26*, 457–470.

Kohn, L. T., Corrigan, J. M., & Donaldson, M. (Eds.). (1999). *To err is human: Building a safer health system.* Washington, DC: Institute of Medicine.

Köhnke, M. D. (2008). Approach to the genetics of alcoholism: A review based on pathophysiology. *Biochemical Pharmacology, 75*, 160–177.

Kolata, G. (2016, May 2). That lost weight? The body finds it. *New York Times*, A1.

Koopmans, G. T., & Lamers, L. M. (2007). Gender and health care utilization: The role of mental distress and help-seeking propensity. *Social Science and Medicine, 64*, 1216–1230.

Kop, W. J. (2003). The integration of cardiovascular behavioral medicine and psychoneuroimmunology: New developments based on converging research fields. *Brain, Behavior and Immunity, 17*, 233–237.

Kop, W. J., Stein, P. K., Tracy, R. P., Barzilay, J. I., Schulz, R., & Gottdiener, J. S. (2010). Autonomic nervous system dysfunction and inflammation contribute to the increased cardiovascular mortality risk associated with depression. *Psychosomatic Medicine, 72*, 626–635.

Kopnisky, K. L., Stoff, D. M., & Rausch, D. M. (2004). Workshop report: The effects of psychological variables on the progression of HIV-1 disease. *Brain, Behavior and Immunity, 18*, 246–261.

Koppel, B. S. Brust, J. C. M., Fife, T., Bronstein, J., Youssof, S., Gronseth, G., … Gloss, D. (2014). Systematic review: Efficacy and safety of medical marijuana in selected neurologic disorders: Report of the Guideline Development Subcommittee of the *American Academy of Neurology, 82*(17), 1556–1563.

Kosok, A. (2006). The moderation management programme in 2004: What type of drinker seeks controlled drinking? *International Journal of Drug Policy, 17*, 295–303.

Koss, M. P. (1990). The women's mental health research agenda: Violence against women. *American Psychologist, 45*, 374–380.

Koss, M. P., Bailey, J. A., Yuan, N. P., Herrara, V. M., & Lichter, E. L. (2003). Depression and PTSD in survivors of male violence: Research and training initiatives to facilitate recovery. *Psychology of Women Quarterly, 27*, 130–142.

Koster, A., Caserotti, P., Patel, K. V., Matthews, C. E., Berrigan, D., Van Domelen, D. R., … Harris, T. B. (2012). Association of sedentary time with mortality independent of moderate to vigorous physical activity. *PLoS One, 7*(6), e37696.

Kottow, M. H. (2007). Should research ethics triumph over clinical ethics? *Journal of Evaluation in Clinical Practice, 13*, 695–698.

Koval, J. J., Pederson, L. L., Zhang, X., Mowery, P., & McKenna, M. (2008). Can young adult smoking status be predicted from concern about body weight and self-reported BMI among adolescents? Results from a ten-year cohort study. *Nicotine and Tobacco Research, 10*(9), 1449–1455.

Kowal, J., & Fortier, M. S. (2007). Physical activity behavior change in middle-aged and older women: The role of barriers and of environmental characteristics. *Journal of Behavioral Medicine, 30*, 233–242.

Kozlowski, L. T., Wilkinson, A., Skinner, W., Kent, C., Franklin, T., & Pope, M. (1989). Comparing tobacco cigarette dependence with other drug dependences. *Journal of the American Medical Association, 261*, 898–901.

Krahn, D. D., Kurth, C. L., Gomberg, E., & Drewnowski, A. (2005). Pathological dieting and alcohol use in college women—A continuum of behaviors. *Eating Behaviors, 6*, 43–52.

Krantz, D. S., & McCeney, K. T. (2002). Effects of psychological and social factors on organic disease: A critical assessment of research on coronary heart disease. *Annual Review of Psychology, 53*, 341–369.

Krantz, G., Forsman, M., & Lundberg, U. (2004). Consistency in physiological stress responses and electromyographic activity during induced stress exposure in women and men. *Integrative Physiological and Behavioral Science, 39*, 105–118.

Krarup, L.-H., Truelsen, T., Pedersen, A., Kerke, H., Lindahl, M., Hansen, L., … Boysen, G. (2007). Level of physical activity in the week preceding an ischemic stroke. *Cerebrovascular Disease, 24*, 296–300.

Krewski, D., Lubin, J. H., Zielinski, J. M., Alavanja, M., Catalan, V. S., Field, R. W., … Wilcox, H. B. (2006). A combined analysis of North American case-control studies of residential radon and lung cancer. *Journal of Toxicology and Environmental Health, 69*, 533–597.

Krieger, N., Chen, J. T., Waterman, P. D., Rehkopf, D. H., & Subramanian, S. V. (2005). Painting a truer picture of US socioeconomic and racial/ethnic health inequalities: The public health disparities geocoding project. *American Journal of Public Health, 95*, 312–323.

Krisanaprakornkit, T., Krisanaprakornkit, W., Piyavhatkul, N., & Laopaiboon, M. (2006). Meditation therapy for anxiety disorders. *Cochrane Database of Systematic Reviews*, Cochrane Art. No.: CD004998, DOI: 10.1002/14651858.CD004998.pub2.

Krishna, S., & Boren, S. A. (2008). Diabetes self-management care via cell phone: A systematic review. *Journal of Diabetes, Science and Technology, 2*, 509–517.

Krishnan-Sarin, S., O'Malley, S., & Krysta, J. H. (2008). Treatment implications. *Alcohol Research and Health, 31*(4), 400–407.

Kristeller, J. L., & Wolever, R. Q. (2011). Mindfulness-based eating awareness training for treating binge eating disorder: The conceptual foundation. *Eating Disorders, 19*, 49–61.

Kröner-Herwig, B. (2009). Chronic pain syndromes and their treatment by psychological interventions. *Current Opinion in Psychiatry, 22*(2), 200–204.

Kronish, I. M., Rieckmann, N., Halm, E. A., Shimbo, D., Vorchheimer, D., Haas, D. C., … Davidson, K. W. (2006). Persistent depression affects adherence to secondary prevention behaviors after acute coronary syndromes. *Journal of General Internal Medicine, 21*, 1178–1183.

Kruger, J., Galuska, D. A., Serdula, M. K., & Jones, D. A. (2004). Attempting to lose weight: Specific practices among U.S. adults. *American Journal of Preventive Medicine, 26*, 402–406.

Kübler-Ross, E. (1969). *On death and dying.* New York, NY: Macmillan.

Kuhnel, J., & Sonnentag, S. (2011). How long do you benefit from vacation? A closer look at the fade-out of vacation effects. *Journal of Organizational Behavior, 32*, 125–143.

Kuk, J. L., & Ardern, C. I. (2009). Influence of age on the association between various measures of obesity and all-cause mortality. *Journal of the American Geriatrics Society, 57*(11), 2007–2084.

Kung, H. C., Hoyert, D. L., Xu, J. Q., & Murphy, S. L. (2008). Deaths: Final data for 2005. *National Vital Statistics Reports, 56*(10), 1–66.

Kuntsche, S., Plant, M. L., Plant, M. A., Miller, P., & Gabriel, G. (2008). Spreading or concentrating drinking occasions—Who is most at risk? *European Addiction Research, 14*(2), 71–81.

Kurland, H. (2000). *History of t'ai chi chu'an.* Retrieved May 16, 2008, from http://www.dotaichi.com/Articles/HistoryofTaiChi.htm

Kyngäs, H. (2004). Support network of adolescents with chronic disease: Adolescents' perspective. *Nursing and Health Sciences, 6*, 287–293.

Laaksonen, M., Talala, K., Martelin, T., Rahkonen, O., Roos, E., Helakorpi, S., … Prätälä, R. (2008). Health behaviours as explanations for educational level differences in cardiovascular and all-cause mortality: A follow-up of 60,000 men and women over 23 years. *European Journal of Public Health, 18*, 38–43.

Laatikainen, T., Critchley, J., Vartiainen, E., Salomaa, V., Ketonen, M., & Capewell, S. (2005). Explaining the decline in coronary heart disease mortality in Finland between 1982 and 1997. *American Journal of Epidemiology, 162*, 764–773.

Lai, D. T. C., Cahill, K., Qin, Y., & Tang, J. L. (2010). Motivational interviewing for smoking cessation. *Cochrane Database of Systematic Reviews 2010*, Cochrane Art. No.: CD006936, DOI: 10.1002/14651858.CD006936.pub2.

Laitinen, M. H., Ngandu, T., Rovio, S., Helkala, E.-L., Uusitalo, U., Viitanen, M., … Kivipelto, M. (2006). Fat intake at midlife and risk of dementia and Alzheimer's disease: A population-based study. *Dementia and Geriatric Cognitive Disorders, 22*, 99–107.

Lake, J. (2007). Philosophical problems in medicine and psychiatry, part II. *Integrative Medicine: A Clinician's Journal, 6*(3), 44–47.

Lake, J. (2009). Complementary, alternative, and integrative Rx: Safety issues. *Psychiatric Times, 26*(7), 22–29.

Lamptey, P. R. (2002). Reducing heterosexual transmission of HIV in poor countries. *British Medical Journal, 324*, 207–211.

Landolt, A. S., & Milling, L. S. (2011). The efficacy of hypnosis as an intervention for labor and delivery pain: A comprehensive methodological review. *Clinical Psychology Review, 31*(6), 1022–1031.

Landrine, H., & Klonoff, E. A. (1996). The Schedule of Racist Events: A measure of racial discrimination and a study of its negative physical and mental health consequences. *Journal of Black Psychology, 22*, 144–168.

Lang, E. V., Benotsch, E. G., Fick, L. J., Lutgendorf, S., Berbaum, M. L., Berbaum, K. S., … Spiegel, D. (2000). Adjunctive non-pharmacological analgesia for invasive medical procedures: A randomised trial. *Lancet, 355*, 1486–1490.

Lang, F. R., Baltes, P. B., & Wagner, G. G. (2007). Desired lifetime and end-of-life desires across adulthood from 20 to 90: A dual-source information model. *Journals of Gerontology Series B: Psychological Sciences and Social Sciences, 62B*, 268–276.

Langa, K. M., Foster, N. L., & Larson, E. B. (2004). Mixed dementia: Emerging concepts and therapeutic implications. *Journal of the American Medical Association, 292*, 2901–2908.

Lange, T., Dimitrov, S., & Born, J. (2011). Effects of sleep and circadian rhythm on the human immune system. *Annals of the New York Academy of Sciences, 1193*, 48–59.

Langer, E. J., & Rodin, J. (1976). The effects of choice and enhanced personal responsibility for the aged: A field experiment in an institutional setting. *Journal of Personality and Social Psychology, 34*, 191–198.

Lápez-Moreno, J. A., González-Cuevas, G., Moreno, G., & Navarro, M. (2008). The pharmacology of the endocannabinoid system: Functional structural interactions with other neurotransmitter systems and their repercussions in behavioral addiction. *Addiction Biology, 13*, 160–187.

Largo-Wight, E., Peterson, P. M., & Chen, W. W. (2005). Perceived problem solving, stress, and health among college students. *American Journal of Health Behavior, 29*, 360–370.

Larun, L., Nordheim, L. V., Ekeland, E., Hagen, K. B., & Heian, F. (2006). Exercise in prevention and treatment of anxiety and depression among children and young people. *Cochrane Database of Systematic Reviews*, Cochrane Art. No.: CD004691, DOI: 10.1002/14651858. CD004691.pub2.

Lash, S. J., Stephens, R. S., Burden, J. L., Grambow, S. C., DeMarce, J. M., Jones, M. E., … Hormer, R. D. (2007). Contracting, prompting, and reinforcing substance use disorder continuing care: A randomized clinical trial. *Psychology of Addictive Behaviors*, 21, 387–397.

Lasser, K. E., Himmelstein, D. U., & Woolhandler, S. (2006). Access to care, health status, and health disparities in the United States and Canada: Results of a cross-national population-based survey. *American Journal of Public Health*, 96, 1300–1307.

Lauerman, J. (2011, January 18). Jobs's cancer combined with transplant carries complications. *Bloomberg*. Retrieved April 20, 2012, from http://www.bloomberg.com/news/2011-01-17/jobs-s-liver-transplant-complicated-by-cancer-carries-risks-doctors-say.html

Laurent, M. R., & Vickers, T. J. (2009). Seeking health information online: Does Wikipedia matter? *Journal of the American Medical Informatics Association*, 16, 471–479.

Lautenschlager, N. T., Cox, K. L., Flicker, L., Foster, J. K., van Bockxmeer, F. M., Xiao, J., … Almedia, O. P. (2008). Effect of physical activity on cognitive function in older adults at risk for Alzheimer Disease. *Journal of the American Medical Association*, 300, 1027–1037.

LaVeist, T. A., Bowie, J. V., & Cooley-Quille, M. (2000). Minority health status in adulthood: The middle years of life. *Health Care Financing Review*, 21(4), 9–21.

Lawler, P. R., Filion, K. B., & Eisenberg, M. J. (2011). Efficacy of exercise-based cardiac rehabilitation post-myocardial infarction: A systematic review and meta-analysis of randomized controlled trials. *American Heart Journal*, 162, 571–584.

Lawrence, D., Mitrou, F., Sawyer, M. G., & Zubrick, S. R. (2010). Smoking status, mental disorders and emotional and behavioural problems in young people: Child and adolescent component of the National Survey of Mental Health and Wellbeing. *Australian and New Zealand Journal of Psychiatry*, 44(9), 805–814.

Lazarou, J., Pomeranz, B. H., & Corey, P. N. (1998). Incidence of adverse drug reactions in hospitalized patients: A meta-analysis of prospective studies. *Journal of the American Medical Association*, 278, 1200–1205.

Lazarus, R. S. (1984). Puzzles in the study of daily hassles. *Journal of Behavioral Medicine*, 7, 375–389.

Lazarus, R. S. (1993). From psychological stress to the emotions: A history of changing outlooks. *Annual Review of Psychology*, 44, 1–21.

Lazarus, R. S. (2000). Toward better research on stress and coping. *American Psychologist*, 55, 665–673.

Lazarus, R. S., & Cohen, J. (1977). Environmental stress. In I. Altman & J. Wohlwill (Eds.), *Human behavior and environment: Advances in theory and research* (Vol. 2, pp. 89–127). New York, NY: Plenum Press.

Lazarus, R. S., & DeLongis, A. (1983). Psychological stress and coping in aging. *American Psychologist*, 38, 245–254.

Lazarus, R. S., DeLongis, A., Folkman, S., & Gruen, R. (1985). Stress and adaptational outcomes. *American Psychologist*, 40, 770–779.

Lazarus, R. S., & Folkman, S. (1984). *Stress, appraisal, and coping*. New York, NY: Springer.

Lazovich, D., Vogel, R. I., Berwick, M., Weinstock, M. A., Anderson, K. E., & Warshaw, E. M. (2010). Indoor tanning and risk of melanoma: A case-control study in a highly exposed population. *Cancer Epidemiology, Biomarkers, and Prevention*, 19, 1557–1568.

Leahey, T. M., Kumar, R., Weinberg, B. M., & Wing, R. R. (2012). Teammates and social influence affect weight loss outcomes in a team-based weight loss competition. *Obesity*, 20(7), 1413–1418.

Leape, L. L., & Berwick, D. M. (2005). Five years after *To Err Is Human*: What have we learned? *Journal of the American Medical Association*, 293, 2384–2390.

Leavy, J. E., Bull, F. C., Rosenberg, M., & Bauman, A. (2011). Physical activity mass media campaigns and their evaluation: A systematic review of the literature 2003–2010. *Health Education Research*, 26, 1060–1085.

Lebovits, A. (2007). Cognitive-behavioral approaches to chronic pain. *Primary Psychiatry*, 14(9), 48–50, 51–54.

Lee, H. S., Engstrom, M., & Petersen, S. R. (2011). Harm reduction in 12 steps: Complementary, oppositional, or something in-between? *Substance Use and Misuse*, 46(9), 1151–1161.

Lee, L. M., Karon, J. M., Selik, R., Neal, J. J., & Fleming, P. L. (2001). Survival after AIDS diagnosis in adolescents and adults during the treatment era, United States, 1984–1997. *Journal of the American Medical Association*, 285, 1308–1315.

Lee, M. S., Kim, M. K., & Ryu, H. (2005). Qi-training (qigong) enhanced immune functions: What is the underlying mechanism? *International Journal of Neuroscience*, 115, 1099–1104.

Lee, M. S., Pittler, M. H., & Ernst, E. (2007a). External qigong for pain conditions: A systematic review of randomized clinical trials. *Journal of Pain*, 8, 827–831.

Lee, M. S., Pittler, M. H., & Ernst, E. (2007b). Tai chi for rheumatoid arthritis: Systematic review. *Rheumatology*, 46(11), 1648–1651.

Lee, P. N., & Forey, B. A. (2006). Environmental tobacco smoke exposure and risk of stroke in nonsmokers: A review with meta-analysis. *Journal of Stroke and Cerebrovascular Diseases*, 15(5), 190–201.

Lee, P. R., Lee, D. R., Lee, P., & Arch, M. (2010). 2010: U.S. drug and alcohol policy, looking back and moving forward. *Journal of Psychoactive Drugs*, 42(2), 99–114.

Leeuw, M., Goossens, M. E. J. B., Linton, S. J., Crombez, G., Boersma, K., & Vlaeyen, J. W. S. (2007). The fear-avoidance model of musculo-skeletal pain: Current state of scientific evidence. *Journal of Behavioral Medicine*, 30, 77–94.

Leger, D., Bayon, V., & de Sanctis, A. (2015). The role of sleep in the regulation of body weight. *Molecular and Cellular Endocrinology*, 418, 101–107.

Lemstra, M., Nannapaneni, U., Neudorf, C., Warren, L., Kershaw, T., & Scott, C. (2010). A systematic review of school-based marijuana and alcohol prevention programs targeting adolescents aged 10–15. *Addiction Research and Theory*, 18(1), 84–96.

Lenssinck, M.-L. B., Damen, L., Verhagen, A. P., Berger, M. Y., Passchier, J., & Koes, B. W. (2004). The effectiveness of physiotherapy and manipulation in patients with tension-type headache: A systematic review. *Pain*, 112, 381–388.

Leo, R. J., & Ligot, J. S. A., Jr. (2007). A systematic review of randomized controlled trials of acupuncture in the treatment of depression. *Journal of Affective Disorders*, 97, 13–22.

Leombruni, P., Pierò, A., Lavagnino, L., Brustolin, A., Campisi, S., & Fassino, S. (2008). A randomized, double-blind trial comparing ser-traline and fluoxetine 6-month treatment in obese patients with binge eating disorder. *Progress in Neuro-Psychopharmacology and Biological Psychiatry*, 32(6), 1599–1605.

Leon, A. S., & Sanchez, O. A. (2001). Response of blood lipids to exercise training alone or combined with dietary intervention. *Medicine and Science in Sports and Exercise*, 33, S502–S515.

Lepore, S. J., Fernandez-Berrocal, P., Ragan, J., & Ramos, N. (2004). It's not that bad: Social challenges to emotional disclosure enhance adjustment to stress. *Anxiety, Stress and Coping*, 17, 341–361.

Lepore, S. J., Revenson, T. A., Weinberger, S. L., Weston, P., Frisina, P. G., Robertson, R., … Cross, W. (2006). Effects of social stressors on cardiovascular reactivity in black and white women. *Annals of Behavioral Medicine*, 31, 120–127.

Leserman, J., Ironson, G., O'Cleirigh, C., Fordiani, J. M., & Balbin, E. (2008). Stressful life events and adherence in HIV. *AIDS Patient Care and STDs*, 22, 403–411.

Lestideau, O. T., & Lavallee, L. F. (2007). Structured writing about current stressors: The benefits of developing plans. *Psychology and Health*, 22, 659–676.

Leung, D. P., Chan, C. K., Tsang, H. W., Tsang, W. W., & Jones, A. Y. (2011). Tai chi as an intervention to improve balance and reduce falls in older adults: A systematic and meta-analytic review. *Alternative Therapies in Health and Medicine*, 17(1), 40–48.

Levenson, J. L., & Schneider, R. K. (2007). Infectious diseases. In J. L. Levenson (Ed.), *Essentials of psychosomatic medicine* (pp. 181–204). Washington, DC: American Psychiatric Publishing.

Levenson, R. W., Sher, K. J., Grossman, L. M., Newman, J., & Newlin, D. B. (1980). Alcohol and stress response dampening: Pharmacological effects, expectancy, and tension reduction. *Journal of Abnormal Psychology*, 89, 528–538.

Levenstein, S. (2000). The very model of a modern etiology: A biopsychosocial view of peptic ulcer. *Psychosomatic Medicine, 62,* 176–185.

Leventhal, H., & Avis, N. (1976). Pleasure, addiction, and habit: Factors in verbal report or factors in smoking behavior? *Journal of Abnormal Psychology, 85,* 478–488.

Leventhal, H., Breland, J. Y., Mora, P. A., & Leventhal, E. A. (2010). Lay representations of illness and treatment: A framework for action. In A. Steptoe (Ed.), *Handbook of behavioral medicine: Methods and application* (pp. 137–154). New York, NY: Springer.

Leventhal, H., Leventhal, E. A., & Cameron, L. (2001). Representations, procedures, and affect in illness self-regulation: A perceptual-cognitive model. In A. Baum, T. A. Revenson, & J. E. Singer (Eds.), *Handbook of health psychology* (pp. 19–47). Mahwah, NJ: Erlbaum.

Levi, L. (1974). Psychosocial stress and disease: A conceptual model. In E. K. E. Gunderson & R. H. Rahe (Eds.), *Life stress and illness* (pp. 8–33). Springfield, IL: Thomas.

Levin, B. E. (2010). Interaction of perinatal and pre-pubertal factors with genetic predisposition in the development of neural pathways involved in the regulation of energy homeostasis. *Brain Research, 1350,* 10–17.

Levin, T., & Kissane, D. W. (2006). Psychooncology—The state of its development in 2006. *European Journal of Psychiatry, 20,* 183–197.

Levy, D., & Brink, S. (2005). *A change of heart: How the people of Framingham, Massachusetts, helped unravel the mysteries of cardiovascular disease.* New York, NY: Knopf.

Lewis, E. T., Combs, A., & Trafton, J. A. (2010). Reasons for under-use of prescribed opioid medications by patients in pain. *Pain Medicine, 11,* 861–871.

Lewis, M., & Johnson, M. I. (2006). The clinical effectiveness of therapeutic massage for muscoloskeletal pain: A systematic review. *Physiotherapy, 92,* 146–158.

Li, G., Zhan, P., Wang, J., Gregg, E. W., Yang, W., Gong, Q., … Bennett, P. H. (2008). The long-term effect of lifestyle interventions to prevent diabetes in the China Da Qing Diabetes Prevention Study: A 20-year follow-up study. *The Lancet, 371,* 1783–1789.

Li, Q.-Z., Li, P., Garcia, G. E., Johnson, R. J., & Feng, L. (2005). Genomic profiling of neutrophil transcripts in Asian qigong practitioners: A pilot study in gene regulation by mind-body interaction. *Journal of Alternative and Complementary Medicine, 11,* 29–39.

Li, T.-K., Hewitt, B. G., & Grant, B. F. (2007). The Alcohol Dependency Syndrome, 30 years later: A commentary. *Addiction, 102*(10), 1522–1530.

Li, Y., Long, H., Chu, L., Liu, F., Tian, T., & He, D. (2015). Studies on the association between Alzheimer's disease and vascular risk factors: Reports from China. *Chinese Journal of Contemporary Neurology and Neurosurgery, 15*(7), 518–523.

Liang, X., Wang, Q., Yang, X., Cao, J., Chen, J., Mo, X., … Gu, D. (2011). Effect of mobile phone intervention for diabetes on glycaemic control: A meta-analysis. *Diabetic Medicine, 28,* 455–463.

Lichtenstein, B. (2005). Domestic violence, sexual ownership, and HIV risk in women in the American deep south. *Social Science and Medicine, 60,* 701–715.

Lieberman, M. A., & Goldstein, B. A. (2006). Not all negative emotions are equal: The role of emotional expression in online support groups for women with breast cancer. *Psycho-Oncology, 15,* 160–168.

Liechty, J. M. (2010). Body image distortion and three types of weight loss behaviors among nonoverweight girls in the United States. *Journal of Adolescent Health, 47*(2), 176–182.

Ligier, S., & Sternberg, E. M. (2001). The neuroendocrine system and rheumatoid arthritis: Focus on the hypothalamo-pituitary-adrenal axis. In R. Ader, D. L. Felten, & N. Cohen (Eds.), *Psychoneuroimmunology* (3rd ed., Vol. 2, pp. 449–469). San Diego, CA: Academic Press.

Lillie-Blanton, M., Maddox, T. M., Rushing, O., & Mensah, G. A. (2004). Disparities in cardiac care: Rising to the challenge of *Healthy People 2010. Journal of the American College of Cardiology, 44,* 503–508.

Lin, Y., Furze, G., Spilsbury, K., & Lewin, R. J. (2009). Misconceived and maladaptive beliefs about heart disease: A comparison between Taiwan and Britain. *Journal of Clinical Nursing, 18,* 46–55.

Lincoln, K. D., Chatters, L. M., & Taylor, R. J. (2003). Psychological distress among Black and White Americans: Differential effects of social support, negative interaction and personal control. *Journal of Health and Social Behavior, 44,* 390–407.

Linde, K., Allais, G., Brinkhaus, B., Fei, Y., Mehring, M., Shin, B., … White, A. R. (2016). Acupuncture for tension-type headache. *Cochrane Database Systematic Reviews.* DOI: 10.1002/14651858.CD007587.pub2

Linde, K., Berner, M. M., & Kriston, L. (2008). St. John's wort for major depression. *Cochrane Database of Systematic Reviews, 2008,* Issue 4. Cochrane, Art. No.: CD000448, DOI: 10.1002/14651858.CD000448.pub3.

Linde, K., Witt, C. M., Streng, A., Weidenhammer, W., Wagenfeil, S., Brinkhaus, B., … Melchart, D. (2007). The impact of patient expectations on outcomes in four randomized controlled trials of acupuncture in patients with chronic pain. *Pain, 128,* 264–271.

Linden, W. (2000). Psychological treatments in cardiac rehabilitation: Review of rationales and outcomes. *Journal of Psychosomatic Research, 48,* 443–454.

Lindsay, J., Sykes, E., McDowell, I., Verreault, R., & Laurin, D. (2004). More than epidemiology of Alzheimer's disease: Contributions of the Canadian Study of Health and Aging. *Canadian Journal of Psychiatry, 49,* 83–91.

Lindstrom, H. A., Fritsch, T., Petot, G., Smyth, K. A., Chen, C. H., Debanne, S. M., … Friedland, R. P. (2005). The relationship between television viewing in midlife and the development of Alzheimer's disease in a case-control study. *Brain and Cognition, 58,* 157–165.

Lints-Martindale, A. C., Hadjistavropoulos, T., Barber, B., & Gibson, S. J. (2007). A psychophysical investigation of the Facial Action Coding System as an index of pain variability among older adults with and without Alzheimer's disease. *Pain Medicine, 8,* 678–689.

Lippke, S., Schwarzer, R., Ziegelmann, J. P., Scholz, U., & Schuz, B. (2010). Testing stage-specific effects of a stage-matched intervention: A randomized controlled trial targeting physical exercise and its predictors. *Health Education and Behavior, 37,* 533–546.

Lippke, S., Ziegelmann, J., & Schwarzer, R. (2004). Initiation and maintenance of physical exercise: Stage-specific effects of a planning intervention. *Research in Sports Medicine: An International Journal, 12,* 221–240.

Lipton, R. B., Bigal, M. E., Diamond, M., Freitag, F., Reed, M. L., & Stewart, W. F. (2007). Migraine prevalence, disease burden, and the need for preventive therapy. *Neurology, 68,* 343–349.

Litten, R. Z., Wilford, B. B., Falk, D. E., Ryan, M. L., & Fertig, J. B. (2016). Potential medications for the treatment of alcohol use disorder: An evaluation of clinical efficacy and safety. *Substance Abuse, 37*(2), 286–298.

Litz, B. T., Williams, L., Wang, J., Bryant, R., & Engel, C. C. (2004). A therapist-assisted Internet self-help program for traumatic stress. *Professional Psychology: Research and Practice, 35,* 628–634.

Liu, H., Golin, C. E., Miller, L. G., Hays, R. D., Beck, C. K., Sanandji, S., … Wengr, N. S. (2001). A comparison study of multiple measures of adherence to HIV protease inhibitors. *Annals of Internal Medicine, 134,* 968–977.

Livermore, M. M., & Powers, R. S. (2006). Unfulfilled plans and financial stress: Unwed mothers and unemployment. *Journal of Human Behavior in the Social Environment, 13,* 1–17.

Livneh, H., & Antonak, R. F. (2005). Psychosocial adaptation to chronic illness and disability: A primer for counselors. *Journal of Counseling and Development, 83,* 12–20.

Livneh, H., Lott, S. M., & Antonak, R. F. (2004). Patterns of psychosocial adaptation to chronic illness and disability: A cluster analytic approach, *Psychology, Health and Medicine, 9,* 411–430.

Llewellyn, A., Simmonds, M., Owen, C. G., Woolacott, N. (2016). Childhood obesity as a predictor of morbidity in adulthood: A systematic review and meta-analysis. *Obesity Reviews, 17*(1), 56–67.

Lloyd-Williams, M., Dogra, N., & Petersen, S. (2004). First year medical students' attitudes toward patients with life-limiting illness: Does age make a difference? *Palliative Medicine, 18,* 137–138.

Lobo, A., Dufouil, C., Marcos, G., Quetglas, B., Saz, P., & Guallar, E. (2010). Is there an association between low-to-moderate alcohol consumption and risk of cognitive decline? *American Journal of Epidemiology*, *172*(6), 708–716.

Locher, J. L., Yoels, W. C., Maurer, D., & Van Ells, J. (2005). Comfort foods: An exploratory journey into the social and emotional significance of food. *Food and Foodways: History and Culture of Human Nourishment*, *13*, 273–297.

Lock, K., Pomerleau, J., Causer, L., Altmann, D. R., & McKee, M. (2005). The global burden of disease attributable to low consumption of fruit and vegetables: Implications for the global strategy on diet. *Bulletin of the World Health Organization*, *83*, 100–108.

Locke, J., le Grange, D., Agras, W. S., & Dare, C. (2001). *Treatment manual for anorexia nervosa: A family-based approach*. New York, NY: Guilford Press.

Loftus, M. (1995). The other side of fame. *Psychology Today*, *28*(3), 48–53, 70, 72, 74, 76, 78, 80–81.

Logan, D. E., & Rose, J. B. (2004). Gender differences in post-operative pain and patient controlled analgesia use among adolescent surgical patients. *Pain*, *109*, 481–487.

Loggia, M. L., Juneau, M., & Bushnell, M. C. (2011). Autonomic responses to heat pain: Heart rate, skin conductance, and their relation to verbal ratings and stimulus intensity. *Pain*, *152*, 592–598.

Lohaus, A., & Klein-Hessling, J. (2003). Relaxation in children: Effects of extended and intensified training. *Psychology and Health*, *18*, 237–249.

Lopez, C., Antoni, M., Penedo, F., Weiss, D., Cruess, S., Segotas, M., ... Fletcher, M. A. (2011). A pilot study of cognitive behavioral stress management effects on stress, quality of life, and symptoms in persons with chronic fatigue syndrome. *Journal of Psychosomatic Research*, *70*, 328–334.

Lotta, L. A., Abbasi, A., Sharp, S. J., Sahlqvist, A.-S., Waterworth, D., Brosnan, J. M., ... Wareham, N. J. (2015). Definitions of metabolic health and risk of future Type 2 diabetes in BMI categories: A systematic review and network meta-analysis. *Diabetes Care*, *38*(11), 2177–2187.

Lotufo, P. A., Gaziano, J. M., Chae, C. U., Ajani, U. A., Moreno-John, G., Buring, J. E., ... Manson, J. E. (2001). Diabetes and all-cause and coronary heart disease mortality among US male physicians. *Archives of Internal Medicine*, *161*, 242–247.

Loukola, A., Wedenoja, J., Keskitalo-Vuokko, K., Broms, U., Korhonen, T., Ripatti, S., ... Kaprio, J. (2014). Genome-wide association study on detailed profiles of smoking behavior and nicotine dependence in a twin sample. *Molecular Psychiatry*, *19*(5), 615–624.

Low, C. A., Stanton, A. L., Bower, J. E., & Gyllenhammer, L. (2010). A randomized controlled trial of emotionally expressive writing for women with metastatic breast cancer. *Health Psychology*, *29*, 460–466.

Lowes, L., Gregory, J. W., & Lyne, P. (2005). Newly diagnosed childhood diabetes: A psychosocial transition for parents? *Journal of Advanced Nursing*, *50*, 253–261.

Lowman, C., Hunt, W. A., Litten, R. Z., & Drummond, D. C. (2000). Research perspectives on alcohol craving: An overview. *Addiction*, *95*(Suppl. 2), 45–54.

Lu, Q., & Stanton, A. L. (2010). How benefits of expressive writing vary as a function of writing instructions, ethnicity and ambivalence over emotional expression. *Psychology and Health*, *25*, 669–684.

Lucas, A. E. M., Smeenk, F. W. J. M., Smeele, I. J., van Schayck, C. P. (2008). Overtreatment with inhaled corticosteroids and diagnostic problems in primary care patients, an exploratory study. *Family Practice*, *25*, 86–91.

Luders, E. (2013). Exploring age-related brain degeneration in meditation practitioners. *Annals of the New York Academy of Sciences*, *1307*, 82–88.

Lundahl, B., & Burke, B. L. (2009). The effectiveness and applicability of motivational interviewing: A practice-friendly review of four meta-analyses. *Journal of Clinical Psychology*, *65*, 1232–1245.

Lundahl, B. W., Kunz, C., Brownell, C., Tollefson, D., & Burke, B. L. (2010). A meta-analysis of motivational interviewing: Twenty-five years of empirical studies. *Research on Social Work Practice*, *20*(2), 137–160.

Luo, X. (2004). Estimates and patterns of direct health care expenditures among individuals with back pain in the United States. *Spine*, *29*, 79–86.

Lustman, P. J., & Clouse, R. E. (2005). Depression in diabetic patients: The relationship between mood and glycemic control. *Journal of Diabetes and Its Complications*, *19*, 113–122.

Lutfey, K. E., & Ketcham, J. D. (2005). Patient and provider assessments of adherence and the sources of disparities: evidence from diabetes care. *Health Services Research*, *40*(6p1), 1803–1817.

Lutz, R. W., Silbret, M., & Olshan, W. (1983). Treatment outcome and compliance with therapeutic regimens: Long-term follow-up of a multidisciplinary pain program. *Pain*, *17*, 301–308.

Lycett, D., Munafò, M., Johnstone, E., Murphy, M., & Aveyard, P. (2011). Associations between weight change over 8 years and baseline body mass index in a cohort of continuing and quitting smokers. *Addiction*, *106*(1), 188–196.

Lynch, H. T., Deters, C. A., Snyder, C. L., Lynch, J. F., Villeneuve, P., Silberstein, J., ... Brand, R. E. (2005). BRCA1 and pancreatic cancer: Pedigree findings and their causal relationships. *Cancer Genetics and Cytogenetics*, *158*, 119–125.

Lyvers, M., Cholakians, E., Puorro, M., & Sundram, S. (2011). Alcohol intoxication and self-reported risky sexual behaviour intentions with highly attractive strangers in naturalistic settings. *Journal of Substance Use*, *16*(2), 99–108.

Lyytikäinen, P., Rahkonen, O., Lahelma, E., & Lallukka, T. (2011). Association of sleep duration with weight and weight gain: A prospective follow-up study. *Journal of Sleep Research*, *20*(2), 298–302.

Ma, Y., Fan, R, & Li, M. D. (2016). Meta-analysis reveals significant association of the 3'-UTR VNTR in SLC6A3 with alcohol dependence. *Alcoholism: Clinical and Experimental Research*, *40*(7), 1443–1453.

MacDonald, G., & Leary, M. R. (2005). Why does social exclusion hurt? The relationship between social and physical pain. *Psychological Bulletin*, *131*, 202–223.

MacDougall, J. M., Dembroski, T. M., Dimsdale, J. E., & Hackett, T. P. (1985). Components of Type A, hostility, and anger-in: Further relationships to angiographic findings. *Health Psychology*, *4*, 137–142.

Macedo, A., Baños, J.-E., & Farré, M. (2008). Placebo response in the prophylaxis of migraine: A meta-analysis. *European Journal of Pain*, *12*, 68–75.

Maciejewski, P. K., Zhang, B., Block, S. D., & Prigerson, H. G. (2007). An empirical examination of the stage theory of grief. *Journal of the American Medical Association*, *297*, 716–723.

Mackay, J., & Mensah, G. (2004). *The atlas of heart disease and stroke*. Geneva, Switzerland: World Health Organization and Centers for Disease Control and Prevention.

MacKellar, D. A., Valleroy, L. A., Secura, G. M., Behel, S., Bingham, T., Celentano, D. D., ... Young Men's Survey Study Group. (2007). Perceptions of lifetime risk and actual risk for acquiring HIV among young men who have sex with men. *AIDS and Behavior*, *11*, 263–270.

Mackenbach, J. P., Stirbu, I., Roskam, J.-A. R., Schaap, M. M., Menvielle, G., Leinsalu, M., ... Kunst, A. E. (2008). Socioeconomic inequalities in health in 22 European countries. *New England Journal of Medicine*, *358*, 2468–2481.

MacLeod, A. K., & Conway, C. (2005). Well-being and the anticipation of future positive experiences: The role of income, social networks, and planning ability. *Cognition and Emotion*, *19*(3), 357–374.

Macrodimitris, S. D., & Endler, N. S. (2001). Coping, control, and adjustment in Type 2 diabetes. *Health Psychology*, *20*, 208–216.

Madsen, K. M., Hviid, A., Vestergaard, M., Schendel, D., Wohlfahrt, J., Thorsen, P., Olsen, J., & Melbye, M. (2002). A population-based study of measles, mumps, and rubella vaccination and autism. *New England Journal of Medicine*, *347*(19), 1477–1482.

Maenthaisong, R., Chaiyakunapruk, N., Niruntraporn, S., & Kongkaew, C. (2007). The efficacy of aloe vera used for burn wound healing: A systematic review. *Burns*, *33*, 713–718.

Mafi, J. N., McCarthy, E. P., Davis, R. B., & Landon, B. E. (2013). Worsening trends in the management and treatment of back pain. *JAMA Internal Medicine*, *173*(17), 1573–1581.

Magura, S. (2007). The relationship between substance user treatment and 12-step fellowships: Current knowledge and research questions. *Substance Use and Misuse*, *42*, 343–360.

Mahar, M. (2006). *Money-driven medicine: The real reason health care costs so much*. New York, NY: HarperCollins.

Maier, S. F. (2003). Bi-directional immune-brain communication: Implications for understanding stress, pain, and cognition. *Brain, Behavior and Immunity, 17*, 269–285.

Maier, S. F., & Watkins, L. R. (2003). Immune-to-central nervous system communication and its role in modulating pain and cognition: Implications for cancer and cancer treatment. *Brain, Behavior and Immunity, 17*, 125–131.

Maizels, M., & McCarberg, B. (2005). Antidepressants and antiepileptic drugs for chronic non-cancer pain. *American Family Physician, 71*, 483–490.

Major, B., & O'Brien, L. T. (2005). The psychology of stigma. *Annual Review of Psychology, 56*, 393–421.

Makary, M., & Daniel, M. (2016). Medical error—The third leading cause of death in the US. *British Medical Journal, 353*(2139). DOI: http://dx.doi.org/10.1136/bmj.i2139

Ma-Kellams, C., & Blascovich, J. (2011). Culturally divergent responses to mortality salience. *Psychological Science, 22*(8), 1019–1024.

Malecka-Tendera, E., & Mazur, A. (2006). Childhood obesity: A pandemic of the twenty-first century. *International Journal of Obesity, 30*(Suppl. 2), S1–S3.

Manchikanti, L., Vallejo, R., Manchikanti, K. N., Benyamin, R. M., Datta, S., & Christo, P. J. (2011). Effectiveness of long-term opioid therapy for chronic non-cancer pain. *Pain Physician, 14*, E133–E156.

Mancini, A. D., Bonanno, G. A., & Clark, A. E. (2011). Stepping off the hedonic treadmill: Individual differences in response to major life events. *Journal of Individual Differences, 32*, 144–152.

Mancini, A. D., Griffin, P., & Bonanno, G. A. (2012). Recent trends in the treatment of prolonged grief. *Current Opinion in Psychiatry, 25*, 46–51.

Mandayam, S. (2004). Epidemiology of alcoholic liver disease. *Seminars in Liver Disease, 24*, 217–232.

Manheimer, E., White, A., Berman, B., Forys, K., & Ernst, E. (2005). Meta-analysis: Acupuncture for low back pain. *Annals of Internal Medicine, 142*, 651–663.

Manimala, M. R., Blount, R. L., & Cohen, L. L. (2000). The effects of parental reassurance versus distraction on child distress and coping during immunizations. *Children's Health Care, 29*, 161–177.

Mann, D. M., Ponieman, D., Leventhal, H., & Halm, E. (2009). Predictors of adherence to diabetes medications: The role of disease and medication beliefs. *Journal of Behavioral Medicine, 32*, 278–284.

Mann, D. M., Woodward, M., Muntner, P., Falzon, L., & Kronish, I. (2010). Predictors of nonadherence to statins: A systematic review and meta-analysis. *The Annals of Pharmacotherapy, 44*, 1410–1421.

Mann, K. (2004). Pharmacotherapy of alcohol dependence: A review of the clinical data. *CNS Drugs, 18*, 485–504.

Manna, A., Raffone, A., Perrucci, M. G., Nardo, D., Ferretti, A., Tartaro, A., … Romani, G. L. (2010). Neural correlates of focused attention and cognitive monitoring in meditation. *Brain Research Bulletin, 82*(1/2), 46–56.

Mannan, H. R., Stevenson, C. E., Peeters, A., Walls, H. L., & McNeil, J. J. (2011). Age at quitting smoking as a predictor of risk of cardiovascular disease incidence independent of smoking status, time since quitting and pack-years. *BMC Research Notes, 4*(1), 39–47.

Manne, S. L., & Andrykowski, M. A. (2006). Are psychological interventions effective and accepted by cancer patients? II. Using empirically supported therapy guidelines to decide. *Annals of Behavioral Medicine, 32*, 98–103.

Manni, L., Albanesi, M., Guaragna, M., Barbaro Paparo, S., & Aloe, L. (2010). Neurotrophins and acupuncture. *Autonomic Neuroscience: Basic and Clinical, 157*(1/2), 9–17.

Manor, O., Eisenbach, Z., Friedlander, Y., & Kark, J. D. (2004). Educational differentials in mortality from cardiovascular disease among men and women: The Israel Longitudinal Mortality Study. *Annals of Epidemiology, 14*, 453–460.

Mantell, J. E., Stein, Z. A., & Susser, I. (2008). Women in the time of AIDS: Barriers, bargains, and benefits. *AIDS Education and Prevention, 20*, 91–106.

Mantzari, E., Vogt, F., Shemilt, I., Wei, Y., Higgins, J. P., & Marteau, T. M. (2015). Personal financial incentives for changing habitual health-related behaviors: A systematic review and meta-analysis. *Preventive Medicine, 75*, 75–85.

Mao, J. J., Palmer, C. S., Healy, K. E., Desai, K., & Amsterdam, J. (2011). Complementary and alternative medicine use among cancer survivors: A population-based study. *Journal of Cancer Survivorship: Research and Practice, 5*(1), 8–17.

Marcus, D. A. (2001). Gender differences in treatment-seeking chronic headache sufferers. *Headache, 41*, 698–703.

Margolis, R. D., & Zweben, J. E. (2011). *Treating patients with alcohol and other drug problems: An integrated approach* (2nd ed.). Washington, DC: American Psychological Association.

Mariotto, A. B., Yabroff, K. R., Shao, Y., Feuer, E. J., & Brown, M. L. (2011). Projections of the cost of cancer care in the United States: 2010–2020. *Journal of the National Cancer Institute, 103*, 117–128.

Markovitz, J. H., Matthews, K. A., Whooley, M., Lewis, C. E., & Greenlund, K. J. (2004). Increases in job strain are associated with incident hypertension in the CARDIA study. *Annals of Behavioral Medicine, 28*, 4–9.

Marlatt, G. A., Demming, B., & Reid, J. (1973). Loss of control drinking in alcoholics: An experimental analogue. *Journal of Abnormal Psychology, 81*, 233–241.

Marlatt, G. A., & Gordon, J. R. (1980). Determinants of relapse: Implication for the maintenance of behavior change. In P. O. Davidson & S. M. Davidson (Eds.), *Behavioral medicine: Changing health lifestyles* (pp. 410–452). New York: Brunner/Mazel.

Marlatt, G. A., & Rohsenow, D. J. (1980). Cognitive processes in alcohol use: Expectancy and the balanced placebo design. In N. Mello (Ed.), *Advances in substance abuse: Behavioral and biological research* (pp. 159–199). Greenwich, CT: JAI Press.

Marlatt, G. A., & Witkiewitz, K. (2010). Update on harm-reduction policy and intervention research. *Annual Review of Clinical Psychology, 6*, 591–606.

Marques, L., Alegria, M., Becker, A. E., Chen, C.-N., Fang, A., Chosak, A., …Diniz, J. B. (2011). Comparative prevalence, correlates of impairment, and service utilization for eating disorders across US ethnic groups: Implications for reducing ethnic disparities in health care access for eating disorders. *International Journal of Eating Disorders, 44*(5), 412–420.

Marquié, L., Raufaste, E., Lauque, D., Mariné, C., Ecoiffier, M., & Sorum, P. (2003). Pain rating by patients and physicians: Evidence of systematic miscalibration. *Pain, 102*, 289–296.

Marsland, A. L., Bachen, E. A., Cohen, S., & Manuck, S. B. (2001). Stress, immunity, and susceptibility to infectious disease. In A. Baum, T. A. Revenson, & J. E. Singer (Eds.), *Handbook of health psychology* (pp. 683–695). Mahwah, NJ: Erlbaum.

Marsland, A. L., Bachen, E. A., Cohen, S., Rabin, B., & Manuck, S. B. (2002). Stress, immune reactivity and susceptibility to infectious disease. *Physiology and Behavior, 77*, 711–716.

Marsland, A.L., Pressman, S.D., & Cohen, S. (2006). Positive affect and immune function. In R. Ader (Ed.), *Psychoneuroimmunology* (pp. 761–779). Elsevier Publications.

Martikainen, P., Valkonen, T., & Martelin, T. (2001). Change in male and female life expectancy by social class: Decomposition by age and cause of death in Finland 1971–95. *Journal of Epidemiology and Community Health, 55*, 494–499.

Martin, C. S., Fillmore, M. T., Chung, T., Easdon, C. M., & Miczek, K. A. (2006). Multidisciplinary perspectives on impaired control over substance use. *Alcoholism: Clinical and Experimental Research, 30*, 265–271.

Martin, P. D., & Brantley, P. J. (2004). Stress, coping, and social support in health and behavior. In J. M. Raczynsky & L. C. Leviton (Eds.), *Handbook of clinical health psychology* (Vol. 2, pp. 233–267). Washington, DC: American Psychological Association.

Martin, P. R., Forsyth, M. R., & Reece, J. (2007). Cognitive-behavioral therapy versus temporal pulse amplitude biofeedback training for recurrent headache. *Behavior Therapy, 38*, 350–363.

Martin, P. R., & Petry, N. M. (2005). Are non-substance- related addictions really addictions? *American Journal on Addictions, 14*, 1–3.

Martin, R., & Leventhal, H. (2004). Symptom perception and health care–seeking behavior. In J. M. Raczynski & L. C. Leviton (Eds.),

Handbook of clinical health psychology (Vol. 2, pp. 299–328). Washington, DC: American Psychological Association.

"Martin Sheen." (2008, May 27). Martin Sheen opens up about drug use. *Associated Press*. Retrieved June 26, 2011, from http://www.military.com/entertainment/movies/movie-news/martin-sheen-opens-up-about-drug-use

Martindale, D. (2001, May 26). Needlework: Whether it's controlling the flow of vital energy or releasing painkilling chemicals, acupuncture seems plausible enough. But does it really work? *New Scientist, 170,* 42–45.

Martinez, F. D. (2001). The coming-of-age of the hygiene hypothesis. *Respiratory Research, 2,* 129–132.

Martins, I. J., Hone, E., Foster, J. K., Sünram-Lea, S. I., Gnjec, A., Fuller, S. J., … Martins, R. N. (2006). Apolipoprotein E, cholesterol metabolism, diabetes, and the convergence of risk factors for Alzheimer's disease and cardiovascular disease. *Molecular Psychiatry, 11,* 721–736.

Martins, R. K., & McNeil, D. W. (2009). Review of motivational interviewing in promoting health behaviors. *Clinical Psychology Review, 29,* 283–293.

Martins, T., Hamilton, W., & Ukoumunne, O. C. (2013). Ethnic inequalities in time to diagnosis of cancer: A systematic review. *BMC Family Practice, 14*(1), 197.

Martinsen, E. W. (2005). Exercise and depression. *International Journal of Sport and Exercise Psychology, 3*(Special Issue), 469–483.

Martire, L. M., Lustig, A. P., Schulz, R., Miller, G. E., & Helgeson, V. S. (2004). Is it beneficial to involve a family member? A meta-analysis of psychosocial intervention for chronic illness. *Health Psychology, 23,* 599–611.

Martire, L. M., & Schulz, R. (2007). Involving family in psychosocial interventions for chronic illness. *Current Directions in Psychological Science, 16,* 90–94.

Martire, L. M., Schulz, R., Helgeson, V. S., Small, B. J., & Saghafi, E. M. (2010). Review and meta-analysis of couple-oriented interventions for chronic illness. *Annals of Behavioral Medicine, 40,* 325–342.

Mason, J. W. (1971). A reevaluation of the concept of "non-specificity" in stress theory. *Journal of Psychiatric Research, 8,* 323–333.

Mason, J. W. (1975). A historical view of the stress field. *Journal of Human Stress, 1* (Pt. 2), 22–36.

Mason, P. (2005). Deconstructing endogenous pain modulation. *Journal of Neurophysiology, 94,* 1659–1663.

Matarazzo, J. D. (1987). Postdoctoral education and training of service providers in health psychology. In G. C. Stone, S. M. Weiss, J. D. Matarazzo, N. E. Miller, J. Rodin, C. D. Belar, … J. E. Singer (Eds.), *Health psychology: A discipline and a profession* (pp. 371–388). Chicago, IL: University of Chicago Press.

Matarazzo, J. D. (1994). Health and behavior: The coming together of science and practice in psychology and medicine after a century of benign neglect. *Journal of Clinical Psychology in Medical Settings, 1,* 7–39.

Mathers, M. I., Salomon, J. A., Tandon, A., Chatterji, S., Ustün, B., & Murray, C. J. L. (2004). Global patterns of healthy life expectancy in the year 2002. *BMC Public Health, 4,* record 66. Retrieved August 9, 2005, from http://www.biomedcentral.com/1471-2458/4/66

Mathur, M. B., Epel, E., Kind, S., Desai, M., Parks, C. G., Sandler, D. P., … Khazeni, N (2016). Perceived stress and telomere length: A systematic review, meta-analysis, and methodologic considerations for advancing the field. *Brain, Behavior, and Immunity, 54,* 158–169.

Matthews, K. (2005). Former president to have scar tissue removed. *Associated Press*. Retrieved June 16, 2005, from http://www.greatdreams.com/political/clinton-heart.htm

Matthews, K. A. (2005). Psychological perspectives on the development of heart disease. *American Psychologist, 60,* 783–796.

Matthews, K. A., & Gallo, L. C. (2011). Psychological perspectives on pathways linking socioeconomic status and physical health. *Annual Review of Psychology, 62,* 501–530.

Matthews, K. A., Gallo, L. C., & Taylor, S. E. (2010). Are psychosocial factors mediators of socioeconomic status and health connections? A progress report and blueprint for the future. *Annals of the New York Academy of Sciences, 1186,* 146–173.

Matthews, K. A., Kuller, L. H., Chang, Y., & Edmundowicz, D. (2007). Premenopausal risk factors for coronary and aortic calcification: A 20-year follow-up in the healthy women study. *Preventive Medicine, 45,* 302–308.

Matthies, E., Hoeger, R., & Guski, R. (2000). Living on polluted soil: Determinants of stress symptoms. *Environment and Behavior, 32,* 270–286.

Matud, M. P. (2004). Gender differences in stress and coping styles. *Personality and Individual Differences, 37,* 1401–1415.

Mausbach, B. T., Coon, D. W., Depp, C., Rabinowitz, Y. G., Wilson-Arias, E., Kraemer, H. C., … Gallagher-Thompson, D. (2004). Ethnicity and time to institutionalization of dementia patients: A comparison of Latina and Caucasian female family caregivers. *Journal of the American Geriatrics Society, 52,* 1077–1084.

Mausbach, B. T., Semple, S. J., Strathdee, S. A., & Patterson, T. L. (2009). Predictors of safer sex intentions and protected sex among heterosexual HIV-negative methamphetamine users: An expanded model of the Theory of Planned Behavior. *AIDS Care, 21,* 17–24.

Mayeaux, R. (2003). Epidemiology of neurogeneration. *Annual Review of Neuroscience, 26,* 81–104.

Mayfield, D. (1976). Alcoholism, alcohol intoxication, and assaultive behavior. *Diseases of the Nervous System, 37,* 228–291.

Maynard, L. M., Serdula, M. K., Galuska, D. A., Gillespie, C., & Mokdad, A. H. (2006). Secular trends in desired weight of adults. *International Journal of Obesity, 30,* 1375–1381.

Mayo-Smith, M. F., Beecher, L. H., Fischer, T. L., Gorelick, D. A., Guillaunce, J. L., Hill, A., … Working Group on the Management of Alcohol Withdrawal Delirium. (2004). Management of alcohol withdrawal delirium: An evidence-based practice guideline. *Archives of Internal Medicine, 164,* 1405–1412.

Maziak, W. (2011). The global epidemic of waterpipe smoking. *Addictive Behaviors, 36*(1/2), 1–5.

Mazić, S., Lazović, B., Delić, M., Suzić Lazić, J., Aimović, T., & Brkić, P. (2014). Body composition assessment in athletes: A systematic review. *Medical Review, 67*(7/8), 255–260.

McCallie, M. S., Blum, C. M., & Hood, C. J. (2006). Progressive muscle relaxation. *Journal of Human Behavior in the Social Environment, 13,* 51–66.

McClave, A. K., McKnight-Eily, L. R., Davis, S. P., & Dube, S. R. (2010). Smoking characteristics of adults with selected lifetime mental illnesses: Results from the 2007 National Health Interview Survey. *American Journal of Public Health, 100*(12), 2464–2472.

McColl, K. E. L., Watabe, H., & Derakhshan, M. H. (2007). Sporadic gastric cancer: A complex interaction of genetic and environmental risk factors. *American Journal of Gastroenterology, 102,* 1893–1895.

McCracken, L. M., Eccleston, C., & Bell, L. (2005). Clinical assessment of behavioral coping responses: Preliminary results from a brief inventory. *European Journal of Pain, 9,* 69–78.

McCrae, R. R., & Costa, P. T., Jr. (2003). *Personality in adulthood: A five-factor theory perspective* (2nd ed.). New York, NY: Guilford Press.

McCulloch, M. (2014). Alcohol: To drink or not to drink. *Environmental Nutrition, 37*(12), 6.

McCullough, M. L., Patel, A. V., Kushi, L. H., Patel, R., Willett, W. C., Doyle, C., … Gapstur, S. M. (2011). Following cancer prevention guidelines reduces risk of cancer, cardiovascular disease, and all-cause mortality. *Cancer Epidemiology, Biomarkers and Prevention, 20,* 1089.

McCully, S. N., Don, B. P., & Updegraff, J. A. (2013). Using the Internet to help with diet, weight, and physical activity: Results from the Health Information National Trends Survey (HINTS). *Journal of Medical Internet Research, 15*(8), e148.

McDaniel, S. H., Belar, C. D., Schroeder, C., Hargrove, D. S., & Freeman, E. L. (2002). A training curriculum for professional psychologists in primary care. *Professional Psychology: Research and Practice, 33,* 65–72.

McDaniel, S. H., & le Roux, P. (2007). An overview of primary care family psychology. *Journal of Clinical Psychology in Medical Settings, 14,* 23–32.

McDonough, M., Jose, P., & Stuart, J. (2016). Bi-directional effects of peer relationships and adolescent substance use: A longitudinal study. *Journal of Youth and Adolescence, 45*(8), 1652–1663.

McEachan, R. R. C., Conner, M., Taylor, N. J., & Lawton, R. J. (2011). Prospective prediction of health-related behaviours with the Theory of Planned Behaviour: A meta-analysis. *Health Psychology Review, 5*, 97–144.

McEwen, A., West, R., & McRobbie, H. (2008). Motives for smoking and their correlates in clients attending Stop Smoking treatment services. *Nicotine and Tobacco Research, 10*, 843–850.

McEwen, B. S. (2005). Stressed or stressed out: What is the difference? *Journal of Psychiatry and Neuroscience, 30*, 315–318.

McEwen, B. S., & Gianaros, P. J. (2010). Central role of the brain in stress and adaptation: Links to socioeconomic status, health, and disease. *Annals of the New York Academy of Sciences, 1186*, 190–222.

McGee, D. L. (2005). Body mass index and mortality: A meta-analysis based on person-level data from twenty-six observational studies. *Annals of Epidemiology, 15*, 87–97.

McGregor, B. A., & Antoni, M. H. (2009). Psychological intervention and health outcomes among women treated for breast cancer: A review of stress pathways and biological mediators. *Brain, Behavior, and Immunity, 23*, 159–166.

McGuire, B. E., & Shores, E. A. (2001). Simulated pain on the Symptom Checklist 90–Revised. *Journal of Clinical Psychology, 57*, 1589–1596.

McHugh, M. D. (2007). Readiness for change and short-term outcomes of female adolescents in residential treatment for anorexia nervosa. *International Journal of Eating Disorders, 40*, 602–612.

McIntosh, C. N., Fines, P., Wilkins, R., & Wolfson, M. C. (2009). Income disparities in health-adjusted life expectancy for Canadian adults, 1991 to 2001. *Health Reports, 20*, 55–64.

McKay, D., & Schare, M. L. (1999). The effects of alcohol and alcohol expectancies on subjective reports and physiological reactivity: A meta-analysis. *Addictive Behaviors, 24*, 633–647.

McKay, J. R., & Hiller-Sturmhöfel, S. (2010). Treating alcoholism as a chronic disease: Approaches to long-term continuing care. *Alcohol Research and Health, 33*(4), 356–370.

McKechnie, R., Macleod, R., & Keeling, S. (2007). Facing uncertainty: The lived experience of palliative care. *Palliative and Supportive Care, 5*, 367–376.

McKee, S. A., Sinha, R., Weinberger, A. H., Sofuoglu, M., Harrison, E. L. R., Lavery, M., … Wanzer, J. (2011). Stress decreases the ability to resist smoking and potentiates smoking intensity and reward. *Journal of Psychopharmacology, 25*(4), 490–502.

McLean, S., Skirboll, L. R., & Pert, C. B. (1985). Comparison of substance P and enkephalin distribution in rat brain: An overview using radioimmunocytochemistry. *Neuroscience, 14*, 837–852.

McLellan, A. T., Lewis, D. C., O'Brien, C. P., & Kleber, H. D. (2000). Drug dependence, a chronic medical illness: Implications for treatment, insurance, and outcomes. *Journal of the American Medical Association, 284*, 1689–1695.

McNally, R. J. (2003). Progress and controversy in the study of post-traumatic stress disorder. *Annual Review of Psychology, 54*, 229–252.

McRae, C., Cherin, E., Tamazaki, T. G., Diem, G., Vo, A. H., Russell, D., … Freed, C. R. (2004). Effects of perceived treatment on quality of life and medical outcomes in a double-blind placebo surgery trial. *Archives of General Psychiatry, 61*, 412–420.

McWilliams, J. M. (2009). Health consequences of uninsurance among adults in the United States: Recent evidence and implications. *The Milbank Quarterly, 87*, 443–494.

McWilliams, L. A., Goodwin, R. D., & Cox, B. J. (2004). Depression and anxiety associated with three pain conditions: Results from a nationally representative sample. *Pain, 111*, 77–83.

Mechanic, D. (1978). *Medical sociology* (2nd ed.). New York: Free Press.

Mehler, P. S. (2011). Medical complications of bulimia nervosa and their treatments. *International Journal of Eating Disorders, 44*(2), 95–104.

Mehta, P., & Sharma, M. (2012). Internet and cell phone based physical activity interventions in adults. *Archives of Exercise in Health and Disease, 2*, 108–113.

Meichenbaum, D. (2007). Stress inoculation training: A preventative and treatment approach. In P. M. Lehrer, R. L. Woolfolk, & W. E. Sime (Eds.), *Principles and practices of stress management* (3rd ed., pp. 497–517). New York, NY: Guilford Press.

Meichenbaum, D., & Cameron, R. (1983). Stress inoculation training: Toward a general paradigm for training coping skills. In D. Meichenbaum & M. E. Jaremko (Eds.), *Stress reduction and prevention* (pp. 115–154). New York, NY: Plenum Press.

Meichenbaum, D., & Turk, D. C. (1976). The cognitive-behavioral management of anxiety, anger and pain. In P. O. Davidson (Ed.), *The behavioral management of anxiety, depression, and pain* (pp. 1–34). New York, NY: Brunner/Mazel.

Melamed, B. G., Kaplan, B., & Fogel, J. (2001). Childhood health issues across the life span. In A. Baum, T. A. Revenson, & J. E. Singer (Eds.), *Handbook of health psychology* (pp. 449–457). Mahwah, NJ: Erlbaum.

Melzack, R. (1973). *The puzzle of pain.* New York, NY: Basic Books.

Melzack, R. (1975). The McGill Pain Questionnaire: Major properties and scoring methods. *Pain, 1*, 277–299.

Melzack, R. (1987). The short-form McGill Pain Questionnaire. *Pain, 30*, 191–197.

Melzack, R. (1992, April). Phantom limbs. *Scientific American, 266*, 120–126.

Melzack, R. (1993). Pain: Past, present and future. *Canadian Journal of Experimental Psychology, 47*, 615–629.

Melzack, R. (2005). Evolution of the neuromatrix theory of pain. *Pain Practice, 5*, 85–94.

Melzack, R. (2008). The future of pain. *Nature Reviews Drug Discovery, 7*, 629.

Melzack, R., & Katz, J. (2001). The McGill Pain Questionnaire: Appraisal and current status. In D. C. Turk & R. Melzack (Eds.), *Handbook of pain assessment* (2nd ed., pp. 35–52). New York, NY: Guilford Press.

Melzack, R., & Wall, P. D. (1965). Pain mechanisms: A new theory. *Science, 150*, 971–979.

Melzack, R., & Wall, P. D. (1982). *The challenge of pain.* New York, NY: Basic Books.

Melzack, R., & Wall, P. D. (1988). *The challenge of pain* (rev. ed.). London: Penguin.

Mercken, L., Candel, M., Willems, P., & de Vries, H. (2007). Disentangling social selection and social influence effects on adolescent smoking: The importance of reciprocity in friendships. *Addiction, 102*, 1483–1492.

Merritt, M. M., Bennett, G. G., Williams, R. B., Sollers, J. J., III, & Thayer, J. F. (2004). Low educational attainment, John Henryism, and cardiovascular reactivity to and recovery from personally relevant stress. *Psychosomatic Medicine, 66*, 49–55.

MH Interview: Ricky Gervais. (2013, March 25). Retrieved from http://www.menshealth.co.uk/living/men/mh-interview-ricky-gervais

Michael, K. C., Torres, A., & Seemann, E. A. (2007). Adolescents' health habits, coping styles and self-concept are predicted by exposure to interparental conflict. *Journal of Divorce and Remarriage, 48*, 155–174.

Michaud, D. S. (2007). Chronic inflammation and bladder cancer. *Urologic Oncology, 25*, 260–268.

"Michelle Obama." (2011, Feb. 8). Michelle Obama: President quit smoking. *HuffPost Politics.* Retrieved June 4, 2011, from http://www.huffingtonpost.com/2011/02/08/michelle-obama-president-_n_82034.html

Michie, S., Abraham, C., Whittington, C., McAteer, J., & Gupta, S. (2009). Effective techniques in healthy eating and physical activity interventions: A meta-regression. *Health Psychology, 28*(6), 690–701.

Michie, S., O'Connor, D., Bath, J., Giles, M., & Earll, L. (2005). Cardiac rehabilitation: The psychological changes that predict health outcome and healthy behaviour. *Psychology, Health and Medicine, 10*, 88–95.

Miech, R. A., Johnston, L. D., O'Malley, P. M., Bachman, J. G., & Schulenberg, J. E. (2016). *Monitoring the Future national survey results on drug use, 1975–2015: Volume I, Secondary school students.* Ann Arbor: Institute for Social Research, The University of Michigan. Retrieved from http://monitoringthefuture.org/pubs.html#monographs

Milam, J. E. (2004). Posttraumatic growth among HIV/AIDS patients. *Journal of Applied Social Psychology*, *34*, 2353–2376.

Miles, L. (2007). Physical activity and the prevention of cancer: A review of recent findings. *Nutrition Bulletin*, *32*, 250–282.

Miligi, L., Costantini, A. S., Veraldi, A., Benvenuti, A., & Vineis, P. (2006). Cancer and pesticides. *Annals of the New York Academy of Sciences*, *1076*, 366–377.

Miller, D. B., & Townsend, A. (2005). Urban hassles as chronic stressors and adolescent mental health: The Urban Hassles Index. *Brief Treatment and Crisis Intervention*, *5*, 85–94.

Miller, F. G., & Wager, T. (2004). Painful deception. *Science*, *304*, 1109–1111.

Miller, G. E., & Blackwell, E. (2006). Turning up the heat: Inflammation as a mechanism linking chronic stress, depression, and heart disease. *Current Directions in Psychological Science*, *15*, 269–272.

Miller, G. E., & Cohen, S. (2001). Psychological interventions and the immune system: A meta-analytic review and critique. *Health Psychology*, *20*, 47–63.

Miller, L. G., Liu, H., Hays, R. D., Golin, C. E., Beck, C. K., Asch, S. M., ... Wenger, N. S. (2002). How well do clinicians estimate patients' adherence to combination antiretroviral therapy? *Journal of General Internal Medicine*, *17*, 1–11.

Miller, M., Hemenway, D., & Rimm, E. (2000). Cigarettes and suicide: A prospective study of 50,000 men. *American Journal of Public Health*, *90*, 768–773.

Miller, N. E. (1969). Learning of visceral and glandular responses. *Science*, *163*, 434–445.

Miller, V. A., & Drotar, D. (2003). Discrepancies between mother and adolescent perceptions of diabetes-related decision-making autonomy and their relationship to diabetes-related conflict and adherence to treatment. *Journal of Pediatric Psychology*, *28*, 265–274.

Miller, W. R., & Rollnick, S. (2002). *Motivational interviewing: Preparing people for change* (2nd ed.). New York, NY: Guilford Press.

Miller, W. R., Walters, S. T., & Bennett, M. E. (2001). How effective is alcoholism treatment in the United States? *Journal of Studies on Alcohol*, *62*, 211–220.

Miller, W. R., Wilbourne, P. L., & Hettema, J. E. (2003). What works? A summary of alcohol treatment outcome research. In R. K. Hester & W. R. Miller (Eds.), *Handbook of alcoholism treatment approaches: Effective alternatives* (3rd ed., pp. 13–63). Boston, MA: Allyn and Bacon.

Milling, L. S., Kirsch, I., Allen, G. J., & Reutenauer, E. L. (2005). The effects of hypnotic and nonhypnotic imaginative suggestion on pain. *Annals of Behavioral Medicine*, *29*, 116–127.

Milling, L. S., Levine, M. R., & Meunier, S. A. (2003). Hypnotic enhancement of cognitive-behavioral interventions for pain: An analogue treatment study. *Health Psychology*, *22*, 406–413.

Mills, N., Allen, J., & Morgan, S. C. (2000). Does tai chi/qi gong help patients with multiple sclerosis? *Journal of Bodywork and Movement Therapies*, *4*, 39–48.

Miniño, A. M., Murphy, S. L., Xu, J., & Kochanek, K. D. (2011, December 7). Deaths: Final data for 2008. *National Vital Statistics Reports*, *59*(10), 1–126.

Mitchell, M., Johnston, L., & Keppell, M. (2004). Preparing children and their families for hospitalization: A review of the literature. *Paediatric and Child Health Nursing*, *7*(2), 5–15.

Mitchell, M. S., Goodman, J. M., Alter, D. A., John, L. K., Oh, P. I., Pakosh, M. T., ... Faulkner, G. E. (2013). Financial incentives for exercise adherence in adults: Systematic review and meta-analysis. *American Journal of Preventive Medicine*, *45*(5), 658–667.

Mitchell, W. (2001). Neurological and developmental effects of HIV and AIDS in children and adolescents. *Mental Retardation and Developmental Disabilities Research Reviews*, *7*, 211–216.

Mittring, N., Pérard, M., & Witt, C. M. (2013). Corporate culture assessment in integrative oncology: A qualitative case study of two integrative oncology centers. *Evidence-based Complementary and Alternative Medicine (eCAM)*, *2013*, 1–8.

Miyazaki, T., Ishikawa, T., Iimori, H., Miki, A., Wenner, M., Fukunishi, I., ... Kawamura, N. (2003). Relationship between perceived social support and immune function. *Stress and Health*, *19*, 3–7.

Moak, Z. B., & Agrawal, A. (2010). The association between perceived interpersonal social support and physical and mental health: Results from the national epidemiological survey on alcohol and related conditions. *Journal of Public Health*, *32*, 191–201.

Mochly-Rosen, D., & Zakhari, S. (2010). Focus on: The cardiovascular system: What did we learn from the French (paradox)? *Alcohol Research and Health*, *33*(1/2), 76–88.

Moen, P., & Yu, Y. (2000). Effective work/life strategies: Working couples, work conditions, gender, and life quality. *Social Problems*, *47*, 291–326.

Moerman, D. (2003). Doctors and patients: The role of clinicians in the placebo effect. *Advances*, *19*(1), 14–22.

Moerman, D. (2011). Examining a powerful healing effect through a cultural lens, and finding meaning. *The Journal of Mind-Body Regulation*, *1*, 63–72.

Moerman, D., & Jonas, W. B. (2002). Deconstructing the placebo effect and finding the meaning response. *Annals of Internal Medicine*, *136*, 471–476.

Moldovan, A. R., & David, D. (2011). Effect of obesity treatments on eating behavior: Psychosocial interventions versus surgical interventions: A systematic review. *Eating Behaviors*, *12*(3), 161–167.

Molimard, M., & Le Gros, V. (2008). Impact of patient-related factors on asthma control. *Journal of Asthma*, *45*, 109–113.

Molloy, G. J., O'Carroll, R. E., & Ferguson, E. (2014). Conscientiousness and medication adherence: A meta-analysis. *Annals of Behavioral Medicine*, *47*(1), 92–101.

Molloy, G. J., Perkins-Porras, L., Bhattacharyya, M. R., Strike, P. C., & Steptoe, A. (2008). Practical support predicts medication adherence and attendance at cardiac rehabilitation following acute coronary syndrome. *Journal of Psychosomatic Research*, *65*, 581–586.

Molloy, G. J., Perkins-Porras, L., Strike, P. C., & Steptoe, A. (2008). Social networks and partner stress as predictors of adherence to medication, rehabilitation attendance, and quality of life following acute coronary syndrome. *Health Psychology*, *27*, 52–58.

Monahan, J. L., & Lannutti, P. J. (2000). Alcohol as social lubricant. *Human Communication Research*, *26*, 175–202.

Mongan, J. J., Ferris, T. G., & Lee, T. H. (2008). Options for slowing the growth of health care costs. *New England Journal of Medicine*, *358*, 1509–1514.

Monroe, S. M. (2008). Modern approaches to conceptualizing and measuring human life stress. *Annual Review of Clinical Psychology*, *4*, 33–52.

Monroe, S. M., & Harkness, K. L. (2005). Life stress, the "kindling" hypothesis, and the recurrence of depression: Considerations from a life stress perspective. *Psychological Review*, *112*, 417–445.

Montgomery, G. H., DuHamel, K. N., & Redd, W. H. (2000). A meta-analysis of hypnotically induced analgesia: How effective is hypnosis? *International Journal of Clinical and Experimental Hypnosis*, *48*, 138–153.

Montgomery, G. H., Erblich, J., DiLorenzo, T., & Bovbjerg, D. H. (2003). Family and friends with disease: Their impact on perceived risk. *Preventive Medicine*, *37*, 242–249.

Moore, J. (2004). The puzzling origins of AIDS. *American Scientist*, *92*, 540–547.

Moore, L. J., Vine, S. J., Wilson, M. R., & Freeman, P. (2012). The effect of challenge and threat states on performance: An examination of potential mechanisms. *Psychophysiology*, *49*(10), 1417–1425.

Moore, L. L., Visioni, A. J., Qureshi, M. M., Bradlee, M. L., Ellison, R. C., & D'Agostino, R. (2005). Weight loss in overweight adults and the long-term risk of hypertension: The Framingham Study. *Archives of Internal Medicine*, *165*, 1298–1303.

Moore, S., Sikora, P., Grunberg, L., & Greenberg, E. (2007). Expanding the tension-reduction model of work stess and alcohol use: Comparison of managerial and non-managerial men and women. *Journal of Management Studies*, *44*, 261–283.

Moorman, J. E., Akinbami, L. J., Bailey, C. M., Zahran, H. S., King, M. E., Johnson, C. A., ... Liu, X. (2012). National surveillance of asthma: United States, 2001-2010. *Vital & health statistics. Series 3, Analytical and epidemiological studies/[US Dept. of Health and Human Services, Public Health Service, National Center for Health Statistics]*, (35), 1–58.

Moos, R. H., & Schaefer, J. A. (1984). The crisis of physical illness: An overview and conceptual analysis. In R. H. Moos (Ed.), *Coping with physical illness: Vol. 2. New perspectives* (pp. 3–25). New York, NY: Plenum Press.

Moran, W. R. (2002, January 31). Jackie Joyner-Kersee races against asthma. *USA Today Health.* Retrieved July 7, 2005, from http://www. usato-day.com/news/health/spotlight/2002/01/31/spotlight-kersee.htm

Morgan, N., Irwin, M. R., Chung, M., & Wang, C. (2014). The effects of mind-body therapies on the immune system: Meta-analysis. *PLoS One, 9*(7), 1–14.

Morgan, W. P. (1979, February). Negative addiction in runners. *The Physician and Sportsmedicine, 7,* 56–63, 67–70.

Morgan, W. P. (1981). Psychological benefits of physical activity. In F. J. Nagle & H. J. Montoye (Eds.), *Exercise in health and disease* (pp. 299–314). Springfield, IL: Thomas.

Morillo, L. E., Alarcon, F., Aranaga, N., Aulet, S., Chapman, E., Conterno, L., … Latin American Migraine Study Group. (2005). Prevalence of migraine in Latin America. *Headache, 45,* 106–117.

Morley, S., de C. Williams, A. C., & Black, S. (2002). A confirmatory factor analysis of the Beck Depression Inventory in chronic pain. *Pain, 99,* 289–298.

Morris, J. C., Storandt, M., Miller, J. P., McKeel, D. W., Price, J. L., Rubin, E. H., … Berg, L. (2001). Mild cognitive impairment represents early-stage Alzheimer disease. *Archives of Neurology, 58,* 397–405.

Morris, J. N., Heady, J. A., Raffle, P. A. B., Roberts, C. G., & Parks, J. W. (1953). Coronary heart disease and physical activity of work. *Lancet, 2,* 1053–1057, 1111–1120.

Morris, L. J., D'Este, C., Sargent-Cox, K., & Anstey, K. J. (2016). Concurrent lifestyle risk factors: Clusters and determinants in an Australian sample. *Preventive Medicine, 84,* 1–5.

Morrison, C. D. (2008). Leptin resistance and the response to positive energy balance. *Physiology and Behavior, 94,* 660–663.

Moseley, J. B., O'Malley, K. P., Petersen, N. J., Menke, T. J., Brody, B. A., Kuykendall, D. H., … Wray, N. P. (2002). A controlled trial of arthroscopic surgery for osteoarthritis of the knee. *New England Journal of Medicine, 347,* 81–88.

Moskowitz, J. T. (2003). Positive affect predicts lower risk of AIDS mortality. *Psychosomatic Medicine, 65,* 620–626.

Moskowitz, J. T., Hult, J. R., Bussolari, C., & Acree, M. (2009). What works in coping with HIV? A meta-analysis with implications for coping with serious illness. *Psychological Bulletin, 135,* 121–141.

Moskowitz, J. T., & Wrubel, J. (2005). Coping with HIV as a chronic illness: A longitudinal analysis of illness appraisals. *Psychology and Health, 20,* 509–531.

Mosley, P. E. (2009). Bigorexia: Bodybuilding and muscle dysmorphia. *European Eating Disorders Review, 17*(3), 191–198.

Motivala, S. J., & Irwin, M. R. (2007). Sleep and immunity: Cytokine pathways linking sleep and health outcomes. *Current Directions in Psychological Science, 16,* 21–25.

Mottillo, S., Filion, K. B., Genest, J., Joseph, L., Pilote, L., Poirier, P., … Eisenberg, M. J. (2010). The metabolic syndrome and cardiovascular risk: A systematic review and meta-analysis. *Journal of the American College of Cardiology, 56,* 1113–1132.

Moussavi, S., Shatterji, S., Verdes, E., Tandon, A., Patel, V., & Ustun, B. (2007). Depression, chronic diseases, and decrements in health: Results from the World Health Surveys. *The Lancet, 370,* 851–858.

Moyer, C. A., Rounds, J., & Hannum, J. W. (2004). Meta-analysis of massage therapy research. *Psychological Bulletin, 130,* 3–18.

Mozaffarian, D., Longstreth, W. T., Lemaitre, R. N., Manolio, T. A., Kuller, L. H., Burke, G. L., … Siscovick, D. S. (2005). Fish consumption and stroke risk in elderly individuals: The Cardiovascular Health Study. *Archives of Internal Medicine, 165,* 200–206.

Mukamal, K. J., Chen, C. M., Rao, S. R., & Breslow, R. A. (2010). Alcohol consumption and cardiovascular mortality among U.S. adults, 1987 to 2002. *Journal of the American College of Cardiology, 55*(13), 1328–1335.

Mulvaney, C., Kendrick, D., Towner, E., Brussoni, M., Hayes, M., Powell, J., … Ward, H. (2009). Fatal and non-fatal fire injuries in England 1995– 2004: Time trends and inequalities by age, sex and area of deprivation. *Journal of Public Health, 31*(1), 154–161.

Murgraff, V., White, D., & Phillips, K. (1996). Moderating binge drinking: It is possible to change behavior if you plan it in advance? *Alcohol and Alcoholism, 31,* 577–582.

Murphy, J. K., Stoney, C. M., Alpert, B. S., & Walker, S. S. (1995). Gender and ethnicity in children's cardiovascular reactivity: 7 years of study. *Health Psychology, 14,* 48–55.

Murphy, M. H., Nevill, A. M., Murtagh, E. M., & Holder, R. L. (2007). The effect of walking on fitness, fatness and resting blood pressure: A meta-analysis of randomized, controlled trials. *Preventive Medicine, 44,* 377–385.

Murray, E., Lo, B., Pollack, L., Donelan, K., Catania, J. White, M., … Turner, R. (2003). The impact of health information on the internet on the physician-patient relationship. *Archives of Internal Medicine, 163,* 1727–1734.

Murray, J. A. (2001). Loss as a universal concept: A review of the literature to identify common aspects of loss in diverse situations. *Journal of Loss and Trauma, 6,* 219–231.

Murtaugh, M. A. (2004). Meat consumption and the risk of colon and rectal cancers. *Clinical Nutrition, 13,* 61–64.

Murthy, P., Kudlur, S., George, S., & Mathew, G. (2009). A clinical overview of fetal alcohol syndrome. *Addictive Disorders and Their Treatment, 8*(1), 1–12.

Must, A., Barish, E. E., & Bandini, L. G. (2009). Modifiable risk factors in relation to changes in BMI and fatness: What have we learned from prospective studies of school-aged children? *International Journal of Obesity, 33*(7), 705–715.

Mustard, T. R., & Harris, A. V. E. (1989). Problems in understanding prescription labels. *Perceptual and Motor Skills, 69,* 291–299.

Muthen, B. O., & Muthen, L. K. (2000). The development of heavy drinking and alcohol-related problems from ages 18 to 37 in a U.S. national sample. *Journal of Studies on Alcohol, 61,* 290–300.

Mutti, S., Hammond, D., Borland, R., Cummings, M. K., O'Connor, R. J., & Fong, G. T. (2011). Beyond light and mild: Cigarette brand descriptors and perceptions of risk in the International Tobacco Control (ITC) Four Country Survey. *Addiction, 106*(6), 1166–1175.

Myers, J. (2000). Physical activity and cardiovascular disease. *IDEA Health and Fitness Source, 18,* 38–45.

Myers, T. C., Wonderlich, S. A., Crosby, R., Mitchell, J. E., Steffen, K. J., Smyth, J., … Miltenberger, R. (2006). Is multi-impulsive bulimia a distinct type of bulimia nervosa: Psychopathology and EMA findings. *International Journal of Eating Disorders, 39,* 655–661.

Myung, S.-K., McDonnell, D. D., Kazinets, G., Seo, H. G., & Moskowitz, J. M. (2009). Effects of web- and computer-based smoking cessation programs. *Archives of Internal Medicine, 169*(10), 929–937.

Nahin, R. L. (2015). Estimates of pain prevalence and severity in adults: United States, 2012. *The Journal of Pain, 16*(8), 769–780.

Nahin, R. L., Barnes, P. M., Stussman, B. J., & Bloom, B. (2009). Costs of complementary and alternative medicine (CAM) and frequency of visits to CAM practitioners: United States, 2007. *National Health Statistics Reports, 18,* 1–16.

Napadow, V., Kettner, N., Liu, J., Li, M., Kwong, K. K., Vangel, M., … Hui, K. K. S. (2007). Hypothalamus and amygdala response to acupuncture stimuli in carpal tunnel syndrome. *Pain, 130,* 254–266.

Naparstek, B. (2007). Guided imagery: A best practice for pregnancy and childbirth. *Journal of Childbirth Education, 22,* 4–8.

Napoli, A. M., Choo, E. K., & McGregor, A. (2014). Gender disparities in stress test utilization in chest pain unit patients based upon the ordering physician's gender. *Critical Pathways in Cardiology, 13*(4), 152–155.

Nash, J. M., McKay, K. M., Vogel, M. E., & Masters, K. S. (2012). Functional roles and foundational characteristics of psychologists in integrated primary care. *Journal of Clinical Psychology in Medical Settings, 19*(1), 93–104.

Nash, J. M., Park, E. R., Walker, B. B., Gordon, N., & Nicholson, R. A. (2004). Cognitive-behavioral group treatment for disabling headache. *Pain Medicine, 5,* 178–186.

Nash, J. M., & Thebarge, R. W. (2006). Understanding psychological stress, its biological processes, and impact on primary headache. *Headache, 46,* 1377–1386.

Nassiri, M. (2005). The effects of regular relaxation on perceived stress in a group of London primary education teachers. *European Journal of Clinical Hypnosis, 6*, 21–29.

Nast, I., Bolten, M., Meinlschmidt, G., & Hellhammer, D. H. (2013). How to measure prenatal stress? A systematic review of psychometric instruments to assess psychosocial stress during pregnancy. *Paediatric and Perinatal Epidemiology, 27*(4), 313–322.

National Alliance for Caregiving in Collaboration with AARP. (2009). Executive Summary of Care Giving in the US, Washington, DC.

National Association for Sport and Physical Education (NASPE). (2002). *Guidelines for infants and toddlers.* Retrieved August 5, 2002, from www.aahperd.org/naspe/template.cfm?template=toddlers.html

National Cancer Institute (NCI). (2016). *The genetics of cancer.* Retrieved October 1, 2016, from https://www.cancer.gov/about-cancer/causes-prevention/genetics

National Center for Complementary and Alternative Medicine (NCCAM). (2009/2014). *Using dietary supplements wisely.* NCCAM Publication No. D426. Revised June, 2014. Retrieved May 17, 2016, from https://nccih.nih.gov/sites/nccam.nih.gov/files/Using_Dietary_Supplements_Wisely_CAM_06-12-2014.pdf

National Center for Complementary and Integrative Health (NCCIH). (2005/2015). *Ayurvedic medicine: In depth.* NCCIH Publication No. D287. Revised January, 2015. Retrieved May 13, 2016, from https://nccih.nih.gov/health/ayurveda/introduction.htm

National Center for Complementary and Integrative Health (NCCIH). (2006/2015a). *Massage therapy for health purposes.* NCCIH Publication No. D327. Revised May, 2015. Retrieved May 28, 2016, from https://nccih.nih.gov/health/massage/massageintroduction.htm

National Center for Complementary and Integrative Health (NCCIH). (2006/2015b). *Tai chi and qi gong: In depth.* NCCIH Publication No. D322. Revised August, 2015. Retrieved May 30, 2016, from https://nccih.nih.gov/health/taichi/introduction.htm

National Center for Complementary and Integrative Health (NCCIH). (2007/2012). *Chiropractic: In depth.* NCCIH Publication No. D403. Revised February, 2012. Retrieved May 26, 2016, from http://nccam.nih.gov/health/chiropractic/introduction.htm

National Center for Complementary and Integrative Health (NCCIH). (2007/2016a). *Acupuncture: In depth.* NCCIH Pub. No: D404. Bethesda, MD: Author. Revised August, 2011. Retrieved May 13, 2016, from https://nccih.nih.gov/health/acupuncture/introduction

National Center for Complementary and Integrative Health (NCCIH). (2007/2016b). *Meditation: In depth. NCCIH Publication No. D308.* Revised April, 2016. Retrieved May 30, 2016, from https://nccih.nih.gov/health/meditation/overview.htm

National Center for Complementary and Integrative Health (NCCIH). (2008/2013). *Yoga: In depth.* NCCIH Publication No. D472. Revised June, 2013. Retrieved May 30, 2016, from https://nccih.nih.gov/health/yoga/introduction.htm

National Center for Complementary and Integrative Health (NCCIH). (2008/2015). *Complementary, alternative, or integrative health: What's in a name?* NCCIH Publication No. D347. Revised March, 2015. Retrieved May 13, 2016, from https://nccih.nih.gov/health/integrative-health

National Center for Health Statistics (NCHS). (2011). *Health, United States, 2010.* Hyattsville, MD: U.S. Government Printing Office.

National Center for Health Statistics (NCHS). (2015). *Health, United States, 2014.* Hyattsville, MD: U.S. Government Printing Office.

National Center for Health Statistics (NCHS). (2016a). *Health, United States 2015: With special feature on racial and ethnic health disparities.* Hyattsville, MD: Author.

National Center for Health Statistics (NCHS). (2016b). National health interview survey early release program. Retrieved August 16, 2016, from http://www.cdc.gov/nchs/data/nhis/earlyrelease/quarterly_estimates_2010_2015_q123.pdf

National Task Force on the Prevention and Treatment of Obesity. (2000). Overweight, obesity, and health risk. *Archives of Internal Medicine, 160*, 898–904.

Nausheen, B., Gidron, Y., Peveler, R., & Moss-Morris, R. (2009). Social support and cancer progression: A systematic review. *Journal of Psychosomatic Research, 67*, 403–415.

Naylor, R. T., & Marshall, J. (2007). Autogenic training: A key component in holistic medical practice. *Journal of Holistic Healthcare, 4*, 14–19.

Nelson, D. E., Jarman, D. W., Rehm, J., Greenfield, T. K., Rey, G., Kerr, W. C. ... Naimi, T. S. (2013). Alcohol-attributable cancer deaths and years of potential life lost in the United States. *American Journal of Public Health, 103*(4), 641–648.

Nelson, H. D., Nevitt, M. C., Scott, J. C., Stone, K. L., & Cummings, S. R. (1994). Smoking, alcohol, and neuromuscular and physical functioning of older women. *Journal of the American Medical Association, 272*, 1825–1831.

Nelson, L. D., & Morrison, E. L. (2005). The symptoms of resource scarcity: Judgments of food and finances influence preferences for potential partners. *Psychological Science, 16*, 167–173.

Nemeroff, C. J. (1995). Magical thinking about illness virulence: Conceptions of germs from "safe" versus "dangerous" others. *Health Psychology, 14*, 147–151.

Nerurkar, A., Yeh, G., Davis, R. B., Birdee, G., & Phillips, R. S. (2011). When conventional medical providers recommend unconventional medicine: Results of a national study. *Archives of Internal Medicine, 171*(9), 862–864.

Nes, L. S., & Segerstrom, S. C. (2006). Dispositional optimism and coping: A meta-analytic review. *Personality and Social Psychology Review, 10*, 235–251.

Nestoriuc, Y., & Martin, A. (2007). Efficacy of biofeedback for migraine: A meta-analysis. *Pain, 128*, 111–127.

Netz, Y., Wu, M.-J., Becker, B. J., & Tenenbaum, G. (2005). Physical activity and psychological well-being in advanced age: A meta-analysis of intervention studies. *Psychology and Aging, 20*, 272–284.

Neumark-Sztainer, D. R., Wall, M. M., Haines, J. I., Story, M. T., Sherwood, N. E., & van den Berg, P. A. (2007). Shared risk and protective factors for overweight and disordered eating in adolescents. *American Journal of Preventive Medicine, 33*, 359–369.

Neumark-Sztainer, D. R., Wall, M. M., Story, M., & Perry, C. L. (2003). Correlates of unhealthy weight-control behaviors among adolescents: Implications for prevention programs. *Health Psychology, 22*, 88–98.

Neville, L. M., O'Hara, B., & Milat, A. J. (2009). Computer-tailored dietary behavior change interventions: A systematic review. *Health Education Research, 24*, 699–720.

Newton-John, T. R. (2013). How significant is the Significant Other in patient coping in chronic pain? *Pain, 3*(6), 485–493.

Ng, B. H. P., & Tsang, H. W. H. (2009). Psychophysiological outcomes of health qigong for chronic conditions: A systematic review. *Psychophysiology, 46*(2), 257–269.

Ng, J. Y. Y., & Tam, S. F. (2000). Effects of exercise-based cardiac rehabilitation on mobility and self-esteem after cardiac surgery. *Perceptual and Motor Skills, 91*, 107–114.

Ng, M. K. C. (2007). New perspectives on Mars and Venus: Unravelling the role of androgens in gender differences in cardiovascular biology and disease. *Heart, Lung and Circulation, 16*, 185–192.

Nguyen, L. T., Davis, R. B., Kaptchuk, T. J., & Phillips, R. S. (2011). Use of complementary and alternative medicine and self-rated health status: Results of a national survey. *Journal of General Internal Medicine, 26*(4), 399–404.

Nicassio, P. M., Meyerowitz, B. E., & Kerns, R. D. (2004). The future of health psychology interventions. *Health Psychology, 23*, 132–137.

Nichols, M., Townsend, N., Scarborough, P., & Rayner, M. (2014). Cardiovascular disease in Europe 2014: Epidemiological update. *European Heart Journal*, ehu299.

Nicoll, R. A., & Alger, B. E. (2004, December). The brain's own marijuana. *Scientific American, 291*, 68–75.

Nied, R. J., & Franklin, B. (2002). Promoting and prescribing exercise for the elderly. *American Family Physician, 65*, 419–426, 427–428.

Nielsen, T. S., & Hansen, K. B. (2007). Do green areas affect health? Results from a Danish survey of the use of green areas and health indicators. *Health and Place, 13*, 839–850.

Nieva, G., Ortega, L. L., Mondon, S., Ballbé, M., & Gual, A. (2011). Simultaneous versus delayed treatment of tobacco dependence in alcohol-dependent outpatients. *European Addiction Research, 17*(1), 1–9.

Nikendei, C., Weisbrod, M., Schild, S., Bender, S., Walther, S., & Herzog, W. (2008). Anorexia nervosa: Selective processing of food-related word and pictoral stimuli in recognition and free recall tests. *International Journal of Eating Disorders, 41,* 439–447.

Niswender, K. D., Daws, L. C., Avison, M. J., & Galli, A. (2011). Insulin regulation of monoamine signaling: Pathway to obesity. *Neuropsychopharmacology, 36*(1), 359–360.

Nivison, M. E., & Endresen, I. M. (1993). An analysis of relationships among environmental noise, annoyance and sensitivity to noise, and the consequences for health and sleep. *Journal of Behavior Medicine, 16,* 257–276.

Nocon, M., Hiemann, T., Müller-Riemenschneider, F., Thalau, F., Roll, S., & Willich, S. N. (2008). Association of physical activity with all-cause and cardiovascular mortality: A systematic review and meta-analysis. *European Journal of Cardiovascular Prevention and Rehabilitation, 15,* 239–246.

Nocon, M., Müller-Riemenschneider, F., Nitzschke, K., & Willich, S. N. (2010). Review article: Increasing physical activity with point-of-choice prompts – A systematic review. *Scandinavian Journal of Public Health, 38,* 633–638.

Noel, N. E., Heaton, J. A., & Brown, B. P. (2013). Substance induced myopia. In P. M. Miller, S. A. Ball, M. E. Bates, A. W. Blume, K. M. Kampman, M. E. Larimer, N. M. Petry ... P. De Witte (Eds.), *Comprehensive addictive behaviors and disorders, Vol. 1: Principles of addiction* (pp. 349–354). San Diego, CA: Elsevier Academic Press.

Nordström, A., Karlsson, C., Nyquist, F., Olsson, T., Nordström, P., & Karlsson, M. (2005). Bone loss and fracture risk after reduced physical activity. *Journal of Bone and Mineral Research, 20,* 202–207.

Nori Janosz, K. E., Koenig Berris, K. A., Leff, C., Miller, W. M., Yanez, J., Myers, S., ... McCollough, P. A. (2008). Clinical resolution of Type 2 diabetes with reduction in body mass index using meal replacement based weight loss. *Vascular Disease Prevention, 5,* 17–23.

Norris, F. H., Byrne, C. M., Diaz, E., & Kaniasty, K. (2001). *The range, magnitude, and duration of effects of natural and human-caused disasters: A review of the empirical literature.* Boston, MA: National Center for PTSD.

Northrup, T. F., Jacob III, P., Benowitz, N. L., Hon, E., Quintana, P. J. E., Hovell, M. F., ... Stotts, A. L. (2016). Thirdhand smoke: State of the science and a call for policy expansion. *Association of Schools and Programs of Public Health, 131*(2), 233–238.

Nouwen, A., Winkley, K., Twisk, J., Lloyd, C. E., Peyrot, M., Ismail, K., ... European Depression in Diabetes (EDID) Research Consortium. (2010). Type 2 diabetes mellitus as a risk factor for the onset of depression: A systematic review and meta-analysis. *Diabetologia, 53,* 2480–2486.

Novack, D. H., Cameron, O., Epel, E., Ader, R., Waldstein, S. R., Levenstein, S., ... Wainer, R. B. (2007). Psychosomatic medicine: The scientific foundation of the biopsychosocial model. *Academic Psychiatry, 31,* 388–401.

Novins, D. K., Beals, J., Moore, L. A., Spicer, P., & Manson, S. M. (2004). Use of biomedical services and traditional healing options among American Indians: Sociodemographic correlates, spirituality, and ethnic identity. *Medical Care, 42,* 670–679.

NPD Group. (2013). *The NPD Group reports dieting is at an all time low.* Retrieved from https://www.npd.com/wps/portal/npd/us/news/press-releases/the-npd-group-reports-dieting-is-at-an-all-time-low-dieting-season-has-begun-but-its-not-what-it-used-to-be/

Nunez-Smith, M., Wolf, E., Huang, H. M., Chen, P., Lee, L., Emanuel, E., ... Gross, C. P. (2010). Media exposure and tobacco, illicit drugs, and alcohol use among children and adolescents: A systematic review. *Substance Abuse, 31*(3), 174–192.

"Obama Admits." (2008, June 10). Obama admits smoking cigarettes in last few months. *ABC News.* Retrieved June 2, 2011, from http://blogs.abcnews.com/politicalradar/2008/06/obama-admits-sm.html

O'Brien, C. W., & Moorey, S. (2010). Outlook and adaptation in advanced cancer: A systematic review. *Psycho-Oncology, 19,* 1239–1249.

O'Carroll, R. E., Dryden, J., Hamilton-Barclay, T., & Ferguson, E. (2011). Anticipated regret and organ donor registration: A pilot study. *Health Psychology, 30,* 661–664.

O'Cleirigh, C., Ironson, G., Weiss, A., & Costa, P. T., Jr. (2007). Conscientiousness predicts disease progression (CD4 number and viral load) in people living with HIV. *Health Psychology, 26,* 473–480.

O'Connor, D. B., & Shimizu, M. (2002). Sense of personal control, stress and coping style: A cross-cultural study. *Stress and Health: Journal of the International Society for the Investigation of Stress, 18,* 173–183.

O'Connor, D. W., Ames. D., Gardner, B., & King, M. (2009). Psychosocial treatments of behavior symptoms in dementia: A systematic review of reports meeting quality standards. *International Psychogeriatrics, 21,* 225–240.

O'Connor, R. J., McNeill, A., Borland, R., Hammond, D., King, B., Boudreau, C., ... Cummings, K. M. (2007). Smokers' beliefs about the relative safety of other tobacco products: Findings from the ITC collaboration. *Nicotine and Tobacco Research, 9,* 1033–1042.

O'Donnell, M. J., Xavier, D., Liu, L., Zhang, H., Chin, S. L., Rao-Melacini, P., ... Diener, H-C. (2010). Risk factors for ischaemic and intracerebral haemorrhagic stroke in 22 countries (the INTERSTROKE study): A case-control study. *The Lancet, 376*(9735), 112–123.

Ogden, C. L., Carroll, M. D., Kit, B. K., & Flegal, K. M. (2012). Prevalence of obesity and trends in body mass index among US children and adolescents, 1999–2010. *Journal of the American Medical Association, 307,* 483–490.

Ogden, J. (2003). Some problems with social cognition models: A pragmatic and conceptual analysis. *Health Psychology, 22,* 424–428.

Ogedegbe, G., Schoenthaler, A., & Fernandez, S. (2007). Appointment-keeping behavior is not related to medication adherence in hypertensive African Americans. *Journal of General Internal Medicine, 22,* 1176–1179.

Oguma, Y., Sesso, H. D., Paffenbarger, R. S., Jr., & Lee, I.-M. (2002). Physical activity and all cause mortality in women: A review of the evidence. *British Journal of Sports Medicine, 36,* 162–172.

Oh, K., Hu, F. B., Manson, J. E., Stampfer, M. J., & Willett, W. C. (2005). Dietary fat intake and risk of coronary heart disease in women: 20 years of follow-up of the Nurses' Health Study. *American Journal of Epidemiology, 161,* 672–679.

Oh, Y.-M., Kim, Y. S., Yoo, S. H., Kim, S. K., & Kim, D. S. (2004). Association between stress and asthma symptoms: A population-based study. *Respirology, 9,* 363–368.

O'Hare, P. (2007). Merseyside, the first harm reduction conferences, and the early history of harm reduction. *International Journal of Drug Policy, 18,* 141–144.

Ohmoto, M., Sakasishi, K., Hama, A., Morita, A., Nomura, M., & Misumoto, Y. (2013). Association between dopamine receptor 2 TaqIA polymorphisms and smoking behavior with an influence of ethnicity: A systematic review and meta-analysis update. *Nicotine and Tobacco Research, 15*(3), 633–642.

Okuda, M., & Nakazawa, T. (2004). *Helicobacter pylori* infection in childhood. *Journal of Gastroenterology, 39,* 809–810.

Olander, E. K., & Eves, F. F. (2011). Effectiveness and cost of two stair-climbing interventions—Less is more. *American Journal of Health Promotion, 25,* 231–236.

Oldenburg, R. A., Meijers-Heijboer, H., Cornelisse, C. J., & Devilee, P. (2007). Genetic susceptibility for breast cancer: How many more genes to be found? *Critical Reviews in Oncology/Hematology, 63,* 125–149.

O'Leary, C. M., Nassar, N., Zubrick, S. R., Kurinczuk, J. J., Stanley, F., & Bower, C. (2010). Evidence of a complex association between dose, pattern and timing of prenatal alcohol exposure and child behaviour problems. *Addiction, 105*(1), 74–86.

Olesen, J. (1988). Classification and diagnostic criteria for headache disorders, cranial neuralgias, and facial pain: Headache Classification Committee of the International Headache Society [Special issue]. *Cephalalgia, 8*(Suppl. 7), 1–96.

Olivardia, R., Pope, H. G., & Phillips, K. A. (2000). *The Adonis complex: The secret crisis of male body obsession.* New York, NY: Free Press.

O'Loughlin, J., Karp, I., Koulis, T., Paradis, G., & DiFranza, J. (2009). Determinants of first puff and daily cigarette smoking in adolescents. *American Journal of Epidemiology, 170*(5), 585–597.

Olsen, P., Elliott, J. M., Frampton, C., & Bradley, P. S. (2015). Winning or losing does matter: Acute cardiac admissions in New Zealand during Rugby World Cup tournaments. *European Journal of Preventive Cardiology, 22*(10), 1254–1260.

Olsen, R., & Sutton, J. (1998). More hassle, more alone: Adolescents with diabetes and the role of formal and informal support. *Child Care, Health and Development, 24*, 31–39.

Olshefsky, A. M., Zive, M. M., Scolari, R., & Zuniga, M. (2007). Promoting HIV risk awareness and testing in Latinos living on the U.S. Mexico Border: The Tu No Me Conoces Social Marketing Campaign. *AIDS Education and Prevention, 19*, 422–435.

Olver, I. N., Taylor, A. E., & Whitford, H. S. (2005). Relationships between patients' pre-treatment expectations of toxicities and post chemotherapy experiences. *Psycho-Oncology, 14*, 25–33.

Oman, R. F., & King, A. C. (2000). The effect of life events and exercise program on the adoption and maintenance of exercise behavior. *Health Psychology, 19*, 605–612.

Ondeck, D. M. (2003). Impact of culture on pain. *Home Health Care Management and Practice, 15*, 255–257.

Operario, D., Adler, N. E., & Williams, D. R. (2004). Subjective social status: Reliability and predictive utility for global health. *Psychology and Health, 19*, 237–246.

Orbell, S., Hodgkins, S., & Sheeran, P. (1997). Implementation intentions and the theory of planned behavior. *Personality and Social Psychology Bulletin, 23*, 945–554.

Orford, J., Krishnan, M., Balaam, M., Everitt, M., & van der Graaf, K. (2004). University student drinking: The role of motivational and social factors. *Drugs: Education, Prevention and Policy, 11*, 407–421.

Organisation for Economic Co-operation and Development (OECD). (2008). *OECD health data 2008: Statistics and indicators for 30 countries.* Paris: Organisation for Economic Co-operation and Development.

Organisation for Economic Co-operation and Development (OECD). (2015). *OECD health statistics 2015.* Retrieved April 29, 2016, from www.oecd.org

Ornish, D., Brown, S. E., Scherwitz, L. W., Billings, J. H., Armstrong, W. T., Ports, T., … Gould, K. L. (1990). Can lifestyle changes reverse coronary heart disease? The Lifestyle Heart Trial. *Lancet, 336*, 129–133.

Ornish, D., Scherwitz, L. W., Billings, J. H., Gould, L., Merritt, T. A., Sparler, S., … Brand, R. J. (1998). Intensive lifestyle changes for reversal of coronary heart disease. *Journal of the American Medical Association, 280*, 2001–2007.

Ortner, C. N. M., MacDonald, T. K., & Olmstead, M. C. (2003). Alcohol intoxication reduces impulsivity in the delay-discounting paradigm. *Alcohol and Alcoholism, 38*, 151–156.

Osborn, C. Y., White, R. O., Cavanaugh, K., Rothman, R. L., & Wallston, K. A. (2009). Diabetes numeracy: An overlooked factor in understanding racial disparities in glycemic control. *Diabetes Care, 32*, 1614–1619.

Osborn, J. W. (2005). Hypothesis: Set-points and long-term control of arterial pressure: A theoretical argument for a long-term arterial pressure control system in the brain rather than the kidney. *Clinical and Experimental Pharmacology and Physiology, 32*, 384–393.

Osborn, R. L., Demoncada, A. C., & Feuerstein, M. (2006). Psychosocial interventions for depression, anxiety, and quality of life in cancer survivors: Meta-analyses. *International Journal of Psychiatry in Medicine, 36*, 13–34.

Øystein, K. (2008). A broader perspective on education and mortality: Are we influenced by other people's education? *Social Science and Medicine, 66*, 620–636.

Ozer, E. J. (2005). The impact of violence on urban adolescents: Longitudinal effects of perceived school connection and family support. *Journal of Adolescent Research, 20*, 167–192.

Ozer, E. J., Best, S, R., Lipsey, T. L., & Weiss, D. S. (2003). Predictors of posttraumatic stress disorder and symptoms in adults: A meta-analysis. *Psychological Bulletin, 129*, 52–73.

Paasche-Orlow, M. K., Parker, R. M., Gazmararian, J. A., Nielsen-Bohlman, L. T., & Rudd, R. R. (2005). The prevalence of limited health literacy. *Journal of General Internal Medicine, 20*, 175–184.

Pabst, A., Baumeister, S. E., & Kraus, L. (2010). Alcohol-expectancy dimensions and alcohol consumption at different ages in the general population. *Journal of Studies on Alcohol and Drugs, 71*(1), 46–53.

Pace, T. W. W., & Heim, C. M. (2011). A short review on the psychoneuroimmunology of posttraumatic stress disorder: From risk factors to medical comorbidities. *Brain, Behavior, and Immunity, 25*, 6–13.

Paffenbarger, R. S., Jr., Gima, A. S., Laughlin, M. E., & Black, R. A. (1971). Characteristics of longshoremen related to fatal coronary heart disease and stroke. *American Journal of Public Health, 61*, 1362–1370.

Paffenbarger, R. S., Jr., Laughlin, M. E., Gima, A. S., & Black, R. A. (1970). Work activity of longshoremen as related to death from coronary heart disease and stroke. *New England Journal of Medicine, 282*, 1109–1114.

Paffenbarger, R. S., Jr., Wing, A. L., & Hyde, R. T. (1978). Physical activity as an index of heart attack risk in college alumni. *American Journal of Epidemiology, 108*, 161–175.

Palm, J. (2004). The nature of and responsibility of alcohol and drug problems: Views among treatment staff. *Addiction Research and Theory, 12*, 413–431.

Palmer, R. H. C., McGeary, J. E., Francazio, S., Raphael, B. J., Lander, A. D., Heath, A. C., … Knopik, V. S. (2012). The genetics of alcohol dependence: Advancing towards system-based approaches. *Drug and Alcohol Dependence, 125*(3), 179–191.

Palombaro, K. M. (2005). Effects of walking-only interventions on bone mineral density at various skeletal sites: A meta-analysis. *Journal of Geriatric Physical Therapy, 28*(3), 102–107.

Pambianco, G., Costacou, T., & Orchard, T. (2007). The determination of cardiovascular risk factor profiles in Type 1 diabetes. *Diabetes, 56*(Suppl. 1), A176–A177.

Panagiotidis, P., Papadopoulou, M., Diakogiannis, I., Iacovides, A., & Kaprinis, G. (2008). Young people and binge drinking. *Annals of General Psychiatry, 7*(Suppl. 1), 1.

Pang, R., Wang, S., Tian, L., Lee, M. C., Do, A., Cutshall, S. M., … Chon, T. Y. (2015). Complementary and integrative medicine at Mayo Clinic. *American Journal of Chinese Medicine, 43*(8), 1503–1513.

Papadaki, A., Hondros, G., Scott, J. A., & Kapsokefalou, M. (2007). Eating habits of university students living at, or away from home in Greece. *Appetite, 49*, 169–176.

Papadopoulos, A., Guida, F., Cénée, S., Cyr, D., Schmaus, A., Radoï, L., … Stücker, I. (2011). Cigarette smoking and lung cancer in women: Results of the French ICARE case-control study. *Lung Cancer, 74*, 369–377.

Papas, R. K., Belar, C. D., & Rozensky, R. H. (2004). The practice of clinical health psychology: Professional issues. In R. G. Frank, A. Baum, & J. L. Wallander (Eds.), *Handbook of clinical health psychology* (Vol. 3, pp. 293–319). Washington, DC: American Psychological Association.

Parchman, M. L., Noel, P. H., & Lee, S. (2005). Primary care attributes, health care system hassles, and chronic illness. *Medical Care, 43*, 1123–1129.

Park, C. (2013). Mind-body CAM interventions: Current status and considerations for integration into clinical health psychology. *Journal of Clinical Psychology, 69*(1), 45–63.

Park, J. (2005). Use of alternative health care. *Health Reports, 16*(2), 39–42.

Parker, C. S., Zhen, C., Price, M., Gross, R., Metlay, J. P., Christie, J. D., … Kimmel, S. E. (2007). Adherence to warfarin assessed by electronic pill caps, clinician assessment, and patient reports: Results from the INRANGE study. *Journal of General Internal Medicine, 22*, 1254–1259.

Parker, M., Schaller, J., & Hansmann, S. (2003). Catastrophe, chaos, and complexity models and psychosocial adjustment to disability. *Rehabilitation Counseling Bulletin, 46*, 234–241.

Parrott, D. J., & Zeichner, A. (2002). Effects of alcohol and trait anger on physical aggression in men. *Journal of Studies on Alcohol, 63*, 196–204.

Parschau, L., Richert, J., Koring, M., Ernsting, A., Lippke, S., & Schwarzer, R. (2012). Changes in social-cognitive variables are associated with stage transitions in physical activity. *Health Education Research, 27*, 129–140.

Pascoe, E. A., & Richman, L. S. (2009). Perceived discrimination and health: A meta-analytic review. *Psychological Bulletin, 135*, 531–554.

Patel, A. V., Bernstein, L., Deka, A., Feigelson, H. S., Campbell, P. T., Gapstur, S. M., Colditz, G. A., & Thun, M. J. (2010). Leisure time spent sitting in relation to total mortality in a prospective cohort of US adults. *American Journal of Epidemiology, 172*(4), 419–429.

Patel, S. R., Ayas, N. T., Malhotra, M. R., White, D. P., Schemhammer, E. S., Speizer, F. E., … Hu, F. B. (2004). A prospective study of sleep duration and mortality risk in women. *Sleep, 27,* 440–444.

Patra, J., Taylor, B., Irving, H., Roerecke, M., Baliunas, D., Mohapatra, S., … Rehm, J. (2010). Alcohol consumption and the risk of morbidity and mortality for different stroke types—A systematic review and meta-analysis. *BMC Public Health, 10,* 258–269.

Patterson, D. R. (2010). *Clinical hypnosis for pain control.* Washington, DC: American Psychological Association.

Patterson, D. R., & Jensen, M. P. (2003). Hypnosis and clinical pain. *Psychological Bulletin, 129,* 495–521.

Paull, T. T., Cortez, D., Bowers, B., Elledge, S. J., & Gellert, M. (2001). Direct DNA binding by BRCA 1. *Proceedings of the National Academy of Sciences of the United States of America, 98,* 6086–6091.

Paulozzi, L., Baldwin, G., Franklin, G., Kerlikowske, R. G., Jones, C. M., Ghiya, N., … Popovic, T. (2012). CDC grand rounds: Prescription drug overdoses—A U.S. epidemic. *Morbidity and Mortality Weekly Report, 61,* 10–13.

Pauly, M. V., & Pagán, J. A. (2007). Spillovers and vulnerability: The case of community uninsurance. *Health Affairs, 26,* 1304–1314.

Paun, O., Farran, C. J., Perraud, S., & Loukissa, D. A. (2004). Successful caregiving of persons with Alzheimer's disease. *Alzheimer's Care Quarterly, 5,* 241–251.

Pavlik, V. N., Doody, R. S., Massman, P. J., & Chan, W. (2006). Influence of premorbid IQ and education on progression of Alzheimer's disease. *Dementia and Geriatric Cognitive Disorders, 22,* 367–377.

Pavlin, D. J., Sullivan, M. J. L., Freund, P. R., & Roesen, K. (2005). Catastrophizing: A risk factor for postsurgical pain. *Clinical Journal of Pain, 21,* 83–90.

Paxton, R. J., Motl, R. W., Aylward, A., & Nigg, C. R. (2010). Physical activity and quality of life: The complementary influence of self-efficacy for physical activity and mental health difficulties. *International Journal of Behavioral Medicine, 17,* 255–263.

Paynter, J., & Edwards, R. (2009). The impact of tobacco promotion at the point of sale: A systematic review. *Nicotine and Tobacco Research, 11*(1), 25–35.

Pearson, B. L., Reeder, D. M., & Judge, P. G. (2015). Crowding increases salivary cortisol but not self-directed behavior in captive baboons. *American Journal of Primatology, 77*(4), 462–467.

Peay, M. Y., & Peay, E. R. (1998). The evaluation of medical symptoms by patients and doctors. *Journal of Behavioral Medicine, 21,* 57–81.

Pedersen, A. F., Zachariae, R., & Bovbjerg, D. H. (2009). Psychological stress and antibody response to influenza vaccination: A meta-analysis. *Brain, Behavior, and Immunity, 23,* 427–433.

Peele, S. (2002, August 1). Harm reduction in clinical practice. *Counselor: The Magazine for Addiction Professionals,* 28–32.

Peele, S. (2007). Addiction as disease: Policy, epidemiology, and treatment consequences of a bad idea. In J. E. Henningfield, P. B. Santora, & W. K. Bickel (Eds.), Addiction treatment: Science and policy for the twenty-first century (pp. 153–164). Baltimore, MD: Johns Hopkins University Press.

Peila, R., Rodriguez, B. L., & Launer, L. J. (2002). Type 2 diabetes, APOE gene, and the risk for dementia and related pathologies. *Diabetes, 51,* 1256–1262.

Pelletier, K. R. (2002). Mind as healer, mind as slayer: Mind-body medicine comes of age. *Advances in Mind-Body Medicine, 18,* 4–15.

Pence, L. B., Thorn, B. E., Jensen, M. P., & Romano, J. M. (2008). Examination of perceived spouse responses to patient well and pain behavior in patients with headache. *The Clinical Journal of Pain, 24,* 654–661.

Penley, J. A., Tomaka, J., & Wiebe, J. S. (2002). The association of coping to physical and psychological health outcomes: A meta-analytic review. *Journal of Behavioral Medicine, 25,* 551–603.

Pennebaker, J. W., Barger, S. D., & Tiebout, J. (1989). Disclosure of traumas and health among Holocaust survivors. *Psychosomatic Medicine, 51,* 577–589.

Pennebaker, J. W., Colder, M., & Sharp, L. K. (1990). Accelerating the coping process. *Journal of Personality and Social Psychology, 58,* 528–537.

Penza-Clyve, S. M., Mansell, C., & McQuaid, E. L. (2004). Why don't children take their asthma medications? A qualitative analysis of children's perspectives on adherence. *Journal of Asthma, 41,* 189–197.

Penzien, D. B., Rains, J. C., & Andrasik, F. (2002). Behavioral management of recurrent headache: Three decades of experience and empiricism. *Applied Psychophysiology and Biofeedback, 27,* 163–181.

People. (2016). Charlie Sheen says most recent rehab stint was a 'relief' after '2,000' tries to quit drinking. *People Magazine.* Retrieved July 3, 2016, from http://www.people.com/article/charlie-sheen-dr-oz-interview

Pepper, J., Emery, S., Ribisl, K., Rini, C., & Brewer, N. (2015). How risky is it to use e-cigarettes? Smokers' beliefs about their health risks from using novel and traditional tobacco products. *Journal of Behavioral Medicine, 38*(2), 318–326.

Pereira, M. A., Kartashov, A. I., Ebbeling, C. B., Van Horn, L., Slattery, M. L., Jacobs, D. R., Jr., … Ludwig, D. S. (2005). Fast-food habits, weight gain, and insulin resistance (the CARDIA study): 15-year prospective analysis. *Lancet, 365,* 36–42.

Peres, M. F. P., Mercante, J. P. P., Tanuri, F. C., & Nunes, M. (2006). Chronic migraine prevention with topiramate. *Journal of Headache and Pain, 7,* 185–187.

Peretti-Watel, P., Constance, J., Guilbert, P., Gautier, A., Beck, F., & Moatti, J.-P. (2007). Smoking too few cigarettes to be at risk? Smokers' perceptions of risk and risk denial, a French survey. *Tobacco Control, 16,* 351–356.

Permutt, M. A., Wasson, J., & Cox, N. (2005). Genetic epidemiology of diabetes. *Journal of Clinical Investigation, 115,* 1431–1439.

Perram, S. W. (2006). The results of 47 clinical studies examined in a 30-year period. *American Chiropractor, 28,* 42–44.

Pert, C. B., & Snyder, S. H. (1973). Opiate receptor: Demonstration in nervous tissue. *Science, 179,* 1011–1014.

Peterlin, B. L., Rosso, A. L., Rapoport, A. M., & Scher, A. I. (2010). Obesity and migraine: The effect of age, gender and adipose tissue distribution. *Headache, 50*(1), 52–62.

Petersen, G. L., Finnerup, N. B,, Colloca, L., Amanzio, M., Price, D. D., Jensen, T. S., … Vase, L. (2014). The magnitude of nocebo effects in pain: A meta-analysis. *Pain, 155*(8), 1426–1434.

Petrie, K. J., Perry, K., Broadbent, E., & Weinman, J. (2012). A text message programme designed to modify patients' illness and treatment beliefs improves self-reported adherence to asthma preventer medication. *British Journal of Health Psychology, 17,* 74–84.

Petticrew, M., Bell, R., & Hunter, D. (2002). Influence of psychological coping on survival and recurrence in people with cancer: A systematic review. *British Medical Journal, 325,* 1066.

Pettman, E. (2007). A history of manipulative therapy. *Journal of Manual and Manipulative Therapy, 15,* 165–174.

Pew Internet. (2012). *Highlights of the Pew Internet Project's research related to health and health care.* Retrieved March 28, 2012, from http://www.pewinternet.org/Commentary/2011/November/Pew-Internet-Health.aspx

Phillips, F. (2005). Vegetarian nutrition. *Nutrition Bulletin, 30*(2), 132–167.

Phillips, J. G., & Ogeil, R. P. (2007). Alcohol consumption and computer blackjack. *Journal of General Psychology, 134,* 333–353.

Phillips, K. M., Antoni, M. H., Carver, C. S., Lechner, S. C., Penedo, F. J., McCullough, M. E., … Blomberg, B. B. (2011). Stress management skills and reductions in serum cortisol across the year after survey for non-metastatic breast cancer. *Cognitive Therapy and Research, 35,* 595–600.

Phipps, E., Braitman, L. E., Stites, S., & Leighton, J. C. (2008). Quality of life and symptom attribution in long-term colon cancer survivors. *Journal of Evaluation in Clinical Practice, 14,* 254–258.

Pho, L., Grossman, D., & Leachman, S. A. (2006). Melanoma genetics: A review of genetic factors and clinical phenotypes in familial melanoma. *Current Opinion in Oncology, 18,* 173–179.

Picavet, H. S. J. (2010). Musculoskeletal pain complaints from a sex and gender perspective. In P. Croft, F. M. Blyth, & D. van der Windt (Eds.), *Chronic pain epidemiology: From Aetiology to Public Health* (pp. 119–126). New York, NY: Oxford University Press.

Pickup, J. C., & Renard, E. (2008). Long-acting insulin analogs versus insulin pump therapy for the treatment of Type 1 and Type 2 diabetes. *Diabetes Care*, *31*(S2), S140–S145.

Pierce, J. P. (2005). Influence of movie stars on the initiation of adolescent smoking. *Pediatric Dentistry*, *27*, 149.

Pierce, J. P., Distefan, J. M., Kaplan, R. M., & Gilpin, E. A. (2005). The role of curiosity in smoking initiation. *Addictive Behaviors*, *30*, 685–696.

Pietiläinen, K. H., Korkeila, M., Bogl, L. H., Westerterp, K. R., Yki-Järvinen, H., Kaprio, J., … Rissanen, A. (2010). Inaccuracies in food and physical activity diaries of obese subjects: Complementary evidence from doubly labeled water and co-twin assessments. *International Journal of Obesity*, *34*(3), 437–445.

Pietinen, P., Malila, N., Virtanen, M., Hartman, T. J., Tangrea, J. A., Albanes, D., … Virtamo, J. (1999). Diet and risk of colorectal cancer in a cohort of Finnish men. *Cancer Causes and Control*, *10*(5), 387–396.

Piette, J. D., Heisler, M., Horne, R., & Caleb Alexander, G. (2006). A conceptually based approach to understanding chronically ill patients' responses to medication cost pressures. *Social Science and Medicine*, *62*, 846–857.

Pike, K. M., Timothy, B., Vitousek, K., Wilson, G. T., & Bauer, J. (2003). Cognitive behavior therapy in posthospitalization treatment of anorexia nervosa. *American Journal of Psychiatry*, *160*, 2046–2049.

Pilote, L., Dasgupta, K., Guru, V., Humphries, K. H., McGrath, J., Norris, C., … Tagalakis, V. (2007). A comprehensive view of sex-specific issues related to cardiovascular disease. *Canadian Medical Association Journal*, *176*(6), S1–S44.

Pimlott-Kubiak, S., & Cortina, L. M. (2003). Gender, victimization, and outcomes: Reconceptualizing risk. *Journal of Consulting and Clinical Psychology*, *71*, 528–539.

Pinel, J. P. J. (2009). *Biopsychology* (7th ed.). Boston, MA: Allyn and Bacon.

Pinel, J. P. J. (2014). *Biopsychology* (9th ed.). Boston, MA: Pearson.

Pinel, J. P. J., Assanand, S., & Lehman, D. R. (2000). Hunger, eating, and ill health. *American Psychologist*, *55*, 1105–1116.

Piñeiro, B., Correa, J. B., Simmons, V. N., Harrell, P. T., Menzie, N. S., Unrod, M., … Brandon, T. H. (2016). Gender differences in use and expectancies of e-cigarettes: Online survey results. *Addictive Behaviors*, *52*, 91–97.

Pingitore, R., Scheffler, R., Haley, M., Seniell, T., & Schwalm, D. (2001). Professional psychology in a new era: Practice-based evidence from California. *Professional Psychology, Research and Practice*, *32*, 585–596.

Piotrowski, C. (1998). Assessment of pain: A survey of practicing clinicians. *Perceptual and Motor Skills*, *86*, 181–182.

Piotrowski, C. (2007). Review of the psychological literature on assessment instruments used with pain patients. *North American Journal of Psychology*, *9*, 303–306.

Pischon, T., Boeing, H., Hoffmann, K., Bergmann, M., Schulze, M. B., Overvad, K., … Riboli, E. (2008). General and abdominal adiposity and risk of death in Europe. *New England Journal of Medicine*, *359*(20), 2105–2120.

Pisinger, C., & Godtfredsen, N. S. (2007). Is there a health benefit of reduced tobacco consumption? A systematic review. *Nicotine and Tobacco Research*, *9*, 631–646.

Pisinger, C., & Jorgensen, T. (2007). Weight concerns and smoking in a general population: The Inter99 study. *Preventive Medicine*, *44*, 283–289.

Plasqui, G., & Westerterp, K. R. (2007). Physical activity and insulin resistance. *Current Nutrition and Food Science*, *3*, 157–160.

Plunk, A. D., Syed-Mohammed, H., Cavazos-Rehg, P., Bierut, L J., & Grucza, R. A. (2014). Alcohol consumption, heavy drinking, and mortality: Rethinking the J-shaped curve. *Alcoholism: Clinical and Experimental Research*, *38*(2), 471–478.

Pole, N., Best, S. R., Metzler, T., & Marmar, C. R. (2005). Why are Hispanics at greater risk for PTSD? *Cultural Diversity and Mental Health*, *11*, 144–161.

Polgar, S., & Ng, J. (2005). Ethics, methodology and the use of placebo controls in surgical trials. *Brain Research Bulletin*, *67*, 290–297.

Polich, J. M., Armor, D. J., & Braiker, H. B. (1980). *The course of alcoholism: Four years after treatment*. Santa Monica, CA: Rand.

Polivy, J., Coelho, J., Hargreaves, D., Fleming, A., & Herman, C. P. (2007). The effects of external cues on eating and body weight: Another look at obese humans and rats. *Appetite*, *49*, 321.

Polivy, J., & Herman, C. P. (2002). Causes of eating disorders. *Annual Review of Psychology*, *53*, 187–214.

Polivy, J., & Herman, C. P. (2004). Sociocultural idealization of thin female body shapes: An introduction to the special issues on body image and eating disorders. *Journal of Social and Clinical Psychology*, *23*, 1–6.

Pollack, M., Chastek, B., Willaism, S. A., & Moran, J. (2010). Impact of treatment complexity on adherence and glycemic control: An analysis of oral antidiabetic agents. *Journal of Clinical Outcomes Management*, *17*, 257–265.

Pollock, M. L., Wilmore, J. H., & Fox, S. M., III. (1978). *Health and fitness through physical activity*. New York, NY: Wiley.

Pomerleau, O. F., & Kardia, S. L. R. (1999). Introduction to the features section: Genetic research on smoking. *Health Psychology*, *18*, 3–6.

Pool, G. J., Schwegler, A. F., Theodore, B. R., & Fuchs, P. N. (2007). Role of gender norms and group identification on hypothetical and experimental pain tolerance. *Pain*, *129*, 122–129.

Poole, H., Branwell, R., & Murphy, P. (2006). Factor structure of the Beck Depression Inventory-II in patients with chronic pain. *Clinical Journal of Pain*, *22*, 790–798.

Pope, C., Mechoulam, R., & Parsons, L. (2010). Endocannabinoid signaling in neurotoxicity and neuroprotection. *NeuroToxicology*, *31*(5), 562–571.

Pope, S. K., Shue, V. M., & Beck, C. (2003). Will a healthy lifestyle help prevent Alzheimer's disease? *Annual Review of Public Health*, *24*, 111–132.

Popham, R. E. (1978). The social history of the tavern. In Y. Israel, F. B. Glaser, H. Kalant, R. E. Popham, W. Schmidt, & R. G. Smart (Eds.), *Research advances in alcohol and drug problems* (Vol. 2, pp. 225–302). New York, NY: Plenum Press.

Popkin, B. (2009). *The world is fat: The fads, trends, policies, and products that are fattening the human race*. New York, NY: Avery/Penguin.

Porta, M., Greenland, S., Hernán, M., dos Santos Silva, I., & Last, J. M. (2014). *A Dictionary of Epidemiology*. Oxford University Press, USA.

Porter, J., & Jick, H. (1980). Addiction rate in patients treated with narcotics. *New England Journal of Medicine*, *302*, 123.

Poss, J. E. (2000). Developing a new model for cross-cultural research: Synthesizing the health belief model and the theory of reasoned action. *Advances in Nursing Science*, *23*, 1–15.

Possemato, K., Ouimette, P., & Geller, P. A. (2010). Internet-based expressive writing for kidney transplant recipients: Effects on post-traumatic stress and quality of life. *Traumatology*, *16*, 49–54.

Poston, W. S. C., Taylor, J. E., Hoffman, K. M., Peterson, A. L., Lando, H. A., Shelton, S., … Haddock, C. K. (2008). Smoking and deployment: Perspectives of junior enlisted U.S. Air Force and U.S. Army personnel and their supervisors. *Military Medicine*, *173*, 441–447.

Pouchot, J., Le Parc, J.-M., Queffelec, L., Sichère, P., & Flinois, A. (2007). Perceptions in 7700 patients with rheumatoid arthritis compared to their families and physicians. *Joint Bone Spine*, *74*, 622–626.

Pouletty, P. (2002). Opinion: Drug addictions: Towards socially accepted and medically treatable diseases. *Nature Reviews Drug Discovery*, *1*, 731–736.

Powell, J., Inglis, N., Ronnie, J., & Large, S. (2011). The characteristics and motivations of online health information seekers: Cross-sectional survey and qualitative interview study. *Journal of Medical Internet Research*, *13*, e20.

Powell, K. E., Paluch, A. E., & Blair, S. N. (2011). Physical activity for health: What kind? How much? How intense? On top of what? *Annual Review of Public Health*, *32*, 349–365.

"Practical Nurse." (2008). Hereditary breast cancer risk overestimated. *Practical Nurse*, *35*(9), 9.

Prapavessis, H., Cameron, L., Baldi, J. C., Robinson, S., Borries, K., Harper, T., … Grove, J. R. (2007). The effects of exercise and nicotine replacement therapy on smoking rates in women. *Addictive Behaviors*, *32*, 1416–1432.

Prejean, J., Song, R., Hernandez, A., Zieball, R., Green, T., Walker, F., … HIV Incidence Surveillance Group. (2011). Estimated HIV incidence in the United States, 2006–2009. *PLoS One*, *6*, e17502.

Pressman, S. D., & Cohen, S. (2005). Does positive affect influence health? *Psychological Bulletin, 131,* 925–971.

Prestwich, A., Perugini, M., & Hurling, R. (2009). Can the effects of implementation intentions on exercise be enhanced using text messages? *Psychology and Health, 24,* 677–687.

Price, D. D., Finniss, D. G., & Benedetti, F. (2008). A comprehensive review of the placebo effect: Recent advances and current thought. *Annual Review of Psychology, 59,* 565–590

Prince, M. (2004). Care arrangements for people with dementia in developing countries. *International Journal of Geriatric Psychiatry, 19,* 170–177.

Prochaska, J. J., Spring, B., & Nigg, C. R. (2008). Multiple health behavior change research: An introduction and overview. *Preventive Medicine, 46,* 181–188.

Prochaska, J. O., DiClemente, C. C., & Norcross, J. C. (1992). In search of how people change: Applications to addictive behaviors. *American Psychologist, 47,* 1102–1114.

Prochaska, J. O., Norcross, J. C., & DiClemente, C. C. (1994). *Changing for good.* New York, NY: Avon Books.

Proctor, R. N. (2012). *Golden holocaust: Origins of the cigarette catastrophe and the case for abolition.* Berkeley, CA: University of California Press.

Purslow, L. R., Sandhu, M. S., Forouhi, N., Young, E. H., Luben, R. N., Welch, A. A., … Wareham, N. J. (2008). Energy intake at breakfast and weight change: Prospective study of 6,764 middle-aged men and women. *American Journal of Epidemiology, 167,* 188.

Puska, P. (2002). Nutrition and global prevention on non-communicable diseases. *Asia Pacific Journal of Clinical Nutrition, 11*(Suppl. 9), S755–S758.

Puska, P., Vartiainen, E., Tuomilehto, J., Salomaa, V., & Nissinen, A. (1998). Changes in premature death in Finland: Successful long-term prevention of cardiovascular diseases. *Bulletin of the World Health Organization, 76,* 419–425.

Puthumana, J., Ferrucci, L., Mayne, S., Lannin, D., & Chagpar, A. (2013). Sun protection practices among melanoma survivors. *Cancer Research, 73*(Suppl. 8), 1365–1365.

Qiu, C., Kivipelto, M., & von Strauss, E. (2011). Epidemiology of Alzheimer's disease: Occurrence, determinants, and strategies toward intervention. *Dialogues in Clinical Neuroscience, 11,* 111–128.

Quartana, P. J., Laubmeier, K. K., & Zakowski, S. G. (2006). Psychological adjustment following diagnosis and treatment of cancer: An examination of the moderating role of positive and negative emotional expressivity. *Journal of Behavioral Medicine, 29,* 487–498.

Quinn, J. F., Bodenhamer-Davis, E., & Koch, D. S. (2004). Ideology and the stagnation of AODA treatment modalities in America. *Deviant Behavior, 25,* 109–131.

Quinn, J. R. (2005). Delay in seeking care for symptoms of acute myocardial infarction: Applying a theoretical model. *Research in Nursing and Health, 28,* 283–294.

Quist, M., Rorth, M., Zacho, M., Andersen, C., Moeller, T., Midtgaard, J., … Adamsen, L. (2006). High-intensity resistance and cardiovascular training improve physical capacity in cancer patients undergoing chemotherapy. *Scandinavian Journal of Medicine and Science in Sports, 16,* 349–357.

Qureshi, A. A., Laden, F., Colditz, G. A., & Hunter, D. J. (2008). Geographic variation and risk of skin cancer in US women. *Archives of Internal Medicine, 168,* 501–507.

Rabin, C., Leventhal, H., & Goodin, S. (2004). Conceptualization of disease timeline predicts posttreatment distress in breast cancer patients. *Health Psychology, 23,* 407–412.

Racine, M., Tousignant-Laflamme, Y., Kloda, L. A., Dion, D., Dupuis, G., & Choinière, M. (2012). A systematic literature review of 10years of research on sex/gender and pain perception–Part 2: Do biopsychosocial factors alter pain sensitivity differently in women and men? *Pain, 153*(3), 619–635.

Ragan, D. T. (2016). Peer beliefs and smoking in adolescence: A longitudinal social network analysis. *American Journal of Drug and Alcohol Abuse, 42*(2), 222–230.

Rahim-Williams, F. B., Riley, J. L., III, Herrera, D., Campbell, C. M., Hastie, B. A., & Fillingim, R. B. (2007). Ethnic identity predicts experimental pain sensitivity in African Americans and Hispanics. *Pain, 129,* 177–184.

Rainville, P., & Price, D. D. (2003). Hypnosis phenomenology and the neurobiology of consciousness. *International Journal of Clinical and Experimental Hypnosis, 51*(Special Issue, Pt. 1), 105–129.

Rainwater, D. L., Mitchell, B. D., Gomuzzie, A. G., Vandeberg, J. L., Stein, M. P., & MacCluer, J. W. (2000). Associations among 5-year changes in weight, physical activity, and cardiovascular disease risk factors in Mexican Americans. *American Journal of Epidemiology, 152,* 974–982.

Rami, B., Popow, C., Horn, W., Waldhoer, T., & Schober, E. (2006). Telemedical support to improve glycemic control in adolescents with Type 1 diabetes mellitus. *European Journal of Pediatrics, 165,* 701–705.

Ramsay, S., Ebrahim, S., Whincup, P., Papacosta, O., Morris, R., Lennon, L., … Wannamethee, S. G. (2008). Social engagement and the risk of cardiovascular disease mortality: Results of a prospective population-based study of older men. *Annals of Epidemiology, 18,* 476–483.

Rapoff, M. A. (2003). Pediatric measures of pain: The Pain Behavior Observation Method, Pain Coping Questionnaire (PCQ), and Pediatric Pain Questionnaire (PPQ). *Arthritis and Rheumatism: Arthritis Care and Research, 49*(S5), S90–S91.

Rasmussen, H. N., Scheier, M. F., & Greenhouse, J. B. (2009). Optimism and physical health: A meta-analytic review. *Annals of Behavioral Medicine, 37,* 239–256.

Ratanawongsa, N., Karter, A. J., Parker, M. M., Lyles, C. R., Heisler, M., Moffet, H. H., Adler, N., Warton, M., & Schillinger, D. (2013). Communication and medication refill adherence: The Diabetes Study of Northern California. *JAMA Internal Medicine, 173*(3), 210–218.

Raum, E., Rothenbacher, D., Ziegler, H., & Brenner, H. (2007). Heavy physical activity: Risk or protective factor for cardiovascular disease? A life course perspective. *Annals of Epidemiology, 17,* 417–424.

Raynor, H. A., & Epstein, L. H. (2001). Dietary variety: Energy regulation and obesity. *Psychological Bulletin, 127,* 325–341.

Rayworth, B. B. (2004). Childhood abuse and risk of eating disorders in women. *Epidemiology, 15,* 271–278.

Read, J. P., Wood, M. D., & Capone, J. C. (2005). A prospective investigation of relations between social influences and alcohol involvement during the transition into college. *Journal of Studies on Alcohol, 66,* 23–34.

Reader, D. M. (2007). Medical nutrition therapy and lifestyle interventions. *Diabetes Care, 30*(Suppl. 2), S188–S193.

Reagan, N. (2000). *I love you Ronnie: The letters of Ronald Reagan to Nancy Reagan.* New York, NY: Random House.

Reas, D. L., & Grilo, C. M. (2008). Review and meta-analysis of pharmacotherapy for binge-eating disorder. *Obesity, 16*(9), 2024–2038.

Reas, D. L., Nygård, J. F., & Sørensen, T. (2009). Do quitters have anything to lose? Changes in body mass index for daily, never, and former smokers over an 11-year period (1990–2001). *Scandinavian Journal of Public Health, 37*(7), 774–777.

Reed, G. M., & Scheldeman, L. (2004). News. *European Psychologist, 9,* 184–187.

Regehr, C., Glancy, D., & Pitts, A. (2013). Interventions to reduce stress in university students: A review and meta-analysis. *Journal of Affective Disorders, 148*(1), 1–11.

Regoeczi, W. C. (2003). When context matters: A multilevel analysis of household and neighbourhood crowding on aggression and withdrawal. *Journal of Environmental Psychology, 23,* 457–470.

Rehm, J., Baliunas, D., Borges, G. L. G., Graham, K., Irving, H., Kehoe, T., … Taylor, B. (2010). The relation between different dimensions of alcohol consumption and burden of disease: An overview. *Addiction, 105*(5), 817–843.

Rehm, J., Patra, J., & Taylor, B. (2007). Harm, benefits, and net effects on mortality of moderate drinking of alcohol among adults in Canada in 2002. *Annals of Epidemiology, 17*(5S), S81–S86.

Reich, A., Müller, G., Gelbrich, G., Deutscher, K., Gödicke, R., & Kiess, W. (2003). Obesity and blood pressure—Results from the examination of 2365 schoolchildren in Germany. *International Journal of Obesity, 27,* 1459–1464.

Reiche, E. M. V., Nunes, S. O. V., & Morimoto, H. K. (2004). Stress, depression, the immune system, and cancer. *Lancet Oncology, 5,* 617–625.

Reid, C. M., Gooberman-Hill, R., & Hanks, G. W. (2008). Opioid analgesics for cancer pain: Symptom control for the living or comfort for the dying? A qualitative study to investigate the factors influencing the decision to accept morphine for pain caused by cancer. *Annals of Oncology, 19,* 44.

Reilly, T., & Woo, G. (2004). Social support and maintenance of safer sex practices among people living with HIV/AIDS. *Health and Social Work, 29,* 97–105.

Reitz, C., Tang, M. X., Manly, J., Schupf, N., Mayeaux, R., & Luchsinger, J. A. (2008). Plasma lipid levels in the elderly are not associated with the risk of mild cognitive impairment. *Dementia and Geriatric Cognitive Disorders, 25,* 232–237.

Rentz, C., Krikorian, R., & Keys, M. (2005). Grief and mourning from the perspective of the person with a dementing illness: Beginning the dialogue. *Omega: Journal of Death and Dying, 50,* 165–179.

Renz, H., Blümer, N., Virna, S., Sel, S., & Garn, H. (2006). The immunological basis of the hygiene hypothesis. *Chemical Immunology and Allergy, 91,* 30–48.

Research and Policy Committee. (2002). *A new vision for healthcare: A leadership role for business.* New York, NY: Committee for Economic Development.

Resnicow, K., Jackson, A., Wang, T., Aniridya, K. D., McCarty, F., Dudley, W. N., … Baranowski, T. (2001). A motivational interviewing intervention to increase fruit and vegetable intake through Black churches: Results of the Eat for Life trial. *American Journal of Public Health, 91,* 1686–1693.

Rethorst, C. D., Wipfli, B. M., & Landers, D. M. (2007). The effect of exercise on depression: Examining clinical significance. *Journal of Sport and Exercise Psychology, 29*(Suppl.), S198.

Reuben, A. (2008). Alcohol and the liver. *Current Opinion in Gastroenterology, 24,* 328–338.

Reuter, T., Ziegelmann, J. P., Wiedemann, A. U., Lippke, S., Schüz, B., & Aiken, L. S. (2010). Planning bridges the intention–behaviour gap: Age makes a difference and strategy use explains why. *Psychology and Health, 25,* 873–887.

Reyes, C., Leyland, K. M., Peat, G., Cooper, C., Arden, N. K., & Prieto-Alhambra, D. (2016). Association between overweight and obesity and risk of clinically diagnosed knee, hip, and hand osteoarthritis: A population-based cohort study. *Arthrtis and Rheumatology, 68*(8), 1869–1875.

Reynolds, S. L., Haley, W., & Kozlenko, N. (2008). The impact of depressive symptoms and chronic diseases on active life expectancy in older Americans. *American Journal of Geriatric Psychology, 16,* 425–432.

Rhee, Y., Taitel, M. S., Walker, D. R., & Lau, D. T. (2007). Narcotic drug use among patients with lower back pain in employer health plans: A retrospective analysis of risk factors and health care services. *Clinical Therapeutics, 29*(Suppl. 1), 2603–2612.

Riazi, A., Pickup, J., & Bradley, C. (2004). Daily stress and glycaemic control in Type 1 diabetes: Individual differences in magnitude, direction, and timing of stress-reactivity. *Diabetes Research and Clinical Practice, 66,* 237–244.

Ricciardelli, L. A., McCabe, M. P., Williams, R. J., & Thompson, J. K. (2007). The role of ethnicity and culture in body image and disordered eating among males. *Clinical Psychology Review, 27,* 582–606.

Richardson, J., Smith, J. E., McCall, G., Richardson, A., Pilkington, K., & Kirsch, I. (2007). Hypnosis for nausea and vomiting in cancer chemotherapy: A systematic review of the research evidence. *European Journal of Cancer Care, 16,* 402–412.

Richardson, K. M., & Rothstein, H. R. (2008). Effects of occupational stress management intervention programs: A meta-analysis. *Journal of Occupational Health Psychology, 13,* 69–93.

Richman, J. A., Cloninger, L., & Rospenda, K. M. (2008). Macrolevel stressors, terrorism, and mental health outcomes: Broadening the stress paradigm. *American Journal of Public Health, 98,* 323–329.

"Ricky Gervais had sausage binge" (2010, April 13). Retrieved from http://www.mirror.co.uk/3am/celebrity-news/ricky-gervais-had-sausage-binge-1685778

Rietveld, S., & Koomen, J. M. (2002). A complex system perspective on medication compliance: Information for healthcare providers. *Disease Management and Health Outcomes, 10,* 621–630.

Riley, J. L., III, Wade, J. B., Myers, C. D., Sheffield, D., Papas, R. K., & Price, D. D. (2002). Racial/ethnic differences in the experience of chronic pain. *Pain, 100,* 291–298.

Riley, K. E., & Kalichman, S. (2015). Mindfulness-based stress reduction for people living with HIV/AIDS: Preliminary review of intervention trial methodologies and findings. *Health Psychology Review, 9*(2), 224–243.

Rimm, E. B., & Moats, C. (2007). Alcohol and coronary heart disease: Drinking patterns and mediators of effect. *Annals of Epidemiology, 17*(S5), S3–S7.

Ringen, P. A., Andreas, M. I., Birkenaes, A. B., Engh, J. A., Faerden, A., Vaskinn, A., … Andreassen, O. A. (2008). The level of illicit drug use is related to symptoms and premorbid functioning in severe mental illness. *Acta Psychiatrica Scandinavica, 118*(4), 297–304.

Ringström, G., Abrahamsson, H., Strid, H., & Simrén, M. (2007). Why do subjects with irritable bowel syndrome seek health care for their symptoms? *Scandinavian Journal of Gastroenterology, 42,* 1194–1203.

Rise, J., Sheeran, P., & Hukkelberg, S. (2010). The role of self-identity in the Theory of Planned Behavior: A meta-analysis. *Journal of Applied Social Psychology, 40,* 1085–1105.

Rissanen, A., Hakala, P., Lissner, L., Mattlar, C.-E., Koskenvuo, M., & Rönnemaa, T. (2002). Acquired preference especially for dietary fat and obesity: A study of weight-discordant monozygotic twin pairs. *International Journal of Obesity and Related Metabolic Disorders, 26,* 973–977.

Ritter, A., & Cameron, J. (2006). A review of the efficacy and effectiveness of harm reduction strategies for alcohol, tobacco and illicit drugs. *Drug and Alcohol Review, 25,* 611–624.

Rivis, A., Sheeran, P., & Armitage, C. J. (2009). Expanding the affective and normative components of the Theory of Planned Behavior: A meta-analysis of ancitipated affect and moral norms. *Journal of Applied Social Psychology, 39,* 2985–3019.

Roberts, B. A., Fuhrer, R., Marmot, M., & Richards, M. (2011). Does retirement influence cognitive performance? The Whitehall II Study. *Journal of Epidemiology and Community Health, 65,* 958–963.

Roberts, S. O. (2002). A strong start: Strength and resistance training guidelines for children and adolescents. *American Fitness, 20*(1), 34–38.

Roberts, W. O. (2007). Heat and cold: What does the environment do to marathon injury? *Sports Medicine, 37,* 400–403.

Robine, J.-M., & Ritchie, K. (1991). Healthy life expectancy: Evaluation of global indicator of change in population health. *British Medical Journal, 302,* 457–460.

Robins, L. N. (1995). The natural history of substance use as a guide to setting drug policy. *American Journal of Public Health, 85,* 12–13.

Robinson, L., Clare, L., & Evans, K. (2005). Making sense of dementia and adjusting to loss: Psychological reactions to a diagnosis of dementia in couples. *Aging and Mental Health, 9,* 337–347.

Robinson, M. E., Gagnon, C. M., Dannecker, E. A., Brown, J. L., Jump, R. L., & Price, D. D. (2003). Sex differences in common pain events: Expectations and anchors. *Journal of Pain, 4,* 40–45.

Robinson-Whelen, S., Tada, Y., MacCallum, R. C., McGuire, L., & Kiecolt-Glaser, J. K. (2001). Long-term caregiving: What happens when it ends? *Journal of Abnormal Psychology, 110,* 573–584.

Robles, D. S. (2011). The thin is in: Am I thin enough? Perfectionism and self-esteem in anorexia. *International Journal of Research and Review, 6*(1), 65–73.

Robles, T. F., Glaser, R., & Kiecolt-Glaser, J. K. (2005). Out of balance: A new look at chronic stress, depression, and immunity. *Current Directions in Psychological Science, 14,* 111–115.

Röder, C. H., Michal, M., Overbeck, G., van de Ven, V. G., & Linden, D. E. J. (2007). Pain response in depersonalization: A functional imaging study using hypnosis in health subjects. *Psychotherapy and Psychosomatics, 76,* 115–121.

Rodin, J., & Langer, E. J. (1977). Long-term effects of a control-relevant intervention with the institutionalized aged. *Journal of Personality and Social Psychology, 35,* 897–902.

Rodin, J., Silberstein, L., & Striegel-Moore, R. (1985). Women and weight: A normative discontent. In T. B. Sonderegger (Ed.), *Psychology and gender* (pp. 267–307). Lincoln, NE: University of Nebraska Press.

Rodriguez, J., Jiang, R., Johnson, W. C., MacKenzie, B. A., Smith, L. J., & Barr, R. G. (2010). The associationof pipe and cigar use with cotinine levels, lung function, and airflow obstruction. *Annals of Internal Medicine, 152*(4), 201–210.

Rodu, B., & Cole, P. (2007). Declining mortality from smoking in the United States. *Nicotine and Tobacco Research, 9*, 781–784.

Roe, S., & Becker, J. (2005). Drug prevention with vulnerable young people: A review. *Drugs: Education, Prevention and Policy, 12*, 85–99.

Roelofs, J., Boissevain, M. D., Peters, M. L., de Jong, J. R., & Vlaeyen, J. W. S. (2002). Psychological treatments for chronic low back pain: Past, present, and beyond. *Pain Reviews, 9*, 29–40.

Roesch, S. L., Adams, L., Hines, A., Palmores, A., Vyas, P., Tran, C., … Vaughn, A. A. (2005). Coping with prostate cancer: A meta-analytic review. *Journal of Behavioral Medicine, 28*, 281–293.

Roger, V. L., Go, A. S., Lloyd-Jones, D. M., Benjamin, E. J., Berry, J. D., Borden, W. B., … American Heart Association Statistics Committee and Stroke Statistics Subcommittee. (2012). Heart disease and stroke statistics—2012 update: A report from the American Heart Association. *Circulation, 125*, e2–e220.

Rogers, C. J., Colbert, L. H., Greiner, J. W., Perkins, S. N., & Hursting, S. D. (2008). Physical activity and cancer prevention: Pathways and targets for intervention. *Sports Medicine, 38*, 271–296.

Rollings, G. (2011, January 1). I smiled as I cut off my arm. I was grateful to be free. *The Sun.* Retrieved February 4, 2012, from http://www.thesun.co.uk/sol/homepage/showbiz/film/3326119/I-smiled-as-I-cut-off-my-arm-I-was-just-grateful-to-be-free.html

Rollins, S. Z., & Garrison, M. E. B. (2002). The Family Daily Hassles Inventory: A preliminary investigation of reliability and validity. *Family and Consumer Sciences Research Journal, 31*, 135–154.

Rollman, G. B. (1998). Culture and pain. In S. S. Kazarian & D. R. Evans (Eds.), *Cultural clinical psychology: Theory, research, and practice* (pp. 267–286). New York, NY: Oxford University Press.

Romeyke, T., & Stummer, H. (2015). Evidence-based complementary and alternative medicine in inpatient care: Take a look at Europe. *Journal of Evidence-Based Complementary and Alternative Medicine, 20*(2), 87–93.

Ronan, G. F., Dreer, L. W., Dollard, K. M., & Ronan, D. W. (2004). Violent couples: Coping and communication skills. *Journal of Family Violence, 19*, 131–137.

Room, R., & Day, N. (1974). Alcohol and mortality. In M. Keller (Ed.), *Second special report to the U.S. Congress: Alcohol and health* (pp. 79–92). Washington, DC: U.S. Government Printing Office.

Rooney, K., & Ozanne, S. E. (2011). Maternal over-nutrition and offspring obesity predisposition: Targets for preventative interventions. *International Journal of Obesity, 35*(7), 883–890.

Roozen, S., Peters, G.-J. Y., Kok, G., Townend, D., Nijhuis, J., & Curfs, L. (2016). Worldwide prevalence of fetal alcohol spectrum disorders: A systematic literature review including meta-analysis, *Alcoholism: Clinical and Experimental Research, 40*(1), 18–32.

Rosal, M. C., Olendzki, B., Reed, G. W., Gumieniak, O., Scavron, J., & Ockene, I. (2005). Diabetes self-management among low-income Spanish-speaking patients: A pilot study. *Annals of Behavioral Medicine, 29*, 225–235.

Rosario, M., Salzinger, S., Feldman, R. S., & Ng-Mak, D. S. (2008). The roles of social support and coping. *American Journal of Community Psychology, 41*, 43–62.

Rose, J. P., Geers, A. L., Rasinski, H. M., & Fowler, S. L. (2011). Choice and placebo expectation effects in the context of pain analgesia. *Journal of Behavioral Medicine.* DOI:10.1007/s10865-011-9374-0.

Rosen, C. S. (2000). Is the sequencing of change processes by stage consistent across health problems? A meta-analysis. *Health Psychology, 19*, 593–604.

Rosenberg, E., Leanza, Y., & Seller, R. (2007). Doctor-patient communication in primary care with an interpreter: Physician perceptions of professional and family interpreters. *Patient Education and Counseling, 67*, 286–292.

Rosenberg, H., & Melville, J. (2005). Controlled drinking and controlled drug use as outcome goals in British treatment services. *Addiction Research and Theory, 13*, 85–92.

Rosenberg, N. L., Grigsby, J., Dreisbach, J., Busenbark, D., & Grigsby, P. (2002). Neuropsychologic impairment and MRI abnormalities associated with chronic solvent abuse. *Journal of Toxicology: Clinical Toxicology, 40*, 21–34.

Rosenberg, S. D., Lu, W., Mueser, K. T., Jankowski, M. K., & Cournos, F. (2007). Correlates of adverse childhood events among adults with schizophrenia spectrum disorders. *Psychiatric Services, 58*, 245–253.

Rosenblatt, K. A., Wicklund, K. G., & Stanford, J. L. (2000). Sexual factors and the risk of prostate cancer. *American Journal of Epidemiology, 152*, 1152–1158.

Rosengren, A., Hawken, S., Ounpuu, S., Sliwa, K., Zubaid, M., Almahmeed, W. A., … INTERHEART Investigators. (2004). Association of psychosocial risk factors with risk of acute myocardial infarction in 11119 cases and 13648 controls from 52 countries (the INTERHEART study): Case-control study. *Lancet, 364*, 953–962.

Rosengren, A., Subramanian, S. V., Islam, S., Chow, C. K., Avezum, A., Kazmi, K., … INTERHEART Investigators. (2009). Education and risk for acute myocardial infarction in 52 high, middle and low-income countries: INTER-HEART case-control study. *Heart, 95*, 2014–2022.

Rosenkranz, M., Davidson, R. J., MacCoon, D., Sheridan, J. F., Kalin, N. H., & Lutz, A. (2013). A comparison of mindfulness-based stress reduction and an active control in modulation of neurogenic inflammation. *Brain, Behavior, and Immunity, 27*(1), 174–184.

Rosenman, R. H., Brand, R. J., Jenkins, C. D., Friedman, M., Straus, R., & Wurm, M. (1975). Coronary heart disease in the Western Collaborative Group Study: Final follow-up of 8 1/2 years. *Journal of the American Medical Association, 233*, 872–877.

Rosier, E. M., Iadarola, M. J., & Coghill, R. C. (2002). Reproducibility of pain measurement and pain perception. *Pain, 98*, 205–216.

Rosland, A., Kieffer, E., Israel, B., Cofield, M., Palmisano, G., Sinco, B., … Heisler, M. (2008). When is social support important? The association of family support and professional support with specific diabetes self-management behaviors. *Journal of General Internal Medicine, 23*, 1992–1999.

Rösner, S., Hackl-Herrwerth, A., Leucht, S., Vecchi, S., Srisurapanont, M., & Soyka, M. (2010). Opioid antagonists for alcohol dependence. *Cochrane Database of Systematic Reviews 2010, 12*, Cochrane Art. No.: CD001867, DOI: 10.1002/14651858.CD001867.pub3.

Ross, M. J., & Berger, R. S. (1996). Effects of stress inoculation training on athletes' postsurgical pain and rehabilitation after orthopedic injury. *Journal of Consulting and Clinical Psychology, 64*, 406–410.

Rosser, B. A., & Eccleston, C. (2011). Smartphone applications for pain management. *Journal of Telemedicine and Telecare, 17*, 308–312.

Rössler, W., Lauber, C., Angst, J., Haker, H., Gamma, A., Eich, D., … Ajdacic-Gross, V. (2007). The use of complementary and alternative medicine in the general population: Results from a longitudinal community study. *Psychological Medicine, 37*, 73–84.

Rossow, I., Grøholt, B., & Wichstrøm, L. (2005). Intoxicants and suicidal behaviour among adolescents: Changes in levels and associations from 1992 to 2002. *Addiction, 100*, 79–88.

Roter, D. L., & Hall, J. A. (2004). Physician gender and patient-centered communication: A critical review of empirical research. *Annual Review of Public Health, 25*, 497–519.

Roth, M., & Kobayashi, K. (2008). The use of complementary and alternative medicine among Chinese Canadians: Results from a national survey. *Journal of Immigrant and Minority Health, 10*(6), 517–528.

Rotskoff, L. (2002). *Love on the rocks: Men, women, and alcohol in post–World War II America.* Chapel Hill, NC: University of North Carolina Press.

Rotter, J. B. (1966). Generalized expectancies for internal versus external control of reinforcement. *Psychological Monographs, 80*(Whole No. 609).

Rozanski, A., Blumenthal, J. A., Davidson, K. W., Saab, P. G., & Kubzansky, L. (2005). The epidemiology, pathophysiology, and management of psychosocial risk factors in cardiac practice: The emerging field of behavioral cardiology. *Journal of the American College of Cardiology, 45*, 637–651.

Rozin, P. (2005). The meaning of food in our lives: A cross-cultural perspective on eating and well-being. *Journal of Nutrition Education and Behavior, 37*(Suppl. 2), S107–S112.

Rubak, S., Sanboek, A., Lauritzen, T., & Christensen, B. (2005). Motivational interviewing: A systematic review and meta-analysis. *British Journal of General Practice, 55*, 305–312.

Rubenstein, S., & Caballero, B. (2000). Is Miss America an undernourished role model? *Journal of the American Medical Association, 283*, 1569.

Rubenstein, S. M., van Middelkoop, M., Assendelft, W. J., de Boer, M. R., & van Tulder, M. W. (2011). Spinal manipulative therapy for chronic low-back pain. *Cochrane Database of Systematic Reviews, 2011*, Issue 2, Cochrane Art. No.: CD008112, DOI: 10.1002/14651858. CD008112.pub2.

Rudd, R. E. (2007). Health literacy skills of U.S. adults. *American Journal of Health Behavior, 31*, S8–S18.

Ruitenberg, A., van Swieten, J. C., Witteman, J. C., Mehta, K. M., van Duijn, C. M., Hofman, A., ... Breteler, M. M. B. (2002). Alcohol consumption and risk of dementia: The Rotterdam Study. *The Lancet, 359*(9303), 281–286.

Rutherford, B. R., Pott, E., Tandler, J. M., Wall, M. M., Roose, S. P., & Lieberman, J. A. (2014). Placebo response in antipsychotic clinical trials: A meta-analysis. *JAMA Psychiatry, 71*(12), 1409–1421.

Rutledge, P. C., Park, A., & Sher, K. J. (2008). 21st birthday drinking: Extremely extreme. *Journal of Consulting and Clinical Psychology, 76*, 511–516.

Rutten, G. (2005). Diabetes patient education: Time for a new era. *Diabetic Medicine, 22*, 671–673.

Ryan, C. J., & Zerwic, J. J. (2003). Perceptions of symptoms of myocardial infarction related to health care seeking behaviors in the elderly. *Journal of Cardiovascular Nursing, 18*, 184–196.

Sääkslahti, A., Numminen, P., Varstala, V., Helenius, H., Tammi, A., Viikari, J., ... Välimäki, I. (2004). Physical activity as a preventive measure for coronary heart disease risk factors in early childhood. *Scandinavian Journal of Medicine and Science in Sports, 14*, 143–149.

Saab, P. G., McCalla, J. R., Coons, H. L., Christensen, A. J., Kaplan, R., Johnson, S. B., ... Melamed, B. (2004). Technological and medical advances: Implications for health psychology. *Health Psychology, 23*(2), 142.

Sabia, S., Marmot, M., Dufouil, C., & Singh-Manoux, A. (2008). Smoking history and cognitive function in middle age from the Whitehall II study. *Archives of Internal Medicine, 168*, 1165–1173.

Sachdev, P., Mondraty, N., Wen, W., & Gulliford, K. (2008). Brains of anorexia nervosa patients process self-images differently from non-self-images: An fMRI study. *Neuropsychologia, 46*, 2161–2168.

Sackett, D. L., & Snow, J. C. (1979). The magnitude of compliance and noncompliance. In R. B. Haynes, D. W. Taylor, & D. L. Sackett (Eds.), *Compliance in health care* (pp. 11–22). Baltimore, MD: Johns Hopkins University Press.

Sackner-Bernstein, J., Kanter, D., & Kaul, S. (2015). Dietary interventions for overweight and obese adults: Comparison of low-carbohydrate and low-fat diets: A meta-analysis. *PLoS One, 10*(10), 1–19.

Sadasivam, R. S., Kinney, R. L., Lemon, S. C., Shimada, S. L., Allison, J. J., & Houston, T. K. (2013). Internet health information seeking is a team sport: Analysis of the Pew Internet Survey. *International Journal of Medical Informatics, 82*(3), 193–200.

Sallis, J. F., Bowles, H. R., Bauman, A., Ainsworth, B. E., Bull, F. C., Craig, C. L., ... Bergman, P. (2009). Neighborhood environments and physical activity among adults in 11 countries. *American Journal of Preventive Medicine, 36*, 484–490.

Samitz, G., Egger, M., & Zwahlen, M. (2011). Domains of physical activity and all-cause mortality: Systematic review and dose–response meta-analysis of cohort studies. *International Journal of Epidemiology, 40*(5), 1382–1400.

Sampson, A., Bhochhibhoya, A., Digeralamo, D., & Branscum, P. (2015). The use of text messaging for smoking cessation and relapse prevention: A systematic review of evidence. *Journal of Smoking Cessation, 10*(1), 50–58.

Samuelson, M., Carmody, J., Kabat-Zinn, J., & Bratt, M. A. (2007). Mindfulness-based stress reduction in Massachusetts correctional facilities. *Prison Journal, 87*, 254–268.

Sánchez del Rio, M., & Alvarez Linera, J. (2004). Functional neuroimaging of headaches. *Lancet Neurology, 3*, 645–651.

Sánchez-Johnsen, L. A. P., Carpentier, M. R., & King, A. C. (2011). Race and sex associations to weight concerns among urban African American and Caucasian smokers. *Addictive Behaviors, 36*(1/2), 14–17.

Sancier, K. M., & Holman, D. (2004). Commentary: Multifaceted health benefits of medical *Qigong. Journal of Alternative and Complementary Medicine, 10*, 163–165.

Sanders, S. (2005). Is the glass half empty or half full? Reflections on strain and gain in caregivers of individuals with Alzheimer's disease. *Social Work in Health Care, 40*(3), 57–73.

Sanders, S. H. (2006). Behavioral conceptualization and treatment for chronic pain. *Behavior Analyst Today, 7*, 253–261.

Sapolsky, R. M. (1997, November). On the role of upholstery in cardiovascular physiology. *Discover Magazine.* Retrieved March 9, 2012, from http://discovermagazine.com/1997/nov/ontheroleofuphol1260

Sapolsky, R. M. (1998). *Why zebras don't get ulcers: An updated guide to stress, stress-related diseases, and coping.* New York, NY: Freeman.

Sapolsky, R. M. (2004). Social status and health in humans and other animals. *Annual Review of Anthropology, 33*, 393–418.

Sartor, C. E., Grant, J. D., Agrawal, A., Sadler, B., Madden, P. A. F., Heath, A. C., ... Bucholz, K. K. (2015). Genetic and environmental contributions to initiation of cigarette smoking in your African-American and European-American women. *Drug and Alcohol Dependence, 157*, 54–59.

Sattin, R. W., Easley, K. A., Wolf, S. L., Chen, Y., & Kutner, M. H. (2005). Reduction in fear of falling through intense tai chi exercise training in older, transitionally frail adults. *Journal of the American Geriatrics Society, 53*, 1168–1178.

Sattler, G. (2005). Advances in liposuction and fat transfer. *Dermatology Nursing, 17*, 133–139.

Saunders, T., Driskell, J. E., Johnston, J. H., & Sales, E. (1996). The effects of stress inoculation training on anxiety and performance. *Journal of Occupational Health Psychology, 1*, 170–186.

Savage, E., Farrell, D., McManus, V., & Grey, M. (2010). The science of intervention development for type 1 diabetes in childhood: Systematic review. *Journal of Advanced Nursing, 66*, 2604–2619.

Sayette, M. A., Kirchner, T. R., Moreland, R. L., Levine, J. M., & Travis, T. (2004). Effects of alcohol on risk-seeking behavior: A group-level analysis. *Psychology of Addictive Behaviors, 18*, 190–193.

Scarborough, P., Matthews, A., Eyles, H., Kaur, A., Hodgkins, C., Raats, M. M., ... Rayner, M. (2015). Reds are more important than greens: How UK supermarket shoppers use the different information on a traffic light nutrition label in a choice experiment. *International Journal of Behavioral Nutrition and Physical Activity, 12*(1), 151.

Scarpa, A., Haden, S. C., & Hurley, J. (2006). Community violence victimization and symptoms of posttraumatic stress disorder: The moderating effects of coping and social support. *Journal of Interpersonal Violence, 21*, 446–469.

Scarscelli, D. (2006). Drug addiction between deviance and normality: A study of spontaneous and assisted remission. *Contemporary Drug Problems, 33*, 237–274.

Schaap, M. M., Kunst, A. E., Leinsalu, M., Regidor, E., Ekholm, O., Dzurova, D., ... Mackenbach, J. P. (2008). Effect of nationwide tobacco control policies on smoking cessation in high and low educated groups in 18 European countries. *Tobacco Control, 17*(4), 248–255.

Schaap, M. M., van Agt, H. M. E., & Kunst, A. E. (2008). Identification of socioeconomic groups at increased risk for smoking in European countries: Looking beyond educational level. *Nicotine and Tobacco Research, 10*(2), 359–369.

Schachter, S. (1980). Urinary pH and the psychology of nicotine addiction. In P. O. Davidson & S. M. Davidson (Eds.), *Behavioral medicine: Changing health lifestyles* (pp. 70–93). New York, NY: Brunner/Mazel.

Schachter, S. (1982). Recidivism and self-cure of smoking and obesity. *American Psychologist, 37*, 436–444.

Schaller, M., Miller, G. E., Gervais, W. M., Yager, S., & Chen, E. (2010). Mere visual perception of other people's disease symptoms facilitates a more aggressive immune response. *Psychological Science*, *21*, 649–652.

Schatzkin, A., Lanza, E., Corle, D., Lance, P., Iber, F., Caan, B., ... the Polyp Prevention Trial Study Group (2000). Lack of effect of a low-fat, high-fiber diet on the recurrence of colorectal adenomas. *New England Journal of Medicine*, *342*(16), 1149–1155.

Schell, L. M., & Denham, M. (2003). Environmental pollution in urban environments and human biology. *Annual Review of Anthropology*, *32*, 111–134.

Schenker, S. (2001, September). The truth about fad diets. *Student BMJ*, 318–319.

Schlenger, W. E., Caddell, J. M., Ebert, L., Jordan, B. K., Rourke, K. M., Wilson, D., ... Kulka, R. A. (2002). Psychological reactions to terrorist attacks: Findings from the National Study of Americans' Reactions to September 11. *Journal of the American Medical Association*, *288*, 581–588.

Schlicht, W., Kanning, M., & Bös, K. (2007). Psychosocial interventions to influence physical inactivity as a risk factor: Theoretical models and practical evidence. In J. Dordan, B. Bardé, & A. M. Zeiher (Eds.), *Contributions toward evidence-based psychocardiology: A systematic review of the literature* (pp. 107–123). Washington, DC: American Psychological Association.

Schmaltz, H. N., Southern, D., Ghali, W. A., Jelinski, S. F., Parsons, G. A., King, K., ... Maxwell, C. J. (2007). Living alone, patient sex and mortality after acute myocardial infarction. *Journal of General Internal Medicine*, *22*, 572–578.

Schmidt-Kassow, M., Deusser, M., Thiel, C., Otterbein, S., Montag, C., Reuter, M., ... Kaiser, J. (2013). Physical exercise during encoding improves vocabulary learning in young female adults: A neuroendocrinological study. *PloS One*, *8*(5), e64172.

Schneider, E. C., Zaslavsky, A. M., & Epstein, A. M. (2002). Racial disparities in the quality of care for enrollees in Medicare managed care. *Journal of the American Medical Association*, *287*, 1288–1294.

Schneider, M. J., & Perle, S. M. (2012). Challenges and limitations of the Cochrane systematic review of spinal therapy. *Journal of the American Chiropractic Association*, *49*(6), 28–33.

Schneiderman, N., Saab, P. G., Carney, R. M., Raczynski, J. M., Cowan, M. J., Berkman, L. F., ... ENRICHD Investigators. (2004). Psychosocial treatment within sex by ethnicity subgroups in the Enhancing Recovery in Coronary Heart Disease clinical trial. *Psychosomatic Medicine*, *66*, 475–483.

Schnittker, J. (2004). Education and the changing shape of the income gradient in health. *Journal of Health and Social Behavior*, *45*, 286–305.

Schnittker, J. (2007). Working more and feeling better: Women's health, employment, and family life. *American Sociological Review*, *72*, 221–238.

Schoenbaum, M. (1997). Do smokers understand the mortality effects of smoking? Evidence from the Health Retirement Survey. *American Journal of Public Health*, *87*, 755–759.

Schoenthaler, A., Allegrante, J. P., Chaplin, W., & Ogedegbe, G. (2012). The effect of patient–provider communication on medication adherence in hypertensive black patients: Does race concordance matter? *Annals of Behavioral Medicine*, *43*(3), 372–382.

Schousboe, K., Visscher, P. M., Erbas, B., Kyvik, K. O., Hopper, J. L., Henriksen, J. E., ... Sørensen, T. I. (2004). Twin study of genetic and environmental influences on adult body size, shape, and composition. *International Journal of Obesity*, *28*, 39–48.

Schroeder, K., Fahey, T., & Ebrahim, S. (2007). Interventions for improving adherence to treatment in patients with high blood pressure in ambulatory settings. *Cochrane Database of Systematic Reviews*, Cochrane Art. No.: CD004804, DOI: 10.1002/14651858. CD004804.

Schroeder, K. E. E. (2004). Coping competence as predictor and moderator of depression among chronic disease patients. *Journal of Behavioral Medicine*, *27*, 123–145.

Schroevers, M., Ranchor, A. V., & Sanderman, R. (2006). Adjustment to cancer in the 8 years following diagnosis: A longitudinal study comparing cancer survivors with healthy individuals. *Social Science and Medicine*, *63*, 598–610.

Schuckit, M. A. (2000). Keep it simple. *Journal of Studies on Alcohol*, *61*, 781–782.

Schulz, K. F., Altman, D. G., Moher, D., and the CONSORT Group. (2010). CONSORT 2010 statement: Updated guidelines for reporting parallel group randomized trials. *Annals of Internal Medicine*, *152*(11), 726–732.

Schulz, R., & Aderman, D. (1974). Clinical research and the stages of dying. *Omega: Journal of Death and Dying*, *5*, 137–143.

Schulze, A., & Mons, U. (2006). The evolution of educational inequalities in smoking: A changing relationship and a cross-over effect among German birth cohorts of 1921–70. *Addiction*, *101*, 1051–1056.

Schüz, B., Sniehotta, F. F., & Schwarzer, R. (2007). Stage-specific effects of an action control intervention on dental flossing. *Health Education Research*, *22*, 332–341.

Schieman, S., Milkie, M. A., & Glavin, P. (2009). When work interferes with life: Work-nonwork interference and the influence of work-related demands and resources. *American Sociological Review*, *74*, 966–988.

Schuh-Hofer, S., Wodarski, R., Pfau, D. B., Caspani, O., Magerl, W., Kennedy, J. D., ... Treede, R. D. (2013). One night of total sleep deprivation promotes a state of generalized hyperalgesia: A surrogate pain model to study the relationship of insomnia and pain. *Pain*, *154*(9), 1613–1621.

Schwartz, B. S., Stewart, W. F., Simon, D., & Lipton, R. B. (1998). Epidemiology of tension-type headache. *Journal of the American Medical Association*, *279*, 381–383.

Schwartz, G. E., & Weiss, S. M. (1978). Behavioral medicine revisited: An amended definition. *Journal of Behavioral Medicine*, *1*, 249–251.

Schwarzer, R. (2008). Modeling health behavior change: How to predict and modify the adoption and maintenance of health behaviors. *Applied Psychology: An International Review*, *57*, 1–29.

Schwarzer, R., Luszczynska, A., Ziegelmann, J. P., Scholz, U., & Lippke, S. (2008). Social-cognitive predictors of physical exercise adherence: Three longitudinal studies in rehabilitation. *Health Psychology*, *27*(S1), S54–S63.

Sclafani, A. (2001). Psychobiology of food preferences. *International Journal of Obesity*, *25*(Suppl. 5), S13–S16.

Sclafani, A., & Springer, D. (1976). Dietary obesity in adult rats: Similarities to hypothalamic and human obesity. *Physiology and Behavior*, *17*, 461–471.

Scott, D. J., Stohler, C. S., Egnatuk, C. M., Wang, H., Koeppe, R. A., & Zubieta, J.-K. (2008). Placebo and nocebo effects are defined by opposite opioid and dopaminergic responses. *Archives of General Psychiatry*, *65*, 220–231.

Scott-Sheldon, L. A., Kalichman, S. C., Carey, M. P., & Fielder, R. L. (2008). Stress management interventions for HIV+ adults: A meta-analysis of randomized controlled trials, 1989 to 2006. *Health Psychology*, *27*, 129–139.

Scullard, P., Peacock, C., & Davies, P. (2010). Googling children's health: Reliability of medical advice on the internet. *Archives of Disease in Childhood*, *95*(8), 580–582.

Searle, A., & Bennett, P. (2001). Psychological factors and inflammatory bowel disease: A review of a decade of literature. *Psychology and Health Medicine*, *6*, 121–135.

Searle, A., Norman, P., Thompson, R., & Vedhara, K. (2007). A prospective examination of illness beliefs and coping in patients with Type 2 diabetes. *British Journal of Health Psychology*, *12*, 621–638.

Sears, S. R., & Stanton, A. L. (2001). Expectancy-value constructs and expectancy violation as predictors of exercise adherence in previously sedentary women. *Health Psychology*, *20*, 326–333.

Sebre, S., Sprugevica, I., Novotni, A., Bonevski, D., Pakalniskiene, V., Popescu, D., ... Lewis, O. (2004). Cross-cultural comparisons of child-reported emotional and physical abuse: Rates, risk factors and psychosocial symptoms. *Child Abuse and Neglect*, *28*, 113–127.

Seegers, V., Petit, D., Falissard, B., Vitaro, F., Tremblay, R. E., Montplaisir, J., ... Touchette, E. (2011). Short sleep duration and body mass index: A prospective longitudinal study in preadolescence. *American Journal of Epidemiology*, *173*(6), 621–629.

Segall, A. (1997). Sick role concepts and health behavior. In D. S. Gochman (Ed.), *Handbook of health behavior research: Vol. 1. Personal and social determinants* (pp. 289–301). New York, NY: Plenum Press.

Segerstrom, S. C. (2005). Optimism and immunity: Do positive thoughts always lead to positive effects? *Brain, Behavior, and Immunity, 19*, 195–200.

Segerstrom, S. C. (2007). Stress, energy, and immunity: An ecological view. *Current Directions in Psychological Science, 16*, 326–330.

Segerstrom, S. C., & Miller, G. E. (2004). Psychological stress and the human immune system: A meta-analytic study of 30 years of inquiry. *Psychological Bulletin, 130*, 601–630.

Seifert, T. (2005). Anthropomorphic characteristics of centerfold models: Trends toward slender figures over time. *Journal of Eating Disorders, 37*, 271–274.

Selkoe, D. J. (2007). Developing preventive therapies for chronic diseases: Lessons learned from Alzheimer's disease. *Nutrition Reviews, 65*(S12), S239–S243.

Selye, H. (1956). *The stress of life*. New York, NY: McGraw-Hill.

Selye, H. (1976). *Stress in health and disease*. Reading, MA: Butterworths.

Selye, H. (1982). History and present status of the stress concept. In L. Goldberger & S. Breznitz (Eds.), *Handbook of stress: Theoretical and clinical aspects* (pp. 7–17). New York, NY: Free Press.

Seow, D., & Gauthier, S. (2007). Pharmacotherapy of Alzheimer disease. *Canadian Journal of Psychiatry, 52*, 620–629.

Sepa, A., Wahlberg, J., Vaarala, O., Frodi, A., & Ludvigsson, J. (2005). Psychological stress may induce diabetes-related autoimmunity in infancy. *Diabetes Care, 28*, 290–295.

Sephton, S. E., Dhabhar, F. S., Keuroghlian, A. S., Giese-Davis, J., McEwen, B. S., Ionan, A. C., … Spiegel, D. (2009). Depression, cortisol, and suppressed cell-mediated immunity in metastatic breast cancer. *Brain, Behavior, and Immunity, 23*, 1148–1155.

Sepulveda, M.-J., Bodenheimer, T., & Grundy, P. (2008). Primary care: Can it solve employers' health care dilemma? *Health Affairs, 27*, 151–158.

Severson, H. H., Forrester, K. K., & Biglan, A. (2007). Use of smokeless tobacco is a risk factor for cigarette smoking. *Nicotine and Tobacco Research, 9*, 1331–1337.

Sevincer, A. T., & Oettingen, G. (2013). Alcohol intake leads people to focus on desirability rather than feasibility. *Motivation and Emotion, 37*(1), 165–176.

Shai, I., Spence, J. D., Schwarzfuchs, D., Henkin, Y., Parraga, G., Rudich, A., … DIRECT Group. (2010). Dietary intervention to reverse carotid atherosclerosis. *Circulation, 121*, 1200–1208.

Shalev, I., Moffitt, T. E., Braithwaite, A. W., Danese, A., Fleming, N. I., Goldman-Mellor, S., … Caspi, A. (2014). Internalizing disorders and leukocyte telomere erosion: A prospective study of depression, generalized anxiety disorder and post-traumatic stress disorder. *Molecular Psychiatry, 19*(11), 1163–1170.

Shannon, S., Weil, A., & Kaplan, B. J. (2011). Medical decision making in integrative medicine: Safety, efficacy, and patient preference. *Alternative and Complementary Therapies, 17*(2), 84–91.

Shapiro, D., Cook, I. A., Davydov, D. M., Ottaviani, C., Leuchter, A. F., & Abrams, M. (2007). Yoga is a complementary treatment of depression: Effects of traits and moods on treatment outcome. *Evidence-Based Complementary and Alternative Medicine, 4*, 493–502.

Shapiro, J. R., Berkman, N. D., Brownley, K. A., Sedway, J. A., Lohr, K. N., & Bulik, C. M. (2007). Bulimia nervosa treatment: A systematic review of randomized controlled trials. *International Journal of Eating Disorders, 40*(4), 321–336.

Sharpe, L., Sensky, T., Timberlake, N., Ryan, B., Brewin, C. R., & Allard, S. (2001). A blind, randomized controlled trial of cognitive-behavioral intervention for patients with recent onset rheumatoid arthritis: Preventing psychological and physical mobility. *Pain, 89*, 275–283.

Shea, M. K., Houston, D. K., Nichlas, B. J., Messier, S. P., Davis, C. C., Miller, M. E., … Kritchevsky, S. B. (2010). The effect of randomization to weight loss on total mortality in older overweight and obese adults: The ADAPT study. *Journals of Gerontology Series A: Biological Sciences and Medical Sciences, 65A*(5), 519–525.

Sheehy, R., & Horan, J. J. (2004). Effects of stress inoculation training for 1st-year law students. *International Journal of Stress Management, 11*, 41–55.

Sheeran, P. (2002). Intention-behavior relations: A conceptual and empirical review. *European Review of Social Psychology, 12*, 1–36.

Sheeran, P., & Orbell, S. (1999). Implementation intentions and repeated behaviour: Augmenting the predictive validity of the theory of planned behaviour. *European Journal of Social Psychology, 29*, 349–369.

Sheeran, P., & Orbell, S. (2000). Using implementation intentions to increase attendance for cervical cancer screening. *Health Psychology, 19*, 283–289.

Sheese, B. E., Brown, E. L., & Graziano, W. G. (2004). Emotional expression in cyberspace: Searching for moderators of the Pennebaker disclosure effect via e-mail. *Health Psychology, 23*, 457–464.

Shen, B.-J., Avivi, Y. E., Todaro, J. F., Spiro, A., Laurenceau, J.-P., Ward, K. D., … Niaura, R. (2008). Anxiety characteristics independently and prospectively predict myocardial infarction in men: The unique contribution of anxiety among psychologic factors. *Journal of the American College of Cardiology, 51*, 113–119.

Shen, B.-J., Stroud, L. R., & Niaura, R. (2004). Ethnic differences in cardiovascular responses to laboratory stress: A comparison between Asian and White Americans. *International Journal of Behavioral Medicine, 11*, 181–186.

Shen, Z., Chen, J., Sun, S., Yu, B., Chen, Z., Yang, J., … Wu, A. Q. (2003). Psychosocial factors and immunity of patients with generalized anxiety disorder. *Chinese Mental Health Journal, 17*, 397–400.

Sheps, D. S. (2007). Psychological stress and myocardial ischemia: Understanding the link and implications. *Psychosomatic Medicine, 69*, 491–492.

Sher, K. J. (1987). Stress response dampening. In H. T. Blane & K. E. Leonard (Eds.), *Psychological theories of drinking and alcoholism* (pp. 227–271). New York, NY: Guilford Press.

Sher, K. J., & Levenson, R. W. (1982). Risk for alcoholism and individual differences in the stress-response-dampening effect of alcohol. *Journal of Abnormal Psychology, 91*, 350–367.

Shere-Wolfe, K. D., Tilburt, J. C., D'Adamo, C., Berman, B., & Chesney, M. A. (2013). Infectious diseases physicians' attitudes and practices related to complementary and integrative medicine: Results of a national survey. *Evidence-based Complementary and Alternative Medicine (eCAM), 2013*, 1–8.

Sherman, D. K., Updegraff, J. A., & Mann, T. L. (2008). Improving oral health behavior: A social psychological approach. *Journal of the American Dental Association, 139*, 1382–1387.

Sherman, K. J., Cherkin, D. C., Hawkes, R. J., Miglioretti, D. L., & Deyo, R. A. (2009). Randomized trial of therapeutic massage for chronic neck pain. *Clinical Journal of Pain, 25*(3), 233–238.

Shernoff, M. (2006). Condomless sex: Gay men, barebacking, and harm reduction. *Social Work, 51*, 106–113.

Sherwood, L. (2001). *Human physiology: From cells to systems* (4th ed.). Pacific Grove, CA: Brooks/Cole.

Shi, L., Liu, J., Fonseca, V., Walker, P., Kalsekar, A., & Pawaskar, M. (2010). Correlation between adherence rates measured by MEMS and self-reported questionnaires: A meta-analysis. *Health and Quality of Life Outcomes, 8*, 99.

Shi, S., & Klotz, U. (2008). Clinical use and pharmacological properties of selective COX-2 inhibitors. *European Journal of Clinical Pharmacology, 64*, 233–252.

Shiffman, S., Balabanis, M. H., Paty, J. A., Engberg, J., Gwaltney, C. J., Liu, K. S., … Paton, S. M. (2000). Dynamic effects of self-efficacy on smoking lapse and relapse. *Health Psychology, 19*, 315–323.

Shiffman, S., Brockwell, S. E., Pillitteri, J. L., & Gitchell, J. G. (2008). Use of smoking-cessation treatments in the United States. *American Journal of Preventive Medicine, 34*, 102–111.

Shifren, K., & Hooker, K. (1995). Stability and change in optimism: A study among spouse caregivers. *Experimental Aging Research, 21*(1), 59–76.

Shimabukuro, J., Awata, S., & Matsuoka, H. (2005). Behavioral and psychological symptoms of dementia characteristics of mild Alzheimer patients. *Psychiatry and Clinical Neurosciences, 59*, 274–279.

Shinnick, P. (2006). Qigong: Where did it come from? Where does it fit in science? What are the advances? *Journal of Alternative and Complementary Medicine, 12*, 351–353.

Shmueli, A., Igudin, I., & Shuval, J. (2011). Change and stability: Use of complementary and alternative medicine in Israel: 1993, 2000 and 2007. *European Journal of Public Health, 21*(2), 254–259.

Siegel, M., & Biener, L. (2000). The impact of an antismoking media campaign on progression to established smoking: Results of a longitudinal youth study. *American Journal of Public Health, 90*, 380–386.

Siegel, M., & Skeer, M. (2003). Exposure to secondhand smoke and excess lung cancer mortality risk among workers in the "5 B's": Bars, bowling alleys, billiard halls, betting establishments, and bingo parlours. *Tobacco Control, 12*, 333–338.

Siegel, R., Naishadham, D., & Jemal, A. (2012). Cancer statistics, 2012. *CA: A Cancer Journal for Clinicians, 62*, 10–29.

Siegel, R. L., Miller, K. D., & Jemal, A. (2016). Cancer statistics, 2016. *CA: A cancer Journal for Clinicians, 66*(1), 7–30.

Siegler, B. (2003, August 6–12). Actress Halle Berry battles diabetes. *Miami Times, 80*(48), 4B.

Siegler, I. C., Bastian, L. A., Steffens, D. C., Bosworth, H. B., & Costa, P. T. (2002). Behavioral medicine and aging. *Journal of Consulting and Clinical Psychology, 70*, 843–851.

Siegman, A. W. (1994). From Type A to hostility to anger: Reflections on the history of coronary-prone behavior. In A. W. Siegman & T. W. Smith (Eds.), *Anger, hostility, and the heart* (pp. 1–21). Hillsdale, NJ: Erlbaum.

Siemiatycki, J., Richardson, L., Straif, K., Latreille, B., Lakhani, R., Campbell, S., … Boffetto, P. (2004). Listing occupational carcinogens. *Environmental Health Perspectives, 112*, 1447–1459.

Sigmon, S. T., Stanton, A. L., & Snyder, C. R. (1995). Gender differences in coping: A further test of socialization and role constraint theories. *Sex Roles, 33*, 565–587.

Silberstein, S. D. (2004). Migraine pathophysiology and its clinical implications. *Cephalalgia, 24*(Suppl. 2), 2–7.

Silveira, H., Moraes, H., Oliveira, N., Coutinho, E. S. F., Laks, J., & Deslandes, A. (2013). Physical exercise and clinically depressed patients: A systematic review and meta-analysis. *Neuropsychobiology, 67*(2), 61–68.

Silverman, S. M. (2008). Lindsay Lohan opens up about recent troubles. *People.* Retrieved March 6, 2008, from http://www.people.com/people/article/0,20181019,00.html

Simoni, J. M., Frick, P. A., & Huang, B. (2006). A longitudinal evaluation of a social support model of medication adherence among HIV-positive men and women an antiretroviral therapy. *Health Psychology, 25*, 74–81.

Simoni, J. M., Pearson, C. R., Pantalone, D. W., Marks, G., & Crepaz, N. (2006). Efficacy of interventions in improving highly active antiretroviral therapy adherence and HIV-1 RNA viral load: A meta-analytic review of randomized controlled trials. *Journal of Acquired Immune Deficiency Syndromes, 43*, S23–S35.

Simonsick, E. M., Guralnik, J. M., Volpato, S., Balfour, J., & Fried, L. P. (2005). Just get out the door! Importance of walking outside the home for maintaining mobility: Findings from the Women's Health and Aging Study. *Journal of the American Geriatrics Society, 53*, 198–203.

Simpson, S. H., Eurich, D. T., Majundar, S. R., Padwal, R. S., Tsuyuki, R. T., Varney, … Johnson, J. A. (2006). A meta-analysis of the association between adherence to drug therapy and mortality. *British Medical Journal, 333*, 15–18.

Sims, E. A. H. (1974). Studies in human hyperphagia. In G. Bray & J. Bethune (Eds.), *Treatment and management of obesity.* New York: Harper and Row.

Sims, E. A. H. (1976). Experimental obesity, dietary-induced thermogenesis, and their clinical implications. *Clinics in Endocrinology and Metabolism, 5*, 377–395.

Sims, E. A. H., Danforth, E., Jr., Horton, E. S., Bray, G. A., Glennon, J. A., & Salans, L. B. (1973). Endocrine and metabolic effects of experimental obesity in man. *Recent Progress in Hormonal Research, 29*, 457–496.

Sims, E. A. H., & Horton, E. S. (1968). Endocrine and metabolic adaptation to obesity and starvation. *American Journal of Clinical Nutrition, 21*, 1455–1470.

Sin, N. L., & DiMatteo, M. R. (2014). Depression treatment enhances adherence to antiretroviral therapy: A meta-analysis. *Annals of Behavioral Medicine, 47*(3), 259–269.

Singletary, K. W., & Gapstur, S. M. (2001). Alcohol and breast cancer: Review of epidemiologic and experimental evidence and potential mechanisms. *Journal of the American Medical Association, 286*, 2143–2151.

Sinniah, D., & Khoo, E. J. (2015). E-cigarettes: Facts and legal status. *International e-Journal of Science, Medicine and Education, 9*(3), 10–19.

Sjöström, M., Oja, P., Hagströmer, M., Smith, B. J., & Bauman, A. (2006). Health-enhancing physical activity across European Union countries: The Eurobarometer study. *Journal of Public Health, 14*, 291–300.

Skinner, B. F. (1953). *Science and human behavior.* New York, NY: Macmillan.

Skinner, T. C., Hampson, S. E., & Fife-Schaw, C. (2002). Personality, personal model beliefs, and self-care in adolescents and young adults with Type 1 diabetes. *Health Psychology, 21*, 61–70.

Slomkowski, C., Rende, R., Novak, S., Lloyd-Richardson, E., & Niaura, R. (2005). Sibling effects on smoking in adolescence: Evidence for social influence from a genetically informative design. *Addiction, 100*, 430–438.

Sluik, D., Buijsse, B., Muckelbauer, R., Kaaks, R., Teucher, B., Johnsen, N. F., … Ardanaz, E. (2012). Physical activity and mortality in individuals with diabetes mellitus: A prospective study and meta-analysis. *Archives of Internal Medicine, 172*(17), 1285–1295.

Slugg, R. M., Meyer, R. A., & Campbell, J. N. (2000). Response of cutaneous A- and C-fiber nociceptors in the monkey to controlled-force stimuli. *Journal of Neurophysiology, 83*, 2179–2191.

Small, B. J., Rosnick, C. B., Fratiglioni, L., & Bäckman, L. (2004). Apoli-poprotein ε and cognitive performance: A meta-analysis. *Psychology and Aging, 19*, 592–600.

Smedslund, G., & Ringdal, G. I. (2004). Meta-analysis of the effects of psychosocial interventions on survival time in cancer patents. *Journal of Psychosomatic Research, 57*, 123–131.

Smeets, R. J., Severens, J. L., Beelen, S., Vlaeyen, J. W., & Knottnerus, J. A. (2009). More is not always better: Cost-effectiveness analysis of combined, single behavioral and single physical rehabilitation programs for chronic low back pain. *European Journal of Pain, 13*, 71–81.

Smelt, A. H. M. (2010). Triglycerides and gallstone formation. *Clinica Chimica Acta, 411*(21/22), 1625–1631.

Smetana, G. W. (2000). The diagnostic value of historical features in primary headache syndromes: A comprehensive review. *Archives of Internal Medicine, 160*, 2729–2740.

Smiles, R. V. (2002). Race matters in health care: Experts say eliminating racial and ethnic health disparities is the civil rights issue of our day. *Black Issues in Higher Education, 19*(7), 22–29.

Smith, C. A., Hay, P. P., & MacPherson, H. (2010). Acupuncture for depression. *Cochrane Database of Systematic Reviews, 2010*, Issue 1, Cochrane Art. No.: CD004046, DOI: 10.1002/14651858.CD004046.pub3.

Smith, C. F., Whitaker, K. L., Winstanley, K., & Wardle, J. (2016). Smokers are less likely than non-smokers to seek help for a lung cancer 'alarm'symptom. *Thorax.* DOI:10.1136/thoraxjnl-2015-208063.

Smith, D. A., Ness, E. M., Herbert, R., Schechter, C. B., Phillips, R. A., Diamond, J. A., … Landrigen, P. J. (2005). Abdominal diameter index: A more powerful anthropometric measure for prevalent coronary heart disease risk in adult males. *Diabetes, Obesity and Metabolism, 7*, 370–380.

Smith, D. P., & Bradshaw B. S. (2006). Rethinking the Hispanic paradox: Death rates and life expectancy for US non-Hispanic white and Hispanic populations. *American Journal of Public Health, 96*, 1686–1692.

Smith, K. M., & Sahyoun, N. R. (2005). Fish consumption: Recommendations versus advisories, can they be reconciled? *Nutrition Reviews, 63*, 39–46.

Smith, L. A., Roman, A., Dollard, M. F., Winefield, A. H., & Siegrist, J. (2005). Effort-reward imbalance at work: The effects of work stress on anger and cardiovascular disease symptoms in a community sample. *Stress and Health: Journal of the International Society for the Investigation of Stress, 21*, 113–128.

Smith, P. H., Kasza, K. A., Hyland, A., Fong, G. T., Borland, R., Brady, K., … McKee, S. A. (2015). Gender differences in medication use and cigarette smoking cessation: Results from the International

Tobacco Control Four Country Survey. *Nicotine and Tobacco Research, 17*(4), 463–472.

Smith, P. J., Blumenthal, J. A., Hoffman, B. M., Cooper, H., Strauman, T. A., Welsh-Bohmer, K., ... Sherwood, A. (2010). Aerobic exercise and neurocognitive performance: A meta-analytic review of randomized controlled trials. *Psychosomatic Medicine, 72,* 239–252.

Smith, T. W., & Ruiz, J. M. (2002). Psychosocial influences on the development and course of coronary heart disease: Current status and implications for research and practice. *Journal of Consulting and Clinical Psychology, 70,* 548–568.

Smyth, J. M., Stone, A. A., Hurewitz, A., & Kaell, A. (1999). Effects of writing about stressful experiences on symptom reduction in patients with asthma or rheumatoid arthritis: A randomized trial. *Journal of the American Medical Association, 281,* 1304–1309.

Snyder, S. H. (1977, March). Opiate receptors and internal opiates. *Scientific American, 236,* 44–56.

Sobel, B. E., & Schneider, D. J. (2005). Cardiovascular complications in diabetes mellitus. *Current Opinion in Pharmacology, 5,* 143–148.

Sobell, L. C., Cunningham, J. A., & Sobell, M. B. (1996). Recovery from alcohol problems with and without treatment: Prevalence in two population surveys. *American Journal of Public Health, 86,* 966–972.

Sola-Vera, J., Sáez, J., Laveda, R., Girona, E., García-Sepulcre, M. F., Cuesta, A., ... Sillero, M. (2008). Factors associated with non-attendance at outpatient endoscopy. *Scandinavian Journal of Gastroenterology, 43,* 202–206.

Soler, R. E., Leeks, K. D., Buchanan, L. R., Brownson, R. C., Heath, G. W., Hopkins, D. H., ... Task Force on Community Preventive Services. (2010). Point-of-decision prompts to increase stair use: A systematic review update. *American Journal of Preventive Medicine, 38,* S292–S300.

Song, F., Maskrey, V., Blyth, A., Brown, T. J., Barton, G. R., Aveyard, P., ... Brandon, T. (2016). Differences in longer-term smoking abstinence after treatment by specialist of nonspecialist advisors: Second analysis of data from a relapse prevention trial. *Nicotine and Tobacco Research, 18*(5), 1061–1065.

Song, M.-Y., John, M., & Dobs, A. S. (2007). Clinicians' attitudes and usage of complementary and alternative integrative medicine: A survey at the Johns Hopkins Medical Institute. *Journal of Alternative and Complementary Medicine, 13,* 305–306.

Song, Z., Foo, M.-D., Uy, M. A., & Sun, S. (2011). Unraveling the daily stress crossover between unemployed individuals and their employed spouses. *Journal of Applied Psychology, 96,* 151–168.

Sont, W. N., Zielinski, J. M., Ashmore, J. P., Jiang, H., Krewski, D., Fair, M. E., ... Létourneau, E. G. (2001). First analysis of cancer incidence and occupational radiation exposure based on the National Dose Registry of Canada. *American Journal of Epidemiology, 153,* 309–318.

Soole, D. W., Mazerolle, L., & Rombouts, S. (2008). School-based drug prevention programs: A review of what works. *Australian and New Zealand Journal of Criminology, 41*(2), 259–286.

Sours, J. A. (1980). *Starving to death in a sea of objects: The anorexia nervosa syndrome.* New York, NY: Aronson.

Speck, R. M., Courneya, K. S., Masse, L. C., Duval, S., & Schmitz, K. H. (2010). An update of controlled physical activity trials in cancer survivors: A systematic review and meta-analysis. *Journal of Cancer Survivorship, 4,* 87–100.

Spiegel, D. (2004). Commentary on "Meta-analysis of the effects of psychosocial interventions on survival time and mortality in cancer patients" by Geir Smedslund and Gerd Inter Ringdal. *Journal of Psychosomatic Research, 57,* 133–135.

Spiegel, D., Bloom, J. R., Kraemer, H. C., & Gottheil, E. (1989). Effect of psychosocial treatment on survival of patients with metastatic breast cancer. *Lancet, ii,* 888–891.

Spiegel, D., & Giese-Davis, J. (2003). Depression and cancer: Mechanisms and disease progression. *Biological Psychiatry, 54,* 269–282.

Spierings, E. L. H., Ranke, A. H., & Honkoop, P. C. (2001). Precipitating and aggravating factors of migraine versus tension-type headache. *Headache, 41,* 554–558.

Spitzer, B. L., Henderson, K. A., & Zivian, M. T. (1999). Gender differences in population versus media body size: A comparison over four decades. *Sex Roles, 40,* 545–566.

Springer, J. F., Sale, E., Kasim, R., Winter, W., Sambrano, S., & Chipungu, S. (2004). Effectiveness of culturally specific approaches to substance abuse prevention: Findings for CSAP's national cross-site evaluation of high risk youth programs. *Journal of Ethnic and Cultural Diversity in Social Work, 13,* 1–23.

Spruijt-Metz, D. (2011). Etiology, treatment, and prevention of obesity in childhood and adolescence: A decade in review. *Journal of Research on Adolescence, 21*(1), 129–152.

Sri Vengadesh, G., Sistla, S. C., & Smile, S. R. (2005). Postoperative pain relief following abdominal operations: A prospective randomised study of comparison of patient controlled analgesia with conventional parental opioids. *Indian Journal of Surgery, 67,* 34–37.

Stacey, P. S., & Sullivan, K. A. (2004). Preliminary investigation of thiamine and alcohol intake in clinical and healthy samples. *Psychological Reports, 94,* 845–848.

Staessen, J. A., Wang, J., Bianchi, G., & Birkenhager, W. H. (2003). Essential hypertension. *Lancet, 361,* 1629–1641.

Stallworth, J., & Lennon, J. L. (2003). An interview with Dr. Lester Breslow. *American Journal of Public Health, 93,* 1803–1805.

Stamler, J., Elliott, P., Dennis, B., Dyer, A. R., Kesteloot, H., Liu, K., ... INTERMAP Research Group. (2003). INTERMAP: Background, aims, design, methods, and descriptive statistics (nondietary). *Journal of Human Hypertension, 17,* 591–608.

Stamler, J., Stamler, R., Neaton, J. D., Wentworth, D., Daviglus, M. L., Garside, D., ... Greenland, P. (1999). Low risk-factor profile and long-term cardiovascular and noncardiovascular mortality and life expectancy: Findings for 5 large cohorts of young adult and middle-aged men and women. *Journal of the American Medical Association, 282,* 2012–2018.

Stampfer, M. J., Hu, F. B., Manson, J. E., Rimm, E. B., & Willett, W. C. (2000). Primary prevention of coronary heart disease in women through diet and lifestyle. *New England Journal of Medicine, 343,* 16–22.

Standridge, J. B., Zylstra, R. G., & Adams, S. M. (2004). Alcohol consumption: An overview of benefits and risks. *Southern Medical Journal, 97,* 664–672.

Stanner, S. A., Hughes, J., Kelly, C. N. M., & Buttriss, J. (2004). A review of the epidemiological evidence for the "antioxidant hypothesis." *Public Health Nutrition, 7,* 407–422.

Stanton, A. L., Revenson, T. A., & Tennen, H. (2007). Health psychology: Psychological adjustment to chronic disease. *Annual Review of Psychology, 58,* 565–592.

Starkstein, S. E., Jorge, R., Mizrahi, R., Adrian, J., & Robinson, R. G. (2007). Insight and danger in Alzheimer's disease. *European Journal of Neurology, 14,* 455–460.

Stason, W., Neff, R., Miettinen, O., & Jick, H. (1976). Alcohol consumption and nonfatal myocardial infarction. *American Journal of Epidemiology, 104,* 603–608.

Staton, L. J., Panda, M., Chen, I., Genao, I., Kurz, J., Pasanen, M., ... Cykert, S. (2007). When race matters: Disagreement in pain perception between patients and their physicians in primary care. *Journal of the National Medical Association, 99,* 532–537.

Stayner, L., Bena, J., Sasco, A. J., Smith, R., Steenland, K., Kreuzer, M., ... Straif, K. (2007). Lung cancer risk and workplace exposure to environmental tobacco smoke. *American Journal of Public Health, 97*(3), 545–551.

Stead, L. F., Bergson, G., & Lancaster, T. (2008). Physician advice for smoking cessation. *Cochrane Database of Systematic Reviews,* Cochrane Art. No.: CD000165, DOI: 10.1002/14651858.CD000165.pub2.

Stead, L. F., Perera, R., Bullen, C., Mant, D., & Lancaster, T. (2008). Nicotine replacement therapy for smoking cessation. *Cochrane Database of Systematic Reviews,* Cochrane Art. No.: CD000146, DOI: 10.1002/14651858.CD000146.pub3.

Steele, C. M., & Josephs, R. A. (1990). Alcohol myopia: Its prized and dangerous effects. *American Psychologist, 45,* 921–933.

Steffen, K. J., Mitchell, J. E., Roerig, J. L., & Lancaster, K. L. (2007). The eating disorders medicine cabinet revisited: A clinician's guide to ipecac and laxatives. *International Journal of Eating Disorders, 40,* 360–368.

Steifel, M. C., Perla, R. J., & Zell, B. L. (2010). A health bottom line: Healthy life expectancy as an outcome measure for health improvement efforts. *The Milbank Quarterly, 88*, 30–53.

Stein, M. B., Schork, N. J., & Gelernter, J. (2008). Gene-by-environment (serotonin transporter and childhood maltreatment) interaction for anxiety sensitivity, an intermediate phenotype for anxiety disorders. *Neuropsychopharmacology, 33*, 312–319.

Steinbrook, R. (2004). The AIDS epidemic in 2004. *New England Journal of Medicine, 351*, 115–117.

Steinhausen, H. C., & Weber, S. (2010). The outcome of bulimia nervosa: Findings from one-quarter century of research. *American Journal of Psychiatry, 166*(12), 1331–1341.

Stelfox, H. T., Gandhi, T. K., Orav, E. J., & Gustafson, M. L. (2005). The relation of patient satisfaction with complaints against physicians and malpractice lawsuits. *The American Journal of Medicine, 118*, 1126–1133.

Stephens, J., & Allen, J. (2013). Mobile phone interventions to increase physical activity and reduce weight: A systematic review. *The Journal of Cardiovascular Nursing, 28*(4), 320.

Steptoe, A., Hamer, M., & Chida, Y. (2007). The effects of acute psychological stress on circulating inflammatory factors in humans: A review and meta-analysis. *Brain, Behavior and Immunity, 21*, 901–912.

Steptoe, A., Wardle, J., Bages, N., Sallis, J. F., Sanabria-Ferrand, P.-A., & Sanchez, M. (2004). Drinking and driving in university students: An international study of 23 countries. *Psychology and Health, 19*, 527–540.

Stetter, F., & Kupper, S. (2002). Autogenic training: A meta-analysis of clinical outcome studies. *Applied Psychophysiology and Biofeedback, 27*, 45–98.

Stevenson, R. J., Hodgson, D., Oaten, M. J., Barouei, J., & Case, T. I. (2011). The effect of disgust on oral immune function. *Psychophysiology, 48*, 900–907.

Stewart, J. C., Janicki, D. L., & Kamarck, T. W. (2006). Cardiovascular reactivity to and recovery from psychological challenge as predictors of 3-year change in blood pressure. *Health Psychology, 25*, 111–118.

Stewart, K. L. (2004). Pharmacological and behavioral treatments for migraine headaches: A meta-analytic review. *Dissertation Abstracts International: Section B, 65*(3-B), 1535.

Stewart, L. K., Flynn, M. G., Campbell, W. W., Craig, B. A., Robinson, J. P., Timmerman, K. L., ... Talbert, E. (2007). The influence of exercise training on inflammatory cytokines and C-reactive protein. *Medicine and Science in Sports and Exercise, 39*, 1714–1719.

Stewart, S. T., Cutler, D. M., & Rosen, A. B. (2009). Forecasting the effects of obesity and smoking on U.S. life expectancy. *The New England Journal of Medicine, 361*, 2252–2260.

Stewart-Knox, B. J., Sittlington, J., Rugkåsa, J., Harrisson, S., Treacy, M., & Abaunza, P. S. (2005). Smoking and peer groups: Results from a longitudinal qualitative study of young people in Northern Ireland. *British Journal of Social Psychology, 44*, 397–414.

Stewart-Williams, S. (2004). The placebo puzzle: Putting together the pieces. *Health Psychology, 23*, 198–206.

Stice, E., Marti, C. N., & Rohde, P. (2013). Prevalence, incidence, impairment, and course of the proposed DSM-5 eating disorder diagnoses in an 8-year prospective community study of young women. *Journal of Abnormal Psychology, 122* (2), 445–457.

Stice, E., Marti, C. N., Rohde, P., & Shaw, H. (2015). Young woman smokers gain significantly more weight over 2-year follow-up than non-smokers. How Virginia doesn't slim. *Appetite, 85*, 155–159.

Stice, E., Presnell, K., Groesz, L., & Shaw, H. (2005). Effects of a weight maintenance diet on bulimic symptoms in adolescent girls: An experimental test of the dietary restraint theory. *Health Psychology, 24*, 402–412.

Stice, E., Presnell, K., & Spangler, D. (2002). Risk factors for binge eating onset in adolescent girls: A 2-year prospective investigation. *Health Psychology, 21*, 131–138.

Stice, E. Rohde, P., & Shaw, H. (2013). *The Body Project: A dissonance-based eating disorder prevention intervention, updated edition—programs that work.* New York, NY: Oxford University Press.

Stice, E., Trost, A., & Chase, A. (2003). Healthy weight control and dissonance-based eating disorder prevention programs: Results from a controlled trial. *International Journal of Eating Disorders, 33*, 10–21.

Stickney, S. R., Black, D. R. (2008). Physical self-perception, body dysmorphic disorder, and smoking behavior. *American Journal of Health Behavior, 32*, 295–304.

Stojanovich, L., & Marisavljevich, D. (2008). Stress as a trigger of autoimmune disease. *Autoimmunity Review, 7*, 209–213.

Stokols, D. (1972). On the distinction between density and crowding: Some implications for future research. *Psychological Review, 79*, 275–277.

Stone, A. A., Krueger, A. B., Steptoe, A., & Harter, J. K. (2010). The socioeconomic gradient in daily colds and influenza, headaches, and pain. *Archives of Internal Medicine, 170*, 570–572.

Stone, A. A., Reed, B. R., & Neale, J. M. (1987). Changes in daily event frequency precedes episodes of physical symptoms. *Journal of Human Stress, 13*, 70–74.

Stone, G. C. (1987). The scope of health psychology. In G. C. Stone, S. M. Weiss, J. D. Matarazzo, N. E. Miller, J. Rodin, C. D. Belar, ... J. E. Singer (Eds.), *Health psychology: A discipline and a profession* (pp. 27–40). Chicago, IL: University of Chicago Press.

Storr, C. L., Lalongo, N. S., Anthony, J. C., & Breslau, N. (2007). Childhood antecedents of exposure to traumatic events and posttraumatic stress disorder. *American Journal of Psychiatry, 164*, 119–125.

Strachan, E., Saracino, M., Selke, S., Magaret, A., Buchwald, D., & Wald, A. (2011). The effects of daily distress and personality on genital HSV shedding and lesions in a randomized, double-blind, placebo-controlled, crossover trial of acyclovir in HSV-2 seropositive women. *Brain, Behavior, and Immunity, 25*, 1475–1481.

Strasser, A. A., Lerman, C., Sanborn, P. M., Pickworth, W. B., & Feldman, E. A. (2007). New lower nicotine cigarettes can produce compensatory smoking and increased carbon monoxide exposure. *Drug and Alcohol Dependence, 86*, 294–300.

Straus, M. A. (2008). Dominance and symmetry in partner violence by male and female university students in 32 nations. *Children and Youth Services Review, 30*, 252–275.

Strazdins, L., & Broom, D. H. (2007). The mental health costs and benefits of giving social support. *International Journal of Stress Management, 14*, 370–385.

Streltzer, J. (1997). Pain. In W.-S. Tseng & J. Streltzer (Eds.), *Culture and psychopathology: A guide to clinical assessment* (pp. 87–100). New York, NY: Brunner/Mazel.

Streppel, M. T., Boshuizen, H. C., Ocké, M. C., Kok, F. J., & Kromhout, D. (2007). Mortality and life expectancy in relation to long-term cigarette, cigar and pipe smoking: The Zutphen study. *Tobacco Control, 16*, 107–113.

Striegel, R. H., Bedrosian, R., Wang, C., & Schwartz, S. (2012). Why men should be included in research on binge eating: Results from a comparison of psychosocial impairment in men and women. *International Journal of Eating Disorders, 45*(2), 233–240.

Striegel-Moore, R. H., DeBar, L., Perrin, N., Lynch, F., Kraemer, H. C., Wilson, G. T., ... Kraemer, H. C. (2010). Cognitive behavioral guided self-help for the treatment of recurrent binge eating. *Journal of Consulting and Clinical Psychology, 78*, 312–321.

Striegel-Moore, R. H., Franko, D. L., Thompson, D., Barton, B., Schreiber, G. B., & Daniels, S. R. (2004). Changes in weight and body image over time in women with eating disorders. *International Journal of Eating Disorders, 36*, 315–327.

Strine, T. W., Mokdad, A. H., Balluz, L. S., Berry, J. T., & Gonzalez, O. (2008). Impact of depression and anxiety on quality of life, health behaviors, and asthma control among adults in the United States with asthma, 2006. *Journal of Asthma, 45*, 123–133.

Stroebe, W., Papies, E. K., & Aarts, H. (2008). From homeostatic to hedonic theories of eating: Self-regulatory failure in food-rich environments. *Applied Psychology: An International Review, 57*, 172–193.

Strong, C. A. (1895). The psychology of pain. *Psychological Review, 2*, 329–347.

Strong, D. R., Cameron, A., Feuer, S., Cohn, A., Abrantes, A. M., & Brown, R. A. (2010). Single versus recurrent depression history:

Differentiating risk factors among current US smokers. *Drug and Alcohol Dependence, 109*(1–3), 90–95.

Stotts, J., Lohse, B., Patterson, J., Horacek, T., White, A., & Greene, G. (2007). Eating competence in college students nominates a non-dieting approach to weight management. *FASEB Journal, 21*, A301.

Stroebe, W. (2008). *Dieting, overweight, and obesity: Self-regulation in a food-rich environment.* Washington, DC: American Psychological Association.

Stroud, C. B., Davila, J., Hammen, C., & Vrshek-Schallhorn, S. (2011). Severe and nonsevere events in first onsets versus recurrences of depression: Evidence for stress sensitization. *Journal of Abnormal Psychology, 120*, 142–154.

Stroud, C. B., Davila, J., & Moyer, A. (2008). The relationship between stress and depression in first onsets versus recurrences: A meta-analytic review. *Journal of Abnormal Psychology, 117*, 206–213.

Stuart, R. B. (1967). Behavioral control of overeating. *Behavior Research and Therapy, 5*, 357–365.

Stults-Kolehmainen, M. A., & Sinha, R. (2014). The effects of stress on physical activity and exercise. *Sports Medicine, 44*(1), 81–121.

Stunkard, A. J., & Allison, K. C. (2003). Binge eating disorder: Disorder or marker? *International Journal of Eating disorders, 34*(Suppl. 1), S107–S116.

Stunkard, A. J., Harris, J. R., Pedersen, N. L., & McClean, G. E. (1990). The body-mass index of twins who have been reared apart. *New England Journal of Medicine, 322*, 1483–1487.

Stunkard, A. J., Sørensen, T. I. A., Hanis, C., Teasdale, T. W., Chakraborty, R., Schull, W. J., … Schulsinger, F. (1986). An adoption study of human obesity. *New England Journal of Medicine, 314*, 193, 198.

Stürmer, T., Hasselbach, P., & Amelang, M. (2006). Personality, lifestyle, and risk of cardiovascular disease and cancer: Follow-up of population based cohort. *British Medical Journal, 332*, 1359.

Su, D., Li, L., & Pagán, J. A. (2008). Acculturation and the use of complementary and alternative medicine. *Social Science and Medicine, 66*, 439–453.

Suarez, E. C., Saab, P. G., Llabre, M. M., Kuhn, C. M., & Zimmerman, E. (2004). Ethnicity, gender, and age effects on adrenoceptors and physiological responses to emotional stress. *Psychophysiology, 41*, 450–460.

Substance Abuse and Mental Health Services Administration (SAMHSA). (2010). *Results from the 2009 National Survey on Drug Use and Health: Vol. 1. Summary of national findings* (Office of Applied Studies NSDUH Series H-38A, DHHS Publication No. SMA 10-4586 Findings). Rockville, MD: National Clearinghouse for Alcohol and Drug Information.

Substance Abuse and Mental Health Services Administration (SAMHSA). (2013, September 9). 18 Percent of pregnant women drink alcohol during early pregnancy. *NSDUH Report: Data Spotlight.* Retrieved from www.samhsa.gov/data/spotlight/spot123-pregnancy-alcohol-2013.pdf

Substance Abuse and Mental Health Services Administration (SAMHSA). (2014). *Results from the 2013 National Survey on Drug Use and Health: Summary of National Findings,* NSDUH Series H-48, HHS Publication No. (SMA) 14-4863. Rockville, MD: Author. Retrieved July 8, 2016, from http://www.samhsa.gov/data/sites/default/files/NSDUHresultsPDFWHTML2013/Web/NSDUHresults2013.pdf

Substance Abuse and Mental Health Services Administration (SAMHSA). (2015). *Behavioral health trends in the United States: Results from the 2014 National Survey on Drug Use and Health* (HHS Publication No. SMA 15-4927, NSDUH Series H-50). Retrieved July 3, 2016, from http://www.samhsa.gov/data/ http://www.samhsa.gov/data/sites/default/files/NSDUH-DetTabs2014/NSDUH-DetTabs2014.pdf, p. 660 Table 2.41A.

Sufka, K. J., & Price, D. D. (2002). Gate control theory reconsidered. *Brain and Mind, 3*, 277–290.

Suls, J., & Bunde, J. (2005). Anger, anxiety, and depression as risk factors for cardiovascular disease: The problems and implications of overlapping affective dispositions. *Psychological Bulletin, 131*, 260–300.

Suls, J., Martin, R., & Leventhal, H. (1997). Social comparison, lay referral, and the decision to seek medical care. In B. P. Buunk & F. X. Gibbons (Eds.), *Health, coping and well-being: Perspectives from social comparison theory* (pp. 195–226). Mahwah, NJ: Lawrence Erlbaum Associates.

Suls, J., & Rothman, A. (2004). Evolution of the biopsychosocial model: Prospects and challenges for health psychology. *Health Psychology, 23*, 119–125.

Sundblad, G. M. B., Saartok, T., & Engström, L.-M. T. (2007). Prevalence and co-occurrence of self-rated pain and perceived health in schoolchildren: Age and gender differences. *European Journal of Pain, 11*, 171–180.

Surwit, R. S., Van Tilburg, M. A. L., Zucker, N., McCaskill, C. C., Parekh, P., Feinglos, M. N., Lane, J. D. (2002). Stress management improves long-term glycemic control in Type 2 diabetes. *Diabetes Care, 25*, 30–34.

Susser, M. (1991). What is a cause and how do we know one? A grammar for pragmatic epidemiology. *American Journal of Epidemiology, 133*, 635–648.

Sutton, S., McVey, D., & Glanz, A. (1999). A comparative test of the theory of reasoned action and the theory of planned behavior in the prediction of condom use intentions in a national sample of English young people. *Health Psychology, 18*, 72–81.

Svansdottir, H. B., & Snaedal, J. (2006). Music therapy in moderate and severe dementia of Alzheimer's type: A case-control study. *International Psychogeriatrics, 18*, 613–621.

Svendsen, R. P., Jarbol, D. E., Larsen, P. V., Støvring, H., Hansen, B. L., & Soendergaard, J. (2013). Associations between health care seeking and socioeconomic and demographic determinants among people reporting alarm symptoms of cancer: A population-based cross-sectional study. *Family Practice, 30*(6), 655–665.

Svetkey, L. P., Stevens, V. J., Brantley, P. J., Appel, L. J., Hollis, J. F., Loria, C. M., … Weight Loss Maintenance Collaborative Research Group. (2008). Comparison of strategies for sustaining weight loss. *Journal of the American Medical Association, 299*, 1139–1148.

Swaim, R. C., Perrine, N. E., & Aloise-Young, P. A. (2007). Gender differences in a comparison of two tested etiological models of cigarette smoking among elementary school students. *Journal of Applied Social Psychology, 37*, 1681–1696.

Sweeney, C. T., Fant, R. V., Fagerstrom, K. O., McGovern, F., & Henningfield, J. E. (2001). Combination nicotine replacement therapy for smoking cessation rationale, efficacy and tolerability. *CNS Drugs, 15*, 453–467.

Swinburn, B. A., Sacks, G., Hall, K. D., McPherson, K., Finegood, D. T., Moodie, M. L., … Gortmaker, S. L. (2011). The global obesity pandemic: Shaped by global drivers and local environments. *The Lancet, 378*, 804–814.

Swithers, S. E., Martin, A. A., Clark, K. M., Laboy, A. F., & Davidson, T. L. (2010). Body weight gain in rats consuming sweetened liquids. Effects of caffeine and diet composition. *Appetite, 55*(3), 528–533.

Sypeck, M. F., Gray, J. J., Etu, S. F., Ahrens, A. H., Mosimann, J. E., & Wiseman, C. V. (2006). Cultural representations of thinness in women, redux: Playboy magazine's depiction of beauty from 1979 to 1999. *Body Image, 3*, 229–235.

Szapary, P. O., Bloedon, L. T., & Foster, B. D. (2003). Physical activity and its effects on lipids. *Current Cardiology Reports, 5*, 488–492.

Szekely, C. A., Breitner, J. C., Fitzpatrick, A. L., Rea, T. D., Psaty, B. M., Kuller, L. H., … Zandi, P. P. (2008). NSAID use and dementia risk in the Cardiovascular Health Study: Role of APOE and NSAID type. *Neurology, 70*, 17–24.

Tacker, D. H., & Okorodudu, A. O. (2004). Evidence for injurious effect of cocaethylene in human microvascular endothelial cells. *Clinica Chimica Acta, 345*, 69–76.

Takahashi, Y., Edmonds, G. W., Jackson, J. J., & Roberts, B. W. (2013). Longitudinal correlated changes in conscientiousness, preventative health-related behaviors, and self-perceived physical health. *Journal of Personality, 81*(4), 417–427.

Takkouche, B., Regueira, C., & Gestal-Otero, J. J. (2001). A cohort study of stress and the common cold. *Epidemiology, 12*, 345–349.

Talbot, M. (2000, January 9). The placebo prescription. *New York Times Magazine,* 34–39, 44, 58–60.

Tamres, L. K., Janicki, D., & Helgeson, V. S. (2002). Sex differences in coping behavior: A meta-analytic review and an examination of relative coping. *Personality and Social Psychology Review, 6*, 2–30.

Tan, J. O. A., Stewart, A., Fitzpatrick, R., & Hope, T. (2010). Attitudes of patients with anorexia nervosa to compulsory treatment and coercion. *International Journal of Law and Psychiatry, 33*(1), 13–19.

Tang, B. M. P., Eslick, G. D., Nowson, C., Smith, C., & Bensoussan, A. (2007). Use of calcium or calcium in combination with vitamin D supplementation to prevent fractures and bone loss in people aged 50 years and older: A meta-analysis. *Lancet, 370,* 657–666.

Tanofsky-Kraff, M., Marcus, M. D., Yanovski, S. Z., & Yanovski, J. A. (2008). Loss of control eating disorder in children age 12 years and younger: Proposed research criteria. *Eating Behaviors, 9,* 360–365.

Tanofsky-Kraff, M., & Wilfley, D. E. (2010). Interpersonal psychotherapy for the treatment of eating disorders. In W. S. Agras (Ed.), *The Oxford handbook of eating disorders* (pp. 348–372). New York, NY: Oxford University Press.

Tardon, A., Lee, W. J., Delgaldo-Rodriques, M., Dosemeci, M., Albanes, D., Hoover, R., … Blair, A. (2005). Leisure-time physical activity and lung cancer: A meta-analysis. *Cancer Causes and Control, 16,* 389–397.

Tashman, L. S., Tenenbaum, G., & Eklund, R. (2010). The effect of perceived stress on the relationship between perfectionism and burnout in coaches. *Anxiety, Stress and Coping, 23,* 195–212.

Taylor, D. H., Jr., Hasselblad, V., Henley, S. J., Thun, M. J., & Sloan, F. A. (2002). Benefits of smoking cessation for longevity. *American Journal of Public Health, 92,* 990–996.

Taylor, E. N., Stampfer, M. J., & Curhan, G. C. (2005). Obesity, weight gain, and the risk of kidney stones. *Journal of the American Medical Association, 293,* 455–462.

Taylor, R., Najafi, F., & Dobson, A. (2007). Meta-analysis of studies of passive smoking and lung cancer: Effects of study type and continent. *International Journal of Epidemiology, 36*(5), 1048.

Taylor, S. E. (2002). *The tending instinct: How nurturing is essential to who we are and how we live.* New York, NY: Times Books, Henry Holt and Company.

Taylor, S. E. (2006). Tend and befriend: Biobehavioral bases of affiliation under stress. *Current Directions in Psychological Science, 15,* 273–277.

Taylor, S. E., Gonzaga, G., Klein, L. C., Hu, P., Greendale, G. A., & Seeman, T. E. (2006). Relation of oxytocin to psychological and biological stress responses in women. *Psychosomatic Medicine, 68,* 238–245.

Taylor, S. E., Klein, L. C., Lewis, B. P., Gruenewald, T. L., Gurung, R. A. R., & Updegraff, J. A. (2000). Biobehavioral responses to stress in females: Tend-and-befriend, not fight-or-flight. *Psychological Review, 107,* 411–429.

Taylor, S. E., Saphire-Bernstein, S., & Seeman, T. E. (2010). Are plasma oxytocin in women and plasma vasopressin in men biomarkers of distressed pair-bond relationships? *Psychological Science, 21,* 3–7.

Taylor, G. H., Wilson, S. L., & Sharp, J. (2011). Medical, psychological, and sociodemographic factors associated with adherence to cardiac rehabilitation programs: A systematic review. *Journal of Cardiovascular Nursing, 26,* 202–209.

Taylor-Piliae, R. E., Haskell, W. L., Waters, C. M., & Froelicher, E. S. (2006). Change in perceived psychosocial status following a 12-week Tai Chi exercise programme. *Journal of Advanced Nursing, 54,* 313–329.

Tedeschi, R. G., & Calhoun, L. G. (2006). Time of change? The spiritual challenges of bereavement and loss. *Omega: Journal of Death and Dying, 53,* 105–116.

Tedeschi, R. G., & Calhoun, L. G. (2008). Beyond the concept of recovery: Growth and the experience of loss. *Death Studies, 32,* 27–39.

Templeton, D. (2008, April 15). Bill Clinton's heart troubles hard to detect, experts say. *Pittsburg Post-Gazette.* Retrieved June 1, 2008, from http://www.post-gazette.com/pg/08106/873418-114.stm

Teo, K. K., Ounpuu, S., Hawken, S., Pandey, M. R., Valentin, V., Hunt, D., … INTERHEART Study Investigators. (2006). Tobacco use and risk of myocardial infarction in 52 countries in the INTERHEART study: A case-control study. *The Lancet, 368,* 19–25.

Terry, A., Szabo, A., & Griffiths, M. D. (2004). The Exercise Addiction Inventory: A new brief screening tool. *Addiction Research and Theory, 12,* 489–499.

Testa, M., Vazile-Tamsen, C., & Livingston, J. A. (2004). The role of victim and perpetrator intoxication on sexual assault outcomes. *Journal of Studies on Alcohol, 65,* 320–329.

Theberge, N. (2008). The integration of chiropractors into healthcare teams: A case study from sport medicine. *Sociology of Health and Illness, 30,* 19–34.

Theis, K. A., Helmick, C. G., & Hootman, J. M. (2007). Arthritis burden and impact are greater among U.S. women than men: Intervention opportunities. *Journal of Women's Health, 16,* 441–453.

Thielke, S., Thompson, A., & Stuart, R. (2011). Health psychology in primary care: Recent research and future directions. *Psychological Research and Behavior Management, 4,* 59–68.

Thomas, J. J., Keel, P. K., & Heatherton, T. E. (2005). Disordered eating attitudes and behaviors in ballet students: Examination of environmental and individual risk factors. *International Journal of Eating Disorders, 38,* 263–268.

Thomas, W., White, C. M., Mah, J., Geisser, M. S., Church, T. R., & Mandel, J. S. (1995). Longitudinal compliance with annual screening for fecal occult blood. *American Journal of Epidemiology, 142,* 176–182.

Thombs, D. L., O"Mara, R. J., Hou, W., Wagenaar, A. C., Dong, H.-J., Merves, M. L., … Clapp, J. D. (2011). 5-HTTLPR genotype and associations with intoxication and intention to drive: Results from a field study of bar patrons. *Addiction Biology, 16*(1), 133–141.

Thompson, O. M., Yaroch, A. L., Moser, R. P., Finney Rutten, L. J., Petrelli, J. M., Smith-Warner, S. A., … Nebeling, L. (2011). Knowledge of and adherence to fruit and vegetable recommendations and intakes: Results of the 2003 Health Information National Trends Survey. *Journal of Health Communication: International Perspectives, 16,* 328–340.

Thompson, P. D. (2001, January). Exercise rehabilitation for cardiac patients: A beneficial but underused therapy. *The Physician and Sportsmedicine, 29,* 69–75.

Thompson, P. D., Franklin, B. A., Balady, G. J., Blair, S. N., Corrado, D., Domenico, E., III, … American College of Sports Medicine. (2007). Exercise and acute cardiovascular events: Placing the risks into perspective. *Medicine and Science in Sports and Exercise, 39,* 886–897.

Thompson, S. H., & Hammond, K. (2003). Beauty is as beauty does: Body image and self-esteem of pageant contestants. *Eating and Weight Disorders, 8,* 231–237.

Thorn, B. E., & Kuhajda, M. C. (2006). Group cognitive therapy for chronic pain. *Journal of Clinical Psychology, 62,* 1355–1366.

Thorn, B. E., Pence, L. B., Ward, L. C., Kilgo, G., Clements, K. L., Cross, T. H., … Tsui, P. W. (2007). A randomized clinical trial of targeted cognitive behavioral treatment to reduce catastrophizing in chronic headache sufferers. *Journal of Pain, 8,* 938–949.

Thun, M. J., Day-Lally, C. A., Calle, E. E., Flanders, W. D., & Heath, C. W., Jr. (1995). Excess mortality among cigarette smokers: Changes in a 20-year interval. *American Journal of Public Health, 85,* 1223–1230.

Thune, I., Brenn, T., Lund, E., & Gaard, M. (1997). Physical activity and the risk of breast cancer. *New England Journal of Medicine, 336,* 1269–1275.

Thune, I., & Furberg, A. S. (2001). Physical activity and cancer risk: Dose-response and cancer, all sites and site-specific. *Medicine and Science in Sports and Exercise, 33,* S530–S550.

Thuné-Boyle, I. C. V., Myers, L. B., & Newman, S. P. (2006). The role of illness beliefs, treatment beliefs, and perceived severity of symptoms in explaining distress in cancer patients during chemotherapy treatment. *Behavioral Medicine, 32,* 19–29.

Thygesen, L. C., Johansen, C., Keiding, N., Giovannucci, E., & Grønbæk, M. (2008). Effects of sample attrition in a longitudinal study of the association between alcohol intake and all-cause mortality. *Addiction, 103,* 1149–1159.

Tice, D. M., Bratslavsky, E., & Baumeister, R. F. (2001). Emotional distress regulation takes precedence over impulse control: If you feel bad, do it! *Journal of Personality and Social Psychology, 80,* 53–67.

Tilburt, J. C., Emanuel, E. J., Kaptchuk, T. J., Curlin, F. A., & Miller, F. G. (2008). Prescribing "placebo treatments": Results of national survey of US internists and rheumatologists. *British Medical Journal, 337,* a1938.

Tindle, H. A., Chang, Y. F., Kuller, L. H., Manson, J. E., Robinson, J. G., Rosal, M. C., … Matthews, K. A. (2009). Optimism, cynical hostility, and incident coronary heart disease and mortality in the Women's Health Initiative. *Circulation*, *120*(8), 656–662.

To, T., Stanojevic, S., Moores, G., Gershon, A. S., Bateman, E. D., Cruz, A. A., … Boulet, L. P. (2012). Global asthma prevalence in adults: Findings from the cross-sectional world health survey. *BMC Public Health*, *12*(1), 204.

Tobar, D. A. (2005). Overtraining and staleness: The importance of psychological monitoring. *International Journal of Sport and Exercise Psychology*, *3*, 455–468.

Todd, J. E., & Variyam, J. N. (2008). *The decline in consumer use of food nutrition labels, 1995–2006*. Washigton, DC: U.S. Department of Agriculture.

Tolfrey, K. (2004). Lipid-lipoproteins in children: An exercise dose-response study. *Medicine and Science in Sports and Exercise*, *36*, 418–427.

Tolfrey, K., Jones, A. M., & Campbell, I. G. (2000). The effect of aerobic exercise training on the lipid-lipoprotein profile of children and adolescents. *Sports Medicine*, *29*, 99–112.

Tolstrup, J. S., Nordestgaard, B. G., Rasmussen, S., Tybjærg-Hansen, A., & Grønbæk, M. (2008). Alcoholism and alcohol drinking habits predicted from alcohol dehydrogenase genes. *Pharmacogenomics Journal*, *8*, 220–227.

Tomar, S. L., & Hatsukami, D. K. (2007). Perceived risk of harm from cigarettes or smokesless tobacco among U.S. high school seniors. *Nicotine and Tobacco Research*, *9*, 1191–1196.

Tomfohr, L. M., Martin, T. M., & Miller, G. E. (2008). Symptoms of depression and impaired endothelial function in healthy adolescent women. *Journal of Behavioral Medicine*, *31*, 137–143.

Toneatto, T. (2013). Natural recovery. In P. M. Miller, S. A. Ball, M. E. Bates, A. W. Blume, K. M. Kampman, M. E. Larimer, … S. A. Ball (Eds.), *Comprehensive addictive behaviors and disorders, Vol. 1: Principles of addiction* (pp. 133-139). San Diego, CA: Elsevier Academic Press.

Torchalla, I., Okoli, C. T. C., Hemsing, N., & Greaves, L. (2011). Gender differences in smoking behaviour and cessation. *Journal of Smoking Cessation*, *6*(1), 9–16.

Torian, L., Chen, M., Rhodes, P., & Hall, H. R. (2011). HIV surveillance—United States, 1981–2008. *Morbidity and Mortality Weekly Report*, *60*(21), 689–693.

Torpy, J. M. (2006). Eating fish: Health benefits and risks. *Journal of the American Medical Association*, *296*, 1926.

Torstveit, M. K., Rosenvinge, J. H., & Sundgot-Borgen, J. (2008). Prevalence of eating disorders and the predictive power of risk models in female elite athletes: A controlled study. *Scandinavian Journal of Medicine and Science in Sports*, *18*, 108–118.

Tortorella, A., Fabrazzo, M., Monteleone, A. M., Steardo, L., & Monteleone, P. (2014). The role of drug therapies in the treatment of anorexia and bulimia nervosa: A review of the literature. *Journal of Psychopathology*, *20*(1), 50–65.

Tousignant-Laflamme, Y., Rainville, P., & Marchand, S. (2005). Establishing a link between heart rate and pain in healthy subjects: A gender effect. *Journal of Pain*, *6*, 341–347.

Tovian, S. M. (2004). Health services and health care economics: The health psychology marketplace. *Health Psychology*, *23*, 138–141.

Travis, L. (2001). Training for interdisciplinary healthcare. *Health Psychologist*, *23*(1), 4–5.

Treiber, F. A., Davis, H., Musante, L., Raunikar, R. A., Strong. W. G., McCaffrey, F., … Vandermoot, R. (1993). Ethnicity, gender, family history of myocardial infarction, and hemodynamic responses to laboratory stressors in children. *Health Psychology*, *12*, 6–15.

Treur, T., Koperdák, M., Rózsa, S., & Füredi, J. (2005). The impact of physical and sexual abuse on body image in eating disorders. *European Eating Disorders Review*, *13*, 106–111.

Trinh, K., Graham, N., Irnich, D., Cameron, I. D., & Forget, M. (2016). Acupuncture for neck disorders. *Cochrane Database Systematic Reviews*, DOI: 10.1002/14651858.CD004870.pub4

Trock, B., Lanza, E., & Greenwald, P. (1990). Dietary fiber, vegetables, and colon cancer: Critical review and meta-analyses of the epidemiologic evidence. *Journal of the National Cancer Institute*, *82*(8), 650–661.

Troxel, W. M., Matthews, K. A., Bromberger, J. T., & Sutton-Tyrrell, K. (2003). Chronic stress burden, discrimination, and subclinical carotid artery disease in African American and Caucasian women. *Health Psychology*, *22*, 300–309.

The truth about dieting. (2002, June). *Consumer Reports*, *67*(6), 26–31.

Tsai, A. G., & Wadden, T. A. (2005). Systematic review: An evaluation of major commercial weight loss programs in the United States. *Annals of Internal Medicine*, *142*, 56–66.

Tsao, J. C. I (2007). Effectiveness of massage therapy for chronic, non-malignant pain: A review. *Evidence-Based Complementary and Alternative Medicine*, *4*, 165–179.

Tsao, J. C. I., & Zeltzer, L. K. (2005). Complementary and alternative medicine approaches for pediatric pain: A review of the state-of-the-science. *Evidence-Based Complementary and Alternative Medicine*, *2*, 149–159.

Tsiotra, P. C., & Tsigos, C. (2006). Stress, the endoplasmic reticulum, and insulin resistance. In G. P. Chrousos & C. Tsigos (Eds.), *Stress, obesity, and metabolic syndrome* (pp. 63–76). New York, NY: Annals of the New York Academy of Sciences.

Tsoi, D. T., Porwal, M., & Webster, A. C. (2010). Interventions for smoking cessation and reduction in individuals with schizophrenia. *Cochrane Database of Systematic Reviews 2010*, *6*, Cochrane Art. No.: CD007253, DOI:10.1002/14651858.CD007253.pub2.

Tucker, J. A., Phillips, M. M., Murphy, J. G., & Raczynski, J. M. (2004). Behavioral epidemiology and health psychology. In R. G. Frank, A. Baum, & J. L. Wallander (Eds.), *Handbook of clinical health psychology* (Vol. 3, pp. 435–464). Washington, DC: American Psychological Association.

Tucker, J. S., Orlando, M., & Ellickson, P. L. (2003). Patterns and correlates of binge drinking trajectories from early adolescence to young adulthood. *Health Psychology*, *22*, 79–87.

Tucker, O. N., Szomstein, S., & Rosenthal, R. J. (2007). Nutritional consequences of weight loss surgery. *Medical Clinics of North America*, *91*, 499–513.

Turk, D. C. (1978). Cognitive behavioral techniques in the management of pain. In J. P. Foreyt & D. P. Rathjen (Eds.), *Cognitive behavior therapy* (pp. 199–232). New York, NY: Plenum Press.

Turk, D. C. (2001). Physiological and psychological bases of pain. In A. Baum, T. A. Revenson, & J. E. Singer (Eds.), *Handbook of health psychology* (pp. 117–131). Mahwah, NJ: Erlbaum.

Turk, D. C., & McCarberg, B. (2005). Non-pharmacological treatments for chronic pain: A disease management context. *Disease Management and Health Outcomes*, *13*, 19–30.

Turk, D. C., & Melzack, R. (2001). The measurement of pain and the assessment of people experiencing pain. In D. C. Turk & R. Melzack (Eds.), *Handbook of pain assessment* (2nd ed., pp. 3–11). New York, NY: Guilford Press.

Turk, D. C., Swanson, K. S., & Gatchel, R. J. (2008). Predicting opioid misuse by chronic pain patients: A systematic review and literature synthesis. *Clinical Journal of Pain*, *24*, 497–508.

Turner, J., & Kelly, B. (2000). Emotional dimensions of chronic disease. *Western Journal of Medicine*, *172*, 124–128.

Turner, J. A., Deyo, R. A., Loeser, J. D., Von Korff, M., & Fordyce, W. E. (1994). The importance of placebo effects in pain treatment and research. *Journal of the American Medical Association*, *271*, 1609–1614.

Turpin, R. S., Simmons, J. B., Lew, J. F., Alexander, C. M., Dupee, M. A., Kavanagh, P., … Cameron, E. R. (2004). Improving treatment regimen adherence in coronary heart disease by targeting patient types. *Disease Management and Health Outcomes*, *12*, 377–383.

Twicken, D. (2011). An introduction to medical qi gong. *Acupuncture Today*, *12*(2), 20.

Twyman, L., Bonevski, B., Paul, C., & Bryant, J. (2014). Perceived barriers to smoking cessation in selected vulnerable groups: A systematic review of the qualitative and quantitative literature. *BMJ Open*, *4*(12), e006414.

Tylka, T. L. (2004). The relation between body dissatisfation and eating disorder symptomatology: An analysis of moderating variables. *Journal of Counseling Psychology*, *51*, 178–191.

Uchino, B. N., Cawthon, R. M., Smith, T. W., Light, K. C., McKenzie, J., Carlisle, M., … Bowen, K. (2012). Social relationships and health: Is feeling positive, negative, or both (ambivalent) about your social ties related to telomeres? *Health Psychology*, *31*(6), 789.

UCLA Cousins Center for Psychoneuroimmunology. (2011). *About us.* Retrieved June 12, 2016, from https://www.semel.ucla.edu/cousins/about

Ullman, D. (2010). A review of a historical summit on integrative medicine. *Evidence-Based Complementary and Alternative Medicine (eCAM), 7*(4), 511–514.

Ulrich, C. (2002). High stress and low income: The environment of poverty. *Human Ecology, 30*(4), 16–18.

UNAIDS. (2007). *AIDS epidemic update, 2007.* Geneva, Switzerland: Joint United Nations Programme on HIV/AIDS.

UNAIDS (2010). *Report on the global AIDS epidemic, 2010.* Geneva, Switzerland: World Health Organization.

UNAIDS (2016). Fact sheet 2016. Retrieved August 16, 2016, from http://www.unaids.org/en/resources/fact-sheet

Unger-Saldaña, K., & Infante-Castañeda, C. B. (2011). Breast cancer delay: A grounded model of help-seeking behavior. *Social Science and Medicine, 72*, 1096–1104.

Updegraff, J. A., Silver, R. C., & Holman, E. A. (2008). Searching for and finding meaning in a collective trauma: Results from a national longitudinal study of the 9/11 terrorist attacks. *Journal of Personality and Social Psychology, 95*, 709–722.

Updegraff, J. A., & Taylor, S. E. (2000). From vulnerability to growth: Positive and negative effects of stressful life events. In J. Harvey & E. Miller (Eds.), *Loss and Trauma: General and Close Relationship Perspectives* (pp. 3–28). Philadelphia, PA: Brunner-Routledge.

Updegraff, J. A., Taylor, S. E., Kemeny, M. E., & Wyatt, G. E. (2000). Positive and negative effects of HIV infection in women with low socioeconomic resources. *Personality and Social Psychology Bulletin, 28*, 382–394.

Urizar, G. G., & Muñoz, R. F. (2011). Impact of a prenatal cognitive-behavioral stress management intervention on salivary cortisol levels in low-income mothers and their infants. *Psychoneuroimmunology, 36*, 1480–1494.

U.S. Census Bureau (USCB). (2011). *Statistical abstract of the United States: 2012* (131st ed.). Washington, DC: U.S. Government Printing Office. Retrieved September 28, 2012, from http://www.census.gov/compendia/statab/

U.S. Census Bureau (USCB). (2014). *Current population survey: 2014 annual social and economic (ASEC) supplement.* Retrieved August 16, 2016, from www2.census.gov/programs-surveys/cps/

U.S. Census Bureau (USCB). (2015). *Current population survey: 2015 annual social and economic (ASEC) supplement.* Retrieved August 16, 2016, from www2.census.gov/programs-surveys/cps/

U.S. Department of Health and Human Services (USDHHS). (1990). *The health benefits of smoking cessation: A report of the Surgeon General* (DHHS Publication No. CDC 90-8416). Washington, DC: U.S. Government Printing Office.

U.S. Department of Health and Human Services (USDHHS). (1995). *Healthy People 2000 review, 1994* (DHHS Publication No. PHS 95-1256-1). Washington, DC: U.S. Government Printing Office.

U.S. Department of Health and Human Services (USDHHS). (1996). *Physical activity and health: A report of the Surgeon General.* Atlanta, GA: Centers for Disease Control and Prevention.

U.S. Department of Health and Human Services (USDHHS). (2000). *Healthy People 2010: Understanding and improving health* (2nd ed.). Washington, DC: U.S. Government Printing Office.

U.S. Department of Health and Human Services (USDHHS). (2003). *The seventh report of the Joint National Committee on Prevention, Detection, Evaluation and Treatment of High Blood Pressure* (NIH Publication No. 03-5233). Washington, DC: Author.

U.S. Department of Health and Human Services (USDHHS). (2007). *Healthy people 2010 midcourse review.* Retrieved August 5, 2008, from http://www.healthypeople.gov/Data/midcourse/

U.S. Department of Health and Human Services (USDHHS). (2008a). *Physical activity guidelines for Americans.* Retrieved February 20, 2012, from http://www.health.gov/PAGuidelines/factsheetprof.aspx

U.S. Department of Health and Human Services (USDHHS). (2008b). *The Secretary's Advisory Committee on National Health Promotion and Disease Prevention Objectives for 2020. Phase I report: Recommendations for the framework and format of Healthy People 2020. Section IV. Advisory Committee findings and recommendations.* Retrieved April 12, 2012, from http://www.healthypeople.gov/2020/about/advisory/PhaseI.pdf

U.S. Department of Health and Human Services (USDHHS). (2010a). *Healthy People 2020.* Washington, DC: U.S. Government Printing Office. Retrieved April 20, 2012, from http://www.healthypeople.gov/2020/

U.S. Department of Health and Human Services (USDHHS). (2010b). *HHS announces the nation's new health promotion and disease prevention agenda* (press release). Retrieved April 10, 2012, from http://www.hhs.gov/news/press/2010pres/12/20101202a.html

U.S. Department of Health and Human Services (USDHHS). (2010c). *How tobacco smoke causes disease: The biology and behavioral basis for smoking-attributable disease: A report of the Surgeon General.* Atlanta, GA: Centers for Disease Control and Prevention.

U.S. Department of Health and Human Services (USDHHS). (2010d). *A report of the Surgeon General: How tobacco smoke causes disease: What it means to you.* Retrieved February 27, 2012, from http://www.cdc.gov/tobacco/data_statistics/sgr/2010/consumer_booklet/pdfs/consumer.pdf

U.S. Department of Health and Human Services (USDHHS). (2014). *The Health Consequences of Smoking: 50 Years of Progress. A Report of the Surgeon General.* Atlanta, GA: U.S. Department of Health and Human Services, Centers for Disease Control and Prevention, National Center for Chronic Disease Prevention and Health Promotion, Office on Smoking and Health.

U.S. Department of Veterans Affairs. (n.d.). Chiropractic services. Retrieved June 12, 2016, from http://www.rehab.va.gov/chiro/

U.S. Public Health Service (USPHS). (1964). *Smoking and health: Public Health Service report of the Advisory Committee to the Surgeon General of the Public Health Service* (PHS Publication No. 1103). Washington, DC: U.S. Government Printing Office.

Vainionpää, A., Korpelainen, R., Leppäluoto, J., & Jämsä, T. (2005). Effects of high-impact exercise on bone mineral density: A randomized controlled trial in premenopausal women. *Osteoporosis International, 16*, 191–197.

Vall, E., & Wade, T. D. (2015). Predictors of treatment outcome in individuals with eating disorders: A systematic review and meta-analysis. *International Journal of Eating Disorders, 48*(7), 946–971.

van Baal, P. H. M., Polder, J. J., de Wit, G. A., Hoogenveen, R. T., Feenstra, T. L., Bohuizen, H. C., … Brouwer, W. B. (2008). Lifetime medical costs of obesity: Prevention no cure for increasing health expenditure. *PLoS Medicine, 5*(2), 242–249.

Van der Does, A. J., & Van Dyck, R. (1989). Does hypnosis contribute to the care of burn patients? Review of evidence. *General Hospital Psychiatry, 11*, 119–124.

van Dillen, S. M. E., de Vries, S., Groenewegen, P. P., & Spreeuwenberg, P. (2011). Greenspace in urban neighborhoods and residents' health: Adding quality to quantity. *Journal of Epidemiology and Community Health. 66*(6), e8.

van Dongen, E. V., Kersten, I. H., Wagner, I. C., Morris, R. G., & Fernández, G. (2016). Physical Exercise Performed Four Hours after Learning Improves Memory Retention and Increases Hippocampal Pattern Similarity during Retrieval. *Current Biology, 26*(13), 1722–1727.

van Hanswijck de Jonge, P., van Furth, E. F., Lacey, J. H., & Waller, G. (2003). The prevalence of DSM-IV personality pathology among individuals with bulimia nervosa, binge eating disorder and obesity. *Psychological Medicine, 33*, 1311–1317.

van Reekum, R., Binns, M., Clarke, D., Chayer, C., Conn, D., & Herrmann, N. (2005). Is late-life depression a predictor of Alzheimer's disease? Results from a historical cohort study. *International Journal of Geriatric Psychiatry, 20*, 80–82.

van Ryn, M., & Burke, J. (2000). The effect of patient race and socioeconomic status on physicians' perception of patients. *Social Science and Medicine, 50*, 813–828.

van Zundert, J., & van Kleef, M. (2005). Low back pain: From algorithm to cost-effectiveness? *Pain Practice, 5*, 179–189.

Varady, K. A., & Jones, P. J. H. (2005). Combination diet and exercise interventions for the treatment of dysilipidemia: An effective preliminary strategy to lower cholesterol levels? *Journal of Nutrition, 135*, 1829–1835.

Vargas, A. J., & Thompson, P. A. (2012). Diet and nutrient factors in colorectal cancer risk. *Nutrition in Clinical Practice, 27*(5), 613–623.

Vartanian, L. R., Herman, C. P., & Polivy, J. (2007). Consumption stereotypes and impression management: How you are what you eat. *Appetite, 48*(3), 265–277.

Veehof, M. M., Oskam, M.-J., Schreurs, K. M. G., & Bohlmeijer, E. T. (2010). Acceptance-based interventions for the treatment of chronic pain: A systematic review and meta-analysis. *Pain, 152*, 533–542.

Veldtman, G. R., Matley, S. L., Kendall, L., Quirk, J., Gibbs, J. L., Parsons, J. M., … Hewison, J. (2001). Illness understanding in children and adolescents with heart disease. *Western Journal of Medicine, 174*, 171–173.

Velicer, W. F., & Prochaska, J. O. (2008). Stages and non-stage theories of behavior and behavior change: A comment on Schwarzer. *Applied Psychology: An International Review, 57*, 75–83.

Velligan, D. I., Wang, M., Diamond, P., Glahn, D. C., Castillo, D., Bendle, S., … Miller, A. L. (2007). Relationships among subjective and objective measures of adherence to oral antipsychotic medications. *Psychiatric Services, 58*, 1187–1192.

Vemuri, P., Gunter, J. L., Senjem, M. L., Whitwell, J. L., Kantarci, K., Knopman, D. S., … Jack, C. R., Jr. (2008). Alzheimer's disease diagnosis in individual subjects using structural MR images: Validation studies. *NeuroImage, 39*, 1186–1197.

Venn, A., & Britton, J. (2007). Exposure to secondhand smoke and bio-markers of cardiovascular disease risk in never-smoking adults. *Circulation, 115*, 900–995.

Verbeeten, K. C., Elks, C. E., Daneman, D., & Ong, K. K. (2011). Association between childhood obesity and subsequent Type 1 diabetes: A systematic review and meta-analysis. *Diabetic Medicine, 28*, 10–18.

Verhagen, A. P., Damen, L., Berger, M. Y., Passchier, J., & Koes, B. W. (2009). Behavioral treatments of chronic tension-type headache in adults: Are they beneficial? *CNS Neuroscience and Therapeutics, 15*(2), 183–205.

Verheggen, R. J. H. M., Maessen, M. F. H., Green, D. J., Hermus, A. R. M. M., Hopman, M. T. E., & Thijssen, D. H. T. (2016). A systematic review and meta-analysis on the effects of exercise training versus hypocaloric diet: Distinct effects on body weight abnd visceral adipose tissue. *Obesity Reviews, 17*(8), 664–690.

Verhoeven, J. E., van Oppen, P., Puterman, E., Elzinga, B., & Penninx, B. W. (2015). The association of early and recent psychosocial life stress with leukocyte telomere length. *Psychosomatic Medicine, 77*(8), 882–888.

Verkaik, R., Van Weert, J. C. M., & Francke, A. L. (2005). The effects of psychosocial methods on depressed, aggressive and apathetic behaviors of people with dementia: A systematic review. *International Journal of Geriatric Psychiatry, 20*, 301–314.

Verma, K. B., & Khan, M. I. (2007). Social inhibition, negative affectivity and depression in cancer patients with Type D personality. *Social Science International, 23*, 114–122.

Vermeire, E., Hearnshaw, H., Van Royen, P., & Denekens, J. (2001). Patient adherence to treatment: Three decades of research. A comprehensive review. *Journal of Clinical Pharmacy and Therapeutics, 26*, 331–342.

Verplanken, B., & Faes, S. (1999). Good intentions, bad habits, and effects of forming implementation intentions on healthy eating. *European Journal of Social Psychology, 29*, 591–604.

Vissers, D., Hens, W., Hansen, D., & Taeymans, J. (2016). The effect of diet or exercise on visceral adipose tissue in overweight youth. *Medicine and Science in Sport and Exercise, 48*(7), 1415–1424.

Veugelers, P., Sithole, F., Zhang, S., & Muhajarine, N. (2008). Neighborhood characteristics in relation to diet, physical activity and overweight of Canadian children. *International Journal of Pediatric Obesity, 3*, 152–159.

Victor, T. W., Hu, X., Campbell, J. C., Buse, D. C., & Lipton, R. B. (2010). Migraine prevalence by age and sex in the United States: A life-span study. *Cephalalgia, 30*, 1065–1072.

Villalba, D., Ham, L. S., & Rose, S. (2011). Alcohol intoxication and memory for events: A snapshot of alcohol myopia in a real-world drinking scenario. *Memory, 19*(2), 202–210.

Viner, R. M., & Taylor, B. (2007). Adult outcomes of binge drinking in adolescence: Findings from a UK national birth cohort. *Journal of Epidemiology and Community Health, 61*(10), 902–907.

Virmani, R., Burke, A. P., & Farb, A. (2001). Sudden cardiac death. *Cardiovascular Pathology, 10*, 211–218.

Visser, M. (1999). Food and culture: Interconnections. *Social Research, 66*, 117–132.

Vitória, P. D., Salgueiro, M. F., Silva, S. A., & De Vries, H. (2009). The impact of social influence on adolescent intention to smoke: Combining types and referents of influence. *British Journal of Health Psychology, 14*(4), 681–699.

Vlachopoulos, C., Rokkas, K., Ioakeimidis, N., & Stefanadis, C. (2007). Inflammation, metabolic syndrome, erectile dysfunction, and coronary artery disease: Common links. *European Urology, 52*, 1590–1600.

Voas, R. B., Roman, T. E., Tippetts, A. S., & Durr-Holden, C. D. M. (2006). Drinking status and fatal crashes: Which drinkers contribute most to the problem? *Journal of Studies on Alcohol, 67*, 722–729.

von Baeyer, C. L., & Spagrud, L. J. (2007). Systematic review of observational (behavioral) measures of pain for children and adolescents aged 3 to 18 years. *Pain, 127*, 140–150.

von Hertzen, L. C., & Haahtela, T. (2004). Asthma and atopy—The price of affluence? *Allergy, 59*, 124–137.

Von Korff, M., Barlow, W., Cherkin, D., & Deyo, R. A. (1994). Effects of practice style in managing back pain. *Annals of Internal Medicine, 121*, 187–195.

von Zglinicki, T. (2002). Oxidative stress shortens telomeres. *Trends in Biochemical Sciences, 27*(7), 339–344.

Vu, K. N., Ballantyne, C. M., Hoogeveen, R. C., Nambi, V., Volcik, K. A., Boerwinkle, E., … Morrison, A. C. (2016). Causal role of alcohol consumption in an improved lipid profile: The Atherosclerosis Risk in Communities (ARIC) Study. *PLoS One, 11*(2), 1–16.

Waber, R. L., Shiv, B., Carmon, Z., & Ariely, D. (2008). Commercial features of placebo and therapeutic efficacy. *Journal of the American Medical Association, 299*, 1016–1017.

Wadden, T. A., Crerand, C. E., & Brock, J. (2005). Behavioral treatment of obesity. *Psychiatric Clinics of North America, 28*, 151–170.

Wager, T. D., Rilling, J. K., Smith, E. E., Sololik, A., Casey, K. L., Davidson, R. J., … Cohen, J. D. (2004). Placebo-induced changes in fMRI in the anticipation and experience of pain. *Science, 303*, 1162–1167.

Wahlberg, A. (2007). A quackery with a difference—New medical pluralism and the problem of 'dangerous practitioners' in the United Kingdom. *Social Science and Medicine, 65*(11), 2307–2316.

Wakefield, A. J., Murch, S. H., Anthony, A., Linnell, J., Casson, D. M., Malik, M., … Walker-Smith, J. A. (1998). RETRACTED: Ileal-lymphoid-nodular hyperplasia, non-specific colitis, and pervasive developmental disorder in children. *The Lancet, 351*(9103), 637–641.

Waite-Jones, J. M., & Madill, A. (2008a). Amplified ambivalence: Having a sibling with juvenile idiopathic arthritis. *Psychology and Health, 23*, 477–492.

Waite-Jones, J. M., & Madill, A. (2008b). Concealed concern: Fathers' experiences of having a child with juvenile idiopathic arthritis. *Psychology and Health, 23*, 585–601.

Wakefield, M., Loken, B., & Hornik, R. (2010). Use of mass media campaigns to change health behaviour. *The Lancet, 376*, 1261–1271.

Walach, H., & Jonas, W. B. (2004). Placebo research: The evidence base for harnessing self-healing capacities. *Journal of Alternative and Complementary Medicine, 10*(S1), S103–S112.

Walcher, T., Haenle, M. M., Mason, R. A., Koenig, W., Imhof, A., & Kratzer, W. (2010). The effect of alcohol, tobacco and caffeine consumption and vegetarian diet on gallstone prevalence. *European Journal of Gastroenterology and Hepatology, 22*(11), 1345–1351.

Wald, H. S., Dube, C. E., & Anthony, D. C. (2007). Untangling the Web—The impact of Internet use on health care and the physician-patient relationship. *Patient Education and Counseling, 68*, 218–224.

Waldrop-Valverde, D., Osborn, C. Y., Rodriguez, A., Rothman, R. L., Kumar, M., & Jones, D. L. (2010). Numeracy skills explain racial differences in HIV medication management. *AIDS and Behavior, 14*, 799–806.

Walen, H. R., & Lachman, M. E. (2000). Social support and strain from partner, family, and friends: Costs and benefits for men and women in adulthood. *Journal of Social and Personal Relationships, 17*, 5–30.

Walker, A. R. P., Walker, B. F., & Adam, F. (2003). Nutrition, diet, physical activity, smoking, and longevity: From primitive hunter-gatherer to present passive consumer—How far can we go? *Nutrition, 19*, 169–173.

Walker, E. A., Mertz, C. K., Kalten, M. R., & Flynn, J. (2003). Risk perception for developing diabetes. *Diabetes Care, 26*, 2543–2548.

Wall, P. (2000). *Pain: The science of suffering.* New York, NY: Columbia University Press.

Waltenbaugh, A. W., & Zagummy, M. J. (2004). Optimistic bias and perceived control among cigarette smokers. *Journal of Alcohol and Drug Education, 47*, 20–33.

Wamala, S. P., Mittleman, M. A., Horsten, M., Schenck-Gustafsson, K., & Orth-Gomér, K. (2000). Job stress and the occupational gradient in coronary heart disease risk in women: The Stockholm Female Coronary Risk study. *Social Science and Medicine, 51*, 481–489.

Wang, C., Bannuru, R., Ramel, J., Kupelnick, B., Scott, T., & Schmid, C. H. (2010). Tai chi on psychological well-being: Systematic review and meta-analysis. *BMC Complementary and Alternative Medicine, 10*, 23.

Wang, C., Schmid, C. H., Rones, R., Kalish, R., Yinh, J., Goldenberg, D. L., … McAlindon, T. (2010). A randomized trial of tai chi for fibromyalgia. *New England Journal of Medicine, 363*(8), 743–754.

Wang, C., Wan, X., Wang, K., Li, J., Sun, T., & Guan, X. (2014). Disease stigma and intentions to seek care for stress urinary incontinence among community-dwelling women. *Maturitas, 77*(4), 351–355.

Wang, C.-W., Chan, C. H. Y., Ho, R. T. H., Chan, J. S. M., Ng, S.-M., & Chan, C. L. W. (2014). Managing stress and anxiety through qigong exercise in healthy adults: A systematic review and meta-analysis of randomized controlled trials. *BMC Complementary and Alternative Medicine, 14*, 1–9. http://www.biomedcentral.com/1472-6882/14/8

Wang, D. D., Li, Y., Chiuve, S. E., Hu, F. B., & Willett, W. C. (2015). Improvements in US diet helped reduce disease burden and lower premature deaths, 1999–2012; overall diet remains poor. *Health Affairs, 34*(11), 1916–1922.

Wang, H.-W., Mittleman, M. A., & Orth-Gomér, K. (2005). Influence of social support on progression of coronary artery disease in women. *Social Science and Medicine, 60*, 599–607.

Wang, H.-X., Leineweber, C., Kirkeeide, R., Svane, B., Schenck-Gustafsson, K., Theorell, T., … Orth-Gormér, K. (2007). Psychosocial stress and atherosclerosis: Family and work stress accelerate progression of coronary disease in women. The Stockholm Female Coronary Angiography Study. *Journal of Internal Medicine, 261*, 245–254.

Wang, J., & Li, M. D. (2010). Common and unique biological pathways associated with smoking initiation/progression, nicotine dependence, and smoking cessation. *Neuropsychopharmacology, 35*(3), 702–719.

Wang, J. L., Lesage, A., Schmitz, N., & Drapeau, A. (2008). The relationship between work stress and mental disorders in men and women: Findings from a population-based study. *Journal of Epidemiology and Community Health, 62*, 42–47.

Wang, S.-W., Shih, J. H., Hu, A. W., Louie, J. Y., & Lau, A. S. (2010). Cultural differences in daily support experiences. *Cultural Diversity and Ethnic Minority Psychology, 16*, 413–420.

Wang, Y. (2004). Diet, physical activity, childhood obesity and risk of cardiovascular disease. *International Congress Series, 1262*, 176–179.

Wansink, B., & Payne, C. R. (2008). Eating behavior and obesity at Chinese buffets. *Obesity, 16*, 1957–1960.

Warburton, D. E. R., Nicol, C. W., & Bredin, S. S. D. (2006). Health benefits of physical activity: The evidence. *Canadian Medical Association Journal, 174*, 801–809.

Ward, B. W., Schiller, J. S., & Goodman, R. A. (2012). Multiple chronic conditions among US adults. *Preventing Chronic Disease: Public Health Research, Practice, and Policy, 11*, 1–4.

Warner, R., & Griffiths, M. D. (2006). A qualitative thematic analysis of exercise addiction: An exploratory study. *International Journal of Mental Health and Addiction, 4*, 13–26.

Warren, C. W., Jones, N. R., Peruga, A., Chauvin, J., Baptiste, J.-P., de Silva, V. C., … Asma, S. (2008). Global youth tobacco surveillance, 2000–2007. *Morbidity and Mortality Weekly Reports, 57*(SS-1), 1–27.

Watanabe, T., Higuchi, K., Tanigawa, T., Tominaga, K., Fujiwara, Y., & Arakawa, T. (2002). Mechanisms of peptic ulcer recurrence: Role of inflammation. *Inflammopharmacology, 10*, 291–302.

Watkins, L. R., Hutchinson, M. R., Ledeboer, A., Wieseler-Frank, J., Milligan, E. D., & Maier, S. F. (2007). Glia as the "bad guys": Implications for improving clinical pain control and the clinical utility of opioids. *Brain, Behavior and Immunity, 21*, 131–146.

Watkins, L. R., & Maier, S. F. (2003). When good pain turns bad. *Current Directions in Psychological Science, 12*, 232–236.

Watkins, L. R., & Maier, S. F. (2005). Immune regulation of central nervous system function: From sickness responses to pathological pain. *Journal of Internal Medicine, 257*, 139–155.

Waye, K. P., Bengtsson, J., Rylander, R., Hucklebridge, F., Evans, P., & Clow, A. (2002). Low frequency noise enhances cortisol among noise sensitive subjects during work performance. *Life Sciences, 70*, 745–758.

Wayne, P. M., Kiel, D. P., Krebs, D. E., Davis, R. B., Savetsky-German, J., Connelly, M., … Buring, J. E. (2007). The effects of tai chi on bone mineral density in postmenopausal women: A systematic review. *Archives of Physical Medicine and Rehabilitation, 88*, 673–680.

Webb, O. J., & Cheng, T.-F. (2010). An informational stair climbing intervention with greater effects in overweight pedestrians. *Health Education Research, 25*, 936–944.

Webb, T. L., Joseph, J., Yardley, L., & Michie, S. (2010). Using the Internet to promote health behavior change: A systematic review and meta-analysis of the impact of theoretical basis, use of behavior change techniques, and mode of delivery on efficacy. *Journal of Medical Internet Research, 12*, e4.

Weems, C. F., Watts, S. E., Marsee, M. A., Taylor, L. K., Costa, N. M., Cannon, M. F., … Pina, A. A. (2007). The psychological impact of Hurricane Katrina: Contextual differences in psychological symptoms, social support, and discrimination. *Behavior Research and Therapy, 45*, 2295–2306.

Weidner, G. (2000). Why do men get more heart disease than women? An international perspective. *Journal of American College Health, 48*, 291–296.

Weidner, G., & Cain, V. S. (2003). The gender gap in heart disease: Lessons from Eastern Europe. *American Journal of Public Health, 93*, 768–770.

Weil, C. M., Wade, S. L., Bauman, L. J., Lynn, H., Mitchell, H., & Lavigne, J. (1999). The relationship between psychosocial factors and asthma morbidity in inner-city children with asthma. *Pediatrics, 104*, 1274–1280.

Weil, J. M., & Lee, H. H. (2004). Cultural considerations in understanding family violence among Asian American Pacific islander families. *Journal of Community Health Nursing, 21*, 217–227.

Weiner, H., & Shapiro, A. P. (2001). *Helicobacter pylori*, immune function, and gastric lesions. In R. Ader, D. L. Felten, & N. Cohen (Eds.), *Psychoneuroimmunology* (3rd ed., Vol. 2, pp. 671–686). San Diego, CA: Academic Press.

Weiner, M. F., Hynan, L. S., Bret, M. E., & White, C., III. (2005). Early behavioral symptoms and course of Alzheimer's disease. *Acta Psychiatrica Scandinavica, 111*, 367–371.

Weingart, S. N., Pagovich, O., Sands, D. Z., Li, J. M., Aronson, M. D., Davis, R. B., … Bates, D. W. (2006). Patient-reported service quality on a medicine unit. *International Journal for Quality in Health Care, 18*, 95–101.

Weinstein, N. D. (1980). Unrealistic optimism about future life events. *Journal of Personality and Social Psychology, 39*, 806–820.

Weinstein, N. D. (1984). Why it won't happen to me: Perceptions of risk factors and susceptibility. *Health Psychology, 3*, 431–457.

Weinstein, N. D. (2001). Smokers' recognition of their vulnerability to harm. In P. Slovic (Ed.), *Smoking: Risk, perception and policy* (pp. 81–96). Thousand Oaks, CA: Sage.

Weir, H. K., Thun, M. J., Hankey, B. F., Ries, L. A. G., Howe, H. L., Wingo, P. A., … Edwards, B. K. (2003). Annual report to the nation on the status of cancer, 1975–2000, featuring the uses of surveillance data for cancer prevention and control. *Journal of the National Cancer Institute, 95*, 1276–1299.

Weiss, J. W., Cen, S., Schuster, D. V., Unger, J. B., Johnson, C. A., Mouttapa, M., … Cruz, T. B. (2006). Longitudinal effects of pro-tobacco and anti-tobacco messages on adolescent smoking suscepti-bility. *Nicotine and Tobacco Research, 8,* 455–465.

Weiss, R. (1999, November 30). Medical errors blamed for many deaths; as many as 98,000 a year in US linked to mistakes. *Washington Post,* p. A1.

Weitz, R. (2010). *The sociology of health, illness, and health care: A critical approach* (5th ed.). Belmont, CA: Wadsworth.

Wells, J. C. K. (2011). An evolutionary perspective on the trans-generational basis of obesity. *Annals of Human Biology, 38*(4), 400–409.

Wells, R. E., Phillips. R. S., Schachter, S. C., & McCarthy, E. P. (2010). Complementary and alternative medicine use among U.S. adults with common neurological conditions. *Journal of Neurology, 257,* 1822–1831.

Wen, C., Tsai, S. P., Cheng, T. Y., Chan, H., T., Chung, W. S. I., & Chen, C. J. (2005). Excess injury mortality among smokers: A neglected tobacco hazard. *Tobacco Control, 14*(Suppl. 1), 28–32.

Wen, M. (2007). Racial and ethnic differences in general health status and limiting health conditions among American children: Parental reports in the 1999 National Survey of America's Families. *Ethnicity and Health, 12,* 401–422.

Wendel-Vos, G. C., Schuit, A. J., Feskens, E. J., Boshuizen, H. C., Verschuren, W. M., Saris, W. H., … Kromhout, D. (2004). Physical activity and stroke: A meta-analysis of observational data. *International Journal of Epidemiology, 33,* 787–798.

Wenzel, S. E. (2006). Asthma: Defining of the persistent adult phenotypes. *Lancet, 368,* 804–813.

West, S. L., & O'Neal, K. K. (2004). Project D.A.R.E. outcome effectiveness revisited. *American Journal of Public Health, 94,* 1027–1029.

Wetter, D. W., Cofta-Gunn, L., Fouladi, R. T., Irvin, J. E., Daza, P., Mazas, C., … Gritz, E. R. (2005). Understanding the association among education, employment characteristics, and smoking. *Addictive Behaviors, 30,* 905–914.

Wetter, D. W., McClure, J. B., Cofta-Woerpel, L., Costello, T. J., Reitzel, L. R., Businelle, M. S., … Cinciripini, P. M. (2011). A randomized clin-ical trial of a palmtop computer-delivered treatment for smoking relapse prevention among women. *Psychology of Addictive Behaviors, 25,* 365–371.

Whang, W., Kubzansky, L. D., Kawachi, I., Rexrode, K. M., Kroenke, C. H., Glynn, R. J., … Albert, C. M. (2009). Depression and risk of sudden cardiac death and coronary heart disease in women: Results from the Nurses' Health Study. *Journal of the American College of Cardiology, 53,* 950–958.

Wheaton, A. G., Perry, G. S., Chapman, D. P., McKnight-Eily, L. R., Presley-Cantrell, L. R., & Croft, J. B. (2011). Relationship between body mass index and perceived insufficient sleep among U.S. adults: An analysis of 2008 BRFSS data. *BMC Public Health, 11*(1), 295–302.

White, S., Chen, J., & Atchison, R. (2008). Relationship of preventive health practices and health literacy: A national study. *American Journal of Health Behavior, 32,* 227–242.

White, V. M., Durkin, S. J., Coomber, K., & Wakefield, M. A. (2015). What is the role of tobacco control advertising intensity and duration in reducing adolescent smoking prevalence? Findings from 16 years of tobacco control mass media advertising in Australia. *Tobacco Con-trol, 24*(2), 198–204.

White, W. L. (2004). Addiction recovery mutual aid groups: An enduring international phenomenon. *Addiction, 99,* 532–538.

Whitfield, K. E., Weidner, G., Clark, R., & Anderson, N. B. (2002). Socio-demographic diversity in behavioral medicine. *Journal of Consulting and Clinical Psychology, 70,* 463–481.

Wider, B., & Boddy, K. (2009). Conducting systematic reviews of comple-mentary and alternative medicine: Common pitfalls. *Evaluation and the Health Professions, 32*(4), 417–430.

Wilbert-Lampen, U., Leistner, D., Greven, S., Pohl, T., Sper, S., Völker, C., … Steinbeck, G. (2008). Cardiovascular events during World Cup Soccer. *New England Journal of Medicine, 358,* 475–483.

Wilbert-Lampen, U., Nickel, T., Leistner, D., Guthlin, D., Matis, T., Volker, C., … Steinbeck, G. (2010). Modified serum profiles of inflam-matory and vasoconstrictive factors in patients with emotional

stress-induced acute coronary syndrome during World Cup Soccer 2006. *Journal of the American College of Cardiology, 55,* 637–642.

Wiley, J. A., & Camacho, T. C. (1980). Life-style and future health: Evi-dence from the Alameda County Study. *Preventive Medicine, 9,* 1–21.

Wilkin, H. A., Valente, T. W., Murphy, S., Cody, M. J., Huang, G., & Beck, V. (2007). Does entertainment education work with Latinos in the United States? Identification and the effects of a telenovela breast cancer storyline. *Health Communication, 21,* 223–233.

Williams, L. J., Jacka, F. N., Pasco, J. A., Dodd, S., & Berk, M. (2006). Depression and pain: An overview. *Acta Neuropsychiatrica, 18,* 79–87.

Williams, M. T., & Hord, H. G. (2005). The role of dietary factors in can-cer prevention: Beyond fruits and vegetables. *Nutrition in Clinical Practice, 20,* 451–459.

Williams, P. G., Holmbeck, G. N., & Greenley, R. N. (2002). Adolescent health psychology. *Journal of Consulting and Clinical Psychology, 70,* 828–842.

Williams, P. T. (2001). Health effects resulting from exercise versus those from body fat loss. *Medicine and Science in Sports and Exercise, 33,* S611–S621.

Williams, R. B., Jr. (1989). *The trusting heart: Great news about Type A behavior.* New York, NY: Times Books.

Williams, R. B., Barefoot, J. C., Califf, R. M., Haney, T. L., Saunders, W. B., Pryor, D. B., … Mark, D. B. (1992). Prognostic importance of social and economic resources among medically treated patients with angio-graphically documented coronary artery disease. *Journal of the American Medical Association, 267,* 520–524.

Williamson, D. A., Thaw, J. M., & Varnado-Sullivan, P. J. (2001). Cost-effectiveness analysis of a hospital-based cognitive-behavioral treat-ment program for eating disorders. *Behavior Therapy, 32,* 459–470.

Willey, J. Z., Gardener, H., Caunca, M. R., Moon, Y. P., Dong, C., Cheung, Y. K., … Wright, C. B. (2016). Leisure-time physical activity associ-ates with cognitive decline The Northern Manhattan Study. *Neurol-ogy, 86*(20), 1897–1903.

Wills, T. A. (1998). Social support. In E. A. Blechman & K. D. Brownell (Eds.), *Behavioral medicine and women: A comprehensive handbook* (pp. 118–128). New York, NY: Guilford Press.

Wills, T. A., Sargent, J. D., Stoolmiller, M., Gibbons, F. X., & Gerrard, M. (2008). Movie smoking exposure and smoking onset: A longitudinal study of meditation processes in a representative sample of U.S. adolescents. *Psychology of Addictive Behaviors, 22,* 269–277.

Wills-Karp, M. (2004). Interleukin-13 in asthma pathogenesis. *Immuno-logical Reviews, 202,* 175–190.

Wilson, B., & McSherry, W. (2006). A study of nurses' inferences of patients' physical pain. *Journal of Clinical Nursing, 15,* 459–468.

Wilz, G., Schinkothe, D., & Soellner, R. (2011). Goal attainment and treat-ment compliance in a cognitive-behavioral telephone intervention for family caregivers of persons with dementia. *GeroPsych: The Jour-nal of Gerontopsychology and Geriatric Psychiatry, 24,* 115–125.

Wimberly, S. R., Carver, C. S., Laurenceau, J.-P., Harris, S. D., & Antoni, M. H. (2005). Perceived partner reactions to diagnosis and treat-ment of breast cancer: Impact on psychosocial and psychosexual adjustment. *Journal of Consulting and Clinical Psychology, 73,* 300–311.

Wimo, A., Jönsson, L., Bond, J., Prince, M., Winblad, B., & Interna-tional, A. D. (2013). The worldwide economic impact of dementia 2010. *Alzheimer's and Dementia, 9*(1), 1–11.

Wing, R. R., Gorin, A. A., Raynor, H. A., Tate, D. F., Fava, J. L., & Machan, J. (2007). "STOP Regain": Are there negative effects of daily weigh-ing? *Journal of Consulting and Clinical Psychology, 75,* 652–656.

Wing, R. R., & Polley, B. A. (2001). Obesity. In A. Baum, T. A. Revenson, & J. E. Singer (Eds.), *Handbook of health psychology* (pp. 263–279). Mahwah, NJ: Erlbaum.

Wingard, D. L., Berkman, L. F., & Brand, R. J. (1982). A multivariate anal-ysis of health-related practices: A nine-year mortality follow-up of the Alameda County study. *American Journal of Epidemiology, 116,* 765–775.

Winter, J. E., MacInnis, R. J., Wattanapaiboon, N., & Nowson, C. A. (2014). BMI and all-cause mortality in older adults:

A meta-analysis. *American Journal of Clinical Nutrition*, 99(4), 875–890.

Winterling, J., Glimelius, B., & Nordin, K. (2008). The importance of expectations on the recovery period after cancer treatment. *Psycho-Oncology*, 17, 190–198.

Wipfli, B. M., Rethorst, C. D., & Landers, D. M. (2008). The anxiolytic effects of exercise: A meta-analysis of randomized trials and dose-response analysis. *Journal of Sport and Exercise Psychology*, 30, 392–410.

Wise, J. (2000). Largest-ever study shows reduction in cardiovascular mortality. *Bulletin of the World Health Organization*, 78, 562.

Wiseman, C. V., Gray, J. J., Mosimann, J. E., & Ahrens, A. H. (1992). Cultural expectations of thinness in women: An update. *International Journal of Eating Disorders*, 11, 85–89.

Wiseman, C. V., Sunday, S. R., & Becker, A. E. (2005). Impact of the media on adolescent body image. *Child and Adolescent Psychiatric Clinics of North America*, 14, 453–471.

Witt, C. M., Brinkhaus, B., Reinhold, T., & Willich, S. N. (2006). Efficacy, effectiveness, safety and costs of acupuncture for chronic pain—Results of a large research initiative. *Acupuncture in Medicine*, 24(S33), 33–39.

Wolff, N. J., Darlington, A.-S. E., Hunfeld, J. A. M., Verhulst, F. C., Jaddoe, V. W. V., Moll, H. A., ... Tiemeier, H. (2009). The association of parent behaviors, chronic pain, and psychological problems with venipuncture distress in infants: The Generation R Study. *Health Psychology*, 28, 605–613.

Wolfgang, M. E. (1957). Victim precipitated criminal homicide. *Journal of Criminal Law and Criminology*, 48, 1–11.

Wolin, K. Y., Yan, Y., Colditz, G. A., & Lee, I.-M. (2009). Physical activity and colon cancer prevention: A meta-analysis. *British Journal of Cancer*, 100, 611–616.

Wonderlich, S. A., Wilsnack, R. W., Wilsnack, S. C., & Harris, T. R. (1996). Childhood sexual abuse and bulimic behavior in a nationally representative sample. *American Journal of Public Health*, 86, 1082–1086.

Wood, P. D., Stefanick, M. L., Dreon, D. M., Frey-Hewitt, B., Garay, S. C., Williams, P. T., ... Haskell, W. L. (1988). Changes in plasma lipids and lipoproteins in overweight men during weight loss through dieting compared with exercise. *New England Journal of Medicine*, 319, 1173–1179.

Woodcock, J., Franco, O. H., Orsini, N., & Roberts, I. (2011). Non-vigorous physical activity and all-cause mortality: Systematic review and meta-analysis of cohort studies. *International Journal of Epidemiology*, 40(1), 121–138.

Woodhouse, A. (2005). Phantom limb sensation. *Clinical and Experimental Pharmacology and Physiology*, 32, 132–134.

Woods, E., Burke, A., & Rodzon, K. S. (2011). Characteristics and correlations between human and pet use of acupuncture: A cross-sectional survey of four clinics. *American Acupuncturist*, 55, 18–27.

Woodward, H. I., Mytton, O. T., Lemer, C., Yardley, I. E., Ellis, B. M., Rutter, P. D., ... Wu, A. W. (2010). What have we learned about interventions to reduce medical errors? *Annual Review of Public Health*, 31, 479–497.

Wooldridge, T., & Lemberg, R. (2016). Macho, bravado, and eating disorders in men: Special issues in diagnosis and treatment. *Psychiatric Times*, 33(5), 1–5.

Woolrich, R. A., Cooper, M. J., & Turner, H. M. (2008). Metacognition in patients with anorexia nervosa, dieting and non-dieting women: A preliminary study. *European Eating Disorders Review*, 16, 11–20.

World Cancer Research Fund/American Institute for Cancer Research (WCRF/AICR). (2007). *Food, nutrition, physical activity, and the prevention of cancer: A global perspective*. Washington, DC: AICR.

World Health Organization (WHO). (2004). *Neuroscience of psychoactive substance use and dependence*. Geneva, Switzerland: Author.

World Health Organization (WHO). (2008a). *The WHO report on the global tobacco epidemic, 2008*. Geneva, Switzerland: Author.

World Health Organization (WHO). (2008b). *World health 2008*. Geneva, Switzerland: WHO Press.

World Health Organization (WHO). (2009). *WHO report on the global tobacco epidemic, 2009: Implementing smoke-free environments*. Geneva, Switzerland: Author.

World Health Organization (WHO). (2011). *WHO report on the global tobacco epidemic, 2011: Warning about the dangers of tobacco*. Retrieved June 14, 2016, from http://www.who.int/tobacco/global_report/2011/en/

World Health Organization (WHO). (2012). *WHO global report: Mortality attributable to tobacco*. Retrieved December 28, 2016 from http://apps.who.int/iris/bitstream/10665/44815/1/9789241564434_eng.pdf

World Health Organization (WHO). (2014). *Global status report on alcohol and health 2014*. Geneva, Switzerland: Author.

World Health Organization (WHO). (2015a). *WHO global report on trends in tobacco smoking 2000–2025*. Geneva, Switzerland: Author.

World Health Organization (WHO). (2015b). *WHO report on the global tobacco epidemic, 2015: Raising taxes on tobacco*. Retrieved June 14, 2016, from www.who.int/tobacco/global_report/2015/en

World Health Organization (WHO). (2015c). *World Health Statistics 2015*. Retrieved April 9, 2016, from www.who.int/gho

World Health Organization (WHO). (2016a). *Global Health Observatory (GHO) data: Overweight and obesity by country*. Retrieved August 6, 2016, from http://www.who.int/gho/ncd/risk_factors/overweight/en/

World Health Organization (WHO). (2016b). *Obesity and overweight: Fact sheet*. Retrieved August 5, 2016, from http://www.who.int/mediacentre/factsheets/fs311/en/

World Health Organization (WHO). (2016c). *World Health Statistics 2015*. Retrieved October 4, 2016, from www.who.int/gho

World Medical Association. (2004). *Declartion of Helsinki: Ethical principles for medical research involving human subjects*. Retrieved February 7, 2008, from http://www.wma.net/e/policy/b3.htm

Writing Group for the Women's Health Initiative Investigators. (2002). Risks and benefits of estrogen plus progestin in healthy postmenopausal women: Principal results from the Women's Health Initiative randomized controlled trial. *Journal of the American Medical Association*, 288, 321–333.

Wu, J.-R., Moser, D. K., Chung, M. L., & Lennie, T. A. (2008). Objectively measured, but not self-reported, medication adherence independently predicts event-free survival in patients with heart failure. *Journal of Cardiac Failure*, 14, 203–210.

Wu, T., Gao, X., Chen, M., & van Dam, R. M. (2009). Long-term effectiveness of diet-plus-exercise interventions vs. diet-only interventions for weight loss: A meta-analysis. *Obesity Reviews*, 10(3), 313–323.

Wyden, P. (1965). *The overweight society*. New York, NY: Morrow.

Xin, L., Miller, Y. D., & Brown, W. J. (2007). A qualitative review of the role of qigong in the management of diabetes. *Journal of Alternative and Complementary Medicine*, 13, 427–434.

Xu, J., Murphy, S. L., Kochanek, K D., Bastian, B. A. (2016). NCHS (2016). Deaths: Final Data for 2013. *National Vital Statistics Reports*, 64(2), 1–118.

Xu, S., Wang, L., Cooper, E., Zhang, M., Manheimer, E., Berman, B., ... & Lao, L. (2013). Adverse events of acupuncture: A systematic review of case reports. *Evidence-based Complementary and Alternative Medicine*, 2013, 1–15.

Xue, C. C. L., Zhang, A. L., Greenwood, K. M., Lin, V., & Story, D. F. (2010). Traditional Chinese medicine: An update on clinical evidence. *Journal of Alternative and Complementary Medicine*, 16(3), 301–312.

Xue, C. C. L., Zhang, A. L., Lin, V., Da Costa, C., & Story, D. F. (2007). Complementary and alternative medicine use in Australia: A national population-based survey. *Journal of Alternative and Complementary Medicine*, 13, 643–650.

Xutian, S., Zhange, J., & Louise, W. (2009). New exploration and understanding of traditional Chinese medicine. *American Journal of Chinese Medicine*, 37(3), 411–426.

Yager, J. (2008). Binge eating disorder: The search for better treatments. *American Journal of Psychiatry*, 165, 4–6.

Yamashita, H., & Tsukayama, H. (2008). Safety of acupuncture practice in Japan: Patient reactions, therapist negligence and error reduction strategies. *Evidence-Based Complementary and Alternative Medicine (eCAM)*, 5(4), 391–398.

Yan, L. L., Liu, K., Daviglus, M. L., Colangelo, L. A., Kiefe, C. I., Sidney, S., ... Greenland, P. (2006). Education, 15-year risk factor progression, and coronary artery calcium in young adulthood and early middle age. *Journal of the American Medical Association, 295*, 1793–1800.

Yan, L. L., Liu, K., Matthews, K. A., Daviglus, M. L., Freguson, T. F., & Kiefe, C. I. (2003). Psychosocial factors and risk of hypertension. *Journal of the American Medical Association, 290*, 2138–2148.

Yang, Z., & Levey, A. (2015). Gender differences: A lifetime analysis of the economic burden of Alzheimer's disease. *Women's Health Issues, 25*(5), 436–440.

Yang, Y., Verkuilen, J., Rosengren, K. S., Mariani, R. A., Reed, M., Grubisich, S. A., … Woods, J.A. (2007). Effects of a taiji and qigong intervention on the antibody response to influenza vaccine in older adults. *American Journal of Chinese Medicine, 35*, 597–607.

Yano, E., Wang, Z.-M., Wang, X.-R., Wang, M.-Z., & Lan, Y.-J. (2001). Cancer mortality among workers exposed to amphibole-free chrys-otile, asbestos. *American Journal of Epidemiology, 154*, 538–543.

Ye, X., Gross, C. R., Schommer, J., Cline, R., & St. Peter, W. L. (2007). Association between copayment and adherence to statin treatment initiated after coronary heart disease hospitalization: A longitudinal, retrospective, cohort study. *Clinical Therapeutics, 29*, 2748–2757.

Yi, H.-Y., Chen, C. M., & Williams, G. D. (2006). *Trends in alcohol-related fatal traffic crashes, United States, 1982–2004* (Alcohol Epidemiologic Data System, Surveillance Report No. 76). Arlington, VA: National Institute of Alcohol Abuse and Alcoholism.

Yin, P., Gao, N., Wu, J., Litscher, G., & Xu, S. (2014). Adverse events of massage therapy in pain-related conditions: A systematic review. *Evidence-based Complementary and Alternative Medicine (eCAM), 2014*, 1–11.

Ylvén, R., Björck-Åkesson, E., & Granlund, M. (2006). Literature review of positive functioning in families with children with a disability. *Journal of Policy and Practice in Intellectual Disabilities, 3*, 253–270.

Yong, H.-H., Borland, R., Hyland, A., & Siahpush, M. (2008). How does a failed quit attempt among regular smokers affect their cigarette consumption? Findings from the International Tobacco Control Four-Country Survey (ITC-4). *Nicotine and Tobacco Research, 10*, 897–905.

Yoshino, A., Okamoto, Y., Onoda, K., Yoshimura, S., Kunisato, Y., Demoto, Y., … Yamawaki, S. (2010). Sadness enhances the experience of pain via neural activation of the anterior cingulate cortex and amygdala: An fMRI study. *NeuroImage, 50*, 1194–1201.

Young, K. A., Gobrogge, K. L., & Wang, Z. (2011). The role of mesocorticolimbic dopamine in regulating interactions between drugs of abuse and social behavior. *Neuroscience and Biobehavioral Reviews, 35*(3), 498–515.

Young, L. R., & Nestle, M. (2007). Portion sizes and obesity: Responses of fast-food companies. *Journal of Public Health Policy, 28*(2), 238–248.

Yu, Z., Nissinen, A., Vartiainen, E., Song, G., Guo, Z., Zheng, G., … Tian, H (2000). Associations between socioeconomic status and cardio-vascular risk factors in an urban population in China. *Bulletin of the World Health Organization, 78*, 1296–1305.

Yuhas, N., McGowan, B., Fontaine, T., Czech, J., & Gambrell-Jones, J. (2006). Psychosocial interventions for disruptive symptoms of dementia. *Journal of Psychosocial Nursing and Mental Health Services, 44*, 34–42.

Yusuf, S., Hawken, S., Ôunpuu, S., Bautista, L., Franzosi, M. G., Commerford, P., … INTERHEART Study Investigators. (2005). Obesity and the risk of myocardial infarction in 2700 participants from 52 countries: A case-control study. *Lancet, 366*, 1640–1649.

Yusuf, S., Hawken, S., Ôunpuu, S., Dans, T., Avezum, A., Lanas, F., … INTERHEART Study Investigators. (2004). Effect of potentially modifiable risk factors associated with myocardial infarction in 52 countries (the INTERHEART study): Case-control study. *Lancet, 364*, 937–952.

Zaarcadoolas, C., Pleasant, A., & Greer, D. S. (2005). Understanding health literacy: An expanded model. *Health Promotion International, 20*, 195–203.

Zack, M., Poulos, C. X., Aramakis, V. B., Khamba, B. K., & MacLeod, C. M. (2007). Effects of drink-stress sequence and gender on alcohol stress response dampening in high and low anxiety sensitive drinkers. *Alcoholism: Clinical and Experimental Research, 31*, 411–422.

Zainal, N. Z., Booth, S., & Huppert, F. A. (2013). The efficacy of mind-fulness-based stress reduction on mental health of breast cancer patients: A meta-analysis. *Psycho-Oncology, 22*(7), 1457–1465.

Zautra, A. J. (2003). *Emotions, stress, and health.* New York, NY: Oxford University Press.

Zehnacker, C. H., & Bemis-Dougherty, A. (2007). Effect of weighted exercises on bone mineral density in post-menopausal women: A systematic review. *Journal of Geriatric Physical Therapy, 30*, 79–88.

Zelenko, M., Lock, J., Kraemer, H. C., & Steiner, H. (2000). Perinatal complications and child abuse in a poverty sample. *Child Abuse and Neglect, 24*, 939–950.

Zhan, C., & Miller, M. R. (2003). Excess length of stay, charges, and mortality attributable to medical injuries during hospitalization. *Journal of the American Medical Association, 290*, 1868–1874.

Zhang, B., Ferrence, R., Cohen, J., Bondy, S., Ashley, M. J., Rehm, J., … Miller, A. (2005). Smoking cessation and lung cancer mortality in a cohort of middle-aged Canadian women. *Annals of Epidemiology, 15*, 302–309.

Zhang, Y., Leach, M. J., Hall, H., Sundberg, T., Ward, L., Sibbritt, D., … Adams, J. (2015, March 11). Differences between Male and Female Consumers of Complementary and Alternative Medicine in a National US Population: A Secondary Analysis of 2012 NIHS Data. *Evidence-based Complementary and Alternative Medicine, 2015*, 1–10.

Zhou, E. S., Penedo, F. J., Lewis, J. E., Rasheed, M., Traeger, L., Lechner, S., … Antoni, M. H. (2010). Perceived stress mediates the effects of social support on health-related quality of life among men treated for localized prostate cancer. *Journal of Psychosomatic Research, 69*, 587–590.

Zhu, J., Su, X., Li, G., Chen, J., Tang, B., & Yang, Y. (2014). The incidence of acute myocardial infarction in relation to overweight and obesity: A meta-analysis. *Archives of Medical Science, 10*(5), 855–862.

Zijlstra, G. A., Rixt, H., Jolanda, C. M., van Rossum, E., van Eijk, J. T., Yardley, L., … Kempen, G. I. (2002). Interventions to reduce fear of falling in community-living older people: A systematic review. *Journal of American Geriatrics Society, 55*, 603–615.

Zimmerman, T., Heinrichs, N., & Baucom, D. H. (2007). "Does one size fit all?" Moderators in psychosocial interventions for breast cancer patients: A meta-analysis. *Annals of Behavioral Medicine, 34*, 225–239.

Zinberg, N. E. (1984). *Drug, set, and setting: The basis for controlled intoxicant use.* New Haven, CT: Yale University Press.

Zolnierek, K. B., & DiMatteo, M. R. (2009). Physician communication and patient adherence: A meta-analysis. *Medical Care, 47*, 826–834.

Zorrilla, E. P., Luborsky, L., McKay, J. R., Rosenthal, R., Houldin, A., Tax, A., … Schmidt, K. (2001). The relationship of depression and stressors to immunological assays: A meta-analytic review. *Brain, Behavior and Immunity, 15*, 199–226.

Zubin, J., & Spring, B. (1977). Vulnerability: A new view of schizophrenia. *Journal of Abnormal Psychology, 86*, 103–127.

Zupancic, M. L., & Mahajan, A. (2011). Leptin as a neuroactive agent. *Psychosomatic Medicine, 73*(5), 407–414.

Zvolensky, M. J., Jenkins, E. F., Johnson, K. A., & Goodwin, R. D. (2011). Personality disorders and cigarette smoking among adults in the United States. *Journal of Psychiatric Research, 45*(6), 835–841.

Zyazema, N. Z. (1984). Toward better patient drug compliance and comprehension: A challenge to medical and pharmaceutical services in Zimbabwe. *Social Science and Medicine, 18*, 551–554.

Zywiak, W. H., Stout, R. L., Longabaugh, R., Dyck, I., Connors, G. J., & Maisto, S. A. (2006). Relapse-onset factors in Project MATCH: The relapse questionnaire. *Journal of Substance Abuse Treatment, 315*, 341–345.

NAME INDEX

SUBJECT INDEX